24.95

Y0-EIL-177

COMPREHENSIVE REHABILITATION NURSING

Edited by

Nancy Martin, R.N., M.A.
Director of Nursing
University of Chicago Hospitals
 and Clinics

Nancye B. Holt, R.N., M.S.
Director of Nursing
Rehabilitation Institute of Chicago

Dorothy Hicks, R.N., M.N.
Chairperson, Continuing Education
 Program
College of Nursing
Arizona State University

COMPREHENSIVE REHABILITATION NURSING

McGraw-Hill Book Company
New York   St. Louis   San Francisco   Auckland   Bogotá
Guatemala   Hamburg   Johannesburg   Lisbon   London
Madrid   Mexico   Montreal   New Delhi   Panama   Paris
San Juan   São Paulo   Singapore   Sydney   Tokyo   Toronto

NOTICE

Medicine is an ever-changing science. As new research and clinical experience broaden our knowledge, changes in treatment and drug therapy are required. The editors and the publisher of this work have made every effort to ensure that the drug dosage schedules herein are accurate and in accord with the standards accepted at the time of publication. Readers are advised, however, to check the product information sheet included in the package of each drug they plan to administer to be certain that changes have not been made in the recommended dose or in the contraindications for administration. This recommendation is of particular importance in regard to new or infrequently used drugs.

COMPREHENSIVE REHABILITATION NURSING

Copyright © 1981 by McGraw-Hill, Inc. All rights reserved. Printed in the United States of America. No part of this publication may be reproduced, stored in a retrieval system, or transmitted, in any form or by any means, electronic, mechanical, photocopying, recording, or otherwise, without the prior written permission of the publisher.

1234567890 DODO 8987654321 0

This book was set in Serif Gothic by Monotype Composition Company, Inc.
The editors were Laura A. Dysart
and Irene Curran;
the designer was Robin Hessel;
the production supervisor was Jenet C. McIver.
The drawings were done by Fine Line Illustrations, Inc.
R. R. Donnelley & Sons Company was printer and binder.

Library of Congress Cataloging in Publication Data
Main entry under title:

Comprehensive rehabilitation nursing.

    Bibliography: p.
    Includes index.
    1. Rehabilitation nursing. I. Martin, Nancy, date II. Holt, Nancye B. III. Hicks, Dorothy J.
[DNLM: 1. Nursing. 2. Rehabilitation—Nursing texts.
WY150 M382c]
RT120.R4C65   610.73'6   80-13432
ISBN 0-07-040611-1

TO

Henry Brognard Betts, M.D., and Dorothy Ranney Donnelley and to the memory of Bertha Evans Brown. Their visionary commitment and leadership have been singularly directed toward the improvement of life for physically disabled persons.

CONTENTS

List of Contributors — xi
Foreword — xv
Preface — xvii

PART ONE CONCEPTUAL AND THEORETICAL CONSIDERATIONS

1 The Value of the Disabled Life — 3
   Edward A. Eckenhoff
2 Reactions of the Nonimpaired to the Physically Impaired — 10
   Gary L. Albrecht
3 Methods of Coping — 21
   Carolyn E. Carlson
4 Help, Helping, and Helplessness — 39
   Carolyn E. Carlson
5 Variables That Influence Compliance — 53
   Margaret A. Williams
6 Variables That Predict Successful Community Reintegration — 69
   Sandra Mock and Jeannette Taylor
7 Sexuality — 85
   Winona Griggs
8 The Threatened Practitioner: Work Under Stress — 100
   Meyer S. Gunther
9 Experiencing Loss — 115
   Hector R. Roché

PART TWO   ASSESSMENT AND MODALITIES FOR MANAGEMENT

10   The Rehabilitation Experience   127
    Henry B. Betts

11   Cognition   136
    Don A. Olson

12   Speech and Language Disorders of Neurological Origin in Adults   149
    Anita S. Halper and Sandra Oslager Glista

13   Chewing and Swallowing   173
    George L. Larsen

14   Urinary Function   186
    Lee Shields

15   Bowel Function   223
    Betty Cannon

16   Assessment and Management of Soft Tissue Pressure   242
    Rosemarie B. King

17   Physical Therapy Assessment   269
    Frederick J. Schneider

18   Functional Living Skills   298
    Beverly J. Ritt and Janie J. McColey

19   Acquired Speech and Language Disorders in Children   340
    Anita S. Halper and Deborah Lynn Korkos

PART THREE   NURSING MANAGEMENT OF SELECTED PHYSICAL IMPAIRMENTS

20   Brain Damage from Stroke   353
    Jennifer McCarthy

21   Brain Damage from Trauma   386
    Betsy Schnek

22   Multiple Sclerosis   400
    Dorothy L. Gordon

23   Spinal Cord Injury: Acute Phase   418
    Dorothy L. Gordon and Margaret M. Stevens

24   Spinal Cord Injury: Postacute Phase   449
    Marjorie A. Boyink and Susan M. Strawn

25   Upper Extremity Amputation   492
    Hildegarde Myers

26   Lower Extremity Amputation   506
    Betty Quinn

27   Third Degree Burns   520
    Verna Cain and Janet A. Marvin

28   Impairment as a Result of Cancer   552
    Susan Hillenbrand Herbst

29   Cardiac Impairment   579
    Mary Doherty and Sue Ann Prato

30   Rheumatic Disease   607
    Linda Mills Hennig

31	Pain as a Result of Physical Impairment Irene B. Alyn	644

PART FOUR THE WORLD OUT THERE

32	Discharge Planning for the Transition from a Health Care Facility to the Community Susan M. Povse and Mary E. Keenan	667
33	Vocational Rehabilitation Patricia Booth and Jack Mason	690
34	Resocialization Betty Goldiamond	697
35	The Environmental Situation Barbara L. Allan and Robert E. Small	728
36	The Future: Commitment to the Disabled? Sandra Mock and Jeannette Taylor	750
37	The Insurance Industry as a Support Structure Helen M. Degner	759
38	Going Back to Work: A Personal Recollection John A. McWethy	766

Index   777

LIST OF CONTRIBUTORS

Gary L. Albrecht, Ph.D.
Associate Professor
School of Public Health
University of Illinois
Chicago, Illinois

Barbara L. Allan, B.F.A.
Visiting Lecturer
University of Washington;
Consultant, Barrier Free Design
Easter Seal Society
Seattle, Washington

Irene B. Alyn, R.N., Ph.D.
Professor of Nursing
College of Nursing
University of Illinois
Chicago, Illinois

Henry B. Betts, M.D.
Executive Vice President and Medical Director
Rehabilitation Institute of Chicago
Chicago, Illinois

Patricia Booth, M.A.T.
Work Evaluator
Vocational Rehabilitation Department
Rehabilitation Institute of Chicago
Chicago, Illinois

Marjorie A. Boyink, B.S.N.
Assistant Director, Nursing Education
Rehabilitation Institute of Chicago
Chicago, Illinois

Verna Cain, R.N.
Discharge Planning Nurse, Burn Center
University of Washington
Seattle, Washington

Betty Cannon, R.N., B.S.N.
Nurse Clinician
Department of Rehabilitation Medicine
Emory University
Atlanta, Georgia

Carolyn E. Carlson, Ph.D., R.N.
Professor and Head
Department of Medical-Surgical Nursing
College of Nursing
University of Illinois
Chicago, Illinois

Helen M. Degner, R.N., M.S.
Rehabilitation Services Director
Employers Insurance of Wausau
Wausau, Wisconsin

Mary Doherty, R.N., M.S.
Clinical Director, Surgery
University of Chicago Hospitals and Clinics
Chicago, Illinois

Edward A. Eckenhoff, M.A., M.H.A.
Vice President and Administrator
Rehabilitation Institute of Chicago
Chicago, Illinois

Sandra Oslager Glista, M.S., CCC-SP
Clinical Supervisor, Speech-Language Pathology
Rehabilitation Institute of Chicago
Chicago, Illinois

Betty Goldiamond, Ph.D.
Social Psychologist
Chicago, Illinois

Dorothy L. Gordon, R.N., D.N.Sc.
Nurse Researcher
Maryland Institute for Emergency Medical
  Service;
Assistant Professor
School of Nursing
University of Maryland
College Park, Maryland

Winona Griggs, M.S.N., R.N.
Director, Nursing Education
Rehabilitation Institute of Chicago
Chicago, Illinois

Meyer S. Gunther, M.D.
Associate Clinical Professor
Departments of Psychiatry, Physical Medicine,
  and Rehabilitation
Northwestern University Medical School;
Staff Physician
Rehabilitation Institute of Chicago
Chicago, Illinois

Anita S. Halper, M.A., CCC-SP
Director, Communicative Disorders
Rehabilitation Institute of Chicago
Chicago, Illinois

Linda Mills Hennig, R.N., M.A.
Consultant, Rehabilitation Nursing
Huntington, West Virginia

Susan Hillenbrand Herbst, R.N., M.S.
Oncology Clinical Specialist
Decatur Memorial Hospital
Decatur, Illinois

Mary E. Keenan, R.N.
Nurse Clinician, Outpatient Department
Rehabilitation Institute of Chicago
Chicago, Illinois

Rosemarie B. King, R.N., M.S.
Assistant Director of Nursing
Rehabilitation Institute of Chicago
Chicago, Illinois

Deborah Lynn Korkos, M.A., CCC-SP
Clinical Supervisor
Speech-Language Pathology
Rehabilitation Institute of Chicago
Chicago, Illinois

George L. Larsen, Ph.D.
Chief Speech Pathologist
Veterans Administration Hospital
Seattle, Washington

Janet A. Marvin, R.N., M.N.
Associate Director, Burn Center
University of Washington
Seattle, Washington

Jack Mason, B.A.
Work Evaluator
Vocational Rehabilitation Department
Rehabilitation Institute of Chicago
Chicago, Illinois

Jennifer McCarthy, B.S.N.
Head Nurse
Rehabilitation Institute of Chicago
Chicago, Illinois

Janie J. McColey, O.T.R.
Clinical Education Specialist
Rehabilitation Institute of Chicago;
Instructor, Northwestern University
Chicago, Illinois

John A. McWethy
Formerly Midwest Editor
Wall Street Journal
Sun City, Arizona

Sandra Mock, A.C.S.W., C.S.W.
Supervisor, Social Work Department
Rehabilitation Institute of Chicago
Chicago, Illinois

Hildegarde Myers, R.N., R.P.T.
Formerly Chief of Physical Therapy
Rehabilitation Institute of Chicago
Chicago, Illinois

Don A. Olson, Ph.D.
Director, Education and Training
Rehabilitation Institute of Chicago
Chicago, Illinois

Susan M. Povse, R.N., M.S.N.
Clinical Specialist
Department of Nursing
Rehabilitation Institute of Chicago
Chicago, Illinois

Sue Ann Prato, R.N., M.S.
Associate Clinical Director, Medicine
University of Chicago Hospitals and Clinics
Chicago, Illinois

Betty Quinn, R.N.
Director of Nursing
Rehabilitation Institute of West Florida
Pensacola, Florida

Beverly J. Ritt, O.T.R.
Supervisor, Occupational Therapy Department
Rehabilitation Institute of Chicago
Chicago, Illinois

Hector R. Roché
Social Worker
Rehabilitation Institute of Chicago
Chicago, Illinois

Frederick J. Schneider, M.Ed., R.P.T.
Director, Physical Therapy Education
Rehabilitation Institute of Chicago;
Associate, Health Sciences and Arts
Northwestern University Medical School
Chicago, Illinois

Betsy Schnek, R.N., M.S.N.
Administrative Nurse Clinician
Medical-Surgical Nursing
University Hospitals of Cleveland;
Assistant Clinical Professor
Case Western Reserve University
Cleveland, Ohio

Lee Shields, R.N., M.S.
Clinical Specialist
Texas Institute for Rehabilitation and Research
Houston, Texas

Robert E. Small, A.I.A.
Professor of Architecture
University of Washington
Seattle, Washington

Margaret M. Stevens, R.N., B.S.
Neurotrauma Nurse Coordinator
Maryland Institute for Emergency Medical
   Service
University of Maryland
College Park, Maryland

Susan M. Strawn, R.N., B.S.N.
Head Nurse
Rehabilitation Institute of Chicago
Chicago, Illinois

Jeannette Taylor, M.S.W., A.C.S.W.
Social Worker
Rehabilitation Institute of Chicago
Chicago, Illinois

Margaret A. Williams, R.N., Ph.D., F.A.A.N.
Professor of Nursing
University of Wisconsin
Madison, Wisconsin

FOREWORD

The underlying theme throughout this book is that of commitment toward improvement of the quality of life of those whom we call disabled. As the citizens of this nation have become more aware of the plight of the physically disabled among us, there has grown a concomitant awareness of the need for enhanced and expanded services, personnel, and facilities directed toward that life-style goal. Although not a new concept, rehabilitation practice has not received from many of the health care disciplines the recognition it deserves for its effectiveness in enabling and assisting persons with disabilities to actualize their fullest potential. Nor has the literature in the relevant professional fields directed much attention to either the philosophy or the practice of rehabilitation, with the result that there is a scarcity of properly prepared personnel. This situation is especially true in nursing. *Comprehensive Rehabilitation Nursing* has been designed to address that problem. It was written with the purpose of assisting nurses perform an essential role in helping the patient/client/family to function in the most effective and satisfying manner possible in a complex world filled with barriers to those who are "different."

A book may be important for its purpose, its content, or its timeliness. This book meets all three criteria. The content covered in this volume is extremely broad in scope, addressing on the one hand the social issues of access and finance and on the other the treatment of specific functional disorders. The approach is both theoretical and practical and in that mode is clearly reflective of the philosophy of rehabilitation. Historically, there have been few books on rehabilitation nursing, and most that were written were very basic, addressing narrow technical issues, and thus were not appropriate for use by baccalaureate students of nursing or by nurses in practice in rehabilitation settings. The present volume, because of its comprehensive approach and the level of its content, meets that need and joins a small, select collection in the rehabilitation nursing literature.

The editors are experienced, expert practitioners of rehabilitation nursing in the areas of clinical practice, administrative management, research, and collegiate teaching. The authors selected by these knowledgeable editors are members of the widely varying disciplines which impact upon practice in the field of rehabilitation. Represented are architecture, sociology, and theology, as well as the many clinical disciplines. The editors wisely decided that to meet its mission of comprehensiveness the book would have to address the multiple, interactive factors that shape the rehabilitation process and critically affect its outcome. Thus the book approaches the rehabilitation process from three perspectives: from that of the client, too often thought of as purely a passive recipient of care, from that of the multidiscipline services provided to the client, and from that of the sociocultural environment impacting upon both. In my view, the chapters that combine those perspectives capture the essence of rehabilitation.

Each of the editors is my professional colleague of many years' standing and my friend. We have worked together and individually to further the practice of rehabilitation nursing, to improve it, to make it more visible to others in the field, and to shape it into an ever more effective component in the process that enables persons with physical disabilities attain a better life. I believe that this book will help students of nursing and rehabilitation nurses reach the goal of improved rehabilitation nursing practice for their clients.

June S. Rothberg,
Ph.D., R.N., F.A.A.N.
Dean, School of Nursing
Adelphi University
Garden City, New York

PREFACE

Our decision to edit *Comprehensive Rehabilitation Nursing* was based in large measure on the opportunity it afforded to include in one nursing text contributions from authors who represent the multiple health care disciplines that work with physically disabled persons. The book is intended for use by baccalaureate nursing students and nurse practitioners. The ultimate intended population, of course, is the physically disabled people with whom nurses work.

We asked our authors to write to the nuts and bolts, to those things that elude and puzzle us, but also to that combination of scientific and human elements that pulls lives together again. The book is divided into four parts. The major thrust of each is as follows.

Part One, Conceptual and Theoretical Considerations, pertains to those concepts and issues that significantly bear on the ability of the patient/client and others (family, health workers) to deal effectively with any permanent or progressive disorder. In this part the contributing authors are from the fields of sociology, psychiatry, nursing, anthropology, health care management, medical social work, and social psychology.

Since any realistic goal setting for severely impaired persons must begin with an accurate assessment of present abilities and losses, we felt it necessary to consider in Part Two, Assessment and Modalities for Management, those assessment tools and modalities most often used by various disciplines working with such patient/clients, particularly in regard to those activities of daily life most frequently affected by disabling conditions. In this part the contributing authors represent the fields of nursing, medicine, speech pathology, and physical and occupational therapy.

As we all know, the job of incorporating nursing goals with goals of other health disciplines into a meaningful 24-hour-a-day patient/client program belongs to nursing. The contributing authors for Part Three, Nursing Management of Selected Physical Impairments, are, therefore, all nurses.

Part Four, The World Out There, considers the disabled person in the process of discharge and after discharge from a health care setting. We examine the world that now exists, what should exist, and possibly what will exist. Contributing authors here represent the fields of architecture, insurance, nursing, vocational counseling, the behavioral sciences, business, and medical social work.

The contributing authors were selected for the unique contribution we believed each could make. While authors were asked to address specific areas, they have approached them in their own ways. You will therefore see a variety of styles and conceptual approaches throughout the text.

We are grateful to our contributors for their work. Special thanks go to Sharon Massey, Mary Lou Hyman, Jennifer McCarthy, and Kimberly Smith. We are particularly fortunate to have had the support and understanding of family and friends throughout the preparation of this book. Finally, we appreciate the support of the James R. Donnelley desk.

Nancy Martin
Nancye B. Holt
Dorothy Hicks

COMPREHENSIVE REHABILITATION NURSING

PART ONE

CONCEPTUAL AND THEORETICAL CONSIDERATIONS

1
edward a. eckenhoff

the value
of the disabled life

INTRODUCTION

Some ancient societies had a quick solution to the problems caused by a handicapped child—they threw the infant off a cliff. The Eskimos dealt with the disabled and aged by leaving them on free-floating ice to die. The Indians placed a poisonous snake in the tent of the disabled and hoped for a swift passing. As shocking as it sounds, these societies could not afford a nonproducing member. A disabled individual was an intolerable drain on the family unit.

In our own country, just 35 to 40 years ago, many of our disabled citizens were being treated in the basements and back rooms of hospitals, hidden from most of us, even from staff. When discharged, if discharged, they were sent home, often very dependent, and were again confined to basements, attics, or single rooms.

As recently as 20 years ago in some sections of this country, spinal cord–injured patients were kept in hospitals on Stryker frames, some for years. A few years before the Stryker frames, as late as 1955, there were patients who were placed in boxes lined with sawdust because of the problem of bowel or bladder incontinence.

In the United States up to about 1940 (before antibiotics), about 75 percent of the spinal cord injury–paralyzed died within a few years. Even today in India, about 80 percent of all spinal cord–injured patients die before they get to the hospital (Rama, Rao, 1978). When hospitalized, they usually survive the critical, acute stages of their injury, but following discharge they often no longer have access to adequate medical attention or rehabilitation. Many die soon after returning to their villages.

What about our society today? What has changed? For one thing, we expend billions of dollars annually to rehabilitate people. Today, 60 percent of spinal cord–injured people in the United States survive and can live almost as long as "normal" people do (Kraus et al., 1976). Many of these people work and are independent. Of course, some still are not. For the first time in history, we have available the knowledge, technical skill, and capacity to confront much of the problem, but although resources and services are available to many, they are not yet available to all. Unequal income distribution, incomplete catastrophic health insurance, and inner-city and rural problems create discrepancies in availability and access to health care, including rehabilitation.

As our health-care system has expanded, so has governmental control. Health-care professionals are experiencing increasing pressure from the public and the government to satisfy the health-care needs of all people, to control costs, and to be most clearly accountable for both. It may seem that as we attempt to be more humanitarian, we develop technology, rules, and regulations that make us appear less humanitarian.

THE STATISTICS

The National Health Education Committee, in its book entitled *The Killers and Cripplers,* shows that in 1970 (the latest year for which they have compiled data on comprehensive disabling conditions) 23,237,000 people suffered disabling conditions which limited activity. This shocking figure represents more than 10 percent of our entire population. It is equal to the combined populations of New York City, Chicago, Los Angeles, Houston, Philadelphia, Detroit, Baltimore, Dallas, Washington, D.C., Cleveland, Indianapolis, and San Francisco (U.S. Bureau of the Census).

Of this figure, 1,613,000 have impairments of the back and spine; 1,515,000 have impairments of the lower extremities; 914,000 have musculoskeletal disorders; and 817,000 suffer paralysis (Nat'l. Health Ed. Committee). These few categories represent only 21 percent of all those with disabling conditions as reported in 1970. A much smaller proportion of the whole, representing less than three-hundredths of 1 percent, is the category of spinal cord injuries resulting from motor vehicle accidents. In the field of rehabilitation, however, significance of percentages has

CHAPTER 1

very little to do with population size. This seemingly insignificant percentage of the totally disabled is very important.

Motor vehicle accidents account for the vast majority of spinal cord–injured patients. Suddenly, an able-bodied person becomes either a fatality or an irreversibly disabled individual. These individuals who once could engage in many different physical activities now no longer can do so. Once the cord is severed or damaged, the patient is left with appendages that don't work and organs that rarely function as efficiently as they once did. Sensation is lost. Of the population at risk, young males between the ages of 16 and 35 appear to be the most frequent victims of such injuries. In 1974 it was estimated that 5315 people suffered spinal cord injuries from motor vehicle accidents alone (Smart and Sanders, 1976).

LIVES VERSUS DOLLARS

When people become severely and irreversibly disabled, are they worth saving? Will the cost for their care in an acute-care hospital, in a rehabilitation hospital, and after discharge be outweighed by the contribution the person can make to society once he or she is discharged from the hospital? Are not these people a significant drain on society and its resources? Can society better channel the billions of dollars into more worthwhile endeavors such as better education, better housing, more aid for the poor, or stronger national defense? Could the monies spent for care of these injured be better channeled into preventing similar injuries? Once a patient has been injured severely, do we let the patient die, then erase guilt feelings by spending the dollars on prevention? The answers are both yes and no, but they are meaningless. Why? Because who is going to make the decision as to which disability category will no longer be paid for? Who is going to make the decision that a certain number of unfortunate people must die annually, even though with present-day medical technology those people could live? These questions and many others have been of concern to the nation but for moral and ethical reasons we continue to spend more for health care, train more people for the delivery of that care, invent and update more diagnostic and treatment equipment, and practice heroic acute-care measures to keep physically impaired people alive.

In 1978 the President proposed this country's first $500 billion budget. Roughly 36 percent, or $181.2 billion, was under the direct control of the Department of Health, Education, and Welfare. This $181.2 billion was spent for social security, education, Medicare, and Medicaid, among the many other programs. In 1978 the Medicare allotment for treating the elderly was nearly $30 billion. In 1977, it was estimated that 65 percent of Medicare appropriation was spent on people who died that same year. Does the justification for spending those billions come from knowing that we, as a society, did all that was possible for these people during the last few months of their lives? If this is the case, then the expenditures for young spinal cord–injured individuals become even more significant. For these individuals, we are no longer talking about a few months or a few years, but the greater portion of their productive lives. We talk about societal value, but most important, we talk about quality of life. As many as 7000 people sustained spinal cord injuries during 1976 and lived to get to the hospital.[1] Most became permanently disabled as a result of that injury.

The families of these disabled people spent hundreds of millions of dollars raising them from birth to young adulthood. Estimates vary, of course, as to how much parents spend on their children, but few would disagree that it is at least $27,000 per child (U.S. Dept. of Agriculture), and usually significantly more. Thus, from a pure cost standpoint, if such patients are allowed to die or are not rehabilitated, the loss is great. Add to this the costs of foregone future productivity. If

---

[1] Figure presented represents joint extrapolation of unpublished 1976 findings of the National Center for Health Statistics and the 1971 18-county northern California study on survival among persons sustaining acute spinal cord injury. (J. F. Kraus and associates, Univ. of California, Davis.)

these patients are not rehabilitated, their chances for productivity are minimal. It has already been mentioned that the predominant age range for spinal cord–injured patients is between 16 and 35. The average male in this age group should have earnings during his career of approximately $594,000. Females of the same age range would average $314,000 (U.S. Dept. HEW, 1975).[2] Add this loss in potential earning power to the money it took to raise each of these people and the economic loss becomes more and more significant.

Finally, the cost of caring for such a disabled, nonproductive person in a nursing home will probably be $235,000 during the remaining 25 to 35 years of life (U.S. Dept. HEW, 1977).[3]

The total direct costs of motor vehicle-related spinal cord injuries in 1974 was estimated to be $248,628,790 or $46,780 per patient and $92,410 per permanently disabled patient (Smart, Sanders). These costs include emergency assistance at the time of injury, initial hospitalization (acute, subacute and rehabilitation), home modifications, vocational rehabilitation, institutional and attendant care, medical equipment and appliances, drugs and medical supplies, rehospitalization, and miscellaneous services and supplies. Keeping in mind the cost of raising the child to young adulthood, estimated potential future earnings, the average age, and the potential costs of future care if not rehabilitated, a spinal cord–injured patient, rehabilitated to the point of productivity and gainful employment, would offer benefits far beyond the cost. The ratio would be about $3 saved for every $1 for care services, assuming regained employment and avoided home care expense are included (Thornton and Harasymiw, 1978). Over and above the moral and ethical implications and the preservation of human resources, rehabilitation would appear to be in the best economic interest of society.

This author assumes that people will continue to become patients, that spinal cord injuries will continue to happen, and that a multiplicity of other disabling conditions will most assuredly require rehabilitation care, particularly rehabilitation nursing care. This book is for the rehabilitation nurse who sees and learns to care for each of these disabled people. Without the rehabilitation nurse, the considerable benefits of rehabilitation would not be realized by the disabled person or society. The rehabilitation team is anchored by nursing concepts and skills, and by the nurse herself or himself.

A CARE ENVIRONMENT—THE REHABILITATION HOSPITAL

The nursing department in any hospital is always the largest department. On the average it expends one-third of the hospital's budget and includes a third of all hospital personnel. It is also usually the department with the most needs, the most gripes, and the highest level of frustration.

Is the nurse the team member to monitor and keep homeostasis among the myriad people working with the rehabilitation patient? Or is this the physician's role? Is it the nurse who maintains an orderly unit with policies and procedures which ensure a comfortable and secure environment for the patient? Or does the nurse provide the cautious, silent visit to the paraplegic's room at 1 A.M. to check whether or not the patient is sleeping comfortably and all is well? The nurse may never quite realize the security represented

---

[2] These figures result from calculation of present value of expected lifetime earnings for men and women aged 25 to 29 performed by Barbara S. Cooper and Wendyce Brody of the Social Security Administration, Division of Health Insurance Studies, U.S. Dept. of Health, Education, and Welfare. They have been adjusted to 1977 wage levels, using as an index the degree of change in average weekly earnings of private nonagricultural workers between 1972 and July 1977, reported by the U.S. Bureau of Labor Statistics. Since Cooper and Brody provided only a field of estimates of varying discount rates for a present value estimate, it was necessary to extrapolate from the relative differences between these figures to arrive at the nondiscounted figures.

[3] Calculated by using the average total monthly charge for routine nursing-care level service for persons under 65 in U.S. nursing homes, as reported by the 1973–74 National Nursing Home Survey. Cost cited was upgraded to reflect 1978 prices by use of the Hospital Service Charges Index of the Bureau of Labor Statistics.

by this visit to the patient who has looked and waited for hours to have someone enter the room.

Patients learn quickly when a shift starts, who is on and who is off, when a nurse is not feeling well, and when a nurse is feeling great. If there is a bit of warmth, a caring response that the patient can elicit, the patient will become an expert at obtaining it and will learn quickly to expect it—perhaps because the need is so desperate.

Sometimes a patient will not seem to understand or appreciate the warmth, caring, or the security the nurse provides. The patient may be depressed, angered, afraid, withdrawn, or even desperately demanding. Patients may lash out and be overcritical because they are frightened in a strange environment.

The hospital is an environment that frequently creates uncertainty. Medicine is not a profession with foolproof processes and guaranteed results. Patients want to know more and more about their condition and the potential outcome, and this desire places pressures on the staff. When answers are not given or are not easy to accept or understand, patients feel anxious.

An additional anxiety is the lengthy, seemingly endless time the patient must spend in the hospital. The average patient in the acute-care community hospital spends 6 to 7 days. In the rehabilitation hospital, a patient may spend months. The patient may never see the same meal twice in a 6-day stay in a community hospital; he or she may see the same menu dozens of times in a rehabilitation hospital.

For the patient in a rehabilitation hospital, the day may begin unappealingly with interruptions by the lab technician, the physician, and an accompanying cadre of residents and medical students, with nurses toileting, seeing the patient through dressing programs, and assisting with eating breakfast.

Millions of other people that same morning are leisurely sipping their coffee, eating toast, and reading the morning newspaper before leaving for the office. The patients were doing just that, every morning, before being admitted to the hospital. But the hospital changes all that. Within a matter of hours, the patients become dependent on an unfamiliar structure and on unknown faces who use an unfamiliar medical language. They do not know if something will cause pain or not, or whether they will be heard or responded to when the need to be heard or responded to arises.

In the hospital environment, patients for the most part find it difficult to decide crucial issues of their own well-being. Burdened by the disintegrative and anxiety-provoking aspects of their illnesses, they do not know how to deal with procedures personally, particularly when they have no idea of the significance of the procedures. They are, or feel they are, at the mercy of the medical staff, the nursing staff, and the policies and procedures set by administration. Their apprehension inevitably inhibits trust and confidence in the hospital and staff. And the nursing department must deal with this lack of trust every hour, 24 hours a day, 168 hours a week.

The nurse often is placed in an intermediary role, answering for the medical staff, the administration, and the various other members of the team, putting out "fires" daily on behalf of all, and acting as a buffer for all. Expected to know it all, the nurse works unending hours, "cares" 24 hours a day, must be prim and proper at all times, and must never talk back or seem disturbed, rustled, or insecure. Not some nurses; *all* nurses. That's what administration, medical staff, patients, patients' families, and the rest of the hospital staff expect of nurses.

CONCLUSION

Patients in rehabilitation facilities are preoccupied with loss; their unimpaired capacities are ignored, and they feel a sudden and massive constriction of life space. They are overwhelmed with their immediate problem, desperately wishing it to be immediately corrected, with maximal attention in minimal time and at minimal expense. Patients, further, find it hard to believe that medicine does not have all the answers. They cannot understand the complexities of hospitals; they do not wish to understand that the people working in the hospitals are caught up in their own problems (whether professional or personal). It is difficult, often impossible, to educate patients to better understand this environment and the caring staff within it. Typically, patients do not want to hear explanations, or accept them. They are in hospitals to get better, regardless of the level of reality of their expectations.

Patients expect the hospital and its staff to render attentive, quality care, and they pay handsomely for that care. Professionals in the hospital environment should exercise the responsibilities and obligations appropriately expected by patients—the responsibilities professionals have been trained for and are paid for.

If nurses allow themselves to be as human as patients, particularly when dealing with patients, and cannot set aside those burdensome human qualities which interfere, then possibly they have been trained for the wrong profession. The rehabilitation nurse has a challenging responsibility because it is the rehabilitation nurse and the department of nursing that make the hospital system work. Further, it is the rehabilitation nurse who assists so greatly in restoring the disabled person.

Speaking from experience as a patient for a long period of time, as a counselor, and as an administrator, the author can unhesitatingly say that nursing is *the* critical service.

When people become patients, they need care, and they continue to be demanding. Most expect too much, hoping for magical, guaranteed results, and expecting all staff to perform at 110 percent constantly. In addition, each staff member in this profession "overexpects" from other members.

Perhaps, in this field, the overexpectation assists in facilitating excellence of care. If this overexpectation can be viewed as *positive,* then with expertise, understanding, and genuine caring, perhaps nurses can gently but firmly ask 110 percent of patients. By this overexpectation patients can be helped to resee their value in this world.

BIBLIOGRAPHY

Kraus, J. F., C. E. Franti, R. S. Riggins, and N. D. Borhani: "Survival Among Persons with Spinal Cord Injury," unpublished research paper presented at the 104th American Public Health Association meeting, Miami Beach, Fla., Oct. 19, 1976, p. 6.

National Health Education Committee: *The Killers and Cripplers,* David McKay, New York, 1976, p. 232.

Rama, Rao: "Accent Talks with Director of India Rehab Center," *Accent on Living,* Winter: 56, 1978.

Smart, C. N., and C. R. Sanders: "The Costs of Motor Vehicle Related Spinal Cord Injuries" (study performed for The Insurance Institute for Highway Safety), Insurance Institute of Highway Safety, Washington, D.C., 1976, pp. 24, 98–99.

Thornton, J. W., and S. J. Harasymiw: "Cost-effectiveness of Rehabilitating the Spinal Cord Injured," paper submitted to the Rehabilitation Institute of Chicago in fulfillment in part of RSA Research Project S-39 (CMOPERS), August 1978.

Thornton, John W., and Jesse F. Kraus and Associates, August 1977 (personal communication).

———, and Donald Smith, National Center for Health Statistics, Hospital Discharge Survey, February 1978 (personal communication).

U.S. Bureau of the Census: "1975 Estimates," in *The World Almanac and Book of Facts,* 1978, p. 194.

U.S. Dept. of Agriculture, *The Cost of Raising a Child, Detail Tables,* CFE (Adm.)-318, September 1971. Based on 1970 data updated to 1977 prices by consumer price index for each category of expense. 1970 data source.

U.S. Department of Health, Education, and Welfare, Public Health Service: "Charges for Care and Sources of Payment for Residents in Nursing Homes," *Vital and Health Statistics, ser. 13,* no. 32, November 1977, p. 9.

———, Social Security Administration: "1972 Lifetime Earnings by Age, Sex, Race and Education Level," by Barbara S. Cooper and Wendyce Brody, *Research and Statistics Note* no. 14, September 1975, p. 4.

2

gary l. albrecht

reactions of
the nonimpaired to
the physically impaired*

INTRODUCTION

We learn to survive and grow in our social world through interaction with other people, continually responding to our own self-expectations and the expectations of others. Most people assume that they will interact with other "normal" people, normalcy in this context being socially defined and culturally specific. For example, virtually everyone we know can process language and communicate verbally. We and our friends have all our limbs and can walk and run. However, each of us can think of situations where these abilities do not exist. Participants in social interaction then tend to feel uncomfortable and express their feelings subtly in strained behavior. This chapter is concerned with one set of these conditions, the reactions of the nonimpaired to the physically impaired, using social interaction as the theoretical context of the analysis. As members of society, individuals act according to specified, socially learned rules. This chapter examines what happens when some of the rules are violated.

The health problems of developed countries are related to chronic diseases (Glazier, 1973). Medical professionals with current knowledge and technology maintain people for years with chronic health conditions who, before the advent of new medical treatment, might have died quickly. As a consequence, the prevalence of serious chronic health conditions is rising in industrial countries. Since this is a relatively recent phenomenon, people are not used to dealing with the effects of chronic health problems. Research has shown that individuals with chronic health conditions often are physically and socially isolated (Albrecht et al., 1976a). Their isolation deprives them of part of their existence and renders them dependent (Scott, 1970); it also deprives the larger society of the benefits of their experience. A major strength of American society has been the diversity of its peoples, and there is a strong American urgency to integrate all citizens into the larger society. Physical and social isolation of minority groups encourages a homogeneous, prejudiced, and naive public that negatively affects the entire society. American values in this regard are so strong that antidiscriminatory laws are being enforced, resulting in settlements for women, children, American Indians, the elderly, and the disabled. Yet, while the powerful sanction of the law is useful, prejudices cannot be legislated away. Social acceptance is the key.

THE IMPAIRED

There is considerable confusion over who the impaired are and where they fit into society. Who gets labeled and who bears the brunt of discrimination is frequently a matter of definition, yet definitions also determine who is eligible for disability benefits. Being identified as impaired is, thus, an important process with far-reaching consequences. The label can change an individual's social definition and place in society.

The distinction between impaired and nonimpaired individuals is not clearly understood by the public. Many people refer to handicap, impairment, disability, functional incapacity, and cosmetically repugnant conditions interchangeably. This usage obscures the bases of prejudice. Handicapism is "a set of assumptions and practices that promote the differential and unequal treatment of people because of apparent or assumed physical, mental, or behavioral differences" (Bogdan and Biklen, 1977). *Handicapism,* a global concept, refers to the prejudicial treatment given to certain minority groups. It is based on labeled stereotypes of behavior, given certain descriptive characteristics of an individual. *Impairments* are anatomical, physiological and/or neurological abnormalities which may or may not be associated with an active pathological condition (Riley and Nagi, 1970). Spinal curvature caused by arrested polio would be one example, and aphasia resulting from a

---

*Research for this chapter was supported by DHEW-SRA grant No. 16 P56809–5–07.

cerebrovascular accident another. Impairment does not necessarily imply a decreased functional capacity. Many people function extremely well with some spinal curvature, a missing little finger, or with slightly decreased lung capacity. *Functional limitation* refers to impairments which restrict the individual in the performance of expected activities, such as dressing, walking, and balancing a checkbook. Haber (1973) refers to these limitations as functional incapacities that affect role performance. *Disability* is a more general term that refers to the limiting effect of a chronic condition on an individual's role performance over time. For example, the Social Security Administration operationally defines disability as a functional incapacity "lasting three months or longer" (Treitel, 1977).

Any impairment can disrupt social interaction. The condition need not have serious physical or mental functional consequences to have far-reaching effects. In fact, there is evidence to show that individuals with little or no functional limitation can suffer catastrophic social injustice if they are labeled (Mercer, 1973). In a classic study of mental retardation, Mercer found that children from lower-social-class backgrounds and minority groups were more likely than white, Anglo, middle- and upper-class children to be labeled mentally retarded and placed in special education classes. The teachers appeared to be relatively unbiased in their referral rates to the school testing service. Rather, discrimination and labeling seemed to occur as a result of using the IQ (intelligence quotient) test almost exclusively as the criterion to determine mental retardation and placement in special education programs. This procedure is problematic since IQ tests appear to be class and culture specific. Once children are labeled as mentally retarded, they find it difficult, if not impossible, to receive the same education as their peers. These educational differences later influence job potential and earnings. Therefore, slight impairments or functional differences, used as a basis for labeling individuals, can have serious social consequences that last a lifetime.

DIFFERENTIAL CONSEQUENCES OF IMPAIRMENTS

How the Impaired Present Themselves

A disrupted social life as a result of impairment is one of the problems of the afflicted individual. Impairments associated with specific diseases, accidents, or genetic conditions have discernible effects on body and mind. Individual adaptation depends on the nature of the impairing condition, the individual's health status, and the available resources, such as family support and insurance coverage. Health professionals give much attention to these variables in the medical care process, but they recognize that impairments are as much a social as a physical condition. While diseases, accidents, and genetic anomalies may physically affect a body part's appearance and function, attributions are typically made of the *person* not the involved organ or body part. The meaning of a specific impairment is in its social context (Albrecht, 1977). Social meanings of the impairment take form through interaction with others in the individual's social space and result in a new social identity for the person. Therefore, the individual's presentation of the impairment and the reactions of others to it are crucial elements in the forging of new social identities. The impaired individual discovers altered behavioral expectations mean a redefined social role. Consequently, his or her perceptions change, as do behavior and performance affected by the new self-identity and expectations. The reactions of the nonimpaired in social interactions mean *everything* to the physically impaired.

Self-perceptions strongly influence the way the impaired present themselves in social situations. Individuals who experience impairment often question their own worth and avoid social contact with others (Shontz, 1978). In a study of women who had mastectomies, Jamison et al. (1978) discovered that nearly one-quarter contemplated suicide at one time or another. A considerable percentage of women in this sample also reported difficulties in emotional adjustment to the impairment. Increased use of alcohol and drugs and diminished social interaction are frequent responses to stress experienced as a result of impairment. People going through these adjustments often think that others have more negative attitudes and feelings toward them than is actually the case (Schroedel and Schiff, 1972).

The ways in which impaired individuals present themselves have substantial effects on how they are treated by others. Traditionally, impaired people are expected to accept the sick role and cooperate with medical advice. The sick role, as articulated by Parsons (1975), assumes that sick persons are exempted from some or all of their normal role responsibilities, are not to blame for their illnesses, want to get well, seek appropriate help for their problems, and cooperate with medical help. Yet, in the case of disability, cooperating with the physician's plan and regimen does not necessarily mean that rehabilitation will be successful. In fact, some patients judged by medical staff as uncooperative and unwilling to complete therapy make remarkable strides in rehabilitation (Albrecht and Higgins, 1977). Furthermore, Scott (1970) shows how blind people who cooperate and receive services from agencies for the blind are made dependent, not rehabilitated. Therefore, being a docile and cooperative patient does not ensure successful rehabilitation as measured by functional improvement. These facts cause a dilemma for knowledgeable impaired persons. Impaired people who assert themselves and actively manage their rehabilitation process may become functionally independent, but they may be labeled hostile, aggressive, and uncooperative. On the other hand, if impaired people passively accept their condition, follow medical advice without question, and rely on others for help, they may be less likely to attain their full functional potential. These problems are compounded by age, race, sex, and social class differences. Independent behavior by adult, white, middle-class males is more accepted than in others because in American society this group is expected to be aggressive, knowledgeable, and decisive (Broverman et al., 1970). Others are more likely to be negatively stigmatized for independence and to be referred to as "a tough, aggressive woman," or "an uncooperative blind client" for trying to succeed as a woman in a male world or as a blind person in a sighted world (Bourne and Winkler, 1978; Scott, 1970). Expectations do influence behavior. Therefore, it is not surprising that "the bulk of evidence suggests that the white males, married and with dependents of middle and upper socioeconomic status, with stable work histories, and engaged in nonmanual, less physically exerting occupations are more likely to return to work (after the onset of disability) than their counterparts" (Brown and Rawlinson, 1977).

Self-directed behavior is extremely important to rehabilitation outcome and to acceptance of the impaired because successful rehabilitation requires intensive patient exertion and exercise. For example, success in physical therapy requires considerable patient effort and self-initiation, but presentation of self must be managed in terms of one's own impairment, race, age, sex, and social class to be effective. A person's role as impaired is defined in an interactive context (Twaddle, 1969). If impaired people take charge and rehabilitate themselves but alienate those around them, they are left functionally independent and alone. The optimal strategy aims at functional independence *and* social involvement, requiring the impaired to have continual contact with the nonimpaired as the rehabilitation process proceeds. The impaired must learn to present themselves effectively in a nonimpaired world or face isolation or confinement to an institution for the impaired. Bloombaum and Gugelyk (1970) clearly made this point in their study of the Kalaupapa leper colony. As part of their treatment for Hansen's disease, lepers were isolated on this Hawaiian island. After they were allowed to leave, many of the impaired elected to remain in the compound or asked to come back because they did not feel comfortable in social interaction with the nonimpaired. Although part of this reaction could be due to the visibility of the impairment, lack of contact with the nonimpaired during treatment did have a lasting effect. The impaired were not able to live comfortably in a nonimpaired world.

REACTIONS OF THE ABLE-BODIED TO THE IMPAIRED

Up to this point, attention has been focused on how the impaired present themselves in a social context. While this is critically important, more is known about the other side of the interaction process: how the able-bodied react to the impaired. Much of the early behavioral science research on the impaired concentrated on attitudes toward the physically disabled. The working assumption of these studies was that attitudes are closely related to behavior. Researchers assumed that if the attitudes of the able-bodied toward the disabled were favorable, behavior toward the disabled would be positive. Careful research has demonstrated that this assumption of correspondence between attitudes and behavior is questionable. In a thorough review of attitude-behavior relations, Ajzen and Fishbein (1977) indicate that attitudes do not always correspond with behavior. Some of the differences are due to inadequate measures and poor research designs. After assessing many studies with inconsistent findings, Ajzen and Fishbein (pp. 912–914) concluded that "strong attitude-behavior relations are obtained only under high correspondence between at least the target and action elements of the attitudinal and behavior entities." The target refers to the person, place, or thing at which the action is directed. The action refers to what was done. Therefore, an attitudes toward hiring the handicapped should be expected to correspond to actual employment of the handicapped if both are measured appropriately. Conversely, an attitude toward living in the same neighborhood as an elderly couple would not be expected to correspond closely to marrying a spinal cord–injured person.

Attitudinal studies are useful in examining the reactions of the able-bodied to the impaired, but this research must be interpreted with care. The correspondence between attitudes and behavior is influenced not only by the similarity of target and action but also by the characteristics of the impaired individual and of the able-bodied group being measured. Results of research using Yuker's Attitude Toward Disabled People Scale (Shaw and Wright, 1970) show that females generally have more positive attitudes toward the disabled than males; positive attitudes are related to acceptance of "different" people; positive attitudes are associated with contact with disabled people of similar social class; positive attitudes are more likely to be found in those with little or considerable education rather than those with a high school education, and these attitudes are positively related to the ego strength and security of the able-bodied (Yuker, Block, Younng, 1970).

Attitudes toward the disabled are generally favorable and relatively stable across groups. Albrecht (1976b) found that a sample of adults on the sidewalk of the Chicago Loop had favorable attitudes toward the disabled but did not have much knowledge about what could be realistically expected from the impaired. However, *initial* reactions toward the physically handicapped are usually less favorable than toward the able-bodied (Richardson, 1976). Harasymiw et al. (1976) discovered considerable consensus among college students, disabled people, professionals, and the general public in their general attitudes toward specific disabled groups such as amputees, paraplegics, cardiac patients, and people with mental illness. These attitudes seem to be formed early in life and remain constant through the adult years. There are consistent perceived differences in attitudes toward people with various types of disabilities. These differences are so powerful that they largely mask effects due to race (Richardson, 1976).

Behavioral Responses of the Able-bodied toward the Impaired

While the study of attitudes toward the impaired is important, behavioral responses determine the nature and type of social interactions between the able-bodied and the handicapped. There is accumulated evidence to show that the able-bodied feel more uncomfortable and place more distance between themselves and individuals with social impairments, such as alcohol and drug problems, than individuals with physical impairments, such as stroke and amputations (Harasymiw et al.). The able-bodied seem to feel most uncomfortable and to place greater social distance between themselves and impaired individuals who are perceived to be responsible for their handicap. In a survey, able-bodied respondents stated that people can stop drinking, taking drugs, or stealing from others, but they are not responsible for their amputations and blindness (Albrecht et al., 1978). Yet, spinal cord-injury accident victims are best able to cope with their disability if they blame themselves for the accident (Bulman, Wortman). Victims who blamed others or felt that they could have avoided the accident were not judged to be coping as well with their disability. Therefore, perceived attribution of responsibility does influence social interaction and the manner in which the disabled cope with their handicaps.

In a series of studies on interpersonal relations between the impaired and nonimpaired, Kleck and his colleagues (Kleck, 1966; Kleck, Ono, Hastorf, 1966) found that able-bodied adults, interacting with a disabled person in a wheelchair, were uncomfortable, inhibited, tended to distort their opinions in ways they felt would be more acceptable to the impaired person, and quickly terminated the interaction. In face-to-face interaction, able-bodied people display less variability in verbal output, exhibit less smiling behavior, show less eye contact, and demonstrate greater motor inhibition with the disabled than with other able-bodied persons (Comer and Piliavin, 1972).

These effects are discovered early in life and occur even between infants and their mothers. In an experimental design study, Kagan et al. (1966) showed three-dimensional human faces to 4-month-old babies. Both normal and distorted faces were presented to the infants. Babies who saw the face with abnormal placement of features reacted with fear and crying. They did not respond this way to the normal face. Similarly, mothers respond with aversion to handicapped children. When mothers are presented with birth-defective children, they react with grief, depression, anger, and shock and initially isolate themselves from their babies. The mothers are uncertain how to behave when faced with this unanticipated event. The usual activities following childbirth are dramatically altered (Richardson).

The visibility of the handicap in part determines the degree to which social interaction with the able-bodied is affected. In a set of experiments, Farina (1966, 1968) showed that reaction of the able-bodied to the disabled is more positive in situations where the physical disability is both serious and visible than in cases where it is moderate and less visible. West (1977) reported that cancer patients with facial disfigurements following surgery adapted well to their visible handicap. These patients returned to work and engaged anew in social activities with colleagues, friends, relatives, and society in general. In general, these patients felt that people treated them no differently from before, but some negative reactions of the able-bodied resulted in feelings of self-consciousness, embarrassment, and anger. The most common negative behaviors perceived by the facially disfigured were staring, avoidance, and mistreatment. Successful adaptation to a highly visible handicap seems largely a product of positive reinforcement from family, friends, and the general public.

Willingness to help the handicapped is also influenced by the visibility of the impairment and the seriousness of the dependency. The public is more willing to help the disabled when the costs are low, perceived satisfaction high, and the need of the dependent person high (Cowan and Inskeep, 1978). These general findings are supported in a large study by Zahn (1973) which showed that the more severely disabled are apt to have better interpersonal relationships with the able-bodied than are the less seriously disabled. An impaired person's ability to get and hold a job was positively associated with interpersonal relations among nonfamily members in Zahn's study. People who were not able to work had better relationships with their spouses and other relatives. Furthermore, communication problems disrupted interpersonal relations both at home and at work. Contrary to expectations, Zahn discovered that those who were sexually impaired had better relationships with their spouses than did those who did not experience sexual dysfunction. In summary, Zahn's results show that ambiguity regarding the degree of impairment has the most negative impact on interpersonal relationships. When impaired people have an ambiguous status, expectations are confused, goals are unclear, and roles are poorly defined. Social interaction under these conditions results in dissatisfaction for all the participants.

REDUCING STRAIN IN SOCIAL INTERACTION

Normalization is a strategy that is used by the chronically ill to define their new social position (Davis, 1961). In successful interaction, role ambiguities must be resolved and clear and realistic expectations must be set. When the able-bodied and the disabled first meet, the interaction is usually strained. Neither knows what to expect. The able-bodied person is withdrawn, afraid to take a risk, or to invest socially, and the disabled person has a fear of rejection. Able-bodied people frequently do not know much about disability or its consequences and consequently have difficulty in responding appropriately to new stimuli in the interactional setting. Normalization is a process that resolves some of these strains. At first the impaired person is usually only superficially accepted. The impaired person is tolerated, but no interactional commitments are made. If meaningful interaction is to occur, the able-bodied and impaired need a basis for communication. Role relationships are typically redefined and new identities are forged. Impaired persons provide information and test their abilities in interactional settings. As able-bodied persons become more familiar with the disabled, they learn to accept the new identities and identify with the disabled. This mutual growth and understanding results in a situation in which the participants no longer treat the handicap as a deviant condition or difference. In fact, when the new identity is accepted, the impairment is not intrinsic in the relationship. The new condition and identity are taken for granted, creating an appropriate response. This process is what Davis refers to as normalization. The new identities and relationships are based on interactional experiences that form realistic role expectations and new rules of conduct.

Strauss (1975) presents a more general model for adjusting to the problems of impairments brought on by chronic diseases or accidents. He argues that chronic illness and disability are conditions to be managed by the individual and those concerned with patient care. The problems to be solved include preventing and managing medical crises, managing of treatment regimens, symptom control, reordering of time to fit the demands of the disability, managing the trajectory (natural history) of the disease process, social isolation, and normalizing and redefining family relationships. Each of these problems in living with chronic illness places stresses on established interaction patterns. Successful management of chronic illness is aided by involving the others in one's life in the rehabilitation process.

Numerous studies have demonstrated that behavior is most effectively changed by altering the contingencies and rewards attached to the desired behavior (Bandura, 1969). In fact, in many instances, the most effective way to change attitudes, perceptions and emotional states is to first change the behavior (Bandura et al.). This is a strong argument for placing handicapped children in classrooms with nonhandicapped children. While this strategy often does produce more positive attitudes toward the disabled by the able-bodied and increases behavioral competencies in the handicapped children, the handicapped still experience rejection. These children are less frequently selected as friends, playmates, and workmates and are more often chosen as least liked by the nonhandicapped

CHAPTER 2   16

children (Richardson). Reducing the social barriers caused by impairment is difficult.

In a series of studies, Albrecht (1976b) investigated how the able-bodied react to the disabled in public places. A white male paraplegic in a wheelchair rolled up to a curb in the Chicago Loop that he could not cross. The paraplegic's position on the sidewalk and the amount of effort expended in trying to get over the curb were systematically controlled in 102 trials. Analyses were done of videotapes of the trials and of pedestrians who were involved in the trials. The paraplegic was helped in less than 5 min in every trial. The more visible the distress, the more quickly the disabled person was helped. Multiple regression analyses revealed that the length of time in receiving help was best explained by the number of people in the crowd (shorter time with more people), curb position (shorter in the middle third of the sidewalk), and degree of distress and initiation of verbal discourse by the helper (shorter when the disabled showed distress). Able-bodied pedestrians who helped were best characterized as perceiving that the disabled paraplegic needed and wanted help, being male, and knowing someone who was disabled. The public had positive attitudes toward the disabled but did not have clear or accurate knowledge about their needs, capacities, and potential. General positive attitudes toward the disabled were not highly predictive of helping behavior. Many impaired people are afraid to venture out alone in public places. This research, however, suggests that the public will be helpful rather than intimidating. It also shows that the public is not knowledgeable about disability and does not know what realistically to expect from the impaired. While this research is informative, the results should not be generalized without further examination.

STRATEGIES FOR REDUCING SOCIAL BARRIERS TOWARD THE PHYSICALLY IMPAIRED

Social integration of the disabled into the community is a major rehabilitation goal contingent upon the way in which the able-bodied and the impaired interact in social situations. The able-bodied are more accepting of the impaired when there is a shared realistic knowledge of expectations, clear self-identities, and defined roles. Usually, the clearer the communication, the more knowledge and direct contact, the more successful the social interaction, the acceptance of the impairment, and the integration of the impaired into the community.

Harasymiw and Horne (1975) found that teachers from school settings that integrated the handicapped into the classrooms had more positive attitudes toward handicapped children than those teachers who taught in nonintegrated school settings. In this study, younger teachers had more favorable attitudes than older teachers. There were no sex differences.

In a study of parental acceptance of a child's diagnosis of mental retardation, Svarstad and Lipton (1977) found that parents were more likely to accept the diagnosis when the communication from health professionals was clear, explicit, direct, explanatory of the problem and its consequences, and contained hard data to confirm the diagnosis. Parental acceptance was not significantly dependent on the characteristics of the parents, the child, or the professional who provided the information. Reaction to impairment is a social process. Successful adjustment requires that the family and work or play groups do as much adaptation as the impaired person. Close contact and open, accurate communication facilitate this process.

Aside from direct contact, videotape and audiotape presentations have been used effectively to break down stereotypes toward the physically disabled and to change attitudes and behavior (Albrecht, 1976b; Donaldson and Martinson, 1977). These tapes have been used to present role models, present different successful adaptive modes, teach patients rehabilitation techniques, and raise sensitive topics such as sexual behavior and financial planning. The use of tapes has been effective with groups of disabled, the impaired and their families, employers, and the general public.

CONCLUSION

This discussion of the reactions of the able-bodied to the impaired has emphasized the reciprocal nature and complexity of the interaction process. The presentation stresses general principles and conceptual approaches that have withstood the test of research. The conclusion will highlight some prescriptions that will help to improve social interaction between the able-bodied and the impaired and to integrate the handicapped into society.

The functional level of the disabled in the community is immediately affected by a combination of social and physical barriers. Attention is being given in many communities to reducing physical barriers, such as inaccessible buses and trains and curbed sidewalks, but less emphasis has been focused on how social and physical barriers reinforce each other. Curbs reinforce social isolation. Isolation produces a lack of public awareness of the problems of the disabled, and lack of awareness translates into few architectural codes designed to produce barrier-free environments. These interrelated sets of barriers need to be attacked as units.

Positive attitudes toward the physically disabled do not necessarily imply accurate knowledge and realistic expectations. In fact, the public has little knowledge about the needs, functional limitations, and potential of the physically disabled. Attitude change is not all that is needed. Instead, the public needs to be specifically educated about the capabilities and potential of the physically disabled. Presently, they do not have the necessary information on which to act.

The disabled should be encouraged to go out in public places. In general, the public has positive attitudes toward the disabled and, if needed, will quickly help them. In this special case, crowds are not dangerous places to be. Public visibility of the disabled is an effective means of providing models to the public. These models increase knowledge and clarify expectations.

The impaired should be taught ways to control other people's reactions to them. Research shows that the responses of the public are highly contingent upon how the public perceives the disabled and how disabled persons present themselves in public. In the full sense, if the disabled person asks for help, he or she will generally receive it.

The disabled should be taught to function alone in public places, not only in institutions or with assistance. The problems confronted in public are different from those encountered in institutions and require other knowledge and skills. Research reveals that both the public and the disabled are uneducated about how and under what conditions the disabled can function in public. The successful impaired person must learn to interact with an ill-informed, perhaps even a biased public.

Adaptation to impairment does not end with discharge from an institution. Adaptation to impairment is an ongoing learning experience based on interaction in a specific physical and social environment. Patients should be clinically followed at home and at work. Rehabilitation professionals should go on site to help in the mutual adaptation process.

Videotapes and films are powerful tools for educating the disabled, their families, employers, rehabilitation staff, and the public about the disabled. These tools can be used repetitively and in diverse settings. Both direct contact and video techniques should be directed toward improving interactions between the able-bodied and the impaired by changing behavior, perceptions, and knowledge. Resourceful implementation of these related strategies could have a substantial impact. Better interaction can lead to a greater public acceptance of the impaired in the community.

BIBLIOGRAPHY

Ajzen, Icek, and Martin Fishbein: "Attitude-Behavior Relations: A Theoretical Analysis and Review of Empirical Research," *Psychol Bull* 84:888–918, 1977.

Albrecht, Gary L.: *Reducing Public Barriers of the Severely Handicapped,* Northwestern Univ., Research Report R-20, Chicago, 1976b.

———: "The Negotiated Diagnosis and Treatment of Occlusal Problems," *Soc Sci Med* 11:277–283, 1977.

———, and Paul C. Higgins: "Rehabilitation Success: The Interrelationships of Multiple Criteria," *J Health Soc Behav* 18:36–45, 1977.

———, Vivian Walker, Judith Levy, and Patricia Vance: "Responses to Disability," a paper presented to the American Sociological Association, Boston, 1979.

———, Dorothy Collins, Jane Nosbisch, Byron Hamilton, Carl Granger, and Therese E. Fitzpatrick: *Severe Physical Disability: Dependency or Potential,* Urban Institute, Washington, D.C., 1976a.

Bandura, Albert: *Principles of Behavior Modification,* Holt, Rinehart & Winston, New York, 1969.

———, Edward B. Blanchard, and Brinhilde Ritter: "Relative Efficacy of Desensitization and Modeling Approaches for Inducing Behavioral, Affective, and Attitudinal Changes," *J Pers Soc Psychol* 13:173–199, 1969.

Bloombaum, Milton, and Ted Gugelyk: "Voluntary Confinement Among Lepers," *J Health Soc Behav* 11:16–20, 1970.

Bogdan, Robert, and Douglas Biklen: "Handicapism," *Soc Pol* 14:19, 1977.

Bourne, Patricia G., and Norma J. Wilker: "Commitment and the Cultural Mandate: Women in Medicine," *Soc Prob* 25:430–440, 1978.

Broverman, Inge K., Donald M. Broverman, Frank E. Carlson, Paul S. Rosenkrantz, and Susan R. Vogel: "Sex Role Stereotypes and Clinical Judgments of Mental Health," *J Consult Clin Psychol* 34:1–7, 1970.

Brown, Julia, and May E. Rawlinson: "Sex Differences in Sick Role Rejection and in Work Performance Following Cardiac Surgery," *J Health Soc Behav* 18:276–292, 1977.

Bulman, Ronnie J., and Camille B. Wortman: "Attributions of Blame and Coping in the Real World: Severe Accident Victims React to their Lot," *J Pers Soc Psychol* 35:351–363, 1977.

Comer, R. J., and J. A. Piliavin: "As Others See Us: Attitudes of Physically Handicapped and Normals toward Own and Groups," *Rehabil Lit* 36:206–221, 1975.

Cowan, G., and R. Inskeep: "Commitments to Help Among the Disabled-Disadvantaged," *Pers Soc Psychol Bull* 4:92–96, 1978.

Davis, F.: "Deviance Disavowal: The Management of Strained Interaction by the Visibly Handicapped," *Soc Prob* 9:120–132, 1961.

Donaldson, Joy, and Melton C. Martinson: "Modifying Attitudes Toward Physically Disabled Persons," *Except Child* 43:337–341, 1977.

Farina, A., C. H. Holland, and K. Ring: "Role of Stigma and Set in Interpersonal Interaction," *J Abnorm Psychol* 71:421–428, 1966.

———, J. Sherman, and J. G. Allen: "Role of Physical Abnormalities in Interpersonal Perception and Behavior," *J Abnorm Psychol* 73:590–593, 1968.

Glazier, W. H.: "The Task of Medicine," *Sci Am* 228:13–17, 1973.

Haber, Lawrence D.: "Disabling Effects of Chronic Disease and Impairment. II. Functional Capacity Limitations," *J Chronic Dis* 26:127–152, 1973.

Harasymiw, Stefan J., and Marcia D. Horne: "Integration of Handicapped Children: Its Effects on Teacher Attitudes," *Education* 96:153–158, 1975.

———, Marcia D. Horne, and Sally C. Lewis: "Disability Social Distance Hierarchy for Population Subgroups," *Scand J Rehabil Med* 8:33–36, 1976.

Jamison, Kay R., David W. Wellisch, and Robert O. Pasnau: "Psychosocial Aspects of Mastectomy: The Woman's Perspective," *Am J Psychiatry* 135:432–436, 1978.

Kagan, J., B. A. Henker, A. Hen-Tov, J. Levine, and M. Lewis: "Infants' Differential Reactions to Familiar and Distorted Faces," *Child Dev* 37:518–532, 1966.

Kleck, R.: "Emotional Arousal in Interactions with

Stigmatized Persons," *Psychol Rep* 19: 12–26, 1966.

———, H. Ono, and A. H. Hastorf: "The Effects of Physical Deviance on Face-to-Face Interaction," *Hum Rel* 19:425–436, 1966.

Mercer, Jane: *Labelling the Mentally Retarded,* Univ. of California Press, Berkeley, 1973.

Parsons, Talcott: "The Sick Role and the Role of the Physician Reconsidered," *Milbank Mem Fund* 53:257–278, 1975.

Richardson, Stephan A.: "Attitudes and Behavior Toward the Physically Handicapped," *Birth Defects* 12:15–34, 1976.

Riley, Lawrence, and Saad Nagi: *Disability in the United States: A Compendium of Data in Prevalence and Programs.* Ohio State University Press, Columbus, Ohio, 1970.

Schroedel, John G., and William Schiff: "Attitudes Towards Deafness Among Several Deaf and Hearing Populations," *Rehabil Psychol* 19: 59–70, 1972.

Scott, R.: *The Making of Blind Men,* Russell Sage Foundation, New York, 1970.

Shaw, Marvin E., and Jack M. Wright: *Scales for the Measurement of Attitudes,* McGraw-Hill, New York, 1967, pp. 480–483.

Shontz, Franklin C.: "Psychological Adjustment to Physical Disability: Trends in Theories," *Arch Phys Med Rehabil* 59:251–254, 1978.

Strauss, Anselm: *Chronic Illness and The Quality of Life,* Mosby, St. Louis, 1975.

Svarstad, Bonnie L., and Helene L. Lipton: "Informing Patients About Mental Retardation: A Study of Professional Communication and Parent Acceptance," *Soc Sci Med* 11: 645–651, 1977.

Treitel, Ralph: *Disability Survey 72: Disabled and Nondisabled Adults,* U.S. Department of Health, Education, and Welfare, Social Security Administration, Washington D.C., 1977.

Twaddle, Andrew C.: "Health Decisions and Sick Role Variations: An Exploration," *Health Soc Behav* 10:105–114, 1969.

West, Dee W.: "Social Adaptation Patterns Among Cancer Patients with Facial Disfigurements Resulting from Surgery," *Arch Phys Med Rehabil* 58:473–479, 1977.

Yuker, Harold E., J. R. Block, and Janet H. Younng: *The Measurement of Attitudes Toward Disabled Persons,* Human Resources Center, Albertson, N.Y., 1970.

Zahn, M.A.: "Incapacity, Impotence and Invisible Impairment: Their Effects upon Interpersonal Relations," *J Health Soc Behav* 14: 115–123, 1973.

3

carolyn e. carlson

methods
of coping

INTRODUCTION

Illness, accidents, medical treatment, and other events that affect a person's physical functioning all have the potential to disrupt the lives of many people. Demands may tax or exceed resources momentarily or for long periods of time. Consider the following situations.

John Jamison is a 35-year-old construction worker who is happily married with a family of four children. The children's ages range from 5 to 13. The Jamisons are buying their home and live comfortably, although they are able to save little money. The lives of all members of the Jamison family were disrupted recently when Mr. Jamison was injured seriously at work when a scaffolding collapsed. He is now paralyzed as a result of an injury to the cervical spinal cord. At present he is unable to move his fingers although he can extend his wrists, and he cannot feel or move anything below the nipple line.

Geri Scott, the nurse who admitted Mr. Jamison to the rehabilitation unit, was responsible for planning his nursing care. Geri Scott is married and has a family which includes her husband and three children. She works 3 days a week because she enjoys nursing as well as the supplementary income. During the past few weeks, Ms. Scott spent less and less time with the Jamisons and finally informed the head nurse that she was going to quit.

At present Mr. Jamison has become very critical of his doctor and of the care he is being given. His wife believes that he is getting good care but tries not to interfere with his angry outbursts. She is having her own troubles at home with the children, who have become very irritable and demanding. The oldest boy, 13, has become more withdrawn, and Mrs. Jamison is concerned that he may be drinking and experimenting with drugs. These are new behaviors for all the children.

Mr. Jamison's injury has disrupted the lives of all the people mentioned. The life of each member of the family has become filled with uncertainty and unpredictability. Even Geri Scott's life seems to be upset, although the cause is not clear. Perhaps the Jamisons' situation has made her recognize her own vulnerability. On the other hand, she may feel helpless because she is unable to change the Jamisons' difficult circumstances. For each person, demands, at least for the time being, seem to exceed resources, and it is fair to say that each one is trying to cope.

Coping is not a simple process. It is highly individual; therefore, the processes and behavior involved in coping are highly variable. Nurses are often in a position to facilitate effective coping.

The purpose of this chapter is (1) to define coping and its functions; (2) to describe steps in and dimensions of coping; (3) to distinguish coping from grief and mourning; (4) to discuss illness-disability and coping; and (5) to present strategies for nursing management.

THE MEANING OF COPING

The word cope, common to the lay and professional vocabulary, refers to attempts to manage difficulties, to work through or around obstacles, or to reduce tension. Although this chapter will not analyze subtle differences in definitions, variations in use do exist in the relationship of the term cope to adaptation, adjustment, defense, and mastery.

COMMON DEFINITIONS

Adaptation, a major concept in biology, refers to regulatory processes or mechanisms that maintain or establish equilibrium in the organism and in organism-environment transactions. *Adjustment,* very similar to adaptation, describes an individual's psychosocial regulatory processes. A distinction is not always made between adaptation and adjustment processes. Also, it is not uncommon for adaptation to be used as a term to encompass all types of regulation or maintenance of stability. Regulatory processes required for adaptation may be major or minor and may occur continuously on behavioral, cellular, systemic, and other levels.

CHAPTER 3

The term *coping* is generally reserved for psychological or psychosocial attempts to maintain or reestablish balance. It is sometimes used to describe small, everyday adjustments, but it is more often used to describe attempts to deal with moderate or major life disruptions.

Defense implies threat or danger and is commonly used to describe unconscious psychologic mechanisms used to combat anxiety or fear. Defense mechanisms, like coping methods, are often subsumed under adaptation and adjustment. Sometimes viewed as types of coping, defense mechanisms may also be viewed as separate. Defense often connotes a distortion of reality.

Mastery, according to some theories, is a goal of personality development. People strive to master their environments or to master things that get in their way.

Stress is a term generally used in conjunction with coping, adjustment, adaptation, defense, and mastery. When demands drain or exceed resources, stress is the condition created in the organism. The demands take many forms. If mastery is a motive, its demands may at times exceed resources.

Whether the desired outcome of adjustment, coping, defense, or adaptation is restoration of some prior state or of mastery, many of the mechanisms or behaviors used to achieve the goal are likely to be the same, at least some of the time. For example, information gathering or the use of resources may be as important as mastery in coping effectively with a crisis.

Definition of Coping

Coping is here defined as the psychosocial processes involved in responding to moderate or severe stress in order to regain or establish balance in a person-environment interaction. It includes perception, cognition, and behavior. A coping style is an individual's characteristic method of reacting to stress and a coping strategy is a particular technique used to deal with a particular stress. Coping strategies thus make up one's coping style.

Needs, Goals, and the Functions of Coping

Why do people try to cope? What are the goals of coping strategies? A review of the sequence of events leading up to attempts to cope may help reveal the functions more clearly.

Everyone has implicit or explicit goals that emerge as a consequence of basic and acquired needs. Through experience, patterns of successful behavior in achieving these individual goals are developed. Behavior that achieves goals is used regularly and predictably.

Since goals reflect biological, psychological, and social needs, individuals develop ways to maintain their biopsychosocial integrity. Although physical, psychological, and social aspects of life are often separated in theory, in reality needs, goals, and behaviors can seldom be categorized as purely physical, psychological, or social. A person's goals generally reflect a need to maintain or establish physical well-being, self-esteem, and desirable and effective interactions with others in the environment. Self-esteem is based on the extent to which self-concept, body image, and behavior patterns match one's own expectations. These expectations are influenced greatly by the expectations of others.

Bryne and Thompson (1972) have described how behavior patterning begins at birth. Crying is one of the first behaviors used to respond to stress. If crying is reinforced by feeding or by relief of some other discomfort, it is likely to be repeated when the same discomfort is experienced again.

Consider the patterning of behavior in your own life. Can you identify patterns that are reasonably consistent and predictable that are used to achieve various goals? Do you have particular ways of meeting needs for rest, food and fluids, for affiliation with others? How do these differ from those around you?

Auger (1976) has described Dorothy E. Johnson's model of eight behavioral subsystems that develop as a human being tries to meet basic needs: ingestive; eliminative; dependency; sexual; affiliative; aggressive-protective; achievement; and restorative. Each has certain goals based on the primary function of the subsystem. For example, the goal of the eliminative subsystem is "to release, let go, get rid of waste products, excess, or nonfunctional matters within the system." The goal of the achievement subsystem is to master and control self and environment sufficiently to obtain desired objects or to meet needs. Ordinarily, when goals are being achieved, the subsystem behavior patterns continue and a dynamic state of equilibrium exists in person-environment interaction.

Behavioral subsystems, along with other goal or need frameworks, can be used by the nurse in assessing important areas of a patient's life. Regardless of the framework used, it is important to recognize that (1) people act to meet needs and to achieve goals; (2) relatively stable patterns of behavior are usually developed; and (3) disruption of patterns results in stress, since both needs and goals are threatened.

Coping is a response to stress. Its primary purpose is to remove the threats to meeting needs and achieving goals. Hamburg and Adams (1967) have identified five functions of coping behavior in patients with severe injuries. Successful coping, they say, keeps stress within manageable limits; maintains self-esteem or feelings of personal worth; restores relationships with significant others; facilitates recovery of physical functions; and contributes to the development of a situation that is personally valued and is socially acceptable after maximum recovery has occurred.

If patterns of behavior were effective prior to disruption, coping methods may be geared to the restoration of those prior patterns. Illness or disability which make former behaviors impossible to perform may interfere with success.

Illness, accidents, hospitalization, and treatment methods all can cause major life disruptions. Even a simple cold can interrupt important transactions between the person and the environment and can threaten needs and goals. Hospitalization can disrupt sexual, affiliative, restorative, ingestive, eliminative, and dependency patterns of behavior, to name only a few. Such disruptions create stress and can deplete the energy necessary for recovery or for therapeutic efforts.

Family, friends, and health professionals may err by overlooking or minimizing disruptions in behavior patterns; however, the opposite may also occur. An individual who does not assess a situation carefully can come to the premature, often erroneous conclusion that a patient with a particular condition has nothing of worth left. Such a conclusion leads to pity, separation of that person from those who do have things of worth, and to other attitudes and behaviors that add stress. Jory Graham, a journalist who has metastatic cancer, pointed out that calling a person a victim isolates that individual from nonvictims. "Pity crumbles the strengths we are trying to find within ourselves and degrades the very real efforts we make to retain our dignity as human beings."

The person who is ill or disabled continues to have personal needs and goals and attempts to cope with disruptions as well as possible. Nurses may be able to prevent some disruptions and to facilitate return to prior patterns of behavior by encouraging attempts to cope. These activities are likely to be more effective if the nurse has a clear understanding of coping and is skillful in each step of the nursing process.

APPROACHES TO COPING CLASSIFICATIONS

Because coping with stress is a subject of concern to theoreticians, members of helping professions, and to all who try to cope with life disruptions, many approaches have been developed. A few of these approaches will be described, along with a model incorporating various aspects of the approaches. A concluding summary will discuss the multiple dimensions of coping style.

Some classify all attempts to respond to stress as attempts to cope; others classify coping as a specific response. Wright (1960), for example, has contrasted coping and succumbing. Hann (1977) has identified three types of coping responses: (1) coping which is based on intersubjective reality and logic, is flexible, and involves purpose and choice; (2) defensive coping, which involves distortion of reality and logic and the covert expression of impulses; it is rigid and compelled; and (3) coping by fragmentation, which involves violation of reality, is automated and ritualistic, and is affectively (emotionally) directed. The latter can be very dysfunctional. Lazarus (1976) has divided coping into two categories: direct action and palliation. Direct action is behavior that aims at dealing with the stressor by changing relationships within the environment. Palliation is an effort to reduce, tolerate, or get rid of the perceived distress, hence to comfort.

Works on coping also differ in terms of whether or not the emphasis is on behavioral or cognitive activity. Lazarus and Haan deal with both. Harvey and Janis and Mann emphasize the perceptual and cognitive aspects of coping, but Moos and Tsu emphasize actions or skills. Others focus on personality attributes and ego operations that are charcteristic of successful copers.

Harvey has described four belief system types (conceptual styles) which indicate ways individuals monitor internal and external environments and also how stimuli or events are received, interpreted, and integrated. A *belief system* is a predisposition to interpret ego-involving events in a certain way. Those who are said to belong to System 1 tend to be very concrete with an undifferentiated and poorly integrated cognitive structure. They are dependent on external authority, intolerant of ambiguity, and have a great need for structure. Their methods and goals are poorly differentiated and they have stereotyped ways of approaching problems. System 2 persons tend to be negative, with an antiauthority, antirule orientation. Cognitive organization is poorly integrated although their cognitive structure is more differentiated than in System 1. The System 2 representative tends to associate lack of structure with distrust, fear of rejection, loss of security, and a feeling of loss of control over the situation. The System 3 individual wants to be liked and tries to establish and maintain relationships that foster mutual dependency, allowing for the manipulation of others. This person's awareness of the self as a causal agent allows for a more differentiated cognitive organization. There is less categorical evaluation, less deference toward authority, and less concern with authority and extrapersonal forces. Instead, there is more concern with peer attitudes, social acceptance, and responsibility. Feedback is important because personal standards are not clearly defined. Finally, the System 4 individual is highly task oriented, seeks information, is highly involved in exploratory behavior, risk taking, and independence. This person has internal standards of conduct and personal criteria for evaluation. Relativism in thought and action, differentiation, and integration are highest in this system. This individual is able to have many points of view and multiple relationships. System 4 individuals are least likely to generalize impressions based on incomplete information; they tend to work for intrinsic rather than extrinsic rewards. System 4 persons have a low need for structure, high tolerance for ambiguity, high ability to differentiate methods from goals, ability to generate multiple ways of achieving a goal, and high ability to change views.

These brief descriptions show differences that would be expected to influence the outcomes of attempts to deal with stress. Persons with System 1 and 2 orientations might act too quickly since they tend to be categorical and to respond in stereotyped ways. The System 4 individual, on the other hand, can tolerate conflicting information, tends to be open to information, and is generally more flexible. In most cases, the System 4 person would seem to have the advantage in handling stress.

Janis and Mann (1976) have developed a framework for viewing patterns of coping when decisional conflict creates the stress. Five patterns of coping have been identified, and each is thought to be associated with particular antecedent conditions and stress levels. *Unconflicted adherence* is a decision to continue what one has been doing and to ignore potential negative consequences of this choice. *Unconflicted*

25   METHODS OF COPING

change reflects an uncritical decision to take whatever new action is most salient or forcefully suggested. *Defensive avoidance* is a decision to evade conflict by rationalizing, procrastinating, putting the responsibility on someone else, or being selectively inattentive to corrective information. In the fourth pattern, *hypervigilance,* the person making the decision searches frantically for a way out of the conflict and tends to be too quick to grab at an apparently promising solution for the present. Long-term consequences are often overlooked. In the extreme form, this pattern is called panic. These four patterns are not considered desirable, although they may occasionally be effective. The most effective pattern of dealing with decisional conflict is *vigilance.* After a careful search for relevant information, the information is assessed in an unbiased way and alternatives are considered carefully before a choice is made. This form of decision making is not effective if danger is rapidly approaching and a decision must be made quickly. Similarities can be seen beween the System 4 methods of functioning and the vigilance pattern in decision making.

Moos and Tsu (1977) have developed a conceptual framework of coping which includes the major coping skills used to deal with certain adaptive tasks. The skills they describe (1) may be used individually, in order, or in combination; (2) are not in themselves adaptive or maladaptive; (3) do not have mental and behavioral distinctions; and (4) can be taught and used flexibly depending on the situation. The seven coping skills described are those that deny or minimize the seriousness of the stress; those that seek relevant information and facilitate the effective use of intellectual resources; skills in requesting emotional support and reassurance from others; abilities to learn procedures related to illness and treatment; skill in setting specific, limited goals; ability to rehearse various potential outcomes; and the ability to find purpose in things that have happened. Just about any activity can be a coping skill if it serves to accomplish the necessary tasks.

Obviously there is much overlap in the various approaches. Despite the fact that the emphasis may vary, all approaches to coping seem to acknowledge the processes of perception, cognition, decision making, and behavior.

COPING MODEL

This coping model, which includes steps of coping and coping style dimensions, is a guide to the assessment of coping style.

STEPS INVOLVED IN COPING

An individual's coping style includes the usual steps taken in reacting to stress, ways of handling each step, and variations in different situations. For example, people who avoid or run away from stressful situations whenever possible have to choose another method when they are kept from running away. Similarly, different strategies are used to cope with moderate and severe stress, physical and mental stress, clear and ambiguous stressors, and the like. Many variables alter the coping process. An individual's techniques or strategies for coping reveal similarities across situations as well as variations in certain circumstances. Both consistencies and variations are important.

The process of coping involves perception, cognition, and behavior as the primary activities. Four basic steps are described below (see Fig. 3-1). Although a sequence is suggested, it is important to realize that the individual is often involved in all activities and steps at a given point in time. Transactions with the environment do not cease just because the person is trying to decide how to deal with a previously perceived stressor.

Step 1 Step 1 is the *initial assessment* of ongoing events. Some call this primary appraisal. The outcome of the assessment with respect to the coping process is either the perception of stress or the perception that no stress exists at

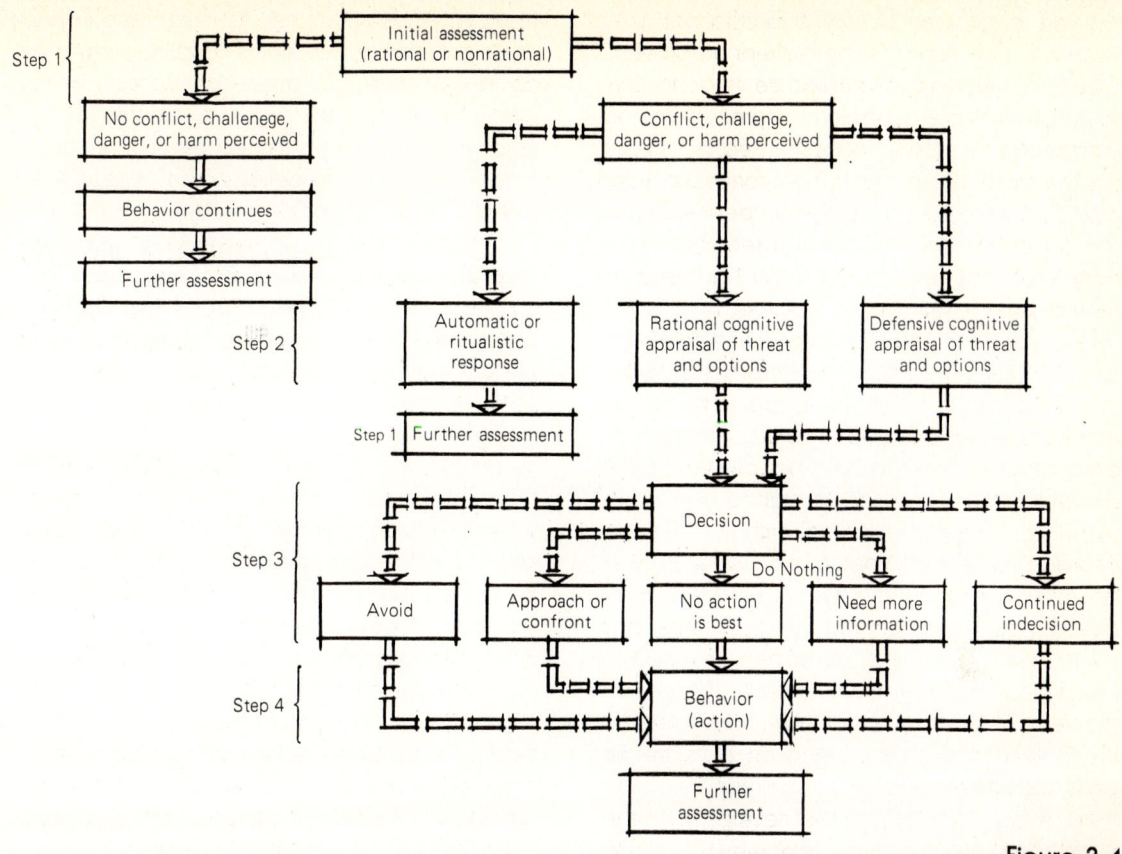

Figure 3-1
Steps involved in coping.

present. Stress may take the form of conflict, challenge, danger, or harm that has already occurred. Harm does not denote only physical harm. It can be any thwarting in the process of goal achievement. Self-esteem drops if one does not live up to expectations of the self or others. Disruption of any goal-achievement activities may be perceived as harm.

Anything that influences an individual's perception can influence Step 1. Perception relies on physiological, psychological, and environmental factors, and accurate perception requires the functioning of sensory systems as well as the higher centers of the brain. Any malfunction of any of these systems can result in distortion of perception. Blind or deaf persons have initial difficulty in perceiving certain types of danger because of their lost sensory modality. Development of compensatory mechanisms is necessary to improve perception.

Psychological defense mechanisms serve to reduce threat through distortion of perception. Defense mechanisms tend to operate automatically in response to anxiety. Anxiety lets a person know that something is wrong. Defense mechanisms can operate to keep anxiety within limits so that problem solving can occur. If the mechanisms are ineffective, panic can result. Also, if overused, or used in the wrong circumstances, defense mechanisms can lead to ineffective problem solving and maladaptive behavior patterns. Detailed descriptions of defense mechanisms, psychosomatic, neurotic, and psychotic patterns of response, are beyond the scope of

27   METHODS OF COPING

this text, but the reader will find information in psychiatric nursing or general psychology texts.

The belief systems described earlier that serve as filters between the internal and external environments can also influence perception during the initial assessment. The System 2 person may be more likely to perceive threat because of a predisposition to suspiciousness. This would be especially true if authority figures were involved.

Finally, stressors may be camouflaged unintentionally or by design. A patient may not be given information that is threatening. A potential attacker may hide a weapon and act friendly. In these cases, a clear picture is not present by the environment and a wrong perception may result.

Step 2 Step 2 of the coping process occurs after the initial assessment results in the perception of stress. During Step 2, at least three processes can occur. First, if the initial assessment resulted in the perception of imminent danger, the person may react in a reflexive, ritualistic, or fragmented way. If a person puts a hand on a burner, a reflex response is initiated and the hand is pulled away. Ritualistic or fragmented responses, on the other hand, are unhealthy responses that may be the result of psychopathology. The perception of reality is not accurate in these instances, and behaviors are often ineffective.

The other two processes that occur during Step 2 involve further appraisal of the situation in order to decide on a course of action. There is a problem; what should be done? Lazarus calls this secondary appraisal. At this stage, the individual assesses what can be done about the danger, threat, or conflict, and what consequences are likely. Some actions may be eliminated as too risky because other individuals may retaliate or because the action is insufficient to combat the stressor. This appraisal can range from a rational, reality-oriented, problem-solving approach to one that is influenced greatly by the defense mechanisms mentioned earlier. It is probably rare for the assessment to be totally rational or totally defensive. It is shown that way in Fig. 3-1 only for emphasis.

Many factors influence this appraisal. An individual's perception of skill in dealing with stress, past experience with stress, repertoire of behavioral skills, perceived urgency, problem-solving skills, motivation to succeed in coping, developmental level, and belief system type are just a few of these factors.

Step 3 Following the second-level assessment, a decision is usually made as to what course of action should be taken. Among the possibilities are (1) to avoid the stressor; (2) to approach or confront the stressor; (3) to do nothing. As shown in Fig. 3-1, the decision to do nothing can be made for several reasons. Doing nothing may seem the most effective way of handling the situation either because nothing is likely to be effective or because the stress will be managed by some other intervening force. The decision may also be based on the realization that more information is needed before the right decision can be made. The decision to seek more information is a decision in itself. If this were a defensive decision, the behavior would be more accurately classified as avoidance. The third reason for a do-nothing choice is continued indecision, which may represent decisional conflict (Janis and Mann).

Step 4 The best decision will be best only if it can be implemented. The range of behaviors that serve the cause of coping is vast, and both approach and avoidance use a variety of behaviors. For example, approach can be managed through direct or indirect, verbal or physical means. The object of approach behavior may be the threatening object itself or some substitute. Substitution is used, for example, by the employee who is angry at his boss but who senses that a direct attack would have dire consequences. The object of attack then becomes his wife, his dog, or some uninvolved object. Substitution can also cause an angry preoccupation by patients with hospital food. Avoidance behavior shows similar variations.

A person who is ill or who, for some other reason, has experienced a change in physical functioning may have great difficulty at Step 4 in the coping process. The perceptual and cognitive processes may be intact, but old behaviors are not available anymore. A young man who formerly handled stress in a physical way and is now quadriplegic experiences such a situation. He must find new ways to deal with stress.

DIMENSIONS OF COPING STYLE

Several dimensions, factors used to describe a person's coping style, are suggested by the four-step coping process. Assessment of these will be helpful to those who want to facilitate successful coping. Most of the dimensions are stated as opposites, and most people's coping styles fall between the extremes. Also, most individuals may be able to change a typical pattern if the situation demands it. The amount of flexibility depends on the ability to consider alternatives, skills, and available resources.

Perceptual and Cognitive Dimensions

Accurate Versus Distorted Perception The degree of accuracy of perception has been discussed above. Neurological deficits and the use of defense mechanisms can result in distorted perceptions and perhaps in unsuccessful coping. It is not easy to measure accuracy of perception because events have different meanings even to people without perceptual distortion. There are a few clues that can be used, however. First, the individual's perceptions can be compared with those of others. If, for example, 90 percent of the people perceive danger when going for surgery, the other 10 percent who say they do not perceive danger might be looked at more closely for reasons for differences in their perception. Agreement of the majority, however, does not automatically signify error or distortion on the part of the minority. The minority may lack information and therefore be unaware of danger. Or they may have *more* information, which results in a different perception. Second, patterns of perception can be observed. Does behavior suggest the involvement of a defense mechanism? Such assessments should be made with caution since the labeling of behavior is seldom useful and behaviors that look defensive may not be.

Consider Mrs. Gabrielli, who is dying of cancer.. Her family doesn't talk about it nor does she. She talks of things she is going to do in the future—traveling she will do, parties she will have, persons she will visit. She has told her doctor she knows that she has little time left.

Many might conclude from Mrs. Gabrielli's behavior that she is denying her situation; however, the facts suggest that she is not. She may have very realistic reasons for not wanting to talk about the terminal nature of her illness. Perhaps she is concerned about discomfort of family members.

A few of the wide variety of thought processes used in coping style dimensions are the following:

Skill in Problem Solving This skill encompasses several characteristics, such as the ability to assess alternatives, the ability to identify resources needed and available, openness to information, flexibility, and locus of control orientation. The contribution of these factors to coping has not yet been determined through research. Problem-solving skill is influenced by the ability to concentrate, by intelligence, short- and long-term memory, belief system type, and other factors.

Spontaneity Versus Careful Planning Some people prefer to take action only after very careful, thorough planning; others prefer a lifestyle that leaves room for considerable spontaneity. Still others plan under some circumstances but behave spontaneously in others. If the individual is familiar with a situation and its demands, a spontaneous response may be very successful. Planning may be needed in less familiar circumstances. Spontaneity does not imply impulsivity, which is discussed under short- and long-range coping.

Spontaneity is often disrupted by illness and disability. Even simple responses that used to be automatic must be planned. The person in a wheelchair can no longer decide to take off to a better climate for the weekend without risk of finding places inaccessible to wheelchairs. Planning may take a lot of fun out of life and may create more tensions that require coping.

Short- Versus Long-Range Coping Time is a vital dimension in determining how to cope. Sometimes short-range coping is more reasonable. There may not be time for long-range considerations in an emergency. Some persons, however, have a short-term focus in nonemergency situations, perhaps caused by a lack of faith in the future or an inability to delay gratifications.

The time dimension is often critical in rehabilitation since much of today's therapy is aimed at long-range rewards or consequences. For some patients, such a delay between work and consequences is quite foreign. Establishment of short-term, meaningful goals may help the therapy.

The long-range view in coping can be problematic, too. Patients may refuse to learn how to care for themselves because when they get home, someone else will do everything for them. Such a situation is difficult for a staff that values independence as well as an individual's right to make decisions about goals and care.

Since all dimensions require observation of behavior, all dimensions can be called behavioral. The following dimensions, however, refer to behavior that occurs during Step 4—implementation—of the coping process.

Behavioral Dimensions

Of the several dimensions that can be assessed from an individual's coping behavior, these are prominent.

Attack Versus Avoidance Although an individual may attack or directly confront some problems or objects and avoid others, a usual pattern can sometimes be identified. Even when a person prefers to avoid or ignore a problem, some circumstances demand attack-or-approach behavior.

A young man avoided most stressful events, including making a decision to do something about his mother who lived alone in the same town. She was in her eighties, very forgetful, was not eating properly, and had become very weak. Neighbors would check on her and let the son know about any problems. When he heard that she was beginning to fall frequently and was becoming incontinent, he could not avoid the problem any longer. He decided to try managing his mother in the home with the help of attendants.

Attack should not be equated with violence, although violence is an extreme form of attack. Attack simply means that the person takes some action against the real threat. Attack against a substitute threat or object involves both attack and avoidance. Direct action that removes the threat may take the form of education or skill development. For example, if the threat is inability to make a living with present abilities, enrolling in college, after hospitalization, to prepare for another type of work would be called attack.

Avoidance can take many forms, too. Defense mechanisms offer ways to avoid the impact of stress. Sublimation may take many forms, physical or mental. Keeping busy to avoid thinking about or doing anything about a problem is a form of avoidance, and many tasks or diversional activities can be used for such avoidance.

Physical Versus Verbal Action This dimension, like the others, can be viewed as a continuum, from high reliance on physical skills to high reliance on verbal skills. Some persons may be equally reliant on both. Illness can disrupt or take away both forms of coping, thus compounding the tasks involved in rehabilitation.

Active Versus Passive Action Coping styles differ in terms of activity and passivity. One who is angry may actively show it verbally or physically, may express it through passive resistance, or may let someone get hurt by not warning of danger.

CHAPTER 3 30

Direct Versus Indirect Action Direct or indirect actions, although they overlap with active and passive actions, are somewhat different. An individual can be active and direct or indirect, or passive and direct or indirect. This dimension is closely associated with attack-avoidance. Direct action is aimed at the stressor. Indirect action may be geared to an improvement of skills that may or may not affect a given stressor; or it can involve action through and around other people, organizations, or structures. For example, a young man, furious at his doctor and other members of the staff, may perceive direct action as too dangerous. He becomes active in organizations designed to change health-care systems. This action may eventually affect the doctor and staff. Indirect action is different from avoidance in that the action taken may eventually influence the perceived stressor.

Passive and indirect action are frequently components of what is labeled manipulative behavior.

Reliance on External Objects

Degree and Type of Reliance on Others Another dimension of coping involves the extent and type of reliance on others in the coping process. The style of some persons is to try to cope with problems alone; others reach out for help. The former may try to work things out alone, then test them out with others.

Reliance on others can take many forms. There may be a preference for a few significant others to help with coping. Or strangers may be preferred for help; or there may be reliance on many people.

Reliance on God is another form of external help that is very important to coping. Beliefs in God and other external powers vary greatly; therefore, an assessment of beliefs is necessary to understand coping style.

Involvement with others takes many forms. The outside person may be a "sounding board," a helper in the problem-solving process, a partner in distraction activities, or a helper with direct attack.

Reliance on Drugs and Other Objects It is important to realize that the objects on which people rely in attempting to cope are not always people. Alcohol, marijuana, tranquilizers, and countless other substances are used in ever-increasing amounts for various reasons. Perhaps, at times, the use of these drugs can make effective problem solving possible by keeping anxiety or pain within manageable limits. Often, however, problem solving doesn't occur because management of anxiety becomes the goal rather than a means to achieve other goals. Drugs are then taken primarily for comfort. Tension management can be a reasonable goal when problem-solving efforts have been exhausted and the tension remains. Is it wrong for the tension to be relieved? Such issues are not easily resolved and cause considerable controversy.

These then are some of the major dimensions of coping. Assessment of an individual on each dimension will provide a relatively clear picture of that person's coping style. The dimensions are summarized in Fig. 3-2.

Factors Contributing to Coping

Many factors that influence coping have already been noted, such as cognitive ability, neurological deficits, belief system type, behavioral repertoire, and internal-external control orientation. Countless factors influence methods of coping. Moos and Tsu name three major categories: background and personal factors; illness-related factors; physical and social environmental factors. These factors are similar to those suggested by Trieschmann (1974) to determine the level of functioning achieved: person, organismic, and environmental variables. Person variables include habits, personality attributes, goals, and attitudes. Organismic variables include illness-related factors and age. Environmental variables include opportunities available, transportation, access to resources, and other external influences.

Successful copers tend to (1) reach out for new experiences, (2) be active when faced with new tasks, and (3) gain pleasure from mastering

DIMENSIONS	SCALE
Perceptual and Cognitive Dimensions	
1. Accurate vs. distorted perception	Accurate ├──────────┤ Distorted
2. Skill in problem solving	High skill ├──────────┤ Low skill
3. Spontaneity vs. careful planning	Spontaneity ├──────────┤ Careful planning
4. Short vs. long-range coping	Short-range ├──────────┤ Long-range
Behavioral dimensions	
1. Attack vs. avoidance	Attack ├──────────┤ Avoidance
2. Physical vs. verbal action	Physical ├──────────┤ Verbal
3. Active vs. passive action	Active ├──────────┤ Passive
4. Direct vs. indirect action	Direct ├──────────┤ Indirect
Reliance on External Objects	
1. Degree of reliance on others	High reliance ├──────────┤ Low reliance
2. Reliance on drugs and other objects	High reliance ├──────────┤ Low reliance

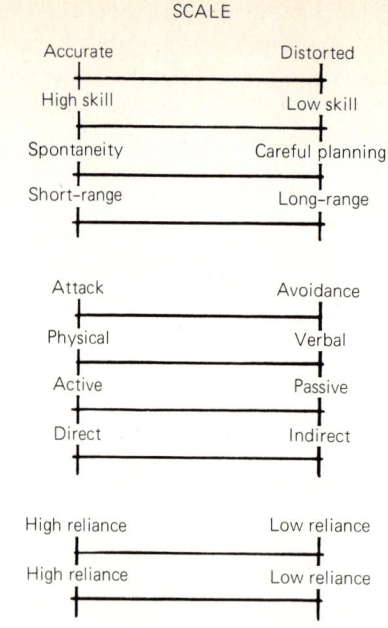

Figure 3-2
Coping style dimensions.

situations (Trieschmann). Lipowski (1970) has stated that the coping strategies chosen by a person with a physical illness are determined by the individual's attitude toward illness, disability, or injury. Illness may be viewed as challenge, enemy, punishment, weakness, relief, strategy (i.e., to get attention), irreparable loss or damage, or as value. Attitudes are especially important to perceptual and cognitive aspects of coping.

Developmental level or age can be very important, both in terms of the threats an illness, disability, or treatment may present and with respect to the coping skills that have been developed. During growth and development, a child has to master various tasks. For example, during adolescence, the individual is faced with establishing identity, determining a future career, developing intimate relationships with members of the opposite sex, along with many other important issues. Illness and disability can disrupt progress in working through these tasks and threaten an already tenuous identity. Body appearance and functioning are of primary concern to the adolescent. Scars, limps, deformities, and loss of function, whether visible or not, are often devastating during this time of life.

Generally, it seems that previous coping methods and coping success are the best predicators of current or future strategies and success in coping. This may not be the case if coping strategies are themselves disrupted by illness, injury, or other circumstances.

Relationship of Coping to Grief and Mourning

In Chap. 9, the process of grief and mourning is described. This process often follows a major crisis or a life-disorganizing event. Such events cause intense stress, disrupt numerous behavior patterns, and lead to instability (disequilibrium) in person-environment interaction.

Coping is very much a part of grief and mourning. Generally, people try to cope with even the most overwhelming events. Descriptions of stages of mourning include coping strat-

CHAPTER 3

egies that are commonly seen during the various periods. The stages are based on observations of many people's responses to life-changing events. They reflect common experiences of many people. Of course, many individual differences occur within and across the stages. Variations in coping style probably account for many of these differences.

The immediate reaction to a highly stressful event is more similar for all people than their later reactions. Shock, the inability to perceive the true meaning of the event, and denial reflect processes that operate to protect the individual and allow life to go on. Denial helps to minimize the impact of the stressful event on the individual's life patterns.

The length of denial and the course that grief and mourning follow probably depend largely on a person's coping style. If an individual tries to cope by avoiding stressful objects or events, denial may be prolonged. During a stage when anger is dominant, individual styles of anger are unique.

Individual coping styles become more apparent as grief and mourning progress. In other words, once a person gets beyond shock and disbelief, his or her usual ways of handling stress are likely to surface.

Although some people deal with multiple crises, the term crisis means that something beyond what is usual has happened to a person. The individual, then, has little experience to call on and few, if any, ways developed for coping with this different event. As the crisis is buffered through denial or other mechanisms, the disruptions caused by the event may look more manageable, and the person begins to call on past experiences and a repertoire of behavior.

In summary, grief and mourning are terms used to describe the sequence of responses that generally follow a stressful event of such magnitude as to cause a major disorganization of life. Usual coping strategies tend to be inadequate to deal with stress of such magnitude. Defenses such as denial minimize the stress for a time. As stress is allowed into consciousness in more manageable forms, former coping patterns will probably be used. It should be remembered, however, that a crisis may lead to the development of new coping styles or strategies.

ILLNESS, DISABILITY, AND COPING

Illness and disability may be the sources of disruption in many goal-directed patterns of behavior. The extent of interference depends on such things as the significance of the goal to the person, the availability of substitute behaviors to incorporate into goal-directed patterns, and the extent of disruption in goal-directed activity. The extent of disruption is not always apparent to the observer, who often is concerned about degrees of loss of function. An objective description of functional loss might be "legal blindness," paraplegia due to complete lesion at T12, or loss of ability to move the left index finger. The observer could list these according to the quantity of functional change.

The person with the change, however, would be likely to describe the change in relation to goals that are disrupted or methods of goal achievement no longer available. To the professional pianist, the loss of function in the left index finger can mean loss of a way to make a living as well as to achieve recognition. Shontz (1975) has identified in body experience seven psychologic functions: (1) an instrument for action, (2) an expressive instrument, (3) a social stimulus, (4) a stimulus to others, (5) a stimulus to self, (6) a sensory register, and (7) a source of drive. These seven functions suggest ways that the body contributes to goal achievement and ways that physical illness and disability can disrupt that achievement. For example, goals that require physical abilities involve the instrument-for-action function. Any disease or other event that alters physical functioning (the instrument) threatens to disrupt equilibrium and therefore increases stress. If a person has a cerebrovascular accident with resultant right hemiplegia and aphasia, at least two psychologic functions of body experience are disrupted, the instrument for action and the expressive instrument.

Illness and disability affect coping in at least two ways. First, they cause various amounts of stress through disruptions in physical, psychological, and social functioning. Unless stress is minimal, coping processes are called upon to restore stability. Second, illness and disability often interfere with usual coping style.

NURSING MANAGEMENT

The overall goals of nursing with respect to facilitating patient coping differ according to such factors as overall treatment goals, the patient's premorbid coping style, and time available to work with the patient. In programs emphasizing physical rehabilitation, goals involving major personality reorganization are seldom realistic or even possible. Such goals, on the other hand, may be primary in a psychiatric setting. The patient's return to a coping style and life-style that approximate the premorbid one is often a considerable achievement. Many health professionals have difficulty settling for goals that involve the patient's return to patterns that may not be the healthiest or the most effective. Yet setting goals beyond or very different from premorbid patterns may lead to certain failure. This is not to say that it is wrong to encourage the development of more effective coping styles. Instead, nurses should try to be realistic in determining what can be accomplished with the resources and time available.

ASSESSMENT

Assessment that facilitates coping includes gathering information about premorbid life-style, coping style, and amount and type of resources available; the extent of current disruption in life-style, coping style, and resources; and current level of stress, coping methods and effectiveness of coping methods.

Assessment of premorbid life-style involves a determination of needs, goals, and of patterns of behavior used to meet or achieve them. The subsystems of behavior described earlier, along with other needs or goals, can be used as guides in this assessment. Such information will provide data about the types of events likely to be disruptive or stressful to the person. Illness or disability sometimes has a minimal effect on usual behavior patterns. In other instances, even small changes in physical functioning have a major impact on goal achievement.

Assessment of premorbid coping style also takes many forms. The steps and dimensions of coping presented earlier in this chapter can be used as a framework for assessing coping style. Information gathered from the patient as well as from persons who know the patient well will help the nurse to get a clear picture of how the individual usually responds to problems and stressful situations. It is seldom easy to get accurate information at first since most people have ideas about the "right way" to behave and may try to create an impression that approximates the socially desirable view. Thus, it may take considerable time, with close attention to subtle clues, to put the picture of the coping puzzle together.

Mr. and Mrs. Collins described their 13-year-old son, Jerry, as a model child who was always obedient, was never in trouble, and did not drink alcohol or smoke. While in the hospital, Jerry seldom obeyed, frequently violated rules, and was found more than once drinking and smoking. Only when a brother came to visit did the staff find out that this was Jerry's usual way of behaving when he was upset. The brother was not as invested in the "ideal image" as were his parents.

As more and more information is gathered, consider the steps of coping and the coping dimensions shown in Fig. 3-2. Can you develop a profile of premorbid coping? The coping dimension framework simply serves as a guide to determine what is already known about a patient and what additional factors may be important. You may find other guides that will work better for you.

The third major part of premorbid assessment concerns resources available to the individual. Here the nurse gathers information about abilities of the patient and about people and circumstances external to the patient that facilitated goal achievement prior to illness or injury. Resources include faith, confidence, skills, money, job or educational opportunities, availability of help with tasks, and people to love and who love in return. The possible resources, too numerous to list here, are critical to goal achievement.

Assessment of the situation includes the factors listed above as well as a comparison of the current situation with premorbid circumstances. Consider how illness or disability has disrupted previous patterns of behavior and coping style. If you don't know about prior patterns, signs of anxiety, fear, or anger are common indicators of stress. Recall that stress results when patterns of behavior are disrupted and goal achievement is threatened in some way. It is important to note the extent to which premorbid coping style is likely to be effective in meeting current demands.

Following the assessment, the nurse develops a list of nursing diagnoses related to stress and coping. It is important that clear terminology be used to achieve mutual understanding among staff.

A great deal of knowledge goes into an assessment: knowledge of age, developmental level, sex, socioeconomic level, ethnicity, religion, pathophysiology, family dynamics, and education. All are helpful in gathering and interpreting information.

PLANNING

Planning is most effective when it is done with the patient since the patient's goals are the most critical aspect of the planning. In the realm of coping, planning includes a determination of goals, of nursing intervention, and of methods to be tried to maintain or improve coping ability. Coping ability can be improved by decreasing stress as well as by increasing coping skill.

The nurse, with the patient, can determine the temporary and long-term demands of the situation that must be coped with in some way, and which dimensions of the prior coping style are still available. Consideration can be given to alternative coping methods or skills that could be developed to meet the demands or to handle problems. Which are most reasonable considering intellectual capacity, goals, age, phases of grief and mourning, etc.? What methods or skills would accomplish the goals with the least amount of change from premorbid coping style?

It is useful to state goals in terms of patient behavior so that achievement of the goals is observable. Consider the following example:

Gloria Stevens, 35 years old, has multiple sclerosis, which was diagnosed 7 years ago. She has been confined to a wheelchair for 3 years. Mrs. Stevens has a 6-year-old daughter living with her. She says her husband divorced her 5 years ago because they couldn't get public aid if they remained married; she says they will be remarried soon and she will have the help she needs at home. She has not been told that her husband has remarried.

In this situation the nurse does not know if the patient is using a denial mechanism since it is not clear what she has been told by or about her former husband. The nurse is concerned with helping Mrs. Stevens find a different way to cope with problems at home since her former husband is not likely to be helping her. Beginning goals might be stated as follows:

By next week, Mrs. Stevens will list the activities of daily living with which she needs assistance. By discharge Mrs. Stevens will describe exactly how she will get the help she says she needs. These descriptions will not include her husband.

Goals can be made more precise as more is learned about available resources.

Once the goals are determined, methods need to be worked out to achieve them. For Mrs. Stevens, the first step may be giving her accurate information about her former husband's ability to help her. If she continues to insist that he will take care of everything, the rehabilitation team may consider having a psychologist or psychiatrist see her and suggest approaches to the home care problems.

Planning does not always involve setting goals and determining methods to help the patient change in some way. If stress can be reduced to a manageable level, an individual's coping mechanism may be sufficient. Often this can be accomplished by acting on the environment rather than the individual. Explaining procedures to be done or changes that have been made in scheduling can prevent stress from building up. Reducing environmental noise, helping family and others cope, and removing distressing people from the situation are all ways of facilitating coping by acting on the environment.

Specific goals set for the patient and methods used to facilitate coping are numerous, but their success is often a consequence of care in planning.

INTERVENTION METHODS

Methods that can be used to facilitate coping are teaching, encouraging problem solving and role playing, modeling, listening, operant conditioning, and altering the environment.

When teaching is used to facilitate coping, it includes any activity that provides the patient with information needed to prevent or reduce stress, to recognize and use resources, or to develop new behaviors for coping. Obviously, teaching overlaps with other intervention methods. The nature of the learner must be considered before determining what to teach and how. Teaching is more effective when the learner can perceive its relevance to personal goals. In other words, not everyone wants to learn in order to stay healthy. A connection may have to be made between being healthy and meeting personal goals.

Mr. Benson was an avid horse-racing fan before his CVA (cerebrovascular accident), subsequent Broca's aphasia, and right hemiplegia. Nurses had difficulty getting him to do anything until they started relating skill development to the possibility of getting back to the racetrack.

By asking questions, making suggestions, reminding the patient of alternatives or resources available, and by pointing out left-out steps, a nurse can encourage problem solving and help the patient do a thorough job at each problem level. Timing of these activities is important. It is difficult to follow logical steps of problem solving when in pain, when concerned about other difficulties, or when there are other distractions.

Role playing can be used to let the patient experiment with behaviors that might be effective in particular problem situations or to practice behaviors that the patient wishes to develop. A young man who was paraplegic said he had had trouble adjusting to the idea of dating after his injury. In such a situation, the patient might role play asking someone for a date, then practice ways of responding to rejection or acceptance. It is helpful for the role player to be as realistic as possible so that the patient is prepared for real situations.

Modeling is the learning of behavior through watching another person's performance. The newly injured quadriplegic who is concerned about coping with the dating situation may benefit from watching someone deal effectively with the same situation. Observation may be in person, through movies, or television. Behaviors that are viewed as successful are likely to be tried. The nurse is often able to refer a patient to persons who might serve as models. Members of Ostomy clubs, Alcoholics Anonymous, Lost Chord clubs, and others serve as models for new members.

Behavior that is followed by a positive reinforcer (reward) tends to be repeated; behavior that is followed by a negative reinforcer (punishment) tends to decrease in frequency. These are both basic principles of learning theory and provide the bases for operant conditioning. It is sometimes difficult to keep from rewarding ineffective behavior or behavior that works against goals of the rehabilitation program. The patient who refuses to go to therapies often gets a great deal of attention from people who try to find out why or who encourage reconsideration. The attention that follows the refusal may serve as a positive reinforcer. If so, the refusals are likely to increase. The person with chronic pain is also often subject to some inadvertent conditioning of pain behavior.

Ann Jones has had increasingly severe pain in her lower back over the past 5 years. Her pain has become the primary topic of her conversation. Hospitalized several times, she has been encouraged each time to go as long as she can between doses of pain medication so that she won't become addicted. By the time she finally takes her pain medication, the pain is very severe. She gets her pain medicine and is told to rest. Pain relief and rest have become positive reinforcers of pain behavior.

Although principles of learning theory can be used to modify patient behavior, there are ethical issues that need to be confronted. Does anyone have the right to control another person's behavior? Who decides what behavior is desirable? Does behavior modification limit freedom or does it increase freedom by providing a greater repertoire of behaviors? What methods of behavior modification are ethical? These are a few of the issues to be considered when behavior modification seems to be a desirable goal.

Coping can often be facilitated by working on aspects of the environment rather than on the patient. Several methods may be effective depending on the circumstances. Stressors may be removed, supports added, or physical barriers removed. Examples of removing stressors include removing noisy distractions to facilitate problem solving, changing patient room assignments when personalities clash or are otherwise stressful, and advising other persons in the environment of the actions the patient finds stressful. Added supports may be physical, social, or economic. Availability of family, friends, physical aids, and financial resources are usually crucial to long-range success in coping. The nurse can coordinate efforts to build in the necessary supports. It is important that the uniqueness of each person be kept uppermost in mind when attempting to provide supports. It is very easy to become routinized in providing supports. Then many needs are unmet.

Finally, numerous physical barriers exist that limit the freedom of the person with a disability. Any restriction of freedom has the potential to disrupt the individual's coping abilities through increasing stress and diminishing coping options. Even though public awareness of physical barriers is increasing, countless barriers remain. Nurses, nursing students, and all members of the health professions can do a great deal to educate individuals and groups about ways to increase accessibility of the environment to all citizens.

Intervention methods should be consistent with a patient's short- and long-term goals and with the resources available to the individual. For example, rewards used to help an individual change behavior are more effective in the long run if they can be used in the home environment also. Guiding a patient to learn to cope through an open and honest expression of feelings when such expression will not be tolerated in the home environment can have unfortunate consequences.

EVALUATION

Progress in goal achievement is the first step in evaluation. If progress in improving coping through changes in the environment or changes in the person is satisfactory, the program of nursing intervention can be continued. If progress does not seem sufficient, several reassessments may reveal the reasons. First, patient problems may not have been assessed accurately in the beginning or the problems may have changed. Plans for nursing care often have to be designed with limited information. As more information becomes available, assessment becomes more accurate and more effective planning is possible. Second, the method of nursing intervention chosen may not be effective either because it is not implemented correctly or because the method is not suited to the person or the problem. If the intervention involves operant conditioning, for example, the chosen reinforcer may not be perceived as rewarding by the patient. Patient teaching is often ineffective because it is given at a time inappropriate to learning or in a way that is not understandable. Based on evaluation, adjustments may be made in any of the steps of the nursing process.

CONCLUSION

The content of this chapter will help the reader recognize situations where stress exists, identify current attempts to cope, compare current options for coping with prior coping patterns, and plan and implement nursing interventions to help the patient manage stress and the return to a life-style that approximates the former one as closely as possible. Achieving a life-style similar to a former one may require finding new ways to meet some needs or to achieve important goals, as well as substitute ways of coping with stress. The steps of coping and the coping dimensions provide guidelines for analyzing coping style and determining aspects altered by illness and disability.

Coping in highly stressful circumstances usually requires help from others. Family members rely on each other and may need outside help if their resources are diminished. The nurse tries to help the patient and family. It is hoped that nurses and other team members will recongize stress in each other and will contribute constructively to coping with situations which are at times overwhelming.

BIBLIOGRAPHY

Auger, Jeanine R.: *Behavioral Systems and Nursing,* Prentice-Hall, Englewood Cliffs, N.J., 1976.

Byrne, Marjorie L., and Lida F. Thompson: *Key Concepts for the Study and Practice of Nursing,* Mosby, St. Louis, 1972.

Grace, Helen, Janice Layton, and Dorothy Camilleri: *Mental Health Nursing: A Sociopsychological Approach,* Wm. C. Brown, Dubuque, Iowa, 1977.

Graham, Jory: "A Time to Live: Make 'Cancer Victim' Taboo," *Chicago Daily News,* January 26, 1978.

Haan, Norma: *Coping and Defending,* Academic Press, New York, 1977.

Hamburg, David A., and John E. Adams: "A Perspective on Coping Behavior," *Arch Gen Psychiatry,* vol. 17, 1967.

Harvey, O. J., and C. Felknor: "Parent-Child Relations as an Antecedent to Conceptual Functioning." In G. A. Milton, and R. A. Hoppe (eds.) *Early Experiences and the Processes of Socialization,* New York, Academic, 1970

Janis, Irving L., and Leon Mann: "Coping with Decisional Conflict," *Am Sci* 64:6, 1976.

Lazarus, Richard S.: *Patterns of Adjustment* (3d ed.), McGraw-Hill, New York, 1976.

Lipowski, Z. J.: "Physical Illness, The Individual and the Coping Processes," *Psychiatry Med* 1, 1970.

Moos, Rudolf H., and Vivien Davis Tsu: "The Crisis of Physical Illness: An Overview," in Rudolf H. Moos (ed.), *Coping with Physical Illness,* Plenum, New York, 1977.

Shontz, Franklin C.: *The Psychological Aspects of Physical Illness and Disability,* Macmillan, New York, 1975.

Silber, Earle, David A. Hamburg, George V. Coelho, Elizabeth B. Murphy, Morris Rosenberg, and Leonard I. Pearlin: "Adaptive Behavior in Competent Adolescents," in R. H. Moos (ed.), *Human Adaptation,* D. C. Heath, Lexington, Mass., 1976.

Trieschmann, Roberta B.: "Coping with a Disability: A Sliding Scale of Goals," *Arch Phys Med Rehabil* 55, 1974.

Wright, Beatrice: *Physical Disability—A Psychological Approach,* Harper & Row, New York, 1960.

4

carolyn e. carlson

help, helping, and helplessness

INTRODUCTION

Help. We all need it. Most of us give it. None can live without it. Illness and disability usually increase the need for help or alter the nature of the help that is needed. The professional nurse can provide the assistance needed or facilitate linking the person in need with the individual, agency, or other resource that can provide help.

Unfortunatley, much help is given on a trial-and-error basis. Helping will be more effective when outcomes of specific actions become more predictable. Theory on help and helping can provide a framework for identifying needs for help, taking action in response to those needs, and conducting research on various aspects of the helping process.

Chapter 3 focused on coping. The coping process is initiated when stress is perceived; stress is perceived when needs are not being met. Individual patterns of behavior to meet needs involve varying amounts of help from sources outside the self. Coping may require the same kind of assistance—a person to listen, provision of needed materials to combat danger, or opportunities for skill development. Helping is an important part of everyday living.

This chapter will discuss equity theory, variables that influence helping in specific situations, helplessness, and the application of these topics to illness, disability, and nursing.

BASIC CONCEPTS

HELP

Help is a simple word used to describe assisting actions. It is also used to request assistance from others. Although help usually implies action, the best help may be the inhibition of certain actions. A request for help to become more independent, for example, often requires that the helper stand back and keep from doing particular things for the person.

It seems useful to consider help as it is viewed by the person giving the help as well as by the one receiving it. Help as perceived by the giver is an overt or covert activity intended to facilitate some outcome for the receiver. Help may be offered to make a goal achievable or to make a task easier. The receiver of help may perceive the intended helping actions quite differently. A given action may facilitate some desired outcomes and take away from or inhibit others. For example, taking over the bathing and dressing of another person who is slow and is struggling to bathe and dress will speed up the completion of those tasks but may make that person feel worthless. If the positive accomplishments facilitated by the helper's actions exceed the negative consequences, the recipient is apt to label the actions as help. If, on the other hand, there are many negative outcomes, the actions will be considered obstacles. Alertness to the needs and goals of the client can increase the effectiveness of offering and giving help and can prevent good intentions from going awry.

HELPING

Helping is the process of providing aid, support, encouragement, money, reward, muscle power, a listening ear, guidance, and the many other forms of assistance used to attain certain outcomes. Effective helping generally requires assessment of needs and the nature of the needs, assessment of actions and resources that might facilitate meeting the needs, and ability and willingness to perform necessary actions.

HELPLESSNESS

Lange (1978) describes helplessness as the syndrome of emotions, cognitions, and actions seen when events cannot be controlled or when nothing can be done to alter a situation. The person has lost control over outside events and is overwhelmed. Helplessness may be transient or temporary, as in various crisis situations, or it may be a chronic syndrome.

DEPENDENCE, INDEPENDENCE, AND INTERDEPENDENCE

The need for help is closely related to the various dependency states. From the time of birth, the human infant is extremely dependent and requires continuous help to survive. The infant's needs are easily recognized by others, and help is usually given.

Normal development involves the progression from dependence to independence and finally to interdependence. Anyone who has watched a child grow realizes how early the quest for independence emerges. Although there is a need to strive for independence, few if any persons ever achieve total independence from others because few physical, emotional, or social needs can be met without the help of others. We need materials grown and manufactured by others, skills and services offered by others, and social interactions, love, and friendship that can only be achieved with others. People, therefore, are to a great extent interdependent.

The nature of interdependence is unique for each pair or larger group of people. For example, one individual may have most needs met by several people or groups; another may rely on one or very few. A person may give to some people and receive from others; however, in close relationships that last for any length of time, there is generally mutual give and take.

Although we are all involved in interdependent relationships, the amount of giving and receiving is often not equal. There are individuals who are excessively dependent on others and tend to receive more than they return. On the other hand, there are those who seem to give more than they receive. It should be pointed out that it is difficult for the external observer to determine the amount of giving and receiving between people since so much depends on individual needs and subtle ways of expressing and meeting needs.

DEVELOPMENT OF HELPLESSNESS

Development and maintenance of interdependence or mutual help relationships is influenced by many factors, whether or not an individual recognizes and responds to the needs of another person.

According to Schmale (1964), feelings of helplessness have their origin in early childhood. The child between 12 and 16 months of age begins to realize his or her dependence on external laws and external objects. Gratification often requires help from others. When it is needed and is not available, helplessness is experienced. Generally the child learns that there are dependable people around for protection and gratification, even though gratification may not be immediate. However, helplessness will be experienced if there is prolonged absence of gratification. Schmale suggests that

> Feelings of helplessness may recur at any time during life whenever there is a loss or threat of loss of an object which is a supplier of immediate gratification and there is no way found for avoiding or overcoming the loss.

Since loss of gratification is perceived as the absence of something that can only be supplied by others, the person feels let down, deprived—helpless.

Helplessness occurs when something necessary for gratification and external to the self is unavailable and the person feels unable to do anything about it. Helplessness is not the same as hopelessness. Hopelessness, as described by Schmale, occurs when an individual experiences defeat or loss of control over the self. Helplessness is oriented to outside events and to objects required for gratification. Hopelessness pertains to the self. Helplessness, therefore, can occur without hopelessness.

Feelings of helplessness include a decreased sense of purpose, self-esteem, and self-confidence; loss of belief in self as a provider of pleasure; and feelings of failure, humiliation, and shame (Goldfarb, 1975). Goldfarb has written that feelings of helplessness result when loss of resources leads to decreased mastery (gratification). Feelings of helplessness bring fear, anger, and attempts to get help. The attempts to get help can be rational or irrational; therefore, helplessness may have numerous manifestations. Consider the coping process described in Chap. 3. Fear and anger, as responses to danger perceived in the environment, may be rational, distorted, or defensive feelings. Rational appraisal is usually followed by rational appeals for help. Less effective appeals are likely to follow distorted perceptions of helplessness.

Helplessness can be a response to loss of control over the environment or loss of predictability of events. Seligman (1976) suggests that helplessness occurs when people learn that gratification does not depend on their behavior, and they give up or fail to try anymore. In other words, when persons learn from experience that what they do does not influence what happens to them, they have no feeling of control over particular happenings. If a little boy is spanked when he does what he is told as well as when he disobeys, he may decide that what he does has nothing to do with getting spanked and that he is helpless in influencing whether or not he will be punished. Although animal studies have shown considerable support for this theory, results of studies with humans have been less conclusive.

Other theories predict different responses to loss of control or loss of freedom. Brehm (1972), in his reactance theory, predicts that when behavioral freedom is lost or threatened, the individual is motivated to attempt to restore the freedom rather than to give up. It is possible to integrate the learned helplessness and reactance theories to explain some of the apparent differences between them (Walster et al., 1976). Two important concepts in the integration are expectation of control and importance.

> If a person expects to be able to control or influence outcomes that are of some importance to him, finding those outcomes to be uncontrollable should arouse psychological reactance. Thus, among individuals who initially expect control, the first few trials of helplessness training should act as a threat to their freedom. They should experience increased motivation to exert control, and improved performance should occur. The more important the uncontrollable outcome, the more reactance should be experienced. But despite his increased motivation to do so, the individual comes to learn through extended helplessness training that he cannot control the outcome. When a person becomes convinced that he cannot control his outcomes, he will stop trying. (Walster et al., p. 308)

An individual who does not expect to have control will not be likely to experience the increased motivation (reactance) and may become helpless rapidly when faced with uncontrollable outcomes. Consider the following examples.

> Dr. Jordan is the president of his own company that has been doing very well. For several years most things have gone the way he wanted them to go. He feels that he has control over just about everything he wants.
>
> Mr. Miller, unable to work much of his life because of chronic health problems, believes that many things are beyond his control. Working depends on his health, and many aspects of his life are influenced by his sporadic income.

In these examples Dr. Jordan has a background that will lead him to expect freedom and control. Mr. Miller will expect little or no control. According to the integrated theory, Mr. Miller would become helpless faster than Dr. Jordan if faced with something important and beyond control. He doesn't expect control so he gives up more readily.

Unfortunately, helplessness is viewed negatively in many social groups. If helplessness is negatively sanctioned, negative emotions are likely to be engendered when helplessness is experienced. All persons, at some time in life, will face situations over which they have little or no control, such as illness, death of loved ones, violent storms, or the price of a dozen eggs. Under such circumstances, the most constructive response may be to do nothing, to simply accept the fact of helplessness, and to adjust to a lack of control. If one acknowledges a helpless state and gives up, negative feelings (i.e., depression) may occur. If, however, giving up attempts to control the uncontrollable frees energy so that it can be used in areas where greater control is possible, gratification may result. Dwelling on helplessness, on the other hand, will probably lead to increased frustration, anxiety, or depression. In other words, feelings associated with the inability to control what happens may be negative, but they need not always be.

WHY DO PEOPLE HELP EACH OTHER?

WHY DO PEOPLE HELP?

After a person discovers that another person needs help, what determines the decision to perform the help-giving acts? Schwartz (1977) offers three explanations: (1) arousal of emotion; (2) activation of social expectations; and (3) activation of self-expectations. In the first case, emotional or emphatic arousal leads to helping, which then decreases the arousal or distress (positive reinforcement). When activation of social expectations occurs, the individual's behavior is motivated by what is socially acceptable in the situation (external reinforcement). On the other hand, if self-expectations are activated, helping behavior can occur without external reinforcement because internalized norms and values that advocate helping or a feeling of moral obligation are aroused. Conformity to self-expectation leads to pride, increased self-esteem, and other positive evaluations of the self. In each case, the individual's experiences are positive following the helping act.

Helping in some instances is reciprocal. A favor is followed by a returned favor or some other repayment. Theories that explain reciprocity behavior help us understand the behavior of ongoing interactions. However, help is often given to strangers. What principles govern helping behavior in situations that do not involve long-term ongoing interactions? Presenting one theory of reciprocity and a model of helping in emergency situations will identify some of the issues involved.

Many theories present the human being as a selfish organism, and the following basic propositions of equity theory have been formulated by Walster, Bercheid, and Walster:

> Proposition I: Individuals will try to maximize their outcomes (where outcomes equal rewards minus costs).
>
> Proposition IIA: Groups can maximize collective reward by evolving accepted systems for "equitably" apportioning rewards and costs among members. Thus, members will evolve such systems of equity and will attempt to induce members to accept and adhere to these systems.
>
> Proposition IIB: Groups will generally reward members who treat others equitably and generally punish (increase the costs for) members who treat others inequitably.
>
> Proposition III: When individuals find themselves participating in inequitable relationships, they become distressed. The more inequitable the relationship, the more distress individuals feel.
>
> Proposition IV: Individuals who discover they are in an inequitable relationship attempt to eliminate their distress by restoring equity. The greater the inequity that exists, the more distress they feel, and the harder they try to restore equity.

Restoration of equity can occur by actually changing the inputs of the participants or by distorting perception of outcomes for the self and for others. In the latter case, psychologic equity is restored since the change is perceptual rather than actual.

What is equitable varies a great deal in different social systems, and although methods used to separate and apportion resources are different, norms are established that maximize collective rewards. These norms are taught to members of the social system.

A relationship is equitable when the person observing (or participating in) a relationship perceives that each participant is receiving relatively equal outcomes from the relationship. Positive and negative outcomes balance out. Inputs to the relationship can be assets or liabilities. An input that is an asset entitles one to rewards; one that is a liability produces negative outcomes.

Consider how equity theory applies to helping relationships. Initially, two persons are involved in an equitable relationship, but if person A helps person B, the relationship may come to be perceived as inequitable. Person B may feel that he or she is profiting more than person A; person A may think that the profit and costs are unequal. According to equity theory, both persons should experience discomfort and try to restore actual or psychologic equity. Intentionality and ability to repay have been found to be important determinants of responses in inequitable helping relationships.

Research on intentionality and ability to repay in inequitable helping relationships has led to two conclusions. First, greater discomfort will be felt and a stronger desire to restore equity will be present when the inequity was produced intentionally than when it happened accidentally. The person who has been helped intentionally has a greater wish to pay back than does one helped unintentionally (Staub, 1976). A patient, for example, might work for a change in hospital policy to allow visitors to stay later in the evening. Although this effort was for the patient, it will, no doubt, be helpful to others. The others will not be likely to experience inequity or to wish to repay under these circumstances. If the patient acts with the specific intent to change a policy for someone else's benefit and the other person is aware of it, inequity and a wish to repay are more probable.

Second, the person with little or no ability to repay (to restore equity) is less likely to try to do so than one who has the ability. The inequity creates discomfort unless it can be justified (psychological equity restored). Walster, Berscheid, and Walster report that people are less likely to ask for help or accept gifts if they cannot pay back. They suggest that acceptance puts the recipient in a position of obligation which is uncomfortable.

Temporary inequities do not create discomfort when members of the relationship know that equity will be restored. In other words, participants in relationships in which rewards and costs are generally equal will not be distressed with short-term periods of disruption in this equality.

Equity theory suggests some basic principles underlying helping behavior that seem to relate primarily to ongoing relationships. Often, help is asked by and given to strangers. Research on altruistic or prosocial behavior provides information about factors that influence helping behavior in nonemergency and emergency situations.

WHY DO PEOPLE HELP IN GIVING SITUATIONS?

Helping, unless done accidentally, requires awareness of the need for help, a decision to help or not to help, and the actual performance of what is needed.

In nonemergency situations which are frequent and are usually pretty well understood, awareness of the need for help occurs in different ways. The person in need can ask for help; the observer may notice that help is needed; or a notice requesting help or some other passive method may be used. It has been found that the potential helper tends to provide less help when the freedom of choice to refuse is threatened. Also, positive-toned, simple requests lead to more helping responses than do negative-toned appeals (Bar-Tal, 1976).

According to Bar-Tal, an emergency situation has five characteristics: (1) there is threat of harm or actual damage to life or property and intervention can be costly, (2) the situation is unusual, (3) demands are unique and the helper needs to have particular skills, (4) the event is generally unanticipated, and (5) the intervention required must be immediate.

Bar-Tal's model for helping in emergency situation is shown in Fig. 4-1 and is similar to the model for nonemergency situations. The first

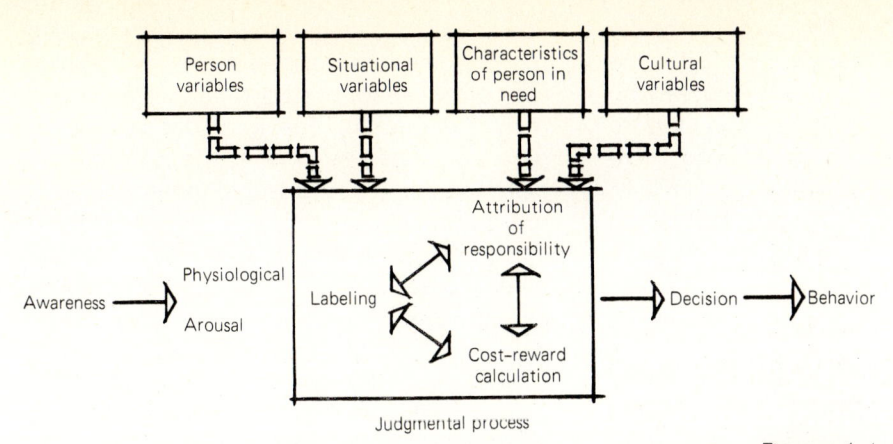

Figure 4-1
Bar-Tal's decision-making model of helping. *(Used with permission from Bar-Tal, Daniel, Prosocial Behavior, Hemisphere, Washington, D.C., 1976, p. 97.)*

phase of the model is awareness. The potential helper encounters a direct or indirect appeal or a situation where there is no appeal but the need for help is obvious. Awareness is followed by physiological arousal (absent in nonemergency situation) and then by the judgmental process. The judgmental process involves three interacting processes. First, the victim labels the situation as an emergency by making the appeal. This labeling is absent from the nonemergency situation. Second, the potential helper judges whether or not the victim is responsible for the thing that has happened or if responsibility is external to the person. Is the person requesting help because of some personal inadequacy or because of factors that are beyond the individual's control? Third, the potential helper does a quick cost-reward analysis. What are the potential costs and rewards for helping and for not helping? Action may be dangerous or take a great deal of time and effort; on the other hand, refusal to help may lead to shame, decreased self-esteem, or other costly consequences. A decision to help or not to help follows the judgmental process along with the associated behaviors (Bar-Tal).

The sequence of events reflected in the model tend to occur very quickly and are thought to be influenced by several sets of variables: (1) variables related to the potential helper's personality traits, age, sex, and race; (2) situation variables such as clarity of the need, degree of need, prior experience helping the person, presence of others, dependency of the person in need, and observation of others helping; (3) characteristics of the person in need such as internal-external control orientation, sex, race, age, appearance, similarity between person in need and the potential helper, and relationship between the persons; and (4) cultural variables, primarily values and norms (Staub). In research on helping behavior, it is often difficult to separate the effects of variables, and there are few findings which are indisputable. See Staub and Chap. 2 by Albrecht for a review of experiments on helping a person in distress.

Equity theory and Bar-Tal's model provide guidelines that can be used in giving and receiving help. Equity theory suggests that it is important for participants in a relationship to monitor rewards and costs and to manage inequities if they want the relationship to continue. In order to do this effectively, each participant in a relationship needs to know how the other is perceiving rewards and costs.

Bar-Tal's model of helping shows the component parts of the process. The potential helper must be aware of the need for help. Since the decision to act is based on several variables and processes, the person needing help can increase the likelihood of getting it by learning more about these variables and processes. Similarly, helpers can aid those in need by understanding the various aspects of the helping process.

ILLNESS AND DISABILITY AND HELPING CONCEPTS

CHANGES IN NORMAL PATTERNS AND HELPLESSNESS

Needs for help change throughout life as a result of changes in goals, demands, and resources. Illness and disability can cause great changes in the nature and amount of help needed from others. In addition, the amount and kind of help that the ill or disabled person can give is often disrupted and relationships that were equitable often become inequitable.

One might expect that severe illnesses, poor prognoses, and loss of body parts and functions commonly would be followed by overwhelming feelings of helplessness. Certainly grieving is common and helplessness is one of the subjective reactions of grief. But few people maintain feelings of helplessness for a long period of time (Carlson, 1974). In a study of life satisfaction following spinal cord injury, 54 men were asked to take the *This I Believe* test (Harvey, 1966) and to write their responses to "This I believe about helplessness." Over half wrote that there was no such thing, that it was all in the mind, relative, that they didn't believe in it, and that much could be done to avoid or lessen it. Helplessness when acknowledged was described as a very negative experience. While some of these responses may have been defensive, others suggested that many of the men had found ways to have considerable control over their lives and did not feel helpless.

Illness and disability may cause serious disruption in control over the environment, and Seligman's learned helplessness model may explain temporary periods of apathy or giving up (Seligman, Klein, Miller). The ill or disabled person may no longer be able to perform the old behaviors that led to desirable consequences, or the old behaviors may now lead to different outcomes. For example, 8-year-old Joey was held in great esteem by his peers for breaking rules at school. Now he's in the hospital. He has few peers and his rule breaking has led to anything but esteem.

Learned helplessness need not persist. If helplessness can be learned, it can also be extinguished. The helpless individual has to learn new ways to affect the environment, to make events more predictable or controllable. Helplessness should diminish as the relationship between action and consequence becomes more clear and reliable.

THE HELPING PROCESS

Basically, in health or when ill or disabled, the requirements for successful receiving or giving of help are the same. First, there is a need. Then the need is made known to someone who can help. The potential helper decides to help or not to help. The person, ill or disabled, who needs help must find people who will help, get them to help, and keep them as helpers. There may be multiple needs with different people required to meet each of them. Some help may need to be given by specialists; other help, of a more general nature, can be provided by many persons.

The Helpers

Family and other significant persons are usually called upon for help when a person becomes ill or injured. They are the major persons in most individual support systems. Caplan identifies eight support system functions of the family. These include being (1) a source of aid and service; (2) a haven for rest and recuperation; (3) a source and validator of identity; (4) a guide and

CHAPTER 4 46

mediator in problem solving; (5) a collector and giver of information about the world; (6) a source of ideology; (7) a feedback guidance system; and (8) a reference and control group.

The first four functions are especially relevant following changes in health or functional abilities. Such practical services as caring for children, shopping, calling people, financial aid, and doing laundry may be needed. Rest and recuperation are high priorities, often facilitated most by persons with whom there is a close relationship. Since identity often becomes diffuse and uncertain during a crisis, the source and validator of identity function is important. Individuals who are closest to the person in crisis usually can provide the most useful information about identity and worth. Finally, significant family and friends often facilitate the problem solving necessary following life-changing events. Persons who are close generally share problems and help each other find and use necessary resources.

Frequently, a crisis that is experienced by an individual is also a crisis for family and intimate friends, and the help needed may be beyond what the support network can provide. The nurse, often in a position to recognize such depletion of resources, can direct individuals to other resources or can facilitate problem solving.

According to equity theory, inequities in helping or in rewards and costs cause tension unless they can be removed psychologically or actually. Illness and disabilities can disrupt relationships that were previously equitable. Role changes and alterations in dependency relationships are two potential disruptions. A husband who finds himself in the role of a primary caregiver or a wife who suddenly becomes the sole means of financial support (because, for instance, the husband has a stroke, is paralyzed, and has Wernicke's aphasia) may for a while believe the inequities are temporary. They may think that equity will be restored when the ill member becomes well or when lost function returns. As time goes on and inequity continues (the wife works and cares for her husband; his condition doesn't change), discomfort is likely to increase in all participants. Equity can be restored if the individuals can develop new patterns of interacting and sharing that will equalize rewards and costs for each member or if the inequities can be justified in some way. The man with the stroke may be able to do some things to help at home, an outside aide may be gotten to take the burden off the wife, or the wife may establish psychologic equity by finding ways to convince herself that the changes in the relationship are adding to her rewards or increasing her husband's costs. For instance, she may tell herself, "He's suffering so much more than I am. I will become a better person from going through this," etc.

Needs for help are seldom met completely by persons in a support network. Professional help may be needed, or help from whoever happens to be available. Regardless of who the helper is, the help (unless accidentally given) depends on the awareness of need, recognition of what is needed, and a decision on whether or not to act. As suggested in Bar-Tal's model, the assessment of costs and rewards of helping or not helping will affect the decision.

Individual skills in recognizing needs vary. Even professionals differ in levels of skill, in the types of needs they recognize, and in needs to which they respond. Social workers, nurses, and physicians, for example, have particular areas of expertise that guide their assessment and intervention, and they should notice needs for help that the untrained observer will miss.

Recognition of the type of help needed is not easy because the help asked for is not always the help required. A patient experiencing discomfort, for example, may request pain medication when the best relief will be obtained through change in position and massage. Sometimes, an individual is unable to ask for help. The inability may stem from lack of awareness of a need for help or from a physical or psychological inability to ask for help. For example, the patient with right hemisphere brain damage and left hemiplegia is often unaware of the physical deficits and does not request help (Chap. 12). The patient with Broca's aphasia may recognize the need for help but be unable to communicate it to others. Finally, an individual who needs to be independent or wishes not to impose on others can hinder or prevent requests for help.

Professional helpers are expected to try to determine the best way to help each patient achieve an individual goal. It is all too easy to develop patterns of helping that meet needs other than those of the patient. For example, it is difficult to watch a person struggle to eat or take a great deal of time and effort to get dressed without having the urge to "help." But the helper who feeds or dresses the patient may be depriving that individual of essential learning, at the same time deriving personal gratification of needs by decreasing frustration or completing work faster. Strangers who see someone on crutches or in a wheelchair may assume, responding to gross cues and perhaps past experience, that the individual needs help. The individuals may not need help at all (see Chap. 2).

As described earlier, the decision to act depends on many variables. Some people may refuse to help if they think the need was brought on by the individual's bad judgment or carelessness. Others may never fail to respond to a need for help. Analysis of rewards and costs of helping or not helping is probably determined by social and personal norms and values, personality characteristics, and circumstances surrounding the need for help, such as danger, ability to avoid the situation, presence of other people, time and energy required, relationship to the person in need, attractiveness of the person needing help, perceived inequities, and many other criteria.

Help can come from sources other than people, although personal assistance is the primary focus of this chapter. The individual's God is often a primary source of help and is the object of many requests for guidance, strength, and other needs. The nurse who acknowledges it as a source can facilitate the use of this help. Frequently a religious leader or a person with similar beliefs can provide support to patients in exercising their beliefs.

The Help Given

The actual help given will depend on the accuracy of assessment of need, the skills of the individual, and the decision to act or not to act. Methods used to offer and provide help can be of critical importance to the receiver. Help is most effective when the recipient is treated with respect, as a person worth helping. Otherwise, the assistance can contribute to loss of self-respect, loss of self-esteem, or to feelings of obligation or indebtedness to the helper. When losses exceed gains, the net result is not help. An assessment of the outcome of helping actions must be based on knowledge of the individual's goals and usual behavior patterns. Changes in verbal evaluations of self-worth or in amount and type of interaction with others may be taken as signs of alteration in self-esteem.

The Recipient of Help

Receiving help often requires awareness of a need, the willingness to receive assistance, and the ability to request help. Help is sometimes given, however, when the recipient is unaware of a need, does not want aid, and does not ask for assistance. For example, in an emergency, the recipient may be unconscious and totally reliant on the action of others.

Individuals differ in their awareness of a need for help. Not everyone is able to determine what the problem is or when help is needed. Sensitivity to one's own needs for assistance influence the kind of help requested. Also, some request help at the first sign of need while others exhaust every personal resource before asking for help. Awareness of need is closely related to the ability to accept help.

Dependence, independence, and mutual dependence were discussed earlier. Individuals differ greatly in the ease with which they can be dependent on others, and previous patterns no doubt influence the perception of equity or inequity in relationships. The person who has taken great pride in being independent is likely to suffer from the inequity in relationships if illness or disability makes dependency on others necessary. Equity may be restored temporarily through psychologic means, such as emphasizing the lack of control anyone has over illness. If, however, independence masked dependency needs, the illness or disability may legitimize asking for help and depending on others on a long-term basis.

Once an individual has determined a need for help, the probability of receiving it can be increased by planning the best way to request it. As Bar-Tal found, requests that are positively toned and which give a person the choice of refusing are more likely to be honored than those that limit freedom or are negatively toned. In other words, demands are less likely to be responded to than requests.

To suggest that there is a "right" way to ask for help in all situations would be oversimplifying a complex issue. Emergencies don't allow time to choose the best way to request aid. A shout, command, or demand may be required to get the attention of others. In nonemergency situations, however, planning is possible. Wording of a request or tone of voice can make a great difference in the responses of potential helpers. Anyone can think of requests that were turn-offs as well as those that aroused an eagerness to help. What characteristics cause the different reactions?

Theories about helping suggest that requests that optimize rewards and minimize costs to the potential helper increase the probability of getting help. First, the person in need should limit the request to what is needed. In other words, no one should ask for more help than is needed. Limiting the request decreases the time and energy required to provide the help. Second, the person asking for help might bargain. For example, "I'll make the phone calls you need to make today if you will do some shopping for me." Bargaining is a way of preventing inequities and is probably most crucial in long-term relationships. Distribution of requests, a third method, is similar to the first. When possible, the potential recipient can spread around requests for help so that no person feels overburdened. This distribution of costs is probably most critical in long-term relationships.

Thus far, discussion has focused on the recipient who needs or wants help. What does the person do when unwanted help is offered? Where bystanders overdo it, are quick to offer help, then refuse to take no for an answer when they have offered assistance, the situation can be very frustrating and demoralizing to the recipient. Such acts may call unnecessary attention to a disability. Rushing up to help someone on crutches cross the street may be an embarrassing attention to the person on crutches. How the individual handles the situation will be determined to a great extent by the amount of stress perceived and by coping style. Blackwell (1978) has described how important it is for a person who has been discredited (has an obvious stigma, for instance) to learn to manage tension in interpersonal situations. Responding to assistance that is not wanted may be an important way to manage tension. Since persons offering help may be embarrassed by a refusal to accept, a young quadriplegic, totally independent in most situations, said that he often accepts help that he doesn't want or need. He does this partly to prevent a scene but also because he fears that if he refuses the help, the potential helpgiver may not offer help to others who really need it.

The recipient of help can increase the likelihood of receiving help from strangers as well as family and friends by considering rewards and costs to all participants including the self. Each situation may have unique characteristics; however, most of them can be analyzed in terms of equity principles. In order for the helping process to be effective, all participants must consider consequences to the self and others of aid or of the refusal to assist.

NURSING INTERVENTIONS

Like any other person, the nurse receives and gives help. In the professional nurse role with patients, the nurse's role is as helper more than recipient. The nurse, ideally, receives much help from other health professionals and also receives social supports.

Help given to clients is often given directly; however, it may be given through others. The nurse can facilitate the helping process as it involves the patient, family, friends, and other resources.

THE NURSE AS THE DIRECT HELP GIVER

Like any other potential helper, the nurse must assess the needs for help and make a decision to help or not to help. A nursing assessment includes an evaluation of the extent to which the patient's basic and acquired needs are met, and includes coping as well as physical needs. Where needs are not being met, the nurse and the patient (together, when possible) set goals for more effective need gratification and select ways to facilitate goal attainment. The most realistic goals are those that will be appropriate in the patient's home environment. This cannot be overstressed. Like anyone else, the nurse is vulnerable to gross unmet needs observed in others. It is easy to give too much, to do too much, or to try to help too much. When the patient leaves or the nurse is no longer able to help, the patient may be worse off than before the help was given.

The nurse's assessment of rewards and costs may be different from those of a lay person or of another professional group. A nurse's expectations differ from those of a physician, physical therapist, speech pathologist, occupational therapist, or nutritionist. Professional expectations influence perceptions of rewards and costs. For example, refusing to help a patient who needs help with something distasteful may represent negligence in the professional nurse role, which would be a much greater cost.

Since nurses have needs that do not disappear when a uniform is put on, "Whose needs am I meeting?" is an important question to keep in mind. The patient who raves about nursing care or who shows rapid progress often receives more time and help than one who is cranky, angry, and regressing, but the latter may have the greater need for help.

Knowledge of needs, the helping process, and the potential pitfalls in both helping and refusing to help will usually facilitate accurate assessment and decision making. Feedback and support from other professionals are also essential for effective helping. Peers can correct each other's distortions.

HELPING OTHERS TO HELP

Often the most effective help a nurse can give a patient is through other people or agencies. In the nursing assessment, which includes resources as well as needs and problems, family, friends, other patients, and agencies are potential sources of needed help. Help may involve referring the patient to particular agencies that offer needed services. Assistance also frequently comes from other patients, staff members, family, and friends.

Caplan (1976, pp. 19–36) has identified general principles to follow in organizing support systems. First, he suggests that persons in need be linked with significant others quickly. Then the professionals should allow them to help each other, intervening only to prevent maladaptive responses. Next, he suggests that persons who are struggling or who need help should not be labeled as deviant or psychologically ill since labels stigmatize and dehumanize the person. The reciprocity of natural support groups is considered superior to professional help since the help is more likely to be viewed as a right rather than a favor. If mutual help groups and networks were organized, people with similar problems could get together. Then victims could become helpers and models for each other. Finally, Caplan suggests that the supporters need to be supported to prevent depletion. These principles apply to the nurse working with the ill, the disabled, and the support systems. In addition to these principles, much teaching about help is necessary.

When family and friends are taught the knowledge and skills they need to give necessary aid, they can be accurate in assessing needs and in offering what is needed. Such knowledge and skill do not guarantee that help will be given when needed. Knowledge of crisis, the rewards and costs of helping, and the principles of equity or reciprocity allow the nurse to anticipate and, it is hoped, to prevent short- and long-term problems in relationships. Patients and family members often can be encouraged to find ways to share helping or to find new, mutually satisfying patterns of relating. Family members may want to or feel obligated to help. If costs exceed rewards, however, resentment is likely to build up and the client may lose important sources of help. Helplessness that occurs because of loss of gratification from external objects sometimes can be prevented by working with patient supports (i.e., family). All members of the health team can contribute to helping family members and clients reduce costs and increase rewards by decreasing the time and energy required for various tasks, by distributing the tasks, and by offering help only when it is actually necessary.

The nature of a patient's belief in God or supernatural powers is an important variable to be considered in planning nursing care and should be part of the assessment of resources.

HELPING THE ONE IN NEED DEVELOP NECESSARY SKILLS

The discussion of helplessness and information about the recipient of help suggests ways that nurses can assist patients to get the help they need. Learned helplessness can be combated by clarifying relationships between client actions and consequences so that consistent outcomes occur after specific behaviors, restoring the patient's belief in personal ability to influence events.

Skill in asking for help includes being able to discriminate necessary from unnecessary assistance, asking only for necessary help, asking in such a way as to maximize rewards and minimize costs to the potential helper, and maintaining equitable relationships whenever possible. A patient can be encouraged to develop strategies for putting others at ease, offering things in return for assistance, making needs clear and unambiguous, and planning for assistance in advance whenever possible. This skill in requesting assistance should lead to receiving needed help.

CONCLUSION

More needs to be learned about helping concepts. Some patients are very effective in getting and maintaining the assistance they need; others are dismal failures. How are they different? Can they learn to be more effective? What are the most useful ways to offer help without causing loss of self-esteem? How can costs of helpers be minimized? If helplessness is learned, what are the most efficient methods of extinguishing the learning? These are but a few important questions about helping.

All people need assistance from others. Reciprocity theories and models for helping in emergency and nonemergency situations offer suggestions for understanding important issues and variables in the helping process. Investigations of various aspects of the process should lead to more effective helping.

BIBLIOGRAPHY

Bar-Tal, Daniel: *Prosocial Behavior,* Hemisphere, Washington, D.C., 1976, p. 97.

Blackwell, Betty: "Stigma," in Carolyn E. Carlson and Betty Blackwell (eds.), *Behavioral Concepts and Nursing Intervention* (2d ed.), Lippincott, Philadelphia, 1978.

Brehm, Jack W.: *Responses to Loss of Freedom: A Theory of Psychological Reactance,* General Learning Press, Morristown, N.J., 1972.

Caplan, Gerald: "The Family as a Support System," in G. Caplan and M. Killilea (eds.), *Support Systems and Mutual Help,* Grune & Stratton, New York, 1976, pp. 19–36.

———: "Organization of Support Systems for Civilian Populations," in G. Caplan and M. Killilea (eds.), *Support Systems and Mutual Help,* Grune & Stratton, New York, 1976, pp. 273–315.

Carlson, Carolyn E.: "Cognitive Structure, Goal Characteristics and Life Satisfaction Following Spinal Cord Injury," doctoral dissertation, University of Colorado, Boulder, 1974.

Goldfarb, Alvin I.: "Depression in the Old and Aged," in Frederic F. Flach and Suzanne C. Draghi (eds.), *The Nature and Treatment of Depression,* Wiley, New York, 1975, pp. 119–144.

Harvey, O. J.: "System Structure, Flexibility, and Creativity," in O. J. Harvey (ed.), *Experience, Structure, and Adaptability,* Springer, New York, 1966.

Lange, Silvia: "Hope," in Carolyn E. Carlson and Betty Blackwell (eds.), *Behavioral Concepts and Nursing Intervention* (2d ed.), Lippincott, Philadelphia, 1978, pp. 171–190.

Schmale, Arthur H., Jr.: "A Genetic View of Affects with Special Reference to the Genesis of Helplessness and Hopelessness, in *The Psychoanalytic Study of the Child,* International Universities Press, New York, 1964, pp. 287–310.

Schwartz, Shalom H.: "Normative Influences on Altruism," in L. Berkowitz (ed.), *Advances in Experimental Social Pscyhology,* vol. 10, Academic Press, 1977, pp. 222–275.

Seligman, M. E. P., D. C. Klein, and W. R. Miller: "Depression," in H. Leitenberg (ed.), *Handbook of Behavior Modification and Behavior Therapy,* Prentice-Hall, Englewood Cliffs, NJ, 1976, pp. 168–210.

Staub, Ervin: "Helping a Distressed Person: Social, Personality, and Stimulus Determinants," in L. Berkowitz (ed.), *Advances in Experimental Social Psychology,* 10, Academic Press, 1976, pp. 222–275.

Walster, Elaine, Ellen Berscheid, and G. William Walster: "New Directions in Equity Research," in L. Berkowitz (ed.), *Advances in Experimental Social Pscyhology,* vol. 9, Academic Press, 1976, pp. 1–42.

Wortman, Camille B., and Jack W. Brehm: "Responses to Uncontrollable Outcomes: An Integration of Reactance Theory and the Learned Helplessness Model," in L. Berkowitz (ed.), *Advances in Experimental Social Psychology,* vol. 8, Academic Press, 1975, pp. 277–336.

5

margaret a. williams

variables that
influence compliance

INTRODUCTION

Compliance is often discussed as "the problem of compliance." Some persons have suggested that it may be more of a problem to health-care providers than to patients. That may be true in many instances; at the same time, when certain self-administered treatment regimens will effectively ameliorate distressing symptoms or prevent complications in long-term rehabilitation, noncompliance may indeed create problems.

There is no doubt that the extent of noncompliance in chronic disorders is high (less is known about compliance in acute disorders). This should not be surprising, since reflection upon one's own behavior in maintaining a healthful style of life usually supports the adage that it is difficult to follow good advice. Because definitions of compliant behavior vary, however, it is nearly impossible to specify overall rates of noncompliance. In the case of long-term self-administration of prescribed medication, the rate is rather consistently estimated at about 50 percent. What the rates are in such matters as compliance with exercise, diet, or special procedural regimens is not known, except for certain small study groups.

This chapter considers the concept of compliance, some cautions in accepting findings from compliance studies, major findings about variables affecting compliance, and the implications for practice. Compliance is a complex phenomenon about which much remains to be known. The evidence, however, about what affects compliance should be incorporated into practice. Much of the literature considers compliance in terms of the patient-physician dyad, although it should be apparent that many care providers are involved in influencing the extent to which patients' behavior coincides with what has been prescribed in the way of medications, diets, special procedures, life-style changes, and the like.

All members of the rehabilitation team should be concerned with developing, with the patient, plans for long-term care and treatment, and for assisting the patient in carrying out those plans so that benefit ensues and a viable life-style can be maintained. With that perspective, compliance for the sake of compliance has no place and the problem of compliance becomes one of how health-care providers can better provide assistance in achieving mutually agreed-upon goals. Some of the forms of assistance are particularly within the realm of nursing, but no attempt will be made here to specify nursing actions as unique from actions carried out by other health professionals.

THE CONCEPT OF COMPLIANCE

The term *compliance* frequently has a negative connotation, conjuring up a picture of patients struggling valiantly to follow a set of arbitrary rules devised by a dictatorial professional. Attempts to avoid negative connotations by substitution of another term or phrase are regularly made. More positive terminology, however, such as "cooperative behavior" or "therapeutic alliance" tends to be cumbersome, and "adherence" is no real improvement over compliance. The use of a term that is unambiguous and carries agreed-upon meaning has undeniable advantages; for the most part, compliance is increasingly accepted as that term. Some persons still restrict its meaning to "how well a person carries out the physician's orders," though such a definition is unduly narrow and furthers the image of a physician decreeing and the patient following. The definition used here is the broader one put forth by the leaders of an influential 1974 Canadian workshop/symposium on compliance. Compliance is defined as "the extent to which the patient's behavior (in terms of taking medications, following diets, or executing other life-style changes) coincides with the clinical prescription" (Sackett and Haynes, 1976). Such a definition allows the patient to be an active participant in deciding the clinical prescription and also allows the clinical prescriptions to be made by nonphysician health professionals.

Compliance with a clinical prescription has as its goal the attainment of some therapeutic objective. An objective might be the loss of 10 pounds, preventing skin breakdown, achieving increased joint movement, reduction of pain, elimination of infection, or the like. When the treatment objective is not attained, several explanations are possible:

1. The diagnosis was incorrect.
2. The treatment prescribed was not the correct or most effective one.
3. The instructions given the person were not clear and the person complied with a partially correct (as understood) prescription.
4. The person did not comply with the instructions.

If the treatment objective is attained, the assumption is generally made that the diagnosis was correct, that the treatment was effective, and that the person followed instructions. This may or may not be true; the objective may have been attained because of some other action that the person took rather than the one prescribed; or the diagnosis may have been wrong and the condition improved in spite of the treatment. The point is that achievement of treatment objectives is not always the result of patient compliance, and lack of success in achievement of goals may be caused by a variety of factors other than patient noncompliance.

The focus in most of the studies on compliance has been on the patient, the implicit assumption being that compliance to a prescribed course of action is the determining factor in attaining the treatment objectives. Thus, large numbers of studies have attempted to ascertain the characteristics of noncompliant versus compliant patients. The characteristics studied have included intelligence, personality attributes, ethnicity, occupation, education, age, sex, marital status, religion, and family organization. Less emphasis has been given to the process by which health professionals attempt to instruct patients and help them to understand and comply with a treatment plan. Similarly, little emphasis has been given to the characteristics of professionals who tend to be successful or unsuccessful in achieving patient compliance. Several studies have looked at situational factors that may affect ability to comply with a treatment plan, such as the cost of prescribed equipment or medication, or the cost and availability of transportation to a clinic, hospital, or doctor's office. A number of studies have also examined the effect of clinic appointment schedules (e.g., long waiting times) or of seeing the same versus different health practitioners at follow-up visits. For the most part, however, the unstated assumption in the bulk of compliance studies has been that noncompliance has been due to patient factors rather than institutional or care-provider factors. The negative connotation imputed to the term has thus been unfortunately reinforced by the considerable number of studies that in implicitly putting the responsibility for complaint behavior on the patient also place the onus for noncompliance in the same place.

EVALUATING COMPLIANCE STUDIES

Health professionals concerned with how best to work with patients to facilitate their participation in arriving at and subsequently complying with a mutually agreed-upon clinical prescription will find a wealth of studies from which to draw information. Four rather simple questions can help to evaluate the appropriateness of the conclusions.

WHO WAS STUDIED?

In many instances, the persons whose extent of compliance is being measured are those who are currently attending a clinic or, less frequently, patients of physicians in private or group practice. To some extent these persons are already compliant; at least they have not dropped out of the system. The number of persons who did drop out of treatment may or may not be noted, and the reasons for dropping out may not be known.

Dissatisfaction with the treatment may have been a reason, but persons may also have moved, then sought care in a new locale, or they may have stopped supervision but not compliance with a regimen. Ideally, all persons who enter into a specific treatment regimen over a period of time should be followed, whether they stay in treatment or drop out. This is especially true if one is interested in the extent of compliance over time. Because a follow-up on all such persons may be inordinately time-consuming and expensive, usually not all members of the group starting treatment are accounted for.

It is also useful to look at the criteria used for inclusion of subjects in the study. A number of subjects, especially potential noncompliers, may have been weeded out on the basis of certain criteria, before the study began. Persons who do not speak English, for example, are frequently excluded if the study involves interviews by the investigator.

It is also important to know whether the subjects are under supervision for preventive treatment, control of symptoms, or rehabilitation. The way in which an asymptomatic person views a regimen that is intended to prevent some future health problem, for example, may be quite different from the way the same person views a plan of treatment that helps relieve existing painful or disabling symptoms.

HOW WERE COMPLIANCE AND/OR NONCOMPLIANCE DEFINED AND MEASURED?

The definition of what constitutes compliance is an especially sticky matter. Are persons noncompliant, for example, if in a home exercise regimen they perform the exercises faithfully four times a day as prescribed, but do not do them correctly? Or, are persons noncompliant who have self-adjusted their medication dosage to twice rather than three times a day, compared with persons who occasionally take the wrong dose of medication but do so faithfully three times a day as prescribed? If the desired therapeutic effect is being accomplished even though the regimen is not followed exactly, should the person's behavior be termed noncompliant? A desired outcome may occur, for example, when an infection is controlled even though the patient took less than the prescribed amount of antibiotic.

If a desirable outcome is considered evidence of compliance, is it certain that the outcome resulted from following a certain clinical prescription or because of other factors? The lifting of a depressive mood can be due to some change in the person's social situation rather than to having faithfully taken prescribed antidepressive agent, and an increase in mobility may be due to new, socially motivating factors rather than to faithfulness in following an exercise regimen.

Compliance with medication schedules is sometimes measured by taking blood samples to determine drug levels or by measuring urinary excretion of the drug, a metabolic by-product, or a tracer substance added to the medication. In carrying out such measures, attention must be paid to the drug's excretion pattern. A urine specimen obtained 8 h after the person took a rapidly excreted drug would yield different results from one taken 2 h after the same drug. Were persons characterized as compliant or noncompliant on the basis of a single test made or were a series of tests run?

Patients' reports of their own compliance are perhaps the most frequently used measure in clinical practice; i.e., the person is asked whether he or she has been following the treatment plan as prescribed. Coupled with astute observation of the person's condition, such information may be adequate and often is all the health practitioner has to rely on. The validity of self-reports has been questioned, however, with comparisons made between them and certain measures such as pill counts or urine tests. In general, such comparisons show that persons tend to overestimate their degree of compliance although those who are most noncompliant usually acknowledge that fact. Physicians have been asked to estimate their patients' extent of compliance. Their estimates have been quite inaccurate, attributing higher degrees of compliance by patients than actually exist. There is no evidence to suggest that other health professionals do any better in making such estimates.

Pill counts are frequently used as a measure of compliance to medication regimens. The person is instructed to bring the medication container along when returning for a checkup, or pill counts are made during a home visit. The amount of medication remaining in the bottle is compared with the amount that should have remained, given the prescription and length of time for which the prescription was made. Theoretically, this measurement should accurately reflect compliance with medication regimens; in practice, remaining contents can be consciously altered by the person, contents may be accidentally spilled and pills lost, or other family members may take part of the medication. Logs have been used for patients to record certain drug-taking or treatment activity; these, of course, are subject to errors in recording and may not report actual behavior. In addition, the instructions actually given to a patient may not coincide with the prescription shown in the medical record, and the number of pills dispensed by the pharmacist may not be the same as stated in the prescription.

Even so "simple" a matter as determining the rate of appointments kept for follow-up purposes as a measure of compliance is not without pitfalls. High rates of missed appointments (in ambulatory care facilities these have ranged from 16 to 44 percent) may not be so much a measure of patients' compliance with instructions about follow-up as they are of the institution's health professionals' communication patterns and accommodation to the needs of the population served.

WERE MEASURES TO IMPROVE COMPLIANCE SUCCESSFUL OR WERE THE PERSONS WHO ADMINISTERED THEM SUCCESSFUL?

Reports of improved compliance following the use of a particular educational, motivational, or reminder strategy will usually attribute the success to the strategy and not to the persons employing it. However, it is wise to question that conclusion. In many instances, the increased attention given to the patients who were subjects in the experimental group may have been the major reason for improved compliance. Certain procedures may also be successful when the person who administers them is a supportive, warm, and interested person; the same procedures used by someone else may be less effective.

HOW WAS COMPLIANCE RELATED TO OUTCOME?

This problem relates to the second question: Is a desirable outcome the result of a certain regimen or of other factors? Further, if a great deal of effort went into improving compliance, and if, indeed, compliance improved but there was relatively little effect on the long-term outcome, then conclusions that attribute "success" to the efforts are questionable. The goal of any effort to enhance compliance with a clinical prescription is to better achieve the therapeutic goal of that prescription, not to improve compliance for itself.

VARIABLES AFFECTING COMPLIANCE

A large number of variables believed to affect compliance have been investigated. Most studies have focused on patient factors rather than on provider or situational factors. This bias in focus may be changing, however. More complex models of compliance are being considered showing effects of one or several fairly easily defined variables such as those of age, sex, social class, marital status, or the like. The associations that have been found between ten variables or classes of variables and compliance will be discussed in this section. The variables are

1. Demographic factors
2. Diagnosis
3. Treatment factors
4. Knowledge of disease and treatment
5. Intelligence and personality
6. Convenience in seeing practitioner
7. Continuity of care
8. Patient-practitioner relationship
9. Social support
10. Beliefs and attitudes.

DEMOGRAPHIC FACTORS

It is now generally acknowledged that there is little association between compliance and the variables of age, sex, marital status, religion, ethnicity, and socioeconomic status with its components of income, occupation, and education. Although the weight of evidence confirms the above findings, there are some who are uneasy about including socioeconomic status in the list because of discrepant results. Some of the evidence indicates, for example, that lower-class persons tend to be more noncompliant relative to taking medications, staying on diets, restricting activity, and keeping return appointments. Those who seek to explain this finding tend to use either financial explanations (the expense involved in taking medications and keeping appointments), attitudinal explanations (the lower class has a subculture of attitudes and value orientations that places health lower in priority than other life matters; the poor are unable to defer gratification and do not plan use of limited resources well), or a "professional distrust" explanation. The latter explanation states that the poor tend to distrust professionals in general and have trouble communicating with them. These latter two explanations rather obviously demonstrate the tendency to interpret noncompliance as the "fault" of the patient because of certain characteristics or "deficiencies" of that person, rather than as a lack of accommodation or use of communication skills by care providers.

Some persons, too, have found that the very young or the very old are exceptions to the statement that age makes no difference. The weight of evidence, however, appears to support the original statement.

As some authors point out, the relevance of demographic factors may be more a matter of who utilizes health-care facilities and providers than in who complies with treatments since almost all compliance studies have been done on persons already in the health-care system.

DIAGNOSIS

The disease or disorder from which a person suffers does not appear to be predictive of compliance or noncompliance. However, most studies of the extent of compliance and of treatment dropout rates have been done with persons having chronic disorders. Compliance among those with acute disorders and time-limited treatments is relatively unknown. Some figures on treatment dropout rates among those with chronic disorders show that such rates are high no matter what the diagnosis. In an extensive review of the subject, dropout rates for general psychiatric clinics are cited at 20 to 57 percent after the first visit; for outpatient treatment of alcoholism at 52 to 75 percent by the fourth session; for methadone maintenance at 7 to 64 percent by 6 months; for inpatient treatment of tuberculosis at 37 to 60.2 percent for those who sign out against advice; and for hypertension at 20 to 50 percent for those dropping out in the first year of treatment, most during the first 2 months (Baekeland and Lundwall).

TREATMENT FACTORS

Studies agree that the more complex the regimen and the greater the degree of behavioral change expected of the patient, the greater is the extent of noncompliance. The highest degree of compliance occurs for treatments or tests administered by hospital or clinic staff, where the type of involvement is more passive and also more visible to staff than is self-care at home. Compliance tapers off as persons are expected to add new habits, such as taking medications or performing self-treatments, and is least where old habits and behaviors must be altered or broken, as in the case of changing dietary habits or stopping smoking. Conclusions about the effect on compliance of duration of treatment generally depend on whether a group was studied from the time treatment was initiated or whether the group had started therapy considerably before initiation of the study, and therefore did not consider previous dropouts. For the most part, however, the conclusion is that the longer treatment continues, the less the degree of compliance. The cost of treatment as a factor in compliance has not been extensively explored, but the tentative conclusion of those who have considered it is that it may not be as important as other matters.

KNOWLEDGE OF DISEASE AND TREATMENT

Whether increased knowledge about a disease and its treatment increases compliance has been a controversial question. The weight of evidence is that increased knowledge by itself does not improve compliance, even though "common sense" would indicate that the two should be positively related. Studies utilizing the soundest methodology show no relationship between extent of knowledge and degree of compliance. The fact that intelligence and educational level are unrelated to compliance appears to support the above conclusion.

One should not presume, on the basis of these findings, that patient education programs have no value. Patients cannot comply with a regimen unless they understand the instructions. What should be carefully looked at, though, is whether patient teaching is simply an imparting of facts and information that health professionals think patients should know, or whether it takes into account personal attitudes, beliefs, life-styles, and support systems, as well as knowledge level. The learning achieved through active participation in an educational program may be quite different from that achieved as a passive recipient of cognitive information. The involvement of family members in educational programs has also tended to be neglected. Certainly the person's "right to know" is an important ethical concept. The implication, however, is that patient education programs, to be successful, must include more than simple facts about a disorder and its treatment.

INTELLIGENCE

As noted in the foregoing discussion, intelligence has been found to bear no relationship to compliance. This finding has important implications since estimates of patients' intelligence often affect management plans. Persons considered to have low intelligence may be omitted from some therapies because it is assumed that they cannot carry out the instructions or restrictions involved. Unfortunately, belief that someone cannot learn often acts as a self-fulfilling prophecy and serves to reinforce caregivers' biases.

When a patient is judged to have a low intelligence level, professionals may, indeed, need to alter their approach. However, since the evidence is that simply learning facts and increasing one's knowledge about a disorder and its therapy do not assure compliance, it would appear that approaches based on assessments other than intelligence should be used with all patients. An understanding, for example, that certain activities will increase mobility, prevent skin breakdown, or prevent pain would not seem to be based on intellect alone.

CONVENIENCE IN SEEING PRACTITIONER

The factor of convenience in seeing the practitioner or health professional is associated primarily with the keeping of appointments and may or may not be associated with actual compliance at home. Persons who do not follow prescribed regimens may still faithfully keep appointments at a clinic, office, or in the home. Conversely, if one is "doing well" on a treatment plan, possible inconvenience, cost or dissatisfaction with the practitioner may cause the person to forego return visits. A belief that "They'll just tell me I'm doing all right" may be operative in many instances.

Most studies relative to appointment keeping focus on patient characteristics to explain rates of broken appointments. A number of studies conclude that low-income persons do not keep appointments as well as middle-class persons. The inconveniences associated with keeping appointments have not always been recognized; they include travel distance, cost of transportation, necessity to take time away from a job, child care, and prolonged waiting time at the appointment site. The factor of waiting time has been shown to be important in appointment keeping, not only at the office or clinic (including the pharmacy), but also between appointments. The person who feels that a visit is necessary within the week but is told it cannot be scheduled for several weeks may understandably make alternative plans.

Ease of communication is also a factor. Persons who do not speak English may not have a family friend or relative to rely upon in making interpretations, and health facilities in multiethnic locales should have skillful interpreters available. Organizations that provide this assistance when needed, that use scheduling compatible with the work schedules of the population served, and that make every effort to avoid prolonged waiting times before and during appointments will predictably have higher rates of kept appointments than organizations that do poorly in these services. This supposes, of course, that persons are also satisfied with their care and their relationship with the health-care providers.

CONTINUITY OF CARE

Persons who receive their care from the same health practitioner are more compliant than those who are treated or examined by different practitioners. The explanation may be a combination of interpersonal comfort, ease of communication, and a saving in time needed to explain problems. The brevity of the usual patient record also detracts from the ease with which another practitioner takes over. Problem-oriented records and flowsheets stating physical findings, lab tests, and medications or treatments are helpful in allowing a practitioner new to the case to grasp the whole picture. These records also assist the person's usual caregiver in following progress.

PATIENT-PRACTITIONER RELATIONSHIP

The relationship between the patient and the health practitioner is one of the more important factors in compliance. This factor is difficult to measure, but that is probably not the reason few studies focus on it as a variable in compliance. The current emphasis on patient characteristics is a probable reason. Studies dealing with the relationship have examined it from the standpoint of patterns and content of communication on the part of the practitioner (usually the physician), patient satisfaction with the encounter, extent to which patient expectations are met, amount of reciprocal interaction between patient and practitioner, and congruity between what the patient thinks he or she is to do and what the practitioner thinks the patient is doing.

In general, the studies have indicated that when the practitioner communicates in a formal, controlling manner, when there is little reciprocal interaction, and when patients' expectations are unmet, compliance is low. One extended study found a basic gap in communication, that is, the use of medical terminology without accompanying explanation, and especially a lack of explicit definitions and expectations for the patient to carry out in the use of prescribed drugs, to be major factors in patient errors with drug usage. The author of that study noted, however, that patients also fail to be explicit when communicating with the physician; they sometimes withhold questions so as not to appear "dumb" and uneducated. Explicit, written, and consistent communication was positively associated with patients' understanding of how to take a medication and their compliance with the advice. It was also concluded, however, that many such communications were neither necessary nor sufficient to achieve patient understanding. In the study, the amount of instruction given did not vary according to patients' characteristics but did vary among the physicians (whose characteristics were not defined). One conclusion reached was that approachability on the part of the physician is a necessary, though not sufficient, condition for patient inquiry (Svarstad, 1974). The same conclusion may be true for other health professionals.

One of the early studies of nurse-run clinics compared with physician-run clinics, though not expressly dealing with compliance, found different communication patterns that suggested reasons for the difference in outcomes between the nurse clinic group and the control group. There were significant reductions in the frequency of symptoms, number of patients visiting physicians outside the institution, and in the rate of broken appointments among nurse-clinic patients. Physicians emphasized technical aspects of diagnosis and management of disease in their processes of care; the nurses described their activities in terms of supporting-role functions. The authors concluded that the latter pattern more consistently fitted the majority of needs of the chronically ill, who comprised the patient population in both clinics (Lewis et al.).

The relationship between patient and practitioner, like any relationship, is complex. It would appear, however, that simple friendliness does not result in subseuqent compliance with advice, although unfriendliness may result in decreased compliance, and that relationships marked by formal and one-sided information giving are not especially successful. Relationships in which the patient is an "engaged" participant, in which he or she is made to feel supported with respect to health problems, and in which expectations of care can be openly dealt with and met insofar as possible would appear to be positive factors in compliance.

SOCIAL SUPPORT

The value of social support as a variable in compliance behavior is increasingly recognized. Cobb defines social support as information belonging to one or more of the following classes:

1. Information leading to belief that the subject is cared for and loved.
2. Information leading to a belief that the subject is esteemed and valued.
3. Information leading to belief that the subject belongs to a network of communication and mutual obligation.

Caplan et al. (1976) used social support, as a working definition, to mean any input directly provided by another person (or group) which moves the receiving person toward desired goals. They made further distinctions between social support, supportive behavior, and supportive relations. Social support referred to input, which would agree with Cobb's definition of social support as a type of information; supportive behavior was defined as the act of providing the input; and supportive relationships referred to a pattern of relations between two or more persons, at least one of them receiving inputs.

Studies using social support as a variable in compliance have quite consistently found that persons who have social support tend to remain in treatment and to follow clinical prescriptions. The previously cited comprehensive review of dropping out of treatment, for example, found that social isolation and/or lack of affiliation were major causes of dropouts in 19 of the 19 studies that used them as variables. Sackett and Haynes (1976) reviewed 21 studies that used variables indicative of social support, such as influence of family and friends, family stability, "good" social environment, and pretreatment home satisfaction. Fifteen of the studies showed a positive relation, and six showed no relationship between these variables and compliance. Considering the problems formerly mentioned in drawing conclusions about compliance, this amount of support for the association would appear substantial.

Several reasons that suggest why social support can lead to compliance include: (1) The person who has feelings of self-competence is more apt to learn information related to personal health; a feeling of social support, in other words, leads to feelings of competence, and learning occurs best under conditions of psychologic success; (2) social support reduces the discomforts of anxiety or depression that often accompany illness; and (3) social support may increase tolerance for stress, at least in those persons who need and can accept the support of others (Caplan et al.).

The effect of social support could conceivably be in the opposite direction; that is, a person might receive support for manipulating a treatment plan or for abandoning it. In any event, as with other factors associated with compliance, social support may be a necessary, but not a sufficient, condition for compliance.

Social support can come from a number of sources, including spouse, other family members, friends, a supervisor at work, members of a work group, or members of a church or community group. Health professionals can be a major source of support, and their demonstrated belief that the patient can accomplish certain goals, that he or she is a valuable person worthy of attention and esteem may be the most effective part of a treatment plan. The educational strategies found to be effective in compliance are those that incorporate some aspect of social support, even if it is only a warm, supportive attitude on the part of the person carrying out the strategy. Such matters are difficult to measure, of course, and emphasize the kernel of truth in the cliché that "*any* method will work so long as (X-person) does it."

In the findings of one study, social support from the spouse was associated with low levels of depression while social support from other sources had no such effect. Self-esteem and compliance were positively correlated. When both self-esteem and social support from physician or spouse were high, compliance reached the highest levels. High self-esteem without social support, however, was associated with the lowest levels of reported compliance. The suggestion was made that patients who feel competent still need someone around who appreciates their efforts (Caplan et al.).

BELIEFS AND ATTITUDES: A COMPLIANCE MODEL

The influence of certain beliefs and attitudes about health and illness are unquestionably important in the extent to which a person will comply with a clinical prescription. Persons, for example, who believe their illness is not especially serious (perhaps contrary to information presented to them) or that the treatment prescribed is ill-advised will undoubtedly forego the plan of treatment much sooner than persons who believe their condition is serious and that the prescribed plan of care will be helpful. The person who, on the basis of past experience, believes that health professionals have little to offer may be reluctant to follow any plan of care. Ever alert to evidence that supports that belief, the person may, on the smallest evidence, drop out of treatment altogether. These examples appear true on a common-sense basis, but it is also probable that they are true only under certain conditions. For example, the person who does not believe in the seriousness of a physical condition may still comply with a regimen if it is fairly simple, does not disrupt usual activities and behavior patterns, and if the compliant behavior is supported by spouse, children, and the health practitioner.

A model that incorporated these more subjective aspects of behavior related to health was first formulated in an attempt to explain preventive health behaviors and was termed the *health belief model*. A number of persons have contributed to the formulation of the model; the history of its development and aspects of its use are included in a monograph edited by Becker.

The model is derived from value-expectancy theory in which behavior is predicted from the value of an outcome to an individual, and from the individual's expectation that a given action will result in that outcome. The model has the following three elements:

1. The individual's evaluation of the particular health condition is determined both by what the person perceives as the likelihood of susceptibility to that particular illness and by perception of the probable severity of the subsequent disease. The result is a subjective state of readiness to take action.
2. The individual's evaluation of the advocated health behavior in terms of its feasiblity and efficacy (i.e., an estimate of the action's potential benefits in reducing susceptibility and/or severity) weighed against estimates of the physical, psychologic, financial, and other costs of, or barriers to, the proposed behavior.
3. A cue to action must occur to trigger the advocated health behavior; this stimulus can be either internal (e.g., perception of bodily states) or external (e.g., interpersonal interactions, mass media communications) (Becker).

Elements of the health belief model, rather extensively tested over a period of years, have provided satisfactory explanations for most findings in the field of preventive health behavior. Because the same elements are presumed to have equal efficacy in explaining compliance behavior, they have been reformulated into a model of that behavior. Such a reformulation takes into account that in compliant behavior the individual's evaluation of the health condition also considers the likelihood of resusceptibility and that an evaluation of the cost/benefit ratio is in terms of the clinical prescription. Figure 5-1 shows the hypothesized compliance model.

The model shows that a person's readiness to undertake recommended compliance behavior is determined by (1) certain motivations, including the salience of health matters in general to that person; (2) the value of a reduction in illness threat to the person, including subjective estimates of susceptibility or resusceptibility as well as experience with past or present symptoms; and (3) the probability that compliant behavior will reduce the threat, based on subjective estimates of the proposed regimen's safety and efficacy. These factors in turn are influenced by (1) demographic factors, such as extremes in age (very young or very old); (2) structural factors, such as the cost, duration, and side effects of the regimen, and the need for new patterns of behavior; (3) attitudes about the health-care staff, their procedures and facilites; (4) interaction with the physician; and (5) certain other factors, such as prior experience with the illness or the regimen, and advice and social pressure from others. The interplay between these factors then determines the likelihood of compliant behavior.

One of the values of the model in practice is that practitioners can "do something about" many of the components. That is, specific actions can be taken to change or modify attitudes and beliefs and to increase positive motivations. A person's belief in a lack of susceptibility to the complications accompanying a chronic disorder or disability may be changed by information communicated about the danger of disregarding behaviors that reduce the possibility of such complications. Several of the modifying and enabling factors are amenable to direct action; that is, regimens can often be simplified, ways to reduce costs of treatment can be investigated, there can be consciousness-raising on interactional aspects of the patient-practitioner relationship, and so forth. The compliance model needs considerably more testing, particularly in its complete form rather than in parts. To date, only one reported study has tested it in its entirety, but the results were supportive of the model (Becker).

IMPLICATIONS FOR PRACTICE

In the foregoing discussion, the major factors known to influence compliance included a number of implications for practice. Now, an attempt

Readiness to undertake recommended compliance behavior

Motivations
Concern about (salience of) health matters in general
Willingness to seek and accept medical direction
Intention to comply
Positive health activities

Value of illness threat reduction
Subjective estimates of:
 Susceptibility or resusceptibility (including belief in diagnosis)
 Vulnerability to illness in general
 Extent of possible bodily harm*
 Extent of possible interference with social roles*
 Presence of (or past experience with) symptoms

Probability that compliant behavior will reduce the threat
Subjective estimates of:
 The proposed regimen's safety
 The proposed regimen's efficacy to prevent, delay, or cure (including "faith in doctors and medical care" and "chance of recovery")

Modifying and enabling factors

Demographic
(very young or old)

Structural
(cost, duration, complexity, side-effects, accessibility of regimen; need for new patterns of behavior)

Attitudes
(satisfaction with visit, physician, other staff, clinic procedures, and facilities)

Interaction
(length, depth, continuity, mutuality of expectation, quality, and type of doctor-patient relationship; physician agreement with patient; feedback to patient)

Enabling
(prior experience with action, illness or regimen; source of advice and referral [including social pressure])

Compliant behavior

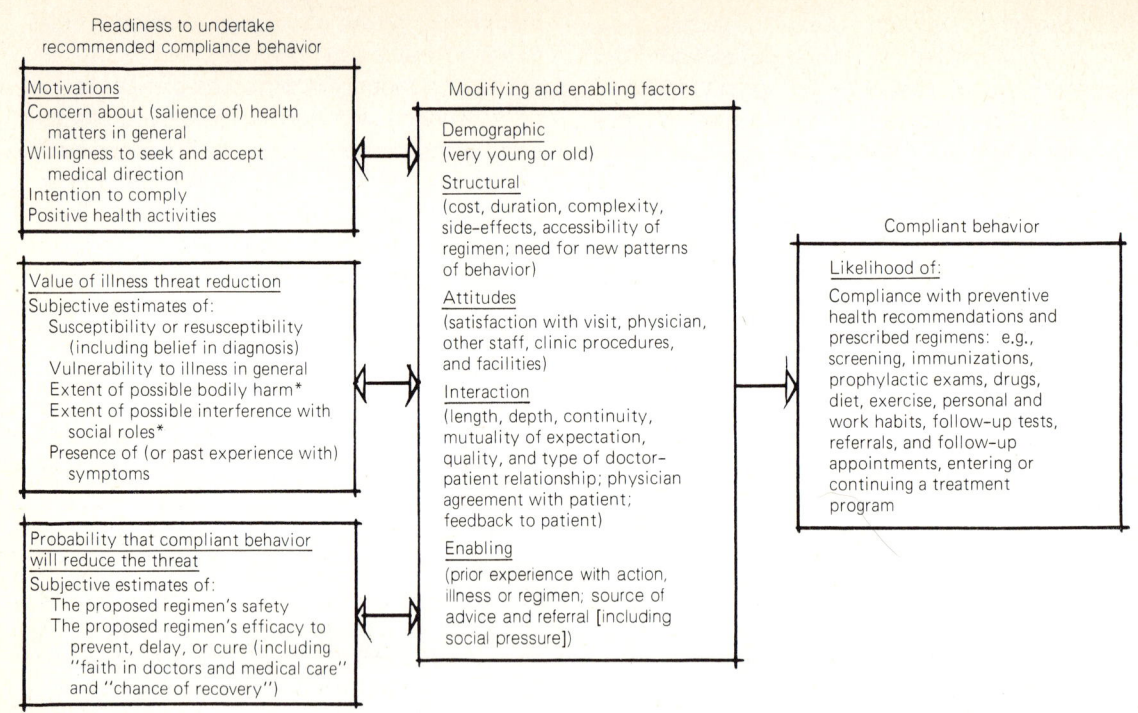

Likelihood of:
Compliance with preventive health recommendations and prescribed regimens: e.g., screening, immunizations, prophylactic exams, drugs, diet, exercise, personal and work habits, follow-up tests, referrals, and follow-up appointments, entering or continuing a treatment program

*At motivating, but not inhibiting, levels

Figure 5-1
Hypothesized model for predicting and explaining compliance. *(From Marshall H. Becker, Sociobehavioral Determinants of Compliance, in D. Sackett and R. B. Haynes (eds.), Compliance with Therapeutic Regimens, Johns Hopkins, Baltimore, 1976, p. 48. Used by permission of the publisher.)*

will be made to pull some of those implications together and expand upon them.

The foremost implication is the need to realistically assess where the patient is with respect to ability to carry out a potential treatment plan. The objective of the assessment is to arrive at attainable, feasible goals and actions with which both the patient and the rehabilitation team are comfortable. Assessment information will include the patient's living situation, daily routines, priorities in life, sources of social support, sources of stress, community facilities and resources including, if the person is employed, those at the place of work. One also needs to know how the patient views the diagnosis; does the patient believe that the diagnosis is accurate? The diagnosis itself may be so threatening that the person rejects it and any clinical prescription related to it. Is there belief that the prescription will be effective, or have similar actions in the past been judged ineffective by the person? How vulnerable does the person perceive himself or herself to be to complications, progression of the illness, or recurrence of the illness? How serious is the illness or disabling condition felt to be? Does the person perceive compliance behavior to have a personal benefit? What are the perceived barriers to action?

The rehabilitation team also needs to carefully assess the clinical prescriptions being considered for the patient. Is a recommended action really effective? If the health professional doubts the efficacy of the prescription, that fact will be evident to the patient, and it is best to honestly state those doubts. If finances are a problem for the patient, could the same goals be attained by some equally effective but less expensive option than the original prescription? Is the clinical prescription being made partially on the basis that it is more convenient for the professionals than another prescription that would involve more time and effort for instruction and supervision? Are all members of the team aware of what each one is expecting of the patient? For example, is the patient ending up with separate instructions from a physician, nurse, occupational therapist, and physical therapist that together constitute an almost overwhelming amount of input and expectation? Is the assessment information gained from the patient actually being used as the base from which to individualize the plan of treatment, or is much of the information recorded but unused?

It should be evident from the discussion on factors influencing compliance that judgments about the person's ability to carry out a clinical prescription should not be based on such variables as assumed intelligence or personality attributes, age, ethnicity, religion, sex, education, income, or occupation. Each person needs to be regarded as having unique needs, capabilities, and motivations, but also as a person with competing demands for time, attention, and material resources.

The care provider's firm conviction of the potential effectiveness of a plan can be a strong motivating factor. When, however, that conviction is expressed as simply telling the patient what to do, there may be problems. In crisis situations, a direct takeover approach is indicated; it may also be indicated in instructing persons in actions to take during most episodes of acute illness. In long-term conditions, however, where substantial changes must be made in lifestyle and a good deal of continued effort is needed to maintain relative health stability, the tendency to tell the person what to do needs to be consciously checked. Ultimately, what persons do about their health condition is their decision; health-care providers cannot make the decision for them. Health-care providers do, however, have the responsibility to provide persons with the information they need to make decisions, to assist persons in access to and use of human and material health-care resources, and to support persons in the often difficult adjustments necessitated by long-term disorders and disabilities. Telling a person what is best is easy to do and rather quickly accomplished. The more complex skills of interviewing, of providing patients with the types and amount of input they can handle at any particular time, of negotiating what is possible, and of being supportive in a way that the other person can accept are less easily learned skills.

Long-range goals may appear to the patient to be impossible to achieve. A breakdown of these goals into a series of short-range or intermediate ones that are more easily achievable can be done with some thought and planning. Persons who have used written contracts with patients as a way to improve compliance have used that strategy purposely and successfully, as have others who use it in an informal one-step-at-a-time approach. Successfully carrying out one behavior leads to feelings of competence in undertaking other behaviors. Contracting with patients is also called behavioral contracting or contingency contracting and stems from behavior modification theory. In systematic employment of the strategy, an agreed-upon reward is given for performance of a specified behavior. The patient and care provider together negotiate a written and signed contract specifying the behavior, the reward, and any conditions, such as time limitation. The behavior specified must be an attainable one so that the patient can feel successful. Another contract is then written for the next step toward the long-range goal. Rewards vary considerably but include such things as being able to spend additional time with the health-care provider and being given certain information, assistance, and items of (limited) monetary value (Streckel and Swain).

Almost everyone recognizes the fundamental soundness of reinforcing desired behavior. What often happens in practice, however, is that such behavior is not commented upon, but undesirable behavior receives attention. The successful use of patient contracts should sensitize care providers to certain values, even though they may reject the actual systematic use of the contracts. These values include finding out what is important to the patient, negotiating agreed-upon goals and means of attaining the goals, and setting up a situation in which the patient can be successful. The recognition of effort is central to success. Such recognition is also undoubtedly a major factor in producing the positive associations found between social support and compliance. Recognition of effort should be appropriate to the extent of that effort and to the person's ability to accept positive input. Overblown and excessive praise can, for example, be distasteful to the individual.

Attention to the need for recognition of effort and the need for social support leads naturally to certain actions such as inclusion of family members or significant others in developing the plan of treatment. Their involvement may spell the difference between the person's following a clinical prescription or abandoning it. Self-help clubs may also be a strong source of support to the patient. Such clubs are usually initiated and conducted by patients, ex-patients, or their families and are not under the control of health agencies, governmental agencies, or professionals. They are usually formed for conditions that have no medical cure and in which there is a substantial residue of impairment after an acute phase is over. Through the provision of education, help with skills, encouragement, and other forms of support, members may help each other maintain appropriate rehabilitation procedures and a consequent viable style of life. Health practitioners who are aware of the existence of such clubs in the community can be a prime referral source.

Health-care providers can express their interest in and support of the patient in other ways besides recognition of individual effort, inclusion of family, and attention to community resources. Respect for the individual is also implicit in the efforts care providers make to set up regimens individually suited to the patient and the situation; in efforts to make access to their services as convenient as possible; to help persons understand the basis for treatment; and, if indicated, to keep in telephone contact with the patient or to make home visits.

The literature is replete with specific suggestions on how to improve compliance; these include educational strategies using a variety of motivational inputs, persuasive communications, programmed instruction, lectures, demonstrations, role playing, counseling, and the like. Numerous strategies have been devised relative to use of medications, such as manipulation of schedules or packaging, use of long-acting versus short-acting forms, distinctive color packaging, calendar-type packaging similar to that used for contraceptive pills, reminders such as check-off charts, provision of free medication, and many others. Little has been published about strategies relative to specific procedures applicable to many rehabilitative regimens. With any specific actions or strategies taken to improve compliance, however, it is well to remember that plans for assisting persons to achieve the goals of a clinical prescription need to be individualized or tailored. In addition, a health-care provider who is successful in working with some patients in achieving the goals may be unsuccessful with other patients. Thus, responsibilities among the rehabilitation team members for furthering compliant behavior may shift according to who is most effective with which patients.

CONCLUSION

Compliance with a clinical prescription that involves extensive behavioral and life-style changes, such as the changes often indicated in long-term rehabilitative regimens, is difficult for most persons. Success in carrying out a plan and achieving therapeutic goals will be based on a variety of factors. Important among these factors is the extent to which members of the rehabilitation team can work with the patient on a mutual, realistic basis to negotiate achievable goals and the means to reach them. Existing stereotypes of potentially compliant patients need to be discarded and more attention given to health professionals' abilities to assess patients' perception of their own situation, the professionals' ability to influence attitudes, beliefs, and behaviors, as well as to transmit information, and their ability to be genuinely supportive to patients and families in a variety of ways. A great deal more knowledge is needed to further the understanding of compliance; however, that fact should not deter anyone from incorporating into practice the considerable amount of existing information.

BIBLIOGRAPHY

Baekeland, Frederick, and Lawrence Lundwall: "Dropping Out of Treatment: A Critical Review," *Psychol Bull* 82:738, 1975.

Becker, Marshall H. (ed.): "The Health Belief Model and Personal Health Behavior," *Health Ed Monographs* 2:326, 1974.

Becker, Marshall H.: "Sociobehavioral Determinants of Compliance," in D. L. Sackett and R. B. Haynes (eds.), *Compliance with Therapeutic Regimens,* Johns Hopkins Univ. Press, Baltimore, 1976.

———, Lois A. Maiman, John P. Kirscht, Don P. Haefner, and Robert H. Drachman: "The Health Belief Model and Prediction of Dietary Compliance: A Field Experiment," *J Health Soc Behav* 18:348, 1977.

Borkman, Thomasina S.: "Hemodialysis Compliance: The Relationship of Staff Estimates of Patients' Intelligence and Understanding to Compliance," *Soc Sci Med* 10:385, 1976.

Caplan, Robert D., Elizabeth A. R. Robinson, John R. P. French, Jr., John R. Caldwell, and Marybeth Shinn: *Adhering to Medical Regimens,* Univ. of Michigan, Institute for Social Research, Ann Arbor, 1976.

Carpenter, James O., and Linda J. Davis: "Medical Recommendations—Followed or Ignored? Factors Influencing Compliance in Arthritis," *Arch Phys Med Rehabil* 57:241, 1976.

Cobb, Sidney: "Social Support as a Moderator of Life Stress," *Psychosom Med* 38:300, 1976.

Gussow, Zachary, and George S. Tracy: "The Role of Self-Help Clubs in Adaptation to Chronic Illness and Disability," *Soc Sci Med* 10:407, 1976.

Hayes-Bautista, David E.: "Modifying the Treatment: Patient Compliance, Patient Control and Medical Care," *Soc Sci Med* 10:233, 1976.

Hertz, Philip, and Paula L. Stamps: "Appointment-Keeping Behavior Re-Evaluated," *Am J Public Health* 67:1033, 1977.

Hulka, Barbara S., John C. Cassel, Lawrence L. Kupper, and James A. Burdette: "Communication, Compliance, and Concordance Between Physicians and Patients with Prescribed Medications," *Am J Public Health* 66:847, 1976.

Hyman, Martin D.: "Social Psychological Determinants of Patients' Performance in Stroke Rehabilitation," *Arch Phys Med Rehabil* 53:217, 1972.

Kasl, Stanislav: "Issues in Patient Adherence to Health Care Regimens," *J Human Stress* 1:5, 1975.

Komaroff, Anthony L.: "The Practitioner and the Compliant Patient," *Am J Public Health* 66:833, 1976.

Korsch, Barbara, Ethel K. Gozzi, and Vida Francis: "Gaps in Doctor-Patient Communication: Doctor-Patient Interaction and Patient Satisfaction," *Pediatrics* 42:855, 1968.

Lewis, Charles E., Barbara A. Resnik, Glenda Schmidt, and David Waxman: "Activities, Events and Outcomes in Ambulatory Patient Care," *N Engl J Med* 280:645, 1969.

Marston, Mary-Vesta: "Compliance with Medical

Regimens: A Review of the Literature," *Nurs Res* 19:312, 1970.

Sackett, David L., and R. Brian Haynes (eds.): *Compliance with Therapeutic Regimens,* Johns Hopkins Univ. Press, Baltimore, 1976.

Streckel, Susan B., and Mary Ann Swain: "Contracting with Patients to Improve Compliance," *Hospitals* 51:81, 1977.

Stimson, Gerry V.: "Obeying Doctor's Orders: A View from the Other Side," *Soc Sci Med* 8: 97, 1974.

Svarstad, Bonnie L.: "The Doctor-Patient Encounter: An Observational Study of Communication and Outcome," doctoral dissertation, Univ. of Wisconsin, Madison, 1974.

6

sandra mock
jeannette taylor

variables that predict successful community reintegration

INTRODUCTION

What is successful community reintegration? Can it be defined and evaluated?

The goal of a program of rehabilitation is for patients to be able to cope with living *outside* a health-care setting. The objective is to enable patients to return to a functional life, to be able to enjoy and experience the present, and to plan for the future and toward specific goals like everyone else. Success must be evaluated not on the basis of health-care professionals' personal value systems but in relation to the patient's individual situation.

Successful rehabilitation outcome, as defined in this chapter, is not the ability to function well within a hospital setting but the ability to do well in the community. Success in a rehabilitation program requires coping skills different from managing one's life in the community. Hospitals expect a certain degree of compliance with difficult, rather rigid regimens, without any assurance about the outcome. Persons who function best in such an environment are those who have elements of dependency, subordination, or conformity in their social relationships and so are willing to adapt and to complete treatment. More assertive, independent persons may have difficulty, be seen as noncompliant, and leave the treatment center sooner than recommended. However, long-term adaptation studies have shown that the more assertive personalities are capable of functioning best within the community.

Successful completion of a rehabilitation program is not necessary for successful community reintegration. However, a programmed approach can be extremely helpful not only for physical upgrading and retraining but also as a process that engages an individual in learning new skills and coping with impairment. What is important is not just doing well within hospital walls but also transferring skills learned in the hospital to both the home and the community. This is a process for which both time and practice are required.

CRITERIA FOR SUCCESS

The criteria for successful rehabilitation outcome must be objective and can be discussed in terms of the following functional standards:

1. The person is in reasonably good health, as evidenced by staying out of the hospital and avoiding medical complications.
2. The person is either caring for herself or himself or, if that is not possible, is taking responsibility for seeing that care is given by someone else.
3. The person, though physically impaired, feels comfortable and able in the home and in the community. This perception is shared by others relating closely to the person. Persons who feel "able" do not value themselves exclusively for what they can do. Rather, they are increasing their ability to have "being" experiences. They are seeking techniques for facilitating being: exploring, manipulating, experiencing, being interested, choosing, delighting, enjoying, organizing, simplifying, being truthful and experiencing truth, being playful, being unique, and being realistic.
4. The person has high self-esteem and is not involved in destructive habits such as excessive eating, problem drinking, or the use of mind-stultifying drugs.
5. The person has a stable support system. Interactions with the support system are not disruptive and do not interfere with function. The person has learned to maintain necessary environmental supports to ensure stability in life.

A successful personal outcome is one that the person accepts as successful and that encompasses individual priorities. The person is or can be productive in one of many different ways, such as returning to work and being financially independent. The person may seek further education or training in order to be able to find and hold a job. Viable options to work and study have meaning and social usefulness—the person may become a volunteer and give service to the larger community, may become involved in organizations and work for social legislation, or may be a valued friend, parent, child, spouse, or lover.

PREDICTING SUCCESSFUL REHABILITATION

Health-care professionals are very concerned about being able to predict successful outcomes. They are increasingly aware of the need to set objective, realistic goals and to make plans with the patient and family to meet these goals.

The human and monetary cost of rehabilitation makes professionals acutely aware of the need for more research in the area of variables that affect rehabilitation outcome in order to build what they learn from research into their practice. The financial costs to society are enormous. They include the costs of acute care, of inpatient and outpatient rehabilitation training and continued care, of recurrent hospitalization and surgeries because of complications, and of nursing homes. Governmental agencies must give supplemental incomes to disabled persons who cannot manage in a family unit or be financially independent. Still another cost is the loss of income tax from persons not able to work.

It is of little use to generalize about personality characteristics or patterns that help physically impaired persons reintegrate themselves into the community following a traumatic injury and rehabilitation experience. Part of the problem is that it is wrong to look at the physically impaired as a group. They are amorphous behaviorally and have about as much in common as a group of persons attending a political caucus. Each individual has different characteristics; life experiences prior to injury and experiences and reactions to impairment also vary widely. Trying to determine direct causative relationships between characteristics and positive outcome is very difficult. Factors cannot be isolated, for they are interrelated. What works for one individual is not necessarily successful for another.

Another question that needs to be reevaluated is: Over what period of time is the outcome successful? For many years, rehabilitation experts talked about patients taking about a year to "adjust" to severe impairment. This is certainly not in keeping with experience. The time differs for different persons. Normally, a young quadriplegic who is 14 years old, still in school, and trying to grow up and cope with adulthood takes longer to adjust than does a mature quadriplegic, 30 years old. On the average, it seems to take 3 to 5 years for a person to develop an adequate coping style and to come to grips with the long-term, permanent nature of disability.

ROLES OF THE SOCIAL WORKER

The social worker on the rehabilitation team functions in the following roles:

1. *Advocate.* Committed to serving individuals who are victims of social injustice.
2. *Mobilizer and broker.* Assembles and energizes existing groups, resources, organizations, and structures to create new ways of dealing with problems that exist or to prevent problems from occurring.
3. *Educator.* Interprets details and implications of roles clients want or are expected to play when there is inadequate role preparation or lack of role perception, provides structured learning experiences, gives information, designs growth experiences, acts as a model, and provides feedback.
4. *Counselor.* Enables client to cope effectively with physical and human environment.

The social worker can be very valuable in the reintegration process in the significant ways suggested here. The treatment team is the most effective tool in serving the patient-family system. A significant staff effort is needed to strengthen and sharpen individual skills and to define better ways of working as a team.

PERSONAL QUALITIES

HELPFUL PREMORBID PERSONALITY TRAITS

How to achieve successful rehabilitation is something that cannot be taught. There are numerous activities and lessons for patients to learn while going through the process, but anyone who is successful realizes that success itself is a variable that defies a logical, prescriptive approach. Like much of life, being successful in rehabilitation results not only from the positives that one brings to the experience but also from luck, risk taking in physical experimentation, and social self-examination and reencountering.

Thomas Harris, the transactional analyst who wrote *I'm O.K., You're O.K.,* tells about a child's response to being the last among several children to put his hand in a cookie jar for an afternoon treat. When the child saw that his cookie was not in one piece, he threw it across the room and cried, "My cookie's broke."

Not being able to control what happens is extremely frustrating. Life is always dealing people broken cookies. It takes time, a process, and some maturity to figure out that the outcome of impairment does not have to be total disaster and waste. What is necessary is a changed perception and acceptance of a different identity. "Broken cookies" can be enjoyed, and the essence of someone does not change because the person is not perfect.

The rehabilitation process starts with some self-confidence and self-investment. Then the patient marshals resources in a special way and gathers the visible knowns and unknowns into a focused activity. A person must have goals and must understand the barriers to achievement of these goals. Successful rehabilitation is very often successful problem solving.

The first problem or task in rehabilitation is learning to cope with the sudden, traumatic change. Many programmed life-style changes evoke emotional responses and problems (adolescence, parenthood, retirement), but the life-style change forced by physical impairment is potentially much more taxing and disorganizing. The desired outcome of this first task is for the patient to regain a comfortable personal equilibrium and to minimize the disorganizing effects of the impairment, as well as the crisis that affected every one of the individual's systems (family, job, and community).

The patient needs to learn to move in space, to become aware of a new body image and sense of self, to accept the possibility of never being able to resume certain roles, and to reassess some priorities and values.

The patient may feel like a person going on a long journey who does not want to go, has no time to prepare, no idea of what the cost will be, and no idea of destination, how long it will take, and how things will be on arrival. The person has never experienced anything like this before and is fearful about the journey. It would be nice to have a trusted family member or friend who would make all the decisions for the traveler or at least come along, but it is the individual's trip, and each person will probably do best if the decisions are self-made entirely or at least in part. The guide may be widely respected and knowledgeable, but the traveler does not know enough at first to ask the right questions or correctly use the help.

Rehabilitation problem solving can be like such a journey because it is problem solving for a future that is uncertain and stressful. The patient may decide at an early stage to take things one day at a time, to set expectations and goals that seem reasonable, to gain information needed for making decisions, and to learn to know the health personnel and other patients. The person with a physical impairment can look at personal characteristics, how they were useful in similar situations, what traits were of value in the past, and what coping skills were used successfully. The patient needs to know that one does not have to begin life all over again. It is important to recognize, assess, and consider strengths and positive life achievements. Patients who bring with them a proven ability to effect changes in life situations and to exercise control over their destinies have a greater chance for success.

A REVIEW OF THE LITERATURE

Literature on rehabilitation patterns and outcomes is problematic and incomplete. There are few longitudinal studies, and the complex nature of patient-family involvement and interdisciplinary treatment has not been addressed. The literature does contain some sociological studies on illness and its treatment, some general population studies, and some short-term studies on rehabilitation within an institutional setting. Because there is considerable governmental interest in the area of rehabilitation outcomes, the assumption is that there will be more research in this area.

High-Risk Factors

In the sociological studies reviewed, an important high-risk factor for predicting illness resolution is low socioeconomic status. Earl Coos (1954), the National Opinion Research Center Study of 1964, and Rosenblatt and Suchman (1964) discovered differences in illness and health care according to social class.

The researchers found that serious illness was more prevalent among the poor; the proportion of serious illnesses in the family, when related to income, was two to three times greater in the low socioeconomic class than in the population as a whole. Those in the lower class (1) had less information about their illness and treatment, (2) had less access to a family doctor, (3) were more skeptical about the medical profession, (4) were more likely to use home remedies, and (5) were more upset and anxious about the same type of illness or disability than persons in the middle or upper socioeconomic classes.

The studies suggest that blue-collar workers and slum tenants encounter barriers which discourage their use of medical services. Among these are language problems, cultural traditions, inconvenience of travel, time spent in care dispensaries, and the impersonality of treatment in some medical centers.

The health-care system in the United States reflects a middle-class orientation that emphasizes individual responsibility, deliberate action to promote health, and active participation in an authoritative, programmed attack on health problems. A whole complex of motivational, value, and life-style divergences has as yet been inadequately addressed in present health-care planning.

Although the studies mentioned were not done specifically in rehabilitation settings, the higher recidivism rates for disabled lower-class persons attest to their problems in successful reintegration into the community. This may relate simply to the inaccessibility of certain options and resources (an individual on public aid may not be able to afford the health-care priorities that were stressed as necessary within the institutional setting), but the literaure suggests that it is more than a funding concern. Social class is also connected with another high-risk variable of rehabilitation outcome called the internal-external locus of control.

The *locus-of-control study* (Rotter, 1966) states that individuals who believe that they have some control over their options in life are called "internals." Those who believe that their lives are controlled by chance, fate, and powerful others are labeled "externals." Externals are less prone than internals to try to control their outcomes or environment. Studies have shown that poor or lower-class children have more feeling than do middle- or upper-class children that fate controls them. Feelings of powerlessness are characteristic of the poor (Chilman, 1966).

This is worthwhile information as it relates to the rehabilitation effort. Persons do not try to change their circumstances and work to effect change if they have a built-in negative expectancy for success. Heider (1958) states that there is a contingency relationship between "can" and "try"—persons do not try if they do not believe they can. Lower-social-class status appears to be conducive to the development of a low expectancy for success. Lefcourt's conclusion, following his 1966 study, was that "perhaps the apathy and what is often described as lack of motivation to achieve may be explained as a result of disbelief that effort pays off."

The high-risk factors that have been discussed are easily identifiable. They should be targeted early, and individual remedial action should be built into treatment approaches.

Factors Predictive of Success in Rehabilitation

Characteristics that are positively correlated with successful rehabilitation outcomes are alert mental status, physical attractiveness, a full and successful preonset life experience and patterns, and a good external support system. Ability to accommodate to change and stress and to adapt to society's reactions are also important.

Mental Status Obviously the patient needs a certain degree of orientation, awareness, and ability to learn. Often personality is temporarily disorganized because of minimal brain damage or because of the patient's reaction to the impairment. If there is no permanent brain damage, the personality may be capable of reintegration. Preexisting coping mechanisms can be used to incorporate what has happened into the original personality structure.

Kelman et al. (1966) followed 58 rehabilitation patients over a 2-year period and found that successful community reintegration was contingent upon the individual's maintenance of health levels and resourcefulness. A 3-month follow-up of stroke patients by Anderson et al. in 1974 showed that early success in community reintegration is related to previous medical condition, time since onset, amount of perceptual loss, and motivation. Kerr (1977) found that level of lesion in spinal cord-injured patients is relatively unimportant in comparison to the psychologic problems of persons who are recidivists.

In some way, the person who has become impaired experiences a period of cognitive disorganization, mourning for loss, crisis, and reshuffling of values and goals that can be equated to the stages an individual goes through in coming to terms with death.

In her book, *On Death and Dying,* Kübler-Ross outlines these stages. The first stage is shock and denial—the person's need to protect the ego from the devastating reality of the trauma. The mind *unmakes* the present so ego pain is not full strength. The reaction is a natural response, a retreat. Everyone does this in coping with negative events and changes, and in many ways the reaction is functional and adaptive.

The next stage is anger, anguish, and rage. The person is angry at others' lack of competence, both real and imagined, wants more and better of everything, and may resent other healthier persons. The individual wants someone to blame for the problem and for personal lack of control over circumstances. Bargaining is related to hope and to some magical thinking about goals and rewards for achieving them. The person makes arbitrary deadlines, thinks "cause and effect," and does some independent testing of limits.

Depression is the stage that usually precedes acceptance. It can occur at any time during the process but apparently does not have to occur in all cases. It is the most difficult response for staff and family to handle; it is natural, even expected, but it can be frightening, temporarily nonproductive, and hard to respond to.

There seems to be great divergence of professional opinion about the helpfulness of this theory. It is easily conceptualized, but one must be cautioned not to take the theory as so scientifically exact that one is unprepared for other possibilities. To believe absolute rules about how people rehabilitate themselves does not allow for the reality that some persons want and need to deny for longer periods of time, that some persons feel or express no anger or depression and do well, and that personality disturbance is more likely to occur when the impaired state, the loss, is mild or marginal than when it is severe (Cowen and Bobgrove, 1966).

Physical Attractiveness and Youth America values youth, beauty, and fitness more than any

CHAPTER 6 74

other country. The attributes appear to be relevant to rehabilitation patients' success in community reintegration. Researchers at the Universities of Michigan and Minnesota have found that physically attractive persons are perceived as being more sensitive, interesting, strong, poised, sociable, sexually warm, and outgoing than less attractive persons. In a study of psychiatric hospital patients, a research team at the University of Connecticut found less attractive patients were hospitalized longer, had fewer visitors, were more likely to suffer relapses, and received less attention from attendants. Other studies show that educated persons identify attractiveness with higher intelligence quotient (IQ), believability, trustworthiness, and achievement. In fact, society rewards more attractive people with higher salaries as well as numerous other benefits.

Of course, attractiveness is probably a circular variable, related to how one feels about oneself and how one chooses to transmit this perception outwardly. However, attractiveness does seem to have special implications for physical impairment. Do attractive patients receive more attention? Are staff more invested in them? Does the community accept them more easily? These questions have not been researched for rehabilitation patients, but they are questions that individuals may have to face themselves.

If one does not or cannot fit into the mainstream of society, in the sense of physical fitness and ability, now that one's body has changed, one has to learn to accept one's difference and the fact that it may limit some alternatives. Every individual has the right to be himself or herself, that is, to accept individual differences and have them accepted by others. To be successful in rehabilitation, one must be able to live up to certain illusions and channel remaining energy into other areas.

Preonset Life Experience and Patterns The person with a physical impairment is very much the same individual as at any other time, only more so. Egocentricity and regression to earlier solutions are basic psychological survival mechanisms, a resource bank that one can draw on without much effort. Because most of the patient's drive and energy is being invested in the process of becoming a functional person, initially there seems to be a protective embrace of psychological status quo, resistance to emotional issues, and a change in values and attitudes. The ethnic origin, cultural values, general success in school, at work, and in interpersonal relationships that a person brings to this crisis of impairment are likely to come into play throughout the rehabilitation process.

The values that an individual lives by are important considerations to adaptation to impairment and community reintegration. The congruency of these values with the dominant values of society and of the institution where the person is receiving rehabilitation is also significant. If the preimpaired person, like American society, is work oriented, moralistic, and places high value on financial success, creative achievement, and the possession of certain commodities, not achieving those values affects a person's self-image. One can be made to feel morally defunct by any inability, temporary or permanent.

Individuals often believe that they are totally responsible for what happens to them. They think that if they work hard and are good persons, they will succeed in life. Injuries can be interpreted by these persons as a sign of wrongdoing by themselves or someone else. Beliefs, of course, can provide comfort as well, but if centered on guilt and angry retribution, they can prohibit the positive thoughts and hope which are needed to sustain persons going through the reentry process. Other unhelpful attitudes that come from value orientation and are not easily changed are that money can buy sufficient expertise and service for a return to former health, that a rehabilitation center should be run like a hotel, the patient always right and the staff completely tolerant of patients' moods and reactions, and that one who is going through this experience has a right to be continually overwrought about the unfairness of life. In reality, there are no "shoulds" or guarantees with long-term human relationships. Professionals are persons who have special knowledge, are clinically trained, and attempt to be therapeutic. Even so, a patient's continued agitation and unresolved anger are likely to have unpleasant consequences for the patient.

The prior life experience, then, is a data base that relates to outcome. A full life experience prior to onset of physical impairment leads one to expect that one has the capacity to achieve and to meet crisis; a short, sheltered, or negative life experience creates a vacuum of expectation and an orientation of dependency (Albrecht, 1976).

The Quality of External Support Systems
Families and other support systems are quite consistent in dealing with persons in their immediate social environment, with institutions, and with medical facility and rehabilitation teams. If a family's normal way of dealing with its environment is known, outcomes of interactions with staff can be predicted. In a study by the social work–social research departments at the Rehabilitation Institute of Chicago (Harasymiw, 1977–1980), it was found that patients who had little social interaction and community involvement prior to onset of physical impairment were perceived as more likely to be unsuccessful in rehabilitation. The degree to which families are cooperative, outgoing, optimistic, and effectively involve themselves in the process of rehabilitation and learning is determined by past experience. How much family involvement affects the outcome of rehabilitation has not yet been documented, but observation and experience indicate that it is an important variable.

Degree of Stress Experienced Stress is a variable in successful rehabilitation. Stress is a psychosocial phenomenon that occurs in everyone's life to some extent. Only when stress reaches crisis proportions, as it does for persons trying to accommodate to physical impairment, is it of concern. Energy is devoted to learning about personal, physical, financial, social, and self-concept changes (as perceived by the individual). Within a given year, beyond a certain point, the greater the stress the higher the risk of illness. When the pressure is too great, what appears to be a matter of energy and physiologic changes triggered by emotional reactions results in a "something's got to give" situation.

In fact, the degree of stress in the external environment may be one of the main issues that affect recidivism of rehabilitation patients. In a 2-year longitudinal study at the Rehabilitation Institute of Chicago, Harasymiw is using a revised version of the Holmes-Rahe stress scale and other techniques to identify stress factors experienced by rehabilitation patients prior to onset of injury and during the following rehabilitation hospital stay. The influence of these factors on the rehabilitation outcome will be evaluated.

FACTORS THAT ADVANCE OR IMPEDE THE REHABILITATION PROCESS

If a group of successfully rehabilitated persons were asked what "got them to where they are today," there would be a number of different answers. Qualities such as persistence, assertiveness, creativity, and imagination seem essential for the hard task of rehabilitation and community functioning. Also, the following three abilities are helpful to patients who are moving through the rehabilitation experience.

1 *Ability to cope with change* is the major issue. This change has made the patient different (deviant in a statistical as well as a social sense). This difference, from the old self and from other persons, is painful to accept. Is it temporary or is it permanent? To be different and to accept a socially unacceptable difference takes an enormous amount of strength. If all persons pick up much of their identity from others, what does this social mirror look like to the impaired person? The rehabilitation movie called *Mimi* shows the socialization constraints and stereotyped expectations that exist around paraplegia. The young woman says that the

biggest task for disabled persons is *not* to accept the identity society offers them. Cogswell describes this ability as stigma management.

Persons who are physically normal and then suffer an accident or illness so that rehabilitation is required often will say how humiliating and draining the experience is. One can easily identify with some of the basic problems by imagining urinating all over oneself at an important social affair. Abstract thought, new learning, and enjoyment are hard if one must concentrate on other, more primal concerns. Prior to rehabilitation, patients often feel they have completely lost control. Valued characteristics have been taken away, and old roles and functions have not yet been replaced by new ones.

2 *Problem-solving ability* is the second most important characteristic needed for successful rehabilitation. The uniqueness and severity of the problems to be resolved in impairment make this skill essential. Persons who, despite disability, can continue to define themselves as "whole" can be successful. There is a strong tendency to equate mobility with personhood. Many persons see paralysis as a vegetable state and seek to infantilize patients because of their wheelchair status. Patients must be seen as human and feel human if they are going to pursue survival issues.

It is important for patients to realize that the rehabilitation experience will be slow, arduous, and uncertain. The ability to be aware of this fact is crucial. Daily frustrations have to be overcome. Naturally, a person may feel depressed, but this has to be accepted as part of the process, recognized as something that may come and go but that is manageable, something one can come through. Depression in these circumstances is not a pathologic state but a normal emotion experienced after loss. It is important that depression not lead to lengthy periods of feeling hopeless or helpless. Being hopeful and realistic at the same time is possible and ideal. The hope that aids survival probably starts out as a desire for cure but changes to a more practical survival hope—that things will get better and that one can "make it." Small physical gains can be miracles to a patient with this kind of mind set.

Assessment of situations is healthy when one can focus on what gains have been made rather than what losses have been suffered. This allows a person to build on strengths that remain and begin to fill in gaps left by impairment problems.

New growth opportunities can be sought, and the socialization process can begin. Socialization is a role-adjustment and learning process during which one sees and tries out new attitudes and behavioral patterns. The process depends upon the character of the disability—length of time, visibility, and expected outcome of the impairment. The patient thinks of self in new ways, sees others who are impaired and yet *able,* and comes to terms with the roles it is possible to play. An example of the value-attitudinal change is that a person who held the view that rugged individualism is "the right way to live" can come to accept the need for social interdependence. The person who can learn and be comfortable with this change is more likely to function successfully in the community. It is necessary to compromise and give up plans about the future that are not possible and to recognize the multitude of other possibilities.

Ambiguity regarding the degree of impairment and the patient's functional status has a negative impact on interpersonal relationships and good problem solving. If the patient knows and is easily perceived as having decreased ability, then it is easier to set up new role expectations and move toward them. When someone is on the fringe of functioning or maintains incongruent goals in relation to expert analysis, what can be expected is unclear and disquieting. In many persons going through rehabilitation, this uncertainty exists and interferes with their wanting to learn new ways to cope. It is also very hard on the family system.

Persons who are impatient, have low frustration tolerance, are hostile, and tend to have angry reactions find these characteristics are barriers to problem solving. Rational behavior, such as not ignoring medical advice or one's own body systems and learning how to engage and keep one's support system well functioning, is part of good problem solving.

3 *The ability to be part of the rehabilitation process and yet be separate from it is* important for long-term success. The patient who is the "good" patient, cooperative and appropriately dependent, may not present problems within the hospital, but submissiveness is not usually helpful in community adaptation. What is helpful is the ability to define one's own goals and motivate oneself.

Motivation is defined here as the continuation of an activity without external reinforcement. Of course, external reinforcement facilitates much of the difficult new learning and the repetition embodied in rehabilitation. But when the external reinforcers are withdrawn, the patient needs to have sufficient sense of purpose to continue the original rehabilitation effort while living in the community.

One way to build reinforcement into patients' experience is to have them define their own goals as early as possible, to help them see the pathways for achieving their objectives, and to evaluate and give feedback about the goals all along the way. Sharing the information creates goal congruency and does not inhibit patients' natural motivations to provide for their own needs.

THE INDIVIDUAL AND SYSTEMS
INDIVIDUAL DYNAMICS

In designing a course to prepare a patient for community reintegration, the first task is to decide on the objectives to be achieved and how to monitor or test the patient's knowledge, practice, and understanding of the goals. With any behavior, there is a continuum, and with a patient the extremes and all the alternatives in between are identified. Where does the patient want to be? What can the patient and the professional do to help the patient move in that direction? For example, after a 2- to 3-month stay in a rehabilitation hospital, useful behavior for the patient could be the ability to do the following:

1. Identify physical care needs, if any, and know how to meet those needs through direct self-care or through the direction of that care.
2. Examine the extent of external support systems, such as family, friends, and social agencies, and the extent to which one will be on one's own, including how to manage this.
3. Learn about factors that influence rehabilitation treatment goals and life goals and learn to be pleasantly assertive instead of passive in goal achievement.
4. Be aware of government and private resources available in the community to help in the maintenance of maximum independence and know how to deal with these resources.
5. Be able to problem solve and be willing to risk trial and error on solutions to some problems; have confidence in personal ability to cope.
6. Be aware of problems—medical, sexual, "entitlement," and emotional disturbance, for instance—that a professional consultant might offer help with; know whom to talk to about these concerns.

One distinctive characteristic of being human and functional in the world is the capacity to

CHAPTER 6   78

understand the past and plan the future, to understand consequences and take action accordingly. Thus, a critical alternative in the process of being fully a functional person is whether one's future is something that "happens" or something one "does" as a result of rational decision making. One problem in rehabilitating people is this area of decision making and control. Perhaps because some people come to, and even leave, rehabilitation not being totally able to control their own lives or problem solve, there is often a tendency to do more, to make more decisions, or to offer more advice than is helpful. Too often health-care professionals rely too much on the "me" and not enough on the "you" solution.

To trust persons to know their own best solutions and not to make value judgments about their behavior is primary to facilitating change and teaching. The questions that must always be asked are: Am I doing something that the patient or family could do? How can I teach them to do it? The goal of community reintegration must always be considered; the need is to teach new skills or ways to handle a world that is not yet made for persons who are physically impaired.

Physical skills and the mastery of the body are of first importance; mastery of the body comes before personality integration in normal development. The lifelong adaptation tasks are usually in the areas of social adaptation, of "making it" in the real world. This is why rehabilitation has to be considered an equal partnership arrangement, with the professional expert in the role of consultant-teacher. Often, in a desire to control outcomes, professionals try to remove critical consequences and to intervene in ways that do not help individuals to be responsible for themselves. Everyone has to experience consequences (though not necessarily to suffer in a negative sense) and to learn to trust in his or her own basic ability to learn.

The individual is a center of various system networks. Within the family, at work, in the community, pursuing interests, and with friends, the person is a hub of numerous actions. When an illness or accident necessitates rehabilitation, the person experiences a crisis. A well-known definition of crisis by Caplan and Parad is: "A crisis is provoked when a person faces an obstacle or threat to important life goals, that is, for a time, insurmountable through the utilization of customary methods of problem solving. It is a period of disorganization and upset, during which time many different abortive attempts at solution are made."

Obviously, physical impairment and rehabilitation are crises, made worse by the fact that there is usually little prior knowledge or preparation for the change. This crisis period is time limited (1 to 6 weeks) and is characterized by tension which changes with the movement of the crisis problem. The crisis can stir up unresolved issues from the past; certainly the issue of dependency-independency can be a basic conflictual area. Emotional states experienced in crisis run the gamut from helplessness, disorganization, confusion, and irrational thoughts to rational problem solving and appropriate effect. Crisis is a time when persons are more amenable to the influence of others and more open to change and reassessment. If intervention can occur during periods of active crisis, the chances of avoiding maladaptation and despair are increased (Lukton).

Professionals not only need to project hopeful attitudes during this time but also to be aware of possible unconscious fears of destructiveness and lack of controls. The best course is to listen to patients' hopes as well as the changes in their hopes over time and to strengthen their self-concept by reflecting their feelings and giving support for achievement toward independence. By telling a patient a projected outcome too early, a professional may force the patient to deal with it prematurely; the professional probably is projecting a personal need to cope rather than helping someone else. Often there is a struggle between meeting one's own and the patient's needs. It is not always possible for a newly impaired person to give positive feedback or motivated performance in response to professionals' efforts. To do a good job in rehabilitation requires being aware of one's own motivations, taking care of oneself emotionally outside the job situation, and not expecting patients and families to take the lead in being rational, knowing exactly what their goals are, or how they can be achieved.

Contradictory advice and a sense of powerlessness may alienate the patient, who then submits to the most powerful expert. Unless individuals feel part of any decision regarding them, they lose part of their will to decide. Sometimes persons in crisis may need to borrow a little of a professional's ego strength and accept a lot of structure in their experience for a time (their own inner coping mechanisms being somewhat out of kilter); the task is to nurture and support, then gradually withdraw and return the control to the person, expecting little in terms of thanks because the professional's part may not even be remembered.

THE FAMILY

The family, the central and basic unit of our social structure, is generally the caretaker in our society; specifically, the female members of the family most often give care.

A family is defined as a collection of persons who live together for some period of time, who develop some strong emotional bonds, who have some operating rules and ways of communication, and who are voluntarily committed to responsibility for one another within this unit. They may or may not be related, and monetary remuneration may or may not be involved.

Family systems are families viewed as holistic functioning units made up of interdependent parts. A change in one unit or person affects the other units as in an electrical system; they react and affect the first unit. This is called a feedback loop. The power for positive or negative feedback and energy use is enormous.

When disability affects one individual, it affects the whole family system of which that person is a part. The effect has to be absorbed into this system if the unit is going to function well again

(Albrecht, 1976). It is even thought that the patient and the family move in a parallel process through the onset of disability, convalescence, and rehabilitation.

In each family, every member has certain behavioral, social, and emotional tasks. In the traditional American family, the father is the breadwinner, the decision maker, and the dealer with large systems. The mother is the homemaker, the provider of emotional support, and the caretaker. The children are growers, developers of skills, and bringers of hope and joy. These roles are understood and determine expectation of behavior. Members may occupy many roles at the same time, and roles may overlap. The end result is that the family functions, effectively or ineffectively, to provide for the basic needs of its members for food, shelter, socialization, identification, love, security, sex, and physical care.

It is important to see an individual as part of this family system—a system that has definite ways of working. If health-care professionals are to succeed with patients, they must understand the uniqueness of the families from which patients come. How did they function prior to disability? What was their life-style? What was the quality of the family relationship? How did they spend time? What were their roles? How did they do their work?

The family is disrupted by crisis. The natural equilibrium, the behavioral synergy pattern is upset. The energy for other tasks is rerouted and focused upon the patient, with hopes that there will be a cure and a return to functioning as when well. But the physically impaired person is removed from the system. The longer the patient is away, the more time other patterns of adaptation have to develop. Roles can remain in limbo only so long. Then families may run into role problems, such as:

1 *Role conflict*—the inability to perform two roles. (One cannot be a totally independent person and a patient at the same time.)
2 *Role ambiguity*—roles not clear. What is expected of the person as a patient or a

family member? Will the patient function as before?
3. *Role strain*—not being able to perform all the role expectations at the same time. (Women whose husbands are in the hospital have to visit, care for the kids, take care of bills, mow the grass, run the business, learn care, and observe therapies.)

Virginia Satir, a noted family therapist and social worker, describes systems as open or closed. An open system is the ideal: it provides for and expects changes from the outside. A closed system provides for and expects little or no change.

An open system offers choices. it depends for its continuing growth on successfully meeting reality. A closed system depends on edict, on law and order, and it operates on and through physical and emotional manipulation and force.

The implication for this family systems theory in rehabilitation is obvious. The families of patients, for the most part, have undergone trauma that results in a family need to face some major changes. The family system is undergoing constant actions, reactions, and interactions. It is searching for feedback, answers, and support. When the hospital system meets the traumatized family system, the result is like that old song, "Something's Gotta Give." The best rehabilitation outcome results from the rehabilitation system's giving.

If the family's system is to survive, it has to maintain or restore four basic components:

1. A purpose. Why did the family system exist before? Is there hope for these purposes or reasons again, or for new purposes?
2. An order to the operating parts. Self-worth and common rules and roles have to take a form, whether a new form or a return to the old form.
3. A means of maintaining basic needs, and an agreement about how this will be done.
4. Ways of dealing with change, including changes from the outside. The rehabilitation system has a time-limited interaction and impact on a family system. The family probably existed for a long time prior to this contact and will go on long after the intervention.

The situation must be quickly assessed:

1. What are the family's goals?
2. What are the rehabilitation institute's goals?
3. What was the quality and quantity of family involvement before illness?
4. What is the potential for this involvement now?
5. What does the family need to know?
6. What does the family want to know?
7. What plans have been made?
8. What kind of follow-up will there be?

There needs to be understanding and consensus from the first day between staff and family if staff members are to be most helpful.

When illness hits a family system, things are really out of control. The power that was totally the family's rests in part in the hands of persons the family depends upon because of reputation, not relationship. There are feelings of alienation and powerlessness. Families need to know what is happening, what they can do, what they can expect, how they can play a part and be in control of their situation. For some persons, the easiest thing to do is to place all their trust in the hands of authority; others cope by intellectually distancing themselves. The health-care professionals' job is to uncomplicate the bureaucracy enough for everyone to have a chance to relate to them. The professionals come from families of their own, families with rules, values, myths that they have lived by for a number of years. These ways of looking at life affect how professionals look at, what they expect from, and how they choose to deal with families. The staff as a whole can subjectively label families as "good" or "bad," and this can affect outcome.

Professionals want involvement in the patients' programs and must guard against inhibiting involvement by negativistic labeling and unclear expectations. Families can gain knowledge on these three levels of understanding:

81 VARIABLES THAT PREDICT SUCCESSFUL COMMUNITY REINTEGRATION

Level I. Observational learning. This is primarily information given with prevention in mind; the family will monitor the care given by the patient to self or the care that some other person gives to the patient, for instance in a nursing home. Support and encouragement are part of this level also; care may need to be given in emergencies.

Level II. Observational and experiential learning. A family member will give care with help or will give total care. That family member needs to know in order to teach others.

Level III. Observational, experiential, and affectiveness. The family member learns care but is emotionally involved with the disabled person. This family needs counseling to accompany the educational experience; it may give long-term care.

The family today is not always available as a resource or client. In Levels I and II, the family is viewed primarily as resource; Level III views the family as client. The family unit and individual members have their needs and priorities. A flexible, open system makes the adjustments, and the disabled member is accommodated. A closed system has more difficulty in dealing with outside systems, is rigid in its patterns and expectations, and therefore is extremely poor at long-term community adaptation.

Many hard issues have to be handled with the family: education about the disability and its implications, duration of immobility or nonfunction, recurrent medical problems and implications, length of life, and potential of fullness of life. In most instances, social workers aim to assist families in understanding, acceptance, and management of the patient's disability.

Families need supportive systems to help with a primary problem of social isolation: desertion by friends and relatives is not uncommon over a long period of time. The primary caretaker is frequently the one who begins to show the symptoms of family stress.

It is important for persons working in rehabilitation to take a close look at themselves as part of a system, the rehabilitation hospital system. Does the health-care system offer choices and facilitate successful coping with reality? Do health-care professionals unwittingly, through rules and communication processes, depend on edict (the doctor's and team's decision is, of necessity, the family's) and law and order (excluding the family from full partnership in decision making) to operate the system? These are not rhetorical questions. They cannot be answered by a simple yes or no. There is something beyond the practical realities; this is the humanness that produces healthy systems.

CONCLUSION

There appears to be no correlation between a specific disability and personality characteristics or personality adjustment. Disability relates to many types of problems over a wide range of differences in age, sex, socioeconomic status, and racial and cultural backgrounds. A particular individual is disabled, but even though each individual is different and unique, all are alike and human.

While disability is a negative life experience to be feared and personally rejected by everyone, it can provide an opportunity for some positive as well as negative experiences. Any number of researchers have shown that the best predictor of favorable response to trauma is a history of previously successful coping ability. The individual may be temporarily disorganized because of crisis and the subsequent stress, but integration of the experience into the self comes from individual work with self and the help of family, friends, the community, and professionals. Some persons make the journey through the rehabilitation experience and into the community by one route, others by a different route. Some of the factors that help people get through more easily and some that retard or impede that progress have been suggested. There are a variety of styles, including ways of moving and pacing oneself.

It is safe to say that no one does it alone; everyone needs other persons.

BIBLIOGRAPHY

Albrecht, Gary L.: "Socialization and the Disability Process," in Gary L. Albrecht (ed.) *The Sociology of Physical Disability and Rehabilitation,* Univ. of Pittsburgh Press, Pittsburgh, 1976, pp. 3–38.

"All things bright for beautiful," *Chicago Tribune,* February 12, 1978, pp. 1–2.

Anderson, Thomas P.: "An Alternative Frame of Reference for Rehabilitation, The Helping Process Versus the Medical Model," *Arch Phys Med Rehabil,* March 1975.

———: Norman Bourestom, Frederick Greenberg, Vida Hildyard: "Predictive Factors in Stroke Rehabilitation," *Arch Phys Med Rehabil* 5:533–45, 1974.

"An Ugly Bias," *Chicago Tribune,* February 12, 1978, pp. 1–2.

Baile, Walter F., and Bernard T. Engel: "A Behavioral Strategy for Promoting Treatment Compliance Following Myocardial Infarction," *Psychosom Med* 40:413, 1978.

Barofsky, Ivan: "Compliance, Adherence and the Therapeutic Alliance: Steps in the Development of Self-Care," *Soc Sci Med* 12:369, 1978.

Berman, Eric: "Regrouping for Survival: Approaching Death and Three Phases of Family Interaction," *J Compar Family Stud* 9:63–87, 1973.

Bromley, J.: "Etraplegia and Paraplegis," A Guide for Physiotherapists; Churchill Livingstone, Edinburgh, 1976.

Caplan, Gerald, and Howard Parad: "A Framework for Studying Families in Crisis," *Social Work* 5:3–16, 1960.

Chilman, C. S.: *Growing Up Poor,* Department of Health, Education, and Welfare, Welfare Administration Publ. 13, 1966.

Cogswell, Betty E.: "Conceptual Model of Family as a Group: Family Responses to Disability," in Gary L. Albrecht (ed.) *The Sociology of Disability and Rehabilitation,* Univ. of Pittsburgh Press, Pittsburgh, 1976.

Coos, Earl: *The Health of Regionsville,* Columbia Univ. Press, New York, 1954.

Cowen, E. L., and P. H. Bobgrove: "Marginality of Disability and Adjustment," *Percep Mot Skills* 23:869–70, 1966.

Epstein, Laura: "Casework Process in Crisis Abatement," *Child Welfare,* 1965.

Fink, Stephen L.: "Physical Disability and Problems in Marriage," *J Marriage Fam,* February: 64–73, 1968.

Fogel, Max L., and Ronald H. Rosillo: "Relationships Between Intellectual Factors and Coping in Physical Rehabilitation," *Rehabil Coun Bull,* December:68–77, 1973.

Frank, Jerome D.: *Persuasion and Healing: A Comparative Study of Psychotherapy,* Schocken, New York, 1974.

Freed, Murray, Henry Bakst, and David Barrie: "Life Expectancy, Survival Rates and Causes of Death in Civilian Patients with Spinal Cord Trauma," *Arch Phys Med Rehabil* 47: 457–63, 1966.

Geis, H. Jan: "The Problem of Personal Worth in the Physically Disabled Patient," *Rehabil Lit* 33(2), 1972.

Hallin, Roger P.: "Follow-up of Paraplegics and Tetraplegics After Comprehensive Rehabilitation," *Paraplegia* June:128–34, 1968.

Harasymiw, S. J. et al.: "Post Rehabilitation Problems and Costs: A Study in Progress," 1977–80, working paper, Rehabilitation Institute of Chicago.

Harris, Thomas A.: *I'm O.K.—You're O.K.,* Harper & Row, New York, 1967, pp. 126–27.

Hartman, Ann: "An Ecological Framework for Assessment and Intervention," Univ. of Michigan, School of Social Work, 1976.

Heider, F.: *The Psychology of Interpersonal Relations,* Wiley, New York, 1958.

Henry, Jules: "Human Obsolescence," in *Culture Against Man,* Random House, New York, 1963.

Kelman, Howard R., Milton Lowenthal, and Jonas N. Muller: "Community States of Discharged Rehabilitation Patients: Results of a Longitudinal Study," *Arch Phys Med Rehabil* 47: 670–75, 1966.

Kerr, Nancy: "Staff Expectations for Disabled Persons: Helpful or Harmful," in J. Stubbins (ed.)

Social and Psychological Aspects of Disability: A Handbook for Practitioners, University Park Press, Baltimore, 1977.

Kozy, Mary: "Family Involvement," unpublished paper, Rehabilitation Institute of Chicago, Chicago, Ill., May 1978.

Kübler-Ross, Elisabeth: *On Death and Dying,* Macmillan, New York, 1969, pp. 38–138.

Kutner, Bernard: "Rehabilitation: Whose Goals? Whose Priorities?" *Arch Phys Med Rehabil,* June 1971.

Lefcourt, H. M.: "Internal Versus External Control of Reinforcements: A Review," *Psychol Bull* 65:208–210, 1966.

Ludwig, Edward G., and Shirley D. Adams: "Patient Cooperation in a Rehabilitation Center: Assumption of the Client Role," in J. Stubbins (ed.) *Social and Psychological Aspects of Disability: A Handbook for Practitioners,* University Park Press, Baltimore, 1977.

Lukton, Rosemary Creed: "Crisis Theory: Review and Critique," *Soc Serv Rev,* 48(3), 1974.

McDaniel, James W.: *Physical Disability and Human Behavior,* Pergamon, 1969.

Mimi, Billy Budd Films, 235 E. 57th St., New York, 1972, 16 mm 12 min.

Moos, Rudaly H., and Vivian D. Tsu: *Coping with Physical Illness,* Plenum, New York, 1977.

National Opinion Research Center, United States Department of Health, Education, and Welfare, Washington, D.C., 1964.

Rosenblatt, Aaron: "Evaluating a Medical Symptom with Paraplegics," *Soc Casework* 41: 128–134, 1960.

Rosenblatt, Daniel, and E. A. Suchman: "The Underutilization of Medical-Care Services by Blue-Collarites," in Arthur Shostak and William Gombey (eds.), *Blue Collar World: Studies of the American Worker,* Prentice-Hall, Englewood Cliffs, N.J., 1964.

Rotter, J. B.: "Generalized Expectancies for Internal Versus External Control of Reinforcement," *Psychological Monographs,* 1966, p. 80.

Satir, Virginia: *Conjoint Family Therapy, A Guide to Theory and Technique,* Science and Behavior Books, Palo Alto, Calif., 1967.

———: *Peoplemaking,* Science and Behavior Books, Palo Alto, Calif., 1972.

Schmidt, James P.: "A Behavioral Approach to Patient Compliance," *Postgrad Med* 65: 219, 1979.

Shapiro, Leon N., and Arthur W. McMahan: "Rehabilitation Statement: Problems of Patient-Staff Interaction," *Arch Gen Psychiatry,* 15, 1966.

Shellhase, Leslie J., and Fern E. Shellhase: "Role of the Family in Rehabilitation," *Soc Casework,* November 1972.

Straicklek, Martin, and Margaret Bonnefil: "Crisis Intervention and Social Casework: Similarities and Differences in Problem-Solving," *Clin Soc Work J.* 2:36–44, 1974.

Strubbins, Joseph: "Stress and Disability," in *Social and Psychological Aspects of Disability: A Handbook for Practitioners,* Univ. Park Press, Baltimore, 1977.

Sussman, Marvin: "Non-Traditional Family Forms in the 1970's," National Council on Family Relations, Minneapolis, 1972.

Trieschmann, Roberta B.: "Living with a Disability: A Proposal for Rehabilitation of the Person with Special Injury," unpublished condensation, integration, and elaboration of ideas generated at the Psychological, Social, Vocational Input Conference, February 25–26, 1971, Phoenix, Ariz. This conference was sponsored by the Special Injury Service, Institute of Rehabilitation Medicine, Good Samaritan Hospital, Phoenix, Ariz.

Tucker, Sherry Jill: "A Psychological Look at Physical Disability," unpublished paper, Family Institute of Chicago, Chicago, Ill., 1977.

Wing, J. K.: "Social and Psychological Changes in a Rehabilitation Unit," *Soc Psychiatry* 1: 21–28, 1966.

7
winona griggs

sexuality

INTRODUCTION

Sexuality is an appropriate concern to be included in the health-care needs of the patient today. Promoting or caring for the total health-care needs of the patient includes sexual health and adjustment and should be an integral part of any health-care and rehabilitation program. This concern for the "total person" is the concern of all health-care disciplines. In attending to all human needs, there are many interdisciplinary aspects of care with resultant ill-defined lines of responsibility in many areas of that care. All too often, sexuality is ignored because of this; or because of the more immediate aspects of care; or because of the biases, prejudices, and ignorances which perpetuate such myths as "the disabled are incapable of sexual activity," "the aged are asexual," and "the adolescent is too young."

This chapter will deal with knowledge about human sexuality—a quality that is present in all persons. Human beings, young and old, able-bodied and disabled, are sexual beings; they are likely to have the same sexual and intimacy needs and to engage in much of the same sexual activity. To assist patients with their sexual concerns and to be a fully participating member of the health-care team, the nurse needs to have accurate information about human sexuality.

SOCIETY'S INFLUENCES

The sexual stereotype in our culture today is the body beautiful, a great physique; physical attractiveness and prowess are equated with being sexually desirable and virile. This concept is perpetuated by the commercialism of sex and the bombardment of our senses, especially visual, with the message that beauty, youth, slimness, and agility, plus underarm Brand-X deodorant, will make one sexually attractive and desirable. This message has created a perverted persuasion in our society that the big turn-on comes from beauty and the fluidity of the body's muscular movements.

Another facet of influence is society's preoccupation with genital sex and sexual performance. "Real sex" is defined solely as penile-vaginal penetration. This norm of our culture is slowly giving way to the influences of the sexual revolution of the 1970s. Hunt's 1974 study of sexual behavior in the 1970s concludes that married people are engaging in a variety of sexual activities with an increase in mouth-breast activity and oral-genital techniques. But the amount of increase is not that encouraging and the death or demise of our preoccupation with genital sex is not complete. The penis and vagina still carry a great deal of the emphasis for "normal" sexual functioning in our society. The other erogenous zones of the body rank second best and are often ignored as pleasurable areas.

The male is the greater victim of our society's preoccupation with sexual performance. For many persons, masculinity is defined in terms of sexual performance. In the dating game, the main object is to "score"—with intercourse and ejaculation being the major accomplishments. The female has not been as pressured in the past with these performance demands, but change may come in the near future with the increasing emphasis on the need to experience orgasm, or now multiple orgasms, for complete sexual satisfaction for both the woman and her partner.

Mass media's interest in sexuality, from *Playboy* to *Good Housekeeping,* has created rising expectations about sexual acts. These rising expectations have placed a considerable burden on sex. Sex is important and good for many people, but it may not be all that important or good for all people at all times. Sexuality is only a part of an individual's personality. Sex is not or may not be the ultimate concern or pinnacle of achievement in everyone's life in spite of the many messages received today, especially by the young and middle-aged, from the mass media. For older persons in our society, the message is just the reverse—sex is not a legitimate concern for them at all.

With the new climate of sexual freedom and permissiveness has come more encouragement and freedom to talk about sex. This has not always been so in our culture. It is still not so for many of the patients, married or unmarried, cared for or encountered in the clinical setting. For many, sex is still not something to talk about publicly. Carefully socialized into most of us, this idea can be the cause of faulty learning and of excessive inhibition in sexual functioning. Women are more often victims of this silence because they have never been encouraged to communicate clearly their sexual needs and feelings. This lack of communication, along with the attitudes that women are passive partners in sex, that sex is dirty, and that the primary role of the woman during sexual intercourse is to satisfy the man, has contributed to a lack of enjoyment and satisfaction and possibly to orgasmic dysfunction. In males, the inhibitions related to open, clear communication have also interfered with the ability to express their sexual needs and feelings. Many males enjoy and need experiences other than sexual intercourse but are inhibited in expressing these needs.

Common faulty assumptions are "If he really loves me, he should know what turns me on and what I like," or "What turns me on and what I like has to be what turns her on and should be what she likes." Each partner expects the other to know or to guess. Serious relationship problems can result, especially if changes in sexual functioning occur as a result of aging, chronic disease, or physical disability. Touching, caressing, kissing, and a feeling of sensuality are all important aspects of sexual functioning; along with open, clear communication, they can be experiences that promote joy, intimacy, and love. Although sex is something that more people are talking about today, many still find it difficult to communicate their feelings and needs to their sexual partners. And although sex is a form of physical communication between partners, verbal communication is a very helpful and needed addition.

These attitudes about body beauty and mobility, sexual performance, sexual expectations, and communication between sexual partners can result in and contribute to sexuality problems.

All certainly have contributed to faulty learning and have influenced what is perceived as "normal" or "good" sex. Persons or experiences that do not measure up to these images or expectations are devalued in our society.

THE HUMAN SEXUAL RESPONSE CYCLE

An area where clear, open communication is important between sexual partners is in their individual response to sexual stimuli and what is sexually satisfying for them. Factual information about the human sexual response cycle in men and women will give people a real understanding about what is happening to them during sexual intercourse. It may also point out reasons why things do not work and may indicate that cooperative efforts of both partners are needed for a mutually satisfying sexual experience. Masters and Johnson, pioneers in this work, are responsible for much of what we know about the human sexual response.

THE MALE SEXUAL RESPONSE CYCLE

There is only one clearly identified pattern in the male sexual response cycle. Variations are mainly related to duration rather than intensity of the response. The first phase is the excitement phase which begins with and depends on responses to sexual stimulation. If the stimulation remains adequate to the individual, the intensity of response usually increases rapidly. Penile erection is the first physiologic response to this effective stimulation. In the excitement phase, erection develops rapidly (within seconds), and full erection occurs very early in this phase. The male may partially lose then rapidly regain the erection several times during a prolonged excitement phase. The ejaculatory control varies. Also, partial or even complete loss of erection may occur as a result of outside interference or interruptions (i.e., loud noise, children, unappreciated remarks) despite continued sexual stimulation.

With the rising sexual tensions, the scrotum loses its relaxed scrotal folds and the testes begin to elevate; complete elevation occurs in the plateau phase. This is very important for a full ejaculatory experience. Other extragenital reactions in the excitement phase are nipple erection in some males and increased muscular tensions with involuntary muscle contractions (myotonia). With the rising tension, the heart rate and blood pressure begin to increase in the excitement phase.

From the excitement phase, the male enters the plateau phase where sexual tensions are heightened; heart rate and blood pressure show related elevations. From here, the male moves fairly rapidly to the orgasmic phase. During the orgasmic phase, there are forceful, expulsive penile contractions which result in forceful ejaculation. The ejaculation is a two-stage, well-differentiated process with prostatic contractions and an awareness of fluid emission and pressure. This is the sensation of orgasm. The orgasmic experience, though, is one of total body involvement with involuntary contractions and spasms of the muscles (myotonia response), involuntary rectal sphincter contractions, and increased cardiopulmonary reactions. The resolution phase develops with the final, nonexpulsive contractions of the penis, and the male experiences a refractory period during which he is unable to respond to restimulation. There is penile detumescence and testicular descent. The cardiopulmonary response returns to normal during the resolution phase.

THE FEMALE SEXUAL RESPONSE CYCLE

The female sexual response cycle is more complex and less predictable. There are at least three different identified patterns of sexual response in the female with an infinite variety possible in the individual female. Intensity as well as duration of response are factors in the individual female's sexual reaction. The female response is definitely a total body involvement with sexual tensions affecting areas other than genital organs or structures. During the excitement phase, there are breast changes with nipple erection and an increase in breast size. Myotonia begins in the excitement phase. Along with the rising tensions, which are the same as seen in the male, the heart rate and blood pressure begin to increase. The first physiologic evidence of sexual response in the female is production of vaginal lubrication which occurs within 10 to 30 s after initiation of any effective sexual stimulation. Other changes are labial engorgement, with skin color changes, and clitoral engorgement. Also, there is lengthening and expansion of the inner two-thirds of the vaginal barrel. The walls of the vagina thicken and change in color from purplish red to a darker purplish hue. Also, the uterus elevates. During the plateau phase, the clitoris retracts under its hood, the labia minora increase in size due to engorgement, and full vaginal expansion takes place, with a marked vascongestion response in the outer third of the vagina. This is known as the orgasmic platform and is preliminary to the orgasmic experience. During the plateau phase, the cardiopulmonary response increases to almost peak levels. The orgasmic phase in the female usually extends over a longer period of time than it does in the male. It begins with expulsive uterine contractions. At the same time, there is the involuntary development of contractions of the orgasmic platform in the outer third of the vagina and of the rectal sphincter. This simultaneous onset of contractions provides the sensations of a total pelvic response. As in the male cycle, the orgasmic experience is also one of total body involvement, with involuntary contractions and spasms of muscle groups (myotonia response), increased cardiopulmonary responses, and more varied heart rate resulting from the variety of orgasmic intensity in the female.

The pattern of sexual response in the female can be quite varied. One pattern is that of gradual progression to the plateau phase, the woman then remaining at the level for an extended period of time before going on to orgasm. Another pattern is gradual progression to the plateau phase and then to a series of orgasms (the multiorgasmic response). Other women progress fairly rapidly to the plateau phase, then without any delay go on to orgasm and immediate and fast resolution. The resolution phase is the involuntary period of tension loss. Women differ from men in that they have the potential for another orgasm at any time during this phase. Women also differ from men in that the sexual response cycle is more easily interrupted at any level. The cardiopulmonary responses return to normal in the resolution phase.

The same sexual response cycle of both males and females is seen in masturbation activity, heterosexual activity, and homosexual activity, the only difference being increased intensity of response with masturbation (Masters and Johnson, 1966).

Adequate knowledge about the human sexual response cycle and ease in communicating sexual needs and feelings during the sex act will increase the potential for fuller sexual satisfaction for both partners. For the sake of what is called normal, though, it must be pointed out that not all of these changes always occur; some depend on individual responses.

FACTORS THAT AFFECT THE SEXUAL RESPONSE CYCLE

Emotions, unappreciated stimuli, and environment have already been mentioned as factors that can influence and/or interrupt the sexual response cycle of both men and women. Anger, noise, distraction, anxiety, fatigue, and even deliberate control are examples of such factors. There are other things that can inhibit sexual arousal and/or completion of the sex act. Both overeating and overindulgence in alcohol will influence the sexual response, and when a regular pattern of such abuse is established, sexual functioning will diminish. With alcohol, many people believe just the opposite, that alcohol facilitates sexual exchanges by lowering inhibitions and thus enhances the sexual seduction. This is true only when the drinking is done in moderation and is confined to social drinking. Alcohol is not a stimulant but a nervous system depressant (Renshaw, 1975). Many men have experienced an episode of impotence for the first time after drinking heavily. Chronic alcoholism creates complex sexual dysfunctioning in both men and women.

Two other major offenders that adversely affect the sexual response are depression and drugs. Clinical depression can decrease libido and sexual performance. If the depression is treated with drugs, these drugs can add to the sexual problem in males by causing impotence. The effect of street drugs (marijuana, hallucinogens, amphetamines, etc.) have not always been objectively studied; therefore, reports vary from accounts of a heightening of what is already there to no better or worse effects. With amphetamines, occasional use can increase sexual interest as part of general cerebral stimulation, and chronic use can decrease libido; there are some reports of sexual dysfunction. In prescription drugs, the major problem drugs are tranquilizers, antihypertensive drugs, anticholinergic drugs, sex hormones, hypnotics, barbiturates, and narcotics. The individual drug's effect is varied and can be dose related. The effect can be any one or a combination of the following effects: changes in libido, inhibition of sexual arousal, impotency, decrease in vaginal lubrication, inhibition or changes in ejaculation, and complete relaxation of the vaginal muscles affecting orgasm (Renshaw, 1978). The influence of drugs has not been all bad, however. Oral contraceptives have had a tremendous effect on sexual functioning in our society by shifting contemporary attitudes regarding sexual behavior and intercourse from procreation to recreation.

Patient education in avoidance or moderation of inhibiting factors will help reduce mishaps in sexual functioning and may prevent sexual problems. With drugs, knowledge about the effects of the drugs and a careful history can help avoid problems in many instances by a suggested change in dosage or a change to a drug which has fewer side effects.

SEXUALITY IN THE LIFE CYCLE

Sexuality is a part of a person's continued development from childhood through the late years, and adult sexuality evolves progressively from all previous experiences during the life cycle. It is a learned behavior, and we all can find somewhere along this continuum our own individually defined sexuality and preferred sexual expressions. Sexuality is a lifetime learning experience for most of us.

A brief summary of sexuality in the life cycle follows, with adolescence, young adult, middle, and late years used as milestones.

ADOLESCENCE

An age definition of adolescence is difficult to establish, but adolescence usually covers the period of life between the ages of 12 through 19. This arbitrarily designated age range has some inherent problems because some adolescents who are between 17 and 19 (and even 16 at times) may be well past this defined stage of adolescence.

In adolescence, the search for an independent identity is the major developmental task. This requires individuals to distance themselves from parents and to form closer alliances with peer groups; they conform to peer attitudes and codes of behavior and appearance. Coupled with the drive toward independence is the adolescent's fear of that drive. It is a time when close, strong adult relationships may be perceived as smothering. It is a period of rapid and unpredictable change, both physical and emotional.

The adolescent is confronted with biological puberty and its tremendous impact on body growth and changes. Sexual urges and abilities emerge. The menarche and breast development have or will begin during this time. Nocturnal emissions as "wet dreams" begin in boys. Curiosity about one's own body and that of the opposite sex intensifies. Sexual experimentation, especially that of masturbation, is a most important activity during this time for obtaining knowledge about the body and as a necessary part of the individual's capacity to deal with pubertal sexuality and the final establishment of sexual identity (Moore, 1976).

During adolescence, there is great anxiety and preoccupation about what is "normal" about one's own body, and because normal is a difficult state to achieve, there is great concern about what is wrong with the body. In some persons, when curiosity has not been great or has been suppressed and validation of what is normal has not occurred, this anxiety and fear of being different or abnormal can extend throughout the life cycle. Betty Dobson tells about her concern when she was growing up that she had deformed genitals; she was 35 before she had the courage to admit this to anyone. Only after comparing her genitalia with pictures of other women did she realize that she was not deformed, funny-looking, or ugly but was perfectly normal in her asymmetry. Boys are similarly concerned about penis size. Locker room validation does not dispel the myths. Factual information about body parts and related myths is needed and should be included in any sex education for boys and girls.

Adolescence may be a very active time sexually, as the increase in illegitimate births, abortions, and the epidemic proportions of the incidence of venereal disease in this age group attest. These problems indicate a need for more available sex education *and* accessible medical services, including contraceptive advice and availability. The latter is very important in terms of preventive health care. The "telling" and/or restrictive approach does not work. Teenagers themselves have confirmed that society's attitudes and restrictions have little to do with their actions. In a study by Sorenson (1973) 69 percent of all boys and 55 percent of all girls answered in the affirmative to the statement: "So far as sex is concerned, I do what I want to do regardless of what society thinks." They will and do engage in sexual activity without accurate information regarding human sexuality, without contraceptives, and without a simple preventive means (the condom) against the spread of venereal

CHAPTER 7 90

disease. Education on human sexuality, preventive health care, and responsible sexual activity should be included in the health care given by all professionals.

Adolescents want and need more than facts about sexuality. They want information about the emotional aspects of sexuality as well. They are concerned about feelings, about love, about the relationships that they are in, about caring for their partners, about having sex with more than one person when they have expressed love for one, and about their popularity. Adolescents are also concerned with the different life-styles and value systems that are being more openly expressed in our society today. Providing accurate information and acceptance of these divergent life-styles and values will help the adolescents make more positive and informed choices about their own sexuality. Many legitimate beliefs, practices, and life-styles can be enriching experiences rather than threatening or shameful ones.

Adolescents stress the importance and need of personal freedom and the need to be treated like adults. Coupled with this freedom must be responsibility. In sex education or counseling, the nurse must stress the adolescents' responsibility for their own bodies, responsibility to others, especially their potential sex partners, and responsibility for their sexual choices.

THE YOUNG ADULT

The young adult period in the life cycle is usually described as ages 20 to 35. Again, this is an arbitrarily designated age range, with the same inherent problems cited under adolescence. There are some 17- and 18-year-olds who may be young adults, and there are some adults who, at the age of 40, may also be young adults.

The young adult is concerned with establishing intimate relationships of long duration. This creates new anxieties. Many problems in these relationships are created by the young adults' anxieties and fears of intimacy and closeness and by the demands of sexual performance. Problems of premature ejaculation due to increased sexual tension and impotency are common in the young adult male, and inability to reach orgasm in the female is a problem.

Marriage may or may not result from these relationships of long duration. Young adults have many life-styles open to them today—singlehood, marriage with or without children, communal living, and gay life-styles that may include long-term commitments. Within these life-styles, sexual expression may include, among other things, masturbation, heterosexual activity, homosexual activity, or group sex. Another possibility is the choice of celibacy. In a society where sex is so greatly emphasized and holds such great expectations, this is often a very difficult choice. The nurse may find it necessary to support this choice and to assure the patient who makes such a choice that it is still possible to feel normal sexually.

Many of the concerns seen in the adolescent may still be present in the young adult. Concern about being normal or adequate in body parts may continue to be a problem. Accurate information about contraception, pregnancy, and venereal diseases may be lacking. Sexual roles based on our society's sex stereotyping of what is masculine and what is feminine behavior may be influential in the development of sexual problems. This stereotyping may inhibit creative sexual activity and may inhibit females or males from communicating their sexual desires. There has been some easing of sex roles, but differentiations in what is considered normal masculine and feminine behavior still exist in the attitudes of many persons and institutions today. This sex stereotyping may be restrictive and harmful not only in the sexual arena but in child rearing.

THE MIDDLE YEARS

The middle years take in a large age group, from ages 35 to 65. During the middle years, there are changes in physical condition and body function which may influence sexual activity. Menopause in women may or may not be a threat representing loss of femininity. To a lot of women, it is a welcome change and, with the fear of pregnancy gone, the woman may experience an increase in sexual drive. The most notable changes in the female sexual response cycle due to aging and the postmenopausal state are changes in the vaginal response. The vaginal walls become tissue-paper thin; the vagina shortens and its expansive ability decreases; lubrication may take longer and may not be entirely adequate. These changes due to aging may result in painful intercourse for the woman who engages in coitus only occasionally. Estrogen replacement may be necessary, but a far better remedy is continued, frequent, and regular sexual activity. There is no age limit to sexual performance at orgasmic response levels in women (Masters, and Johnson, 1966).

Changes in the middle-aged male's normal sexual response may be interpreted as a loss in performance power and may create increased anxiety about diminishing masculinity. The most notable and sometimes problematic changes are changes in erection, ejaculation, and the refractory period. The older male (particularly after age 60) is slower to attain an erection, needs more direct stimulation, and may not attain a full erection until immediately prior to orgasm. Once erection is achieved, though, the older man can engage in intercourse over a longer period of time without ejaculation. The female sex partner may enjoy this prolonged phase because it may coincide better with her needs and she may experience multiple orgasms. Another change is in the ejaculation experience which diminishes in intensity and duration, with seepage at times rather than the expulsion of fluid. This change may cause a reduction in the sensual experience. As the demands to ejaculate lessen, the older man may be completely satisfied with few ejaculations regardless of the number of opportunities or sexual demands of his partner. After ejaculation, there is a rapid return to presexual tension levels and the refractory period for the aging male is prolonged, up to 12 to 24 h or longer (Masters and Johnson). All these changes do not have to mean the end of sexual activity. If properly understood and worked with, the sexual experience can still be pleasurable and satisfactory for both partners. Because the man may need more direct and prolonged stimulation, this may be an opportunity for the couple to become more creative in their sexual activities.

Sexual incompatibility may also be noticed in a relationship at this time. The middle-aged male tends to experience a decrease in sexual drive with the female experiencing the opposite, which may create sexual tensions within the relationship. Also, demands of work and family may have depleted the couple's ability to experience fun and playfulness in their sexual activities. The couple may now experience an emptiness in their relationship which is hard to counteract.

These physical changes and related feelings can and do cause sexual problems, but the major cause is usually in the marital relationship (Ficher, 1976). Chronic, long-term incompatibility in the marriage may surface at this time in the form of sexual dissatisfaction and dysfunction. The sexual problem is only the presenting problem. Inadequate communication about feelings, sexual needs, and marital adjustments may contribute to or intensify these sexual problems. Extramarital relationships, impotency, complaints of infidelity, and orgasmic dysfunction may be common problems during this stage of the life cycle. However, all sexual problems that do occur are not the result of the relationship. The great incidence of chronic diseases, particularly diabetes and alcoholism, in this age group may have a direct influence on sexual drive and/or potency. Nor do sexual problems always occur. Many middle-aged persons actually experience greater sexual satisfaction. They have remained lovers and have strengthened their relationships over the years. Others, whose relationships have suffered from stresses and strains, are able to renegotiate their marriages, to relearn how to have fun again with each other, and to be more creative in their sexual activities.

The nurse can allay fears and prevent a lot of sexual dysfunction by providing accurate information about menopause, about the normal changes in the sexual response cycle that occur with age, and, most of all, about the fact that sexual interest and activity are more dependent on previous experience and level of activity than age. In women, it depends mostly on an intact marriage and previous enjoyment in sexual experiences (Pfeiffer and Davis, 1972). All this information allows for acceptance and adaptation to the expected changes in the middle years.

THE LATE YEARS

The age designation for the beginning of the late years is presently 65. Contrary to the myth that sex ceases after middle age, sexual needs do persist through the life cycle. Old people have many of the same needs of intimacy and sexual expression found in the earlier ages. Investigators, such as Newman and Nichols (1960) and the Duke University studies (Pfeiffer et al., 1968), have indicated that well over 50 percent of persons over 60 years of age are sexually active and report engaging in sexual intercourse with some frequency. Only at about age 75 is there a significant decline in sexual activity. The sharp escalation of illness and physical dysfunction at this age is the major reason for giving up sexual activity. Women who remain sexually active throughout their lives do not experience this decline in sexual activity but may give it up because of the lack of a suitable and healthy partner.

The findings of these studies and similar ones, plus the work of Masters and Johnson, confirm the fact that age is not a major factor in experiencing or expressing one's sexuality. What is important is the constancy and regularity of sexual activity, especially in early and middle age. It is equally important to understand that not all older persons will remain sexually active, and some older persons may not have been sexually active in their earlier years. There is a wide spectrum of individual differences in sexual interest in the late years, and there may be many reasons for choosing or not choosing to be sexually active. Older persons have many of the same choices of life-styles and sexual expression as noted in the earlier periods of the life cycle. With society's changing attitudes, it should be noted that options such as communal living and homosexual relationships may be viable and recognizable choices as answers to the problem of the great number of older women without men.

Sexual issues and problems that may be seen in the late years are anxiety about diminishing sexual function, which may be seen as a threat to intimacy and self-worth; a decrease in self-esteem due to society's attitudes about the aged in general, specifically the labeling or treatment of them as asexual; depression, which affects sexual functioning by decreasing the sexual drive and potency capabilities of the male; impotency due to chronic disease or drugs used in the treatment of medical illnesses; and loss of privacy due to changes in living conditions, such as the need to live with children or in nursing homes.

Nurses who are able to discuss sexual issues and concerns openly and realistically with the older person can do much to dispel the sexual myths and ignorance of our society, even those of the older person.

This need for nurses to be able to discuss sexual issues and concerns openly and factually extends throughout the entire life cycle. Armed with accurate information about sexuality in the life cycle and with an awareness of self-sexual values, preferences, and biases, the nurse can, through appropriate intervention, contribute to a person's total health and prevent the unwanted intrusion of self-held values into the teaching or counseling situation with the patient.

SEX VERSUS SEXUALITY

Sexual functioning refers only to the physiological response to psychic or physical stimulation which can occur alone or with another person. Mainly, it involves engaging in sexual intercourse with orgasm and consequent release of tension being the primary goal. However, many persons confuse this limited area of sexual functioning with sexuality. When their sexual functioning—the ability to engage in intercourse—is threatened or changed, such persons have a difficult time making the necessary adaptations to maintaining or seeking a pleasurable relationship. They tend to confuse their loss of physical functioning with their sexuality.

Sexuality is much more than sexual intercourse and is expressed in other ways. Sexuality is the combination of feelings, attitudes, and behaviors that express being a man or being a woman. It encompasses the way we view and think about ourselves, the way we dress, sensuality, and relationship patterns. A woman who has a physical disability has expressed it better: "Sexuality is an integral part of living. It involves the total person in a loving, giving and receiving relationship. The expression of love can involve touching, and not necessarily sex. There are ways of expressing sex without having physical agility. I would emphasize sex as a part of the self-concept, but not the only or most important aspect" (Shaul et al., 1978, p. 57).

This emphasis on the broader concept of sexuality is important to all persons, able-bodied and disabled, young and old. Nurses should be aware that all persons have sexuality; for some, it may be the key part of who they are. Nurses should help patients expand their concepts of sexuality beyond sex to the other experiences and pleasures in a relationship. In addition, nurses should realize that people can and do limit the ways in which they function sexually and engage in relationships. Sexuality for some may be "feeling good" about being a man or woman; it may be a concern about appearance and grooming; or it may be the satisfaction found in everyday relationships with others. How one's sexuality is expressed is the choice of the individual.

EXPRESSIONS OF SEXUALITY

As the choice of sexual expression takes many forms and encompasses different life-styles, nurses may be confronted with choices that are different from their own. Today, because of changes in our society, people are more open about discussing varying life-styles and manners of sexual expression and experimentation.

More people are engaging in sexual intercourse regularly and at a younger age. More young people and old people are living together without getting married. Because of increasing evidence, contrary to myths, that older people who are in reasonably good health and still interested in life maintain a high level of sexual activity, nurses cannot assume that couples are living together solely for economic reasons. Other single, older persons who do not live together may maintain dating patterns. Nurses must be aware that sex may be an issue, whether a patient is married or single, and therefore it is an important subject to cover in the patient interview.

Also, today when a patient begins to discuss sexual problems, the nurse cannot assume that the concern is always in the context of a heterosexual relationship. Many persons whose sexual preferences are for partners of the same sex are more open about their relationships, more willing to "expose" themselves to gain health information and education. This change may not be so much the result of a decrease in fear of exposure as an increase in a positive personal feeling that homosexuality is a legitimate and satisfying choice for some people. The sexual concerns and problems for the person with a homosexual orientation may not be very different from the problems of persons with heterosexual orientations. Because of the tendency toward more variety and sexual experimentation, there may be nothing remarkable or unique in these sexual practices except that the two partners are of the same sex. Many of these relationships are of long duration with commitments of the same quality as in close heterosexual marriages. Often, this fact is overlooked or ignored when a nurse cares for one partner of the couple.

A sexual activity that still causes feelings of uneasiness and concern is masturbation. The women's movement and new books advocating the legitimacy of self-pleasuring have done much to increase awareness that masturbation is an acceptable and normal sexual option for both men and women, but this attitude is not shared by all persons (including some nurses). There is still a great deal of guilt and disapproval attached to masturbation, even in the most liberated persons. Nurses may have to examine their own feelings and biases about this practice, because masturbation may be not only a healthy outlet for increased sexual tensions but even a prescribed way for persons to get to know their bodies and what is sexually satisfying to them. Nurses may be helpful by accepting and giving patients permission to engage in masturbation if it is an acceptable practice for the individual concerned.

Questions or fears of normalcy may be raised by these and other forms of sexual expression and experimentation. The concern may be felt by the nurse as well as the patient. Sexual satisfaction, which consists of giving as well as receiving pleasure, can be accomplished in many ways; what is comfortable and acceptable to both partners is normal. This is an important concept since narrow attitudes about what is normal may inhibit the patient's ability to make necessary changes in sexual activity when disease or physical disability dictate; or nurses may be inhibited from giving permission and adequate information and suggestions.

SELF-CONCEPT AND SEXUALITY

Self-concept is made up of many things that we value or do not value about ourselves. Some things hold more significance and value than others and are more vital to essence as a person, but two vital parts of the concept of self are *identity* and *body image.* Identity is generally expressed by labels—man, woman, housewife, carpenter, executive, mother, etc. Sexuality, an integral part of personality, is a central characteristic of this identity and is incorporated into self-concept and thus body image. Circumstances that influence or endanger sexuality can and do have similar effects on self-concept. In addition, self-concept or self-esteem influences ability to accept or express sexuality, and even more important, the ability to love and be loved.

Body image is a complex conceptual profile of facts and perceptions about the body (Ritchie, 1973). It is an image of self and includes physical appearance, inner feelings, how other people act or react (or one's interpretation of how they react or do not react), and identification with the norms of society. These basic ideas and attitudes of a person toward his or her body go beyond mental image and are reflected in the person's life-style, influencing relation to environment and the whole world. A person's body image is the central core of self-concept and is closely associated with feelings of worth, of being valued, of feeling good about self, and of being accepted. Continuously developing and changing, body image slowly adapts to imposed changes from the self, from outside forces, and from aging.

Nurses who care for patients with changes in body image caused by disease or physical disability are aware that the changes can cause a major identity crisis. This fact has also been documented in the literature (Moos, 1977; Singh, and Magner, 1975). In some respects, as a result of change in appearance or an alteration or loss of body functions, the person experiences the self as a "different person." There is now a distorted appearance, a disfigurement, a body that does not function normally, the result of an event that occurred in an instant and has to be dealt with through a remaining lifetime. As a result of this catastrophic event, the person finds that those external and objective factors that formerly contributed to self or body image are lost or altered. Now, instead of being 6 ft 3 in in height, he finds that he is 4 ft 9 in a wheelchair. Now, instead of being sure-footed and agile on a wilderness trail, she finds that she cannot get to the trail because she is dependent on her wheelchair. Now, instead of being "solid and well built" with bulging muscles, he finds that his muscles have atrophied from disuse as a result of paralysis. She finds that instead of paying her compliments about her beautiful hands, people now stare at them because of the deformity caused by rheumatoid arthritis.

With previous changes in body image, the individual had found support from the social norms and value systems of self, family, and close friends helpful in assisting the adaptation to changes. Now, when the changes are due to a deformity, a disfigurement, or a nonfunctioning body part, the individual will find less support. This is because our society so clearly communicates a negative opinion about disability. The disabled person is looked upon as odd, pitiful, and different from other people.

The newly disabled person also may have previously held these negative opinions; having acquired a disability, that person must now view the changed self negatively. With increasing awareness of the permanence and reality of the disability, the individual must now incorporate the disability into body image and redefine that image to take in these losses or changes. This is the identity crisis. (Andreasen and Norris, 1977). Personal values must be clarified and possibly changed. Life-styles may have to be changed or adapted. The family who has viewed disability negatively and has placed a high value on physical attractiveness and wholeness will also face a crisis (Brodland and Andreasen, 1977). They must also make changes in their value systems in order to adapt to and to aid the disabled individual. This is crucial as the disabled individual will be greatly influenced by how those closest to him or her are able to handle the disability. In addition, the reestablishment of old roles is vital to the recovery of a sense of sameness and continuity of self.

Because identity and body image are closely associated with sexuality, the identity crisis can also precipitate problems in sexuality. Questions from the patient will soon surface, whether spoken or unspoken, about whether he or she is still a sexual being and can be valued as such. The actual physical changes or dysfunctions related to the sexual system will prompt some of the questions about sexual performance, but other questions will be related to tthe person's feelings of self-worth and body image problems. For many patients, it is the latter that will exercise the major influences on sexuality and sexual functioning.

Besides physical changes, the disease or disability may also impose other changes, changes in occupational and family roles. Loss of occupation or ability to work as a result of the disease or disability can become highly problematic in a production-oriented society where the worth or value of a person is determined or influenced by productivity—"what one does." For the patient who has derived a major source of personal identity from an occupational role, this additional loss as well as the need of an altered future occupation can contribute to and magnify the identity crisis. This loss of work may necessitate role changes within the family unit as well, perhaps precipitating problems in sexuality because of the common stereotyped masculine and feminine roles in our society. The man who believes his manliness is evidenced in being the provider, who sees dependency, housework, the raising of children, and cooking as being "women's work," and who incorporates these ideas into his identity as a man can experience problems with his sexuality if dependency or role changes are necessary. The woman who believes her womanliness is shown by being a wife, a mother, and the manager of the house and home can experience problems when she is unable to fulfill these roles because of a disability. As previously stated, masculine-feminine stereotyping may be easing in our total society today as the result of the so-called sexual revolution and the problems of male unemployment. Many women have had to become the sole financial resources for their families. However, permanent, imposed role changes that influence or threaten a person's identity still create sexuality problems for many patients. This threat is not exclusively felt by the patient; the family may also feel threatened. The spouse or sexual partner may not be able to accept the physical changes or the role changes. There may be a feeling of helplessness or of threat to the family's social position because of the social and financial losses, actual or perceived. Also, such seemingly minor changes as a need for position change during sexual intercourse can be unacceptable for either or both partners because of masculine and feminine stereotyping. This seems to be more of a problem for the injured male, though, presenting more of a threat to his male image.

The effect that the disability has on a person's body image, self-concept, and therefore, sexuality will depend on many things among which will be the amount and type of dysfunction, the visibility of the disability, the personality and value system of the person, and how much that person internalizes the values of his culture or society, the characteristics and extent of the identity crisis, and the resources available to resolve this identity crisis. Needless to say, all of these are not amenable to the nurse's intervention. What is important, and goes beyond the physical care dimension, is the nurse's sensitivity to the psychologic effects of the disability, an awareness and sensitivity to how routine nursing actions can contribute to the patient's and family's positive valuation of the patient as a sexual human being. As stated previously, persons who have a physical disability report that their major problems with sexuality are directly related to body image problems. The patient must rebuild a self-image to feel proud and good about; with a disability, this often means a shift from "what a person does" to "who a person is." It also highlights the professional person's task of helping the patient regain as much normalcy in life as existed prior to disease or disability (Sha'ked, 1978).

NURSING RESPONSIBILITY IN SEXUAL HEALTH CARE

The starting place for the nurse in providing sexual health care for patients is at the point of self-examination. The most important beginning is for nurses to understand and become comfortable with their own sexuality. Nurses are also affected by the negative attitudes of society and their own life experiences and develop their own attitudes toward sexuality from these influences. Many nurses may view patients with a physical disability as asexual; they may avoid bringing up the subject of sex with the older patient because of their own feelings and embarrassments; or they may believe that patients with chronic illnesses have a lot more to think about than sexual matters. Nurses must examine and clarify the feelings, beliefs, and values about sexuality and sexual functioning that trigger such attitudes and inhibitions. This will facilitate the development of understanding and acceptance of sexuality in themselves and, it is hoped, in others. Nurses who are able to free themselves from the usual set sexual stereotyping and who realize the possibility of differences in sexual practices are better prepared to provide sexual health care to all of their patients.

Nurses may need to educate themselves to the common and different sexual practices and life-styles in our society and to learn to contain their own sexual hangups and values. A result can be a greater comfort level with the patient's sexuality, with nurses more open in discussing sexual concerns with patients who have different sexual preferences and practices. Above all, the control of their own values and the acquisition of knowledge about human sexuality will elevate the nurse's practice from the level of intuition or opinion giving to the level of permission giving (Annon, 1976).

The level of comfort the nurse feels concerning sexual matters is important in providing effective sexual health care. When the nurse feels comfortable in sex-related conversations with patients with the language of sex and with sexual content, the subject of sex will be brought up more frequently by the professional and will be dealt with more effectively when brought up by the patient. It is the professional's lack of ease in talking about sexual matters that accounts for the common misbelief that the patient should bring up the subject and that sex should not be discussed until the patient initiates it. Sexual health-care needs should be treated as the rest of the patient's needs are treated, and questions about sexuality should be included in the patient interview or other interactions. Initiation of the subject by the nurse who is comfortable with it can facilitate the patient's talking about concerns or problems. The patient may not always be brave enough to bring up the subject. The nurse has many opportunities to open up the issue of sexual health care—when taking the initial history, when dealing with other losses, such as motor or sensory, or when providing counseling on contraceptive needs.

Beyond acquiring a comfort level with their own sexuality, nurses must have knowledge about human sexuality. This includes knowledge of anatomy and physiology of the sexual organs, psychosexual development, typical male and female sexual attitudes and behaviors in our society, and sexual variations among people. The nurse must also know how specific diseases and disabilities and their treatment affect sexual functioning. As sexuality is an extremely sensitive and private area of most persons' lives, nurses must increase their skill and ease in communication and listening in order to assist patients with their sexual problems and concerns. Nurses must know their own limitations in the area of sexual health, and, if necessary, refer the patient to a sex therapist or some other knowledgeable person when a higher level of intervention is called for or if the nurse has personal biases or limitations that interfere with working with the patient.

A very effective model for handling sexual problems or concerns of patients has been adapted from the P-LI-SS-IT Model developed by Annon (1976) and used in many human sexuality programs. Recently this model was further adapted for application to nursing practice (Mims, Swenson). The P-LI-SS-IT Model outlines attitudes, knowledge, and skills needed by the nurse or health-care worker at four different levels of intervention or approach, each building on the preceding level, in resolving sexual problems. As the four ascending levels require increased professional skills, the model offers the advantage that practitioners can practice at their level of competence. The four levels are: Permission-Limited Information-Specific Suggestions-Intensive Therapy. An explanation of the model with a more extensive outline of the knowledge and behavior required at each level as well as illustrative examples, can be found in the articles by Annon and Mims and Swenson. This model has been used successfully by all levels of health-care workers, from health aides to physicians.

CONCLUSION

In rehabilitation, part of the goal of the nurse's interactions with patients is to give the patient input that will assist in the building of positive self-images and strong feelings of self-worth. The nurse should attempt to convey a positive feeling about the patient's body. This will go a long way in assisting the patient to incorporate the imposed body changes into a new and positive body image. Also, the nurse needs to be able to help patients gain insights into their value systems. A most effective way to do this is through the use of value clarification techniques. Finally, the outcome of sex education or counseling is to have the patient develop responsibility for a sexuality based on individual values and choices.

A word of caution may be called for, and that is that sex is not new nor is it a newly identified health problem. It has just risen to our conscious level of total patient care. Nurses should not go overboard in trying to identify sexual problems when there are none. However, it is extremely important to understand that sexuality is an integral part of everyone's personality and that with a disability, adjustments to that disability must include a sexual dimension (Berkman et al.). The person with a disability has the same right to satisfy sexual needs in the same manner as other people.

BIBLIOGRAPHY

"Adolescent Sexuality," *J Clin Child Psychol,* 3:2–70, 1974.

Andreasen, N. J. C., and A. J. Norris: "Long Term Adjustment in Adaptation Mechanisms in Severely Burned Adults," in Rudolf H. Moos (ed.), *Coping with Physical Illness,* Plenum, New York, 1977, pp. 149–166.

Annon, Jack S.: "The PLISSIT Model: A Proposed Conceptual Scheme for the Behavioral Treatment of Sexual Problems," *J Sex Educ Ther,* 2:1–15, 1976.

Berkman, Anne H.: "Sexuality: A Human Condition," *J Rehabil,* January-February: 13–15, 1975.

———, Rae Weissman, and Maxwell H. Frielich: "Sexual Adjustment of Spinal Cord Injured Veterans Living in the Community," *Arch Phys Med Rehabil,* 59:29–33, 1978.

Brodland, G. A., and N. J. C. Andreasen: "Adjustment Problems of the Family of the Burn Patient," in Rudolf H. Moos (ed.): *Coping with Physical Illness,* Plenum, New York, 1977, pp. 167–176.

Coletta, Suzanne S.: "Values Clarification in Nursing," *Am J Nurs,* 78:2057, 1978.

Comfort, Alex: *A Good Age,* Crown, New York, 1976.

Dobson, Betty: *Liberating Masturbation,* Body Sex Designs, New York, 1974, pp. 23–25.

Erikson, Erik H.: *Childhood and Society,* 2d ed., Norton, New York, 1963.

Ficher, Ida V.: "Sex and the Marriage Relationship," in Wilbur W. Oaks, G. A. Melchiode, and I. Ficher (eds.), *Sex and the Life Cycle,* Grune & Stratton, New York, 1976, pp. 81–86.

Griggs, Winona: "Sex and the Elderly," *Am J Nurs,* 78:1352–1354, 1978.

Hunt, Morton: *Sexual Behavior in the 1970s,* Playboy Press, Chicago, 1974.

Masters, William H., and Virginia E. Johnson: *Human Sexual Response,* Little, Brown, Boston, 1966.

Mims, Fern H., and Melinda Swenson: "A Model to Promote Sexual Health Care," *Nurs Outlook* 26:121–125, 1978.

Moos, Rudolf H. (ed.): *Coping with Physical Illness,* Plenum, New York, 1977.

Moore, William T.: "Genital Masturbation and Adolescent Development," in Wilbur W. Oakes, G. A. Melchiode, and I. Ficher (eds.), *Sex and the Life Cycle,* Grune & Stratton, New York, 1976, pp. 53–66.

Newman, Gustave, and Claude E. Nichols: "Sexual Activities and Attitudes in Older Persons," *JAMA* 173:33–35, 1960.

Pfeiffer, Eric, and G. C. Davis: "Determinants of Sexual Behaviorism in Middle and Old Age," *J Am Geriatric Soc,* 20:151–158, 1972.

———, A. Verwoerdt, and H. S. Wang: "Sexual Behavior in Aged Men and Women," *Arch Gen Psychiatry* 19:753–758, 1968.

Renshaw, Domeena: "Sexual Problems of Alcoholics," *Chicago Med.* 78:433–436, 1975.

———: "Drugs and Sex," *Nurs Care* 11:16–19, 1978.

Ritchie, Judith: "Schilder's Theory of the Sociology of the Body Image," *Maternal-Child Nurs J* 2:143–153, 1973.

Sha'ked, Ami: "Editorial," *Sexuality and Disability* 1:3–5, 1978.

Shaul, Susan, Jane Bogle, Julia Hale-Harbaugh, and Ann D. Norman: *Toward Intimacy,* 2d ed., Human Sciences, New York, 1978, p. 57.

Singh, Silas P., and Tom Magner: "Sex and Self: The Spinal Cord Injured," *Rehabil Lit* 36:2–10, 1975.

Sorenson, Robert C.: *Adolescent Sexuality in Contemporary America,* World Pub., New York, 1973.

Ustal, Diane B.: "Values Clarification in Nursing: Application to Practice," *Am J Nurs,* 78:2058–2063, 1978.

Woods, Nancy F.: *Human Sexuality in Health and Illness,* 2d ed., Mosby, St. Louis, 1979.

8

meyer s. gunther

the threatened practitioner: work under stress

INTRODUCTION

It is axiomatic that the more severe the patient's illness, the more complex it is to treat, the more uncertain will be its outcome. Demands upon the staff, demands that tax physical energies, emotional equanimity, and intellectual capabilities will be greater. These factors are intensified in rehabilitation medicine where the illness is profound and severe, treatment programs are highly individualized, achievements are uncertain, and patient-staff contacts are long, complex, and intimate. In many ways, these illnesses are massively distressing to patient, staff, families, and to society in general. This chapter will offer some of the reasons why these burdens are especially acute for the nursing service. It will explore the manner in which this distress affects the nursing staff, how it influences their work with patients, what it means to them, and how nurses have learned to manage this distress.

Nurses are universally idealized in fantasy, depreciated in practice. Lip service is paid to the vital importance of their nurturing, caretaking, and guarding responsibilities. In practice, limited trust and little faith are accorded the nursing service in the exercise of the independent judgment and thoughtful decision making required for constructive discharge of their responsibilities. Furthermore, nursing's inherited sociopsychological burden of being a "woman's field" managed predominantly by male doctors has provided a fertile backlog of distrust and resentment which add immeasurably to the psychologic burdens of nurses in any specialty—especially in rehabilitation.

The chapter's topics include the problem of unrecognized resistance to perception and understanding experiences; some elementary psychological presumptions necessary for understanding all human beings; the unique work role and psychologic position of the nursing department in the spectrum of rehabilitation services; the evidence of nursing services distress, direct and indirect; and some preliminary efforts at understanding the origin, meanings, and management of this distress.

THE PROBLEM OF UNRECOGNIZED RESISTANCE

The leading area of human experience which has, for most of mankind's history, stubbornly resisted scientific investigative efforts is that of the mind's inner psychologic workings, not readily available to simple objective inspection from the outside. That human beings should have difficulty in perceiving exactly how they themselves work is no surprise. To utilize a simple idiom, "The eye has trouble seeing itself." People are notoriously more perceptive of behavior or emotional malfunctioning in someone else than they are of the same malfunctioning within themselves.

There are two ways to study the behavior of other human beings. One is by standing as an observer in a social field watching the interaction of the subject with other subjects, recording externally verifiable objective observations. The observer stands outside and at some distance from any of the participants. For many years this has been the accepted stance of psychology as a science. A second observational stance, which allows more information to become available, is that of the empathic observer. The empathic observer attempts, through certain carefully controlled semiconscious cognitive processes, to sample what it feels like to be within the experiencing self of the patient, and uses this temporary selective merger with the patient's self for the purpose of gathering data.[1]

The material for many of the observations, inferences, and tentative hypotheses in this chapter have been gathered by the author as an empathic participant-observer in the rehabilitative setting. Over the past 18 years, an average of 8 h a week has been spent in a major rehabilitation hospital interviewing individual patients, conducting psychiatric staffings, and meeting once a week with nursing units and other

---

[1] This ability to temporarily feel what it is like to be inside somebody else's skin is fundamental to psychoanalytic depth psychology, and its elaboration in recent years owes much to the works of Heinz Kohut (1971, 1972).

101   THE THREATENED PRACTITIONER: WORK UNDER STRESS

departments in informal, free-for-all seminars. Many thousands of informal individual conversational contacts with nurses at all levels in the department have occurred around everyday issues such as patient management, staff feelings, the meanings of the work, and solutions to innumerable problems.

The difficulties in unrecognized resistance to understanding lie not merely in the problems of collecting the data and organizing it coherently, but also in attempting to spell out its multiple meanings through various layers of inference. There are two particular difficulties, among many others, in the way of attempting to evolve explanations of meaning regarding human beings. The first is the threat of anxiety. People are made anxious by many kinds of threats, such as uncertainty about the future; current overwhelming danger or stress; personal insecurity; excessive demands; and unbearable conflicts of motives or goals. At a more intimate level, there is the psychologic threat that the conscious mind is not really in control of all bodily and mental processes. Finally, people have been made anxious when they are not able to understand the world outside their bodies, that is, the world of nature and natural phenomena which they might wish to influence. To cite an example, the initial reception accorded the findings of Copernicus, Galileo, or Darwin verifies how threatened human beings feel when confronted with the fact that they may not really understand or be in control of their worlds.

SOME ELEMENTARY PSYCHOLOGICAL CONCEPTS

In this section the need for a set of organizing constructs, utilized as scaffolding to help in medical work, will be briefly described. This will be followed by a few specific presumptions which constitute a useful scaffolding for thinking about human beings and their experience in the therapeutic arts.

UNCONSCIOUS MENTAL PROCESSES

What we know of the workings of the mind at a level of consciousness is only a small part of the totality of mental processes. Although we know the contents of individual thoughts, feelings, or reactions, we know virtually nothing of the mechanism or process by which particular thoughts emerge into consciousness, or the manner in which certain ideas are created, connected, or evolved. We know even less of the ultimate motivating forces which may operate at an unconscious level. Yet there is a great deal of indirect evidence from dream research, from the study of psychoneurotic symptoms and hypnosis, and from the study of daydreams, which suggests that all sorts of mental activities go on below the level of consciousness, day and night, without our awareness. For instance, at night a mother sleeps soundly despite street noises, but awakens instantly when her newborn infant, asleep in the next room, begins to breathe differently. Or a patient "forgets" his appointment with the social worker, if the subject of the meeting happens to be discharge planning. Or the very disturbed quadriplegic dreams of flying, unaided, over the countryside, simply by using the magic of "thought power."

THE COMPLEXITY OF HUMAN MOTIVATION

Whether we are talking about moral value systems, the tendency of the human mind to make orderly sense of the world, the desirability of various forms of gratification, the pressure for achievement, or the satisfaction of a host of wishes, human motivation remains as complex, varied, and individualized as human nature itself. The enormous array of differing motives makes it virtually impossible to offer an absolutely reliable explanation of underlying motivational forces simply by observing a similarity in individuals' overt behaviors. For instance, the compliant patient who dutifully follows instructions regarding a medical regimen of pills, exercise, and diet may simply be too frightened to disobey, to challenge the authorities, or too disorganized in thinking to do anything other than drift with the tide.

THE NEED FOR OTHER HUMAN BEINGS

From child development studies, it is evident that a child, in order to survive, to grow, to stabilize, and to flower, requires a context of emotionally responsive human beings (Spitz, 1923). All human beings need one another not merely for sensual gratification or the fulfillment of pleasure wishes, but for confirmation, validation, and maintenance of the intactness, wholeness, and value that comprise the unique, essential self. If one experiences total deprivation of contact with other human beings, such as that of the prisoner in solitary confinement or the Arctic explorer in utter isolation, companions are hallucinated. The human personality cannot survive, intact, when totally alone; it requires emotionally responsive, reactive people for contact, for stimulation, and for confirmation of the essential meaning of existence. All nurses have had the experience of seeing a patient's entire mood and personality change from despair, disorganization, and apathy to reasonable optimism and orderly activity simply because a particular nurse comes on duty.

The are two other concepts specific to rehabilitation patients which are essential in understanding the psychologic context in which physicians, nurses, and allied health personnel work. The first is massive psychic trauma; the second is the difficult-to-label process by which people meet major stress or loss, a process which involves several phases, one of them, inevitably, regression.

MASSIVE PSYCHIC TRAUMA (Krystal, 1968)

This term was originally applied to the experiences of German concentration camp survivors. It refers to life stresses which prove so intellectually overwhelming and emotionally draining that the individual undergoes drastic permanent personality changes which may be the equivalent of psychotic experience—and yet, for technical reasons, the changes do not constitute a true psychosis. In rehabilitation patients (Gunther, 1971), the concept of massive psychic trauma can be considered in any situation of human illness or accident where the following three conditions are met. First, the onset is so sudden, unexpected and overwhelming that the victim has no conceivable preparation for it out of ordinary life experience. Second, the psychologic consequences of the physical lesion itself and its devastatingly life-threatening and life-altering aspects have two significant influences upon personality: (1) the individual's nuclear expectations, ambitions, and ideals may not be capable of realization; and (2) the individual's body image[2] must undergo changes. Thus, two mental structures vitally involved in self-esteem must, in consequence of the physical trauma to the body, be reorganized and changed; the psychologic process that brings about the necessary changes is complex, painful, and lengthy. Third, the lesion produces such permanent visible residues that neither its existence nor its meaning in terms of dramatically altered role functions can be denied. Such information is readily discernible by an outside observer. The traumatic amputation of an arm in a slicing machine would constitute massive psychic trauma as defined by these three criteria; a recovered coronary occlusion, however, might not meet all three of the criteria.

LOSS AND "WORKING THROUGH" PROCESSES

Since World War II, there have emerged in the psychiatric literature many efforts attempting to

---

[2] Body image (Schilder, 1934) refers to the total experimental picture that the individual has of his or her own body in terms of its visual appearance, its contours, and its sensory and emotional feelings, as if standing both inside it and outside it as an observer.

explain the experience of major human stress, especially the manner in which people deal with the loss of vitally important objects (Pollock, 1969; Kübler-Ross, 1968; and Horowitz, 1976). Generally speaking, loss hypotheses all involve some sort of phasic process concepts, that is, the individual is presumed to undergo a series of different emotional experiences that occur in a predictable, interconnected progression. Typically, an initial phase of disbelief, disorganization, and denial is followed by one of depletion and hopelessness; then comes some experience of "working through" in which the victim gradually comes to terms with the meaning of the loss, reintegrates, and returns to normal. All these phasic hypotheses seem to involve an implication that somewhere along the way the individual works down the ladder of psychological development, relating to the world in the way in whch he or she dealt with it and experienced as a child. The process is called *regression*, a return to a time in life when things were simpler, safer, and more predictable—hence, more manageable. If one were to observe a rehabilitation patient carefully through hospitalization, one might identify a series of different phases characterized by different learning tasks, different emotional demands on the staff, and different neuroticlike troubles and reactions (Gunther, 1971, 1977). These phases are summarized below, utilizing the model of spinal cord injury.

Traumatic Disruption

Traumatic disruption occurs from the moment of the injury or the first few hours in the emergency room until transfer to the trauma unit. There is a quickly developing, acute emotional disruption in which the individual is intellectually dulled and slowed, emotional controls are poor, and he or she is either depressed and withdrawn or labile and flighty. Capacity for involvement with the environment, as well as for understanding what has happened, is dramatically diminished. However, as the individual undergoes physiologic stabilization (often after surgical intervention from which there is recovery) that person shifts into the second phase.

Shallow Stabilization

This phase lasts from the time of arrival in the trauma unit or acute cord-injury center until the individual "recovers" over several weeks. Perceptual and cognitive capacities return to normal, emotional controls stabilize, and the person gradually becomes interested in self and what is happening, but with a bland or dulled energy level. During this period, a dependent and idealizing relationship (Kohut, 1971) is developed with the doctors and nurses who are taking care of the patient—a situation which facilitates the origin of a very persistent fantasy: through their simple reassurance and exemplary efforts, the individual becomes certain that everything will turn out okay, that is, that there will be a return to a situation of preillness normalcy. This stable state continues until dramatic changes occur, initiated frequently as the result of transferral to the rehabilitation hospital, which carries with it a variety of painful and overstimulating confrontations. This change introduces the third phase.

Destabilization and Denial

In the rehabilitation hospital, a variety of experiences tend to shake the patient's fantasy of restitution. The patient is confronted in a physical therapy gymnasium by other patients busily and vigorously engaged in all sorts of strange activity. This stirs many aggressive anxieties and conflicts in the patient. There are patients in all stages of rehabilitative treatment. None of them seem to be in the process of magical restoration to preillness normalcy. It dawns on the new patient that this illness may be serious and permanent, and that if anything useful is going to happen, it will depend 75 percent on the patient's own efforts and 25 percent on the efforts of the staff. At this point, the former subtle denial returns more vigorously than ever, but it is now focused on denial of the seriousness and permanence of the illness, denial of its implication of changes in life, and above all, denial of the need for actively assertive work on the patient's part. The patient may, in addition, institute a variety of secondary adaptations such as hopeless apathy or an actively suicidal depression; "accidentally" inflicted physical damage to the body, such as reinfection of vulnerable areas; or paranoid or magical ideas and expectations regarding the causes or cures for the illness. Inevitably, however, such defensive solutions usually begin to melt around the second or third month of hospitalization and the patient slips into the depths of a profound melancholia. The fourth phase follows.

Depression and Working Through to a Reorganized Self

At this point, the patient has little energy, is hopelessly depressed and moody, or is withdrawn and apathetic. Above all, the patient is disinterested in rehabilitative work, demanding guarantees of successful outcome, and even then, being unwilling to do more than a brief, perfunctory job at assigned tasks. In addition, there may be some aggressive testing of the staff's limit setting, including swearing or negativistic, defiant behavior. Inevitably, the patient makes insistent demands on the staff for their emphatic, selfless responsiveness, and even for implicit limit setting. Staff are required to maintain the patient's hope for a better self in the future, that is, for a life which seems worthy, meaningful, and even pleasurable. All this is to counter the desperate feeling, "I have no body, I have no capabilities, I am worthless, I am hopeless. My life is over."[3]

Through a great many back-and-forth transactions with the staff, involving their persistent efforts to support, to respond, and to encourage, the patient begins to climb out of this apathetic, hopeless depression. The staff's responsive "hanging in there" provides a holding environment (Winnicott, 1953) which can be absorbed and with which the patient can make some identification. Concurrent with a shift in interest to the new body, and even the acquisition of the tiniest role skill, the patient starts to climb back up and begins to think of self as "different but not worthless." At this point the patient has begun what eventually will become a lifelong struggle to build, maintain, modify, and express the reorganized self with its altered values, expectations, and competencies.

THE NURSING SERVICE AND ITS WORK

THE ORDINARY MEDICAL REHABILITATION FUNCTIONS OF THE NURSES

Patients come to a rehabilitation hospital after having been ostensibly rendered medically stable. For instance, if they have undergone back surgery, the spine may not be fully stabilized but the healing is well enough along so that a physical medicine program may be initiated. If they have had urinary or pulmonary infections or GI (gastrointestinal) tract problems, these should be controlled, requiring minimal medical management. However, this generalization has to be qualified. There is a principle in developmental psychology which states that newly developed structures are most vulnerable to disruption when their stability is newest. Throughout the course of rehabilitation treatment, patients' physiological stability remains relatively fragile and can be disrupted easily. Cardiovascular decompensations may occur in the elderly who have had strokes; metabolic, biochemical disruptions may occur in the young cord-injured as a result of refusal to eat or drink for several days; urinary tract or bronchial infections and skin disorders may occur in individuals who become careless in their ordinary self-maintenance. Because most rehabilitative treatment begins earlier these days than formerly, patients present themselves for service in a state of fragile stability in the context of a chronic, but latent, vulnerability. Given that situation, what are the tasks of the nursing service?

---

[3] The manner in which these states of hopeless depression alternate with rage at the world, especially a tendency to lash out at those who have shown even a minimum of emotional concern, is illustrated vividly by Jon Voight's portrayal of the paraplegic veteran in the movie *Coming Home*.

The nursing service is responsible for the maintenance of the patient's ordinary well-being through the soundness of general nursing care, and through alertness to minimal, barely discernible signs that something may be going wrong. They must seek to anticipate and thwart any particularly disturbing events in the patient's life, no matter what the origin. Consequently, an appropriately hovering observational responsibility is a major everyday rehabilitation function of the nurse with this seriously vulnerable patient population.

The second responsibility occurs when something major does go wrong. At this point, the rehabilitation nurse shifts from being a rehabilitation specialist to being a generalist. A host of problems must be addressed, an equivalent in medicine to that of general practice—treatment of skin, gastrointestinal, metabolic, digestive, urinary tract, bronchial pulmonary, and other systemic disorders.

The third function of the nursing service is more subtle and complex. This is the responsibility for managing in a balanced, often compromised way, the large variety of demands, stresses, and responsibilities that a rehabilitation program places upon the patient. Decisions have to be made regarding such things as assignment and allocation of energies for the patient, what time of the day and under what circumstances a particular patient will do better at which therapy, and the like. Granted that some of these decisions are shared with the medical managers, at a tactical level a number of the issues become the day-to-day responsibility of the nurse. Frequently, therefore, the nursing service may be at odds with the wishes of other services where matters of departmental convenience and efficiency are involved. But for the nursing service, some sense of patients' overall well-being becomes the ultimate guiding principle. There are no simplistic formulas such as "maximal improvement throughout," or selective upgrading in one role function at the expense of all others. The nursing service thus become the ultimate patient advocate in the hospital situation—a role shared with the physician but unique in its own point of view.

There is one seemingly ordinary psychological function of the nursing service which, in reality, is as vital as any therapeutic activity performed in rehabilitation. The echelon relationship of the nursing service to the other rehabilitation services tends to place nurses in the position of being the most regular recipients of patients' broad concerns about themselves and their well-being. As the most consistently and most immediately available resource, the rehabilitation nurse is the professional toward whom the patients direct their most painful of all questions: "Is there any hope for me? Will I get better?" Without becoming superior and patronizing, defensively aloof, or flooding the patient with overstimulating information, the nursing service must field all of these painful questions by patients while maintaining a predictable optimal responsiveness. In doing so, they rely on their optimistic, straightforward, earnest concern with patients' well-being as a bastion of generalized hope for ultimate improvement, if not for cure. Thus, the almost weekly confrontation with the question, "Wouldn't *you* feel like killing yourself if you were paralyzed like me?" requires the tact and resourcefulness born of successful experience in the management of these predictable crises. It also requires a significant degree of personal equanimity and considerable psychologic sophistication.

SPECIAL CIRCUMSTANCES, PROBLEMS, AND NEEDS

In addition to the previous considerations, there are several particular circumstances unique to nurses and their functions which produce a different set of experiences and pressures from those occurring in other nursing situations. These things have to do with three considerations: the echelon arrangement of services; that is, the manner in which nursing service stands in relation to other therapeutic services; the emotional burdens produced by a relationship of chronicity, intimacy, and extensive physical dependence; and the personal developmental position of most young nurses in relation to the complex, emotional demands of the emotionally regressed patients in the rehabilitation situation. Many of the brain-damaged, cord-injured, and cerebrovascular-accident patients are physically quite helpless. The ordinary role behaviors involving body management and body functions of which most adults are capable have been temporarily, if not permanently lost. Such patients physiologically regress to a state of helplessness like that of a very young child. Furthermore, the steps necessary for the maintenance of elementary physical well-being, like eating, toileting, and bathing, will therefore require direct body handling including, oral, genital, and anal orifice manipulation. These body demands have a predictably recurrent pattern. Nurses and nursing assistants are placed in transactional relationships of intensely personalized intimacy, but without the mitigating effect of the affectionate ties normally present in parent-child relationships—and usually with insufficient didactic preparation or adequate psychologic support to meet such disturbing demands. These circumstances, arising from legitimate nursing care demands of very helpless patients, may stir the caretakers with residual remnants of unresolved experiences left over from their own developmental histories. Whether such experiences—conflicting wishes, anxieties, disappointments, guilts—are unconscious and forgotten or partly conscious, they are nonetheless available to be reawakened as a source of endless trouble. Much will depend on how maturely integrated the nurses are, that is, whether or not a reasonably stable consolidation of the adult self has been achieved.

Many young adults at 21 do not have a consolidated self and a harmonized pattern of mature values, capabilities, and ambitions. Yet nurses are expected to behave and respond as if they had the maturity of persons 10 years older. As an example, a young nurse whose heterosexual experience has consisted of one unsatisfactory if not frightening love affair and whose sexuality is still conflicted and inhibited, may have a dreadful time if she is forced, in an emergency, to catheterize a male patient, especially if a set of gloves is not available. On the other hand, a 30-year-old married woman with two young children would probably not find the demand so disturbing. As a second example, a young woman required to provide ordinary nursing care to an incompletely incapacitated elderly woman with stroke, who is only now beginning a rehabilitation program and who may have certain presenile, infantile qualities, may be particularly distressed if she is in the process of sorting out her feelings toward prematurely senile parent.

The other issue involved relates to the manner in which most rehabilitation hospitals organize their services. Certain of the departments, such as occupational therapy, physical therapy, and speech therapy, may be considered teaching services: that is, patients go to those departments in order to learn elements of old (or new) role functions, built upon special neuromuscular training. Similarly, a number of programs such as recreational therapy and the behavioral science modalities are set up as important but extra programs. The nursing service, on the other hand, is unique—and fundamental. It is a court of last resort for the patients: that is, it is the place where patients are sent back when they become too fatigued, too upset, or too "something" to function on the teaching services. In addition, it is the service where patients go at the end of the working day in much the same way an able-bodied individual from the world of work returns home at the end of vocational activities. Thus, the nursing service becomes a combination of home base, the sheltering family, and a respite from the burden of the day's activities, a place where one may go to relax or to be soothed and restored. For that reason, nurses are looked on as substitute parents or comforting figures toward whom the patients direct many of their burdened, regressed, exhausting emotions incurred through the course of an active rehabiliration day. By the late afternoon or early evening, the nursing service becomes the focus of many of these needs which children at a latency or preadolescent age focus on their families when they return from school. And yet, the nursing service itself has nowhere to send the patients when the patients become "bombed out" on the nursing unit. In addition, the nursing unit is the place where certain family-based social controls are negotiated: that is, responsibility for a reliable pattern of meals, bedtime, baths, passes, and overall appropriate social behavior is established. Becoming the focus of innumerable supportive and parenting needs not only is a very specific conscious drain on nurses' emotional energies and personality resoruces, but it stirs residues of distressing psychologic elements from the developmental background of the nurses themselves.

THE EVIDENCE FOR THE THESIS OF DISTRESS

THE NURSES' OVERT COMPLAINTS

Perhaps the easiest way to become aware of nurses' distress is to listen carefully to the complaints which they verbalize. These are not the formal problems listed on the psychiatric consultant sheet, although certainly one can read behind and into these reports of patients' problems some evidence of the requester's distress. These are the attitudes, feelings, and concerns which emerge in the course of an informal curbstone consultation, the "coffee" contacts that a familiar, trusted consultant who has been a part of the hospital scene for years will have with fellow professionals. The methods for utilizing such complaints for the purpose of data inferences have been detailed in much greater length elsewhere (Gunther, 1977), but can be summarized briefly.

Nurses, as well as other professionals, complain about patients' lack of motivation and energy, their disinterest, even resistance, to engaging in therapies. Cognitively, patients are seen as "overconcerned" with their own illnesses, preoccupied in the wrong way with their bodies. They are believed to be irrationally overconcerned about the permanence or the extent of their bodily changes, or to irrationally deny their significance. Nurses complain about patients' provocative verbal assaults. Nurses resent as unfair patients' endless demands for reassurance, and their inability to respond positively even after the reassurance is given. Nurses appear surprised by patients' gross negativism, their hopeless depression with all of its behavioral and affective qualities, their "irrational" psychoneurotic symptoms. Persistent attitudes of helplessness, confusion, or intellectual disorganization are equally resented. Nurses complain in particular about patients' unwillingness to respond to moral persuasion, sweet reason, and other simple rational explanations when these are used for motivation. There are complaints about the unwillingness of patients to accept nurses as benevolent authorities or arbiters of appropriate behavior, so there are inevitable clashes regarding diet, medication, reporting to therapies on time, coming back from passes drunk, etc.

Each time these kinds of behavior recur, they are viewed as unexpected, unfair, and unmanageable. They are not expected or accepted as an inevitable part of the everyday psychopathology of the rehabilitation situation, and, certainly, they are not in any sense understood in terms of their depth of origin. The expressions by nurses of anxiety, outrage, helplessness, oversensitivity, and intellectual misunderstanding suggest a preconscious message: "We are being traumatized and we resent it!" This situation is further complicated and rationalized by another attitude. Often nurses complain about the failures of other services; they feel, "Our burdens have been exaggerated because other professionals have let us down." Other services may be viewed as inadequate in their understanding, their empathy, and their professional function. What is so obviously unrecognized is that seriously regressed patients often split their relationships with people, especially along the lines of good and bad, or mature and immature. Thus certain attitudes and feelings—literally parts of one's basic self—are turned toward one service while different parts of one's self are turned toward other services.

INDIRECT EVIDENCE

There are several simple ideas available from these observations which seem both self-evident and clear-cut in their implications for nursing service distress. (1) There is a great deal of misunderstanding of elementary psychological constructs—things which might constitute the basics of a first course in "dynamic medical psychology"—symptom formation, unconscious motivation, conflict, stress, regression, and the like. (2) There is considerable difficulty in learning from simple seminar discussions, let alone from formal lecture series. There seem to be a host of resistances which interfere with the spontaneous ability to absorb and integrate new information and new solutions. It seems to take literally years to acquire a set of tools for understanding and doing which enables one to deal with many varieties and forms of difficult patient-management problems. (3) Personnel look endlessly for simple, moralistic techniques, as if all the motivating forces should be at a conscious level and operate reasonably. (4) There is a tendency to guard oneself against empathy, that is, the temporary semicognitive immersion in the subjective experience of someone else's self in order to obtain an impression, diagnostically, of the complex emotions and attitudes which the patient is experiencing at the moment. Even though the virtues of empathy are endlessly extolled by authorities and teachers, there is considerable resistance to opening oneself, as if that kind of data-gathering experience were inevitably painful.[4] (5) There seems to be a peculiar orientation, perhaps reflective of rehabilitation in general, which equates rehabilitation care with cure. Patients' complaints of malfunctioning, suffering, or emotional distress are viewed with a kind of "action" orientation so that many of the solutions for patient distress involve eliminating it, not managing it. A similar attitude occurs toward conflicts about the more social issues such as passes, floor behavior, reporting for therapies, and the like. It is as if all these things are either/or problems that are not so much managed by compromise as "cured" by elimination. One wonders whether or not these staff attitudes may represent defenses against anxiety at least as much as a striving for laudatory, humanistic medical ideals.

One peculiar piece of evidence, part inference, is that nurses confess a tendency to take "mental health days" increasingly when they are forced to work with certain kinds of patients, or they do this more frequently when working in a rehabilitation institute than in other medical settings. They speak of the difficulty of "closing the door at night" when they go home, of carrying the feelings and burdens of their patients with them.

Finally there is an erratic but suggestive statistic on the employment situation, a bimodal distribution curve of length of employment. Many nurses leave at the end of the winter, staying less than 1 year. Another group stays perhaps twice as long, leaving about a year and a half after starting. The smallest group stays 3, 4 or 5 years, moving both horizontally and vertically into more responsible, independent, but, in certain ways, less therapeutically demanding work.

Another group alternates periods of 1 to 2 years at work with an absence of an equivalent amount of time; it repeats this cycle three or four times. Implicit in all these patterns of behavior is the fascinating possibility that nurses experience an inevitable process of burning out or wearing out of their therapeutic energies and optimism. Sometimes such a loss process is overcome or removed by time and respite—but sometimes not.

---

[4] Some reasons for this resistance to empathy, as well as the detailed descriptions, are given in the recent psychiatric literature (Kohut, 1971, 1972).

THE BURDENS OF UNDERSTANDING: MEANING, ORIGIN, AND MANAGEMENT

SIMPLE INFERENCES

Whenever one deals with people, their personalities and their behaviors, it is possible to devise an infinite number of explanations to answer questions of meaning and motivation. If the complexities of a series of social roles imposed through a combination of professional, educational, and institutional factors are added, then the field of explanation is further expanded. Rather than trying to cover and evaluate every possible explanation, let us seek psychologically sophisticated, situationally derived factors which are organized around two different levels of inference, keeping in mind that the goal is to explain why nurses appear so threatened.

Relatively self-evident explanations are derived from the descriptive data, involving a process of inference at a modest level. Second, more abstract explanations involve hypothesized factors more distant from the observational data. Two broad questions are relevant to this second level: (1) What within human personality is being stimulated by the situation of work on a rehabilitation service; and (2) what within the actual circumstances of rehab, in the objective sense, makes it inevitable that the work will be uniquely burdensome? All the factors to be discussed are interconnected and linked in various ways, but for didactic purposes they will be presented as if they are clearly separated. In the operational clinical situation, they are obviously not that separated.

First, it is self-evident that nurses appear traumatized. They act and react as if the burden of patient-care demands, as well as the emotions stirred up within them, are too much to handle all at once, at least to handle maturely and adaptively. This quality of being traumatized or overstimulated is most apparent at two times: very early when the nurse first meets the patient, before it is possible to know much about the patient's personality or to experience the patient other than in the sense of a damaged or handicapped person. This is the time when the actual physical sight of the damaged body and the demands for intimate care may well be the stimuli producing the traumatic state.

There is a second time, toward the middle phase of rehabilitation, when the patients, severely regressed, are placing unusual emotional demands on their caretakers in the form of special relationships called regressive narcissistic transferences.

Severely fragmented, regressed, and depressed rehabilitation patients enter into emotional relationships that are reminiscent of young adult schizophrenics or adolescents undergoing identity-diffusion reactions. But even in this most distressing middle phase, rehabilitation patients are seldom psychotic. Nevertheless, it is as if the patient were saying to the staff member, "My body is in pieces. My life is in pieces. My personality is worthless." At this point, nurses receive demands for reassurance: they are asked to exert control, lend energy, and to offer hope that one day the patient can be whole, worthy, and capable. Rehabilitation nurses, like the nurses on a psychiatric unit, are utilized by patients as a source of "glue" to hold a shattered personality together or to initiate a reintegration. To feel that one has no control or no influence over how one's body works or how one's mind thinks is massively anxiety-provoking; it induces its victims to turn toward caretakers in a truly desperate way. Feelings of being utterly helpless, utterly lost, utterly without hope are among the most frightening and disturbing that anyone can have. But the enormous emotional pressure such feelings generate is turned, typically, on nurses and doctors rather than on the teaching therapists. Often, the caretaking person feels reduced to a series of mere functions to serve the self of another person, no longer an independent separate center for the initiation of feelings and action. Indeed, the object of such special demands feels he or she has no existence except as part of the self of the poor suffering victim. One patient said to a nurse, "You are here for me only. You have no existence outside of what I expect of you and how I experience you. You belong to me." Such expressions are not selfishness in the volitional sense of a consciously immoral act, but they flow from the primitive level to which the self-organization of the patient has regressed (Kohut, 1972).

WHAT IS THE ULTIMATE MEANING OF NURSES' DISTRESS?

As has been said previously, the unique physical circumstances and special demands of rehabilitation work predispose staff members to become victims of the kinds of burdens described above. However, if we look to the deep inner psychological makeup of all human beings, there are two predisposing vulnerabilities (based, in turn, on hidden or unconscious residues of our own developmental experience) that have some immediate relevance in explaining these problems.

The first of these is the issue of massive body damage and the fear all of us carry that such a disaster might conceivably happen to us. It is very difficult when first meeting a seriously damaged patient not to make an immediate massive automatic identification represented by the phrase, "There but for the grace of God go I." This is instantly and automatically negated by, "Thank God that isn't me." The fear that one may not be invulnerable to physical damage (or aging) represents the intrusion of an unwelcome truth which will suffer the fate of immediate denial when it approaches consciousness, especially in young persons. When one is confronted in a persistently overstimulating way by such a threat, it is inevitable that a complex series of internal psychologic defenses will be erected to keep those ideas out of mind, to quiet the anxiety accompanying them, and at the same time diminish the external source of their stimulation. Some of the difficulties with learning, with empathy, and with establishing workable relationships (that is, use of defenses such as isolation, moralization, intellectualization—techniques that constitute part of the inevitable coping devices of people in medicine and nursing—often rationalized as "Scientific Objectivity") can be explained as maladaptive efforts to cope with conflicts over body damage anxiety.

The second vulnerable predisposition, especially focal in explaining staff's reactions to the psychically regressed, emotionally fragmented, and physically damaged patients, is the area of our feelings and attitudes about ourselves, and our inner experiences in contrast to our feelings about others. These constructs, comprising a "psychology of the self," concern the manner in which people organize, stabilize, and express the inner nature of their own personalities (Kohut, 1971, 1972). All human beings have an essential core consisting of a value system, ambitions, and certain talents and energies arranged in a unique scheme which characterizes and identifies that person. This unique core has a continuity over time and a persistence of arrangement so that outside observers easily recognize and distinguish each particular person from others. In this area of feelings lie such things as self-esteem and self-worth, the expectations and pleasures in performance success, the capacity to value others and their approval, etc. Also involved are disappointment with failure to perform successfully or to meet goals and difficulties in valuing others whose goals and ideals are dramatically different. Especially serious is the tendency to feel humiliated and anxious when one's differences or limitations are exposed to others. In the positive sense, such feeling about the self may be expressed through creativity, humor, and the capacity to be empathic. If one has come to a fully mature adult consolidation of personality, particularly the nuclear self elements, including their imperfections, limits, and vulnerability, then one can face the world of differences, of disappointment, of performance difficulties—even the transience of human existence—with a reasonable degree of equanimity. However, when human beings relate to others as if they were merely a part of themselves, there will be trouble if one's self is consolidated, or if one's own self-organization carries significant, unrecognized, and conflict-ridden residual vulnerabilities. Those who work in the rehabilitation field tend to "see" in the disintegrated selves of some patients fears at a very deep level arising from within the depths of themselves about themselves. Thus there is once again raised in our minds the specter that, "I, too, could become as disintegrated and primitive or childish a self as that other person has become, were I to undergo such a trauma."

MANAGEMENT, OR WHAT HELPS

If, after this long explanation, it were possible to provide detailed, reliable, foolproof prescriptions for the management of one's own anxieties and distress, as well as those of patients, then medicine, particularly psychiatry, would have become a precise and exact science instead of being a mixture of art and science. Unfortunately, human nature is exceedingly complex. Variable clinical situations are often overdetermined, and no two human transactions involving different people ever work exactly the same way. With the rather elementary knowledge of these matters available, the best that can be offered are a series of ideas and constructs which might be utilized as tools to manage the many issues. These suggestions can be divided into three broad categories. The first is educational suggestion; the second is suggestions in the direction of improved emotional support or psychotherapeuticlike help; the third is managerial support.

Educational Activities

Educational activities in the form of episodic ongoing in-service training can take many forms—short lecture courses or lengthy, more intensive educational encounters involving visiting experts and scholars. A particularly useful device for educational activities may be built around the ongoing, informal, semistructured, small-group model in which the content of material relates to the kinds of problems with self, patients, and fellow staff members which are encountered almost daily. To be effective, the level of discussion should proceed from the more clinical and familiar to the less clinical, more abstract, and less familiar. Such small-group educational enterprises are best led by a staff member who is knowledgeable and experienced in both rehabilitation and psychologic matters, and who is an accepted member of the institution's staff. The success of such educational enterprises depends on the ultimate ability of the educator and the group to tune in on one another and to evolve a relationship of confidence, trust, reliability, and usefulness.

The payoff from such enterprises is more than simple education. In the course of this kind of group activity, one shares personally distressful feelings about encounters with patients or other staff members, feelings of disappointment, discouragement, and anxiety about the nature of rehabilitation work. This sharing is invaluable because it legitimizes the social normalcy of such feelings and because it provides an opportunity for group sharing, group understanding, and group solutions to the burdens which such feelings impose.

Among the many useful subjects serving as key organizing constructs in such groups discussions is the crucial concept of the *self as a diagnostic tool,* the idea that the self involved in a relationship of confidence with another human being is an invaluable source of information regarding the nature of that other person's experience. In addition, the self may well be a prime therapeutic tool in constructively influencing the patient in the most difficult phases of experience. To learn to use the self as that kind of a tool requires a good deal of experienced practice, along with a preliminary presumption of reasonably good contact with inner feelings, including the more distressful feelings, such as one's own limitations. Without the use of that tool, the ability to be an effective worker in a rehabilitation setting will be limited.

Therapeutic Suggestions

Among the standard suggestions in the category of therapeutic suggestions for the more troubled rehabilitation worker is individual psychotherapy of one form or another. Certainly this is available to anyone, yet experience shows it is taken by relatively few members of the rehabilitation team. The solution of group psychotherapy, particularly the kind often manipulated into existence through institutional management pressure (via the disguise of "training"), is an effort to influence rehabilitation workers in a seductive and coercive manner. Few such "voluntary" enterprises seem truly constructive because psychotherapeutic encounters under the aegis of management inevitably limit the ability of the participants to be open and comfortable and therefore to use the experience constructively.

Managerial Support

There is a form of intervention, however, which is not only ethical but which is highly effective: upper-echelon management's direct support to rehabilitation workers on the firing line. This refers not only to the director of the department of nursing, but to the top managers such as the medical director, business director, and the president of the hospital. Their willingness to spend a day a month floating around the nursing floors, sitting in on conferences, offering support simply through lending their presence, their interest, and their concerned involvement and curiosity would be of great benefit to the daily workings of the nursing service.

Finally, a more distant support factor is in the background: sensitive hospital management, placing the long-term humanistic well-being of patients and staff foremost and offering patients the best circumstances to heal themselves. A sensitive management attempts to make conditions of the work environment for the nursing service favorable, effective, and facilitative. If the hospital is not effectively managed, humanistically oriented, and dedicated to the goal of optimal rehabilitation opportunity, if instead it has only a technological orientation or a cost-accounting orientation, none of the preceding suggestions will do much good. Under those circumstances, the nursing service will continue to be threatened, distressed, and will be ultimately less effective.

CONCLUSION

Psychologically unschooled nurses and other rehabilitation personnel have the inherent capacities, both intellectual and emotional, to make more out of their experience than they believe they can. Most rehabilitation personnel are reasonably well-endowed human beings who grew up in relatively normal family circumstances, are not excessively encumbered with neurotic limitations, and, given appropriate opportunity, have the capacity to develop usable empathic competencies. If management provides a supportive working atmosphere and if the ancillary behavioral science individuals give reasonable guidance and support, rehabilitation nurses can learn effective solutions for managing their patients and can also find ways of dealing with their own inner feelings and distress—a distress to which any dedicated staff is going to be subjected as the inevitable price of truly constructive work with seriously damaged patients.

BIBLIOGRAPHY

Gunther, M. S.: "Psychiatric Consultation in a Rehabilitation Hospital: A Regression Hypothesis," *Compr Psychiatry* 12:572–577, 1971.

————: "The Threatened Staff: A Psychoanalytic Contribution to Medical Psychology," *Compr Psychiatry* 18:385–397, 1977.

Horowitz, M.: *Stress Response Syndromes,* Jason Aronson, New York, 1976.

Kohut, H.: *The Analysis of The Self,* International Universities Press, New York, 1971.

———: "Thoughts on Narcissism and Narcissistic Rage," *Psychoanal Study Child* 27: 360–400, New York Times Press, New York, 1972.

Krystal, H.: *Massive Psychic Trauma,* International Universities Press, New York, 1968.

Kübler-Ross, E.: *On Death and Dying,* Macmillan, New York, 1968.

Pollock, G. H.: "Mourning and Adaptation," *Int J Psychoanal* 42:341–361, 1969.

Schilder, P.: *The Image and Appearance of the Human Body,* International Universities Press, New York, 1950.

Spitz, R. A.: "Hospitalism," *Psychoanal Study Child* 1:57–74, 1945.

Winnicott, D. W.: "Transitional Aspects and Transitional Phenomena," *Int J Psychoanal* 34:89–97, 1953.

9
hector r. roché

experiencing loss

INTRODUCTION

Loss is experienced in many different ways and to different degrees. In the interest of brevity, this discussion of loss is limited to only a few of the contributors to the field. Regardless of the description of the experience of loss, this author would argue that health professionals play a significant role in assisting the patient through the process. This assisting may be as simple as listening—with all our senses.

Dr. Elizabeth Kübler-Ross has studied the experience of loss as it relates to death and the dying process. Because of her research, our culture and our health care system have been shown that death does not just happen; before death there is a process called *dying*.

Physical disability also involves loss and is accompanied by an adjustment process. It is important for us to grasp the meaning of loss so that we may better understand the people who are our patients and how we may relate to them. We must meet them in their hearts, in their minds, and in their souls; we must take part in their experience. There will always be unresolved frustrations. If our goal for patients is complete recovery, we cannot win. Physical disability is different from death in that way. In death there is a clear end; physical life as we know it ends. Much of the pain, grief, and suffering comes either before death (as part of the dying process) or as part of the final resolution of death. Those who work with the physically disabled are involved with people who are at the beginning of a long adjustment process; although their future is life, at the moment of loss many may have preferred death. James Agee understood:

> If there had to be such an accident, this was pretty certainly the best way. That with such a thing, a concussion, he might quite possibly have been left a hopeless imbecile . . . the rest of his life, and that could have been another forty years as easily as not. Or maybe only a semi-invalid, laid up just now and then, with terrific recurrent headaches, or spells of amnesia, of feeble-mindedness . . . If he'd lived, he'd have probably been a hopeless cripple . . . an idiot, or a cripple or a paralytic. Because another thing a concussion can do, is paralyze. Incurably. Those aren't fates you can prefer for anyone to dying. Least of all a man like Jay, with all his vigor, of body and mind too, his independence. . . . (Agee, 1967.)

The poignant truth is that some patients, and their families, do prefer death to life as a "hopeless cripple." Others, in adjusting to the disability and a new life-style, discard the thought as not appropriate for them. Yet others, because of guilt and shame and all those emotions attached to preferring death to life, unconsciously suppress the desire.

This chapter will consider some of the differences and similarities in loss and the psychosocial/emotional process as it related to death and to physical disabilities.

DEATH AND DYING

Much has been written and discussed about grief and mourning in the process of loss as it relates to death and dying. Dr. Kübler-Ross, a pioneer in this sensitive field, learned much from her patients, and through her they have taught us as well. They have taught us how to pay attention, to listen, to hear, to remain sensitive to their needs and not run away. They have also given us some guideposts to help us recognize where they are coming from and what they are experiencing. Dr. Kübler-Ross has taken these guideposts and developed a five-stage process to help us to look and help us to see. The five stages are (1) denial, (2) rage and anger, (3) bargaining, (4) depression, and (5) acceptance (Kübler-Ross, 1969). We shall see that the process as it relates to physical disability is not too dissimilar from this process.

Denial "No, not me." Jim Hall has been told he is dying. He refuses to accept this as a fact. He informs the doctor that it must be the wrong chart, the wrong room, certainly the wrong patient. He contemplates calling friends and relatives to inform them of the lie, to deny the

CHAPTER 9 116

lie and denounce the liar, and to be reassured that it is a lie, but he chooses not to share the news and refuses to speak of it with anyone. For Jim this denial is essential to his physical and emotional health; it allows him to absorb this blow, this insult, this shock to his being.

Rage and Anger "Why me, doctor? Why me, mother? Why me, God? What did I do to deserve this?" Anger. "Why me, God?" No answer. Rage. Jim singles out his doctors and God for particular anger. He views God as arbitrarily imposing death sentences, singling out some of us unjustly.

Bargaining "Yes, me—but..." Jim makes promises and strikes deals with God for at least some more time and maybe even a reversal of the death sentence. He contacts his minister. This is not atypical. People who have not prayed in years or can't remember the last time they spoke with their minister, rabbi, or priest now use them in search of a pardon, a reprieve. As Dr. Kübler-Ross points out, "What they promise is totally irrelevant, because they don't keep their promises anyway" (Kübler-Ross, 1969).

Depression Jim now acknowledges the news to be the truth, reality. He withdraws, retreats into a private place to regroup, to reflect. It is a time of grief; a time for mourning and reflecting on a life filled with other losses, disappointments, wrongs committed, things said and done, and things unsaid and left undone. Jim begins to resolve his past in his own mind, to answer some of his own questions, to finish up his own business.

Acceptance In working through the stage of depression, Jim has become able to accept his fate. There is a sense of victory, although the feeling is relatively emotion-free. It is recognition that the end is in sight. It is the victory of finding peace.

No, there is no legislation mandating every dying person to experience death in this way. If there were, dying people would ignore it anyway. They attempt to maintain control as long as possible. Patients also may tend to vacillate in and out of these stages, get stuck in some, never experience others. They stay depressed longer than they should; become too angry for their own good; continue to deny their fate; or, after appearing to have attained some level of acceptance, regress to a state of denial. What can we do? How can we help? The answer is simple; doing it is more difficult. The answer is to *listen*.

PHYSICAL DISABILITIES

As mentioned earlier, the process of adjustment as it relates to physical disability is similar to that in dying. In death, life itself is lost. What, then, is lost in physical disability? Physically patients may lose sensation, skin integrity, bowel and bladder function, sexual function. Cognitively they may lose the ability to speak, read, write, comprehend. They may lose words from their vocabulary or the ability to use them appropriately. They may lose the memory of things in the distant past, things of the moment, or tasks learned from one minute to the next. Functionally there may be loss of the ability to walk or of the use of the arms. A person who is now a patient may no longer be able to dress, to eat, or to bathe. Socially there may be loss not only of one's job but of the skills required to do that job, as well as avocational skills, the ability to play and to learn. Patients may lose the ability to relate to family, friends, and environment. They may lose their self-image, sense of self-worth, self-esteem, and sexuality. They lose independence and the ability to control their own destiny.

Schwemmer and Kramer (1975), in their study of the rehabilitation process, identify four stages in adjustment: (1) acute disorganization, (2) assessment, (3) mourning, and (4) reentry.

In the first stage those patients interviewed expressed feelings of high anxiety, great fear, and disbelief. They often reported feeling confused and in a state of shock. They begin to question: "Has this really happened to me?" "Why me, God... why me?"

After a time the patients passed into a period

of assessing what had happened to them. They were able to give an accurate history of the cause of their disability. They recognized and identified changes in function (physical, intellectual, emotional). On an emotional level they experienced anger and self-disgust and were depressed. They denied, bargained, and held to a "magic hope" for spontaneous recovery or a medical miracle (a new drug, a new surgical procedure).

Early in the next stage, mourning, the patients continue to experience the anger and depression apparent in the assessment stage. However, there came a new awareness of the losses involved and an attendant mourning for those losses. The patients then entered what Schwemmer and Kramer term a "therapeutic depression." They began to accept their most probable future and to engage themselves more fully in the rehabilitation program.

In the final stage, the patients resolved the therapeutic depression of the mourning process and began to experience more positive feelings about self and the future. They accepted role changes for themselves, those in the family, and others in their environment.

On the basis of her research, Kerr (1961) formulated a five-stage framework to describe the adjustment process. As with the other processes described, it is important to remember again that these categories are not mutually exclusive, nor does every patient pass through the stages in the given order. Kerr's five stages are (1) shock—"This isn't me"; (2) expectation and recovery—"I'm sick, but I'll get well"; (3) mourning—"All is lost" (4) defense A (healthy)—"I'll go on in spite of it"—or B (neurotic), use of defense mechanisms to deny; and (5) adjustment—"It's different but not bad."

Shock In the first stage patients cannot or will not comprehend that there is something wrong with their bodies, even to the extent of denying the data that confirm the diagnosis. As a result they may not initially exhibit the anxiety we might expect. They have successfully protected themselves from the impact of the news so as not to take the full brunt of the trauma. As the reality of the diagnosis sets in, they may become numb and dazed. They begin to exhibit anger and hostility toward their caregivers, blaming them for the situation. As the evidence mounts up and patients recognize on some level that denial of that evidence is not emotionally healthy, they move into the next stage.

Expectation of Recovery Patients will acknowledge that, in fact, something is wrong, that there is disability. At the same time they maintain a belief in full recovery, that all that is required is time and hard work. Their perception of the future includes a whole body, free of restrictions, limitations, and, indeed, disability. Each improvement is viewed as existing somewhere on the continuum which has disability at one end and complete recovery at the other. There is often another more insidious "road to recovery"—"the road to Mecca." Patients may embark on a pilgrimage which takes them to a variety of health care facilities, in search of the place that will effect recovery. They will not engage in activities designed to help them function with disability.

Mourning More time passes. Patients go on an evening-out trip or go home for the weekend. They suddenly find themselves in a position where the reality of the permanence of the disability can no longer be ignored or denied. No longer are they certain that they will actually walk out of the hospital. Future plans no longer make any sense in light of the new awareness; no longer do they believe that they will get well.

Now this person who is our patient believes that all is lost. Among the losses in this stage are self-worth and self-esteem. Thoughts of suicide are not uncommon. All at once such patients are angry and hostile, resigned and withdrawn. They complain and vilify, they seclude themselves in their room. They grieve for and nourn the loss of those things most important to them. They rope off physical and emotional areas upon which no one is to tread. No trespassing . . . this is my time, my place, my space . . . this is my mind, my heart, my soul . . . this is my loss. Eventually, as the patients are ready to let us in, we can assist and facilitate passage through this stage. We can provide situations which will enhance chances for successful endeavors to which they can relate. Kerr points out that some goals may not be viewed as positive for some patients. It should be noted that patients are also dealing with losses related to pride and the capacity to fight and cope with stressful situations. They may castigate themselves for having lost the drive and determination which was so important.

Defense As patients score some successes and have an opportunity to exhibit drive, pride, and self-esteem, they may be able to develop a healthy defense to cope with the disability. They recognize that the disability does, in fact, exist, but now they find the internal resources to go on in spite of it. Physical return, functional improvements, increased levels of independence are placed in proper perspective. Patients are anxious to find means to adapt their life to the disability.

On the other hand, some patients may become entrenched in a denial system which can be further immobilizing. While a patient's premorbid personality characteristics and previous experience with crisis play a role in how he or she copes with this crisis, environmental factors also play a key role in the adoption of denial as a coping mechanism.

Caring, loving, and concerned relatives and friends may, because of their own needs to deny the reality, reinforce those parts of the patient which are whole and normal. They insist that the patient look on the bright side. They want to talk about how it will be when everything is all right, when the patient is whole again. As a result, patients are compelled to conceal the disability or negate the impact of the loss of certain functions. They are not permitted and, in turn, will not permit themselves to acknowledge the disability. Such patients are in a dilemma. They are aware that they are disabled, but they and those around them are unable to acknowledge it and thus to cope with it.

Adjustment In the adjustment stage, patients are able to accept the disability as part of themselves. They do not define themselves as the disability, but the disability is one of many things they are.

One question often asked concerning adjustment to disability is How long. How long should someone be depressed, how long should we permit people to deny, how long should they be angry or hostile, how long before they finally accept? What we must recognize is that each patient has his or her own timetable which may have nothing to do with our efforts, our interventions, our own hopes for the patient. While we provide key elements in helping the patient cope with this period of crisis and adjustment, we also tend to bring our personal and professional experiences into every new situation. By the nature of what we do and because we are helpers, we are vulnerable to our patients' fears, anxieties, hopes, and aspirations. Here is a plea to remain open and vulnerable to patients, being careful not to impose our own needs upon them.

CASE PRESENTATIONS

So now you have seen the process. What separates the process, the stages, the words from the experience of loss is the people. The people who become our patients. The families who are confronted with crisis, trauma, tragedy. The community which sees one of its members crippled. The doctors and nurses charged with caring for the medical needs of these people. The therapists who will assist them in learning new ways to perform lost functions. The counselors who will try to help the patient and family through the psychological and emotional obstacle course toward adjustment. The team who will work collectively to make the whole greater than the sum of its parts. The individual members of that team who will help one another deal with their own issues, their own feelings about the patient, about disability, about their own mortality and fragility. Like our patients, we do not have to be in this alone.

The following case studies have been drawn from the author's experience. In reading these cases, keep a number of questions in mind. What do we expect from the people who are our patients? What do we expect from their families? What do we expect from ourselves? Where is that common ground upon which we can meet our patients and their needs and our own needs and feelings to facilitate adjustment? Where do we fit into these experiences?

Jim

The Smiths are the most "average" American family you could hope to find. Jack has worked for the railroad for more than 25 years, having just been promoted to yard foreman. Jesse has been an active participant in the lives of her children, as well as maintaining her own area of interests. In their 25 years of marriage, they have raised three children. One son is a local police officer. Karen, the only daughter, recently married and now lives in the same community the Smiths have lived in for virtually their entire lives.

And then there is Jim. Until today Jim was a member of the high school swim team, working toward his third palm of Boy Scout merit badges. He was a good student and good athlete and the family comedian. Jim was all these things until, during a camping trip, the tree limb upon which he was balancing gave way. Jim suddenly found himself lying in the grass, unable to move, having difficulty breathing, barely able to call out to his father for help. Jack felt his stomach tighten into a knot as he approached Jim. He could see Jim was in an awfully queer position, acting terribly strange.

Time is interminable and yet so abrupt. Three long hours ago they left for the hospital. Three short hours ago Jim was still climbing trees. Now the doctors speak the words "broken neck," explain the meanings of severed spinal cord, quadriplegia. The Smiths don't hear a word. When will Jim be up and around again?

"It's nighttime," Jim thinks to himself. "It's awfully dark in here." He can make out the figures of other hospital beds in his room in the glare from the naked bulb in the hall. Suddenly he remembers and is struck with fear. "I'm in the hopsital ... the accident ... where are my mother, my father? I can't move my legs. What's going on here? I have a headache. I can't lift my hand to my head. I can't breathe. What's happening to me? Someone help me, someone please ... *nurse!!!*"

Jim began to hallucinate after this experience. He watched himself fall from the tree in slow motion. He experienced the impact of the fall and the inability to breathe all over again. The psychiatrist said Jim was frightened, confused, disoriented.

Jack and Jesse are busy assuring friends that Jim will be all right, all the time not allowing themselves to believe the reality of what has happened to them. They are angry at the doctor, frustrated by everything he has to say but mostly they are scared.

All the Smiths' emotions come in a jumble. They cannot sort out what happened or what it is they are feeling. They are overwhelmed with the entire episode. "My God, what has happened to us?"

Joanie

Joanie is a 23-year-old woman who was diagnosed as having multiple sclerosis 3 years ago. Until recently her condition has been stable. In the past month, however, she has experienced an exacerbation that has left her unable to walk, dependent on her family for care. Now it has put her back in the hospital. When I first met Joanie, she still fully expected to get better. Buoyed by her knowledge of multiple sclerosis and the many documented cases of remission, she often informed me of her plans for the future, which included school, a job, a family of her own, and no disability to interfere with any of these plans.

During the course of her hospitalization I watched and listened as denial and "magic hope" began to erode and she could no longer avoid the reality with which she was confronted. I watched her bargain as she requested more therapy, more work, so she could do what was necessary to get better. I was involved in her discussions with the physicians as she requested a different medication regimen or surgery. I was there as she became increasingly angry at her doctors and nurses, whom she perceived as the cause of her condition or at least of her not getting better.

Joanie then became defiant of those in authority. More than once she refused all medication, all care, all therapy. "Go to hell, world. Go to hell, me." I don't think I had ever known or have known since anyone who was as angry as Joanie for as long a time. It wasn't until subsequent admissions that she and I were able to talk about her experience of loss of function, her loss of self.

Gary

Gary was a pretty wild kid in deed as well as reputation. He liked to cut school, enjoyed going drinking with his friends, loved to fight with his father. Tell him black, he'd say white; tell him no, he'd insist yes. Tell him don't, and he's likely to ride atop a moving freight train just for the thrill of it and lose a leg and injure his spinal cord.

During his stay at the rehabilitation center, Gary had been able to laugh and joke and kid his way through therapy while holding on to the belief that he would be a whole person again. The loss of his leg has almost been secondary to his paraplegia to this point, and he has focused on regaining movement in his other leg, as well as regaining control over his bowel and bladder function. But it has been 3 months now, and nothing has come back yet. He is suddenly hit with the reality of his paralysis and the impact of the loss of his leg as well. His quick wit becomes sarcasm, becomes anger, becomes hostility. A sense of worthlessness, of uselessness, begins to set in. Too many people to have to deal with, too many emotions inside waiting to burst out. Got to get away.

Gary proceeds to alienate all those close to him. He argues with his family to keep them at home, frustrates his nurse by demonstrating poor self-care, causing skin ulcers, and thus keeping her at a distance. Hence he successfully provides himself with his own time and his own space to be depressed and to mourn his losses. He's lost one leg and the use of the other as a result of the injury to his spine. He can no longer be a member of the swim team, no longer run around with his friends as he used to. "No one'll know me, I'm not the same person I was. I don't even resemble me. I'm stuck at home now; no moving out after graduation for me. I've really blown it, haven't I?"

Those who loved Gary had not run away. They stuck it out and were around when he needed someone to listen to him, someone off whom he could bounce his reality testing, his questions about who he was and what he could be. Slowly but surely Gary was able to accept his new body and adapt his perceptions about himself to allow for new goals, new plans for the future. He mobilized his internal resources and those of the people around him so that he could return to a regular school. The struggle was difficult, not just because the school system was tough to fight but because of the fragility of his acceptance of his disability and where that left him in the scheme of things. He was able to say, "If I can go on in spite of my disability, then the school system can accept me in spite of it." And they did, and he won.

Carl

Not everyone comes out of the mourning process with the same positive results as Gary. Carl, who was similarly disabled, came out of the depression more defiant and better defended against the reality of his disability than before. He was angrier and more determined not to be disabled and not to do anything that would reinforce his recognition of his disability. Carl's parents transferred him to another rehabilitation facility where they felt everyone would not be so negative about his chances for recovery. The last we heard of Carl he had been sent home, not having ever been able to engage in a rehabilitation program to help him adapt to his disability.

Lena

Initially Lena was something like Carl in that she left the rehabilitation center after her first admission without having achieved the level of function anticipated for her. Lena was in her senior year of high school at the time of her accident, and she had plans for her future. Before the injury Lena danced, painted, and sang, but mostly she wanted to go into nursing, and, in fact, had been accepted by a large midwestern university for the coming fall.

During her first admission Lena struggled with her family, her physicians, her nurses, and always with herself. She worked hard, tried to understand, tried to accept, but never quite got over the hump. Eventually she left the rehabilitation center and went to live with her brother. Lena needed a vacation from hospitals. Her circuits were just overloaded.

During her stay at home she had an opportunity to assess her disability and where it fitted into her life.

121 EXPERIENCING LOSS

She returned a year later, determined to work hard on learning how to live with her disability. She was prepared to go on in spite of her disability. Along with her continued ambivalence about herself, however, she had to struggle with her family's inability to accept her as she was. She was able to use her newfound resolve to get her past the headaches, the weariness, and the frustrations that had thwarted her before and help her family understand and adjust.

The one concept not really addressed in the case studies presented is acceptance or adjustment. Both Lena and Gary were able to mobilize their inner resources and get on about the business of their lives. The lists of professionals who are physically disabled also attests to the fact that people do adjust.

But what do we mean when we speak of acceptance? I would like to raise a provocative question here. Is there such a thing as unconditional acceptance? Do we ever give up the hope that we will have our miracle or that someone will yet come up with the magic drug or surgery that will restore us to our previously experienced selves? I would like to share a conversation I had with Lena on yet another admission for functional upgrading, an admission in the spring of the year she was to enter college.

I received a message informing me that Lena was very upset and wanted to speak with me. As I sat down next to her she began to tremble and then to cry as I'd never seen her cry before. "You won't believe what I tried to do today. Two years after my injury, I can't believe it. I tried to get up and walk. I was up in physical therapy and was having trouble with my transfers. I started to get frustrated and angry, and all of a sudden I put my hands on the side of my wheelchair and tried to push off and get up and walk." She calmed down after a while and sat there quietly for a few minutes. She began again, "I've spent the better part of the last 2 years of my life convincing myself, learning, believing that I am who I am in spite of my injury, that I count even if I can't walk. It's all a lie." And she began to cry again.

We sat and talked for a while, and she related what she was feeling and what she was experiencing. She felt that she had lost everything that she had learned about herself, all the ground she had covered. Later she began to talk about plans for moving into her own apartment just off campus and all the anxieties that prospect was raising. As we settled into a conversation about her future, we both learned that she was just plain scared—about school, her own apartment, the rest of her life. We tried to put all these feelings into perspective.

Yes, by anyone's yardstick, Lena had adjusted and made a successful reentry into her social milieu. But Lena has accepted her disability and herself, just as we all accept ourselves, with all our insecurities and questions of self-worth intact. And the experience goes on.

CONCLUSION

We've briefly seen the family and how they play a role in the experience of loss, and a fuller description of the family as a support structure is given elsewhere in this section. However, there is an important point which must be made here: the family is a patient, too. We tend to view the family as a resource for our patient in much the same way we might view public aid or a community service agency. But if we look at the role the patient may have played in the family and how the disability affects performance of that role and forces other family members to fill that role; if we watch closely as parents visit their children and husbands their wives and see their hurt; if we watch as some family members, usually children, get lost in the shuffle of the trauma (the hospital visits, the family restructuring); if we listen and hear, we recognize that the family passes through the same process as our patient and maybe without the same supports.

The rehabilitation team plays an important role in this process for the patient, for the family, and for its members. If we are viewing the patients as part of a larger context which is affected by the trauma to the patient, we must include ourselves as part of that larger system with which the family now interacts. You will find yourself caught up in the experience of many of your patients. It is important that you recognize that—not so that you can avoid it, but so that you can find ways to cope with it yourself and not rob your patients or yourself of the experience of mutual growth. Look to your fellow team members for support, for guidance, for help in understanding your own responses to what you are experiencing.

BIBLIOGRAPHY

Agee, James: *A Death in the Family,* Grossett & Dunlap, New York, 1967.

Kerr, Nancy: "Understanding the Process of Adjustment to Disability," *J Rehabil* 27: 16–18, 1961.

Kübler-Ross, Elisabeth: *Death: The Final Stage of Growth,* Prentice-Hall, Englewood Cliffs, N.J., 1975.

———: *On Death and Dying,* Macmillan, New York, 1969.

Schwemmer, Cullen, and Robert Kramer: "Stages of the Rehabilitation Process," unpublished. Marionjoy Rehabilitation Hospital, Wheaton, Ill. 1975.

PART TWO

ASSESSMENT AND MODALITIES FOR MANAGEMENT

10

henry b. betts

the rehabilitation experience

INTRODUCTION

Success for patients in the rehabilitation experience is largely determined by the degree to which the coalition of health professionals dedicated to working with those patients can function effectively as a unit. The following factors are important to this team effort:

1. Technical skills
2. Leadership
3. Individual ego strength but not dominance by any team member
4. Administrative backup
5. Motivation, industriousness, and philosophical commitment to the cause of the disabled

The nurse's position is the most complicated because she or he is the pivotal member of the team, but the physician is the leader and the final authority. As a physician, I should perhaps say that, on the basis of my experience, I believe this is a fact, not an expression of my own ego.

Patients spend more time with nurses than with any other health professional. The nurse is the keeper of the home, that is, where the patients sleep, keep belongings, meet with friends and family, and spend most of their time meditating, worrying, and applying skills learned in other therapies.

The nurse becomes host or hostess, mother or father, teacher, disciplinarian, friend, and confidant. Patients and nurses can seldom escape from one another. There are only a few scheduled times when nurses and patients are not together. They are always reunited at least for the hours chosen for bed rest. No health professional on the team other than the nurse has such prolonged periods of being directly responsible for patients.

Author's note: This chapter is an expression of personal beliefs based on personal experiences. It is presented from the frame of reference provided by the ways in which we strive to function at the Rehabilitation Institute of Chicago. The views may or may not represent those in other settings—none the less, for me they work.

REHABILITATION TEAM MEMBERS

The team in a totally comprehensive rehabilitation setting is made up of a diversity of persons. The team members are physicians, nurses, physical therapists, occupational therapists, recreational therapists, speech pathologists, social workers, psychologists, vocational counselors, and patients. Because the responsibilities of nurses on the rehabilitation team are discussed at length throughout this book, they will not be treated in detail here except in reference to the leadership role.

PHYSICIANS AND NURSES

The physician is the team leader. He or she should be trained in rehabilitation and is usually a physiatrist, although some neurologists, orthopedists, internists, and neurosurgeons function in this role. Whatever their specialty, physicians serve most effectively when they devote full time to the practice of rehabilitation. These full-time physicians become the final authority relative to the treatment of patients. They are responsible for ordering drugs, obtaining consultations, and writing orders for therapy, as well as for catalyzing and coordinating work of all team members. The physicians have final moral and legal responsibility for the patients.

The physician and the nurse have in common the problem of managing a group of persons all directing their attention to the patient. The physician directs a variety of nurses and allied health professionals. The nurse may direct other nurses as well as aides, orderlies, and ward clerks. Although housekeepers, elevator operators, and dietary workers are not directly responsible to the nurses, all these persons must be made to feel part of the alliance. Neither the nurse nor the physician can succeed simply by "directing" (ordering). Success of the team is dependent very much on the physician's and nurse's leadership ability as well as their actual scientific skill.

A major problem in rehabilitation medicine is that very little in their educational experience

CHAPTER 10   128

teaches health professionals how to manage or lead. They are frequently placed in leadership situations immediately out of school, with little preparation and no experience. Fortunately, some programs in medicine and nursing have now begun to cover management problems.

Professionals soon discover that it is necessary to delegate a great deal to others. Effectiveness in delegation of responsibility depends on the following:

1. Knowledge of the scientific facts
2. Understanding of the skills of the person to whom the task is delegated
3. Genuine respect for other individuals and for their ability and motives
4. Ability to listen
5. Simple good manners, such as habitually saying "please" or "thank you" when appropriate
6. Decisiveness
7. Ability and willingness to explain what others do not understand
8. Sufficient ego strength to admit mistakes and, when wrong, to correct an error
9. Willingness to ask the advice of others when necessary
10. Willingness and ability to set an example of competency and industriousness

There are more subtle characteristics, some indefinable. Some leaders with innate charisma bring out the best in all persons around them. Other brilliant scientists with good leadership skills convey confidence and strength even though they lack charisma. They can encourage persons around them to work and can utilize those persons to the utmost. Those leaders usually combine genuine caring, industriousness, imperturbability, and willingness to admit the limits of their knowledge. The first of these four characteristics—caring—is probably innate, but the other three can be learned.

Several characteristics can be totally disastrous for a leader attempting to manage a team: insecurity, self-righteousness, and condescension. An insecure person is likely to compensate in an irrational, unpredictable way and to disparage other team members in an effort to elevate his or her own self-esteem. Someone like this is unpleasant to work for or with, and morale suffers.

Self-righteousness, a characteristic not uncommon among persons in the medical field, interferes with medical treatment and with team morale. Self-righteousness implies a lack of humility and sensitivity. Both qualities are needed by anyone treating a patient, that is, by every team member. Self-righteous persons collaborate poorly because they have difficulty seeing others' points of view and cannot admit to being wrong.

Condescension is all too prevalent in medicine. Condescension irritates patients and has a disastrous effect on team members. Patients are infuriated by the "now shall we take our bath?" approach. In more subtle ways, tone of voice and gestures, as well as words, can convey condescension. Patients do not want to be treated like children (even if they are children) or as inferiors. Nor do team members. In some instances, condescension results from trying too hard. In this era, people are especially aware of the struggles on the part of women and minority groups. Some persons self-consciously and ineffectively try to be ingratiating to individuals with whom they may actually be uncomfortable or about whom they feel guilty. Their motives—wanting to be helpful and to "relate"—may be excellent, but they fail completely to achieve the desired result.

As previously stated, nurses must manage not only other nurses on their unit but also the aides and orderlies. Often these workers have been in the institutions longer than the nurses in charge. In some respects, they may know more about the details of patient care than the nurses initially do themselves. There may be differences in race and background between nurses, who still are likely to be white, and aides and orderlies, who frequently may be members of minority groups. A high degree of maturity is necessary to maintain the leadership role in such situations.

Nurses have to lead personnel responsible for the most intimate aspects of patient care, dealing with patients' fluctuations in motion and motivation. This can be extremely difficult and exhausting and may present a need for considerable counseling.

Nurses as leaders must have an underlying respect for their personnel. The latter are probably paid considerably less than nurses but have difficult and important jobs to perform. Nurses must exhibit no prejudice nor should they feel it in their hearts. If they do, it will become evident in moments of pressure. They must demonstrate proper care and be willing and strong enough to demand that each person perform to his or her maximum skill in offering the patient exactly what is needed. These leaders must not be intimidated by older and/or more outspoken personnel. They must be extremely sensitive to the strenuous and emotionally draining nature of the work of their subordinates.

Most importantly, nurses must be willing to reward financially (if possible), verbally, and by demeanor high levels of performance by people who work for them. Expressions of recognition should be offered both privately and publicly. Wherever possible, new and innovative ideas put forward by personnel should be absorbed into the system and the innovator given the credit. Less experienced nurse leaders may think that in order to move ahead they must take credit for all the good things that occur on their unit. They fail to realize that they can receive no greater credit than the recognition that their staff is industrious, clever, innovative, compassionate, and productive.

All members of the staff—nurses, aides, orderlies—must have a chance to display good skills and ideas to other team members. This can be done in conference, on rounds, or sometimes in special situations.

Earlier, I stated that the nurse is the pivotal member of the team. It is more accurate to say that the nursing team members are the pivot of the total team. A nurse in a rehabilitation setting who cannot get the most from subordinates by inspiration and leadership will not demonstrate great expertise and, most importantly, will not offer maximum care to patients.

The rehabilitation experience then is influenced very strongly by the leadership and management skills of the team leaders. The physician supervises the entire team, and the team nurse supervises several persons. Other team members may also have some supervisory responsibilities. For instance, physical therapists frequently collaborate with physical therapy aides and assistants and occupational therapists with occupational therapy aides.

It cannot be overemphasized that every team member is important to the success of a patient's treatment. Each team member should express in his or her own particular way admiration for the work of the other members and be attentive to their work and to their findings. The physician must play no favorites and must encourage all team members to express themselves, allowing no more time to one than to another. Compliments should be given freely whenever deserved, but the physician must try to avoid focusing on one perhaps particularly talented person. The shyer and less talented can be encouraged to become more secure and more productive by recognition of what they do accomplish.

A school of thought to which I do *not* adhere suggests that competition among team members is an important motivator. Certainly, a sense of competitiveness is present in almost everyone to varying degrees. Indeed, some persons develop great abilities and struggle to reach great heights simply because they want to be better than everyone else. To have on one's team someone with extraordinary talent and such a will to succeed can be very useful. If, however, concomitantly the person cannot bear to see anyone else succeed, is arrogant in success, puts his or her own goals above everyone else's goals, and is insensitive to the emotional needs of other team members, the results are disastrous. Every team member should want to achieve individual excellence. There are guidelines to such achievement, however, other than comparison to others and a need for competition. I believe that one can strive for a pure objective of high competency without trying to outdo someone else and in this way can be more valuable than the sheer competitors, who frequently are divisive and difficult to deal with.

At the risk of sounding frivolous, I propose that the work of a team together should be "fun." Team members deal with serious and admittedly tragic situations and patients. But to dwell continually on tragedy can be oppressive and eventually unproductive, whereas concentrating on the positive features in patients, team members, and the rehabilitation process is stimulating and exhilarating. The positive features of individual personalities should be encouraged and allowed expression. Humor, especially, should be encouraged and treasured.

In a comprehensive rehabilitation setting, each team member has specific functions with which all the other team members must be familiar. Team members need to understand one another as individuals and attempt to appreciate each one's ability, foibles, personality, and style.

PHYSICAL THERAPISTS

The physical therapists are the major strengtheners and exercisers. They may work with patients individually or in groups. Physical therapists deal with ambulation and other forms of mobility, bracing, and modalities such as heat, hydrotherapy, diathermy, ultrasound, paraffin, ultraviolet, and electrical stimulation. They implement prescriptions for braces, prostheses, wheelchairs, and other devices. Activities of daily living taught by physical therapists may include transferring, toilet activities, wheelchair use, and ambulation.

OCCUPATIONAL THERAPISTS

Occupational therapists train patients in activities of daily living related to dressing, eating, hygiene, and other aspects of self-care, as well as to household and domestic activities. These therapists also utilize various crafts and activities that may strengthen and enhance function and coordination. They may teach skills, such as typing, that not only increase independence but also may, or may not, lead to a vocation. For example, a patient may be taught to use a loom to exercise shoulder and arm muscles even though he or she has no thought of weaving as a career. Occupational therapists teach the implementation of hand splints and assistive devices such as those useful in dressing and eating. Also they do muscle and sensory evaluation and retraining. Sometimes they use special techniques, such as brushing and stroking.

RECREATIONAL THERAPISTS

All work and no play makes all of us very dull. There is no reason to assume that patients are an exception and that continual work and exercise alone can contribute to their happiness and satisfaction. Recreational therapists must determine the individual interests of a patient and try to make it possible for her or him to pursue interests in hobbies, sports, games, and other forms of diversion. Many opportunities are available within the institution, in special areas, or in the nursing unit. Perhaps even more significant is that therapists can help patients find recreational interests outside the hospital in the community. Patients may go to movies, plays, museums, sporting events, and community affairs in which able-bodied people also participate. Thus, patients obtain immediate gratification in the form of entertainment and are reminded that they will not be in a protected environment forever. They can learn how to overcome problems that may arise when they again live in the community. They have opportunities to "carry over" activities of daily living learned in the hospital environment.

SPEECH PATHOLOGISTS

Speech therapists retrain patients with articulation, hearing, and language problems. A patient may deal with an individual therapist or with groups and may use various machines for practice in relearning communication skills.

SOCIAL WORKERS

Handicapped people have problems in rejoining family and community life. Understanding and "treatment" of family members are absolutely essential if a given patient is to achieve maximum independence. Also, certain insights into a patient can only be obtained from family and friends. These are the areas with which social workers deal. Also, these workers counsel patients about problems with their families and help them find appropriate solutions.

PSYCHOLOGISTS

Obviously, if people become disabled, they develop psychological problems. For example, if someone suddenly becomes quadriplegic but does *not* become depressed, a psychological problem exists. In the case of brain-damaged patients, organic components must be considered. The psychologist on the team must appraise such factors, treat patients appropriately, and interpret findings and therapy to team members. Psychologists advise other team members about how to deal with patients during various phases of adjustment. They may need to interpret to team members their own capabilities and methods of coping with issues.

VOCATIONAL COUNSELORS

The work ethic in the United States is still alive and well. Directing disabled persons to jobs is a significant issue. They, in most instances, must be prepared early to recognize that an eventual goal is job placement or further education. Testing and interviewing permit patients' skills and motivations to be determined. Placement in appropriate jobs may then be possible.

CHAPLAIN

Even though there is not a preponderance of people today who feel that they are "religious," somehow when disaster strikes, the matter of religion and God recurs in the minds of most of those affected. Relative to the disabled population, the issues are likely to revolve around matters of miracle thinking; whether the onset of the disability represents retribution for some implied "sins"; matters of guilt relative to not having "pleased" God; and, of course, the inevitable question of "why" a God of goodness and kindness would allow such terrible things to occur. These are obviously complex issues, and it is absolutely essential to have a chaplain involved, one who has a broad ecumenical and sophisticated approach. It is important that he or she have a good knowledge of psychology; however, the primary thing is to understand well the matters of theology, dogma, and the Bible to which patients will be referring directly and unconsciously.

PATIENTS

The most important team member is the patient. The days when the patient was a passive partner are gone. No longer can blind faith be assured, nor should it be expected. As professionals, we all know our own inadequacies. Eventual success for patients in rehabilitation lies in their own hands; their destinies are within themselves. We give only tools for patients to use in trying to accomplish *their* goals. Patients should be led into this awareness gradually but early. If they long continue to feel that our supposed miraculous ways will make everything all right, they face shattering disillusionment, which can be extremely traumatic. Patients must be involved in planning their programs and learn in detail about their disabilities, the ways of accomplishing their goals, and the options available to them.

THE TEAM'S WORK

The success for the patient and the joy for the therapists relate very strongly to the degree to which diverse persons, the team members, can understand one another intellectually and emotionally. Each person needs to carry out her or his given task, of course, but with an eye and an ear to the segments of therapy that are the provinces of the others. For the nurse, this is more vital than for any other professional. If the physical therapist has trained a patient to transfer, the patient should probably be encouraged to practice transfer on the nursing unit and not be lifted into bed. If the occupational therapist has taught the patient to eat independently, nurses and aides should not feed the patient. If the psychologist has discovered some significant psychodynamic process, the nurse must know about it because much of the "acting out" occurs on the nursing unit, and patients probably talk more to employees there than in any other place. If the nursing department is treating a pressure sore, all other departments must take this into account when carrying out their activities with the patient.

How can this communication occur? How can information be exchanged? How can team members come to know and respect one another?

1. The physician must make rounds in physical and occupational therapy and on the nursing unit, accumulating information and transmitting it to appropriate individuals.
2. Written reports that become part of the chart should be read by all team members.
3. Informal contact, both directly and by telephone, is needed concerning new and/or especially significant developments in respect to a patient.
4. Informal social gatherings of team members are valuable.
5. Conferences should be the main means of accomplishing cohesion and exchanging facts and ideas.

At the conferences held each week, all team members discuss the progress and problems of every patient currently being treated. Here the physician's leadership ability must be displayed. The appropriate exchange of information must be assured. The following needs to be accomplished:

1. *Goal setting:* Specific goals for patients must be set by the entire team, with each member aware of the others' roles in accomplishing these goals. Goals must be reevaluated regularly so that the team can determine whether they are still realistic and/or whether they have been accomplished. Specific goals are important. Without them, it is too easy for the rehabilitation process to be prolonged unnecessarily. All professionals in the field can easily find themselves unrealistically proceeding with a plan and a program that meet their own needs for success but fail to represent valid goals for the patient.
2. *Presentations of findings in evaluations and in the process of therapy:* Every team member must learn to explain, as concisely and eloquently as possible, to other professionals the procedures that are being carried out. Too much detail is ponderous and irrelevant, so team members must develop skill in understanding the audience and outlining only what is essential.
3. *Documentation for referring physicians, agencies that will be following the patients, and third-party payers:* The proceedings of a conference must be documented in writing in terms that will be meaningful and valid for all persons concerned.
4. *Provision of an opportunity to enhance morale:* The physician directing the conference must be especially sensitive to the individuals participating. Shy members must be encouraged, and those who monopolize must be held in check. If a team member seems discouraged, depressed, or burdened by professional or personal problems, the physician must note this and give special attention to that person. Staff members with humor or ebullient personalities should be encouraged to let these qualities buoy the other members of the team. In addition to dealing with the facts about the patient, the leader must attend to more subtle aspects, being prepared to compliment and encourage when indicated and to note a need for

criticism, although a team member should be criticized at a later time and in private.
5 *Communication with patient and family:* There is no universal agreement as to whether patients or their families should be allowed to attend a conference. There is no question that the team members need to be more skillful in order to report directly to such a diversified audience. The team has what appears to be more complete freedom of discourse with only colleagues present. But the reality is simpler than it seems. It is actually quite rare for a comment to be made in a conference that a patient should not hear. Information concerning definite poor progress should not be discussed for the first time in conference. Such matters should be broached carefully and in private by the patient's physician and others and not mentioned starkly in a crowded room.

Some team members fear exhibiting disagreement in front of patients, but in reality the intervention of the patient in the discussion can frequently be helpful. The advantage is that the patient feels more of a participant in planning and decision making, an absolute essential in the rehabilitation process. Also, the conference is usually—or should be—an impressive display of talent and concern. Invariably, this is reassuring to the patient.

Some team members may worry that they will display their weaknesses or inadequacies at the conference. They are living with an illusion if they believe that such human characteristics can be hidden from the patients no matter how hard they try. In rehabilitation, the patients are very likely to gradually see us as we really are. If they attend conferences, it is unlikely that any visions of perfection will be shattered.

CONSULTANTS

There are physicians other than the attending one who are involved in the care of the patient, although the degree to which they become involved with the team varies. At the Rehabilitation Institute of Chicago, the consultant most actively and successfully involved with staff is the psychiatrist. Psychiatrists see patients but also meet with groups of nurses and team members to discuss problems concerning individual patients as well as to discuss issues of psychodynamics for the staff itself.

Consultants are called in at the request of the attending physician. It is important for the well-being of patients and for the sense of security of the whole team that such requests be made appropriately and expeditiously. It should certainly be well understood that cardiac problems should be treated by a cardiologist, that moderate to severe pressure sores should be evaluated by a plastic surgeon, that accute episodes in children should be treated by a pediatrician, and that most patients with spinal cord injuries should be followed by a urologist. Consultants usually advise the attending physician, who then orders the appropriate treatment.

FOCUS OF THE REHABILITATION EXPERIENCE—THE PATIENT

It perhaps seems unnecessary to remind any health professionals that in the rehabilitation experience, the patient must be the central object of focus. The actual human beings who are the patients must be observed and understood in relation to their total life structure and pattern. This means that the rehabilitation workers must understand not only the patients but also the family, sometimes the friends, the community, the religion, and all significant alliances and relationships the patients may have. Only then can appropriate and reasonable goals be set and achieved.

If this seems obvious, I must mention that there is no special magic or purity in the souls of those who work in health fields. Good character, industriousness, and kindness may appear to be more prevalent among health professionals than in the general population, but still some persons lack insight or ability in ways that can be detrimental to the well-being of the patients.

The rehabilitation experience can be more exciting and fulfilling than any other medical field, but it can be painful because, to be successful, one must do continual self-exploration. Rehabilitation team members must be sure that the goals set are for the patients and not really for themselves and that their behavior is indeed related to patients' needs, not simply designed to achieve elevation in the team hierarchy or to satisfy their own egos. Sometimes, these selfish goals can coincide with the best interests of the patients. It is necessary to know when this is so and when it is not.

CONCLUSION

This chapter has presented an overview of those persons involved in the rehabilitation experience. The task is complicated by the seriousness of its purpose, the range, degree, and mix of skills required, and the diversity of personalities assembled. The rewards are immeasurable.

11
don a. olson

cognition

INTRODUCTION

DEFINITION

Cognition has been defined as "the process of knowing or perceiving." This relatively simple dictionary definition in no way prepares the nurse, physician, or allied health worker for the problems of cognition in brain-damaged patients. Further, in the field of psychology, cognition has for years been left at essentially a philosophical level of understanding. There are literally hundreds of psychologic theories that are of great interest to the clinician but may have no relevance to an understanding of the relearning, perceiving, understanding, and knowing functions of a patient who has had a brain injury or a stroke.

A key word to understanding cognition in brain-damaged patients is reorganization. Cognitive abilities are redefined and reobtained as patients reorganize themselves physically, intellectually, emotionally, socially, and vocationally. The nurse and other health practitioners are interested in assisting patients to reorganize themselves in the most effective manner in order to maximize the cognitive potential they possess.

IMPLICATIONS FOR NURSING

As health practitioners who continually seek a scientific basis for clinical approaches to patients, nurses need appropriate knowledge so that they can devise the proper treatment for each patient and give needed encouragement, opportunity, and protection so the patient can succeed in the rehabilitation process. Evaluation of a brain-damaged patient's cognitive abilities and behavior is critical to the overall planning and eventual functioning of the patient. A nurse trained to observe the functional activities of the patient may be able to evaluate the patient's cognitive functioning more adequately than those professionals who depend solely on formal test measures. The more nurses know and understand about brain-damaged patients, the more efficient they will be as observers.

Early writings on brain-damaged individuals frequently stated that such patients demonstrated catastrophic behavior. When the behavior was analyzed, its cause was more frequently the interaction between the health practitioner and the patient than organic conditions. A lack of understanding by nurses of brain-damaged patients and their learning functioning often affects patients' total adjustment and their eventual rehabilitation accomplishments. The individuality and the particular problems of each patient must be understood by the health practitioner if the patient is to succeed in any rehabilitation program. Again, the nurse who is in constant contact with patients is the one with the best opportunity to achieve this understanding.

BRAIN TRAUMA/STROKE AND FUNCTIONING

When one reviews the literature on cognition and brain trauma, confusion and disagreement are evident. The medical view of the patient emphasizes the significance of the life-or-death situation but frequently does not consider the chronic implications of brain trauma. Disagreements within the fields of psychology, neurology, speech pathology, and other disciplines concerned with brain-damaged individuals contribute to the health practitioners' confusion. Unfortunately, at the end of all this confusion are the patients. Whether brain damage has resulted from trauma or from a stroke, the patients previously functioned in a variety of ways with a variety of skills which may or may not be available to them now. The nurse attempts to relate medical findings on a patient to the cognitive functions that the patient demonstrates. To do this, it is necessary to understand all the processes by which the patient receives sensory input and how that sensory input is transferred, reduced, elaborated, stored, recovered, and eventually used for life and living.

The brain-injured individual is a complicated individual. Another key word to understanding is *individuality*. Although clinicians attempt to categorize disabilities and understand the psychology of each disability, nurses cannot lose track of the unique aspects of each human being and the unique skills, past learning experiences, environmental, social, and family influences that have made that individual.

Patients suffering from brain trauma and those who have had various types of strokes present somewhat similar yet very different syndromes. Clinically, individuals with head injuries make a better recovery than those suffering from various types of strokes or cerebrovascular incidents. The recovery stages may be similar, but the individual with brain trauma frequently goes through the recovery stages more rapidly and reaches higher levels of reorganization following the trauma than does the stroke patient or the patient with a cerebrovascular accident.

Kertesz and McCabe state " . . . posttraumatic aphasia seems to have a more benign course, and somewhat surprisingly dramatic spontaneous recovery was noted. One of our young patients was considered a global aphasic, but recovered to a mild anomic state, a phenomenon not seen in infarcts and other vascular lesions with this extent of initial language development. Complete recovery was seen in more than half of the traumatic cases." Hebb has been instrumental in the neurophysiological and neuropsychological approach to understanding recovery of cognition and to understanding disorganization and development. Hebb's theory of homeostasis further gives important understanding to the controls an individual must maintain in attempting to regain learning and cognitive functioning. Each individual must find a "comfort level" for reorganization, a level that does not overstimulate or overfatigue the neuromechanism. A primary factor the nurse needs to understand in observing and evaluating the brain-damaged patient is the patient's response to all learning situations. Specifically, it is necessary to determine the level at which the patient can react comfortably and does not show signs of overstimulation of fatigue.

An individual's brain injury has been observed clinically to go through several stages of recovery.

Stage 1 Following the trauma, the patient's total system is essentially in shock, and it is impossible to observe the effects of input and output. The question is whether the patient will live or die. The primary need is for medical and nursing expertise and management to maintain life and prevent complications. Luria stated in 1963 that recovery from brain trauma is hypothesized as being the diminution of shock to the brain system and spontaneous recovery, the substitution of new areas for destroyed or damaged areas of the brain, or a total reorganization of cellular structure. The length of time that the patient takes to move from one stage to the next is frequently an important indicator of eventual potential and prognosis. The time spent in Stage 1 appears to be critical in determining the eventual level which the patient's cognitive functioning will achieve.

Stage 2 The patient appears to be in touch with self, if not with the environment. Close observation of the patient reveals a recognition and an awareness of self in this new and frightening setting. During this stage, the patient's fear and anxiety and the extent of injury can prevent further progress.

Stage 3 The patient shows signs of comprehension and understanding. The receptive ability of the patient may be on a one-word level and in a one-to-one situation. That is, the nurse may say "water," and the patient may understand "water" and give a nod or some eye motion that indicates awareness and need. If the nurse says, "Do you want water?" at this stage, the sentence may be far more than the patient can understand. The ability to comprehend and to understand increases slowly. Frequently it goes from one word with a gesture to one word alone, to short phrases, to sentences, and from one-to-one situations to understanding of family members, and eventually to comprehension of small groups.

The receptive and comprehension capabilities of the patient are a strong indicator of the prognosis for language and learning functioning.

CHAPTER 11   138

The nurse should be especially alert to the patient's ability to understand and to the patient's frustration or success in the variety of situations in the hospital setting. There may be little or minimal expressive or spoken language at this stage of recovery.

Stage 4 Patients may be able to express themselves in slow labored speech or may be able to express themselves with a few simple nouns. Other patients may be totally unable to express themselves orally because of motor involvement of the oral musculature. However, observation of the patients will reveal more intact inner speech but difficulty in oral expression. All levels and types of expression should be accepted and encouraged. Nurses should attempt to relate to patients in the same manner they would have related to them before the stroke. The more quiet and controlled is the nurse's speech, the more comfortable will patients feel in their attempts to communicate.

Stage 5 The fifth and final stage in recovery is the highest level the patient can achieve. Higher cognitive functioning, such as reading, spelling, arithmetic, and writing, may be present. These higher cognitive functions need a strong basis of receptive and expressive language and greatly depend on successful passage through the early recovery stages. Further, these levels of cognitive function require considerably more neurological organization and motivation on the patient's part. The patient's interest in any of these higher language functions is in itself an extremely encouraging sign. It must be understood, however, that recognizing words or family members' names on get-well cards is far different from understanding a newspaper article or being able to read a brief article in a magazine. It is necessary to observe the different levels of reading, writing, spelling, or arithmetic to determine the patient's cognitive abilities.

In the management of patients with brain trauma or stroke, a continuing error of the health practitioner is the tendency to overstimulate them. A patient is delayed in passing through the stages of recovery far too frequently because of poor management, the confusion and noise in the large hospital setting, the intrusion of large numbers of health personnel, the overwhelming concern of family members, and frequent visits by too many friends. In many cases, the patient is completely frustrated. A structured environment, in which restimulation can occur at a concrete, slow rate that is comfortable for the patient, results in more rapid recovery and higher levels of attainment following brain trauma.

Four basic deterrents to the redevelopment of cognitive skills in the individual with head injury are:

1. Neurological dysfunction
2. Sensory deprivation
3. Experiential deprivation
4. Emotional disorganization

All four factors are interrelated, and the nurse must be aware of the potential of the patient in each of these areas.

1. *Neurological dysfunction* must be evaluated to determine the degree medically and functionally. Time is a major factor. The patient who recovers rapidly following the cerebral accident frequently is the best candidate for long-range improvement in cognitive skills. However, recent clinical observation has shown that individuals with brain injury do continue to improve in cognitive ability many years after the cerebral insult. The amount and location of the neurological damage will, of course, be important factors in type and degree of involvement demonstrated by the patient.

Sensory deprivation can be as dramatic as visual and hearing problems or as subtle as a lack of sensation in parts of the body. Such problems disturb the patient and contribute to inability to attend to tasks.

Experiential deprivation is of even more concern. Brain damage resulting from trauma and stroke isolates individuals. Because of the isolation, stimulation needed for relearning is limited. Frequently, staff in the acute hospital or in the long-term care center, and the family of the stroke or trauma victim, are confused by the patient's speech, language, and learning. They may prefer to have little contact, and the patient is often shuttled to an isolated spot in the hospital, long-term care center, or home. Lack of appropriate and structured stimulation can be as debilitating and damaging as overstimulation, which was discussed earlier.

Emotional disorganization must also be considered. The patient is frightened, anxious, and confused by a new status. The length of time this confusion, fear, and anxiety last partly determines how well cognitive functioning redevelops.

The nurse must understand that the patient who incurs a cerebrovascular incident due to embolism, aneurysm, other systemic problems, or severe head injury presents a disruption of the major aspects of functioning, physically, intellectually, communicatively, socially, and emotionally. Of great importance is the patient's ability to take in information and to process needed skill knowledge. The reorganization of information and processing for the patient can be better understood if the nurse is aware of the stages of redevelopment. Each stage necessitates structured input and guarding against overstimulation. If the nurse can assist in bringing the patient through Stage 1 to Stage 2, then up the recovery ladder by an understanding of unique and individual responses to at first very limited and structured stimuli, the prognosis for recovery is improved.

ASSESSMENT OF COGNITION

INFORMAL EVALUATION

The nurse must be particularly aware of patients' individual medical problems and symptoms. The general medical condition of patients following a stroke greatly affects their ability to function in cognitive areas. For example, patients frequently complain of headaches or pain, which can affect motivation and the patients' ability to respond to cognitive activities. Dr. John Eisenson has described the brain-damaged adult as being "inefficient" in the ability to respond to cognitive areas. This inefficiency is frequently the result of medical aspects as well as of the symptomatology which develops from the brain trauma. Factors such as the motor involvement resulting from the cerebrovascular incident, seizures, and the effects of medication affect the patient's ability to respond. When the nurse is aware of all of these factors, much of the nursing behavioral analysis and informal testing of the patient can be even more significant than formal test measures.

The patient's ability to respond to cognitive areas can be determined by an informal evaluation of ability to understand. For example, it should be noted whether the patient can understand gestures, vocal inflections, and facial expressions. The nurse is alert to the patient's response to single words and to simple sentences about the environment and to an awareness of and ability to follow conversations with the family. Further, the nurse can investigate the patient's basic cognitive ability if the patient can communicate by gesturing effectively and by using appropriate facial expressions and automatic words. When the patient reaches a level of being able to use "yes" and "no" correctly, that patient is showing improvement and progression through the stages of recovery. Obviously the sooner the patient uses single words, incomplete sentences, or brief telegraphic-type speech the better. When the patient shows ability to converse, interest in reading, and interest in hospital activities, the nurse is aware of important information regarding cognitive functioning which can be applied in a formal test situation.

The nurse who attempts to understand the patient's cognitive abilities not only investigates the area of intelligence but also formally evaluates some of the special disabilities resulting from a cerebrovascular incident, along with personality, educational achievement, and vocational interests and aptitudes.

The medical history provided by the physician, the informal observation provided by the nurse, and the results of formal testing form the basis

CHAPTER 11   140

for the evaluation of a patient's cognitive potential.

FORMAL TESTING

The nurse must be aware of the factors that may affect the patient's ability to take formal tests. The fatigue factor is a major consideration. Patients suffering from brain damage can be tested only for very short periods of time. The patient with brain damage has difficulty in attending to and concentrating on the kinds of tasks presented in formal psychological and cognitive testing. Anxiety, fatigue, tension, and ability to concentrate must all be considered and evaluated by the health practitioner before the patient is subjected to formal testing, or at least before the results of formal testing are taken seriously.

It is also important that the patient rest properly before taking any tests and that the environment be free from distraction, noise, and visual confusion.

Formal tests of intelligence may be administered to establish the patient's intellectual capacity and function. After brain trauma, the tests can be helpful, indicating the degree of deterioration, the type of impairment, and the emotional reaction the patient has to the changed intellectual function. Observation of the patient as the test is taken is frequently more important than the test scores themselves. The patient's response to tests and the ability to handle test items, the degree of frustration demonstrated, the amount of anxiety, and the length of time it takes to complete tasks may, in the long run, be more important to the health practitioner than the actual test results. However, formal tests such as the Wechsler Adult Intelligence Scale can provide information to assist the health practitioner. This test, like all formal tests, has its limitations because of the problems that frequently result from brain trauma, that is, communication problems or motor problems that make it difficult for the patient to respond, to point to, or manipulate pieces of a puzzle or blocks or objects that are part of these tests.

The Vineland Maturity Scale is a tool which should not be neglected and should be available to the nursing staff. The scale evaluates the patient's level of functioning in self-help, motor ability, communication, self-direction, and other areas of significance to cognitive functioning. Tests result in a "social quotient" that is helpful in determining a developmental level of the patient's functioning in everyday activities.

The psychologist evaluating a patient with brain trauma can use formal tests of intelligence. A neuropsychological evaluation is of primary importance for a total understanding of the patient and the patient's cognitive potential. The health practitioner must work closely with the neuropsychologist in order to understand what the various test measures mean. The health practitioner must be very careful not to regard an isolated score as an indication of the patient's true potential. Frequently, the test result reflects only the patient's ability to respond to the test at a particular time. The test result may or may not be an exact indication of the patient's potential for learning or of eventual intellectual level.

Tests which can evaluate special disabilities or special areas relating to brain trauma and brain injury are frequently needed. The brain-damaged individual may have difficulty in the areas of memory, reasoning, judgment, and visual and auditory perception. These areas can be evaluated informally, but formal tests can be provided as part of a neurologic evaluation. Among the classic tests is the Bender Visual-Motor Gestalt Test. It consists of nine geometric forms, each drawn in black on a small white card. The patient is asked to copy each of the forms on a sheet of unlined paper, using a pencil. The test is used as a screening device to indicate the presence of several levels of regression, organic brain pathology, or social and emotional problems. As in all tests with adult brain-damaged patients, the patient's reaction to the test is of primary importance. Therefore, the health practitioner is wise to note the comments, the nonverbal interaction, and other responses the patient may give to the test.

Patients suffering from brain trauma frequently

show more problems in immediate and short-term memory than they do in long-term memory. Memory is, however, one of the least understood neurological and psychological phenomena. Emotional or organic factors, as well as anxiety, depression, and other factors, greatly affect the patient's response to memory test items. The Detroit test of learning has many simple memory tests for both auditory and visual evaluation. Sections of the Wechsler and other test batteries are also helpful in the evaluation of memory. Discussion with the patient, who is requested to recall daily activities or events which happened a week ago or immediately following the stroke, can be beneficial to the health practitioner attempting to evaluate a patient's degree of memory dysfunctioning.

In some settings, patients with traumatic brain injury and/or stroke are submitted to tests of personality, such as the Rorschach Projected Drawing Test and the Thematic Aperception Test. These tests are known to be of small use with patients having limited involvement and therefore are almost valueless for use with patients having brain injury. Traumatic brain injury causes a release of inhibitions, and part of the rehabilitative and recovery process is in regaining inhibition and self-control. Observation of improvement with time in personality areas is frequently a more fruitful indication of recovery than is formal personality testing. Authorities working with brain-damaged individuals believe that, clinically, the best information about personality adjustment of the patient can be obtained through interviews with friends and family members and through observation of the patient in training and rehabilitation settings.

MOTOR AND GNOSTIC ABILITIES

Brain trauma frequently results in hemiplegia and/or hemiparesis. This aspect of the patient's posttraumatic syndrome is often observed in the form of either a flaccid body part or a developing spastic body part. Lack of function is attributed to paralysis due to the brain damage, and recovery varies greatly from patient to patient.

Less well understood are motor deficits and knowledge deficits because the patient's inability to carry out a function solely as a result of brain dysfunction is not purely a motor deficit. The terms *apraxia* and *agnosia* have been given by the medical profession to this type of malfunctioning. Aphasia, which frequently results from brain trauma or cerebrovascular incident, was described earlier in this chapter in more detail. Aphasia is predominantly a language disorder, but since it is rarely confined simply to the language processes, it involves the entire individual. It permeates the patient's intellectual, psychological, social, vocational, and emotional makeup. Aphasic, apraxic, and agnostic factors are closely intermingled and are difficult to diagnose as separate entities. In apraxia, the patient may not be able to use the oral musculature, arm, hand, or leg in a purposeful and intended way. There is no paralysis per se, but the patient is unable to carry out the motor act. For example, the patient may not know how to appropriately use a washcloth. The patient may grasp the fork or spoon and not know what to do with it. In the area of speech and language, there may be difficulty in finding the correct location for specific speech sounds. Apraxia can also affect the patient's ability to gesture or pantomime. Agnosia is frequently found in patients with receptive difficulties, but apraxia is related to an impairment of perception or expression of symbols. In agnosia, the patient has difficulty in evaluating objects or representations of objects. The patient does not recognize objects and simply does not know what they are.

Motor and gnostic difficulties can confuse the nurse and give a poorer impression of the patient's functioning levels than is, in fact, warranted. Close observation of and feedback from the patient will reveal problems of this nature and separate them from other brain and learning disabilities.

THOUGHT, THINKING, ACTING

As stated, brain injuries do not always result in disturbances of intellectual activity such as retardation or loss of functional behavior areas. The great majority of brain-damaged individuals have the potential to restore active thinking following injury. Appropriate nursing care, medical care, therapy, a supportive family, and a stimulating environment are critical to the reestablishment of active thought, thinking, and acting following brain trauma. The individual with physical limitations can still be alert, can contribute to society, and enjoy a high quality of life. Clinical impressions of restoration of active thinking suggest that the most recovery goes on in the first year following the cerebral insult, but clinical observations have documented changes and improvements in thought, thinking, and acting in patients many, many years following these cerebral incidents.

Importantly, some severe brain traumas result in global problems and general retardation. However, this does not happen in the majority of cases. More than likely, the nurse will observe in the patient a reduction in spontaneous thought, a reduction in abstract thinking, and an overall inefficiency in thought, thinking, and acting processes.

A patient may present no immediately observable disturbances in mental functions. There may be good articulation of words, good understanding of what people are saying, perhaps even an ability to read and write; however, closer discussion may reveal that the patient has great difficulty in thinking and that it takes an extraordinary amount of time to organize thinking and thoughts for appropriate response and action. Neurologically we do not know the mechanism of actively flowing thought. However, clinical evidence has suggested that a reorganization of functional support systems for thinking and thought is possible following brain trauma.

Observation of the patient's thinking and thought processes is relatively easy. The nurse, encouraging the patient to relate an incident and a story, may observe that the patient cannot do it alone but can do it with some assistance; that is, if the nurse gives the patient a beginning word and completes a sentence, the patient is assisted in development of the narrative. This practice and stimulation is frequently productive for the patient and assists in restoring active thinking. An active speech and therapy program for this type of patient is always profitable.

The nurse may stimulate patients' thought processes through encouraging them to discuss their immediate environment, their families, and the daily schedule they are involved in. Patients need to look for points of support in their environment and with the people they talk with. As they once again become active in the speech and language area, they are more able to lay the foundation for reorganizing the active flow of thought which was beyond their capacity at the beginning recovery stages.

SPEECH AND LANGUAGE

Human speech is a complex functional system. Cortical areas attributed to speech functioning occupy a large portion of the left hemisphere. Communication and speech ability themselves are a source of mental stimulation. A human being has a basic need to communicate and gains much pleasure and mental stimulation from the practice of communication itself. Individuals with brain injury need sufficient time to organize their thought processes for verbalization. The speech and language potential observed may increase if the nurse gives the patients maximum time to speak, does not interrupt them, and does not confuse them by attempting to give them the words the nurse thinks they want to say. Language potential may also be greater if the nurse accepts the level of communication patients are capable of at that specific time. Further, responding to all patients in an adult fashion and with the dignity they deserve can do much to further elicit speech. Speech is encouraged when the nurse speaks to patients in a normal voice and responds to them much as to peers and colleagues.

Patients with brain trauma frequently do not learn because they are not put in appropriate situations for relearning. For example, patients placed in a nursing home may be alone much of the time, or they may be with patients who do not talk or communicate, or they may not have the benefit of good role models to follow in speech and language. Brain trauma impedes the natural communication process. Patients are confused; speech and language are difficult. They therefore, often withdraw readily from speech and language situations. The nurse must slowly and with great care reintroduce them to language and speech through one-to-one language situations, comfortable group situations, and eventually to the regular activities of the nursing home. Placing patients in front of a noisy television set can be overwhelming and overstimulating. Placing them next to talkative and interested fellow patients can serve as the needed stimulus for alert, interested patients. The nurse must constantly be cautious about overstimulating brain-damaged patients. The goal is to provide a setting which produces the maximum stimulation that patients can take at that point in their recovery.

HIGHER LANGUAGE FUNCTIONING

It is imperative that all diagnostic studies be completed so that a total plan can be made for a patient's rehabilitation. These studies include the medical diagnosis, the psychological study, and therapeutic evaluations. Further, measurements in the areas of higher language functioning, such as reading, writing, spelling, and arithmetic, are frequently needed.

Many tests are available, but, again, informal tests can prove to be the most beneficial. A patient's interest in the newspaper, attempts to read the headlines, and, more important, ability to comprehend what has been read can be easily ascertained by the nurse.

Many tests must be adapted for the brain-damaged individual. For example, the Wide Range Achievement Test is brief and a good, effective screening measure. However, it is presented in very small print; sometimes the size of the letters must be increased so that the patient can truly be evaluated. As well as being simple and quickly administered, the test screens some of the simplest to some of the most complex levels of achievement in reading, spelling, and arithmetic. The test is standardized so that it provides age norms, grade norms, and quotients similar to intelligence quotients; the norms are broadly applicable. Again, the nurse must understand that the scores are indicative only of the patient's ability to perform at that particular time; they do, however, suggest the level of comfort and efficiency in reading, spelling, and arithmetic.

The importance of this type of testing varies with the interest or capability of the patient. Not all patients are equally interested in reading, spelling, or arithmetic functioning. An accountant who had a recent head injury will be greatly frustrated by lack of ability. Motivation and response to other therapeutic measures may be enhanced by an understanding of limitations in the areas of arithmetic, spelling, and reading, and by observation of some progress in these areas.

MOTIVATION FOLLOWING DISTURBANCE OF COGNITION

Disturbance of brain function does not show consistent recovery in all patients. Patterns vary in patients suffering from a cerebrovascular incident or a stroke, as well as in patients suffering from brain trauma as a result of accident or injury. In some cases, cognitive functioning is restored rapidly and only minimal residual problems are revealed through formal and informal testing. In other patients, cognitive delays occur for extended periods of time. And in many cases, permanent limitations of cognition occur which affect the patient's social, emotional, language, and adjustment capabilities.

The patient who shows initiative is the most encouraging patient for health practitioners. The patient who is anxious to improve, who desires rehabilitation, and is anxious for therapy is not only encouraging to health practitioners but also will probably demonstrate more gain of cognitive ability over time. The self-starting patient is the desired patient. Indications of this ability are yet another evaluation the nurse can make to determine readiness for therapy and for more complicated sensory and motor input for the patient.

Many factors affect the patient's motivation. The amount of brain damage revealed through medical testing, the degree and number of physical and secondary medical factors which may or may not persist, and the age of the patient all must be considered. It is hypothesized that the brain of a younger person has more recovery powers and can compensate more effectively than can the more aged patient. However, other less well-defined areas may also affect recovery.

Motivation of the patient toward recovery is as yet understood only in a limited manner. Critical aspects affecting motivation may be summarized as follows:

1. The patient with self-motivation and self-starter abilities is a better candidate for a rehabilitation program and will no doubt achieve greater gains in the program.
2. Motivation sometimes is easier to instill in the patient who was a well-adjusted individual before the accident; that is, the patient whose premorbid psychologic structure was one of organization, direction, and self-motivation will probably also be the better candidate for reorganization and regrowth of cognitive ability and skills.
3. Motivation is frequently influenced by the timing of therapies to promote cognitive functioning. Early intervention of physical, occupational, and speech therapy can give the patient immediate support and contribute to the development of self-motivation.
4. The patient who has strong family support and continued interest of family members will be better motivated for cognitive development. Family support must be encouraged to be supportive in accepting the patient at the current level of recovery.
5. Motivation is greatly affected by the patient's own past interest in and response to cognitive functioning. The patient who was a well-read and highly verbal person will frequently be more motivated than the one who was previously not interested in learning functions.

Cognition, however, must be considered both a verbal and nonverbal activity, and aspects of both verbal and nonverbal learning must be evaluated. If the nurse or therapist can find areas of reorganization and relearning in which the patient can be successful, a basis for future cognitive development can be established.

In medical, nursing, and allied health support of the patient, the attempt is to assist and to reorganize remaining skills, to redevelop lost skills, and to make progress in recovery in a step-by-step redevelopment. Individual involvement in this process is critical, and the patient's motivation and interest in the recovery process must be understood.

RESEARCH NEEDS

With brain injuries and strokes occurring more frequently and in much younger patients, medical, allied health, and nursing research in the area is critically needed in order to maximize the potential of patients. Nurses could consider research in the following areas, as they relate specifically to the relearning ability of patients with brain injuries.

Clinical Research and Clinical Documentation The nurse is in an excellent position to document (1) scheduling as it relates to the patient's ability to handle cognitive aspects of the environment, (2) the effects of the environment on patients and their learning abilities; and (3) the effects of a coordinated team approach on the patient's ability to learn. The overstimulation of the hospital rehabilitation setting that results from confused scheduling, lack of coordination between team members, and confusion in the environment can adversely affect the patient's recovery and ability to relearn.

Stages of Recovery Observation by nurses and allied health workers has suggested that recovery from brain damage goes on for a much longer period of time than was previously thought. The nurse frequently is in a position to observe changes in patients when they return for re-evaluations. Evaluations of cognitive aspects should be considered not only during the early months of the patient's recovery but also a year or two after the original brain insult.

The nurse who sees the patient on a regular basis is in a better position than other rehabilitation workers to observe the diminution of psychological factors, such as withdrawal symptoms, unrealistic euphoria, perseveration, and echolalia, which are secondary effects of brain damage but which directly affect relearning. Working with the psychologist and the physician, the nurse can contribute much to the understanding of the basic deterrents to normal relearning and cognitive functioning..

Understanding Motivation and Self-initiation for the Brain-Damaged Individual Brain injury adversely affects the patient's self-motivation and self-initiation of cognitive tasks. Neurological dysfunctioning is a factor, but patients also need psychological support, some more than others.

The nurse, aware of many of the aspects of brain injury which contribute to poor learning, has an opportunity to document this information and provide important clinical findings. These can be highly relevant to a patient's overall recovery and eventual ability to handle learning more comfortably.

CONCLUSION

Understanding the cognitive abilities of the brain-damaged individual is difficult. Disagreement among professionals concerning types of intervention and therapies which will assist the redevelopment of cognition causes confusion. The nurse is in a unique position to help the patient to develop cognitive functioning to the maximum. The nurse's understanding of the patient's age, physical condition, sensory integrities, language abilities, years of past schooling, emotional and motivational factors may be more significant than the results of formal tests.

The main goal for all patients is to become functioning social beings. This can be achieved only if all diagnostic areas are integrated. One professional alone cannot comprehensively evaluate cognition. The team approach has been shown through the years to be the most effective means for such an evaluation. The medical findings, the neurologic findings, and the informal observational findings must be coordinated so that it is possible to plan a rehabilitation program that will result in an increased ability to relearn.

Health practitioners deal with many factors when they work with patients with brain trauma, stroke, and aphasia. Their concern is with the nature of the problem as it affects the individual and with how each patient can relearn lost abilities. In daily contacts with the patient, nurses must constantly observe how the problem appears to be affecting the individual's ability to learn. A cerebrovascular incident results in a loss of ability to function. Some areas may be totally lost, but other areas can compensate for loss. All levels of learning are affected—verbal deficiency, nonverbal deficiencies, and symbolic and nonsymbolic areas. Patients may have difficulty with speaking, reading, writing, arithmetic, spelling, counting, comprehending what is said to them, or recognizing objects.

The multiple aspects of loss of ability to function must be considered as rehabilitation for the patient is planned. Nursing care, physical therapy, speech pathology, and the maintenance of health are all part of the plan for the patient. The potential for rehabilitation is the level of cognitive functioning an individual is capable of reaching under specific conditions. The nurse needs to understand the variables, such as the specific characteristics of impairments, the underlying pathology for functional limitations, the residual capabilities, and the prognosis for improvement. The patient's understanding of the problem, reaction to it, and motivation are also highly important. Further, environmental conditions, family support, and other areas affect the patient's recovery in cognitive functioning.

The nurse can be a primary resource for the identification of learning problems and so assist the patient to become a more efficient learner. More importantly, the nurse can help determine the patient's readiness for growth of cognitive ability by skilled observation of behavior. The patient will be more able to achieve maximum development of cognitive ability when the nurse understands the uniqueness of that patient and that patient's learning ability, learning pattern, and learning levels.

BIBLIOGRAPHY

Ault, Ruth L.: *Children's Cognitive Development,* Oxford Univ. Press, New York, 1977.

Chernigovskĭy, V. N., and Donald B. Lindsley (eds.): *Interoceptors,* American Psychological Assn., Washington, D.C., 1967.

Cunningham, Michael: *Intelligence, Its Organization and Development,* Academic Press, New York, 1972.

Eisenson, J.: "Language Rehabilitation of Aphasic Adults: Some Observations on the State of the Art," *Folia Phoniatr* 29(1):61–83, 1977.

Elkind, David, and John H. Flavell: *Studies in Cognitive Development,* Oxford University Press, New York, 1969.

Estes, W. K. (ed.): "Attention and Memory," in *Handbook of Learning Cognitive Processes,* vol. 4, Laurence Erlbaum Associates, Hillsdale, N.J., 1976.

Gainotti, Guido, and Camello Tiacci: "The Relationships Between Disorders of Visual Perception and Unilateral Spatial Neglect," *Neuropsychologia* 9:451, 1971.

Gardner, Howard: "The Loss of Language," *Hum Nature* 76: March 1978.

———: *The Shattered Mind,* Knopf, New York, 1975.

Glista, Sandra, Anita Halper, and Kayte Nowikowski: "Language Rehabilitation in Patients with Non-Dominant Hemisphere Lesions," paper presented at the Convention of the Illinois Speech and Hearing Association, 1977.

Goldstein, Kurt: *Aftereffects of Brain Injuries in War,* Grune & Stratton, New York, 1942.

Gurdjian, E. S.: *Head Injury from Antiquity to the Present with Special Reference to Penetrating Head Wounds,* Charles C Thomas, Springfield, Ill., 1973.

Hebb, D. O.: "Physiological Learning Theory," *J Abnorm Child Psychol* 4(4):309–314, 1976.

Hilgard, Ernest R.: *Theories of Learning,* Appleton-Century-Crofts, New York, 1948.

Hirschberg, Gerald G., Leon Lewis, and Patricia Vaughan: *Rehabilitation,* 2d ed., Lippincott, Philadelphia, 1976.

Hooper, Reginald: *Patterns of Acute Head Injury,* Williams & Wilkins, Baltimore, 1969.

Kertesz, Andrew, and Patricia McCabe: "Recovery Patterns and Prognosis in Aphasia," *Brain* 100:1, 1977.

Kimura, Doreen: "Temporal Lobe Damage," *Arch Neurol* 8:264–271, 1963.

Klocke, Joleen: "The Role of Nursing Management in Behavioral Change of Hemiplegia," *J Rehabil* 24: July-August, 1969.

Kreitler, Hans, and Shulmith Kreitler: *Cognitive Orientation and Behavior,* Springer, New York, 1976.

Langley, L. L.: *Homeostasis: Origins of the Concept,* Dowden, Hutchinson & Ross, Stroudsberg, PA, 1973.

Lezak, Muriel D.: *Neuropsychological Assessment,* Oxford University Press, New York, 1976.

Luria, A. R.: *Cognitive Development: Its Cultural and Social Foundations,* Harvard University Press, Cambridge, Mass., 1976.

———: *Restoration Function After Brain Injury,* Macmillan, New York, 1963.

McLaurin, Robert L.: *Head Injuries—Proceedings*

Miller, George A.: *Language and Communication,* McGraw-Hill, New York, 1951.

Neisser, U.: *Cognitive Psychology,* Appleton-Century-Crofts, New York, 1967.

Newcombe, F., and W. Ritchie Russell: "Dissociated Visual Perceptual and Spatial Deficits in Focal Lesions of the Right Hemisphere," *J Neurol Neurosurg Psychiatry* 32:73–81, 1969.

Ornstein, Robert: "The Split and the Whole Brain," *Hum Nature* 76: May, 1978.

Reitman, Walter R.: *Cognition and Thought,* Wiley, New York, 1966.

Sarbin, Theodore R., Ronald Taft, and Daniel Bailey: *Clinical Inference: Cognitive Theory,* Holt, Rinehart & Winston, New York, 1960.

Sarno, John E., and Martha Taylor Sarno: "The Diagnosis of Speech Disorders," *Med Clin North Am* 53(3):561–573, 1969.

Schroeder, Oliver, Jr. (ed.): "The Head: A Law-Medicine Problem," *Proceedings of the Institute of Law-Medicine,* Western Reserve University, Cleveland, Ohio, 1957.

Strub, Richard L., and F. William Black: *The Mental Status Examination in Neurology,* Davis, Philadelphia, 1977.

Travis, Lee Edward (ed.): *Handbook of Speech Pathology,* Appleton-Century-Crofts, New York, 1957.

Weinberg, Joseph, Leonard Diller, Wayne A. Gordon, Louis Gerstman, Abraham Lieberman, Phylis Lakin, Germaine Hodges, and Ora Ezrachi: "Visual Scanning Training Effect on Reading-Related Tasks in Acquired Right Brain Damage," *Arch Phys Med Rehabil* 58:479–486, 1977.

Wicklund, Robert A., and Jack W. Brehm: *Perspectives on Cognitive Dissonance,* Wiley, New York, 1976.

12

anita s. halper
sandra oslager glista

speech and
language disorders
of neurological
origin in adults

INTRODUCTION

The utilization of speech and language is a "distinctively human ability to express new thoughts and to understand entirely new expressions of thought, within the framework of an 'instituted language' . . ." (Chomsky, 1968). Total loss of communicative ability alters a person's life, the interaction with others, self-image, and professional and psychological well-being immeasurably. Imagine, if you can, that you have lost your ability to communicate. Imagine that you can no longer understand what your spouse is saying or what the person next to you has just uttered. Try to envision an existence in which you cannot express ideas or desires, a life devoid of human interaction. If you can possibly conceive of this world of silence, isolation, and confusion, perhaps then you will appreciate the difficulties faced by the communicatively impaired individual.

The purpose of this chapter is threefold: first, to describe and define the speech and language problems that result from neurological injury; second, to describe the assessment procedures and general therapy techniques employed by the speech-language pathologist to evaluate speech and language; and third, to discuss management techniques that can be implemented by the nursing staff and taught to family members for carry-over into the home environment. It will include definitions of aphasia and dysarthria and will delineate the symptomatology for these disorders as well as for patients with right brain damage. The problem of counseling the patient and family toward acceptance of the communication impairment will be addressed.

NORMAL LANGUAGE AND SPEECH

LANGUAGE AND SPEECH

An understanding of normal speech and language processes is a prerequisite to conceptualizing the specific deficit areas that occur in the communication problems that will be described later. Language may be defined as a systematic set of symbols that are used for conveying needs, ideas, or feelings. Throughout the chapter, auditory comprehension, speech or oral expression, reading, writing, and gestures are all considered to be components of language. Speech and language are not viewed as synonymous terms and, therefore, are not used interchangeably. Speech is one aspect of language and may be defined as the communication of needs, ideas, or feelings in spoken words. The essential features of any language system of which speech is a component are phonemes, morphemes, syntax, and semantics. Phonemes are the distinctive sounds of speech such as *p* and *b*. Morphemes refer to the smallest unit of meaning within a word. All monosyllabic words, such as *so* and *to*, are single morphemes, but they are whole words. Some morphemes are prefixes and suffixes, such as *pre-* and *-ly*, while others such as *s* denote plural, possession, or verb tense. All morphemes contribute to the meaning of the word. Syntax or grammar refers to rules for structuring and ordering words within a sentence. Semantics is concerned with the meanings conveyed by words.

Normal language depends upon the effective functioning and integration of the receptor, central, and effector processes. The receptors receive the auditory or visual stimuli at the level of the ears or eyes. The stimuli are then coded into patterns of impulses which, after recoding and processing, arrive at the appropriate primary sensory areas of the cortex. These impulses are then coded into meaningful stimuli within the central processor. A response is subsequently activated by one of the effectors for speech, writing, or gestures in the motor areas of the cortex (National Institute of Health and Public Health Service, 1969).

NORMAL SPEECH PRODUCTION

Speech production requires the coordination of respiratory, laryngeal, pharyngeal, palatopharyngeal, lingual, mandibular, and labial musculature. Although it has not been possible to determine the exact number of muscles necessary for speech production, Lenneberg indicates that well over 100 muscles must be controlled centrally. "Since the passage from any one speech sound to another depends ultimately on differences in muscular adjustments, fourteen times per second, an 'order must be issued to every muscle,' whether to contract, relax, or maintain its tonus" (Lenneberg, 1967, pp. 91–92). Thus, the production of even a single word requires complex neuromuscular interaction.

A breath stream, produced by the expiratory muscles, is vibrated, interrupted, and shaped by a series of valves throughout the speech mechanism. Darley, Aronson, and Brown (1975) charted the flow of air through the laryngeal valve which vibrates the air and provides the dimensions of pitch, intensity, and quality of voice. The second valve consists of the posterior pharynx and velum or palatopharyngeal valve which may modify the resonating qualities of the speech sounds and provide the added dimension of nasality when appropriate. Further interruption or shaping of the air flow occurs at the lingual and labial valves as these articulators move in conjunction with each other, the teeth, and the hard palate in the oral cavity to produce recognizable vowels and consonants. The sounds are sequenced into words, phrases, and sentences using prosodic elements such as varying intensity, pitch, and rate, which provide the rhythmical patterns of our speech. Thus, the production of normal speech requires the coordination of these essential components of neuromuscular functioning.

APHASIA

BRIEF HISTORICAL REVIEW

Although loss of speech has been documented in the literature since the time of the ancient Egyptians (3000 and 2500 B.C.), it was only in the latter 19th century that the primary ideas reflected in current theories of aphasia were first postulated. In 1861, Paul Broca described a patient who understood speech but could not verbalize. Broca termed this disorder *aphemia* and concluded that it resulted from a lesion of the third frontal convolution (Schuell et al., 1964).

Carl Wernicke followed in 1874 by publishing his work on aphasia entitled, "The Symptom-Complex of Aphasia: A Psychological Study on an Anatomical Basis." He advocated the scientific study of aphasia and proposed a comprehensive theory of the neurological analysis of language functioning and dysfunctioning. He remains renowned for his descriptions of sensory (Wernicke's) aphasia resulting from a temporal lobe lesion and for his theories concerning other disorders, including conduction aphasia, pure word blindness, and pure word deafness among others (Geschwind, 1967b).

In contrast to Broca and Wernicke, who upheld the view that particular functions rely on specific parts of the brain, Hughlings Jackson felt that more empirical study was necessary before generalizations could be made about behavior, and specifically about speech and language. He postulated that aphasia was not a loss of words, but a loss of ". . . the ability to express relationships through 'propositions'. . . ." Henry Head (1963) thought of aphasia as an impairment in "symbolic formulation and expression." Jackson and his student Head remain noteworthy for their emphasis upon precise and objective observations of aphasic behavior (Schuell, 1964).

Goldstein (1948) studied the brain-damaged patient after World War I and advocated what he termed the "organismic approach to aphasia." His viewpoint emphasized *"that every individual speech-performance is understandable only from the aspect of its relation to the function of the total organism in its endeavor to realize itself as much as possible in the given situation"* [italics are Goldstein's]. He is also noted for distinguishing between concrete and abstract language and the respective impairment of each in aphasia.

Weisenburg and McBride (1964) contributed

to the study of aphasia through their comprehensive examinations of patients. On the basis of their study, they formulated four general groups of aphasics classified according to language behaviors: predominantly expressive, predominantly receptive, expressive-receptive, and amnesic.

After World War II, numerous investigators continued to study aphasia in an increasingly systematic manner. Wepman, Eisenson, and Luria are representative of modern investigators who developed evaluation procedures, expanded theoretical and behavioral observations, and researched the effectiveness of treatment. But it is beyond the scope of this chapter to further elucidate the historical and theoretical perspectives of aphasia. The interested reader is referred to the original sources listed in the bibliography.

DEFINITIONS OF APHASIA

Throughout its history, aphasia has had many and varied definitions depending upon the theoretical stance of the definition's author. But, "... agreement among aphasiologists and clinicians who have experience with aphasic patients in recognizing or identifying a person as aphasic, is likely to be much greater than their agreement as to definitions of aphasia or to the *essence* of aphasic involvement" (Eisenson, 1971, p. 1219). This can be corroborated by a speech-language pathologist who evaluates patients with language disorders daily. Aphasia is an acquired language disorder which may affect comprehension of speech, oral expression, reading comprehension, and written expression. Since language is a component of mathematics, handling money and performing arithmetic calculations may also be disturbed (a condition often referred to as acalculia). Hildred Schuell, who devoted most of her professional career to the study of aphasia diagnosis and therapy and who is one of the most acclaimed contributors to the study of aphasia, defined it as a general language deficit. While she was the chief of the aphasia section of the Minneapolis Veteran's Administration Hospital, Schuell et al. defined aphasia as a "general language deficit that crosses all language modalities and may or may not be complicated by other sequelae of brain damage ... the language deficit itself is characterized by reduction of available vocabulary, impaired verbal retention span and impaired perception and production of messages, perhaps second to impairment of the first two dimensions" (Schuell et al., 1964, p. 113).

Another point of view is that of Harold Goodglass and Edith Kaplan, who do not think that aphasia is an impairment of general language capacity. They feel that "aphasia refers to the disturbance of any or all of the skills, associations and habits of spoken or written language, produced by injury to certain brain areas which are specialized for these functions" (Goodglass and Kaplan, 1972, p. 5).

Classification System

Goodglass and Kaplan adhere to classical terminology to describe aphasia. This diagnostic classification system, easily understood among professionals within a medical setting, retains descriptive behavioral observations. The following presentation of the aphasic syndromes, according to Goodglass and Kaplan, includes a supplementary discussion of global aphasia.

The major division between the aphasic syndromes is based on the characteristics of oral expression. Generally, speech is nonfluent or halting when the locus of the lesion producing the aphasia is anterior to Rolando's fissure, or prerolandic. But when the speech is fluent and marked by paraphasia, the lesion is suspected to be posterior to Rolando's fissure. Thus, the major aphasic syndromes may be grossly categorized as either nonfluent (Broca's) or fluent (Wernicke's, anomic, and conduction).

Broca's Aphasia Broca's aphasia usually results from a lesion in the third frontal convolution of the left hemisphere, which has been referred to as Broca's area or as Brodmann's area 44 (see Fig. 12-1). Because of the proximity of Broca's area to the left motor cortex, it has been estimated that approximately 80 percent of Broca's

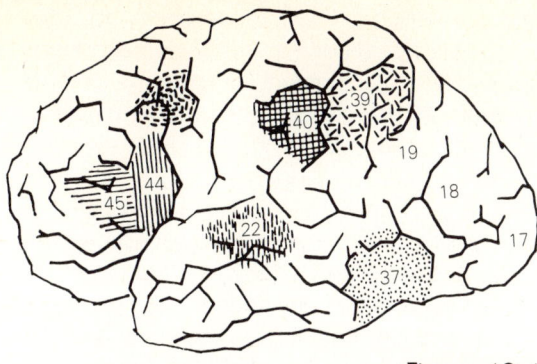

Figure 12-1
The lateral surface of the brain, showing the location of some of the areas related to language: 22, the auditory association cortex related to auditory aphasia or word deafness; 37, area of visual-auditory association; 39, angular gyrus; 40, supramarginal gyrus. Area 44 and the adjoining part of 45 approximately define Broca's motor speech area. *(Adapted from Elizabeth C. Crosby, Tryphena Humphrey, and Edward W. Lauer, Correlative Anatomy of the Nervous System, Macmillan, New York, 1962.)*

aphasics have an accompanying right hemiplegia or hemiparesis (Brown, 1972). Other aphasiologists have referred to Broca's aphasia as verbal aphasia (Head, 1963), motor aphasia (Goldstein, 1948), efferent motor aphasia (Luria, 1966), and expressive aphasia (Weisenburg, McBride, 1964). Despite the assorted nomenclature, one can discern definite similarities in the symptomatology described by each of these authors.

Broca's aphasia is differentiated from other aphasias by the presence of apraxia of speech and agrammatism, and is characterized by word-finding or word-retrieval problems. Canter (1973) defines apraxia of speech as "an impairment of motor speech encoding due to cerebral injury, which is characterized by disturbances of speech initiation, transitionalization, and phoneme selection. It is seen most commonly as part of the symptom-complex of Broca's aphasia. It is distinguishable from dysarthria (due to upper or lower motor neuron disease) and from fluent paraphasic speech (observed in many aphasic patients with posterior cerebral lesions)." The speech may sound nonflowing and halting with frequent misarticulations. Speech often lacks melodic contour or intonation. The person's speech may be limited to overlearned, automatic phrases such as "okay" and "no" or to profanity because of the inability to initiate speech sounds.

Researchers such as Trost and Canter (1974) have examined the articulatory errors characteristic of apraxia of speech and described the error patterns. In the population of 10 Broca's aphasics with apraxia of speech that they studied, they found that substitutions, additions, and compound errors made up the majority of apractic errors on single consonants. Some examples of these articulation errors are *b* for *p* (a sound substitution), *sl* for *s* (a sound addition), and *sw* for *sh* (a compound error). Further, they found that vowels are produced more accurately than isolated consonants and the consonant blends are the most difficult. However, the same speech muscles which cannot produce speech sounds without great effort or struggle can perform involuntary vegetative movements, such as elevating the tongue tip to the rugae for food retrieval, normally and with no difficulty. Infrequently, a pure apraxia of speech without concomitant dysfunction in the other language modalities or in syntax and word recall can be manifested. Although it is relatively rare, pure apraxia of speech may be observed as a residual of an initial Broca's aphasia.

A second symptom of Broca's aphasia is agrammatism, which has been described as telegraphic speech. Speech resembles a telegram and consists of isolated or small groups of substantive words, such as nouns and verbs, without the presence of function words, such as *to, in, of, the,* and *is.* An example of this is "Man store" to communicate "The man is going to the store." In addition to apraxia of speech and agrammatism, the patient may also experience word-finding or word-retrieval problems. This symptom, sometimes referred to as anomia, may be present in all aphasias, regardless of type, but not necessarily to the same degree nor with the same effect on different classes of words. The anomia in the Broca's aphasic affects substantive as well as grammatical words.

As previously mentioned, in severe cases of Broca's aphasia, speech may be absent. However, as recovery occurs, single-word and short-phrase responses may become available. Elementary grammatical forms such as simple declarative statements tend to return, with repetition being produced better than spontaneous speech attempts. Articulation will be clearer and agrammatism will be reduced in repetition of longer grammatical units. In less severe cases, the speech repertoire may consist of short phrases and simple grammatical structures. The absence of complex grammatical structures and apraxia of speech affecting intonation may persist.

In relation to speech, auditory comprehension is relatively good. There may be no difficulty comprehending single words or short messages such as, "Comb your hair." But difficulty in understanding longer, more complex units such as, "Before you go to dinner, wash your hands and take your medicine," may occur. Specifically, Brown states that "patients will err on complex yes/no questions, particularly those involving adverbs such as before and after, e.g., 'Do you have lunch before breakfast?' and they will have difficulties with passive-active transformation, e.g., 'With the pen touch the spoon,' to 'Touch the spoon with the pen'." (p. 113). Similarly, reading comprehension may be relatively well spaced, with difficulty again occurring for longer printed matter.

Last, writing usually mirrors speech attempts and may be as severely or more severely impaired than speech. Spontaneous writing may be limited to writing of the patient's name and a few single words. This is caused by deficits in recall of written symbols and words, rather than the use of the nondominant left hand. When additional written language is present, it, too, is typically characterized by agrammatism. As a component of written expression, spelling can be impaired because of inability to recall the graphic symbols or letters in the word. Occasionally, an individual patient uses written expression in lieu of, or as a supplement to, oral expressive attempts. However, reliance on this mode of expression is not possible for most Broca's aphasics.

Along with the speech and language symptoms of the Broca's aphasic, depression, anger, and frustration may occur. These behaviors are understandable if one considers how heavily we rely on oral communication to relate thoughts and feelings and how devastating it must be to be suddenly deprived of this avenue of expression. Benson discusses these behaviors in more detail in his article entitled, "Psychiatric Aspects of Aphasia." He states, "The feeling of being locked in, of knowing what he wants to say [the aphasic patient] but being unable to say it, can produce a severe sense of frustration, a complex emotional state which is particularly common in aphasia" (Benson, 1973, p. 560). He considers anger an important component of the aphasic's frustration and gives as examples outbursts of physical hostility such as shouting or pushing away food. He notes that these behaviors are most often directed toward persons who have a close relationship with the aphasic.

Benson further states that frustration may have positive implications and be indicative of self-awareness of the problem and a desire to take steps toward remediation. However, the frustration may lead to depression in some individuals, become a deterrent to rehabiliattion, and require professional intervention. In addition, this depression may indicate an incapability to contend with the significant change in life-style. However, it is not known whether this depression is attributable to a reaction to the aphasia or to an inherent aspect of the left frontal lobe damage (Strub and Black, 1977).

Wernicke's Aphasia Wernicke's aphasia, the most common fluent aphasia, results from a posterior lesion. Goodglass and Kaplan state that the lesion associated with Wernicke's aphasia is usually in the posterior portion of the first temporal gyrus of the left hemisphere. Strub and

Black indicate that the lesion is more likely to be in this area when auditory comprehension is severely impaired. They also feel that if single word comprehension is adequate, then the lesion is more likely to involve the parietal lobe. Because of the location of the lesion, these patients typically do not have a right hemiplegia, but may have a hemiparesis or sensory loss. However, for the same reason, the lesion may extend into the visual cortex, often resulting in a transient homonymous hemianopsia. Other researchers have referred to Wernicke's aphasia as syntactic aphasia (Head, 1963), sensory aphasia (Goldstein, 1948), acoustic aphasia (Luria, 1966), and receptive aphasia (Weisenburg and McBride, 1964).

The two major symptoms of Wernicke's aphasia are impaired auditory comprehension and feedback and fluent or hyperfluent well-articulated paraphasic speech. These, along with an impairment in repetition, differentiate Wernicke's aphasia from the other fluent aphasias. The auditory comprehension of individuals with Wernicke's aphasia varies in degree of severity. For example, some are unable to comprehend even single words while others break down with complex directions. But unlike the Broca's aphasic who becomes aware of comprehension deficits, these patients are often unaware of their lack of understanding, at least in the early stages.

This lack of awareness is also reflected in the patient's expressive attempts. The speech is well articulated with good speech melody and may be produced at a rate that is normal or faster than normal. The speech lacks content because of these self-monitoring deficits in addition to word-finding problems, and consists of many function words such as *one, this, his, of,* and *is*. This results in what has been termed extended English jargon, defined as connected speech consisting of English words, but having little content or meaning. One patient, when asked to describe breakfast, said, "I had one of these, you know, a thing like this of one you have too." Some patients exhibit what is termed neologistic jargon, defined as connected speech consisting of neologisms (meaningless words) interspersed with some English words. In response to the question, "What did you do for a living?" the patient responded, "I was the hypum . . . the ead of it, the read of it . . . for my hyput . . . for the people." The more severe the aphasia is, the more likely the patient is to exhibit extended English jargon or extended neologistic jargon. The patient is most often unaware of these errors and subsequently cannot self-correct.

Single-word paraphasic errors are present in the speech and generally can be categorized according to type. A verbal paraphasic error is the substitution of one word for another, such as *cloud/daughter*. As the patient progresses, in-class substitutions occur, such as *wife/daughter*. Literal paraphasias are the fluent substitutions, additions, or transpositions of sounds within a word, such as *toulder/shoulder* or *nuffles/knuckles*. Neologistic paraphasias are the substitutions of a meaningless word that contains the phonemes of the speaker's native language, such as *vilafilim/leaf* or *nickwer/hammock*. Errors are not necessarily as random as they might appear, but seem to be based upon either phonetic or semantic associations during the word-retrieval process (Burns and Canter, 1977). These paraphasic errors are also reflected in the patient's attempts to repeat.

In contrast to the Broca's aphasic's speech, which is agrammatic, syntax is described as paragrammatic. Grammar is incorrect and "there is usually free use of complex verb tenses, embedded subordinate clauses, and other departures from simple declarative word order" (Goodglass and Kaplan, p. 59). Overuse of auxiliary verbs and conjugation of nouns may be present, as in "The run is boying."

Reading comprehension is usually impaired but severity varies. In some patients, this modality is better preserved in relation to other modalities, but this is highly individual since in other patients reading skills will be as impaired, if not more so than the other language modalities. Writing is always impaired and the level of severity is usually consistent with or worse than speech. Although the patient may continue to use the dominant hand for writing, occasionally the writing mirrors the fluency and the paraphasia of the speech, i.e., "Raiding year wrring out tending to no nout goind art noting to using. The not using are really readed are year after are go are gooded."

As previously mentioned, a concomitant symptom of Wernicke's aphasia may be unawareness of the language difficulty. This is particularly true in individuals whose comprehension is more severely impaired. These patients may appear euphoric in relation to the level of severity of their language problems. Wernicke's aphasics seldom exhibit frustration until recovery and awareness of errors occurs. Benson states that a paranoid reaction may occur in patients whose comprehension, unawareness, and unconcern are all severe. The patient thinks people are talking about him and are "out to get him" because he cannot understand. Thus, the Wernicke's aphasic's reaction is in marked contrast to that of the Broca's aphasic and may be more of a deterrent to language rehabilitation.

Conduction Aphasia Conduction aphasia results from a posterior lesion that occurs deep to the supramarginal gyrus and which affects the arcuate fasciculus. The arcuate fasciculus is a fiber which is postulated to carry information from Wernicke's to Broca's area (Geschwind, 1965). This type of aphasia has also been termed central aphasia (Goldstein, 1948) and afferent motor aphasia (Luria, 1966).

The speech of a conduction aphasic is typically fluent and marked by literal paraphasia, although verbal and neologistic paraphasia may occur. A symptom of the syndrome is a disturbance in repetition that is not commensurate with the fluency of the spontaneous speech nor the relative normalcy of auditory comprehension. Repetition is particularly deficient for polysyllabic words and less common and longer sentences. In repeating the sentence "the vat leaks," the patient's first attempt was "the vast leats," which he immediately attempted to correct with "no, the van leats." However, single familiar words and phrases as well as numbers may be repeated well. Unlike the Wernicke's aphasic who may or may not be aware of speech errors, the conduction aphasic recognizes mistakes and attempts constant corrections which may only lead to further literal paraphasic errors. While auditory comprehension is preserved, deficits in reading comprehension can be exhibited. The impairment in writing may range from the inability to produce any single words to only occasional spelling errors. Because their error awareness is intact, patients with conduction aphasia often display frustration when unable to correct their own errors. This, however, does not interfere with their vigilant persistence to succeed.

Anomic Aphasia Anomic aphasia occurs as a result of posterior cerebral damage, often caused by a temporal-parietal lesion which may involve the area of the angular gyrus (Goodglass and Kaplan). Strub and Black indicate that lesions in other areas of the dominant hemisphere may produce an anomic aphasia, but that a more severe impairment is usually caused by damage either to the parietotemporal area or to the second and third gyri. Other aphasiologists have referred to anomic aphasia as nominal aphasia (Head), amnesic aphasia (Goldstein), and semantic aphasia (Wepman and Jones).

The predominant symptom of anomic aphasia is word-finding problems in the context of fluent, grammatically correct speech (Goodglass and Kaplan). The oral expression lacks content (substantive) words and consists of many function words, such as **one, this, his, is,** and **of.** Some patients are able to produce circumlocutions easily for words which elude them. One patient, when asked, "Where did you go to school?" responded with, "Well, it wasn't here, it was over there, you know, across the ocean. Not in France or Italy, but the one with a queen." In more severe anomics, rate of speech may be reduced also because of the pervasive word-finding problems. Because of the prevalence of anomia in all the aphasic syndromes, much research has been devoted to its analysis (Goodglass, Klein, Carey, and Jones, 1966; Geschwind, 1967a).

Auditory comprehension is generally good, although the patient occasionally does not understand and rejects a word that is supplied when unable to produce it himself. A study by Goodglass, Gleason, and Hyde (1970) revealed that anomic aphasics' comprehension of isolated nouns and verbs is significantly poorer in relation to their overall level of comprehension. The level of severity in both reading and writing is quite variable, and may range from mild to severe. Although there is little documentation specific to the accompanying behavioral symptoms of anomic aphasia, clinical observations reveal the frequent presence of depression, frustration, and anger similar to Broca's aphasia.

Global Aphasia Global aphasia results from a large lesion that affects both Broca's and Wernicke's areas. Sequelae usually include an accompanying right hemiplegia or hemiparesis. These patients have no consistent functional skills in any of the language modalities. Understanding of speech or written information and written expression may be absent. The speech of some patients is limited to the use of a meaningless recurrent utterance, such as, "bibobobibobobo." Some patients present the symptoms of a global aphasia following the immediate onset of aphasia during their acute hospitalization. However, as the patient recovers and cerebral edema diminishes, remission of many of the severe symptoms occurs and a residual aphasia is observed, often of a Broca's or anomic type. Clinical observations indicate that behavioral symptoms vary from euphoria to depression.

Transcortical Aphasias The transcortical aphasias, including transcortical sensory, motor, and mixed, occur less frequently than the other aphasia syndromes. They are most commonly caused by anoxia secondary to decreased cerebral circulation and occlusion of the carotid artery. "The lesions causing transcortical aphasia are extensive crescent-shaped infarcts within the border zones between major cerebral vessels (e.g., within the frontal lobe between territories of the anterior and middle cerebral arteries)" (Strub and Black). Broca's and Wernicke's areas and the connections between them are usually spared but are cut off from other areas of the brain (Goodglass and Kaplan). The shared symptoms of the transcortical aphasias is relatively intact repetition in relation to all other language skills.

Transcortical motor aphasia is produced by an anterior border zone lesion. These patients have comparatively good auditory comprehension and reading skills in addition to being able to repeat. However, they do not initiate spontaneous speech and have difficulty organizing responses. Once speech is produced, it is fairly well articulated. Transcortical sensory aphasia results from a lesion in the posterior border zone which produces a syndrome similar to Wernicke's aphasia; speech is fluent and paraphasic, and comprehension is impaired. However, unlike Wernicke's aphasia, repetition is good, even for lengthy unfamiliar sentences. A third transcortical aphasia combines the symptoms of both transcortical motor and sensory aphasias and is caused by a lesion affecting both the anterior and posterior border bones. Comprehension and reading are impaired. Speech is marked by lack of spontaneity, intact repetition, and echolalia, that is, the repetition of all comments and questions that are directed toward the patient. Generalizations about the behavior of transcortical aphasics cannot be made because of the low incidence rate.

EVALUATION PROCEDURES

In evaluating the aphasic patient, the speech-language pathologist usually assesses the four language modalities: (1) auditory comprehension, (2) oral expression, (3) reading comprehension, and (4) written expression. In some patients, gestural expression and comprehension, ability to handle money, and arithmetic calculations may also be tested. Tasks ranging from simple to complex are presented in each of these areas. An audiologic evaluation which assesses the pure tone thresholds of hearing acuity and speech discrimination is an integral segment of the evaluation process for aphasics and all other patients with speech and language disorders. When a decrease in hearing acuity is detected, the audiologist may administer additional audiological tests and/or refer the patient directly to an otologist.

A variety of commercially produced tests are available for the assessment of aphasia. Test selection is often based on the clinician's theoretical viewpoint of language and aphasia. The most frequently used aphasia tests are summarized below.

Boston Diagnostic Aphasia Examination The Boston Diagnostic Aphasia Examination was developed by Harold Goodglass and Edith Kaplan in 1972. The authors indicate that this test was designed to correlate language-test findings with prexisting aphasic syndromes identified by neurologists. The test battery can be administered in 1 to 3 h and consists of an evaluation of the four major language modalities with supplementary tests for further psycholinguistic evaluation, in addition to the assessment of arithmetic functioning, apraxias, finger agnosias, and right-left orientation. Test items are based on a hierarchy of difficulty ranging from the simplest to most difficult tasks, and provide a solid basis for the development of a treatment program. For example, single words (from a variety of semantic classes), body parts, 1- to 5-step commands, and sentences and paragraphs varying in length and complexity of content and sentence structure are examined in the evaluation of auditory comprehension and oral expression as well as the accuracy of response. At the conclusion of the evaluation, a profile of test scores can be completed on which patterns emerge which will assist in the differential diagnosis of the aphasic syndromes.

Minnesota Test for Differential Diagnosis of Aphasia This test was developed by Dr. Hildred Schuell after many years of revisions; it was published in 1965. Schuell felt a need to develop a test which was uniform and would permit comparison among aphasic patients, analysis of specific symptoms, and determination of progress. At the time it was developed, it was the most comprehensive aphasia test available and included items to assess auditory disturbances, visual and reading disturbances, speech and language disturbances, visuomotor and writing disturbances, and disturbances in numerical relations and arithmetic processes. Its subtests are designed to measure not only the area of impairment, but also the level of severity in each area. Administration of all subtests may take longer than other batteries, but the results are highly specific and detailed, providing an invaluable basis for treatment.

Porch Index of Communicative Ability The Porch Index of Communicative Ability (PICA) was developed by Bruce Porch in 1967. Porch felt that a tool for assessing aphasic behavior must have high reliability and should quantify responses rather than simply record pass/fail. As a result, he developed a 16-point multidimensional scoring system which includes the variables of accuracy, responsiveness, completeness, promptness, and efficiency. The test consists of 18 subtests which measure gestural, verbal, and graphic abilities. Responses are rated using the multidimensional scale and are then recorded on a test profile. An overall score is obtained by averaging all of the subtest means and is considered by Porch to be the best index of the patient's general communication ability. The PICA also allows the examiner to plot a recovery curve, useful for predicting progress.

Functional Communication Profile The Functional Communication Profile (FCP) was developed by Martha Taylor Sarno and copyrighted in 1963. It measures language ability in the areas of movement, speaking, understanding, reading, and other. Each patient serves as an individual norm; thus a normal rating indicates performance at the same estimated level of proficiency as prior to the onset of aphasia. The test measures common and familiar language behaviors, such as speaking on the telephone and handling money, in a natural setting rather than a structured clinical test situation. Forty-five language behaviors are rated on a nine-point scale from zero to normal. An overall percentage score can be obtained. The FCP is intended for use by speech-language pathologists who evaluate many aphasic patients per year, and is to be used only in conjunction with additional language testing.

Other Additional Aphasia Tests Many other aphasia tests are commercially available for use by the speech-language pathologist. Although the following list is not all inclusive, it is representative of additional tests that are available: *Examining for Aphasia* (Eisenson, 1954); *Language Modalities Test for Aphasia* (Wepman and Jones, 1961); *Neurosensory Center Comprehensive Examination for Aphasia* (Spreen and Benton, 1969); and *The Token Test* (DeRenzi and Vignolo, 1962). For a more in-depth evaluation of reading, mathematics, etc., supplementary tests drawn from educational sources may be selected and administered depending upon the specific needs of the patient. Efforts continue to be made in the development of more valid and meaningful evaluative techniques. An example is *Communicative Ability in Daily Living* (Holland, 1977) which measures patients' communicative abilities in their daily lives.

TREATMENT OF APHASIA

Prognosis and Candidacy for Treatment

Candidacy for treatment and prognosis for improvement are determined upon completion of the aphasia test battery. The speech-language pathologist not only analyzes and interprets the results of language testing, but also considers other factors such as the patient's medical stability and readiness for therapy before treatment is initiated. Overall prognosis for language recovery is dependent upon numerous variables which may positively or negatively affect the patient's progress in reacquiring functional communication.

Prognostic indicators include the following:

1. Severity of aphasia: A patient with a mild to moderate aphasia with residual functioning in all language modalities has a better prognosis than does a global aphasic. The global aphasic may derive questionable value from direct speech-language treatment, but may require psychologic and social intervention (Sarno, Silverman, and Sands, 1970; Schuell, Jenkins and Jiménez-Pabón, 1964).
2. Time between onset and initiation of therapy: Initiation of therapy within the first 6 months of onset is a positive factor. This capitalizes on the period of spontaneous recovery which is generally considered to occur within 2 to 6 months. Early intervention prevents the establishment of inappropriate and ineffective compensatory techniques and the development of frustration and depression. However, this should not rule out therapy for those patients who do not fall into this category and have never received treatment.
3. Etiology: Patients whose problems are due to traumatic causes are thought to progress more readily and to a higher level than those whose deficits are due to cerebrovascular origin. Similarly, patients who have a single lesion are thought to improve more quickly than those with multiple lesions unless the single lesion is in the temporoparietal region (Eisenson, 1964).
4. Age: Youth has a positive effect on the progression of skills.
5. Educational level and intelligence: Although supporting data are inconclusive, educational level, intelligence, former occupation, and social status should be considered.
6. Awareness and self-correction skills: Perhaps most importantly, patients who recognize their own errors have a better prognosis than those who cannot.

Yet each patient is unique. Caution must be exercised in the application of these factors so as not to limit, without justification, the individual's hope for recovery.

Efficacy of Treatment

Studies of the value of treatment have addressed the issues and interrelationships of the severity and type of aphasia, spontaneous recovery period, and length of treatment (Schuell, Jenkins, and Jiménez-Pabón; Sarno, Silverman, and Sands). Vignolo (1964) analyzed the effect of direct language therapy with 69 aphasics in a retrospective study. He concluded that speech and language treatment does have a positive and specific effect on aphasics, particularly when treatment is begun between 2 and 6 months from onset and when the treatment lasts for more than 6 months. Early intervention by the speech-language pathologist affords the patient psychologic support and promotes the development of the patient's "active participant" role in the rehabilitation process (Eisenson).

Intervention Techniques

Formal speech and language treatment programs may be carried out individually or in a group, but all are tailored to meet the individual level of impairment, immediate communication needs, and preillness vocational and avocational interests of the patient. Consideration must also be given to the patient's premorbid speech and language abilities and idiosyncrasies, including cultural, ethnic, and educational variations. For example, a speech-language pathologist would not expect a patient who had been illiterate to read after becoming aphasic.

Similarly, the speech-language pathologist exercises discretion in deciding whether to stimulate the use by bilingual or multilingual patients of a native or most frequently used language. The research in recovery of aphasia in polyglots is not conclusive regarding which language returns first or why one may appear at a superior level. Obler and Albert (1977) suggest that age at onset of the aphasia is influential in determining the language which is better preserved. They indicate that in the young or middle-aged polyglot, the language most recently used has a greater chance of returning; in the older patient, recovery is more dependent on chance. Thus, the speech-language pathologist restimulates previously established language skills and does not attempt to teach new ones.

While there are a great variety of approaches to aphasia therapy, in all cases treatment is a stimulation process rather than an educative one (Schuell, Jenkins, Jiménez-Pabón, 1964; Wepman, 1953). But aphasics cannot be expected to learn at the same rate nor to have the same level of achievement as do normal speakers (Carson, Carson, Tikofsky). Aphasics tend to learn at a slower rate with limitations on the retention of information. However, the use of principles of therapeutic management that are consistent with learning theory is basic to therapy. Measurable realistic goals reflecting the patient's needs are established, and a hierarchy of multimodality tasks is followed to achieve these goals. The use of meaningful and appropriate stimuli, high successful-response ratios, and effective positive and negative reinforcement are instrumental in achieving success.

Since there are characteristic language mechanisms underlying the various aphasic syndromes, specific therapeutic approaches can be applied to each and are briefly described below.

Auditory Comprehension The reestablishment of comprehension skills is essential to the initiation of treatment and to the reacquisition of abilities in all other language modalities. The identification of single familiar objects or pictures, following simple one- or two-component directives, and answering simple yes or no questions form the most basic activities in this modality. Manipulation of the rate, syntactic, and semantic complexity of messages rebuilds the patient's ability to comprehend normally. At more advanced levels, directing the patient to listen to news broadcasts or television or radio shows may be the best stimulation for improved auditory attention, retention, and integration.

Oral Expression The development of oral expression or speech is often the major therapeutic goal an aphasic patient envisions. This is probably due to the overt loss of speech and the resulting frustration experienced by the patient.

Therapy concentrates on the reestablishment of some form of expression as soon as possible.

In the case of a Broca's aphasic with apraxia of speech, the speech-language pathologist may direct the patient to simultaneously imitate, repeat, and spontaneously produce phonemes, syllables, words, phrases, and finally sentences. Maximal cues are provided initially by the speech-language pathologist in the form of auditory, visual, or graphic stimuli and are gradually withdrawn. Another apraxia treatment procedure described by Sparks et al. (1974) is call Melodic Intonation Therapy (MIT). The MIT approach uses systematic levels of increasingly difficult tasks involving "sung intonation of propositional sentences in such a way that the intoned pattern is similar to the natural prosodic pattern of the sentence when it is spoken" (Sparks et al.).

It is rare for a treatment program not to include therapy tasks geared toward improving word-retrieval skills, regardless of the type of aphasia. Exercises aimed at rebuilding associations between words may consist of completing open-ended sentences (e.g., "I cut with a ____."), describing objects in terms of function and physical attributes, and generating definitions. Through the use of role play and internalization of association cues, carry-over into functional situations can be achieved.

Wepman (1976) cautions the speech-language pathologist not to place inordinate emphasis upon strict and static techniques that may inhibit creativity and sensitivity. He postulates that aphasia is an impairment of thought and hence therapy should focus upon the "embellishment of thought rather than on the specific elements of linguistics either expressive or receptive" (Wepman, 1976, p. 131). He advocates the use of an indirect approach called thought-process stimulation that encourages thinking about ideas other than the patient's own speech. He feels this may generate the need for and the production of language.

Reading Comprehension and Written Expression These two language modalities are not necessarily included in all treatment programs. The individual patient's needs, interests, and premorbid abilities are taken into consideratoin before initiating therapy. Yet when it is deemed appropriate, treatment for reading comprehension and written expression become essential. For some patients, progress in these modalities may be paramount to their return to a vocational setting. As in the other language modalities, therapy begins at the patient's level of breakdown in each area and follows a hierarchy of development.

For example, reading comprehension may proceed from single words to phrases, sentences, and multiple paragraphs of varying syntactic and semantic complexity. Emphasis is placed upon the selction of reading materials that are of interest to the patient and that may provide a source of recreation. In written expression, the patient may be encouraged initially to copy single words that are being stimulated in oral expressive tasks. Retraining the patient to produce a signature or to utilize written expression as a supplement to oral expression is a goal. Patients functioning at a higher level may redevelop spelling and sentence-formulation skills.

RIGHT BRAIN–DAMAGED PATIENTS

CLINICAL DESCRIPTION

The previous discussion has been limited to patients with aphasia resulting from lesions in the dominant hemisphere of the brain. But what about the patient with a lesion in the nondominant hemisphere, that is, right brain damage with an associated left hemiphlegia? Does this population demonstrate any communication impairment? Sarno and Sarno (1969) described a nonaphasic language disorder present in patients having right-sided brain damage as having cognitive and perceptual deficits with symptoms including persisting disorientation and confusion, impaired visual and auditory memory for recent events, poor judgment, and concrete thinking. Sarno (1975) feels that speech-language pathologists do not treat this communication disorder because of its relationship to cognition; yet no suggestion is made as to who should intervene. It is the authors' opinion that speech-language pathologists should take an active role in the rehabilitation of this population because of their training in language, behavior modification, perception, attention, and memory.

Clinically, in addition to the above-mentioned problems, these patients also exhibit impulsivity, reduced and fleeting visual and auditory attention spans, and difficulty in organizing and putting information into sequence. All these factors reduce the individual's ability to utilize language skills. The presence of visual-perceptual deficits further affect language functioning. Weinberg et al. (1977) propose that visual neglect and the associated inability to scan the environment adequately are the major impairments underlying the visual-perceptual problem in this population. Difficulty in recognizing familiar persons, confusion about whereabouts, and inability to remember the month and year may all be manifested. Attention span for a specific task may be as little as a minute or two, and distractibility from both visual and auditory stimuli within the environment further confounds the problem. The patient may not remember eating breakfast or having been to physical therapy. Because of the visual neglect of the left side, a man may shave only the right side of his face or eat only what's on the right side of the plate. The patient may adequately participate in a simple conversation about himself or herself or the immediate environment but be unable to attend when more complex and lengthy topics are introduced. Speech may be disorganized, excessive, concrete, and unrelated to the topic at hand. Thus, in contrast to aphasia, this is not a symbolic disorder, but rather a disorder in which cognitive and perceptual deficits reduce the patient's efficiency in utilizing language skills.

EVALUATION AND TREATMENT

Although standard tests for the evaluation of aphasia are available, no such tools have been produced for assessment of the right brain-damaged patient. In this absence, a battery of tests including a visual-perceptual test, selected subtests in each language modality chosen from standardized aphasia tests, and academically related language tests (reading, mathematics) are administered. In addition, behaviors pertinent to this population are observed and measured. Weinberg et al. suggest neuropsychological evaluation of facial recognition, digit span, object assembly, and picture completion from the Wechsler Adult Intelligence Scale, in addition to evaluation of reading, math, and visual scanning, among others. Some of the same prognostic factors that apply to the aphasic population can be applied to this group, such as age at time of onset, etiology, and extent of lesion. Those patients with emerging error awareness and self-correction ability appear to have a better prognosis than those who are totally unaware of their errors.

As with the aphasic patient, treatment may take many forms but is consistent with learning theory and is individualized according to the patient's needs and interests. The foci of the treatment programs are manipulating the environment from structured to less structured, increasing attention span, orienting the patient to time, place, and person, and improving visual-perceptual skills, including left-sided awareness, through utilization of linguistic materials. For example, in a patient whose base-line attention span of 2 minutes detracted from performance in all areas, therapy was initiated by establishing a goal of visual attention for 10 min. The cogent factor was to isolate a relatively simple and unfrustrating task in a particular area and gradually to increase its length and complexity. It has been the authors' experience that one of the most important outcomes of speech-language treatment with this population is that the patient's improved task orientation and increased attention span allow more effective participation in other therapies. The improvement additionally results in an increase in the effectiveness and efficiency of the patient's utilization of language skills.

DYSARTHRIA

DEFINITION OF DYSARTHRIA

Dysarthria refers to a group of disorders affecting either single or combined motor control of respiration, phonation, articulation, resonance, and prosody resulting from peripheral or central nervous system damage. It is due to paralysis, weakness, or incoordination of the oral musculature and is not due to a symbolic language disturbance, as in aphasia, or a perceptual, cognitive disturbance, as in right brain damage. Darley, Aronson, and Brown (1975) provided a major contribution to the evaluation and diagnosis of dysarthria in their discrete analyses of muscle function and acoustic characteristics, and in their systematic classification of symptoms according to neurologic damage. By analyzing the deviant speech and voice characteristics, they identified clusters of acoustic patterns which emerged as typical of each dysarthria (Darley, Aronson, and Brown, 1969). The severity of the dysarthria may vary from mild to severe depending on the extent of the neurologic damage.

DIFFERENTIAL DIAGNOSIS OF DYSARTHRIA

Flaccid Dysarthria Flaccid dysarthria is due to a lower motor neuron disorder and usually results in hypotonia and weakness of the speech musculature; this may be generalized or limited to a specific structure depending upon the cranial nerve involement. It is associated with disorders such as bulbar palsy, specific cranial nerve palsies, such as hypoglossal palsy and myasthenia gravis. The predominant characteristics of the speech include hypernasality, often accompanied by nasal emission, audible inspiration, a breathy voice with monotonous pitch, and short phrases.

Spastic Dysarthria Spastic dysarthria, associated with pseudobulbar palsy, is due to upper motor neuron disorders which result in hypertonicity (spasticity) and disintegration of movement patterns rather than paralysis of isolated muscles. Due to the bilateral innervation of the cranial nerves, unilateral lesions of the cortex usually do not result in a permanent dysarthria. Spastic dysarthria is thus caused by multiple or bilateral cerebrovascular accidents (CVAs), multiple sclerosis, congenital cerebral palsy, and traumatic brain injury, among others. Voluntary muscle movement is slow and weak with limited range of excursion. Articulation is imprecise and produced at a reduced rate, and a harsh or strained/strangled voice quality, sometimes accompanied by pitch breaks, is typically observed. The voice is usually low, monopitch, and monoloud with reduced stress.

Ataxic Dysarthria Ataxic dysarthria occurs as a result of damage to the cerebellum and may be due to trauma, strokes, multiple sclerosis, and toxicity, among other causes. The oral musculature is hypotonic and movements are slow, inaccurate, and dysrhythmic. Coordination between speech production processes (e.g., respiration and phonation) may be disturbed. Articulation is imprecise with inconsistent, nonsystematic breakdown of consonants and vowels. Syllables within words and words are produced with equal stress, and unstressed words are also emphasized. Phonemes and the intervals between them are prolonged. Rate is reduced and the voice may be harsh with monopitch and monoloudness.

Hypokinetic Dysarthria Hypokinetic dysarthria results from a disorder of certain parts of the extrapyramidal system, as seen in Parkinsonism. Characteristics of muscle movement include rigidity, reduced range, force of motion, and a hypernormal rate of repetitive movements, while individual movements remain slow. The predominant acoustic characteristics include monopitch, reduced stress, and reduced intensity. There are short rushes of speech with inappropriate silences; voice quality may be breathy and/or harsh, and articulation is imprecise.

Hyperkinetic Dysarthria Hyperkinetic dysarthria resulting from disorders of the extrapyramidal system refer essentially to two categories of dysarthrias—predominantly slow hyperkinetic and predominantly quick hyperkinetic—depending upon the speed of involuntary movements observed. These dysarthrias may form a continuum of movement from quick to slow.

Quick Hyperkinesias Quick hyperkinesias, as seen in chorea, are characterized by rapid, abnormal, involuntary movements that may or may not be sustained briefly. In chorea, all aspects of respiration, phonation, resonance, articulation, and prosody are impaired, but the distinguishing feature of this disorder is the random interruption of these functions. Articulation irregularly breaks down. There are intermittent periods of hypernasality, harshness, breathiness, and fluctuating intensity. Prosodic elements include excess and equal stress and inappropriate silences.

Slow Hyperkinesias Slow hyperkinesias, as seen in dystonia, are characterized by slow, involuntary, and distorted movements and postures that are sustained for variable intervals before relaxation. These affect respiration, articulation, phonation, and prosody. The acoustic characteristics of dystonia (slow hyperkinetic) resemble those of chorea (quick hyperkinetic) in articulation, prosody, and phonation. In dystonia, however, rate may be slow as compared with a varying rate in chorea.

Mixed Dysarthria The dysarthrias may occur in pure form, or more than one may be present in the same patient, observed in amyotrophic lateral sclerosis, which results in a spastic-flaccid type of dysarthria, or multiple sclerosis, which may have both spastic and flaccid components. Mixed dysarthrias occur when more than one motor system is affected or in patients who have had strokes, tumor, trauma, or degenerative diseases when the nervous system damage is a result of multiple or diffuse lesions.

EVALUATION PROCEDURES

The evaluation of a dysarthria patient includes an assessment of oral musculature and an analysis of acoustic characteristics of speech. Unlike commercial aphasia tests, dysarthria evaluations per se have not been published; however, formats for the examination of oral muscle structure and function are presented in the professoinal literature (Darley, Aronson, Brown, 1975).

The evaluation commences with the examination of the oral musculature at rest. The structure and symmetry of facial, labial, lingual, mandibular, and palatopharyngeal musculature are observed. The presence or absence of atrophy, fasciculations, tremor, or other involuntary movements is noted. Muscle function is measured on both a voluntary and reflexive level. Chewing and swallowing behaviors are observed to ensure the patient's adequacy or efficiency in maintaining an oral diet.

Reflexes such as the gag reflex are elicited, not only to determine the potency of a specific muscle group for voluntary speech production and vegetative functioning, but also to assist in differentiating the varying motor systems involved. The assessment of voluntary muscle function is central and essential to the differential diagnosis of dysarthria. Individual and repetitive muscle movements are evaluated along five parameters: muscle sterngth, rate, range, accuracy, and tone. This evaluation is accomplished by asking the patient to perform actions such as lip closure, tongue tip elevation, and rapid repetition of movements or syllables involving the structures, such as "puh-tuh-kuh."

The amount and duration of muscle contraction is reflective of strength and is important in sustaining movements such as velopharyngeal functioning during speech. Rate of movement essentially means the speed with which contractions are carried out and contributes primarily to prosodic elements in speech. Range of motion refers to consistent muscle excursion to a target that also adds to prosody and clarity of speech. Precision or accuracy is the coordination of strength, speed, range, direction , and timing of muscle movement and influences articulation and phonation. Muscle tone is the resistance that a relaxed muscle displays to movement and may affect phonation by either its decrease or increase. Thus, impairment of any of these parameters will affect the normal production of speech and result in deviant acoustic characteristics.

The evalutaiton continues with the recording of a speech sample consisting of conversational speech and an oral reading passage. The patient's speech can be analyzed along 38 dimensions that have been isolated and described by Darley, Aronson, and Brown (1969). Such factors as loudness level, hypernasality, rate, reduced stress, imprecise consonants, and voice quality are defined. The severity and interaction of all these factors determine the overall level of intelligibility of functional speech as judged by the listener. In addition, the patient's articulation may be further assessed by the use of articulation tests that are commercially available and allow a more finite analysis of phoneme production. In some instances, further examination by an otolaryngologist may be indicated, as in the case of a patient with a voice disorder where it is necessary to rule out pathology, and for treatment procedures such as Teflon injection into a paralyzed vocal fold. Last, it may be necessary for the speech pathologist to evaluate chewing and swallowing, since these, too, may be affected in conjunction with oral motor dysfunction (see Chap. 13). The synthesis of oral muscle-function findings and the cluster of acoustic characteristics that emerge from the patient's speech result in the differential diagnosis of the dysarthria.

TREATMENT OF DYSARTHRIA

Although multiple dysarthrias exist, general treatment principles apply to most diagnostic categories. Speech treatment is aimed toward improving the features of respiration, phonation, articulation, prosody, and resonance. The rationale for development of a treatment program is based on a thorough understanding of the muscle mechanisms underlying the acoustic production. Whatever the methods employed, the ultimate goal is increased intelligibility of functional speech, which may be obtained either through improved muscle functioning or compensation. However, in patients with severe dysarthrias or progressive diseases, this goal may be unrealistic, and maintenance of existing functions is all that may be expected. Thus, the prognosis for improvement is largely dependent upon the severity of the muscle dysfunction.

Respiration The synchronization of quick inhalation and controlled slow exhalation of the airstream is essential for speech production. Respiration can be directly treated by teaching the patient about the process of respiration itself, by showing the patient how to coordinate and synchronize inhalation and exhalation, and by instructing the patient in relaxation techniques. To either increase a patient's phonic breath support or to decrease a patient's air wastage, treatment is directed toward appropriate phrasing of syllables and words in a more proficient manner. After establishing consistent diaphragmatic breathing, the patient is taught to take another breath at intervals in an utterance synchronized with prosodic elements and air supply. For example, instead of stating, "I/ went/ to/ my/ daugh/ ter's house/ last/ week/ end," the patient is instructed to anticipate appropriate breath control before speaking and to say, "/I went to/ my daughter's/ house/ last weekend." Further, improvements in articulatory and phonatory valving indirectly contribute to more efficient use of the airstream so that speech is audible and intelligible.

Phonation Components of the patient's voice, including pitch, intensity, and quality, are dependent upon laryngeal valving and are directly related to the approximation or the amount of tension in the vocal folds. The increase or decrease in vocal fold tension, then, is a primary mechanism in achieving optimal loudness, pitch, and voice quality. For example, a patient with a breathy voice, attributed to inadequate vocal fold approximation, might be instructed to increase laryngeal tension by simultaneously pushing against the wheelchair and phonating. Thus, laryngeal muscle tone and vocal fold approximation are increased, improving quality and intensity of voice. On the other hand, a pateint with a strained/strangled voice quality, attributed to hyperadduction of the vocal folds, may be trained to decrease tension through the application of relaxation techniques. By external massage of the larynx, by assuming a relaxed posture, or by practicing progressive relaxation, a patient's laryngeal tension may be decreased which, in effect, improves voice quality. Voice quality may also be altered by either increasing or decreasing loudness and pitch until the optimum loudness and pitch are discovered for the individual patient. Although therapy may, for example, emphasize achieving optimum pitch, intensity and voice quality will also be affected because of their interrelationship and their interdependence upon muscle tone, air pressure, or air flow.

Articulation Since articulation errors are prevalent in most dysarthrias, articulation therapy is common and may be crucial to improving overall intelligibility. In the more severely affected patient, passive, active, and resistive exercises of the lingual and labial musculature may precede articulation therapy in order to increase the strength and mobility of the articulators. The use of biofeedback has also been explored as a means to modify hypertonicity, thus improving muscle function for speech, although its application to date is limited (Netsell and Cleeland, 1973). A number of techniques may be employed to improve consonant and vowel production. These include reducing rate of speech to accommodate the impaired articulators, exaggerating each syllable of an utterance by overarticulating, and drilling on individual phonemes in isolation, single words, sentences, and connected speech.

Resonance Without adequate closure of the velopharyngeal mechanism, hypernasality and nasal emission may result. Thus, production of phonemes requiring oral air pressure or oral air flow (e.g., *s, sh, p*) may be nasalized and subsequently distorted or omitted as a result of inadequate valving. Treatment stresses auditory and kinesthetic discrimination of oral versus nasal production. The patient is asked to focus upon air flow through the oral cavity. More severly affected patients may require direct stimulation of the palatal musculature either by palatal massage or through the use of a palatal prosthesis.

Prosody Prosodic features, such as intonation or stress, can be manipulated primarily through varying loudness and pitch. For example, pitch is elevated in asking questions. Loudness and pitch variations may be lost or equalized in dysarthrias so that speech becomes monoloud and monopitch. By teaching the patient to increase or decrease loudness or pitch, stress patterns are established and prosody can be reinstated. The immediate and concrete feedback of audio- or videotapes is instrumental in coordinating the above procedures and in integrating all these aspects of speech production.

Alternate Communication Systems Severely dysarthric patients may not develop intelligible speech despite intensive therapeutic efforts. Therefore, alternate means of communication are vital and can be developed to meet the language and physical capabilities and individual needs of the patient. An alphabet or word communication board may be fabricated by the speech-language pathologist which enables the patient to either spell a word or point to a phrase which indicates desires or needs. Electronic communication systems, which are commercially produced, may also be obtained. One example is a scanning system which patients can activate with very limited movement. The device allows the patient to select and indicate a symbol or message on a display board with a light or arrow. Modern technology has allowed these devices to become increasingly available so that patients who may never again speak can communicate.

MULTIPLE SPEECH AND LANGUAGE DISORDERS

Aphasia, dysarthria, and symptoms of right brain damage may coexist in patients with multiple or diffuse lesions. Diagnosis and treatment of these patients demand the establishment of priorities by the speech-language pathologist. Immediate establishment of a viable means of communication and consideration of the patient's chief complaints are taken into account in the development and ordering of therapy. For example, if a patient has a severe anomic aphasia and a mild ataxic dysarthria, treatment of the anomia outweighs the dysarthria because of its disproportionate interference with functional expression.

NURSING MANAGEMENT OF THE COMMUNICATIVELY IMPAIRED

The key to management of a patient with a communication impairment is an understanding of the individual's problem and how they affect daily functioning in the environment (hospital, rehabilitation center, nursing home, etc.). Nursing cooperation is an intrinsic component of successful carry-over of speech and language skills from clinical to real life settings. In conjunction with the speech pathologist, the nurse can implement management techniques in the nursing unit and can educate the patient and family.

While a nurse should never be expected to assume the role of a speech-language pathologist, a general idea of the person's strengths and weaknesses in the various language modalities should be formulated through knowledge of the speech and language disorders just described. The prime consideration in dealing with a communicatively impaired patient is to treat the person as an adult at all times. There is a tendency to react as though the patient is a child because of the communication problem. "Accept him as he is and for what he is, remembering that he needs your help in his adjustment to the situation. While he must never be placated with false hopes of complete recovery, he must be praised and encouraged for each accomplishment" (Halper, Baker, Worcester).

The nurse can anticipate that the patient may cry, laugh, or swear without control and often without provocation, particularly in the early stages. On these occasions, the patient requires quiet reassurance and redirection of attention to either another task or another topic. Unpredictable inconsistencies in the patient's performance and communication attempts can be expected to occur and to contribute further to emotional lability. However, by stabilizing the environment through the use of familiar personal items (e.g., family photographs, a watch) and the establishment of a routinized daily schedule, lability and behavioral inconsistencies can be controlled and may be decreased.

The nurse can influence the patient's attitude toward and adjustment to the communication loss by accepting and emphasizing what the patient actually is capable of expressing. In so doing, positive feelings about self are accentuated, and withdrawal from social interaction or the environment is diminished. This supportive approach enhances the patient's ability to again be able to make choices and decisions and to actively participate in nursing care and in the rehabilitative process.

APHASIA

The aphasic patient with comprehension problems is often aware of and sensitive to nonverbal communication such as facial expressions, body position, and tone of voice. Even though the actual meaning of a statement may be positive, if the tone of voice and facial expression convey impatience or intolerance, the patient may react and respond to the latter. While fragments of conversation may be understood, the full meaning may elude the patient so that an incorrect reply is given. Because of fragmentary understanding, family members and staff need to exert care regarding the content of conversations when the patient is present. Comprehension can be facilitated by limiting background noise such as the radio, television, and loudspeaker. Monitoring the number of visitors and the flow of staff further reduces conflicting external stimuli. Speech may need to be inhibited in patients who exhibit hyperfluency or jargon, since this, too, interferes with reception of a message or command. By speaking in brief sentences at a reduced rate, and by including only pertinent information, the patient's likelihood of understanding speech is augmented. By rephrasing a statement rather than shouting, and by supplementing directions with gestures, information can be made more readily available to the patient.

Just as the patient's comprehension can be facilitated, so can expression be fostered by the nurse. After a brief period of observation, the nurse can predict the type and level of response the patient can produce and can phrase questions to the patient accordingly. Rather than asking the patient who has no speech, "Who came to visit you last night?" a perceptive nurse might say, "Did your wife come to visit you last night?" This simple rephrasing allows the patient to respond by a headshake and promotes successful communication.

Similarly, the nurse's knowledge of the individual patient's level of frustration is vital to the creation of a tension-free atmosphere. For example, the patient who has inconsistently available speech may require a longer time to respond; the listener need not immediately supply the word for which the patient is searching. Sometimes it is necessary to accept a wrong response since the patient may be deterred from further attempts if repeatedly corrected. By not interrupting the patient, not anticipating the response, and not talking for the patient, communication is encouraged.

Several techniques are available to help the patient convey ideas. Asking the patient to describe the word searched for in terms of physical attributes, location, or use often aids in the retrieval of the sought-after word. Can the patient write the word or tell what letter it begins with? Ask the patient to show what is needed by pointing or gesturing if possible. Finally, if it is possible to guess what the patient is attempting to say, supply the word and ask the patient to repeat it if possible. If all else fails, let the patient know that it is not possible to understand. The pretense of understanding only leads to frustration and failure for both the nurse and the patient. At times, silence and a reassuring handclasp may prove to be the most meaningful expression.

RIGHT BRAIN-DAMAGED

The same guidelines described for the communicatively impaired patient in general apply to the right brain-damaged patient. Exerting control over the environment by structuring and minimizing auditory and visual stimulation permits the patient to better attend to the task at hand. Avoiding rapid movement around the patient, accentuating visual reference points in the room such as doorways and furniture, and routinizing schedules may decrease the patient's confusion. The use of a calendar and clock in the room rebuilds the patient's orientation to time.

One-sided neglect occurs in both right- and left-sided brain-damaged patients but is more common in the left hemiplegic patient with right brain damage. Rearranging the environment to utilize the right visual field maximizes the patient's performance. For example, foods and silverware can be placed on the right side of the table so the patient can more successfully handle self-feeding. By keeping the unimpaired side toward the action, unless therapists are specifically working with the impaired side, the patient does not become isolated and can subsequently participate in therapy and care more efficiently. When staff members are heightening the awareness of the neglected side or neglected visual field, frequent reminders may redirect the patient's attention and lead to eventual awareness and compensation. Impulsivity may be extinguished by encouraging the patient simply to slow down as well as by breaking up tasks into a specified number of small steps, supplementing all directions with simple and repeated verbal cues if necessary. Regardless of the task involved, immediate and positive feedback given frequently will help the patient recognize errors and alter performance.

DYSARTHRIA

The act of feigning comprehension of the aphasic patient's speech also applies to the dysarthric population. The techniques used by the speech-language pathologist in treatment can be adopted by the nurse to improve intelligibility of the patient's speech. Asking the patient to slow down and exaggerate each word improves precision of articulation. Having the patient rephrase and shorten the intended message increases the probability of understanding. Request the patient to write or gesture ideas that are not understood. Finally, if all of these methods are unsuccessful or if the patient has no intelligible speech, the nurse may have to construct a simple alphabet or word board in the absence of a speech-language pathologist.

PATIENT AND FAMILY COUNSELING AND EDUCATION

Counseling and education of the patient and family are an ongoing and integral part of the total management of communication problems. Though there are many stages and these may differ from patient to patient and from family to family, the purpose remains alleviation of anxiety. Reassuring the patient and family that the patient is still the same individual, along with explaining the nature of the disorder, dispels fear of the unknown. Once therapy has begun, the patient and family need to be counseled concerning the expectations and duration of therapy and they should be advised of the personal commitment necessary for full participation in the treatment process.

It is hoped that this involvement will reduce the omnipresence of impossible or unrealistic aspirations. With the guidance of a supportive speech-language pathologist, the patient and family can gradually learn to cope with the communication loss and accept the fact that a complete cure is not to be expected. If the services of a speech-language pathologist are not available, the nurse can direct the family to the American Speech-Language-Hearing Association or to state speech and hearing professional associations for a listing of services. In some cases, it may be necessary to enlist the support of a social worker, psychologist, or psychiatrist to tackle obstacles connected with the patient's and family's adjustment to each other and the communication loss. Once in the community, the patient and family can join a local stroke club, when available, for social, educational, and supportive activities. Information regarding these clubs can be received through either the American Heart Association or local branches.

Bibliotherapy provides another means of educating and counseling the family. Many books and pamphlets describing communication problems are available. These are directed toward the layperson and can be used to reinforce what the speech-language pathologist or nurse is teaching. Personal accounts written either by a person who has a communication loss or those close to such persons are also available and can prove illuminating to the family and comforting to the patient. Annotated bibliographies of these sources and audiovisual materials can be obtained from the American Heart Association, the American Speech-Language-Hearing Association, and the National Easter Seal Society for Crippled Children and Adults.

Addresses

American Speech-Language-Hearing Association
10801 Rockville Pike
Rockville, Maryland 20852

American Heart Association
44 East 23rd Street
New York, New York 10010

National Easter Seal Society for Crippled Children and Adults
2023 Ogden Avenue
Chicago, Illinois 60612

CONCLUSION

The management and rehabilitation of adults with speech and language disorders of neurological origin is interdependent upon the respective and integral roles of the speech-language pathologist and nurse. Reestablishment of communication restores an individual's sense of self-worth as well as improving relationships with others.

All those concerned with speech and language continue to investigate normal processes and disorders. Specifically, research is being conducted to correlate aphasia diagnosis with the results of computerized tomography. Investigators have hypothesized that the type and severity of aphasia may be predicted on the basis of computerized tomography results (Naeser and Hayward, 1977). Others have pointed to the necessity for further study of speech and language performance in the normal aging process (Hutchinson and Beasley, 1976). This process is particularly critical because it has been estimated that 11 percent of the population of the United States is 65 or over, and this percentage is increasing (Oyer and Oyer, 1976). Also, since this age group is vulnerable to neurological disease, the data will be invaluable in differentiating normal deterioration from disorders of speech and language in the geriatric population.

BIBLIOGRAPHY

Benson, D. Frank: "Psychiatric Aspects of Aphasia," *Brit J Psychiatry* 123:555–566, 1973.

Benton, Arthur: "Problems of Test Construction in the Field of Aphasia," *Cortex* 3:32–58, 1976.

Boone, Daniel R.: *The Voice and Voice Therapy,* Prentice-Hall, Englewood Cliffs, N.J., 1971.

Brookshire, Robert H.: *An Introduction to Aphasia,* BRK Publishers, Minneapolis, Minn., 1973.

Brown, Jason: *Aphasia, Apraxia and Agnosia,* Charles C Thomas, Springfield, Ill., 1972.

Burns, Martha S., and Gerald J. Canter: "Phonemic Behavior of Aphasic Patients with Posterior Cerebral Lesions," *Brain and Language* 4:492–507, 1977.

Canter, Gerald J.: "Dysarthria, Apraxia of Speech and Literal Paraphasias: Three Distinct Varieties of Articulatory Behavior in the Adult with Brain Damage," presented at the American Speech and Hearing Association Convention, Detroit, Mich., 1973.

Carson, Daniel, Florence E. Carson, and Ronald Tikofsky: "Learning Characteristics of Adult Aphasics," *Cortex* 4:92–112, 1968.

Chomsky, Noam: *Language and Mind,* Harcourt Brace World, New York, 1968.

Darley, Frederick L., Arnold E. Aronson, and Joe R. Brown: "Clusters of Deviant Speech Dimensions in the Dysarthrias," *J Speech Hearing Research* 12:462–496, 1969.

———, ———, ———: Differential Diagnostic Patterns of Dysarthria, *J Speech Hear Res* 12:246–269, 1969.

———, ———, ———: *Motor Speech Disorders,* Saunders, Philadelphia, 1975.

De Renzi, Ennio and Luigi A. Vignolo: "The Token Test: A Sensitive Test to Detect Receptive Disturbances in Aphasics," *Brain* 85:665–678, 1962.

Eisenson, Jon: *Adult Aphasia: Assessment and Treatment,* Prentice-Hall, Englewood Cliffs, N.J., 1973.

———: "Aphasia: A Point of View as to the Nature of the Disorder and Factors That Determine Prognosis for Recovery," *Int J Neurol* 4:287–295, 1964.

———: "Aphasia in Adults: Basic Considerations," in Lee Edward Travis (ed.), *Handbook of*

Speech Pathology and Audiology, Prentice-Hall, Englewood Cliffs, N.J., 1971.

———: *Examining for Aphasia,* Psychological Corp., New York, 1954.

Fowler, Roy S., and W. E. Fordyce: *Stroke: Why Do They Behave That Way?* American Heart Association, New York, 1974.

Geschwind, Norman: "Disconnexion Syndromes in Animals and Man," *Brain* 88:273–294, 585–644, 1965.

———: *Selected Papers on Language and the Brain,* Reidel Pub., Boston, 1974.

———: "The Organization of Language and the Brain," *Science* 170:940–944, 1970.

———: "The Varieties of Naming Errors," *Cortex* 3:97–112, 1967a.

———: "Wernicke's Contribution to the Study of Aphasia," *Cortex* 3:449–463, 1967b.

Glista, Sandra O., Anita S. Halper, and Kayte C. Nowikowski: "Language Rehabilitation in Patients with Non-Dominant Hemisphere Lesions," presented at the *Illinois Speech and Hearing Association* Convention, 1977.

Goldstein, Kurt: *Language and Language Disturbances,* Grune & Stratton, New York, 1948.

Goodglass, Harold, Jean Berko Gleason, and Mary R. Hyde: "Some Dimensions of Auditory Language Compression in Aphasia," *J Speech Hear Res* 13:595–606, 1970.

———, Barbara Klein, Peter W. Carey, and Kenneth J. Jones: "Specific Semantic Word Categories in Aphasia," *Cortex* 2:74–89, 1966.

———, and Edith Kaplan: *The Assessment of Aphasia and Related Disorders,* Lea & Febiger, Philadelphia, 1972.

Halper, Anita S., Ellyn J. Baker, and Carol S. Worcester: "Communication Problems of the Stroke Patient," *Nurs Homes* 16:16–19, 1967.

Head, Henry: *Aphasia and Kindred Disorders of Speech,* Hafner, New York, 1963.

Heart Facts, American Heart Association, New York, 1977.

Holland, Audrey: "Communicative Ability in Daily Living: Its Measurement and Observation," presented at the Academy of Aphasia, Montreal, Quebec, Canada, 1977.

Hutchinson, John M., and Daniel S. Beasley: "Speech and Language Functioning Among the Aging," in Herbert J. Oyer and E. Jane Oyer (eds.), *Aging and Communication,* University Park Press, Baltimore, 1976.

Lenneberg, Eric H.: *Biological Foundations of Language,* Wiley, New York, 1967.

Lieberman, Philip: *Speech Physiology and Acoustic Phonetics,* Macmillan, New York, 1977.

Luria, Alexksandr Romanovich: *Higher Cortical Functions in Man,* Basic Books, New York, 1966.

———: "Factors and Forms of Aphasia," in A. V. S. De Reuck and Maeve O'Connor (eds.), *Disorders of Language,* Little, Brown, Boston, 1964.

Naeser, Margaret, and Robert W. Hayward: "Correlation Between Size and Density of CT Scan Lesion Sites and Severity of Aphasia in Stroke Patients," presented at the Academy of Aphasia, Montreal, Quebec, Canada, 1977.

Netsell, Ronald, and Charles S. Cleeland: "Modification of Lip Hypertonia in Dysarthria Using EMG Feedback," *J Speech Hear Disord* 38:131–140, 1973.

Obler, Lorraine K., and Martin L. Albert: "Influence of Aging Recovery for Aphasia in Polyglots," *Brain and Language* 4:460–463, 1977.

Oyer, Herbert J., and E. Jane Oyer (eds.): *Aging and Communication,* University Park Press, Baltimore, 1976.

Porch, Bruce E.: *Porch Index of Communicative Ability,* Consulting Psychologists Press, Palo Alto, California, 1967.

Sarno, Martha Taylor (ed.): *Aphasia: Selected Readings,* Prentice-Hall, Englewood Cliffs, N.J., 1972.

———: "Disorders of Communication in Stroke," in Sidney Licht (ed.), *Stroke and Its Rehabilitation,* Waverly Press, Baltimore, 1975.

———, Marla G. Silverman, and Elaine Sands: "Speech Therapy and Language Recovery in Severe Aphasia," *J Speech Hear Res* 13:607–623, 1970.

Sarno, John E., and Martha Taylor Sarno: "The Diagnosis of Speech Disorders in Brain Damaged Adults," *Med Clin North Am* 53: 561–573, 1969.

Schuell, Hildred, James J. Jenkins, and Edward Jiménez-Pabón: *Aphasia in Adults,* Harper & Row, New York, 1964.

———: *Differential Diagnosis of Aphasia with the Minnesota Test,* University of Minnesota Press, Minneapolis, 1965.

Skelly, Madge: "Aphasic Patients Talk Back," *Am J Nurs* 75:1140–1142, 1975.

Sparks, Robert, Nancy Helm; and Martin L. Albert: "Aphasia Rehabilitation Resulting from Melodic Intonation Therapy," *Cortex* 10: 303–316, 1974.

Spreen, Otfried, and Arthur L. Benton: *Neurosensory Center Comprehensive Examination for Aphasia,* Univ. of Victoria, Victoria, B.C., Canada, 1969.

Strub, Richard L., and F. William Black: *The Mental Status Examination in Neurology,* F. A. Davis Company, Philadelphia, 1977.

Trost, Judith, and Gerald Canter: "Apraxia in Patients with Broca's Aphasia: A Study of Phoneme Production Accuracy and Error Patterns," *Brain Lang,* 1:63–80, 1974.

U.S. Department of Commerce: *Resource Materials for Communication Problems of Older Persons,* Washington, D.C., prepared by the American Speech and Hearing Association Committee on Communication Problems of the Aging, 1975.

U.S. Department of Health, Education, and Welfare: *Human Communication and Its Disorders—An Overview,* National Institutes of Health and Public Health Service, Bethesda, Maryland, 1969.

Vanderheiden, Gregg C., and Kate Grilley (eds.): *Non-Vocal Communication Techniques and Aids for the Severely Physically Handicapped,* University Park Press, Baltimore, 1977.

Vignolo, Luigi: "Evaluation of Aphasia and Language Rehabilitation: A Retrospective Exploratory Study," *Cortex* 1:344–367, 1964.

Weinberg, Joseph, Leonard Diller, Wayne Gordon, Louis Gerstman, Abraham Lieberman, Phyllis Lakin, Germaine Hodges, and Ora Ezrachi: "Visual Scanning Training Effect on Reading-Related Tasks in Acquired Right Brain Damage," *Arch Phys Med Rehabil* 58:479–486, 1977.

Weisenburg, Theodore, and Katherine E. McBride: *Aphasia: A Clinical and Psychological Study,* Hafner, New York, 1963.

Wepman, Joseph M.: "A Conceptual Model for the Process Involved in Recovery from Aphasia," *J Speech Hearing Disord* 18: 4–13, 1953.

———: "Aphasia: Language Without Thought or Thought Without Language," *ASHA* 18: 131–136, 1976.

———, and Lyle V. Jones: *Studies in Aphasia: An Approach to Testing,* Education-Industry Service, Chicago, 1961.

Zemlin, Willard R.: *Speech and Hearing Science,* Prentice-Hall, Englewood Cliffs, N.J., 1968.

13
george l. larsen

chewing
and swallowing

THE PROBLEM OF DYSPHAGIA

The human pharynx is the common pathway for both feeding and respiration. Swallowing separates the two. The disorder of swallowing, called *dysphagia*, leads to two major health crises, malnutrition and aspiration. Dysphagia can occur at all ages. In the infant, congenital, natal, and developmental disorders, including cleft lip and palate and cerebral palsy, may cause dysphagia. Poliomyelitis and brain stem glioma are the more common disease etiologies. From preadolescence to middle age, neoplastic disease affecting the brain stem, bacteria and virus causing the Guillain-Barré syndrome, and the demyelinating diseases are more frequent causes. In mature years, the vascular diseases leading to bulbar and pseudobulbar palsy and Parkinsonism with its unknown cause are seen most commonly.

Less frequently seen but significant in causing dysphagia are postdiphtheritic paralysis, botulism, peripheral nerve involvement, and the myopathies and dermatomyositis. Head trauma may result in bulbar or superior bulbar palsy. Surgical reconstruction of the mouth and its contents causes a special form of swallowing disorder.

Considering the multitude of etiologies of dysphagia, it would appear more economical in a discussion of swallowing disorders to review normal swallowing in some detail, look at the effect of disease, trauma, or revision of the mechanism involved upon swallowing, and then develop a management or rehabilitation plan based on this understanding.

NORMAL ANATOMY AND PHYSIOLOGY

Normal swallowing requires intellectual awareness of the bolus to be introduced, functional, facial, intraoral, and laryngopharyngeal musculature, and an intact nervous system to mediate sensations and musculature behavior intellectually and reflexly.

Deglutition may be conveniently divided into three major processes. The first step is the buccopharyngeal stage, or that process in which a bolus is placed through the lips on to the tongue. The tongue tip rises to the palate, and the muscles of the cheeks and base of the tongue work the food to the rear of the mouth and the pharynx. The second stage is the pharyngeal stage. The pharynx is a common passageway for food passing down the esophagus and for air passing through the larynx and trachea. To prevent food from entering the larynx and choking the individual, this structure is drawn up to the base of the tongue, and the tongue moves backward and meets the larynx. The vocal cords approach each other tightly, and all inspiration and expiration momentarily cease. The upward movement of the larynx during swallowing can be felt or seen readily. If by grasping this structure between thumb and finger its elevation is prevented, swallowing cannot take place. Conversely, if the larynx is gently elevated, the swallow reflex will be stimulated. As the bolus is propelled toward the esophagus, the cricopharyngeus muscle, which serves as an upper esophageal sphincter by sympathetically induced tonic contraction, is relaxed and pulled open. The relaxation is produced by a parasympathetic stimulus carried by the vagus nerve, and the sphincter is passively pulled open by the action of laryngeal elevation and tilting. Contraction of the pharyngeal constrictors in a stripping-like wave drags the bolus finally into the esophagus. It is the action of the pharyngeal constrictors that prepares the esophagus for the final reflexive stage of swallowing.

The third stage of swallowing is the esophageal stage. The food bolus is carried between the pharynx and stomach by peristaltic movements and gravity. A primary peristaltic wave begins the stripping-like action of the pharynx, which spreads into the body of the esophagus and over the lower sphincter to evacuate the swallowed bolus into the stomach.

Five cranial nerves are involved in the act of swallowing, namely the Vth, VIIth, IXth, Xth, and XIIth. Taste is one of the nervous system's input to the reflex center in the medulla that helps the act of swallowing. Taste is picked up by fibers from cranial nerves VII, IX, and X that stream into the solitary nucleus. Taste buds in different parts of the mouth, including the tongue, palate, and epiglottis, pick up salty, sour, sweet, and bitter taste. This results in a flow of saliva which further spreads the sensation of taste, resulting in the nuances of flavor, and increases the stimulation of the taste buds.

It is important to remember that we begin life with about 9000 taste buds and end up with less than half by the age of 60 or so. This helps to explain in part some of the difficulties that may be associated with oral intake in geriatric centers.

The cortex plays a role in taste. With the cortex, we make decisions as to what we consider palatable or unpalatable, and we can make decisions as to whether to accept or reject whatever is in our mouth. The importance of the cortex is further appreciated when one realizes the influence that the sight, smell, and attractiveness of food has on salivation.

Chewing milks more saliva from the salivary glands, mixing it with the bolus to trigger the reflex in the oropharynx that we call swallowing. In chewing, the jaw is normally kept closed in opposition to gravity, but tactile stimulus of food particles against gums, upper and lower teeth, and the anterior part of the hard palate evokes reflex inhibition of the closing muscles, the temporalis and masseter. This is accomplished via the Vth cranial nerve and the reflex pattern in the solitary nucleus in the medulla oblongata. This nerve also relays sensations of heat, cold, and pain.

Opening of the jaw is followed by rebound closing, which, if food is still in the mouth, again stimulates opening. Thus the rhythmic act of chewing continues at an involuntary level. Obviously, there is input to chewing from the cortex, since we can regulate this behavior at will. That is, we can speed or slow the process, or we can initiate or inhibit it as a result of influence from the cortex.

As mentioned, chewing is responsible in part for salivation and moisture in the mouth. Without moisture in the mouth, it is extremely difficult to swallow and is impossible to swallow in rapid succession.

Although the swallow reflex takes only 1 to 2 s, it is a complex behavior that must be studied in detail when it is disturbed in order to develop a treatment plan.

DIFFERENTIAL DIAGNOSIS OF DYSPHAGIA

In discussing the differential diagnosis, we will not be concerned with gastrointestinal disease nor with those nutritional disorders secondary to psychiatric impairment. Our discussion of the differential diagnosis of dysphagia will include swallowing disorders secondary to mechanical impairment in the mouth, paralyzed muscles, or intellectual disturbances interfering with the ability to eat normally.

In evaluating the patient with dysphagia, it is important to look beyond the etiologic diagnosis and try to classify the patient's disorder functionally; that is, determine whether it is a disorder of manipulating the bolus, a disorder of sensation, a disorder of glottic closure, of cricopharyngeal relaxation, or some other type of disorder. When attempting to make this evaluation, it is important in taking the history to ascertain whether there has been nasal regurgitation, hoarseness, or aspiration. The patient who speaks as though talking through the nose may, in fact, have a paralyzed palate and/or oropharynx. A hoarse voice suggests partial paralysis of the Xth cranial nerve, which is important to deglutition. If the patient coughs a second or two after attempting to swallow either liquid or solid, there may be pooling at the upper end of the larynx in an area called the pyriform sinus. This is revealed by indirect laryngoscopic examination and is called the "pooling sign," which is consistent with an impairment in the normal processes of deglutition.

The patient may develop signs of dehydration because of self-imposed restriction of intake due to fear of choking. Radiographic evidence of aspiration may be present, or an unexplained spiking temperature may be the first indication of an aspiration pneumonia.

To effectively implement a treatment plan directed toward the rehabilitation potential of patients with swallowing problems, one must be able to determine the specific disability. There is little difficulty in evaluating the patient who has had physical alteration of the deglutitory mechanism. If the surgery or trauma has involved only the lip, then the patient may only be distressed by sialorrhea. If more than the anterior third of the tongue has been removed, then the patient may have difficulty moving the bolus from the anterior to posterior oropharynx where the reflex may sweep it into the esophagus. If the palate alone is affected, then the patient's concern may be nasal regurgitation.

The patient with paralytic dysphagia has lesions in the lower motor neuron system, which will result in muscle weakness and impairment of oral reflexes relative to the extent and site of lesion in the brain stem or cranial nerves. When the muscles of the face and mouth are palpated, they will be soft and silky. The reflexes in the mouth are tested by stimulating, with a gloved finger or applicator, the right and left sides of the uvula on the soft palate, the right and left sides of the oropharynx that is easily visualized, and the right and left sides of the base of the tongue. When stimulating each of these areas, one observes for the so-called gag reflex. In paralytic dysphagia, the reflex will be diminished or absent, depending on the site and extent of the lesion. The patient's speech will be impaired, depending on the extent of the muscle weakness. As mentioned earlier, indirect laryngoscopy will allow one to assess the relative strength of the vocal cords, and hence the cough reflex, and will also reveal whether there is debris in the vallecula and pyriform sinus referred to as the pooling sign.

The single most critical evaluation, which can be done at bedside, is the assessment of the laryngeal elevation. In the healthy individual, if you place a finger on top of the thyroid cartilage of the larynx and the person swallows, the finger will be deflected as the larynx elevates. If the finger is placed in the slight depression between the thyroid cartilage and the hyoid bone and slight pressure is exerted, the larynx may not elevate in the patient who has weakness of the muscles used in elevating the larynx in the normal swallow. The patient with dysphagia who understands the task will attempt to elevate the larynx but will not be able to deflect the finger. This weakness may be caused by either lower motor or upper motor neuron disease. Laryngeal elevation should also be tested by having the patient swallow a sip of water or a spoonful of ice chips. This will demonstrate whether aspiration is present, whether the larynx elevates normally, and whether there is nasal reflux. Also at this time, one must assess the competency of the cough reflex, for dysphagia rehabilitation cannot proceed if there is not a protective cough.

The general condition of the patient has to be ascertained as well. Certainly, the patient who is extremely debilitated or terminal is not a candidate for rehabilitation or rehabilitative surgery but simply must be given the most practical means of alimentation. Laboratory studies are usually limited to routine evaluations with the exception of cine-esophagram. This is almost universally available and is extremely helpful in determining the role of the cricopharyngeus and whether achalasia is present. Cricopharyngeal achalasia is described when a cricopharyngeus muscle does not relax and open in coordinated effort with the elevation of the larynx and the push of the bolus by the base of the tongue. This results in an incomplete swallow, leaving part or all of the bolus remaining in the hypopharynx. Special tests that are sometimes indicated include Tensilon tests for myasthenia and skin-muscle biopsy for dermatomyositis. These will not be discussed here because they relate to the etiologic diagnosis and are usually in the province of the neurologist.

The patient with pseudobulbar dysphagia will have spastic muscles of the face and oropharynx and hyperactive reflexes as a result of the loss of inhibitory influence from the cortex. To understand this patient, one must recall that the brain is biologically programmed so that the left hemisphere assumes responsibility for communication and the right hemisphere is responsible for intellectual activity involving motor planning. When the hemispheres are functioning optimally, the person is said to have the ability to solve the problems of everyday living appropriate to the level of maturity. The patient with damage to the left hemisphere has deficits in understanding the spoken word and in the ability to speak and has difficulty reading and writing. The problem is referred to as aphasia. This patient will often become overwhelmed and confused if eating and conversing are attempted simultaneously. It is possible for aspiration to occur with attempts to coordinate these two activities.

The patient with damage to the right hemisphere has difficulty solving problems that require action. The problem is called apraxia. The deficit may be in ideational apraxia, where the patient cannot conceive of a plan; it may be constructional apraxia, wherein the patient knows what to do but cannot organize the steps involved to solve the tasks; it may be visual apraxia, wherein a combination of visual perceptual disturbance and visual sequencing disturbance frustrates attempts; or it may be a combination of all of these. In eating, the patient will have difficulty figuring out how to get the food from the tray to the mouth, how much to chew, and when to swallow. Such patients are easily misjudged, and expectations may be excessive if verbal skills are intact.

A bedside screening psychometric test may be devised to help determine whether or not the patient with pseudobulbar dysphagia has sufficient perceptual or language impairment that also contributes to the disorder of swallowing. Draw a square, a cross, and a triangle on a sheet of paper and ask the patient to copy these figures without removing the pencil from the paper (Fig. 13-1). Observe how the patient manipulates the pencil, whether or not the patient knows how to proceed with the task, and then observe the characters that are copied. If the patient has perceptual disturbance severe

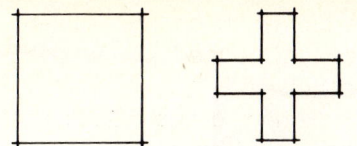

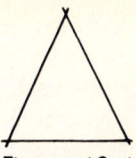

Figure 13-1
Language and perception screening. The subject is instructed as follows: (1) Copy the figures. (2) Name the figures. (3) Spell the names of the figures. (4) Repeat "He shouted the warning!" (5) Explain the meaning. (6) Write the sentence.

enough to interfere with the ability to eat, the corners of the square or the corners of the triangle may not meet, and the patient will most likely have the greatest difficulty with the cross. Typically, one of the legs of the cross will be absent or exaggerated in proportion to the others, or the patient will demonstrate a perseverative type of pattern where only a portion of the cross is drawn in a staircase-type fashion (see Fig. 13-2). These figures may then be used to assess simple language function. The patient is asked to name each figure and spell the name aloud. If the patient cannot do this or makes severe errors in the attempt, then there may indeed be language impairment sufficient to interfere with swallowing. If the patient is able to perform this simple task, the patient is then asked to write the name of each figure. If successful at this, the patient is asked to repeat the sentence "He shouted the warning" and then to explain what the sentence means. If the patient says it means, "Look out," this is a correct answer but may represent concrete thinking. If the patient is able to fabricate a complicated story demonstrating the meaning of the sentence, it is unlikely that there is language impairment sufficiently severe to cause swallowing difficulties.

The combination of a history of swallowing disorders, a competent physical examination of swallowing mechanism, and a screening assessment of the psychological functions that may disturb swallowing should lead the practitioner to the development of a rehabilitation program.

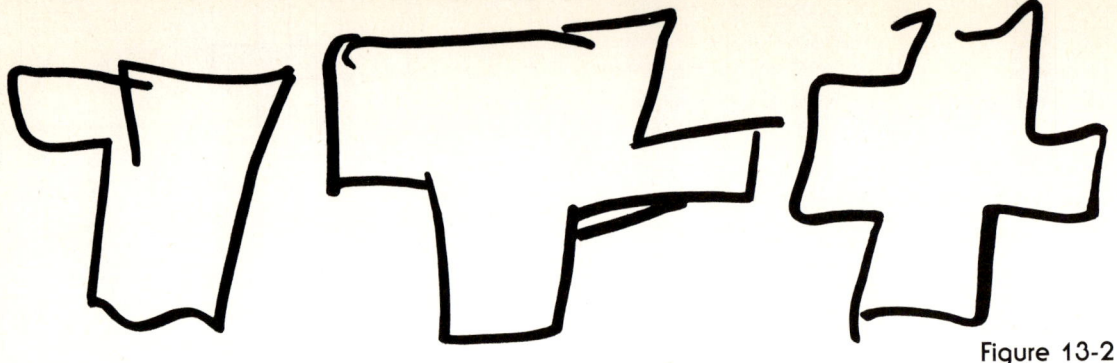

Figure 13-2
Samples of perceptual disturbance.

See Fig. 13-3 for a guideline of the physical examination.

REHABILITATION OF DYSPHAGIA

In the rehabilitation of the patient with a swallowing disorder, one must realize from the outset that considerable time and effort will be expended. To help the patient with disordered swallowing requires time, basic knowledge of what is involved in the swallowing act, and the ability to evaluate the disorder so that an appropriate program may be developed. And, although it has been stated earlier, it bears repeating that the patient must have a protective cough reflex before any program of rehabilitation is instituted.

MECHANICAL DYSPHAGIA

The patient who has difficulty moving the bolus from the anterior to the posterior mouth needs mechanical assistance to place the bolus where the reflexes will move it through the hypopharynx and into the esophagus. Some may require the passage of a stomach tube, performed either by themselves, by a nurse, or by a family member. If this is done several times a day, it is recommended that a very soft silastic feeding tube be used, such as the Keofeed stomach tube available from the Health Development Corporation of Palo Alto, California.

A septo-syringe may be used with a short piece of surgical tubing attached. The length of the surgical tubing should be the same as the distance from the posterior lip to the uvula, or where the uvula should be if it has been amputated. This device will place a bolus sucked up into the syringe and then released in the mouth at the most desirable place to prevent drooling and to assure swallowing.

A glossectomy spoon with a bladelike plunger, which is described in Fig. 13-4, may be used to push soft food off of the spoon when it is placed deep into the mouth. The foods used must be soft enough so that what is remaining of the tongue can crush it against the pharyngeal wall and assure that it is swallowed. Examples of such foods are Jello, custard, and mashed potatoes.

A further complication for the patient with mechanical dysphagia may be the formation of thick, ropy secretions that occur from infrequent swallowing and possibly from the drying effect of salivary gland damage or radiation. In this case, it is sometimes helpful to liquefy the secretions with papain, which is a proteolytic enzyme made from the papaya fruit. This enzyme attacks the protein chain of the saliva, liquefying it and making it easier to swallow or to wipe out of the mouth. Papain is available in most drugstores. It is important to remember to dissolve the papain tablet in the mouth approximately 10 min before feeding time to liquefy the secretions. The tablet should not be swallowed whole, as it is a mild diuretic and so must

```
NAME: _____ SSN: _____ DATE: _____

1. HISTORY:
    Chief complaint: _____
    _____
    Duration: _____ Frequency: _____
    Exacerbating factors: _____
    Solids, semisolids, liquids: _____

2. ASSOCIATED SYMPTOMS:
    _____ Obstruction (Pt. point to level)
    _____ Nasal regurgitation
    _____ Mouth odor
    _____ Aspiration
    _____ GE reflux (heartburn)
    _____ Hoarseness/speech
    _____ Pain
    _____ Weight loss
    _____ Pneumonia

3. HEALTH HISTORY—CURRENT MEDICATIONS:



4. PHYSICAL EXAMINATION:
    _____ General ENT_____
    _____ Masseter/Temporalis_____
    _____ Tongue strength and deviation_____
    _____ Palate elevation_____
    _____ Pharyngeal MM_____
    _____ Indirect laryngoscopy _____ Before swallow_____
                                _____ After swallow_____
    _____ Test swallow (H₂O) other specify_____
    _____ Laryngeal elevation_____
    _____ Coughing_____
    _____ Aspiration_____
    _____ Nasal regurgitation_____
    _____ Voice_____
    _____ Obstruction_____
    _____ Oral retention_____
```

Figure 13-3
Dysphagia worksheet.

be dissolved in order to liquefy secretions. If papain is not available, meat tenderizer made from the papaya enzyme may be used by rolling a lemon glycerin swab in the meat tenderizer and then applying this inside the oral cavity, again about 10 min before feeding time.

The patient who has undergone a supraglottic laryngectomy presents a special case wherein the protective mechanism of the larynx has been modified and the danger of aspiration is great. This patient will have greatest difficulty with liquids, as they spill easily into the modified larynx. This patient should be taught to sit upright while attempting to eat, with the chin slightly

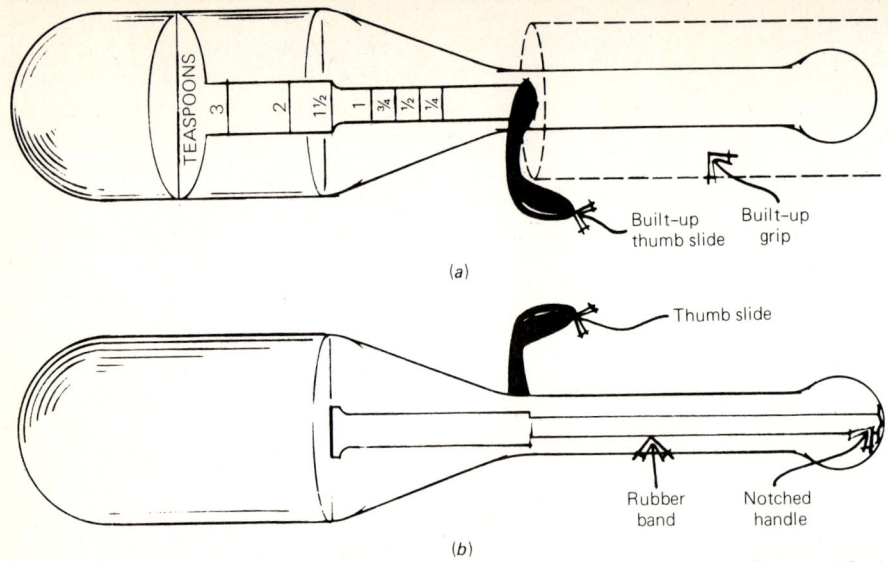

Figure 13-4

Glossectomy spoon, (a) top and (b) bottom. A commercially available measuring spoon can be adapted for use by patients with dysphagia mechanica. These modifications include: (1) A built-up "thumb slide" so that the spoon can be gripped with one hand and the slide pushed forward with the thumb. Using aluminum with a rubberized coating has proved successful. (2) In order to allow the plunger to glide forward and return automatically to a set position, a notch can be made at the back of the handle so that a rubber band can be attached to the notch, run beneath the handle, and attached below the thumb slide. (3) A built-up grip can be fabricated out of stainless steel, aluminum, or orthoplast and spot-welded or glued to the existing handle. This built-up grip is positioned so that the thumb slide is stopped by the grip at a point where $1^1/_2$ teaspoons is measured in the spoon. This allows for an average bolus of food to be placed into the spoon for each bite. The built-up grid should be left open at least $1/4$ in along the bottom to allow for replacement of the rubber bands.

flexed toward the chest so as to provide the most suitable anatomic route into the esophagus and to help use the tongue as a partial protection for the larynx. The patient must be taught to take a breath, swallow the bolus, and then exhale forcefully. When reviewing normal swallowing, one realizes that this is what should be happening anyway, and it is only necessary to reinforce this as a willful action. The purpose, of course, is to clear any remaining food or fluid that may have entered the laryngeal aditus following deglutition. The patient should first practice using ice chips, for if the patient does aspirate some of the ice, the clean water will be easily tolerated by the lungs in small amounts. Once ice chips can be successfully swallowed, then the patient should move on to foods that hold together in a single consistency. Included among these are foods such as soft-boiled eggs or ground meat mixed with gravy.

CHAPTER 13   180

DYSPHAGIA PARALYTICA

In addition to making a differential diagnosis, the practitioner will want to carefully assess the muscles of deglutition in dysphagia paralytica. If the reflexes are totally absent and the tongue and oropharynx, as well as the muscles that elevate the larynx, are paralyzed, then rehabilitation effort will be futile. In this situation, bypass surgery is warranted, and this is discussed later in the chapter.

Rehabilitation of the patient with partial dysphagia paralytica involves strengthening the muscles that are partially functional. Since the patients with dysphagia paralytica have an increased danger of aspiration and aspiration pneumonia, the technique used to strengthen the muscles must avoid the danger of having the patient aspirate. The feeding tube used orally is an excellent means of stimulating the muscles. A #14 or #16 Levine-type tube may be introduced into the mouth and the patient talked through the process of swallowing it orally. If these patients can use their hands, and particularly if they can sit in front of a mirror, have them guide the tube down themselves while receiving encouragement. If not, the tube should be placed in the center of the tongue, guided below the uvula, and passed into the esophagus with the patient's chin slightly flexed so as to provide the best route. The tube will stimulate the swallowing muscles as the patient is encouraged verbally to try to swallow as it is being passed. A particular advantage of using the feeding tube is that it can be readily retrieved if it should get into the larynx and trachea. Since the patient is likely to require a formula several times a day, there is the additional advantage of exercising the patient's muscles the same number of times. Once the tube is in the stomach, the formula can, of course, be given, as well as medications and fluids. In this way, the patient's nutrition is maintained during the rehabilitation process, and the patient also observes the gains being made in swallowing. If the patient requires further strengthening of the swallowing muscles, then the feeding tube may be increased in size up to a #18 French. If it is still necessary to strengthen the deglutitory muscles further, then a soft, rubber, mercury-filled esophageal dilator may be used, although seldom has this been necessary once the patient is succesful in swallowing the #18 French feeding tube. When the patient has developed sufficient strength to swallow the feeding tube, then the practitioner may introduce ice chips, for if they are aspirated, they will be reasonably well tolerated. Patients with dysphagia paralytica may have their intellectual processes intact. In this case, the patient should be encouraged to identify the bolus in the mouth by its texture, pressure, and temperature and to think about swallowing to gain support from the cortex. It is important to observe or palpate the larynx gently to witness the elevation for each swallow. The larynx must elevate completely before the next bolus of ice chips is introduced. When the patient no longer aspirates or chokes on the ice chips, nutritious items may be introduced that stimulate the senses of taste, texture, pressure, and temperature as much as possible. Foods like medium-boiled eggs, sliced canned peaches, and cottage cheese prepared in gelatin that has been doubled in strength or halved in water work very well. When patients are successful with these textures, they should be able to swallow anything they can chew.

Many practitioners assume that soft foods like apple sauce or puree will be easier for the patient to swallow. One must be careful not to confuse the ability to chew with the ability to swallow. Foods with textures like that of apple sauce and puree fall apart in the mouth and may be partially aspirated as well as partially swallowed. In addition, these textures meet only a minimum of the senses necessary to trigger the swallow reflex.

In order to facilitate the oral administration of medications to patients with dysphagia paralytica, it is recommended that ½-in cubes of stiffened gelatin be prepared by the dietitian, with the tablet or capsule imbedded in it for swallowing. If the gelatin is not tolerated, then cubes of ripe watermelon or a spoonful of jelly may work well.

PSEUDOBULBAR DYSPHAGIA

Patients with cortical damage will have been assessed for intellectual involvement. These patients have intact palatal ad pharyngeal reflexes when stimulated externally, but the palate may not elevate on phonation. If such a patient has a feeding tube in place, increased gagging and choking may ensue, for the reflexes are frequently hyperactive. If a feeding tube is in place, nausea may occur during feeding, not because of the formula, but because of the minor vibrations sent through the tube as the formula passes through, triggering the hyperactive gag reflex.

Patients with pseudobulbar dysphagia frequently have more difficulty with liquids than with solids because the liquids do not stimulate the sensory mechanisms in the mouth. The indirect laryngoscopic exam usually shows pooling in the pyriform sinus, and radiographic studies and cine-esophagrams are usually normal.

Consideration must be given to whether the lesion is in the right or the left side of the brain. If it is in the left and speech is impaired, patients will become overwhelmed and confused if eating and talking are attempted simultaneously. Also, these patients may be unable to proceed in an eating task if there is conversation going on around them, even though it may not be directed at them personally. Such patients are best managed by having them sit upright, bringing the food to them, and demonstrating what is expected of them, perhaps accompanied by one-word commands. The important thing is to not overwhelm them with verbal input at the same time they are eating, as this frequently results in overloading the damaged cerebral circuitry, and the patients may cease to perform. If the lesion is in the right side of the brain, resulting in perceptual disturbances, the patient will have difficulty figuring out how to get the food from the tray to the mouth, how much to chew, and when to swallow. This patient needs to be talked through each stage of eating without demonstration. The steps required need to be broken down into the smallest units possible. After each verbal command is given, time should be allowed for it to be executed before the next command in a series is given. This may have to be done for every meal, especially during the acute stages of brain damage. If a routine and unchanging schedule is maintained, these patients may eventually be able to feed themselves and may be helped by being able to refer to a written checklist.

In the geriatric patient, it is not unusual to see bilateral cortical lesions that result in pseudobulbar dysarthria as well as pseudobulbar dysphagia. In such cases, the patient's speech may seem reasonably intelligible but will be hypernasal. The relative influence of aphasia or perceptual disturbance must be carefully assessed to determine how to manage the patient most efficiently.

In addition to determining the most appropriate psychological manipulation for the patient, management also involves increasing the stimuli of texture, temperature, and taste and allowing for the latency that may occur between the stimulus and the response to swallow. Again, patients must be taught not to attempt to swallow at the same time that other activities may be competing for their attention. Patients should concentrate on the task of swallowing volitionally rather than attempting to depend on the reflexes. These patients will be most successful if they are sitting up in a straight-backed chair and encouraged to keep the neck slightly flexed. In order to increase the influence of intellectualization on swallowing, the patients may be encouraged to hold their breath momentarily when they swallow. The person caring for the patient should observe the elevation or feel the elevation of the larynx for each swallow, making sure that it has occurred before introducing the next bolus or sip. The standard bolus is 15 cm for each separate swallow. It is important not to overload the mouth, for swallowing is inefficient if overloaded, and the patient may aspirate. Fluids and solids should be presented separately. Never use fluids to "wash the bolus down," as this will result in coughing and maybe aspiration.

If the patient with pseudobulbar dysphagia has a feeding tube in place, it should be removed during attempts at rehabilitation, for it is difficult to swallow around the tube. It is possible in many instances, but it does increase the burden on the patient, and there is some chance of directing the bolus into the larynx and trachea if it catches on the tube.

If the patient requires tube feeding to maintain nutrition during the rehabilitation process, it is recommended that the orogastric route be used whenever possible, as this provides both stimulation and exercise to the deglutitory mechanism.

BYPASSING SWALLOWING

When conservative management of diet manipulation or deglutitory muscle rehabilitation has failed or if tube feeding is required during rehabilitation attempts, a surgical bypass procedure should be considered. It is advantageous not to have the tubes in the nasopharynx when the therapist is trying to rehabilitate swallowing. The feeding tube may not only be uncomfortable but it also creates bulk around which an oral bolus must pass in an already decompensated mechanism.

Rehabilitative surgery falls into three categories. The first is corrective surgery, such as nerve grafting for the patient with a facial paralysis. Unfortunately, it is almost never possible to restore normal physiology to the patient with dysphagia. In this group of patients, either compensatory surgery, which further modifies the normal physiology to improve the overall function, albeit with some sacrifice, or bypass syrgery, which simply substitutes a totally different mode of functioning, must be considered. Examples of compensatory surgery would be cricopharyngeal myotomy, Teflon vocal cord injection, and such adjunctive procedures as tympanic neurectomy to control sialorrhea. The third category, bypass surgery, includes such procedures as laryngeal diversion, glottic closure, pharyngostomy, esophagostomy, gastrostomy, and jejunostomy. Each of these has its advantages.

Both laryngeal diversion and glottic closure totally separate the alimentary and respiratory tracts. They allow oral feeding, but there is loss of laryngeal speech. Both are potentially reversible. Pharyngostomy is usually performed through the pyriform sinus and is probably the simplest method of managing the patient who is going to be dependent upon tube feeding for a long time. Its main disadvantage has been frequent difficulty in tube changing. In some patients, the tube, when passed into the stoma, tends to go up rather than down, resulting in distress to the patient and possible introduction into the larynx. Esophagostomy is generally preferred as the standard procedure. This involves making an esophageal-cutaneous anastomosis, which will remain lined with epithelium and will allow both simple tube changing and removal of the tube between meals if the patient or the attendants desire. The advantages of this procedure are that it is cosmetically acceptable, being low in the neck; the tube can be left out between meals; skin care is easier than with gastrostomy; the patient can be fed in an upright position, taking advantage of gravity and making use of the GI tract; and the stoma, while semipermanent, can be closed as an outpatient procedure. Gastrostomy, while probably the most popular procedure for long-term alimentation in the United States, is superior to esophagostomy only in situations where esophageal surgery per se is contraindicated. These would include esophageal obstructions, the presence of tumor, heavy doses of irradiation in the neck, or a superior vena cava syndrome. Jejunostomy is perhaps superior to gastrostomy in some instances, and it is especially useful in the patient who has problems with gastroesophageal reflux. This occurs most frequently in patients who are obese, bedridden, and have a hiatus hernia. These patients will do poorly with either gastrostomy or esophagostomy because of constant reflux, and the only real solution is to place the feeding tube distal to the pylorus. A jejunostomy is ideal for this.

Some patients with dysphagia are considered for tracheostomy, although dysphagia is not among its indications. Tracheostomy should be a last resort, used only when the patient with dysphagia or aspiration requires a vigorous pulmonary toilet or ventilatory support. One of the most frequent complications of tracheostomy, even in the otherwise normal patient, is dysphagia caused by the tethering of the laryngotracheal complex and failure of laryngeal elevation. If pharyngeal airway maintenance and laryngeal valving are adequate, tracheostomy can usually be avoided.

DIETARY CONSIDERATIONS

The daily basal caloric requirement for an adult man is about 1500 cal per 24 h. This energy is needed for muscle tone and to maintain basal, circulatory, respiratory, digestive, glandular, and cellular activity. For the amount of work required to move, sit up, cough, and the like for the person who is otherwise on complete bed rest, approximately 2000 cal per day are needed, and for one restricted to ambulation in the hospital room, the requirement is roughly 2250 calories per day. The patient undergoing rehabilitation will have to be assessed carefully for nutritional requirements, especially if the patient has dysphagia. This patient may not be able to indicate a level of thirst. Adequate intake of fluids is an extremely important part of the dysphagic patient's care. Inadequate or excessive body fluids can cause cerebral symptoms and exaggerate symptoms that are already there from the basic disease. If the patient with dysphagia undergoes rapid behavioral changes, then a review of the fluid intake is necessary to rule out this influence when swallowing is not normal.

It is beyond the scope of this chapter to review nutritional needs or the composition of institutional formulas. However, the patient with dysphagia may have difficulties with some foods, while others may improve the outlook of the rehabilitation. Uncooked milk, that is, milk and ice cream, frequently cause the formation of phlegm. The phlegm makes it more difficult to swallow a bolus, and the patient may have a sense of strangulation. Creamed soups and puddings are acceptable because the milk has been brought to a boiling point, and the heat apparently breaks down the protein chains that contribute to the phlegm. Soft foods may be easy to chew, but if they are sticky, they will be difficult to swallow. Examples of this are mashed potatoes, soft, fresh, white bread, and bananas. To make these foods acceptable, bits of meat and gravy should be mixed liberally with the potatoes. Bread should be allowed to sit at least overnight and is often better tolerated if toasted. There appears at first glance to be a contradiction in this statement, but if one realizes that chewing toast or a cracker manipulates it into a bolus acceptable to the oropharynx, it is understandable why drier breads and crackers are easier to swallow. Extremely dry foods can also present a problem, however, and they need to be moistened. Gravy can be added to potatoes and meat, and crackers may be dipped in tea or coffee. Slippery foods, such as canned fruits, are easier to swallow, and they hold together well in the oropharynx, but they may be difficult to control in the mouth for mastication or if there has been surgical revision of the oral contents. Pureed foods provide insufficient texture for stimulation and may fall apart in the mouth and be partially aspirated. Liquids or foods without flavor or with flavor that the patient dislikes may cause an inadequate stimulation to the deglutitory reflex. For example, a patient may aspirate tap water but be able to drink chilled orange juice.

When determining what nutrients to give the patient, it is worthwhile to review the normal anatomy and physiology of deglutition and to consider how to increase the properties of texture, temperature, and flavor.

CONCLUSION

As the population increases in age and as the survival rate of patients improves, rehabilitation practitioners will be increasingly exposed to the challenge of the patient with dysphagia. To understand swallowing disorders, it is essential to have a foundation in the normal anatomy and physiology of this activity. A careful evaluation of the swallowing function is needed to differentiate between mechanical dysphagia, in which there is damage to oral contents, paralytic dysphagia, in which there is disease in the lower motor neuron system, and pseudobulbar dysphagia, in which the upper motor neuron system is impaired. The treatment depends on the type of disorder present.

A basic tenet in the concept of rehabilitation is to make full use of remaining assets and to minimize liabilities. In some cases where swallowing is totally impaired, the rehabilitation specialist must be willing to look at alternative routes of alimentation.

BIBLIOGRAPHY

Acquarelli, Mario J.: "Cervical Esophagostomy," *Arch Otolaryngol* 96:November 1972.

Donner, M. W., and M. L. Silbiger: "Cinefluorographic Analysis of Pharyngeal Swallowing in Neuromuscular Disorders," *Am J Med Sci* 251(5): May 1966.

Fleming, Susan et al.: "The Patient with Cancer Affecting the Head and Neck: Problems in Nutrition," *J Am Diet Assoc* 70: April 1977.

Habel, M. A., and J. E. Murran: "Surgical Treatment of Life-endangering Chronic Aspiration Pneumonia," *Plast Reconstr Surg* 49, 1972.

Heimburger, Robert F., and Ralph M. Reitan: "Easily Administered Written Test for Lateralization of Brain Lesions," *J Neurosurg* 18(3), 1961.

Larsen, G. L.: "Conservative Management for Incomplete Dysphagia Paralytica," *Arch Phys Med Rehabil* 54 (4): April 1973.

———: "Rehabilitating Dysphagia: Mechanica, Paralytica, Pseudobulbar," *J Neurosurg Nurs*, July 1976.

Lindeman, R. C., "Diverting the Paralyzed Larynx: A Reversible Procedure for Intractable Aspiration," *Laryngoscope* 85, 1975.

Montgomery, W. W.: *Surgery of the Upper Respiratory System*, vol. 2, Lea & Febiger, Philadelphia, 1973.

———, "Surgery to Prevent Aspiration," *Arch Otolaryngol* 101, 1975.

Paparella, M. M., and D. A. Shumrick: Otolaryngology, vol. 1: *Basic Sciences and Related Disciplines*, Saunders, Philadelphia, 1973.

Phillips, M. M., and T. R. Hendrix: "Dysphagia," *Postgrad Med* 50:4, 1971.

Pitcher, J. L.: "Dysphagia in the Elderly: Causes and Diagnosis," *Geriatrics*, 23(10): October 1973.

Seaman, W. B., "Pharyngeal and Upper Esophageal Dysphagia," *JAMA* 235(24): June 1976.

Stevens, K. M., and R. C. Newell: "Cricopharyngeal Myotomy in Dysphagia," *Laryngoscope* 77(4): April 1967.

14
lee shields

urinary function

INTRODUCTION

Becoming wet because of a leakage of urine is among the most embarrassing circumstances a person beyond 4 years of age can face. Conversely, being unable to urinate when necessary is one of the most painful events that can be experienced. Urologic complications associated with urinary incontinence or retention of urine are among the most dangerous and life-threatening of clinical problems.

Urologic dysfunction can involve every age group. For the child with urinary incontinence, participation in school activities may be limited to requesting a teacher of the homebound. For adults, particularly those in vocations requiring long hours of sitting in one area—e.g., secretaries, business executives—urinary incontinence may be extremely limiting and disruptive. Travel by airplane can be complicated, and for the retired person, even grocery shopping can be delayed for fear of incontinence.

Urologic problems are considered a very personal and private calamity. If the problem cannot be managed, it can lead to isolation from family and friends. Every activity of daily living can be interrupted, and the problem can cause fear of the company of others at home, school, or work.

Philosophy of Care

Nurses involved in rehabilitation should recognize the right of those with disability to achieve and maintain acceptable forms of urinary bladder emptying. The philosophy of the nurse should include consideration of the patient's unique personality and individual desires. Nursing observations are valuable contributions in assessing psychosocial, vocational, and physical problems related to the patient's genitourinary disorder. An efficient nurse can help the patient and family maintain regimens involved in urologic treatment. An ingenious and creative nurse can assist patients to temporarily or permanently modify their form of urinary drainage as indicated and to make adjustments in their life-style, while maintaining a healthy self-image. A forward-looking nurse can help in preparing the patient and family to follow a urologic self-care regimen in anticipation of discharge from the rehabilitation setting to home and community.

The prevention of metabolic and infectious complications in persons with disorders of the urinary system is vital to decreasing mortality and morbidity in the disabled. Satisfactory renal and urinary bladder function are essential ingredients of independence, the end goal of rehabilitation.

Goals

Urologic nursing care, within the overall nursing care goals, must be presented to the patient and family in terms they can comprehend and use in making decisions about care and goal setting. The primary goal is to deliver quality urologic care. Associated subgoals are (1) to prevent adverse effects from urologic nursing intervention, (2) to help the patient adapt to the urologic disorder, (3) to help the patient maintain a pharmocologic regimen compatible with therapeutic and personal goals, (4) to maintain fluid and electrolyte balance, (5) to teach the patient and the family about the disorder and its manifestations, (6) to control infections, (7) to help the patient to achieve and maintain a functional bladder or acceptable substitute, and (8) to keep the patient free from preventable adverse effects of urologic catheterization procedures (*Standards of Urological Nursing Practice*, 1977).

Assessment

Urologic dysfunction is a problem for a significant portion of the world's population. Its origin can be congenital, gynecological, psychological, traumatic, or neurogenic in nature. Problems can arise from a broad range of disabling conditions that include myelomeningocele, diabetes mellitus, stroke, arteriosclerosis, pernicious anemia, multiple sclerosis, poliomyelitis, spinal or cerebral tumors, and trauma. Not limited only to the urinary tract, the problems accompanying urologic dysfunction may affect the entire body. At no time can the patient's "plumbing" ever be disassociated from the mind, the internal organs, and the exterior.

Collection of sufficient information about the

patient's past and present urologic health status is essential to formulation of an individualized plan of care. The first information is usually collected from patient and family interviews. Such information will indicate the patient's ability to verbalize physical symptoms related to urinary function and give insight into mental and emotional responses to the effects of the disorder.

Information is gathered over time and should expand with each contact. Data particularly pertinent for urologic assessment are compiled within these guidelines:

1. General history and anticipated goals
    a. Reason for past and current evaluation (medical condition)
    b. Previous urologic care
    c. Length of time available for evaluation and nursing care
    d. Patient expectations
    e. Discharge plans and available resources
2. Current status and support structures
    a. Self
        (1) Gender, age, and weight (determine form of bladder emptying, urine-collection devices, and ability to achieve self-care)
        (2) Dietary and fluid intake (volume, times, preferences, mineral content)
        (3) Bowel elimination (method, sphincter tone, effectiveness)
        (4) Autonomic dysreflexia
        (5) Skin lesions
        (6) Medications, allergies (especially drug-resistant organisms, response, knowledge of medications)
        (7) Vital signs (baseline information to assess side effects of autonomic-system drugs)
        (8) Patient's role in society: single, husband or wife, etc.
        (9) Occupation (effects of incontinence)
        (10) Social interests and activities (self-care needs)
        (11) Mental status (level of information for decision making; sense of time; reliability; motivation for self-care; anxious, depressed, suicidal; communication skills)
        (12) Functional ability (dominant hand, dexterity, mobility, strength, length of arms, appliances and braces, type of clothing worn)
        (13) Sexual characteristics (maturational level, sex drive, alterations in sexual function)
            (a) Female (vaginal discharge, menstrual history, use of tampons or sanitary napkins, contraceptives)
            (b) Male (contraceptives, concerns about fertility)
        (14) Sleep patterns (disrupted by incontinence or care needs)
        (15) Pain and relation to urologic function
        (16) Financial status and relation to cost of care and home-care needs
    b. Family and significant others
        (1) Available for teaching
        (2) Social environment (family expectations for patient, their rest and sleep patterns if living with patient; joint problems associated with urologic care)

For each urologic complaint identified as a problem by the patient, a review of the onset and precipitation factors should be conducted. With pertinent information-seeking questions in mind, the interview may be conducted along with the physical examination. To facilitate recall, the written tool can be checked frequently and overlooked questions added.

GENERAL CONSIDERATIONS

The bladder normally functions as a reservoir for storage of urine for the person in a continent state, and a voluntary method of emptying is used. Cerebral control over the detrusor muscle and the periurethral striated muscles, levator ani, and muscles of the urogenital diaphragm achieve urinary continence. During most of the waking and sleeping hours there is a persistent bombardment of impulses from the pudendal motor nerves to the urinary sphincters to stay closed so that no urine leakage occurs (Caldwell, 1975).

The anatomic integrity of the brainstem reticular formation to the spinal cord is necessary for a coordinated detrusor reflex capable of producing complete bladder emptying. Distinguishing information in a urologic assessment includes:

- Bladder sensation of overdistention and temperature change
- Perineal sensation
- Anal sphincter tone and reflexes
- Frequency and 24-h pattern
- Volume
- Incontinence
- Initiation of voiding, control and facilitation used
- Voiding flow rate, size and force of stream
- Residual urine volume
- Composition and physical properties of urine
- Resting bladder pressure and filling pressure
- Bladder tone as shown by intravesical pressure at low volumes
- Maximum intravesical pressure; contraction; pattern of pressure, volume relationships, and changes
- Bladder capacity
- Neurologic lesion type, location, and extent

The perineal (saddle) and perianal area are checked for sensation. If there is a defect in perineal feeling of touch or pinprick, there may be a similar defect in bladder sensation. A person with normal bladder function senses distention with bladder filling and temperature changes, is aware that the bladder is full, and can perceive an urge to void. Because saddle skin sensation (perineal and perianal area) corresponds to the S2–S6 segments that receive sensory impulses from the bladder, the response to touch or pinprick is informative.

The condition of any stomas present should be noted. The anal sphincter tone and the bladder's motor innervation may be estimated when inserting a suppository and can suggest the degree of spasticity.

Inspection of the male genitalia includes evaluation of the condition of the foreskin and description of any urethral discharge. During examination of the female, the size and condition of the labia, the location of the urethral meatus in comparison to the clitoris and vagina, and the presence of any discharge should be noted.

The type and condition of urine-collecting devices, if used, are noted. Positioning should be determined if scrotal edema is anticipated for patients in negative nitrogen balance.

Identification of allergies to soap or collecting-device materials may avoid skin complications. Confluent redness alone or with scattered small pustules, erosions, or papules on the upper thighs and anogenital area without involvement of the creases may indicate prolonged contact with urine. Fungal infection is often found along with body warmth, tight clothing, obesity, and rubbing from extremity spasms. Excess moisture may cause superinfection by yeast or viruses. To identify yeast (moniliasis), look for deep redness and excess moisture in skin folds, creases, or scrotum. Large, moist warts (condylomata acuminata) may interfere with urination and with intercourse (Cohen and Glass, 1978; Parrish, 1975).

Spasms in the legs, particularly when the bladder is full, should be noted. Hyperactive deep tendon reflexes may suggest detrusor activity.

UROLOGIC ASSESSMENT FACTORS

Changes in the volume of excreted urine are usually related to the efficiency of renal function, along with variations in the intake of fluids and foods, the metabolic rate, and the amount of exercise. Most patients in rehabilitation settings experience alterations in these factors. Gross examination of urine output is easily accomplished and may be a valuable indicator of renal function. Reference information can be gained by recording the time and volume of fluid intake and urine output for 48 h.

The simplest of intake and output records becomes crucial to accurate diagnosis. Nurses should be particularly watchful of patients with solitary functioning kidneys. True anuria may result from shock or ureteral obstruction, as from calculi or tumor growth.

Excessive volumes of urine (usually more than 1500 mL within a 24-h period in an adult of normal size and weight) can occur late in certain forms of chronic renal disease when the tubular reabsorption mechanism is damaged and ability to concentrate urine is impaired (Brundage, 1976). This is not to be confused with frequent urination, which patients may perceive as high urine output. An accurate record of 24-h output, with volume and time intervals, is essential to discover the cause of polyuria.

Patients to whom forcing fluids has been stressed, who develop psychogenic habits of drinking water by the pitcherful, can easily produce more than 2000 to 3000 mL in 24 h. If they are experiencing additional stress in cold temperatures or taking thiazide diuretic medication, the output can be excessive.

Urinary Incontinence

Urinary incontinence has been characterized as involuntary loss of urine through the lower urinary tract sufficient to be socially or hygienically unacceptable (Caldwell, 1975). Different types of urinary incontinence are caused by varied pathologic conditions.

Overflow (paradoxical) incontinence occurs when the bladder is overstretched, creating internal pressure higher than that of the urethral sphincter. There is a constant dribble of urine. The cause may be either neurogenic dysfunction or an obstruction to urine outflow, with subsequent decompensation of the detrusor muscle. If there is no sensory defect, urine retention with overflow incontinence is painful.

Urge incontinence results from uncontrollable detrusor contractions. The patient may feel an urge to void frequently and inappropriately and may be wet at night. Bladder inflammation, stones, and tumors can cause strong sensory impulses to reach the central nervous system which overcome the usual inhibition and result in micturition. Loss of cerebral inhibition of the micturition center, as seen in patients with cerebrovascular accident (CVA), lowers the volume at which there are marked detrusor contractions.

Reflex incontinence is present when involuntary reflex produces spontaneous voiding. If a spinal cord lesion is complete, there is usually no sensation of bladder fullness; there may be a vague feeling of abdominal pressure.

Stress incontinence is the loss of urine caused by a rise in intraabdominal pressure. The patient may be wet only with straining. The causes include an incompetent bladder neck and weak urethral and pelvic floor muscles and supporting ligaments. The degrees of stress incontinence are designated as Grade 1, leakage of urine when straining at rest; Grade 2, leakage when moving abruptly; and Grade 3, leakage when lying in bed (Caldwell, 1975).

Initiation of Voiding and Control of Urine

Assessment of the patient's past and present voiding habits is important. One factor to consider is how the patient initiates micturition. Must strain be used? Is Credé manual expression used to help start the stream? Is intraabdominal pressure or the Valsalva maneuver used to help empty the bladder?

The way in which the patient controls the bladder emptying is informative. Normally, the stream can be stopped and restarted at will within 8 to 10 s if there is no significant embarrassment. What is the force and arching of the stream? What is the size of the stream, and is there prolonged dribbling at termination? Is there complete emptying of the bladder? There should be less than 30 mL of residual urine, unless there is significant pain with voiding.

SPECIFIC DIAGNOSTIC MEASURES

Composition and Physical Properties of Urine

The measurement of specific gravity determines the weight of dissolved solutes in the urine. With the development of chronic renal disease, early loss of tubular reabsorption can be measured as less concentrated urine with a low specific gravity.

The density of urine may be increased by sediment of mucus, pus, or blood which can be identified by microscopic examination. Frothy urine may indicate abnormal protein excretion from chronic pyelonephritis. Bleeding may accompany trauma, stones, tumor, or acute cystitis, especially with fungal infections.

Changes in the color of urine from the normal clear yellow to darker amber is not an indicator of concentration. Grossly different variations in color that persist can be significant and require identification by qualitative laboratory tests.

The acidity or alkalinity of urine is determined by its hydrogen ion concentration. Alkaline urine may occur after meals high in dairy products, citrus fruits, and vegetables, when the kidney delivers bicarbonate ions into the urine to buffer the hydrochloric acid formed in the stomach during digestion. Because most diets are high in protein foods that are metabolized to acid end products, the urine is usually acidic. Failure to acidify the urine may occur with hypercalciuria and nephrocalcinosis.

Upon standing, urine decomposes urea into ammonia, which has a characteristic odor. Foul odors usually result from urinary tract infections caused by coliform bacilli. *Escherichia coli* infections give a fishlike smell. Asparagus eaters know the aroma of methylmercaptan in the urine (Macleod, 1976).

The presence or absence of **bacteriuria** must be determined. Acute and chronic inflammation of the urethra, bladder neck, or trigone frequently produce white blood cells in excess of one or two per high-power field, even though the urine is sterile. Urine culture, preferably by clean-catch specimen, is required to identify the infecting organisms. A true infection (significant bacteriuria) is usually said to exist when the colony count from a single culture is over 100,000 organisms per milliliter, with bacteria and pus cells miscroscopically present in a clean-catch specimen. If the specimen is obtained by catheterization, the presence of more than 1000 colonies is considered to constitute a significant infection (Kunin, 1974).

Serum creatinine and *creatinine clearance* tests are used to determine glomerular filtration. The serum creatinine is usually reliable as a measure of glomerular filtration because only a minute amount of this substance is secreted by the renal tubules into the urine. If there is sufficient back pressure on the kidneys to interfere with glomerular filtration, the test report would show a rise in the creatinine level, with variations for sex and age (Winter and Morel, 1977). Because it is possible to get falsely elevated values with laboratory determination, a 24-h creatinine clearance test is carried out simultaneously, especially for patients who appear healthy but become confused or disoriented. The 24-h measurement gives the amount of creatinine that can be cleared by the kidney in 1 min. One of the earliest signs of renal infection, prior to fever, nausea, and vomiting, is a decrease in creatinine clearance.

Radiologic Indicators

Assessment of urine production efficiency is not complete until radiologic results are available. The preliminary films (plain, or scout, film; flat plate) are used for initial visualization of radiopacities that might represent renal or bladder stones and for inspection of the bony structures.

Excretory urography is used to rule out kidney stones, tumors, large cysts, pylonephritis, or hydronephrosis. If the patient is able to void during filming, a picture of the bladder neck and urethra may be obtained. Post-voiding films provide rough estimates of the amount of contrast dye left in the bladder (residual urine volume) after voiding. This may permit visualization of stones in the lower ureters that may have been masked by a distended bladder.

Special radiologic tests such as *renal sonography* and *arteriography* may be done to differentiate mass lesions of the kidney, especially prior to surgery. *Nephrotomograms* are always taken to confirm proper position of nephrostomy tubes with insertion and changes.

Cystograms may be performed to rule out vesicoureteral reflux, define the size, shape, and capacity of the bladder, and observe for tumors or calculi. A retrograde urethrogram may demonstrate urethral strictures, diverticula, or fistulas. A voiding *cine cystogram* under fluoroscopy is frequently used to study the bladder and urethra during voiding.

Urodynamic Studies

Neurourodynamic procedures with sophisticated electronic equipment are being used more extensively to evaluate neuromuscular function of the bladder detrusor and urethra. Physical observations combined with information gathered from graphic results of these tests have proved to be valuable diagnostic tools in the evaluation of urinary incontinence. Properly conducted urodynamic studies usually carry no significant risk. Patients need to know how the procedure will be carried out before each test. They should be reassured about the measures to prevent complications, such as administration of appropriate antibiotics at least 24 h before testing, sterile techniques used, and careful operation of the electronic instruments. They should know that the procedures are not unduly painful. Children are often given light anesthesia or premedication before the study. Excessive movement must be avoided during the tests, because it produces artifacts on the graphic recordings that make interpretation of findings difficult.

Measurement of urinary flow rate, gas cystometry, integrated sphincter electromyelography, and *urethral pressure profiles* are the studies most widely used by major rehabilitation centers to differentiate anatomic obstruction from neurogenic dysfunction. These tests give useful diagnostic information on recurrent urinary tract infection of unknown etiology, retention with high residual volumes, vesicoureteral reflux of undertermined cause, and frequency and urgency (Bradley et al., 1974).

If the patient is capable of voiding, the urinary flow rate may be measured before cystometry. The patient voids into a specially constructed commode chair equipped with flow sensors. The flow sensors determine the rate, which is plotted against time by the recorder unit. An average urinary flow rate is approximately 20 mL/s. When urine flow is measured simultaneously with measurement of intravesical pressure and intrarectal pressure, it is possible to determine whether voiding is caused by detrusor reflex or abdominal straining.

Cystometry measures bladder pressures under varying stages of filling and emptying. The normal bladder is capable of stretching to accommodate increasing bladder volumes, while at the same time maintaining only a small internal pressure rise (intravesical resting bladder pressure). Bladder filling pressure at rest is initially 5 to 15 cm water pressure. As the adult bladder fills to 150 to 250 mL, the detrusor smooth muscle relaxes to accommodate the larger volume, the intravesical pressure stays approximately the same during filling of sufficient duration, and there is usually a sense of fullness in the suprapubic area. When the bladder accumulates the normal peak urine volume (250 to 400 mL in adults; 150 to 200 mL in children), a sense of urgency to void is usually apparent.

Earlier procedures utilized simple manometers to measure the bladder's pressure response to increased volume. The fluid (usually physiologic saline) is instilled into the bladder at a regulated rate. Contemporary cystometers employ carbon dioxide gas as the filling medium, which allows performance of the test in less time, with less discomfort to the patient. Since gas may not seem as physiologic to the bladder as liquid, it may help the patient to know that most of the newer machines have pressure safety valves to prevent overstretching.

The urologist may check the *bulbocavernosus*

CHAPTER 14   192

reflex upon completion of the cystometrogram. With the Foley catheter balloon still inflated and a gloved finger in the rectum, the urologist gently but suddenly tugs on the catheter. The stimulus or similar squeezing of the male glans or female clitoris produces a contraction of the anal sphincter around the motionless finger in the anal canal if the S2-4 reflex arcs are intact.

Before the Foley catheter is removed, the bladder's sensitivity to temperature may be checked by an ice water test to determine the status of detrusor contractility. After the Foley balloon is deflated, 90 mL of saline or Suby's solution cooled to 38°F (approximately 3°C) is instilled rapidly into the catheter. If the cold water is expelled spontaneously within 1 min, the test is said to indicate detrusor contraction.

Sphincter electromyography determines the level of muscular activity in the pelvic floor. To achieve complete bladder emptying during micturition, the external urinary sphincter must open (relax). To maintain a dry state between voidings, this external striated sphincter must stay closed (reflex contracted). Because the urinary external sphincter is linked with the muscles of the pelvic floor, the electrical activity of the latter during micturition is analogous to that of the external urinary sphincter.

It is preferred that sphincter electromyography be performed simultaneously with cystometry when equipment permits. With increased bladder filling, normal persons demonstrate greater electromyographic activity. When the detrusor reflex contraction occurs and the periurethral striated external sphincter is voluntarily relaxed, activity is diminished.

The *urethral pressure profile* measures pressure within the urethra as it leaves the bladder at the bladder neck, along the urethra past the external sphincter to the meatus. Urethral competence is essential to urinary continence. The two major sites of control are the internal sphincter (bladder neck) smooth muscle and the external sphincter striated muscle. The measurements identify and differentiate the sites of urethral resistance to urine outflow by distance and position along the urethra. This is particularly helpful in obstruction or incontinence that are difficult to diagnose and treat.

PATHOPHYSIOLOGIC CONCEPTS AND GENERAL MANAGEMENT

TREATMENT GOALS

The three primary urologic goals in the management of neurogenic bladder dysfunction are (1) to achieve a state of dryness satisfactory to the patient, (2) to preserve renal function, and (3) to avoid urologic complications. Approaches to therapy include regulation of fluid intake, bladder programs using individualized voiding and emptying regimens, manual voiding facilitation techniques, intermittent self-catheterization, external sphincterotomy, indwelling catheters, and urologic surgical techniques. These are used according to the needs of each type of neurogenic bladder. Pharmacologic agents used include cholinergic, anticholinergic, adrenergic, adrenolytic, and skeletal spasmolytic agents.

Selection of therapy is often determined by the philosophy, training, and experience of the patient's physician. Availability of specialized facilities or outpatient follow-up is also a factor. Essential for follow-through of the program instituted are the personal traits of the patient and significant others, the home and work environments, and the financial status for long-term assistance.

NEUROGENIC BLADDER DISEASE

The term *neurogenic bladder disease* refers to bladder dysfunction resulting from lesions of the central or the peripheral nervous system. In the past few decades extensive research in neurophysiology and neuropharmacology, combined with technologic advances in biomedical engineering, have brought new dimensions to the understanding of micturition. Newer knowledge has pointed out the complexity of synchronized bladder neck opening with detrusor contraction during normal voiding (Grabner and Tanagho, 1975).

Shock-phase Variation of Neurogenic Bladder Spinal injury is a frequent cause of neurogenic dysfunction. After sudden extensive trauma to the central nervous system, such as spinal cord injury, or after severe exacerbation of neurologic disease, the bladder may exist in a state of "shock" for days to months.

In spinal cord injury the patient is unable to walk and the extremities are flaccid. The degree of cortical perception of sensory stimuli from other areas of the body may cause variable reaction to sensation in the perineal area. The patient has no voluntary control of urination and has high residual volumes and complete urinary retention. Bladder capacity is grossly increased. The cystometrogram shows low bladder filling pressure. There are no detrusor contractions and almost no bladder tone. The physician will feel no bulbocavernosus reflex or involuntary anal sphincter contraction (Wear, 1974).

Reflex Neurogenic Bladder Patients who most often demonstrate this type of bladder are those with quadriplegia and paraplegia with injury above the T12 vertebrae and sparing of damage to the reflex arc. Neurologic causes of this lesion are spinal fracture-dislocation with compression, hematoma or transection of the cord, tumors invading the cord, multiple sclerosis, syringomyelia, and pernicious anemia. Patients are incontinent, with a voiding pattern that is involuntary, spontaneous, and gushing; they cannot voluntarily initiate voiding. Voiding can often be triggered by external stimuli.

Catheterizations to measure residual urine volume yield over 50 mL and often up to 200 mL initially. Postvoiding residual volumes are high; there is lack of coordinated or balanced voiding, that is, failure of the detrusor to contract adequately to overcome resistance at the internal or external urinary sphincters. The voided stream varies with the intensity of the detrusor contraction and the degree of urethral resistance.

The cystometrogram shows prominent detrusor contractions. Bladder capacity is decreased, usually to less than 300 mL. There is a positive bulbocavernosus reflex, and anal sphincter tone is increased.

Autonomic Hyperreflexia (dysreflexia) Autonomic hyperreflexia is an altered physiologic response that can never be ignored. It is a medical emergency that can result in death if immediate and appropriate treatment is not received. Autonomic hyperreflexia is abnormal hyperactive reflex activity as a result of an interrupted spinal cord. Up to 85 percent of patients with spinal cord injuries above the T7 cord segment can experience autonomic hyperreflexia in some degree (Snow et al., 1977-78). Patients with injuries at or below T7 usually demonstrate milder physiologic alteration (Moeller and Scheinberg, 1973).

Autonomic hyperreflexia is most often set off by stimuli resulting from stretching the bladder, rectum, or pelvic viscera. Urinary catheterization, infection, or bladder calculi can elicit hyperreflexia, as can stimulation of the skin below the spinal lesion, as from pressure on the glans penis or urethra. Extensive infected pressure sores can cause exaggerated autonomic responses. Patients can develop hyperreflexia from bladder distention during urodynamic studies.

The syndrome is set in motion by afferent sensory impulses, which are transmitted from the bladder mucosa through the pelvic and hypogastric nerves into the spinothalamic tracts, where they ascend to the level of the cord injury. This stimulation results in hyperactive reflex motor outflow from intact neurons in the lateral horn cells, most of which are emitted from T5–11 segments of the cord (Shea et al., 1973). This sympathetic hyperactivity is said to cause an exaggerated outpouring of norepinephrine from adrenergic nerve endings in the blood vessels and internal sphincter smooth muscle. This outflow stimulates arteriolar spasm, vasocontraction below the level of cord injury, and subsequent hypertension (Wurster and Randell, 1975). The vasomotor center receives recognition of the excitatory impulses from the baroreceptors of the carotid sinus, aortic arch, and cerebral vessels via the IXth and Xth cranial nerves (Shea et al., 1973). The vasomotor center of the medulla attempts to compensate for the hypertension by slowing the heart rate by stimulation of the vagus nerve. At the same time blood vessels above the cord injury dilate. This produces redness and splotchiness of the skin, predominantly seen on the face, neck, and chest; profuse sweating and a feeling of intense internal heat may be present (Kurnick, 1956). Vasodilatation can also cause nasal congestion and blurred vision. Thus vasodilatation develops above the level of injury and vasoconstriction below the lesion.

This compensatory effort is unsuccessful in lowering blood pressure, since the spinal damage blocks the vasomotor impulses below the level of injury so that compensatory vasodilatation cannot occur in lower body parts (Shea et al., 1973). When the spinal lesion is above T7, severe persistent paroxysmal hypertension occurs, with extremes of systolic blood pressure as high as 300 mmHg and increases of diastolic readings up to 175 mmHg.

The patient usually complains of a throbbing headache. Onset is sudden and often located in the occipital region. The patient is obviously apprehensive, frightened, and anxious, often demanding the care of both the nurse and the physician. The signs of dysreflexia may range from simple flushing of the skin and mild perspiration to more severe forms with profuse sweating, sudden drastic rise in blood pressure, slow pulse, excruciating headache, shaking chills, extreme nervousness, and a feeling of impending doom. In the worst form, convulsions, cerebrovascular accident, respiratory arrest, and myocardial failure occur.

The onset of signs and symptoms varies with completeness of the spinal injury and the level of the lesion. Persons who have complete transection of the cord feel symptoms only above the level of injury. A patient who has an incomplete lesion may experience burning in the penis or discomfort in the suprapubic or abdominal areas.

Hyperreflexia demands prompt evaluation and proper care by the nursing and medical staffs. The first and most important nursing action is so simple it may be easily forgotten in the midst of panic. Unless the patient's spinal injury is unstable or cervical traction is being maintained, *orthostatic hypotension* can effectively lower the blood pressure at the start. This is easily accomplished by raising the patient's head to a 45° angle. The dizziness, pallor, and loss of consciousness due to orthostatic hypotension, for which the head is lowered, should never be confused with the symptoms of dysreflexia.

The next immediate step is to determine the cause of the hyperreflexia and to remove the stimulus. While attempting to detect the cause and offer treatment, blood pressure monitoring every 3 to 5 min must continue. The physician must be notified immediately if the blood pressure continues to rise.

When dysreflexia results in severe hypertension with a diastolic pressure above 120 mmHg, drugs that act as antagonists to acetylcholine to prevent it from stimulating the receptors are indicated. These include intramuscular (IM) or intravenous (IV) administration of the ganglionic blocking agent hydralazine hydrocholoride. Its peak action occurs within 10 to 80 min and lasts for 4 to 6 h. In case extreme hypotension should result, an antidote such as araminol bitartrate should be kept ready (Taylor, 1974). Some physicians advocate the use of trimethaphan camphor sulfonate 0.1% solution in 5% dextrose and water by slow IV drip (Snow et al., 1977–78).

Oxygen may be necessary should signs of respiratory distress appear. A cardiac monitor may be indicated until vital signs are stable. Urine output should be measured hourly until the patient's condition has stabilized.

Daily preventive measures are of prime importance. Nursing observations must note how often hyperreflexia develops, and the events preceding its occurrence must be determined. Recurrent bladder overdistention should be recognized early and controlled. If the patient is on an intermittent-catheterization program, immediate catheterization is indicated for obvious, palpable bladder distention. If the patient has an indwelling catheter, kinking or obstruction should be suspected. Tight clothing may cause a pinched Foley catheter. Rather than attempting vigorous irrigation, catheters that are obviously plugged should be replaced. Local anesthetic applications (Xylocaine ointment into the urethra, Pontocaine 1/4% solution in 30-mL bladder instillations) may be used to prevent impulses arising at the mucosa from reaching the spinal cord. Local anesthesia will not, however, stop the dysreflexia triggered by excitation of the stretch receptors in the detrusor (Snow et al., 1977–78).

Preventive medication for patients with chronic recurrent dysreflexia includes phenoxybenzamine hydrochloride (Dibenzyline). Phenoxybenzamine blocks the alpha-adrenergic receptor sites and prevents the released norepinephrine from exerting its stimulatory effect.

When a patient experiences an episode of hyperreflexia, the medical record should be labeled so as to alert all staff of the potential. Patients should be taught to recognize signs and symptoms in order to prevent episodes or act appropriately should one develop. They should have written and verbal instructions in the steps necessary to interrupt the causative stimuli. They must understand the mechanisms involved in order to teach others. This is especially important in episodes of acute hyperreflexia which occur outside the hospital setting.

Autonomous Neurogenic Bladder This type of neurogenic bladder results from damage to the conus medullaris or cauda equina at or below the T12 vertebra, causing loss of the reflex arc. Impairment of the detrusor reflex may result when trauma, tumors, or demyelinating plaques interrupt the cord pathways between the sacral gray matter and the pontomesencephalic reticular formation.

Children born with myelomeningocele most often exhibit an autonomous bladder, although some may have reflex activity. Persons with herniated nucleus pulposus or those who undergo radical pelvic surgery may experience an autonomous neurogenic bladder.

Urinary incontinence is by overflow when there are high residual volumes (over 200 mL) caused by organic or functional obstruction. If there is extensive damage to motor innervation of the striated muscles of the pelvic floor (little intraurethral resistance), the patient may use Credé expression and straining to achieve low residual volumes. This incontinence is usually total and continuous and requires an external collecting device.

The cystometrogram shows no detrusor contractions. Bladder capacity varies but may be increased beyond 500 to 1000 mL. If cord pathways are interrupted, perineal and bladder sensation are absent or impaired. Usually there is flaccid anal sphincter tone and no bulbocavernosus reflex.

Some patients may be able to empty the bladder by using external pressure (Credé method) or by increasing intraabdominal pressure through straining. Transurethral sphincterotomy may be necessary if sphincter resistance is present. If the latter is not completely effective, intermittent self-catheterization is often recommended.

Motor Paralytic Neurogenic Bladder The cause of this type of neurogenic bladder is usually small localized lesions at S2–4 parasympathetic motor fibers to the bladder. It may occur from pressure on the motor nerves by trauma, tumor, or a herniated nucleus pulposus; from damage incurred with Landry-Guillain-Barré syndrome; or from poliomyelitis.

There is normal perineal and bladder sensation. This bladder type is similar to an autonomous type in that there is overflow incontinence and voiding requires straining and external pressure. The cystometrogram demonstrates no detrusor contractions. Bladder capacity is markedly increased beyond 500 mL, with consistently high residual volumes. The bulbocavernosus reflex is usually present to some degree.

If the cause of dysfunction is temporary, management is aimed at preventing bladder overdistention by intermittent catheterization. When the condition is permanent, self-catherization is preferred when possible. If a transurethral sphincterotomy is performed, Credé expression may be effective.

Sensory Paralytic Neurogenic Bladder This type of neurogenic bladder is less common and is seen most often in peripheral neuropathy secondary to diabetes mellitus, tabes dorsalis, or pernicious anemia. The picture is similar to that of the motor paralytic in that bladder muscle tone is considerably decreased. It should be remembered that impaired sensation can result in progressive stretching and decompensation of the bladder. Although there is no motor damage, impaired motor power is a secondary effect. Perineal sensation varies with the type and extent of the neurologic lesion but is usually impaired. The voiding pattern shows that urination is infrequent (as seldom as once or twice in 24 h).

A bladder retraining program involving regular emptying may be effective in preventing overdistention if decompensation and atonicity are not advanced. If residual urine is significant, a cholinergic agent may be used to improve urination and recompensate the detrusor. If the latter fails, particularly if incomplete bladder emptying is accompanied by infection, incontinence, or deteriorating renal function, intermittent self-catheterization may be indicated.

Mixed Neurogenic Bladder This type of bladder produces a combination of signs characterizing an autonomous neurogenic bladder and low-pressure detrusor contractions. Incontinence is from involuntary detrusor contractions; bladder sensation is usually weak to absent. Residual volume and bladder capacity vary with the effectiveness of emptying when using Credé expression. Perineal sensation is usually present, although reflex is decreased.

Persons with incomplete lesions from sacral cord tumors or myelodysplasia may demonstrate mixed neurogenic bladder. A patient with multiple sclerosis who becomes bedbound may develop a "shock" bladder, similar to the autonomous type, and proceed to a reflex neurogenic bladder with exacerbation, whereas on remission an uninhibited bladder is typical.

The type of neurogenic dysfunction determines the treatment. If incontinence is not present and the patient can empty completely and achieve sterile urine, no therapy may be indicated. Titrated doses of anticholinergic drugs may be given to alleviate bothersome leakage of urine. When the upper tracts are normal but there is recurrent cystitis, administration of antimicrobial medication may be necessary. If the bladder cannot empty completely, cholinergic drugs may reduce residual volumes. Intermittent self-catheterization may be indicated when there is dysfunction of both the bladder and the urethra associated with urge and overflow incontinence. If self-catheterization is not possible, a Foley catheter or urinary diversion may be suggested. For males, transurethral sphincterotomy and an external collecting device may be necessary (Lapides et al., 1971). Anticholinergic medication should not be used concomitantly with cholinergic drugs. Ephedrine sulfate may increase the tonicity of alpha-adrenergic–innervated urethral smooth muscle and improve stress incontinence.

Uninhibited Neurogenic Bladder Infants and young children whose nervous systems are not yet developed demonstrate this bladder type. Persons with cerebral vascular accidents, multiple sclerosis, tumors, or trauma to the brain often develop this type of bladder. Cortical and subcortical lesions in the pathways between the frontal lobes and the pontomesencephalic reticular formation can interfere partially or totally with voluntary control of the micturition reflex accompanied by decreased bladder capacity. Bladder capacity may be as low as 100 mL.

Sensation is usually normal; in fact, the patient perceives distention at a low volume. Unless there is organic obstruction, there should be little residual urine, usually less than 30 mL. The voided stream is normal. The cystometrogram shows uninhibited detrusor contractions, with intravesical pressure rising in proportion to the volume of filling. The bulbocavernous reflex is positive, and the patient can voluntarily contract the anal sphincter.

The problems of the individual patient determine the form of therapy. If the major problem is urge incontinence, moderate restriction of fluids, regulated voiding, and anticholinergic medication may be sufficient. Recurrent urinary infection requires the use of antibacterial agents. The confusion and disorientation so frequently associated with head trauma or cerebrovascular accident contribute to incontinence, as the sensory signals are ignored or the patient is unable to follow through on signals. It is essential, therefore, to utilize timed voiding and reinforce the habit of voiding regularly. In order for these to be effective, the patterns of incontinence must be assessed.

Pharmacologic Treatment

Drugs that stimulate alpha-adrenergic receptors can relieve stress incontinence due to mild sphincter insufficiency. Ephedrine sulfate, pseudoephedrine hydrochloride, and phenylpropanolamine hydrochloride are alpha-adrenergic drugs that stimulate the bladder neck (Diokno and Taub, 1975). Conversely, agents that block alpha-adrenergic receptors relax the bladder neck.

COMPLICATIONS

Urethral Strictures Meatal stenosis and urethral papillomas can be noted as obstructions when a catheter is being inserted. Fistulas and strictures may result from traumatic catheterization or cystoscopy that produces bleeding, an indwelling Foley catheter, the introduction of a foreign body, or a periurethral abscess that heals with subsequent fibrosis. Nonoperative treatment consists of periodic dilatation with bougies. Operative treatment includes meatotomy, internal urethrotomy, and simple excision.

Prostatic Hypertrophy Aged males may have hypertrophy of the prostate. If the median lobe is hypertrophied, it may stretch and elevate the bladder neck. With median-lobe hypertrophy there may be difficulty in passing a straight catheter. Coudé-tip curved catheters are often of value in catheterizing without trauma.

Bladder Outlet Dysfunction A poor urinary stream, residual volumes of more than 100 mL, and persistent urinary infections suggest bladder outlet obstruction, such as detrusor sphincter dyssynergia. This occurs when detrusor contraction effects a reflex contraction of the external urinary sphincter, with resulting incoordination of bladder emptying. The expulsive power of the detrusor can overcome some functional obstruction at the bladder outlet, but it will eventually be unable to compensate fully. A pharmacologic approach may help to lessen detrusor sphincter dyssynergia. When this is unsuccessful, external sphincterotomy will decrease the tension caused by clonic activity of the periurethral striated muscle. External sphincterotomy is thought to prevent secondary bladder neck hypertrophy and may be necessary in patients with incomplete high spinal cord injury. The procedure may cause a constant dripping of urine, necessitating an external collecting device. Transurethral resection of the bladder neck is performed on patients with low incomplete lesions. Removing tissue from the posterior bladder neck may lead to retrograde ejaculation and is undesirable in young male adults.

A defect in bladder innervation for an indefinite period will result in mechanical changes in the bladder smooth muscle. In an attempt to compensate for resistance to expulsion, the detrusor thickens and hypertrophies like the muscle of a weight lifter. As the interfacing muscle fibers enlarge, the mucosa between the muscle bands protrudes from the constant high pressure (trabeculation). As the problem remains, the open spaces become larger and weaker until they bulge more, like a hernia (diverticuli). If the obstruction is not corrected, total bladder atonicity can result, with urine retention.

The urinary stasis promotes infection and stone formation. Smaller diverticuli resolve spontaneously when the obstruction is corrected and infection is controlled. Excision may be necessary for those persisting with infection.

Vesicoureteral Reflux The decompensated bladder with increased intravesical pressure can cause regurgitation of urine into the ureters. Trabeculation of the bladder may change the oblique angle at which the ureters traverse the bladder muscle or may mechanically obstruct the ureteral orifice. Vesicoureteral reflux is often a complication of spinal cord injury. Degrees of reflux are designated as follows: Grade I, minimal, into the lower ureter only; Grade II, complete, reaching into the renal pelvis and calyces but without dilatation of the ureter or pelvicalyceal system; Grade III, marked, extending to the kidney with dilatation of the upper urinary tract; and Grade IV, massive, with pronounced hydroureteronephrosis and renal damage (Pelosof et al., 1973). Increased intravesical pressure, particularly with voiding, in high spinal cord lesions can result in reflux and renal damage.

For these reasons, nursing care is directed toward maintaining unobstructed urine outflow regardless of the artificial drainage. Likewise, no action should be taken that could increase the intravesical pressure. Urologic nursing care must be evaluated in terms of accomplishing these two outcomes. An example of an action that must be evaluated is the frequency of procedures to assure constant patency of urinary outflow. Catheter irrigations should be performed only on the order of the physician in patients with reflux.

Hydronephrosis This is an obstruction at the ureteropelvic junction resulting in distention of the renal pelvis and calyces. It can be secondary to obstruction, infection, reflux, and neurogenic factors. Progressive hydronephrosis can even occur silently in spinal cord–injured patients with sterile urine and in the absence of reflux (Pelosof et al., 1973).

Uncorrected back pressure can lead to renal failure with considerable renal damage before it is discovered. When there is enough back pressure on the kidneys to press on the intrarenal blood vessels, the nephrons become ischemic and urine production decreases. Monitoring urine output is essential to detection and treatment. As the back pressure increases beyond the pressure of glomerular filtration, urine secretion from the affected area stops. It is after hypertrophy and dilatation with diminished thickness of the renal parenchyma that the most damage to renal tissue results.

Changes in the resistance to the outflow of urine can develop several years after neurologic injury. Treatment must decrease the resistance to urine outflow and restore free urine drainage.

Infectious Uropathy Neurologic bladder dysfunction and obstruction significantly increase the residual volume. Persons who require rehabilitation frequently undergo catheterization and instrumentation of the bladder. Catheterization within an institutional setting is a prime mode for the introduction of resistant nosocomial bacteria into a previously sterile urine. If the bladder cannot empty itself of this initial injection of bacteria, within minutes to hours the urine is full of multiplying organisms. Bladder overdistention and increased intravesical pressure are believed to impair blood circulation to the tissues, decrease the antibacterial components reaching the bacteria, and interfere with the structural integrity of the tissues (Kracht and Buscher, 1974). When vesicoureteral reflux is occurring, the stream of bacteria flows to the kidneys with the potential for pyelonephritis. The adequacy of host resistance and of bladder and renal defense mechanisms and the virulence of the organisms determine the extent of the infection.

Renal complications frequently stem from lower urinary tract infections in persons with neurogenic bladder dysfunction. Renal disease continues to be the primary cause of death in spinal cord–injured patients. Preventing the entrance of dangerous nosocomial microorganisms into the urinary tract, particularly by safe catheter technique, and helping the patient to achieve a small residual volume serve to improve the prognosis and quality of life for the disabled person.

Calculous Uropathy A urinary stone, or calculus, is an abnormal collection of mineral salts and other substances. Inorganic materials in the urine precipitate and gather around a nucleus. The nucleus, or center, of a stone may be bacteria, desquamated cells, phosphate or oxalate crystals, or a foreign body such as the balloon of a Foley catheter.

Knowledge of the factors influencing urinary tract stone formation helps to understand the approaches to treatment. The problem of urinary stone disease is complex and surrounded by controversial and opposing etiologic theories and methods of management. A clear perception of the relations between predisposing conditions is difficult but necessary before developing a plan of intervention.

Metabolic factors Stone formation most often occurs in spinal cord–injured patients within the first few years after immobility. During this initial period there is increased calcium excretion in the urine (Claus-Walker et al., 1973). Calculus formation has been thought to be directly related to the hypercalciuria accompanying immobility; but if this were so, after the patients become active again and a normal excretory rate for calcium is regained, stone growth should cease. Some investigators have observed that calculus formation continued even when paralyzed patients progressed quickly to use of a wheelchair and physical activity. It would appear that conditions other than hypercalciuria, immobility, and hyperparathyroidism are responsible for calculus formation in the urinary bladder (Claus-Walker et al., 1973).

Calcium excretion is related to changes in the volume of an immobilized person's extracellular fluid. Concentrations of urine electrolytes vary in that sodium, potassium, and magnesium concentrations in the urine are significantly lower in paralyzed persons. This is believed to be due, in part, to increased fluid intake and output. A low urine output of sodium and potassium may also be enhanced by heavy perspiration (Claus-Walker et al., 1973). It is suggested that lower concentrations of sodium and potassium, particularly in the presence of urinary stasis, inflammation, and infection, favor crystalline formation of bladder calculi when the matrix is present (Lapides et al., 1971).

During the initial period of immobility there is incomplete bladder emptying in those with neurogenic bladder dysfunction. Higher volumes of urine remain in the bladder for longer periods of time, and there is greater likelihood of inflammation of the bladder mucosa. Loose cells dislodged by mucosal irritation become the nucleus for the precipitation of calculus-forming substances. With infected urine the pH is often alkaline, producing even more irritating effects on the bladder mucosa. Thus the factors predisposing to calculus formation in the bladders of paralyzed patients include stasis of urine and mucosal inflammation induced by hypotonic, alkaline, or infected urine, particularly in the presence of an indwelling urethral catheter.

Infection When stagnant urine becomes infected, bacteria can form a nucleus upon which calcium or other salts are precipitated. Some infection-causing bacteria in urine are more apt to potentiate calculus formation than others. Urea-splitting organisms are particularly apt to cause stone formation, so much so that "infection stones" are referred to as "urease stones." Bacteria that produce the enzyme urease are almost all *Proteus* species and some strains of *Pseudomonas, Klebsiella, Staphylococcus,* and *Escherichia coli.* The urease splits the urea, which causes alkalinity, hyperammoniuria, bicarbonaturia, and carbonaturia. This favors precipitation of calcium phosphate. This unusual supersaturation of the urine leads to the formation of carbonate-apatite crystals and magnesium ammonium phosphate (struvite). Struvite is believed to be the predominant component of infection stones. Infection-caused bladder stones that form on the balloons of indwelling catheters are removed by cystoscopy. Unless the indwelling urethral catheter can be eliminated, the stones tend to recur and potentiate recurrent infections (Griffith et al., 1978).

Clinical signs Calculus formation eventually leads to secondary problems. Movement of a bladder stone when the patient's position is changed may trigger profuse sweating that is not controlled by medication. An increase of spasms in the bladder and lower extremities may also occur. These are early signs in detecting stone formation while the calculi are perhaps still small in size.

Hematuria may be microscopic, but if there is a jagged stone, irritation may produce visibly gross bleeding. Otherwise bladder calculi may be completely free of associated symptoms. A patient with sensation may experience voiding discomfort when the calculus exerts pressure on the more sensitive bladder trigone. The majority of calculi are detected by x-ray. Small calculi may be passed on voiding or with catheterization. In order to determine the proper treatment, the stones should be saved for analysis (Rous, 1976).

Management Earlier mobilization, irrigation by fluid intake, better control of urinary tract infection, and intermittent catheterization have reduced the incidence of renal stone formation in paraplegics to less than 20 percent.

Surgical removal may not be well tolerated in debilitated and aging persons, but if the size, infection, and obstruction increase significantly, it may be necessary to operate to remove the stone. There is a high rate of recurrence of renal stones after surgical removal. If a stone fragment remains, recurrence is likely. In spite of the potential complications, surgical removal is usually recommended if the patient is neurologically healthy and physiologically prepared (Kracht and Buscher, 1974).

The preferred form of treatment for renal lithiasis is correction of obstructions and urinary stasis followed by surgical removal of calculus material. Long-term suppressive therapy is usually instituted following antibiotic therapy. Follow-up care at 3- to 6-month intervals is vital to the longevity of persons with renal lithiasis and infection. Various means of prophylaxis must be maintained to control metabolic problems sometimes so severe as to be referred to as "stone cancer."

For those with recurrent nonoperable stones, the aims of treatment are to lower the concentration of precipitating particles, to increase their solubility, and to inhibit their crystalline growth. Conservative treatment measures include increased mobility and physical activity as tolerated, restricted diet, regulated fluid intake, and specific pharmocologic agents. The type of stone characteristic for the individual patient determines the medical management and nursing intervention.

The degree of patient activity can have a direct effect on calculus formation. In the immobile patient who lies in the supine position for lengthy periods, the dependent renal calyces can fill with stagnant urine. Nursing actions include alterations of position with frequent turning and active as well as passive exercises and weight bearing within the limits of the patient's capacity.

Maintenance of a dairy-food intake of less than a quart of milk daily has been recommended to establish a baseline should hypercalciuria require further restriction. Persons who drink excessive amounts of milk and absorbable alkali can usually avoid hypercalcemia by reducing milk and alkali intake to normal dietary levels. Urinary calcium levels can be lowered somewhat by reducing the calcium intake, but this alone is not effective in preventing stone formation.

It is believed that although the total daily output of calcium may be increased, a high fluid intake enables the kidneys to handle the extra calcium excretion, so that the concentrations of calcium and oxalate in the urine remain low (Burr, 1972). It is common practice to encourage patients who are recurrent stone formers to drink more than 3 L per day—some suggest 5 L—producing a rapid washout of crystalline precipitates.

Other physicians consider forcing fluids to be detrimental if they dilute the acidity of the urine or the concentration of infection-suppressant drugs. A distinction should be made between the patient who is managing with an indwelling urinary catheter and one who has spontaneous voiding with or without intermittent catheterization. In patients who have Foley catheters, the urine never remains in the bladder long enough to reach higher concentrations, so suppressant drugs will not be effective.

If infection is not caused by bacteria which produce urease, concurrent administration of a systemic agent such as ascorbic acid or ammonium chloride may be instituted to augment urinary acidification (Burr, 1972).

Summary of Nursing Measures There is incomplete agreement about various programs to interrupt the process of calculous nephropathy, and studies continue to search for the most effective treatment.

NURSING RESPONSIBILITIES IN CLINICAL MANAGEMENT

BLADDER TRAINING

Nursing action is based on a thorough understanding of the patient's background, physical limitations, types of bladder problems, and subsequent urologic complications, the acceptability of the method of incontinence management, and the extent of the patient's awareness and ability to cooperate.

Bladder training refers to emptying the bladder at scheduled hours subsequent to intake of a determined amount of fluid over a 24-h period. The patient with spinal cord lesion and neurogenic bladder dysfunction is often taught to control bladder emptying by one or more manual facilitation techniques, with intermittent catheterization frequently used as an adjunct. For patients who have small-capacity bladders, a period of clamping the catheter may be advocated to increase the bladder capacity, thus lengthening the intervals between bladder emptying. Some patients with bladder capacities as low as 50 mL who have worn Foley catheters for up to 20 years can, with the aid of pharmacologic agents, progress from hourly clamping or catheterization to 4-h intervals. Such a program is tedious and time-consuming, but if the patient is sufficiently motivated the end result can be personally and socially rewarding.

Prior to establishing the written plan for bladder training, a preassessment must be completed. The type of incontinence and the patient's readiness must be determined before taking action.

Fluid Intake The patient's pattern of fluid intake and preference for specific liquids must be determined. Limited and erratic intake of fluids signals a need to explain the program at the outset. A variety of preferred fluids should be easily accessible during the training period. Diuretics such as caffeine-containing drinks usually necessitate bladder emptying within as short a time as $1/2$ h, depending on the volume ingested, time for digestion, and renal function. Fluids in an amount of 200 mL every 2 h are offered and recorded throughout the waking hours from 6 A.M. to 8 P.M.

Daily routines should be determined and encouraged from the onset. This serves to promote more lasting follow-through. A minimum frequency would be emptying upon arising in the morning, before and after meals, before physical or sexual activity, and at bedtime, at intervals of about every 3 to 6 h.

Voiding should occur frequently enough to prevent bladder overdistention as well as incontinence. Thus critical voiding times must take into consideration the patient's bladder capacity. A person with a small capacity of less than 100 mL must obviously empty more often, depending on the intake: approximately 1 to 2 h subsequent to drinking, assuming normal renal function. Initially, bladder emptying is carried out as often as every 2 to 3 h and once or twice during the night if necessary as a prophylaxis against retention and bladder overdistention. At night, the urinal or a bedside commode must be left within reach. Efforts must be made to control nocturia, as the need to awaken at night is a major cause of disintegration of family rapport.

Accessibility to toilet and commode facilities is often the determining factor of success for patients who attempt manual voiding facilitation without catheterization. Unless they can consistently and easily transfer to a commode in a place of privacy, the effectiveness they may achieve in complete bladder emptying using facilitation techniques will be of little use. The nurse must help the wheelchair patient to consider this potential drawback from the outset. At the same time, the nurse can help the patient explore all available facilities. If ample facilities are not available in the home, work, and social setting, intermittent self-catheterization with drainage into artificial drainage containers may be easier and less time-consuming.

Mobility When mobile patients can sit on a toilet, the urine flow can be sustained more easily if the body is tilted forward so that the bladder neck is in the most dependent position. If a wheelchair-to-commode transfer is desirable, it is essential that the bed, wheelchair, and commode be of similar heights. The patient will need to have enough arm strength to open and lower clothing with easy exposure to the perineum.

Clothing Women have found wraparound skirts and two-piece dresses to be an advantage over slacks. If buttons and zippers are a problem in pants openings, replacing them with Velcro can reduce the effort of opening to a slight pull, with just a touch to refasten. Men sometimes find boxer shorts easier to loosen. When voiding facilitation techniques for reflex neurogenic bladders are being used, light clothing should be worn to protect the skin against fingernail scratches.

Behavioral Approach The psychological approach used must be sensitive to the feelings of patients and enhance their dignity and sense of self-worth. Patients should be helped by family and staff to engage in the program as active participants.

Family members and significant others are vital in helping the patient to see positive points of progress. Nursing personnel involved in the program must be convinced of the patient's potential for progress. They must assist the patient with the program when it is appropriate for the patient, not when it is convenient for the nurse. The initial investment of time will eventually reduce the amount of time spent throughout the rehabilitation period.

Voiding Facilitation Techniques

Manual voiding techniques are used at periodic intervals to initiate voiding and to facilitate more complete bladder emptying in patients with neurogenic bladder secondary to spinal cord lesion.

Contraindications The specific facilitation techniques indicated for the patient must be thoroughly explored. A small, contracted bladder may necessitate facilitated voiding so frequently that the procedure becomes impractical. Manual facilitation procedures can create high pressure within the urinary tract, which may be undesirable in patients with high residual volumes, bladder outlet obstruction, and reflux with persistent urinary tract infection or calculi. It has been suggested that manual voiding facilitation may elicit dyssynergic activity at the external sphincter during detrusor contraction in patients with a reflex type of neurogenic bladder.

The patient needs sufficient arm and hand strength to perform the procedures. Obesity can diminish the facilitated stimuli reaching the bladder wall. Extra heavy thighs are a particular problem for females wishing to catheterize themselves from a wheelchair, because they cannot spread the thighs enough to gain easy access to the urethra. If the patient is not ready to engage in the program consistently every day, attempting a voiding facilitation program can be frustrating for all concerned. The patient must fully understand the program and want to accept the requirements.

Selection of Facilitation Method Urologic studies to determine the bladder type, extent of reflex activity, urethral pressures, and rate of urine flow can help to suggest the appropriate method. Measuring the expulsive power generated by the facilitation techniques during testing gives an indication of potential success. Inappropriate facilitation techniques started before there is a reasonable chance of success may frustrate the patient. Some techniques require that the patient possess transfer skills and adequate finger strength. The requirements for selection of methods can be described in terms of the type of neurogenic bladder.

Techniques for reflex neurogenic bladder Successful facilitation in patients with reflex neurogenic bladder dysfunction requires (1) evidence of bladder reflex activity of sufficient pressure, (2) insignificant bladder outlet resistance, (3) bladder capacity adequate to retain urine at least 2 to 3 h, and (4) sufficient hand strength, particularly at the ulnar edge.

Timed voiding is especially important because the reflex bladder is more easily stimulated by distention. The patient must adhere to a schedule of facilitation that follows fluid intake approximately 1½ to 3 h after drinking. The patient should allow approximately 10 min for bladder emptying using trigger techniques. The following procedure describes trigger facilitation techniques which stimulate the voiding reflex in this type of bladder.

1. Have patient assume a half-sitting position (45° angle) for self-stimulation. The abdomen must be relaxed to allow the stimulation to reach the bladder. The supine position is easier for stimulation by another person.
2. Hips should be flexed. Patients may later progress to voiding in a wheelchair, bedside commode, or toilet. Flexion of the hips shortens the muscles and reduces the tendency toward spasms.
3. Demonstrate application of pressure as light blows, with hand lifted away from the abdomen in the intervals. Tapping is aimed directly down into the bladder wall, with quick, abrupt, local blows or pushes of force (not traumatic to the skin), at a rate of 7 to 8 times per 5 s. This helps achieve sufficient abruptness and force and has less tendency to induce spasms. Flatly applied tapping is not so effective, because it causes a lesser degree of stretch.
4. Use only one hand, shifting site of stimulation over bladder area to find the most successful sites. Patients with defective function of the hand muscles may use the ulnar edge of the hand.
5. Stimulation should continue until a good stream appears (a maximum of 50 single pressures). In some patients there may be no response until stimulation is stopped.
6. After a minute, the stimulation is repeated until emptying proceeds in 3 to 6 s.
7. One to two series (of 50 single blows) of stimulation without response signifies that nothing more will be expelled.

If the above is ineffective, perform each of the following one by one for 2 to 3 min each. Wait 1 min between facilitation attempts. (1) Stroke medial thighs in area along the adductor magnus. (2) Pinch abdomen above inguinal ligaments. (3) Pull pubic hairs (do not pull hairs out!) (4) Massage penoscrotal area. (5) Pinch posterior aspect of glans penis.

If little or no micturition results from any of the above, sterile intermittent catheterization every 4 h, clean self-catheterization every 2 to 3 h, or continuous Foley drainage should be resumed as ordered by the physician.

Techniques for autonomous neurogenic bladder Facilitation techniques for persons with autonomous neurogenic bladder dysfunction consist in manual or muscle-induced expression of urine in the absence of parasympathetic control of the bladder. These techniques increase the intravesical bladder pressure enough to overcome closure at the external sphincter.

In order for facilitation to succeed in these patients there must be (1) absence of bladder outlet obstruction; (2) absence of abdominal muscle resistance; (3) sufficient finger, palm, or fist strength; (4) adequate balance for wheelchair sitting or commode transfers; and (5) absence of severe coronary artery disease. The abdominal muscles must be trained to be effective for abdominal straining. Abdominal muscle resistance may interfere with sufficient relaxation for manual pressure. The patient must be able to transfer to and from the commode in a functional length of time, undress, and maintain a sitting position for straining (preferably on a toilet) and must have the finger strength and dexterity to sustain stretch of the anal sphincter if this is employed.

The following procedures describe facilitation techniques for persons with an autonomous type of neurogenic bladder. They include steps related to abdominal straining, the Valsalva maneuver, the Credé method, anal sphincter stretch, and use of corset.

1. Have patient lower clothing and assume a sitting position on a bedpan or transfer to a bedside commode or toilet.
2. Ask patient to lean forward upon the thighs. For patients with a high thoracic lesion, place a belt around the thighs.
3. Buckle trouser belt so that thighs remain abducted when patient leans forward. This is particularly useful for females. Patients with high thoracic lesions may tumble forward.
4. Instruct patient to contract abdominal muscles if possible and to strain or "bear down." Push-ups and bending forward may be helpful. Lighting a cigarette (if allowed) and mental concentration may be useful for some.
5. Instruct patient to hold breath while straining (Valsalva maneuver). If possible, encourage patient to hold strain or breath until urine flow stops, wait 1 minute, then strain again as long as possible. Wait 1 minute between voidings. Forced expiration against a closed glottis should not be practiced by persons with severe coronary artery disease, because it causes the circulatory system to be momentarily engorged with blood under high pressure. Encourage patient to continue until no more urine is expelled.
6. Instruct patient to place hands flat just below umbilical area, then place one hand on top of the other, firmly pressing downward and inward toward the pubic arch (Credé method). Some patients find using the palm or the fist more effective. Repeat six to seven times or until no more urine can be pressed from the bladder. Suggest that patient wait a few minutes before repeating the technique. This allows the bladder to conform to the volume of urine inside by inherent ability of the bladder muscles to contract. Do not use Credé method if there is known reflux.
7. Instruct patient to place one gloved hand behind the buttocks, then insert one or two lubricated fingers into the anus just far enough to enter the anal sphincter. Tell patient to spread fingers apart or pull them in the posterior direction in order to gently stretch the anal sphincter and hold it distended. Caution the patient against spreading the rectal lining, because this may stimulate a bowel movement. If the maneuver is successful, the anal and urethral sphincters should relax. With the second hand, male patients should guide the glans penis toward the water and away from the toilet bowl to prevent its touching the edge. Touching the head of the penis to the commode surface can cause a bulbocavernosus reflex that will close the external sphincter and stop the stream. Ask the patient to bear down, void, and listen to the urine striking toilet water in order to know when voiding is complete. Ask patient to take a deep breath and hold it while straining. This helps to open the bladder neck, which may help the bladder contract. Warn patient to continue regular bowel program even if defecation occurs during sphincter stretch. If a bowel movement is induced, it is usually too small for complete bowel evacuation.
8. If abdominal muscle strength is not adequate to produce satisfactory intrabdominal pressure, suggest that the patient wear a lumbosacral corset. Have patient draw corset straps snug.

Measure amount of urine expelled and volume voided with facilitation. Record the time of voiding facilitation and techniques tried, noting those most successful and the position assumed. Chart the amount of urine expelled with facilitation and the amount with intermittent catheterization.

EXTERNAL URINE-COLLECTING DEVICES

One of the most challenging responsibilities for rehabilitation nurses is to provide each patient with a means of keeping the genitalia dry when urine leakage and subsequent skin irritation are problems.

Males

External urinary drainage appliances are being used increasingly by men who are able to empty their bladder satisfactorily by spontaneous voiding but are unable to predict or control urination. An external collecting device is needed by men who are undergoing intermittent catheterization to reeducate the reflex-type bladder to function as a conduit. Men with an uninhibited type of neurogenic bladder find an external collecting device helpful, particularly at night, during bladder retraining.

Numerous external catheter designs are available, and it is beyond the scope of this chapter to discuss each. With proper attention to instructions and associated warnings, each patient can find the best collecting device and method of management. One style and one procedure will never be satisfactory for all men.

There are some men and some boys whose penis is so short and retracted that it is unwise for them to attempt to wear an external collecting device. These men can sometimes learn self-catheterization and be given anticholinergic agents or adrenergic drugs to relax the bladder and strengthen the internal urinary sphincter in order to achieve dryness.

The design and construction of devices is important to maximum effectiveness. Proper selection, application, and care of an external collecting device should accomplish the following objectives:

1. Provide unrestricted urine drainage without pooling of urine about the penile shaft
2. Prevent urine leakage between the penile skin and the sheath of the device
3. Prevent skin irritation, swelling, ulceration, and urethral fistula
4. Allow easy and convenient application to standard drainage tubing, connectors, and collection bags
5. Provide reusability with low cost

Proper fit should provide snug adherence to the skin to prevent backwash of urine, but not so tight as to interfere with circulation, particularly during sporadic reflex erectile stretching. Most brands currently available are supplied in small and large sizes. Children require a smaller size and modification of design to allow sealing against the skin around the base of the penis. Several brands use a diaphragm base with a urine-proof seal attaching it to the skin around the penis. A suspensory is adjusted over it and around the waist to give a snug fit.

The so-called Texas-style external catheter consists of a 2-in plastic connecting tube inserted into the punctured collection end of a rolled condom and sealed by a $1/2$ in-long inner tube. If the individual has no anatomic problems of fit and is conscientious in checking the placement at periodic intervals, this design is satisfactory. It is simple and can be self-made at a low cost. The primary disadvantage of the Texas style condom catheter is its tendency to twist at the connection, resulting in ballooning of the condom with urine and subsequent leakage. To prevent this, frequent observations are necessary to assure that the condom hangs straight down from the penis without twisting.

Addition of a reusable funnel-shaped semirigid adapter of insert material has helped to solve the problem of twisting. If a funnel insert is used, the condom must be stretched tightly over the funnel to prevent urine from collecting between the condom and the funnel adapter. Newer disposable external catheter designs incorporate a rounded reinforced tip into the one-piece construction that also serves to prevent twisting, if properly applied. The larger rounded funnel area has a reserve capacity for the initial surge of urine. It channels the flow of urine away from the skin through a large-diameter connector tube.

Getting an external collecting device to stay on and not leak is sometimes a real challenge, but with guidance, instruction, encouragement, and occasional trial and error it is possible to find an effective system. The method of application must be individualized to allow efficient attachment. One method of application is by adhesives. Adhesives used most frequently include surgical cement, glue, and sprays. Removal, cleansing of the skin, and reapplication at least every other day to maintain the seal and prevent skin irritation are required. Patients should observe for allergic skin reactions with the first few uses, especially if previous contact allergies are known. With allergic patients, it is advisable to test the product elsewhere on the skin.

Powder or lubricating jelly on the sheath or skin to help the condom slide on easier should be used with caution, because the powder can cake and irritate the skin. Ointments containing petroleum should not be used, because they can interact with the sheath material and cause skin irritation. Strips of stretchable adhesive-backed tape may be used to overlap the top rim of the condom if difficulty has been experienced in getting the condom to adhere. When tape is used it should always be spiraled down over the shaft from the rim in nonoverlapping spirals. Tape should never be applied circularly around the penis, because if applied too tightly it can act as a tourniquet, especially if the patient experiences reflex erections. Only tape that stretches should be used—never adhesive, silk, or paper tape! One manufacturer supplies rubber straps with buttons to hold the condom on the penis. If these are used, caution should be used to observe the skin for abrasive irritation and pressure sores, and they should never be applied too tightly. There are also designs that assemble into a suspensory support made like a jockstrap. Care must be taken to prevent excessive pulling from side to side about the thighs to reduce friction along the edges and in the creases. Tension in the fit can be avoided by the use of measuring guides supplied by the manufacturer.

Skin care and hygiene must be meticulous. It is important to check the condom at convenient intervals during the day and at night to ensure that it is draining satisfactorily and is not twisted. Signs of redness from continued wetness or from allergic reaction to materials should be watched for. The collecting device should be removed at the first sign of excessive swelling. Swelling, rash, redness, and skin irritation usually require removal of the external collector and bed rest to permit drying and healing. Elevating the penis on a folded linen roll helps reduce swelling. If cool applications are ordered, cover the icebag and never place it directly on the skin, particularly that of the scrotum. Cool applications should never be left on for periods longer than 20 min.

Persons in whom the foreskin repeatedly becomes irritated and inflamed may require circumcision. If the skin becomes severely ulcerated, surgical debridement may be necessary. The patient will require intermittent catheterization or an indwelling urethral catheter until healing is complete. If the base of the penis becomes eroded, suprapubic drainage may be necessary to allow closure of the fistula.

Replace the condom every day, or at least every other day, to prevent a buildup of large numbers of bacteria around the external urethral meatus. This serves to decrease odor and skin breakdown. The condom and cement or tape can be gently peeled off as one unit to avoid tearing the skin. Colorless nonabrasive solvents may be used to remove the cement and tape marks. The penis and groin should be washed thoroughly with gentle soapsuds. Thorough rinsing ensures that no soap is left in the skin folds. If pubic hair grows onto the shaft of the penis, a strip of skin can be carefully shaved to allow the cement or tape to adhere more effectively.

The skin should be dried gently by soft patting, then exposed to air, preferably for 15 to 30 min.

While airing, the penis can be placed in a urinal to catch spontaneous voiding. If extremity spasms may tip the urinal, the penis can be propped on a rolled towel and covered lightly with a soft cloth or diaper. It is helpful to remove the external catheter at night to allow longer periods of airing.

Females

No satisfactory external collecting device has been developed for females. Various designs have evolved, but they have been ineffective, uncomfortable, and unsightly.

The problems that confront designers of female urine-collecting devices are many. Obviously, there is no part protruding from the female urethra to which a collection device can be attached. The location of the urethral orifice varies anatomically, sometimes being so recessed within the skin folds that it is difficult for the female herself to find it. When a female is sitting, the urethral meatus is located posteriorly below the level of the perineum. This may create a problem in reaching the urethra. The voided stream of urine from the female is often erratic.

The simplest and most frequently used devices are diapers or sanitary pads. These quickly become saturated with urine and uncomfortable. Incontinence panties are commercially supplied or homemade. It is tiresome to maneuver incontinence panties through and around leg and hip braces for changing. Some patients sew Velcro strips along the sides, and many companies construct both reusable and disposable liners with Velcro fasteners. It is important not to let incontinence panties cause soggy, irritated skin in the groin and the creases around the thighs. One manufacturer has constructed a special incontinence pad that looks like a sanitary pad but is made of layers of resilient white cotton wool backed with polyethylene to allow dispersal of the fluid before absorption. It is said to hold up to three times more fluid. This is worn in close-fitting sanitary briefs. Regardless, padded panties are a reminder of childhood and are particularly embarrassing if the garments require frequent changing by others.

Much investigation has been carried out to design a female appliance that fits over the urethra. Most of the devices lie externally and require pressure exerted inwardly to achieve a tight seal between the collection rim over the urethra and the adjacent skin. Some are designed with a vaginal insert for location and anchoring purposes. The vaginal edges are not desirable, however, in aged women with senile vaginitis, in whom pressure sensitivity and erosion of the vulva's soft tissue can be marked.

Whichever design and method of construction proves most satisfactory, it is obvious that no one device will manage all the types of incontinence-related problems. Several sizes will certainly be required, but not so many as to complicate production techniques and make the cost prohibitive.

Until an acceptable external collecting device is invented, many physicians continue advocating the use of an indwelling urethral catheter. Actually, these are usually tolerated with fewer complications in women than in men. Unfortunately, calculi still form about the balloon. In addition, many sexually active females dislike having intercourse while a Foley catheter is in place, even when it is taped to one side.

In the next section, another alternative will be discussed. Intermittent self-catheterization, for many females, may be the preferred method of management.

INTERMITTENT CATHETERIZATION

Intermittent catheterization is widely accepted by many spinal cord–injury centers throughout the world as the preferred method of initial bladder management (Pearman, 1971). It is recommended as the immediate form of treatment until it can be determined whether sufficient detrusor reflex activity will ensue. It is generally agreed that most spinal cord–injured patients can become catheter-free through intermittent catheterization. This can be true even when the patient has managed with an indwelling catheter for varying lengths of time

CHAPTER 14

(Lindan and Bellomy, 1975). A survey of one group of patients demonstrated a success rate of 75 to 80 percent (Shields, 1975). Intermittent catheterization has been used for patients with incontinence or retention due to causes other than traumatic spinal cord injury. It is of special importance to children with meningomyelocele. After they reach 4 to 7 years of age, it enables them to be dry and to wear panties or briefs like other children.

The advantages of intermittent catheterization are many. For the patient who can achieve spontaneous voiding, intermittent catheterization serves the following purposes:

- Maintains the functional capacity of the bladder by subjecting it to alternate filling and rapid emptying with a rhythm similar to that of normal micturition
- Provides a low-pressure physiologic means of urinary drainage until such time as reflex voiding is satisfactory
- Decreases the bladder infection, stones and fibrosis, periurethral abscesses, and urethral strictures which often accompany long-term Foley catheterization, particulary in males
- Supports a feeling of independence by eliminating the indwelling urethral catheter

Patients who cannot sufficiently empty the bladder may use self-catheterization to reduce residual volume. Such patients can usually stay dry between catheterizations with the aid of pharmacologic therapy and can thus be free of urinary collecting devices and appliances.

The patient must fully understand the program beforehand. Initiation of the intermittent catheterization program, variations in method, and progress and termination of the program must be thoroughly explained to the patient or significant others in consistent and meaningful terms. In addition to medical and social preassessment planning and determination of pharmacologic regimes, the frequency and progression of the catheterizations, the regulation of fluids, the catheterization procedure, infection surveillance, and the control of complications are vital elements of an intermittent catheterization program.

Frequency

In America, life-styles that include high-pressure jobs and urban social functions have contributed to the practice of holding urine in the bladder for long periods. In contrast, rural and some European and Asian customs continue to allow people to empty the bladder at the first sensation of pressure.

Variables that make individualizing the frequency of intermittent catheterization important are inconsistent urine output and fluid intake and uneven distribution of bacteria in the urine, which can occur when a calculus or diverticulum is present. Generally, when bladder function is completely areflexic, catheterizations are performed every 4 to 6 h, day and night. Nursing personnel should palpate the suprapubic area for overdistention every 2 h between catheterizations, particularly during the first week of the program. Sometimes catheterized urine volumes consistently exceed 400 mL during the night.

It is known that the kidneys excrete larger volumes of urine as a result of hemodynamics. Hydrostatic pressure equalizes when the patient is supine, when approximately 11 percent of the blood leaves the legs and goes to the thorax, enhancing venous return. The heart works approximately 30 percent harder in the supine position than in the sitting position, with the result that cardiac output, stroke volume, and heart rate increase progressively as the patient remains bedridden. When the atria and great veins become overfilled with blood, volume receptors in these vessels cause strong renal reflexes which increase excretion of urine. Signals are also sent to the hypothalamus to reduce the output of antidiuretic hormone (ADH), which causes the kidneys to lose extra quantities of water. Consequently, the urine output of some patients may double at night, in which case the frequency of intermittent catheterization should be increased to 2 to 3 h or the amount of fluids reduced.

Catheterization Procedures

The return of adequate reflex bladder activity is favorably influenced by the avoidance of overdistention and chronic infection. When intermittent catheterization is performed at regular intervals using meticulous sterile technique, the likelihood of overdistention and significant bacteriuria is minimized (Pearman, 1976). The incidence of urinary infection is generally lower with the use of single catheterizations with sterile technique than with use of an indwelling catheter. Although the use of intermittent catheterization usually effects sterile urine for long periods of time, it is possible that urinary infections may occur.

Maintenance of a good blood supply to the urethra, bladder, ureters, and kidneys by avoiding increased pressures from overdistention is thought to be the key to preventing urinary tract infection. It has been observed that an indwelling catheter previously well tolerated can provoke sepsis within minutes if it becomes obstructed and allows the bladder to overdistend markedly, allowing bacteria in the urine to spread into the bloodstream. Likewise, intermittent catheterization can be equally dangerous if bacteria gain access when the patient is catheterized and the bladder is allowed to overdistend afterward, before the next catheterization.

Hospitals employ different procedures for intermittent catheterization, but the requirements of the technique are that it be nontraumatizing and as sterile as possible. Essential steps for the procedure are a modified surgical handwash before and after and adequate disinfection of the skin with an iodophor solution, unless allergy is apparent. Thorough lubrication of the catheter and gentle insertion are important to prevent trauma to the urethra.

Spasms of the external sphincter, diverticuli, or strictures may prevent passage of the catheter. If resistance is met at the external sphincter of the male, gentle pressure should be maintained on the catheter for a few minutes to allow the muscle to relax. After resistance diminishes and while the penis is kept gently stretched upward and toward the abdomen, insertion can be tried again. If it is still unsuccessful, the physician should be notified. When resistance is met, never jab, force, or push the catheter in harder. The male urethral lining is quite delicate and can be easily injured.

Sterile technique is essential for preventing cross-contamination with resistant infections between patients; but catheterization using sterile equipment is usually impractical and too expensive to continue in the home, at work or school, or for travel. Intermittent self-catheterization using a *clean technique* is easier to carry out and maintain in the routines of daily living. It can be taught to selected patients just prior to discharge from the hospital or by the outpatient service. It has been shown that sterile urine can be obtained and maintained if the neurogenic bladder is emptied frequently and completely enough to prevent development of high pressure within the bladder by overdistention (Shields, 1975). The use of clean, but not aseptic, technique is satisfactory in preventing infection, since bacteria gaining access to the bladder on the catheter are inhibited by the bladder's host resistance, and bacteria are regularly washed out. This is not true if the catheterizations are not frequent enough to prevent high bladder pressures and overstretching, which can eventually lead to cystitis, pyelonephritis, and sepsis.

Male patients who are quadriplegic can succeed in learning nonsterile intermittent self-catheterization. A greater amount of time is spent in lubricating the catheter and catheter insertion, but the final results are rewarding. Some males who are quadriplegic have used an adapted device to substitute for lack of pinch, which fits into a universal cuff palmar band. This does not require strength, grasp, or fine finger coordination. It must be realized that before beginning self-catheterization with a C6–7-level male quadriplegic, there must be consideration of his medical stability, urologic status, neurologic condition, upper extremity potential, and personal committment.

The way the patient is taught to perform self-catheterization determines the success of the program. Patients must be motivated and want to follow a self-care schedule. It is helpful to discuss a typical weekday schedule of the patient, based on the times at which he or she most often awakens, drinks liquids, travels to and from work or school, and retires. A sample daily record can be devised to illustrate when the patient would probably need to catheterize. The patient is asked to keep a similar daily record of intake, urinary output with catheterizations, and episodes of uncontrolled wetness, for approximately a month. This helps to establish an acceptable schedule. However, the patient must be instructed in how to alter the schedule to allow flexibility for special occasions and weekend hours. The time schedule should not be strict and unbending, since this would take away the freedom the program offers.

Once the program is discussed thoroughly with the patient and questions answered concerning the ramifications for the individual patient, the practice session of actual catheterization technique can proceed. A list of equipment includes the following:

Females

Genitourinary anatomic model for visual illustration
Written instructions
Clear plastic catheter
Mentor female catheter (#14 French diameter, 6-in plastic)
Bardic Util-Catheter
Metal female catheter with curved tip
Examples of carrying containers such as paper towels, plastic bag, compact, cosmetic case, wallet, toothbrush case, etc.
Containers for collecting and measuring urine, such as paper cups, plastic measuring containers, etc.
IV catheter extension tubing (optional)
Betadine skin cleaner or Septisol foam for hand washing while in the hospital
Betadine swabs for metal disinfection while in the hospital
Mirror (first few times only)

Optional items
Betadine solution for soaking catheters
Shallow tray for soaking catheters
Underpads to protect clothing or linen
Washcloth and towel for cleansing
Door signs and bedside screens to assure privacy
Gooseneck lamp or lantern
Sterile gloves for instructor's hands

Males

Genitourinary anatomic model for visual illustration
Written instructions
Clear soft plastic catheter
Bardic Util-Catheter (#14 French diameter)
Robnel or soft red rubber catheters (#14 French diameter or smaller for children; feeding tubes #5 French or larger may be used for children and cut to the desired length)
Examples of carrying containers such as paper towels, plastic bag, wallet, toothbrush case, etc.
Lubricating jelly, water-soluble, for lubricating catheter

Other items are similar to those for females.

Several teaching sessions may be needed. The first demonstrations are usually easier with the patient in bed or on an examining table. Later sessions may be needed to master the procedure from the wheelchair or on the toilet. The major teaching steps are as follows:

Review importance of regular, frequent emptying of the bladder. Using visual aids, point out that decreased blood flow to the bladder wall weakens its resistance to infection and that an overstretched bladder can cause the slowing of blood circulation to the bladder wall.

Stress necessity for frequent catheterization rather than sterility. The more often a bladder is emptied, the greater the washout effect and the fewer the bacteria left in the bladder to multiply.

Be aware of the patient's level of understanding and psychological acceptance before proceeding. His or her success will depend on being motivated and wanting to follow a self-care schedule.

Provide for privacy.

Ask patient to wash hands with soap while in the hospital. Extra hand washing with a stronger cleanser is important to prevent the patient from acquiring a hospital-induced urine infection.

Procedure for Females   Have patient remove panties and expose genital area. Have patient assume a semisitting position with thighs spread apart and heels touching in order to maintain exposure of urinary opening. Depending on patient's degree of balance and functional ability, she may sit or squat on commode with full part of hips forward but not so far as to lose balance. She may sit in wheelchair facing toilet with one foot on toilet seat. Assist patient to position mirror at the best angle to visualize the perineum.

If necessary, instructor may wear sterile gloves to demonstrate remaining steps:

> Ask patient to open catheter package. (Lubrication of catheter for females is optional but is usually not necessary because of natural secretions in the female urethra.)
>
> Explain to patient that even should her circumstances while outside the hospital make it impossible for her to cleanse urethral meatus, she should not postpone catheterization beyond the prescribed time. Emptying the bladder takes priority over cleansing and other activities.
>
> Urge patient not to get angry—this can be self-defeating. Suggest that she not try the procedure when she is nervous; rather, she should do something else and then come back to it, starting from the beginning.
>
> Tell her to apply pressure with the third finger and palpate the urethral opening until she is certain she can feel the urethra without looking. Show her in mirror the location of the urethral opening in relation to the clitoris above it (usually easier to feel) and the vagina below. Point out any protrusions of skin near the meatus that may help in feeling the indentation of the meatus. If she has difficulty finding the urethra, she may put two fingers or a tampax into the vagina to help avoid getting into the wrong area, but this is usually unnecessary.
>
> Ask her to release the pressure and raise the third finger but to keep the other fingers in place. At the same time, with her right hand holding the catheter about $1/2$ in from the tip, have her direct it toward the urethra by tilting it upward. During insertion some women have a tendency to point the catheter downward rather than upward toward the pubis. If using a coudé-tip catheter, the curved tip should be inserted upward following the natural curve of the urethra. If resistance to insertion is met with spasm, waiting a few seconds to minutes and taking a few deep breaths may help relax the sphincter.
>
> If patient has trouble getting urine stream to reach toilet from a wheelchair, a piece of extension tubing may be connected to the catheter with an adapter.
>
> Show patient how to apply gentle pressure over bladder (Credé method) before removing catheter. Patients with reflux should not be allowed to use this method unless specifically ordered by the physician.
>
> Because vacuum is formed, there will be urine in the catheter until air gets into the it to break the vacuum, so tell patient to pinch tip of catheter and hold it upward when removing it, to avoid soiling clothes.
>
> Once catheter is removed, let patient wipe

intralabial area with water-moistened washcloth to remove lubricant, antiseptic, and leaked urine. Urge her to dry area thoroughly before redressing.

Instruct patient to record on a bladder training flow chart, while in the hospital and during first month at home, the amount of urine obtained, in order to evaluate progress. Record how well the patient carried out the steps of self-catheterization procedure and any difficulties encountered.

Procedure for Males Instruct patient to squeeze lubricant onto sterile gauze or onto inner wrapper of catheter. This is readied for lubrication of catheter prior to insertion. If patient is uncircumcised, instruct him to push back the foreskin before cleansing. Ask patient to open catheter package, remove catheter, and lubricate entire length of catheter, lubricating tip of catheter especially well. While in the hospital, an unopened sterile catheter should be used each time.

The remainder of the procedure is the same as that for females.

Infection Control While practicing in the hospital, the patient uses a sterile catheter each time. The patient is instructed on how to reuse the catheters at home. After removing the catheter, show the patient how to wash the outer surface of the catheter with the same soapsuds used to lather hands. Afterward the inside and outside of the catheter are rinsed with clear water while rinsing hands. No disinfecting solution is recommended. The nurse can show the patient how to dry the catheter with a paper towel and store it in a clean, dry condition in a paper towel, plastic bag, or carrying case.

Infection surveillance and control measures are ongoing. Urine specimens are collected twice weekly for colony counts. Readings of more than 100,000 colonies signal a need for a sensitivity report. Signs of urinary infection are reported promptly to the physician and recorded. Patients utilizing clean self-catheterization are taught to use a urine screening device at least monthly or whenever signs of urine infection are present. Recurrent infections occur in occasional patients undergoing intermittent catheterization, but when effectively treated with antibiotics, most, if catheter-free, can achieve sterile urine by the time of discharge.

Problems and Complications

Problems and possible complications must be carefully monitored. A failure to develop spontaneous voiding, high residual volumes, lack of patient cooperation and motivation—particularly with regard to fluid restriction—persistent urinary tract infection, calculi, and too small a bladder capacity necessitating too-frequent catheterizations are problems that interfere with attempts to become catheter-free. Decreasing manual dexterity is a problem for patients with progressive disabilities. Inability to adjust to the procedural requirements and routine can become a problem for mothers of young, hyperactive children and for adolescents.

While intermittent catheterization appears successful within the first year of management, recent data suggest harmful effects for some persons after a long catheter-free period. When acute complications interfere with normal ingestion of fluids and an intravenous regime is necessary, an indwelling catheter may be inserted for several days until oral fluid intake can be resumed.

The length of time the patient may undergo intermittent catheterization in the hospital varies with the type of neurogenic bladder and the goal of the program. For spinal cord–injured patients, the time required to achieve satisfactory function varies from a few days to several weeks. Patients with an areflexic detrusor or detrusor sphincter dyssynergia may continue for months. Extended periods of intermittent catheterization in the hospital can become frustrating for patients. The cost of sterile intermittent catheterization supplies alone may reach into the thousands of dollars. For these reasons, more attention is being directed to earlier recognition of patients in whom intermittent catheterization may not be successful in establishing an early catheter-free status (Perkash, 1976). Urologic surgical intervention for these patients is discussed in a later section.

INDWELLING CATHETERIZATION

Although the use of an indwelling urethral catheter has potential hazards, there are valid indications for its use. Appropriate reasons for utilizing indwelling urethral catheters include (1) provision of continuous urinary drainage for malfunctioning bladders, (2) monitoring of urine output in acutely ill patients, (3) provision of postoperative continuous bladder drainage, and (4) instillation of medications or diagnostic contrast media. If indwelling catheters are used wisely and properly, these objectives can be achieved without serious complications.

Urinary tract infections account for almost one-half of all nosocomial infections in the United States, and the indwelling catheter is the leading cause (Shields, 1975). Since chronically disabled patients with neurogenic bladder dysfunction are predisposed to urinary tract infection and urologic complications, every effort should be made to institute optimal care and to utilize the best equipment available to reduce the incidence of hospital-acquired urinary tract infection and catheter-related complications. Factors that influence the development and control of urinary tract infection are the condition of the urethra and bladder, the patient's overall resistance to infection, the initial catheterization technique, and subsequent care of the indwelling catheter and its drainage system.

Bladder Defense Mechanisms The normal bladder has its own mechanisms for resisting infection within the mucosal lining of the bladder wall. Frequent emptying is known to wash out bacteria and ward off infection (Hinman and Cox, 1966). An indwelling catheter is a foreign body that provides a continuous portal of entry for bacteria that can overcome the bladder's resistance. Rates of urinary tract infection and urologic complications are higher in the critically ill, debilitated, or elderly patient (Garibaldi et al., 1974).

Catheterization Technique

Initially, infection may result from bacteria introduced by the catheter. *Strict* sterile technique should be observed. Despite effective skin disinfection, pathogenic bacteria inhabit the distal section of the urethra and can be pushed into the bladder. Urethral instillation of an antiseptic gel or solution before catheterization may be recommended (Dale, 1975).

Less urethral irritation may occur when catheters made of newer, inert materials are used. The most widely used Foley catheter is made of rubber or latex. This material can absorb up to 40 percent of its own weight in water. This reduces the lumen diameter and increases the external diameter, with perhaps greater irritation to the urethral wall. Consequently, latex catheters usually require changing every 1 to 2 weeks (Wastling, 1974). Polyvinylchloride and Teflon catheters have a smaller outside diameter while maintaining the same lumen diameter. Silastic catheters (made from a medical grade of silicone) and silicone-treated catheters are less apt to kink and are easily inserted but may bubble, peel, and crack. Silicone is thought to be non-reactive to human tissue and nonporous.

For males, a catheter no larger than a #16 French should be used routinely; for females, up to #18 French may be recommended. If bladder spasms cause leakage around the catheter, the remedy is not a larger size; instead, the physician may consider pharmacologic treatment of the bladder spasms. To combat urine leakage, balloons should not be inflated beyond 8 to 10 cm^3. The additional pressure of the balloon resting on the bladder neck may trigger increased spasms and urine leakage. Larger, 30-cm^3 balloons should be used only as a tampon to control hemorrhage.

Coudé tip catheters may be indicated for those in whom straight catheter insertion is made difficult by an elevated bladder neck or enlarged prostate. Special skill is required to use these catheters. Catheterizations requiring the use of equipment such as filiform catheters and followers, stylets, catheter guides, or sounds are not nursing procedures and should be done only by a specially trained urologist. There is danger of severe trauma, such as perforation of the urethra or bladder, with introduction of any hard or inflexible equipment through the urethra.

Meatus Care Bacteria may also enter at the junction of the catheter and meatus by way of secretions. This route of infection may be significant because of closeness to the bladder, as compared to the distance from the collecting bag.

Thorough cleansing of the meatus, distal catheter, and perineum twice daily with a proved skin cleanser capable of lathering is recommended. Topical ointments may be applied to the meatus around the catheter; however, antimicrobial agents in creams are effective only for up to 24 h after application (Kunir, 1974). Recleansing is recommended before application is repeated. If an iodophor ointment is applied to the meatus, a light, self-stick sanitary pad may be used by women to prevent discoloration. Gauze pads may be positioned loosely about the penis within the briefs of males. Lotions with an alcohol base dry the skin and should be avoided. Powders are not recommended because they can cake and cause irritation in skin folds.

Taping the Catheter To decrease catheter irritation to the urethral mucosal lining, the catheter must be anchored so that it does not pull or place pressure on the meatus and bladder neck. For the male, positioning the penis downward for long periods increases pressure and friction by the catheter on the urethra at the penoscrotal junction, where a sharp anatomical bend is present. Constant friction at this point may cause inflammation, infection, abscess formation, and development of a fistula. If the penis is maintained in an upright position by taping the catheter to the suprapubic abdominal wall, this penoscrotal angle is lessened, the pressure point eliminated, and the potential for diverticulum formation reduced.

For male patients wearing a corset while sitting, taping the catheter upward on the suprapubic area is not desirable if it pinches off the catheter at the site of taping. The catheter may be taped to the thigh while sitting and retaped to the suprapubic area when supine for extended periods.

For females, the catheter is taped to the inner aspect of either thigh. The site of taping should be rotated. This is particularly important for females with severe lower extremity spasms that cause excessive rubbing on the labia and catheter.

Care of the Urine-collecting Systems Bacteria also gain access to the bladder by moving through the lumen of the catheter or via air bubbles traveling upward from the urine in the drainage tubing or collecting bag. An indwelling catheter connected to an open container provides direct entry into the bladder for pathogenic bacteria within 24 h.

Bacteria multiply in closed drainage systems as well as in open ones. Organisms may be excreted in small numbers from adjacent tissues or introduced with disconnection or with emptying of the collecting bags through the drain spout. When the drainage system is disconnected frequently, the drainage tubing and collecting system should be changed daily to prevent induced ascending infections. A strictly closed bedside urine-collecting system should be initiated and maintained for patients who are bedridden because of acute illness, spinal instability, or surgical operations. The drainage tubing and collecting bag are changed only when there is accumulated sediment, leakage, inadvertent contamination, or odor or when a new catheter is inserted.

Urine specimens are obtained by aspiration through the catheter if a latex or latex-coated self-sealing catheter is used. For nonresealing pure silicone catheters, the specimen must be withdrawn from a urine-sampling port built into the drainage tubing distal to the catheter connection. Caution must always be exercised when clamping the drainage tubing for urine-specimen accumulation. The patient should be observed continuously when the catheter is clamped. Irrigations are not routinely performed. When there is decreased urine flow near the time for change, the entire catheter and collection system should be replaced. If unexpected irrigation is necessary to dislodge debris or clots, the catheter and drainage tubing must be handled with strictly sterile technique during disconnection. If irrigation does not improve urine flow or if gross contamination of the catheter and collecting system occurs, the physician should be notified.

Urine and air must not be allowed to reflux into the bladder, because urine in the collecting bag is usually contaminated. The entire urine-collection system should drain by gravity. Collecting bags detached from the bedside to be lifted above the level of the bladder must have the tubing pinched to prevent backflow of urine into the bladder.

For patients in active phases of rehabilitation who have not been successful in bladder retraining and have resumed continuous urethral drainage, the Foley catheter may be connected to a leg-bag drainage system during the day. These patients are usually dressed and out of bed during normal waking hours. Sterile extension tubing, 6 to 18 in long, allows placement of the leg bag on the thigh or calf while at the same time preventing excessive tension on the catheter. The patient can more easily empty the leg bag and reduce its visibility under clothing if it is positioned on the calf of the leg. Leg bags should be large enough to accumulate urine for up to 2 h before requiring drainage. Most leg bags are supplied in a small size, 200 mL, for children and a medium size of 500 mL and large size of 800 mL for adults.

Many brands of leg bags have flutter valves to prevent reflux of urine and bacteria. These must be checked often to assure that they are functioning satisfactorily. Excessive pressure on the flutter valve from overfilling or improper placement can cause failure of the valve and reflux of urine into the bladder. Leg-bag straps should not be placed so tightly that they act as a tourniquet. Even applied loosely, they may tighten as the leg bag fills and cause excessive constriction or strangulation.

Various custom drain spouts of longer lengths and special release mechanisms are available to allow independent emptying by quadriplegics. These provide individual methods of operation, depending on the patient's upper-extremity strength and coordination, dexterity, use of hand splints, extent of reach, degree of sitting balance, and ability to resume the upright position after hip flexion. The type of clothing preferred and accessibility to a toilet or other means of disposal are also considered when determining the method of leg-bag emptying.

SURGICAL INTERVENTION

The nursing care needs of the patient with urologic disease who requires surgical intervention are similar to those of other surgical patients. It is suggested that the reader refer to surgical nursing texts for routine care following urologic surgery. The care of patients with disability who face a urologic operation demands special knowledge and understanding of the urologic procedure. Beyond this, the effects of the urologic operation on rehabilitation efforts must be considered.

The patient will have many fears related to the decision to consent to surgery and changes in life-style that may be required after the operation. Males may fear sterility or impotency. The nurse who projects confidence in the urologic procedure and genuine interest in the patient's adjustment will be able to make the patient feel in control of the care. When the patient and family are given the necessary knowledge before, during, and after surgery and trust those providing the care, the stress level will be reduced and the patient will be able to participate in the postoperative course to a greater extent.

Another responsibility of the rehabilitation nurse is to assess indicators of stress that may become a barrier to the patient's postoperative recovery. If there is excessive psychological stress associated with the operation, the patient may awake in extreme anxiety or with anger or depression. An increased potential for acute confusion may exist subsequent to surgery on the genital organs; approximately 5 to 7 percent can experience acute confusion following urologic surgery. The elderly, particularly men who undergo prostatectomy, are more susceptible to postoperative confusion. Patients with impaired visual acuity, loss of hearing, and imposed immobility are especially prone to sensory deprivation. Patients with seizure disorders may have seizures followed by an acute state of confusion in the postoperative period (Mesulam and Geschwind, 1976).

Prior to surgery the patient needs to know the usual postoperative care measures, so that the postoperative routines will not be entirely unexpected and frightening. Preoperative teaching should include the site of the surgical incision, which will determine the extent of shaving and skin preparation. The patient should be told, no later than the day before surgery, what to expect: the presence of intravenous solutions, tubes and the usual length of insertion time, and ventilatory measures with or without assistive devices. Special urinary drainage equipment specific to the patient should be readied and made available. Foam padding or positioning aids should be planned with the patient to prevent skin breakdown if prolonged convalescence is expected.

A wide variety of urologic operations may be performed on patients undergoing rehabilitation. Urethral surgery to repair strictures may involve a simple excision and anastomosis or, for larger strictures, a two-stage repair. A meatotomy may be performed to correct meatal stenosis. Circumcision may be performed on patients who have difficulty maintaining external condom catheter drainage.

Suprapubic Procedures

Suprapubic cystostomy is preferred as an alternative to intermittent catheterization in some rehabilitation centers.

Suprapubic catheters are used to temporarily or permanently bypass the urethra in order to prevent or treat penoscrotal abscess with fistula or diverticuli formation and epididymitis. Some patients who experience considerable difficulty in maintaining an external catheter may choose the easier upkeep of a suprapubic catheter. Those who want greater sexual freedom prefer a suprapubic catheter to an indwelling urethral catheter. Where technical manpower and financial resources for labor and supplies are unavailable for intermittent catheterization, a percutaneous suprapubic cystocatheter may make possible intermittent aspiration of urine. The bladder urine may be kept sterile for as long as 5 weeks when this form of aspiration is carried out every 6 h (Fam et al., 1978). An aseptic method of cystostomy with a trocar connected to a cystostomy catheter, then to a closed urinary drainage system, is also used for spinal cord–injured patients (Namiko et al., 1978).

As with urethral catheters, the suprapubic tube provides a route for bacteria to ascend into the bladder. The steps to minimize the incidence of urinary tract infection with a suprapubic catheter are the same as those suggested for an indwelling urethral catheter.

Implantable Incontinence Device

Another alternative to catheterization has emerged over the last decade: the inflatable artificial sphincter developed by Brantley Scott (Scott et al., 1974). It is a silicone sleeve implanted around the urethra above the pelvic floor and connected to a series of one-way valves. A silicone tube connects the sleeve to a spherical silicone bag with a one-way valve, which is implanted into the right side of the labium of the female or scrotum of the male. Another one-way valve connects this bag to a reservoir, which connects by a third one-way valve by silicone tubing to another silicone bag placed on the left side of the labium or scrotum. The second silicone bag is attached to the artificial sphincter by a fourth one-way valve silicone tube section. By pressing one of the silicone bags, fluid is forced from the bag to the reservoir. When pressure on the bag is released, fluid is drawn from the sphincter, the sphincter cuff decompresses, and voiding occurs. When voiding is complete, the patient squeezes the bag on the opposite side, which inflates the sphincter cuff and prevents leakage of urine. Fluid is drawn from the reservoir to refill the bag when the pressure on the second bag is released. The pressure against the urethra is kept at a safe level by built-in mechanisms.

The artificial sphincter can prevent incontinence even with an increase of intraabdominal pressure, as in straining. The nurse must be aware of the presence of this expensive mechanical sphincter in patients; urethral catheterization should not be performed on them.

Transurethral Operations

Transurethral operations performed on male spinal cord–injured patients include sphincterotomy and transurethral resection of the prostate. Indications for sphincterotomy are (1) prolonged intermittent catheterization in complete lesions (more than 20 weeks); (2) vesicourethral reflux in complete transections; (3) high residual urine and severe autonomic dysreflexia; (4) upper tract changes with sustained high intravesical pressure and spastic sphincter; (5) overdistended (atonic) or areflexic bladder, with inability to open the bladder neck on voiding-cystourethrographic studies at least 3 months after the injury; and (6) repeated urinary tract infections with high residual urine and difficulty in emptying the bladder (Perkash, 1976).

External sphincterotomy has been successful in relieving bladder outlet obstruction in 60 to 74 percent of patients with upper motor neuron lesions (Shellhammer et al., 1974). Unfortunately, total incontinence has been a sequel to external sphincterotomy using traditional procedures. Young male patients fear the procedure because it may cause urine leakage during sexual intercourse. It is also difficult for them to change external collecting devices without soiling their clothing.

Surgical division of the external sphincter is performed to relieve resistance to urine outflow at the striated urethral sphincter in patients who have bladder sphincter dyssynergia. Detrusor sphincter dyssynergia is considered the most important reason for surgical intervention in spinal cord–injured patients with upper motor neuron lesions. When the bladder neck fails to open sufficiently during voiding or becomes compromised by hypertrophy, sphincterotomy may be performed early during rehabilitation to prevent more extensive hypertrophy or obviate the need for transurethral resection of the bladder neck.

A majority of patients recover their erectile ability postoperatively, some after a month, but there are some who suffer a permanent decrease in potency. Interruption of blood supply to the corpora is thought to be involved during division of the autonomic nerves in lateral areas of the urethra. Consequently some surgeons place the incision in an anterior position to avoid postoperative impotence (Nanninga et al., 1977). Transurethral resection of the bladder neck is preferred for spinal cord–injured patients with lower motor neuron lesions who cannot void satisfactorily by straining or by use of the Credé method (Fam et al., 1978).

Nursing care required for patients who undergo transurethral surgery is comparatively simple and similar to non-spinal cord–injured persons. On removal of the Foley catheter, the patient may undergo intermittent catheterization for several days to weeks until the residual urine volume is less than 100 mL (Perkash, 1976). Irrigation of the urethral catheter is needed only if it is not draining well and should be carried out only on the physician's order. Extra caution should be exercised when introducing irrigating solution into patients with a small neurogenic bladder. If the returning solution is less than the volume instilled, the physician should be notified. In persons with a reflex type of neurogenic bladder, the nurse must observe for signs of dysreflexia; should they appear, irrigation should be stopped and, again, the physician notified.

Urinary Diversion

In the last decade, more extensive evaluations of urinary diversion have been reported, suggesting that the incidence of upper urinary tract damage following ileal conduit is greater than initially anticipated (Schmidt et al., 1973; Schoenberg et al., 1977; Shapiro et al., 1975). Prior to intermittent catheterization, supravesical diversion was considered by many to be the safest approach to management of upper urinary tract deterioration caused by inadequate bladder emptying, reflux, and ascending infection. The development of improved external urinary collecting systems and stoma appliances and the expertise of enterostomal therapists has served to make living with such a diversion tolerable.

Many children and adults who undertook management by ileal conduit or vesicostomy are returning for revision and follow-up evaluation of their stomas and devices. The enterostomal therapist has become a valuable consultant and should be contacted for solutions to problems the rehabilitation nurse may be unfamiliar with. The care of ostomies is an important area of expertise for rehabilitation nurses. It is a specialty within a specialty, about which more and more is being written, and it is beyond the scope of this chapter.

Wearing a bag for urine collection is not as desirable as near-normal bladder emptying if the latter is possible. More recently, patients with myelomeningocele and traumatic paraplegia with large-capacity neurogenic bladders, for whom intermittent catheterization and ileal loop procedures have not been satisfactory, have found a continent vesicostomy to be a more successful form of management. An anterior flap of the bladder wall is formed into a valvelike intussusception which leads to a stoma on the anterior abdominal wall. It is a totally reversible procedure, in that ureterovesical junctions are left intact and the ability of the bladder to act as a reservoir is preserved (Schmeider et al., 1977). Another advantage is that it requires no external appliance from which urine can leak. A suprapubic catheter and stomal tube is maintained in the diversion for approximately 6 weeks after the operation to avoid premature breakdown of the suture line. When healing is complete, the suprapubic tube and later the stomal tube are removed. Intermittent catheterization of the stoma is begun at 2-h intervals and gradually increased to every 6 to 8 h. This procedure may increase the number of private settings in which catheterization can be performed. Catheterization is carried out in a sitting or supine position with #14–18 catheters.

Problems encountered in initial use include reduction of the intussesception after the initial operation, early dissolution and dehiscence if absorbable sutures were used, inadequate length of the intussusception to handle the bladder's hydrostatic pressure, stomal stenosis, intermittent bacteriuria, and bladder calculi secondary to extruded nonabsorbable sutures.

PATIENT RESPONSIBILITIES AND ONGOING UROLOGIC CARE

The patient with neurogenic bladder dysfunction will always have potential urologic problems. During rehabilitation patients must acquire information and skills to help them adapt to new ways of bladder emptying. Rehabilitation helps to assess what is possible compared with emptying the bladder normally and what is not possible. Urologic patient education should facilitate the change to an altered form of urination. Patient and family teaching programs should be part of the discharge planning and should be initiated upon admission. Basic for all patients with neurogenic bladder dysfunction is an overview of urinary tract anatomy and physiology, with an explanation of terminology that is understandable to the individual patient. A number of excellent written instructions are available as guides for home care.

The Spinal Injury Learning Series (SILS) is an example of a comprehensive system for presenting prescribed and organized information to spinal cord–injured patients and their families in rehabilitation settings. Instruction is provided by full-time professionally trained persons to groups of 8 to 10 patients. The learning specialist possesses skills in group dynamics, interpersonal communication, methods of reinforcement, feedback, and motivation. The SILS Bladder Program consists of six sessions: an introduction and pretest, "How Urine Is Made," "Your Bladder and Spinal Injury," "Bladder Infections," "Dysreflexia," and a review and posttest. The purpose of this program is to provide information and images in a structured, sequential manner that will enable a spinal cord–injured person to maintain a healthy bladder program.

The patient should be taught to recognize urologic problems of urinary retention, symptomatic urinary tract infection, urinary tract stones, and signs of dysreflexia and should be instructed in the first actions to take upon recognizing such problems. Some specialists teach the patient and significant others how to perform catheterization in case of urinary retention. Rather than forgo catheterization in rural areas or undergo catheterization at the hands of inexperienced personnel, the conscientious patient (or significant other) can be trained. Under the direct guidance of a qualified instructor the procedure should be practiced on a training mannikin and on the patient. Written procedural steps should be given for study purposes. This can be mastered before release on weekend passes and before discharge.

Prior to discharge, the primary rules and practices to be followed to maintain optimal bladder emptying in the most satisfactory manner should be reviewed. To avoid urologic problems, patients should be familiar with the names, strength, and dosage of the urologic medications they are taking; they should put this information in writing and keep it on their person. They should know why and how long they will be taking the medication and should be encouraged to follow the prescribed regimen. They should be able to give an accurate account of drug allergies. It is important that they know their residual volume and when it was last checked. They should know when their last kidney x-rays were made, whether they were normal, and whether stones were observed.

They are advised to see their doctor or urologist at least four times a year for urine culture and residual urine measurement and once yearly for plain x-ray of the kidney, ureter, and bladder, with blood studies (CBC, BUN, and creatinine) performed at the same time. The procedures most often taught to patients are the insertion, changing, and care of Foley catheters, intermittent catheterization, and, for males, application of external catheters. Patients should have the name of a physician, urologist, or primary urologic nurse whom they can call any time a danger sign appears, such as stoppage of urination, urinary retention, high fever and feeling sick, bloody urine, abdominal pain, severe headache with sweating and chills, or swelling or abscess of the scrotum; providing patients with the name and telephone number of a resource person gives a sense of security. A simple telephone conversation can frequently prevent small and large urologic difficulties.

Not all those with urologic problems are intelligent, capable, and willing patients who have learned all that is required for safe urologic care. There are those who demonstrate little desire to engage in self-care, who do not empty the bladder as taught or do not catheterize as recommended. If they are fortunate they may have a conscientious significant other who will be a stimulus. There are those, however, whose families consider them a burden and a nuisance. It is these unfortunate ones who can most appreciate a home care coordinator and the Visiting Nurse Association. These nurses can provide insight into potential problems the patient may experience at home, such as inaccessibility of toilet facilities. Follow-up home visits by a visiting nurse may provide continuing home care supervision and assistance when needed.

The patient with neurogenic bladder dysfunction must be followed carefully for those events which lead to accelerated deterioration of renal function. To the extent possible, the patient with neurogenic bladder dysfunction should strive to maintain a dry, low-pressure, sterile urinary drainage system. The maintenance of urinary tract function is vital to life and to the patient's rehabilitation program.

BIBLIOGRAPHY

Bradley, William E., Gerald W. Timm, and F. Brantley Scott: "Innervation of the Detrusor Muscle and Urethra," *Urol Clin North Am* 1:13, 1974.

———, ———, and ———: "Neurology," *Urology* 4:767, 1974.

Brundage, Dorothy J.: *Nursing Management of Renal Problems,* Mosby, St. Louis, 1976.

Burr, R. G., "Urinary Calcium, Magnesium Crystals and Stones in Paraplegia," *Paraplegia* 10:56, 1972.

Caldwell, K. P. S.: *Urinary Incontinence,* Grune & Stratton, New York, 1975.

Claus-Walker, Jacqueline, et al.: "Electrolytes in Urinary Calculi and Urine of Patients with Spinal Cord Injuries," *Arch Phys Med Rehabil* 54:112, 1973.

Cohen, Stephen, and Geraldine K. Glass: "Skin Rashes in Infants and Children," *Am J Nurs,* June 1978, p. 1.

Dale, Gilbert A.: "Iatrogenic Urinary Infections," *Urol Clin North Am* 11:475, 1975.

Diokno, A. C., and M. Taub: "Ephedrine in Treatment of Urinary Incontinence," *Urology* 5:624, 1975.

Fam, B. A., et al.: "Experience in the Urologic Management of 120 Early Spinal Cord Injury Patients," *J Urol* 119:1, 1978.

Garibaldi, R. A., et al.: "Factors Predisposing to Bacteriuria during Indwelling Urethral Catheterization," *N Engl J Med* 291:215, 1974.

Grabner, P., and Emil A. Tanagho: "Urethral Responses to Autonomic Nerve Stimulation," *Urology* 6:52, 1975.

Griffith, Donald P., et al.: "Acetohydrozamic Acid: Clinical Studies of a Urease Inhibitor in Patients with Staghorn Renal Calculi," *J Urol* 119:13, 1978.

Hinman, Frank, and Clair Cox: "The Voiding Vesicle Defense Mechanism: The Mathematical Effect of Residual Urine and Voiding Interval on Volume of Bacteriuria," *J Urol* 86:491, 1966.

Kracht, H., and H. K. Buscher: "Formation of Staghorn Calculi and Their Surgical Implication in Paraplegics and Tetraplegics," *Paraplegia* 12:101, 1974.

Kunin, Calvin M.: *Detection, Prevention and Management of Urinary Infections,* Lea & Febiger, Philadelphia, 1974.

Kurnick, N. B.: "Autonomic Hyperreflexia and Its Control in Patients with Spinal Cord Lesions," *Ann Intern Med* 44:678, 1956.

Lapides, Jack: "Neurogenic Bladder: Principles of Treatment," *Urol Clin North Am* 1:93, 1974.

——— et al.: "Clean Intermittent Self-Catheterization in the Treatment of Urinary Tract Disease," *Trans Am Assoc Genitourin Surg* 63:92, 1971.

Lindan, Rosemary, and Virginia Bellomy: "Effects of Delayed Intermittent Catheterization on Kidney Function in Spinal Cord Injury Patients: A Long-Term Follow-up Study," *Paraplegia* 13:55, 1975.

Macleod, John: *Clinical Examination,* Churchill Livingston, New York, 1976.

Mesulam, Marek-Marsel, and Norman Geschwind: "Disordered Mental States in the Postoperative Period," *Urol Clin North Am* 3:201, 1976.

Moeller, B. A., and D. Scheinberg: "Autonomic Dysreflexia in Injuries below the Sixth Thoracic Segment," *JAMA* 224:1295, 1973.

Namiko, Tokujuro, Hiroyo Ito, and Kosaku Yasuda: "Management of the Urinary Tract by Suprapubic Cystomy Kept under a Closed and Aseptic State in the Acute Stage of the Patient with a Spinal Cord Lesion," *J Urol* 119:359, 1978.

Nanninga, John B., Joel S. Rosen, and Vincent J. O'Connor, Jr.: "Transurethral External Sphincterotomy and Its Effect on Potency," *J Urol* 118:395, 1977.

Parrish, John A.: *Dermatology and Skin Care,* McGraw-Hill, New York, 1975.

Pearman, J. W.: "Urological Results of All Traumatic Cases Admitted to the Royal Perth Hospital Spinal Unit during the Period February 1, 1968 through December 31, 1969," *Proc Veterans Adm Spinal Cord Inj Conf* October 5–7, 1971, p. 115.

———: "Urological Follow-up of 99 Spinal Cord Injury Patients Initially Managed by Intermittent Catheterization," *Brit J Urol* 48:297, 1976.

Pelosof, H. V., F. R. David, and R. E. Carter: "Hydronephrosis: Silent Hazard of Intermittent Catheterization," *J Urol* 110:275, 1973.

Perkash, Inder: "An Attempt to Understand and to Treat Voiding Dysfunctions during Rehabilitation of the Bladder in Spinal Cord Injury Patients," *J Urol* 115:36, 1976.

Rous, Stephan N.: *Urology in Primary Care*, Mosby, St. Louis, 1976.

Schellhammer, P. F., H. R. Hackler, and R. C. Blunts: "External Sphincterotomy: Rationale for the Procedure and Experience with 150 Patients," *Paraplegia* 12:5, 1974.

Schmeider, Keith M., Roberta E. Reid, and Bernard Fruchtman: "The Continent Vesicotomy: Clinical Experiences in the Adult," *J Urol* 117:571, 1977.

Schmidt, J. D., et al.: "Complications, Results and Problems of Ileal Conduit Diversions," *J Urol* 109:210, 1973.

Schoenberg, Harry W., et al.: "Changing Attitudes toward Urinary Dysfunction in Myelodysplasia," *J Urol* 117:50, 1977.

Scott, F. B., W. E. Bardley, and G. W. Timm: "Treatment of Urinary Incontinence by Implantable Prosthetic Urinary Sphincter," *J Urol* 112:75, 1974.

Scott, Michael B., and James W. Morrow: "Phenoxybenzamine in Neurogenic Bladder Dysfunction after Spinal Cord Injury: II, Autonomic Dysreflexia," *J Urol* 109:483, 1978.

Shea, J. D., et al.: "Autonomic Hyperreflexia in Spinal Cord Injury," *South Med J* 65:869, 1973.

Shapiro, S. R., R. Lebowitz, and A. H. Colodny: "Fate of 90 Children with Ileal Conduit Urinary Diversions a Decade Later: Analysis of Complications, Pyelography, Renal Function and Bacteriology," *J Urol* 114:289, 1975.

Shields, Lee: "Use of Intermittent Catheterization in Spinal Cord Injury," *Selected Presentations from the Proceedings of the National Paraplegic Foundation Convention*, 1975.

Snow, J. C., et al.: "Autonomic Hyperreflexia during Cystoscopy in Patients with High Spinal Cord Injuries," *Paraplegia* 15:331, 1977–78.

Standards of Urological Nursing Practice, American Nurses' Association, 1977.

Taylor, A. G.: "Autonomic Dysreflexia in Spinal Cord Injury," *Nurs Clin North Am* 9:717, 1974.

Wastling, Geoffrey: "Long-Term Catheterization," *Nurs Times* 70:17, 1974.

Wear, John B., Jr.: "Cystometry," *Urol Clin North Am* 1:487, 1974.

Winter, Chester C., and Alice Morel: *Nursing Care of Patients with Urological Disease*, Mosby, St. Louis, 1977.

Wurster, R. D., and W. C. Randell: "Cardiovascular Responses to Bladder Distention in Patients with Spinal Transection," *Am J Physiol* 227:1288, 1975.

15
betty cannon

bowel function

INTRODUCTION

Bowel function, though not often openly discussed, is an area of private concern to each individual. During developmental years, bowel training becomes a focus. Progress in achievement of control is equated with success and signals that one is grown-up. Emphasis on bowel function diminishes during teenage and adult years as physical growth, emotional growth, and achievement become prime concerns. In later years bowel function reemerges as a focus. By this time, the concern has shifted from control to the issue of regularity. Advertisements promoting products that prevent constipation and imply that a daily bowel movement is essential for normalcy tend to heighten this bowel consciousness.

When disease or disability results in incontinence, the emotional impact can be devastating. Fecal incontinence is as significant a problem for the patient as the disability itself. The patient with lack of bowel control is frequently embarrassed and hesitant to discuss the problem. Many people seldom think about their bowel habits and less often talk about them, even with family members. The sensitive nurse recognizes that discussion of bowel function, diminished bowel control, and the necessity for others to perform what may be perceived as unpleasant tasks are potentially humiliating experiences.

Incontinence is a counterpart of many neuromuscular disorders. It can be seen in multiple sclerosis, traumatic head injury, stroke, spina bifida, transverse myelitis, spinal cord tumors, and traumatic injury to the spinal cord. Whenever the function of the central nervous system (CNS) is impaired, bowel function may be altered.

Control of incontinence is possible. Management of the problem through an in-depth assessment of bowel function and implementation of a patient-centered bowel program is a vital nursing function in rehabilitation. The net effect of all other rehabilitation efforts may be negated if bowel control is not established. The nurse must convey the attitude that success is expected and that the patient will gradually assume partial or complete responsibility for bowel function. Most important the patient's life-style need not be drastically altered.

THE BOWEL PROGRAM

A bowel program is a planned approach to the regulation of incontinence. It is based on the nursing assessment and is designed specifically for the type of bowel dysfunction exhibited. The objective is to produce a planned, predictable, bowel movement.

To achieve success the program must be consistent, practical, and convenient. Through consistent bowel stimulation, predictable habits are established. Consistency of follow-though is *crucial* to regulation. The program must be practical so that it can be easily carried out, on a long-term basis, by the patient or the primary caregiver. It must be mutually planned, patient-centered, and must be in concert with future plans and potential physical abilities. Can the program initiated in the rehabilitation setting be followed at home? It must be convenient in terms of integration into day-to-day life rather than consuming huge blocks of time. Can the patient achieve elimination in a half hour, or must the patient stay home because this is bowel program night? Active patient-family participation and a problem-solving approach in dealing with the bowel program enhance successful regulation.

Though the program is planned by the nurse and patient, the involvement of the entire rehabilitation team is desirable. Each discipline can contribute to achievement of bowel control. The speech therapist may develop a communication board to enable the patient to make defecation needs known. The physical therapist facilitates muscle strength and toilet transfers. Occupational therapy may assist with dressing training. The dietitian may obtain the nutrition history and provide diet instruction. Everyone should be familiar with the bowel program and participate as it progresses.

NORMAL BOWEL FUNCTION

Innervation The gastrointestinal (GI) system is largely made up of smooth muscle. The intestines consist of single and multiunit smooth cells. The membrane potential of the single unit cells is similar to that of the heart muscle. These cells characteristically show "pacemaker" activity. In addition, single-unit cells function through their own intrinsic (originating entirely within the gut) nerve supply. The multiunit cells of the colon are stimulated by the extrinsic (in the spinal cord, outside the gut) nerves of the autonomic nervous system (ANS). Because the single-unit cells can function without an extrinsic nerve supply, it is difficult to interrupt nervous stimulation and bowel function.

The ANS mediates the nervous innervation of the GI system. Parasympathetic fibers emerge from the brainstem and exit through the cranial nerves and the sacral (S2-S3-S4) spinal cord. These fibers terminate in the stomach and ascending colon, and the descending colon and rectum respectively. They increase peristalsis and inhibit the external anal sphincter. The external anal sphincter is a striated, voluntary muscle that depends upon an extrinsic nerve for tone and contractibility. Electromyographic studies demonstrate that the external sphincter is one of the few striated muscles that constantly contracts even while in the 'resting state' (Staas and DeNault, 1973).

Sympathetic fibers originate in the thoracolumbar area of the spinal cord. Nerves controlling bowel activity exit the cord from the T6–L3 vertebral levels and terminate in the stomach, colon, and rectum. Sympathetic stimulation somewhat slows peristalsis and contracts the internal anal sphincter, an *involuntary* smooth muscle. The internal sphincter can function fully even when completely isolated from an extrinsic nerve supply. Studies have demonstrated that the internal sphincter is an area of high pressure in contrast to the rectum. This provides a safeguard against the loss of small amounts of fecal material which might collect in the anal canal (Staas and DeNault).

Motility Segmentation and peristalsis move fecal material through the small intestine. Segmentation, a ringlike contraction of the intestinal musculature, chops and mixes the contents. It combines with peristalsis, a wavelike contraction that slowly propels fecal material through the small intestine.

Propulsion in the large intestine is sluggish. *Haustral contractions* and *mass movement* are the prevailing forces. Haustral contractions resemble segmentation but are more severe and involve larger segments of the intestinal musculature. These contractions roll fecal material over and over exposing it to absorption of water by the mucosal lining of the colon. Mass movement is a contraction of an extensive portion of the colon that serves to pack the rectum with feces. This distends the rectum and the urge to defecate is felt. Mass movements occur only two to three times a day following food intake.

Defecation Normally, the residue from a given meal is defecated in 24 to 48 h. Naturally, this pattern varies from person to person. A daily bowel movement certainly is not necessary. Elimination may occur twice a day, every other day, or every third day. The consistency of the stool is far more important than the frequency of elimination.

Defecation is the end result of mass peristaltic movements stimulated by food entering the stomach (gastrocolic reflex) and filling of the duodenum (duodenocolic reflex). These reflexes are generally strongest after the very first meal of the day.

The S2-S3-S4 parasympathetic fibers have a very specific function in defecation. As the rectum is distended by feces, stretch receptors are stimulated. Sensory fibers transmit this signal to the sacral segment of the spinal cord. A reflex signal returns to the rectum via sacral motor fibers. Thus, defecation may result from this *spinal reflex* alone. Coinciding with this reflex response is transmission of a nerve impulse to the brain that makes one aware of the urge to eliminate. Defecation can occur without this transmission and subsequent awareness, but the result is fecal incontinence.

The act of defecation requires strength and tone in the following muscle groups: abdominal, pelvic, internal and external anal sphincter. Actual elimination is initiated with an inhalation followed by an exhalation against a closed glottis and by tightening of the abdominal muscles. This is known as the *Valsalva maneuver*. The resulting increase in intraabdominal and intrathoracic pressures forces fecal material into the rectum. Relaxation of the pelvic muscles and both anal sphincters permits the rectum to empty.

Variables Affecting Elimination Elimination is directly related to the type and quantity of food and fluid ingested. Typically, the American diet consists of foods which are high in carbohydrates and low in fiber. The result is decreased gastric motility and constipation. High fiber foods promote motility and add bulk to the stool. Fresh fruits, dried fruits, fresh vegetables (especially greens and celery), and whole grain bread facilitate normal elimination. Fats are known to absorb slowly. Milk and milk products inhibit motility while alcohol and coffee stimulate it. Adequate fluid intake softens the stool. The size of the food particle is another variable. Smaller particles are eliminated faster than larger particles. Clinical studies have demonstrated that the water-holding capacity of food particles significantly affects stool consistency. Coarse bran, oranges, apples, carrots, and brussels sprouts have a high water-holding capacity and promote stool that is bulky and easily passed.

Other factors affecting elimination are muscle strength, activity, stress levels, life-style, and age. Muscle strength determines the position one can assume to defecate, the quality of intraabdominal pressure, and the actual maintenance of fecal continence. Exercise and activity increase the transit time of food and stress inhibits motility. Ignoring the urge to defecate is common when a life-style is fast paced, time is precious, and appointments must be kept. The aged person is generally less active. In addition loose dentures may interfere with mastication. Or a limited income may prohibit selection of healthful food items.

ALTERED BOWEL FUNCTION

Damage to the CNS interrupts nervous pathways between the brain, spinal cord, and GI system. Bowel control as well as bowel function may be compromised. The degree to which control and function are altered depends on the location and extent of the lesion. In instances of spinal cord injury, an additional factor is whether the lesion is complete or incomplete.

You will recall from previous discussion that it is difficult to destroy bowel *function* (see Normal Bowel Function above in this chapter). It is commonly thought that intestinal motility is depressed following CNS insult. One study demonstrated that destruction of the lumbrosacral spinal cord segments results in exaggeration of segmentation contractions. This slows movement toward the anus of intestinal contents, resulting in increased water absorption and hard stools. However, the precise effect of CNS damage on GI function as well as GI response to various laxatives, stool softeners, and foods is an area of poor documentation and deficient clinical research.

Voluntary bowel *control* is altered when motor and sensory pathways are compromised. Fecal incontinence occurs when one or all of the following is impaired: cerebral control (an awareness of urge and ability to inhibit defecation), anal sphincter control, and anal sphincter sensation.

Neurogenic is a term that describes bowel function when CNS damage has occurred. It can be thought of as the initiation and regulation of bowel function without mediation by the cerebral cortex—in other words, without cerebral control.

Sensory and motor tests can be utilized to define the type of neurogenic bowel dysfunction. It is helpful to understand the significance of such tests and to utilize them to assess and plan bowel programs.

Saddle sensation is a perianal sensation that is elicited by response to pinprick or light touch. It indicates intact sensory function at the sacral spinal cord level.

The *bulbocavernous reflex*, which is relayed through somatic pudendal nerves, also indicates intact sacral cord function. This reflex consists of a *palpable* contraction of the bulbocavernous and ischiocavernous muscles and a *visible* contraction of the external anal sphincter. This response is stimulated by squeezing the penis or clitoris. Positive bulbocavernous reflex indicates that reflex bowel function may be expected to return after the period of spinal shock.

The *anal reflex* is also relayed through somatic pudendal nerves. It involves a *visible* contraction of the external anal sphincter in response to pinprick of the adjacent skin. A positive reflex generally is a predictor that reflex bowel function will return following spinal shock.

There are five neurogenic bowel dysfunction classifications (Table 15-1). Only three are commonly seen in rehabilitation settings and these—uninhibited, reflex, and autonomous neurogenic—will be discussed.

Uninhibited Neurogenic Dysfunction

Lesions in the brain are usually associated with brain trauma, brain tumors, cerebrovascular accidents, multiple sclerosis, and cerebral palsy. An upper motor neuron lesion (UMNL) exists, in anatomical terms, when CNS damage occurs above the C1 vertebral level. Cortical and subcortical levels of the brain are affected. There is no sensory loss, bowel sensations are not impaired, saddle sensation is normal, the bulbocavernous reflex is normal or increased, and fecal incontinence is present.

Table 15-1

Levels of Neuraxial Dysfunction Affecting Defecation

BOWEL FUNCTION	LEVEL IN NEURAXIS	POSSIBLE ETIOLOGY	UPPER MOTOR NEURON LESION	LOWER MOTOR NEURON LESION	SENSORY LOSS	SADDLE SENSATION	BULBO-CAVERNOUS REFLEX	FECAL INCONTINENCE
Uninhibited neurogenic	Cortical and sub-cortical	CVA, MS, brain tumors, brain trauma	+	0	0	Normal	Normal or increased	Present—associated with sudden urge
Reflex neurogenic	Spinal cord above conus medullaris	Trauma, tumor, vascular disease, MS, syringomyelia, pernicious anemia	+	0	+	Diminished or absent	Increased	Present—occurs without warning or during reflex
Autonomous neurogenic	Conus medullaris or cauda equina	Spina bifida, trauma, tumor, intervertebral disk	0	+	+	Diminished or absent	0	Present—may be continuous or may occur during stress

BOWEL FUNCTION

Table 15-1 (continued)

Levels of Neuraxial Dysfunction Affecting Defecation

BOWEL FUNCTION	LEVEL IN NEURAXIS	POSSIBLE ETIOLOGY	UPPER MOTOR NEURON LESION	LOWER MOTOR NEURON LESION	SENSORY LOSS	SADDLE SENSATION	BULBO-CAVERNOUS REFLEX	FECAL INCONTINENCE
Motor paralytic	Anterior horn cells or S2, S3, S4 roots (ventral)	Poliomyelitis, intervertebral disk, trauma tumor	0	+	0	Normal	0	Rare, except in widespread disease
Sensory paralytic	S2, S3, S4 roots (dorsal), cells of origin or dorsal horns of spinal cord	Diabetes mellitus, tabes dorsalis	0	0	+	Diminished or absent	Normal, decreased or absent	Rare, except in advanced stages

Source: William E. Staas, Jr. M.D. and Phyllis M. DeNault, R.N. "Bowel Control," *American Family Physician* 7:1, 1973.

Reflex Neurogenic Dysfunction

Lesions above the T12–L1 vertebral level are generally associated with multiple sclerosis, quadriplegia, or high thoracic level paraplegia. An upper motor neuron lesion is present, there is sensory loss, bowel sensation is impaired, saddle sensation is diminished or absent, the bulbocavernous reflex is increased, and fecal incontinence is present.

Autonomous Neurogenic Dysfunction

Spinal cord lesions at or below the T12–L1 vertebral level are usually associated with paraplegia and spina bifida. A lower motor neuron lesion (LMNL) exists. An LMNL occurs when S2-S3-S4 nerve fibers are damaged. Saddle sensation is diminished or absent and there is no bulbocavernous reflex; fecal incontinence is present.

ASSESSMENT OF BOWEL FUNCTION

The most logical place to begin to develop an effective bowel program is with an assessment. This may sound obvious, but it is just as obvious that many bowel programs are managed on a trial-and-error basis. In part, this is because there is a dearth of information about altered bowel function. In part, it is because comprehensive assessments are not utilized as the starting point. Knowledge of normal and altered bowel function, combined with a complete assessment, enhances a rational and scientific approach to management.

Key assessment areas are physical status, bowel history, nutrition history, and functional skills. Much of the needed information can be extracted from the history and the physical and admission assessments of interdisciplinary team members. Additional information must be elicited by patient interview, direct observation, and physical examination.

Physical Status (see Table 15-2) Consider the total picture, not just the bowel history or the incontinence manifested. What is the physical status of the patient today? What is the current neurological status? The etiology of the disability? The location and extent of the lesion? Answers to these questions indicate the type of bowel

Table 15-2

Summary of Bowel Assessment Elements

PHYSICAL STATUS	BOWEL HISTORY	NUTRITION HISTORY	FUNCTIONAL SKILLS	PATIENT-FAMILY UNIT
Etiology of disability	*Preonset Habits*	*Preonset Habits*	Sitting balance	Learning readiness:
Level of lesion	Frequency	Cultural diet pattern	Toilet transfer method	stage of adaptation
Extent of lesion	Time of day	Family meal routine	Hand & finger function:	coping ability
Activity level	Stool consistency	Foods causing:	eating	sexuality
Spinal cord shock	Color of stool	flatus	oral hygiene	feelings about incontinence
Spinal stability	Amount of stool	diarrhea	clothing	knowledge of anatomy
Muscle strength	Stimulation methods	constipation	toilet paper suppository	Family structure
Communication	Medication usage	Type fluid intake	Adaptive devices needed	Finances
Age	Enema usage	Amount fluid intake	Potential for increased function	Discharge plans
Weight	Episodic diarrhea			Home bathroom accessibility
GI problems:	Episodic constipation			
stress ulcer		*Disability-related*		
hemorrhoids	*Disability-related*	Appetite		
impaction	Type of bowel dysfunction	Food preference		
diarrhea	Bulbocavernous reflex	Fluid preference		
constipation	Saddle sensation	Nourishment state		
	Anal reflex	Average fluid intake		
	Incontinence onset	Average food intake		
	Deviation from normal pattern	Chewing ability		
	Current management	Swallowing ability		
	Date of last bowel movement	Denture fit		
		Teeth condition		
		Ability to feed self		

dysfunction. The type of bowel dysfunction points to the appropriate bowel program.

What is the level of activity? Is the patient on bedrest? Does the patient dress, do range of motion, transfers?

Following injury to the spinal cord, the normal activity of the cord is depressed. This is known as **spinal cord shock.** During the shock period, sacral reflexes important to bowel control are suppressed. There is tonic paralysis of the rectum. The recovery period varies in length, and management differs according to the stage of bowel recovery. Is the patient still in spinal cord shock?

Spinal stability determines activity permitted and positions that can be assumed for defecation. The bowel program may progress through different stages as spinal stability and safety permit. When the patient is on a Stryker frame

BOWEL FUNCTION

and immobilized by Crutchfield tongs with traction, management is aimed at maintaining peristalsis, soft stool consistency, and prevention of impactions rather than absolute establishment of continence.

The presence or absence of strength in key muscle groups affects the ability to sit in an upright position, the degree of physical activity, and the force that can be exerted to facilitate defecation. Will stool softeners be needed temporarily? Is muscle strength likely to improve?

Determine if the patient is truly incontinent or is having accidents due to an inability to communicate a need for toileting. Does the young child have a vocabulary adequate to communicate? What signals have the parents learned are meaningful? Is the brain-damaged patient able to understand staff when asked about the need to go to the bathroom? Is the yes and no response of the aphasic patient inconsistently reliable? Does the patient use a special word, perhaps an incorrect one, to indicate need? Does the patient understand written words better than spoken words?

Aging and degeneration of joints decrease activity levels. Liver changes decrease absorption of fats. Intestinal motility is slowed. Aging and concurrent medical problems should be assessed for their relationship to bowel function. In the instance of a young child, the ability to identify body parts signals readiness for toilet training.

Obesity limits physical activity, especially in the presence of a disability. What is the relationship of the patient's body weight to the variables affecting elimination?

Consideration needs to be given to GI problems that should be treated before a bowel program can be effective. If hemorrhoids are present, a decision must be made about the type of diet and medication necessary to produce the desired stool consistency. Is it wise to use a stimulant suppository in this case?

Diarrhea must be evaluated and the cause determined. A fecal impaction should always be ruled out as the cause. Are the liquid stools due to the irritation of hard and dry feces in the colon? Does the patient receive antibiotic medication? Is this contributing to the diarrhea?

Constipation in a disabled population is generally due to decreased muscle tone, fatigue, inactivity, and deterioration of or deficit in nervous innervation. This can be managed through an appropriate bowel program. But, constipation is also related to fundamental beliefs and habits. When organic causes have been excluded, personal habits must be given further investigation. Does the patient assume it is necessary to have a daily bowel movement? What has the patient taken to produce this? Is it possible the colon has given up as a result of being ignored and abused too often? Does assessment indicate that intensive teaching about the effects of food, fluid, and activity on bowel function is needed?

Bowel History (see Table 15-2) Data obtained from assessment of preonset bowel habits is used to plan a program that duplicates previous elimination patterns. Where these habits are healthful, they should be honored. Where they are contrary to proper bowel function, it is wise to invest in patient education and to facilitate change. With what frequency did bowel movements occur? At what times? Was the stool hard, soft, or loose? What was the amount and color? What was done to stimulate defecation? Exercises, hot beverages, prune juice, and other foods are often utilized. Can the same stimulation methods be used now? What routine and prn medications were taken? Were laxatives used routinely? Were enemas used habitually? Did antihypertensives or narcotics inhibit bowel function? What foods and emotions precipitated diarrhea? Was constipation an infrequent or continuous problem? How does the patient define diarrhea and constipation? Does the definition coincide with the nurse's?

Disability-related information is used to plan a program specifically for the neurologic dysfunction exhibited. Is the type of bowel function uninhibited, reflex, or autonomous? Is the bulbocavernous reflex absent, normal, or increased? Is saddle sensation normal, diminished, or absent? Is the anal reflex present? When did the incontinence begin? (Multiple sclerosis exemplifies a disease in which incontinence may not coincide with the onset of the disability.) How has the bowel pattern since the disability deviated from what was normal? What medication and method of stimulating elimination is currently in use? Is it effective? Is it appropriate for the specific type of bowel dysfunction? When was the last bowel movement? Is a fecal impaction present?

Nutrition History (see Table 15-2) Assessment of preonset habits reveals food preferences and the nutritional adequacy of the diet. It also sheds light on the sufficiency of the diet as it pertains to elimination. Dietary measures are one of the most important elements of a bowel program. Is the patient accustomed to meals containing fiber, natural laxatives, and enough fluid? Is the diet excessive in starches and greasy foods? Does the patient understand the relationship between foods eaten and GI response?

Cultural diet patterns may contribute to or detract from a successful bowel program. Although not all members of a given ethnic group will hold fast to their cultural food patterns, it is wise to evaluate them during assessment and planning. Failure to do so may result in a bowel program that works well within the confines of the institution but becomes unregulated when foods prepared in the home are eaten. Does the patient need to be encouraged to include new or less-favored foods in the diet in order to achieve a regulated bowel program?

Eating the same amount of food for each meal helps to promote a regular bowel pattern. What is the family meal routine? Which meal is the heaviest? Is breakfast always skipped? When are snacks eaten? Does the family fast on religious holidays?

Foods that caused flatus, diarrhea, and constipation before the onset of disability are likely to create the same response now. Once identified, these foods can be avoided.

Fluid intake of 2500 to 3000 mL a day is necessary to maintain soft stool consistency. What type and amount of fluid does the patient drink?

Disability-related data are used to establish dietary measures that meet current nutritional needs and facilitate regular bowel patterns. Has the patient's appetite changed? What types of food and fluid are liked? What can't be eaten on a regular basis? What is the patient's state of nourishment? What is the average daily intake of food and fluid? Does lack of sensation and paralysis of the tongue and facial muscles interfere with the ability to chew and swallow? Is dysarthria present? Following a stroke, dentures are often too loose. Do ill-fitting dentures affect the ability to chew food well? Fruits, especially those with skins, and vegetables are principal sources of fiber. Are these foods avoided because of uncomfortable dentures? Mouth care is often neglected during the acute stage of illness. As a result, dental caries and abscesses are frequently a problem in rehabilitation settings. Does the condition of the teeth affect the appetite and food selection? What is the patient's ability to eat without help? Those who are independent often select foods based on what is easily speared by a fork or carried to the mouth by a spoon. Are fresh salads avoided? Can the patient peel an orange or cut into a slice of cantaloupe? Those who require assistance with eating often eat faster and chew less well than they normally would. Digestion is slowed when this situation exists.

Functional Skills (see Table 15-2) In this instance, functional skills pertain to toileting activities. Sitting upright on a toilet enables the force of gravity to assist in expelling stool. How safe is the patient's balance when sitting? Does the hemiplegic fall to one side? Would guardrails beside the toilet permit the patient to grasp and maintain balance? Would a backrest on the toilet improve sitting posture? Is the quadriplegic's trunk balance made safer with the extra support offered by a bedside commode? Is it possible for the patient to transfer to a toilet at all? Does manual dexterity and motor coordination present a barrier to manipulation of toilet paper and clothing? Can a suppository be inserted independently? Mechanical devices for the purpose of suppository insertion and digital stimulation are commercially available. Would such an adaptive device enable the patient with impaired finger function to achieve independent bowel care? Last, assess the potential for improvement in functional skills so that progressive changes in the bowel program are anticipated and planned.

Patient-Family Unit (see Table 15-2) The impact of the disability from the perspective of the patient and the patient's family must be assessed before any in-depth teaching of bowel control is initiated. Are they ready to learn? Keep in mind that family members are likely to be adjusting to the disability at a slower pace than the patient. During periods of denial, instructive information may not be processed and repetition will be necessary. When depression occurs, a lack of follow-through of previously learned skills should be anticipated. It is wise to be prepared to provide emotional support and to assume responsibility for the bowel program when the patient is having difficulty coping. Readiness to learn is also affected by sexuality, feelings about incontinence, and basic knowledge of anatomy. At what level should the nurse begin teaching? When the patient is not able to manage the bowel program independently, the family structure should be assessed. Which family member is best able to assume this responsibility? What is that person's relationship to the patient? Will performing bowel care interfere with the relationship with the patient? What is the patient's financial situation? Is the program designed to be within the patient's means? What does the patient plan to do at the time of discharge? What can the nurse do to arrange a program that is appropriate for the patient's future plans? How accessible is the home bathroom? Can the patient afford to remodel? Will the program in the rehabilitation setting be architecturally feasible in the home?

MANAGEMENT OF NEUROGENIC BOWEL DYSFUNCTION

Regulation of fecal incontinence is best managed by a well-planned bowel program. Active participation, on the part of the patient, in establishing a tailor-made program must be encouraged from the onset. The specific type of bowel dysfunction and data obtained through the assessment determine the initial bowel program. This plan should be altered as the patient's status changes and progresses. Such alterations are necessary in order to achieve predictable bowel movements. Common sense indicates that changes in a program should be implemented one at a time so the effect can more accurately be evaluated. It is wise to observe the bowel plan for at least 3 days before making additional changes. Documentation and accurate recording of the approach and the result are vital. Without detailed bowel records, trial-and-error management is inevitable. (See sample record in Chap. 24.)

Physical exercise, high fluid intake, high fiber foods, and a consistent habit time are necessary components of *all* bowel programs (see Table 15-3).

Physical Exercise Physical exercise prevents constipation and sluggish bowel response. The decreased activity level experienced by those with a physical disability is less of a deterrent to healthful bowel function when activities of daily living (ADL) are performed without assistance from others. Dressing, transfers, and propelling a wheelchair are examples of ADL. When subjected to prolonged bed rest, the patient should continue to carry out as many activities as possible (hiking hips off the bed, turning, bathing, range of motion) in an effort to prevent decreased intestinal motility and constipation.

High Fluid Intake The relationship between fluid intake and stool consistency has been previously discussed. A minimum intake of 2000 mL a day helps to keep stool soft; 3000 mL a day is desirable. When fluids must be restricted

Table 15-3

Neurogenic Bowel Dysfunction and Management

LEVEL OF LESION	DYSFUNCTION CLASSIFICATION	CEREBRAL CONTROL	SPHINCTER CONTROL	INCONTINENCE PICTURE	BOWEL PROGRAM	POTENTIAL PROBLEMS
Spinal cord, above T12–L1 vertebral level	Reflex automatic UMNL	Absent	Absent	Infrequent Sudden Unexpected Occurs without warning	Physical exercise High fluid intake High fiber foods Consistent habit time Suppository program Digital stimulation Stool softener prn	Impaction Autonomic dysreflexia
Spinal cord, at or below T12–L1 vertebral level	Autonomous flaccid LMNL	Absent	Absent	Frequent Induced by physical exercise	Physical exercise High fluid intake High fiber foods Consistent habit time Suppository program Valsalva Manual removal prn	
Brain	Uninhibited UMNL	Decreased	Decreased	Frequent or infrequent Urgency	Physical exercise High fluid intake High fiber foods Consistent habit time Prune juice Stool softener prn Suppository prn	Constipation

Source: American Journal of Nursing Company, adapted and expanded from the Student Syllabus—*The Neurologically Disabled Patient,* 1977.

and intake drops below 3000 mL daily (perhaps due to bladder training), high fiber foods, foods high in water content, and natural laxatives may be added to the diet to maintain the desired stool consistency.

High Fiber Foods Foods that are resistant to hydrolysis by digestive enzymes in the GI tract are called high fiber. Therefore, these foods are not completely digested. Fiber adds bulk to the stool and promotes normal peristalsis. The chief sources of fiber are whole grain cereals and breads, green vegetables, nuts, and fruits with skin and seeds. (See Variables Affecting Elimination earlier in this chapter.) Foods prepared with refined flour and sugar are common in an American diet. They contribute nothing to good bowel response. It is thought that fiber may also have a cathartic effect. Brans and shredded wheat are good examples. Unprocessed bran is easily added to cereals, meat loaf, sauces, and other foods and will act as a natural laxative. Prune juice has long been used for this purpose. Large quantities of prune and orange juice, however, should be avoided as the stool may become too loose. It is wise to introduce fiber into the diet gradually. Begin with whole grain bread and cereal, then add cooked fruit and vegetables before progressing to raw fruit and vegetables. Dietary measures are extremely valuable in obtaining soft stool consistency and preventing constipation. Attempt to achieve effective bowel response by dietary means before introducing stool softeners and laxatives. In the long run, a healthful diet is more beneficial and certainly less costly than continuous use of medications.

Consistent Habit Time Ignoring the urge to defecate is a common cause of irregularity in the nondisabled population. In the presence of neurogenic bowel function this urge must be stimulated as well as heeded if bowel regulation and control are to be accomplished. Establishing a consistent habit time for elimination is critical. A consistent habit time introduces an element of rigidity that is difficult to accept. But clinical experience has demonstrated that the stimulation method must take place at the same hour every time it is scheduled in order to develop prompt bowel response. Consistent timing of the stimulation will achieve the goal of a bowel movement within 30 min. Failure to establish and follow a consistent schedule will result in constipation, impaction, and delayed bowel response. When planning a bowel program, the preonset habits as well as anticipated plans at discharge are important considerations. In a rehabilitation setting, the daily therapy schedule must also be considered. There will be instances when establishing bowel control must rank as a higher priority than early morning therapies or evening recreation activities.

Management methods specific to the type of bowel dysfunction will now be considered.

Reflex Neurogenic (see Table 15-3) Spinal cord lesions above the T12–L1 vertebral level are classified as reflex bowel function. Automatic and UMNL are other terms used to describe this type of bowel dysfunction. The nervous pathways between the brain and spinal cord are interrupted. The extent of the interruption depends on whether the injury is complete or incomplete. Cerebral control of defecation is absent and voluntary control of the anal sphincter is absent. However, the S2–S3–S4 nerve segments remain intact. Thus it is possible to develop a stimulus-response type of bowel control that capitalizes on the intact spinal reflex arc. Feces in the rectum create distention and the bowel reflexly empties. Fecal incontinence is present but occurs infrequently as anal sphincter tone is maintained by parasympathetic innervation through the sacral segment of the spinal cord. (See Innervation earlier in this chapter.)

The thrust of this bowel program is to initiate a stimulus that will reflexly move feces into the rectum for predictable elimination. During spinal cord shock, tonic paralysis of the gut exists and the anal sphincter has flaccid tone. Bowel simulation during the shock period consists of small, properly administered enemas. Flaccid anal tone may interfere with retention of the enema solution. A baby bottle nipple attached to the enema tubing makes an effective shield against involuntary solution return.

When bowel sounds improve, when physical activity increases, and when oral food can be tolerated, the bowel stimulation method progresses to administration of rectal suppositories. These develop a purposeful stimulus-response bowel movement. Suppositories containing bisacodyl are the strongest. They should be used initially to trigger reflex elimination. Although these products are safely used with adults, they may be too strong for children. A glycerin suppository or one-half of a bisacodyl suppository are alternatives for children.

The frequency and time of suppository administration should reflect the preonset habits. It is common practice to proceed with a daily suppository until a reliable bowel pattern is identified. A consistent pattern of a large, soft bowel movement on one day and a small, soft bowel movement the next day signals that an every-other-day suppository program is appropriate. Certain individuals may be able to progress to an every-third-day program, provided stool consistency remains soft. The potential for fecal impaction as a result of infrequent elimination must always be considered. As a general rule, it is safest to allow no longer than 3 days to elapse without bowel stimulation.

Progression from a bisacodyl to a glycerin suppository, and finally to digital stimulation (DS) alone, occurs when the current program has been effective for 3 weeks. The terminal goal is DS as the only stimulus necessary to produce reflex elimination. This goal may not be achieved during the time the patient is in the rehabilitation setting. Efforts to reach the goal should continue long after discharge. DS may, from the onset of bowel training, be effective as the primary stimulation method. DS is also used in conjunction with rectal suppositories. For example, DS is performed when a suppository has not produced a bowel movement within 15 to 20 min. This procedure may be repeated several times.

An accidental bowel movement occurring on the day a bowel program is planned does not preclude following through with the scheduled program. The stimulation method still needs to be carried out at the regular time to facilitate a predictable and purposeful reflex action.

Stool softeners may be necessary components of initial bowel programs. They assist in elimination when abdominal muscle strength is weak or paralyzed. Products containing sodium methylcellulose, casanthranol, and dioctyl sodium or calcium sulfosuccinate are commonly used.

Autonomic dysreflexia is a potential problem for patients with spinal cord lesions above the T6 level (above the splanchinic outflow). Bladder distention seems to be the most common cause. However, rectal stimulation and bowel distention often precipitate this sympathetic response. Symptoms of dysreflexia can be experienced with suppository insertion, digital stimulation, and passage of feces through the rectum. It is important to have baseline blood pressure and pulse readings so the normal range is known. Measuring blood pressure and pulse before, during, and after anorectal stimulation is valuable in identifying autonomic dysreflexia. Application of Nupercainal Ointment on the rectum 5 min before suppository insertion or digital stimulation is helpful in preventing the symptoms.

Autonomous Neurogenic (see Table 15-3) Spinal cord lesions at or below the T12–L1 vertebral level are classified as producing autonomous bowel function. Flaccid and LMNL are other terms that describe this type of neurogenic bowel. As in reflex bowel function, communication of nervous impulses to the brain is compromised. The extent to which this is true pivots around whether the injury is complete or incomplete. Cerebral control of elimination is absent. Voluntary control of the anal sphincter is absent. Because the lesion directly involves the S2–S3–S4 nerve segments, the activity of the spinal reflex arc is destroyed. Signals are not transmitted to or from the spinal cord and reflex emptying of the bowel is absent. Fecal incontinence is frequent, often induced by the stress of physical exercise because the external anal sphincter lacks tone and offers little or no resistance against stool in the rectum. (See Innervation earlier in this chapter.) Incontinence is especially evident when stool consistency is too soft.

Establishing control for this type of bowel function is extremely difficult. In nursing literature, management methods ranging from enemas and manual removals to suppository programs are suggested. Use of enemas beyond the period of spinal cord shock is inadvisable because of the great potential for mechanical injury to the colon. Manual removals stretch the anal sphincter and continuous usage decreases the tone of the already incompetent sphincter. Theoretically, rectal suppositories should be ineffective because the S2–S3–S4 reflex arc is absent. However, actual experience has shown that suppository programs do result in bowel control.

The purpose of this bowel program is twofold. Stool consistency must be very firm and the distal colon must be kept empty. Dietary bulk and bulk-forming medications such as Dialose Plus and Metamucil are valuable in developing a stool consistency that is firm yet not hard. Dulcolax and Vacuetts suppositories effectively stimulate defecation. Lack of anal sphincter tone may result in oozing following anal stimulation. Insertion of a small amount of Nupercainal Ointment into the rectum nullifies the residual action of the suppository. The frequency and timing of suppository administration is identical to that outlined for reflex bowel programs. It is well to be aware that patients tend to want a hard stool consistency. This desire seems to be based on a realistic fear of incontinence and embarrassment. Thus, constipation and fecal impaction are prevalent in autonomous bowel function. It is more sensible to prevent incontinence through the daily use of a suppository to evacuate the distal colon than to develop hard stool and risk impaction and atony of the colon.

Valsalva maneuver (see Defecation earlier in this chapter) augments the suppository program. Digital stimulation is not useful for this type of bowel function as the sacral spinal reflex arc is absent.

Manual removal of stool does not contribute to the goal of planned predictable bowel movements and should not be a standard component of the bowel program. Manual removals should be used with discretion. The presence in the rectum of hard stool that cannot be expelled is an example of legitimate usage.

Uninhibited Neurogenic (see Table 15-3) CNS lesions above the C1 vertebral level are classified as unhibited bowel function. UMNL is a synonymous term. The sacral nerve segments are not damaged, and perianal sensation remains intact. Transmission of impulses through the sacral reflex arc and to the brain is not interrupted, but the deficit is in the ability of the brain to interpret sensory impulses to defecate. Cerebral awareness of the urge to defecate is decreased, and this decreased ability to perceive sensory input results in decreased voluntary control of the anal sphincter. Defecation is not inhibited. Involuntary elimination occurs as a result of the sacral reflex arc acting alone. Fecal incontinence is accompanied by a feeling of urgency.

In addition to promoting bowel regularity, the thrust of this program is to help the patient focus attention on elimination. Means of promoting regularity have been discussed. (See Variables Affecting Elimination earlier in this chapter.) A consistent pattern of food intake and a consistent habit time are essential. The habit time should be planned to augment gastrocolic reflexes. Helping the patient to the toilet 30 min after each meal directs attention to elimination at a time when there is likely to be a bowel response. This also allows staff to detect a reliable defecation pattern. The frequency of toileting is decreased when the patient communicates, verbally or nonverbally, the need to eliminate. Behaviors such as restlessness or picking at the rectum should not be overlooked as they indicate mental awareness of rectal sensation. In the absence of functional speech, these signals are important modes of communication. Large doses of praise following appropriate communication help the patient recognize success.

Prune juice assists in establishing a regular schedule of elimination. It should be given 8 to 12 h before defecation is planned. Four ounces is a common but arbitrary amount. Based on individual response, the amount and time of administration are adjusted.

Stool softeners may be necessary during the acute stage of recovery. Colace, Doxidan, and Surfak are examples of frequently used emollient fecal softeners. Their use should be temporary. When food and fluid intake and physical activity are well tolerated, stool softeners may be replaced by high fiber foods.

Rectal suppositories help to establish a consistent habit time, heighten rectal sensations, and increase awareness of the urge to eliminate. Glycerin suppositories are generally strong enough to be effective in uninhibited bowel function. Again, the frequency of administration is based on preonset bowel habits. Through daily use, a consistent evacuation schedule may be achieved. When the patient begins to have consistent bowel movements and demonstrates awareness of the need to use the toilet, the frequency of administration should be changed. A suppository given every third day, if there is no spontaneous bowel movement, is then appropriate. Suppository usage should be a temporary management method. Unless the extent of brain damage is severe, continence and control can be achieved through compliance with the four basic components of all bowel programs.

Digital stimulation is not recommended because many patients who fall into the uninhibited bowel function classification have intact rectal sensation and DS is painful. Valsalva maneuver should be used with discretion. Straining to eliminate raises the blood pressure above normal. Because many stroke patients are hypertensive and have cardiovascular diseases, this danger must be recognized.

Constipation is a potential problem. The most frequent causes are irregular bowel habits and decreased colon motility. Implementation of the above bowel program greatly assists in preventing the problem.

FACTORS FACILITATING REGULATION

Privacy During elimination, privacy deserves mention as an important factor in achieving bowel regulation. Knowing that sounds and smells are being emitted and that someone may open the cubicle curtain at any moment makes relaxation extremely difficult. Getting the patient out of bed, onto a toilet, and into a bathroom with the door closed are important psychologic considerations. If a bedside commode is used, try to roll it into a bathroom or similar secluded area.

Positioning Sitting upright is stressed for its value in facilitating gravity and the expulsion of stool. Simulating this position when a bedpan must be utilized is a definite challenge. Time should be taken first to position the buttocks and the bedpan at the point where the mattress bends when the head of the bed is elevated. Slouched postures should be avoided. Pillows placed behind the back and under the knees promote the upright position and provide comfort. If the head of the bed cannot be elevated, it is important to bridge the hips, knees, and legs to limit sacral pressure exerted by the bedpan. Spinal cord–injured patients should never use a bedpan. An incontinent pad is a safe and satisfactory alternative. Bedpans should be abandoned for all patients as soon as getting out of bed is medically safe.

A squatlike position (knees slightly higher than the hips) apparently increases abdominal pressure and assists the passage of stool. Hospital toilets and padded shower chairs are often so high that the legs are left dangling. A footstool should support the feet and elevate the knees. When sitting balance permits, the patient can lean forward toward the thighs to further increase abdominal pressure.

Raised toilet seats should be used for those who have difficulty transferring on and off a standard toilet seat. Paraplegics who wish to avoid the expense of a commode chair and who have the upper extremity strength to transfer may find a raised toilet seat suitable. The distance between the raised seat and the toilet rim is such that rectal stimulation and cleansing can be accomplished.

Intraabdominal Pressure Increasing intraabdominal pressure when muscles are debilitated or paralyzed helps force feces into the rectum and speeds up bowel action. The Valsalva maneuver, described earlier, is a technique effective for many quadriplegics and paraplegics. Instruct the patient to breathe in deeply and bear down or strain. Performing this exercise while doing a push-up from the toilet seat often produces better results. Massage of the abdomen, proceeding from the right groin upward across the abdomen and downward to the left groin, stimulates and hastens the defecation process. Abdominal massage is a simple technique effective for all types of disabilities.

Oral Medications There are many instances when stimulant laxatives, emollient softeners, or bulk-forming medications may be indicated. It is imperative that the nurse be well informed about the severity, site, mechanism of action, and the dosage required for effective results. Management of bowel programs is a nursing function in most rehabilitation settings. The nurse must be knowledgeable about a wide variety of bowel medications in order to initiate or even suggest a medication order. The use of medications is not to be considered a cure for hard stools or constipation. Furthermore, prolonged usage can be habit forming. The knowledgeable nurse recognizes this and strives to restore normal bowel function and promote bowel regulation by emphasizing diet, fluid, and exercise.

Numerous medications interfere with bowel function. Narcotics, antihistamines, tranquilizers, some antacids, anticholinergics, adrenergic agents, and muscle relaxants may result in constipation. Assessing the total medication regimen is a part of establishing and maintaining a successful bowel program.

Rectal Suppositories Vacuettes suppositories exert action by releasing carbon dioxide, thus creating pressure in the colon. The release of carbon dioxide is initiated by lubricating the suppository with water immediately prior to insertion. Use of a petroleum lubricant renders the suppository ineffective. This mild-strength suppository is commonly used if abdominal cramping is experienced from other types of suppositories. Some rehabilitation centers successfully use this suppository in the bowel programs for LMNL.

Glycerin suppositories mechanically irritate the rectum, and the bowel responds by secreting fluid that lubricates the feces. It usually takes 30 min for this suppository to work, but the time required varies from person to person. The irritant property that stimulates defecation is also irritating to the mucous membranes, so prolonged usage may cause injury to the tissue. Glycerin is thought to be a suppository of moderate strength.

Bisacodyl suppositories exert action by coming in contact with the mucosa of the rectum. Stimulation of sensory nerve endings results in reflex contractions of the colon, and elimination follows. The fact that this is a *contact* suppository is emphasized. If the suppository is inserted into a mass of feces, there will be little or no bowel movement. Prior to insertion of the suppository, the patient should be positioned on the left side with the right thigh raised toward the chest. The rectum should be checked for the presence of stool. If stool is present, an amount adequate to ensure placement of the suppository against the bowel wall should be removed. The suppository is inserted, pointed end first, into and beyond the anal sphincters, then the end of the suppository is pushed sideways to contact the mucosa of the colon. Results generally occur in 15 to 20 min. Bisacodyl suppositories are generally considered strong stimulants.

Digital Stimulation The technique of manually distending the anal sphincter and stimulating the anal wall to produce reflex elimination is called digital stimulation. It may be used in several ways. The primary use is to establish reflex-response defecation patterns by inserting a finger, rather than a suppository, into the rectum. It is also used to trigger a bowel movement when a suppository has yielded poor results. Another use is to ensure complete emptying of the colon following a bowel movement.

The index finger is gloved, lubricated, and gently inserted into the rectum. The finger is moved in a circular motion against the anal sphincter wall. Stimulation continues until the internal sphincter muscle relaxes. This may take 30 s or 1 to 2 min. When the sphincter is relaxed, the finger is removed and time is allowed for reflex peristaltic contractions to produce evacuation. The procedure may be repeated if necessary.

COMMON COMPLICATIONS

Constipation Constipation may be organic in origin and this cause should always be eliminated. However, a frequent cause in patients with neuromuscular diseases is sluggish movement of feces through the colon. Bowel programs are planned to develop bowel habits and prevent the problem from occurring.

Constipation means abnormally hard stool that is difficult to pass through the rectum. The stool is very dry since it is retained in the distal colon for long periods and more fluid than normal has been absorbed. It is important that the patient and the nurse avoid confusion by discussing the meaning of constipation. There are patients who insist they are constipated when they do not have a daily bowel movement. It should be clarified that the frequency of elimination is not as relevant as the consistency and form of the stool.

The patient and the patient's family should be taught signs that warn of constipation. Slight loss of appetite, abdominal discomfort, and a hard or distended abdomen are common symptoms. Spinal cord–injured persons with lack of abdominal sensation may experience discomfort referred to other parts of the body and may also feel unusually nervous. Once a bowel program has been established and regulated, the patient should be instructed to watch for evacuation of stool that is hard, stool that is small in amount, leaking of loose stool; and passing poorer results than usual.

The physician should be consulted for treatment of constipation. Laxatives and enemas are generally utilized. Enemas can lead to autonomic dysreflexia in spinal cord injuries above the T-6 level, and this hazard needs to be considered.

Impaction Overloading of the colon or rectum with a mass of feces that blocks movement of stool toward the anus is impaction. The warning signs of an impaction are the same as for constipation. If oozing of loose stool occurs, the patient should always be examined for the presence of an impaction. Seepage of loose stool may mean that liquid stool is passing around a fecal mass in the rectum or colon. Impacted stool may be removed manually, followed, if necessary, by an enema. The bowel program may then need to be altered to prevent future occurrence.

Diarrhea This frequent passage of watery stool is often caused by a GI disturbance. When the patient is on an established and regulated bowel program and diarrhea occurs, it is important to search for the cause. Clinical experience has shown that ingestion of spicy foods and large amounts of fruit juices can disrupt a well-regulated program. Certain antacids and antibiotics may contribute to diarrhea or loose stools. Another cause that should be ruled out is a fecal impaction.

Autonomic Dysreflexia A potential risk for those who have a spinal cord injury above the T6 level, autonomic dysreflexia is manifested by severe hypertension, bradycardia, throbbing headaches, diaphoresis, "goose bumps," nasal stuffiness, and flushing of the skin over the face, neck, and chest. Nursing management of dysreflexia caused by fecal impaction or rectal stimulation is the same as that for dysreflexia caused by the bladder. Initial actions are directed toward *immediate* lowering of the blood pressure. Placing the patient in a sitting position helps to accomplish this. The blood pressure and pulse should be monitored every 3 to 5 min. Removing the irritating stimulus (feces) is more complex than eliminating the cause of bladder dysreflexia. Insertion of a finger through the rectum distends the rectum further and causes the blood pressure to climb higher. The physician must be notified. Manual removal of stool should not be attempted until the symptoms have lessened. Nupercainal Ointment should be inserted into the rectum 10 min prior to manual evacuation. Establishment of an appropriate and effective bowel program greatly assists in decreasing the frequency with which this complication occurs.

CONCLUSION

Reestablishing bowel control is an integral component of the total rehabilitation process. No member of the health team can offer the patient as much in this area as the nurse. Bowel programs that are practical, convenient, and that develop consistent habits contribute significantly to the process of assisting patients resume their former life-style.

Bowel programs must be individualized to be effective. Programs planned on the basis of a comprehensive assessment of the patient's physical status, bowel and nutrition history, functional skills, and the many factors affecting the patient-family unit result in positive outcomes. Physical exercise, high fluid intake, high fiber foods, and establishment of a consistent habit time should be components of all bowel programs.

Responsibility for the management of the bowel program should be assumed by the patient as soon as possible. Nurses must invest heavily in patient education if the patient is to be truly in control of the management of the bowel program. Opportunities to practice skills and apply knowledge must be provided as often as possible. Supervised learning experiences within the rehabilitation setting and home visits lead to confidence and independence. Written information about bowel function in general, the program for the specific patient, and warning signs of complications, as well as how to manage them, must be provided as a source of reference when questions and problems arise following discharge from the rehabilitation setting.

There is very little information available in nursing literature that is pertinent to the effects various neuromuscular disorders have on bowel function. References pertaining to nursing management of incontinence show that approaches vary from one rehabilitation setting to another. Research on altered levels of bowel function, as well as management, is desperately needed to strengthen the scientific base from which nurses operate.

BIBLIOGRAPHY

Benson, John A.: "Simple Chronic Constipation-Pathophysiology and Management," *Postgrad Med* 57:1, 1975.

Boroch, Rose Marie: *Elements of Rehabilitation in Nursing,* Mosby, St. Louis, 1976.

Corman, M., M. Veidenheimer, and J. Coller: "Cathartics," *Am J Nurs* 75:2, 1975.

Darlington, Roy C.: "Laxative Products," in *Handbook of Nonprescription Drugs,* American Pharmaceutical Association, Washington, 1977.

Goodman, Jay, Jane Pang, and Alice N Bessman: "Dioctyl sodium sulfosuccinate—An Ineffective Prophylactic Laxative," *J Chronic Dis* 29:1, 1976.

Pepper, Ginette: "The Person with a Spinal Cord Injury—Psychological Care," *Am J Nurs* 77: 2, 1977.

Robinson, Corrine H., and Marilyn R. Lawbe: *Normal and Therapeutic Nutrition,* Macmillan, New York, 1977.

Stass, William E., and Phyllis DeNault: "Bowel Control," *Am Fam Physician* 7:1, 1973.

Schickendanz, Ruth H., and Pamela D. Mayhall: *Restorative Nursing in a General Hospital,* Charles C Thomas, Springfield, Ill. 1975.

Thompson, W. G.: "Constipation and Catharsis," *Can Med Assoc J* 114:10, 1976.

16
rosemarie b. king

assessment and management of soft tissue pressure

INTRODUCTION

Prevention and management of soft tissue necrosis has long been the subject of discussion and research. In addition to being a source of anguish and contributing to long hospitalization for the patient, pressure sores affect health professionals through feelings of guilt and frustration over management of this complication. The purpose of this chapter is to examine the effects of pressure on soft tissue as well as the current concepts in prevention and management of pressure sores.

Although much is known about pressure sore etiology and pathophysiology, translation of this knowledge into actions to prevent soft tissue necrosis is inconsistent. A major focus of this chapter is on preventive aspects of skin care. It is the nurse who, along with the patient, performs the most critical role in prevention. If pressure sores are to be prevented, nurses must accept responsibility for early and continuous assessment as well as for implementation of current knowledge.

TERMINOLOGY

The terms *decubitus ulcer* and *bed sore* are commonly used in discussions of soft tissue necrosis, but these are imprecise terms. "Decubitus," from the Latin *decumbere,* means lying down. "Bed sore" also implies that soft tissue necrosis occurs as a result of being in bed. However, many surfaces may create pressure over a bony prominence, such as an x-ray or operating table, a wheelchair cushion, an orthosis or prosthesis, or a shoe. Thus the terms "decubitus" and "bed sore" do not include the source of the pathologic condition, which is **pressure.** Pressure sore is more descriptive and will be used throughout the chapter to refer to soft tissue necrosis. Pressure sore can be defined as an area of cellular necrosis, usually over a bony prominence that has been subjected to pressure in excess of capillary pressure for a period of time sufficient to cause cell death.

HISTORICAL PERSPECTIVE

Bailey has described scientific efforts attempted since the sixteenth century to determine the etiology and management of pressure sores. Although numerous causes for soft tissue necrosis have been postulated, pressure has long been identified as a major factor (Bailey, 1967). Only in the past 50 years has extensive research expanded our knowledge about the effects and management of soft tissue pressure. Studies on capillary pressure, predisposing factors, equipment to equalize body weight, and soft tissue response to pressure have yielded significant results.

Treatment of pressure sores has ranged from the application of carrot and turnip or bread and charcoal poultices to current management, which includes application of topical enzymes, surgical repair, and highly sophisticated equipment to provide pressure relief. Too often, treatment and devices have been used without thoughtful consideration of rationale and examination of beneficial effects. In recent years, more critical attention has been focused on evaluation of treatment techniques and support systems. Numerous regimens have come and gone, but such time-honored and proven nursing techniques as bridging bony prominences and regular turning remain significant in prevention and treatment of pressure sores.

POPULATION AT RISK

Despite knowledge gained from research and experience, pressure sores continue as a serious potential complication for many patients. Medical advances have resulted in a population increasingly at risk to develop skin breakdown. Greater life expectancy with the potential for periods of immobility resulting from illness or injury has increased the risk in the geriatric population. Survival of the severely injured and those with debilitating chronic illness has also increased the number of persons living with nutritional, sensory, circulatory, and mobility impairments. These individuals are frequently in need of extensive rehabilitation services. Pressure sores may have occurred while the person was comatose or critically ill prior to the active rehabilitation phase. Prevention of soft tissue necrosis and healing of existing skin breakdown can occur if the nurse understands the dynamics and management of pressure on soft tissue. This knowledge must also be imparted to the patient.

EFFECTS OF PRESSURE

Pressure compresses the skin and the layers of subadjacent tissue between bone and an external firm surface, creating ischemia to the localized area. Vasodilation occurs when the pressure is released, resulting in reactive hyperemia which can be observed on the skin as a flushing accompanied by increased local temperature. The flow of blood to the formerly anoxic tissues removes toxic materials and restores nutrition to the cells. Hyperemia is a compensatory mechanism following ischemia from pressure. The reaction is proportional to the duration of the pressure (Lewis, 1925). Normally, discomfort from pressure is perceived; the individual moves, hyperemia occurs, and no cell damage is evident. This cycle repeats itself constantly even in sleep. Any situation that interferes with the sensation of pressure and/or the ability to move places the person at greater risk to develop cell damage.

Studies have shown that capillary pressures range from 12 mmHg to 32 mmHg (Landis, 1930). Several investigators have demonstrated that pressure in excess of capillary pressure is the cause of cellular necrosis (Brooks, 1953; Husain, 1953; Kosiak, 1959; Groth, 1942). It is generally accepted that vascular obstruction with ischemia is responsible for soft tissue changes secondary to pressure.

Normally, human beings tolerate pressure far in excess of 20 to 30 mmHg over bony prominences when sitting, lying, or standing. However, this pressure is intermittent. Kosiak demonstrated that intermittent relief of pressure for 5-min periods prevented change in tissue. In contrast, injury occurred when the same amounts of constant pressure were applied for a 3-h period (Kosiak, 1961). The same investigator also demonstrated an inverse relationship between the intensity and the duration of pressure in the development of soft tissue necrosis (Kosiak, 1959). Therefore, high pressures should be exerted only for brief periods of time, while pressures near or below capillary pressure can be applied for longer periods. When planning and giving care, the nurse must consider that moderate pressure over prolonged time can produce as much or more damage than intense pressure applied for a brief interval. Pressure of 60 to 70 mmHg have been shown to produce pathologic changes in less than 1-h (Trumble, 1930; Kosiak, 1959; Husain, 1953). Pressures exerted when sitting or lying on most surfaces exceed these figures. It is obvious that some patients will be at risk to develop skin breakdown if automatically placed on the routine "every 2-h" turn schedule, while this timing will be adequate for others.

DISTRIBUTION OF PRESSURE

An understanding of pressure distribution over the body surface is useful to control the intensity of pressure to which soft tissue is subjected. As a result of the skeletal configuration, soft tissues covering bony areas are subjected to greater compression than are other body surfaces (Fig. 16-1). Lindan's studies on distribution of pressure revealed that the prone position resulted in more evenly distributed weight than did other positions. The knees and chest wall experienced the highest pressures in the prone position. Pressures were higher over the greater trochanter in the lateral position and higher over the ischial tuberosities while sitting, that is, 75 to 95 mmHg. The surfaces on which these readings were taken were varied, and comparisons were made. A more pliable surface increased the area of contact, and pressure readings were lower (Lindan et al., 1965). Another study of pressure in the sitting position revealed measurements as high as 300 mmHg (Kosiak et al., 1959). This study

CHAPTER 16   244

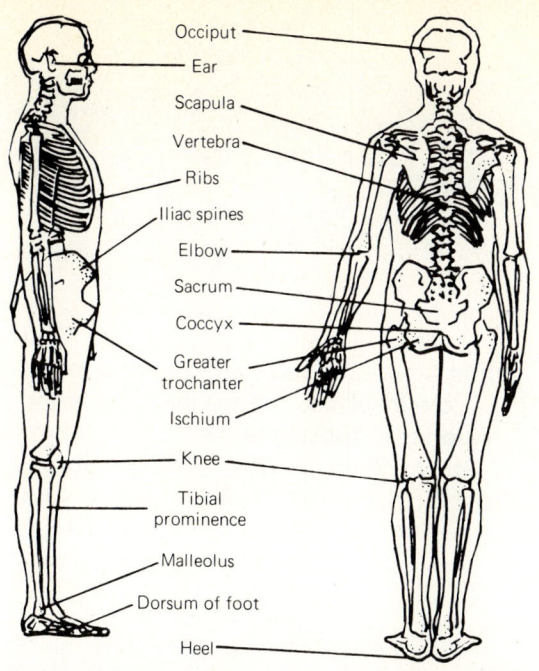

Figure 16-1
Major bony prominences. Soft tissue covering these prominences are more subject to necrosis because of the higher pressure exerted.

Figure 16-2
(A) Compression of soft tissue between sacrum (*a*) and firm mattress (*b*). (B) Foam mattress distributes the compression force over larger area of sacrum (*a*) and mattress (*b*). (Redrawn from Reichel, S. A.: "Shearing Force as a Factor in Paraplegia," JAMA 166(7):762, 1958. Copyright 1958 American Medical Association. Used with permission.)

demonstrated a marked decrease in pressure with the use on a 2-in foam cushion. Figure 16-2 illustrates tissue compression on a surface of foam rubber and on a firm mattress. Trumble demonstrated that even distribution of body weight in the recumbent position would result in pressures of 17 mmHg over all body surfaces (Trumble, 1930). Thus, pressures over all bony prominences would be below capillary pressure. This is the principle of support systems such as water and air beds that have been developed in recent years.

In further support of the findings on pressure distribution, the ischium, sacrum, greater trochanters, and heels are the most common sites of tissue necrosis. Structural changes such as scoliosis or high above-knee amputation place additional stress over certain bony prominences and must be considered when equipment is prescribed and sitting tolerances determined.

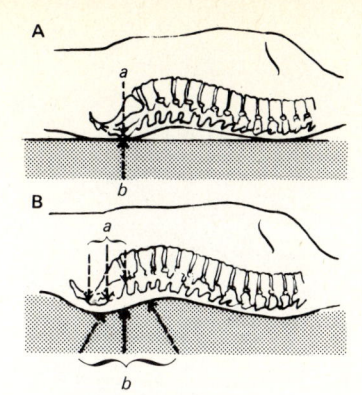

PATHOGENESIS OF PRESSURE SORES

The studies summarized above demonstrate that protracted pressure in excess of capillary pressure over bony areas will produce ischemia of skin and underlying tissues. The amount and duration of the pressure exerted are significant determinants of the degree of ischemia and resultant cellular necrosis.

Relief of pressure following prolonged soft tissue compression results in leakage of cells from damaged vessels, accumulation of edema fluid, dilatation of local blood vessels, and migration of inflammatory cells. Continued application of pressure and sustained ischemia beyond this point interferes with cellular metabolism, which may lead to necrosis of fat, fibrous tissue, muscle, and even bone (Shea, 1975).

CLASSIFICATION OF PRESSURE SORES

A useful classification of pressure sores has been developed to identify and communicate the

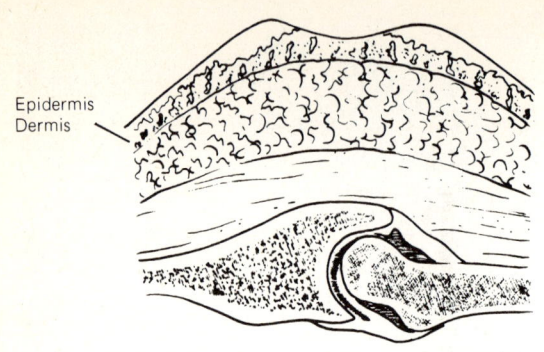

Figure 16-3
Schematic drawing of a Grade I pressure sore. The partial thickness ulceration is limited to the epidermis. Inflammatory reaction affects all soft tissue. *(Redrawn from Shea, J. D.: "Pressure Sores: Classification and Management," Clin Orthop 112:91, 1975. Used with permission.)*

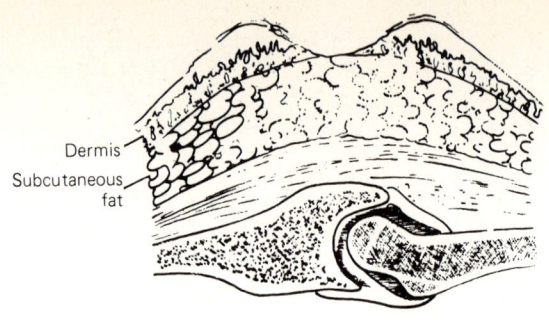

Figure 16-5
Grade II pressure sore. All soft tissue layers are involved. The full thickness lesion extends to subcutaneous fat. *(Redrawn from Shea, J. D.: "Pressure Sores: Classification and Management," Clin Orthop 112:92, 1975. Used with permission.)*

extent of involvement (Shea, 1975). This classification is more precise than such terms as "superficial," "mild," or "extensive." In this system, sores are classified as Grades I through IV and closed.

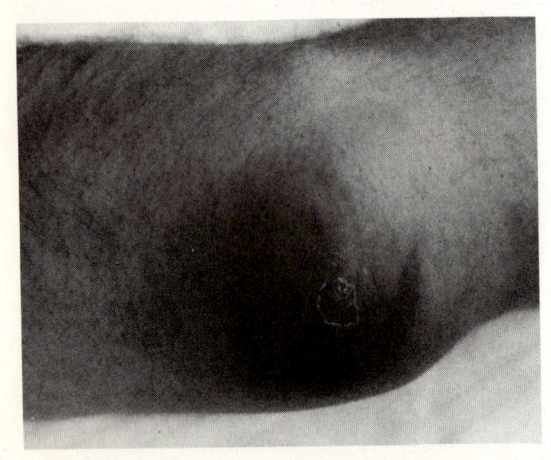

A Grade I sore appears as an area of irregular swelling and induration associated with heat and erythema over a bony prominence (Figs. 16-3 and 16-4). Continued application of pressure results in an ulceration involving the epidermis and exposing the dermis. Although not clinically evident, the underlying layers of soft tissue

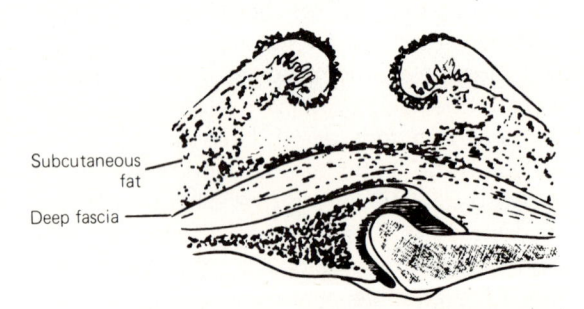

Figure 16-4
Clinical representation of a Grade I pressure sore illustrates erythema, induration, and ulceration of the epidermis. *(Used with permission of the Rehabilitation Institute of Chicago.)*

Figure 16-6
Grade III pressure sore. Progression of the ulceration is deeper with extensive involvement of fat. Deep fascia limits the ulceration. Note undermining of the skin and muscle, periosteum, and joint involvement. *(Redrawn from Shea, J. D.: "Pressure Sores: Classification and Management," Clin Orthop 112:94, 1975. Used with permission.)*

undergo an acute inflammatory reaction. Immediate implementation of preventive measures, especially pressure relief, is essential, since this lesion is reversible.

A Grade II pressure sore develops when the above reaction is intensified by intense or prolonged pressure. The ulceration extends through the epidermis and dermis to subcutaneous fat. The result is a shallow, full-thickness ulcer in which inflammatory and fibrotic changes are more pronounced (Fig. 16-5). Healing will produce a relatively unstable scar. It is imperative to prevent progression to this stage.

Continued application of pressure will result in a Grade III pressure sore with a full-thickness defect extending through subcutaneous fat (Fig. 16-6). Deep fascia limits the depth of the sore, but undermining and distortion of muscle by swelling and inflammation occur. Fluid and protein are lost from the wound. Capsular swelling and synovial effusion develop in nearby joints. Prolonged hospitalization with intense nursing care is necessary to manage pressure relief and wound care and to improve the patient's systemic condition.

Grade IV pressure sores are characterized by penetration of deep fascia and rapidly progressing undermining. All soft tissue structures are necrosed, and bone can be identified at the base of the ulceration (Figs. 16-7 and 16-8). The patient may have multiple skin breakdowns and be dehydrated, anemic, and toxic. Prolonged hospitalization and interference with rehabilitation and life-style result. When extremities are involved, amputation may be necessary. The Grade IV stage can be fatal.

Closed sores occur with repeated pressure for prolonged periods often combined with shearing forces resulting in necrosis in subcutaneous fat. There is no obvious skin ulceration. The result is a bursalike cavity filled with necrotic debris. These sores are most frequently seen over the ischium and trochanter. Clinically, skin appears pigmented, thickened, and may eventually rupture (Shea, 1975). Sinography is recommended to identify these sores early so that aggressive treatment can be started (Putnam et al., 1978).

Prevention of pressure sores such as those described consists of three components: assessment of the patient, management of factors predisposing to pressure sore development, and patient education.

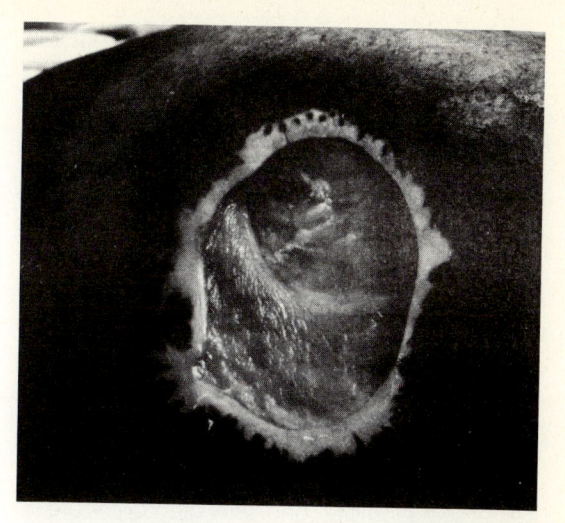

Figure 16-8
Clinical representation of Grade IV pressure sore. Necrosis of all underlying soft tissue has occurred. The patient had multiple infected sores and eventually required extensive plastic surgery. *(Used with permission of the Rehabilitation Institute of Chicago.)*

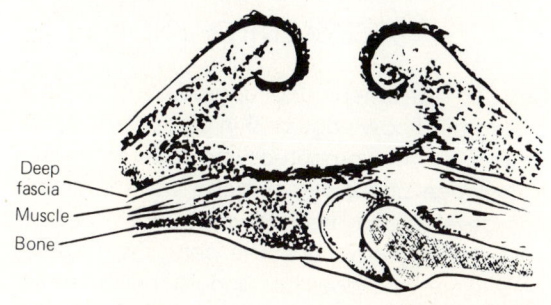

Figure 16-7
Grade IV pressure sore. All soft tissue structures have been necrosed. Bone and joint structures are also affected. *(Redrawn from Shea, J. D.: "Pressure Sores: Classification and Management," Clin Orthop 112:96, 1975. Used with permission.)*

247 ASSESSMENT AND MANAGEMENT OF SOFT TISSUE PRESSURE

ASSESSMENT

GENERAL ASSESSMENT

Initial and continued assessment of the patient by the nurse is paramount to prevention of soft tissue necrosis. General skin condition (presence of lesions and/or scar tissue, cleanliness, elasticity, skin moisture, and the presence of edema) is assessed on admission to the hospital or during outpatient or community health nurse contact. Special attention to elderly patients is necessary, as the incidence of pressure sores acquired during hospitalization is higher in this group. Skin changes, such as thinning of epidermis and decreased elasticity, and skin oils contribute to the susceptibility of the elderly to pressure sores.

During assessment, it is essential to critique the current plan of care. Should the turning schedule be revised? Are mattress and wheelchair cushion appropriate and in satisfactory condition? What is the patient's skin response to the turning schedule? How long does the hyperermic response last? Are hygiene and measures to maintain skin lubrication adequate? If a pressure sore has developed after discharge, how is the patient managing it? Are measures to eliminate pressure adequate? If a sore occurred, what were the circumstances surrounding its development? Adequacy of assistance available in the home, the current social support system, and the emotional status of the patient must be evaluated. A significant routine assessment incorporates visual and tactile skin inspection for the flushing and increased temperature associated with the hyperemic response.

ASSESSMENT OF PREDISPOSING FACTORS

Assessment of factors predisposing to pressure sore development will assist in creating individualized strategies to decrease risk of soft tissue breakdown. Adequate assessment will foster more appropriate use of equipment and personnel. The following clinical factors are commonly recognized as predisposing to tissue necrosis:

1. Nutritional deficits
   a. Hypoproteinemia
   b. Avitaminosis
   c. Weight loss
2. Anemia
3. Incontinence
4. Mobility impairment
5. Sensory impairment (mental status and sensation)
6. Infection/febrile status
7. Muscle atrophy
8. Edema
9. Dry skin
10. Vascular tone
11. Social-emotional factors

Nurse investigators have used combinations of the above factors to devise various rating scales to identify patients at high risk to skin breakdown (Norton, 1975; Williams, 1972; Gosnell, 1973). These rating scales based on predisposing factors were found to be useful in predicting individuals who would develop pressure sores. The refinement and standardization of such an assessment tool would be a significant contribution to the prevention of pressure sores.

ASSESSMENT OF KNOWLEDGE

Regular assessment and upgrading of patient and family knowledge of skin care are critical in prevention. The amputee who lacks adequate knowledge about skin hygiene and inspection can develop skin breakdown that will interfere with use of a prosthesis. The person with spinal cord injury who does not understand the need for routine skin inspection and pressure relief is more at risk to develop serious pressure sores, as well as other complications such as burns. When working with adolescents, the youngster as well as the parents are included in this process. Table 16-1 indicates areas to be assessed in patient

Table 16-1

Assessment of Knowledge of Skin Care

FACTOR	KNOWLEDGE	SKILLS	EQUIPMENT
Sitting tolerance	Safe tolerance How to increase		
Turning schedule	Factors that affect bed or wheelchair tolerance Knows schedule	Turns self or directs others Positions prone	Side rails Firm mattresses with 2-in or special mattress if indicated
Wheelchair pressure relief	Frequency Foot plate position	Able to do pushups or other pressure relief	Loops or other wheelchair adaptation if indicated
Equipment	Maintenance	Able to fill cushion or mattress and to check adequacy of filling	
Skin inspection	Pressure points Frequency of inspection Abnormal signs, i.e., redness, blistering rash, abrasions, open lesions Whom to contact if skin problem occurs What to do if problem occurs	Checks skin visually or directs others Able to palpate for temperature changes in skin	Mirror (one or two as indicated)
Positioning	Protection of pressure points	Positions self or directs others Able to bridge	Pillows Foam blocks Foot board, splint, or other devices if indicated
General skin care	Nutrition/fluids Skin lubrication Care of red areas Effect of pressure on soft tissue Foot care, control of edema Effect of sensory loss Prevention of burns, rashes, bruising, shearing, avoid friction	Cuts toenails correctly Applies skin lubricant Applies support hose and/or position to control edema	

and family knowledge of skin care. Not all items will be applicable to each patient; decisions are based on assessment of the individual and understanding of patient education principles outlined elsewhere in the text.

COMMUNICATION OF THE PLAN OF CARE

A written plan of care must be available and communicated to all nursing personnel as well as to other disciplines. For example, the therapists should know the patient's sitting tolerance and whether specific activities should be modified or delayed because of susceptible skin. Physical therapist, nurse, and physician work closely in patient education, in carry-over of skin care skills such as wheelchair push-ups, and in evaluation of devices issued to equalize pressure. The nursing plan of care should include sensation, lesions present and treatment, turning and sitting tolerance and schedule, level of independence and knowledge of skin care, teaching plan, special positioning techniques, degree of supervision or reinforcement needed, and goals of care. Early patient involvement in setting goals and assisting in planning care is desirable. Assessment of patient readiness is dependent upon knowledge of the principles of learning and an understanding of the process of adapting to disability.

MANAGEMENT OF FACTORS WHICH PREDISPOSE TO PRESSURE SORE DEVELOPMENT

MANAGEMENT OF PRIMARY FACTORS

Factors that contribute to pressure sore development are numerous. Recognition of their role in the pathogenesis of soft tissue necrosis and management of these factors are critical to prevention. The primary factors are external and, to a great degree, controllable through the interventions discussed.

For ease of discussion, these elements are separated into primary and secondary factors. Primary factors are pressure, shearing, friction, moisture, and heat. Figure 16-9 is a diagram of the relationship between many of the primary and secondary factors in the pathogenesis of pressure sores.

Pressure

Pressure is the most significant of the primary factors. Indeed, without pressure there would be no sore. An individual program to control pressure must consider the person's body structure, amount of soft tissue over bone, and presence of scar tissue, as well as distribution of pressure and resources available.

Pressure will vary according to body structure and deformities. Certain bony prominences such as sacrum and heel have minimal soft tissue covering, and thus these areas tolerate less pressure than others. Scar tissue, being inelastic, decreases tolerance to stress and pressure. The following measures are required to control pressure and its effects:

1. Regular pressure relief
2. Skin inspection
3. Maintenance of mobility
4. Correct utilization of mattresses and seating devices

Regular Pressure Relief This is accomplished through turning in bed and performing push-ups or weight shifts when sitting. Without this ingredient, prevention is not feasible. "Turn every 2 h" is commonly found on nursing care plans, but the origin of the 2-h guideline is obscure. This may be a reasonable schedule for some patients to maintain skin integrity. For others, however, notably those identified as having one or more of the secondary predisposing factors, 2-h turns would soon result in tissue necrosis. Turn schedules must be individualized to the patient or they are worthless. Patient comfort and hyperemia are the guidelines utilized in determining the schedule. A patient should *never* be repositioned

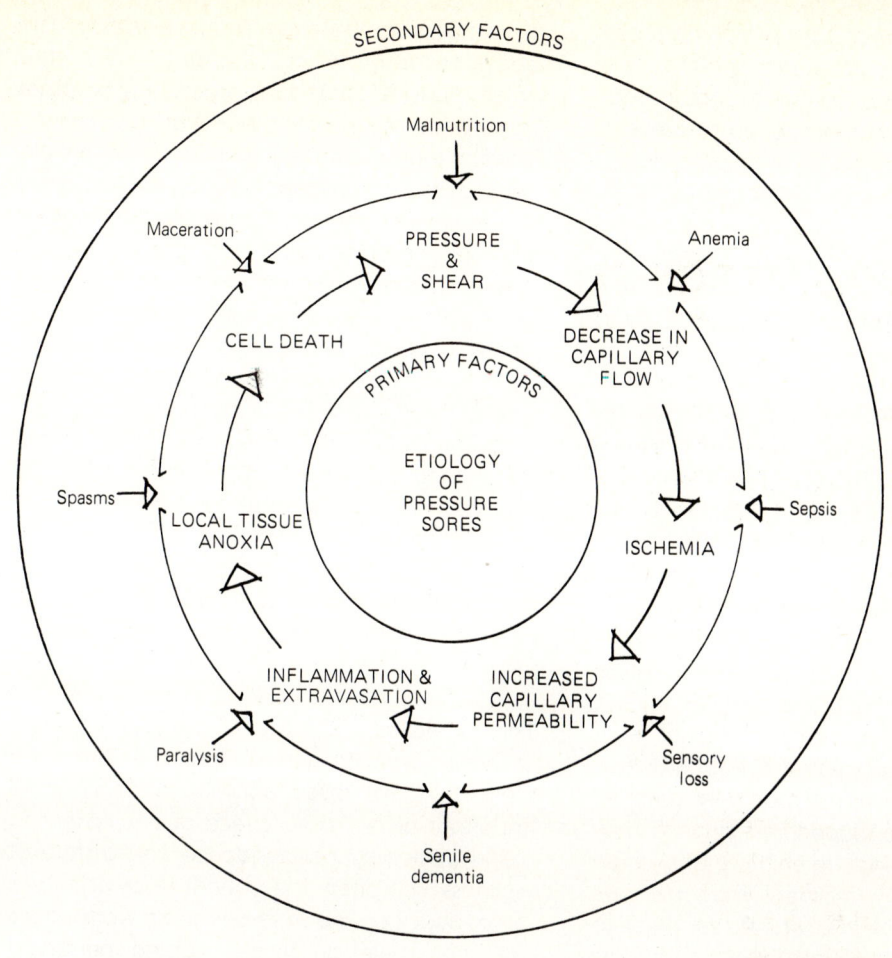

Figure 16-9

The etiology of pressure sores is a dynamic process, as illustrated by this diagram of the primary and secondary factors involved. *(Redrawn from Enis, J., and A. Sarmiento: "The Pathophysiology and Management of Pressure Sores," Orthop Rev 2:26, October 1973. Used with permission.)*

over a bony prominence where hyperemia has not resolved. In such a situation, bridging can be utilized to permit the patient to be turned to all four positions.

A technique that can be used as an adjunct to turning involves small shifts of 20 to 30°. Bridging bony prominences will add to the effectiveness of minor body shifts. This technique could be considered for the patient who requires frequent repositioning and yet who awakens when completely repositioned and cannot return to sleep. Since the prone position tends to distribute pressure more evenly with the exception of high pressure on the knees, proning can be utilized to equalize pressure and to allow longer periods of rest, especially when the patient is at home. Proning is best begun in the hospital for short periods and gradually increased, since patients may be initially frightened and uncomfortable in this position.

ASSESSMENT AND MANAGEMENT OF SOFT TISSUE PRESSURE

Bridging pressure areas with pillows or foam blocks is a technique long utilized by nurses and has been found to be adequate in many situations. Adequate pillows are needed to prevent pressure over the bridged area. If pillows are improperly positioned, pressure will be applied to the bony prominence rather than to soft tissue areas such as thighs. Figure 16-10 illustrates the relief of pressure over heels and sacrum, the points of greatest pressure in the supine position. Adaptation of this procedure to the lateral or prone position is readily accomplished. Since this technique does not eliminate pressure over all areas, skin inspection and turning remain essential. A disadvantage to bridging is the difficulty a family member may have in positioning the patient at home. Practice in the hospital and trials on weekend passes will reveal whether bridging will be practical for home use.

The wheelchair-bound patient who has anesthetic skin and/or paralysis must integrate the habit of pushing up by using arms or shifting weight through other movements such as leaning sideways or forward. Without regular wheelchair pressure relief, ischial tuberosity pressure sores will occur. The dependent patient may need physical assistance to shift weight, or an adapted wheelchair (recliner) may be prescribed. It is necessary to do wheelchair pressure relief every 15 to 20 min because of the intensity of point pressure over the ischium. Local heat and moisture can also be minimized through pressure relief. Proper wheelchair prescription is of considerable importance in prevention. The feet should rest gently on the foot plate so that weight is transmitted to posterior thighs rather than concentrated on the ischial tuberosities. Footrests that are too high will increase pressure loading on the ischium. Armrest placement should be such that part of the body weight is borne on the arms.

Posting and communicating individualized turning schedules and wheelchair-sitting schedules are necessary until the individual is upgraded to maximum time and is reliable. Increasing time in bed or wheelchair position should be a gradual, carefully monitored process. For example, a turning schedule can be increased by 30 min and the skin response assessed for two or three nights. An effort should be made to increase schedules to reasonable limits to enable the patient to reengage in life-style activities upon discharge from the hospital or rehabilitation facility.

Skin Inspection Skin inspection replaces the loss of tactile "warning system" for those with anesthetic skin. For these patients, a mirror is as important as any other piece of equipment to aid in achieving independence and a state of wellness. Too often, the patient relies on others for feedback on the state of skin or, worse, does not check skin at all. All nursing personnel working with the patient are responsible for including skin checks as a routine when the individual arises and retires. This must become

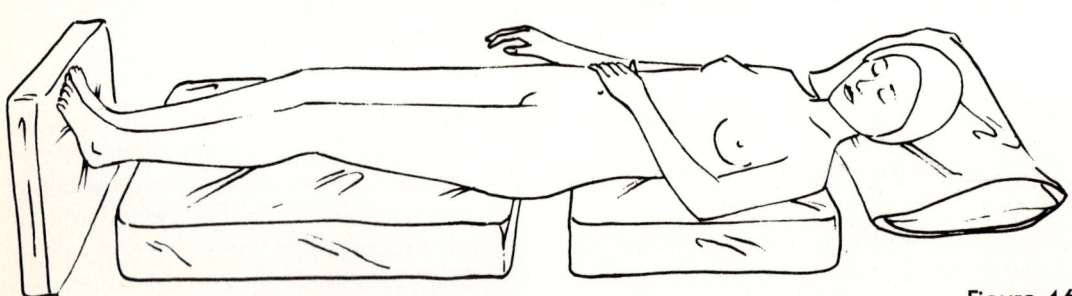

Figure 16-10
Bridging in supine position. Bony prominences are freed of pressure (or bridged) by supporting the body above and below the area on foam blocks or pillows. Note that heels and sacrum are free of pressure.

a lifetime habit if skin is to remain intact. During the interim when turning schedules and wheelchair tolerance are being upgraded, skin inspection is done after each turn and upon return to bed from the wheelchair. The patient can use a mirror for self-inspection. Along with inspection, palpation for increased skin temperature should be done and should be taught to the patient. Tactile measurement of local tissue response to pressure can be obtained by palpating for warmth with the dorsum of the fingers. This routine can be taught to most patients with sensory deficits. Comparison of temperature to a noninvolved area should be done. Tactile assessment of hyperemic responses in dark-skinned individuals is necessary, as visual assessments can be difficult. In addition, patient and staff education includes areas to check and observations to be made as well as frequency of skin inspection. Observations include noting edema, redness, bruises, rashes, blisters, lesions, and other unusual signs such as boils or roughness. Length of hyperemic response must also be noted in order to make decisions about turning and sitting tolerance. Skin inspection is critical. If not done, a lesion could occur over the ischium during the day; if undetected at night and the next morning, it could quickly evolve into a Grade III sore, whereas skin checks could have halted progression at the Grade I level when an erythemic response was present. Examples of patient populations for whom routine skin checks should be done are individuals with diabetes, amputation, spinal cord injuries, and multiple sclerosis and elderly patients immobilized for any reason.

Maintaining Mobility This is a significant aspect of prevention, especially for the geriatric population. Mobility not only alters weight-bearing areas but also adds to overall health, well-being, and alertness, which are necessary to prevention of pressure sores.

Shearing

Shearing forces have been implicated as a causal factor in pressure sore development. Elevating the head of the bed more than 30° but less than

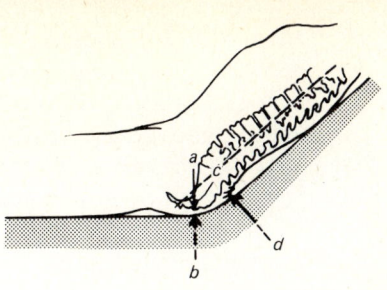

Figure 16-11
Head of bed raised to about 30°. Compressive force acts between sacrum (*a*) and mattress (*b*). Shearing force acts in direction indicated by (*c*). Wrinkling of skin (*d*) is external indirect evidence of shearing forces on soft tissues. (Redrawn from Reichel, S. A.: "Shearing Force as a Factor in Paraplegia," JAMA 166(7): 762, 1958. Copyright 1958 American Medical Association. Used with permission.)

90° causes the trunk to slide toward the foot of the bed. The sacrum and firmly attached deep fascia also slide down, while sacral skin stays in the same position as a result of friction (Fig. 16-11). Shearing is concentrated in the deeper portion of superficial fascia, causing stretch and angulation of blood vessels in the region. The result is thrombosis and subsequent ischemic necrosis. It has been stated that undermining of tissue is secondary to shearing, as large portions of the blood supply are cut off (Reichel, 1958). Shearing forces must be considered as a significant contributor to pressure sores and can be prevented by limiting the amount of time in this position and by supporting the feet against a foot plate or foot board or by elevating the bottom of the bed (not the knee gatch) to prevent sliding.

Friction

Friction, the rubbing of one surface against another, can result in abrasion of the skin. Dinsdale found that friction increases susceptibility of skin to breakdown. Friction does not cause ischemia but rather applies mechanical pressure to the epidermis (Dinsdale, 1974). Spasticity is one source of friction; control of friction through positioning and padding is necessary. Care must be taken to avoid sliding the patient across sheets or doing sliding-board transfers with bare skin in contact with the board. If hyperemic areas occur, they should not be massaged, since this adds friction to already compromised tissue.

Moisture

Several authors have implicated moisture and maceration in pressure sore pathogenesis (Guttman, 1955; Schell & Wolcott, 1966; Bailey, 1967). Recently increased attention has been directed toward determining the role of relative humidity in the etiology of soft tissue necrosis. Since plastic mattress covers and underpads are often used, especially in the immobile patient, dissipation of moisture is impeded. A recent study revealed that control of room temperature and use of terry toweling and sheepskin had a positive effect on local humidity (Brattgard et al., 1976). The type of clothing worn can also affect skin moisture. Patients such as those with spinal cord injury who sit in wheelchairs for long periods should be informed about the benefits of cotton underwear in dissipating moisture. Obviously, frequent turning, push-ups, and reduced use of non-vapor-permeable mattress and cushion covers are advised.

Local Heat

Elevated local temperature increases metabolic needs and thus increases the need for oxygen, the supply of which is already compromised. Monitoring of room temperature, frequent turns, and wheelchair push-ups are necessary to control local skin temperature. Brattgard found that plastic and rubber foam cushions increased local skin temperature. Flotation pads also increased temperatures, but not until after 3 to 4 h of continuous use (Brattgard et al., 1976). Similar findings were reported by Fisher and associates. It is thought that the fluid properties carry heat by convection away from the body and toward the center of the cushion (Fisher et al., 1978).

MANAGEMENT OF SECONDARY FACTORS

Secondary factors contributing to the development of pressure sores can be classified as those which are physiological/metabolic, physical and psychosocial.

Physiological/Metabolic Factors

Protein Deficiency This has been implicated as a secondary factor in pressure sore etiology. Mulholland believed that protein malnutrition caused a change in tissue character so that smaller amounts of pressure for shorter periods of time resulted in tissue necrosis (Mulholland et al., 1943). Negative nitrogen balance resulting from immobility predisposes to tissue edema, which further compromises the supply of nutrients to cells. The role of vitamin C in prevention is not known. It is known that ascorbic acid is necessary to form collagen which is needed for wound healing (Fulgham, 1977).

Marked weight loss, which often occurs with chronic illness and severe disability, results in a decreased amount of subcutaneous tissue, thus reducing the mechanical padding between skin and underlying bone. Creative approaches may be required to ensure adequate protein, vitamin, and caloric intake; protein-sparing foods are needed in adequate amounts. Further research on the importance of each of the above deficiencies is warranted.

Anemia Anemia has frequently been implicated in pressure sore development, but authors do not agree on the significance of this factor. Decreased delivery of oxygen to cells as a result of anemia causes embarrassment of cellular metabolism, which could add to susceptibility of tissue to pressure effects.

Infection This is frequently considered significant in pressure sore etiology. One study that examined the relationship of predisposing factors to pressure sore development revealed a higher incidence among those persons with elevated temperatures (Gosnell, 1973). Febrile states associated with infection contribute to cellular deficiency because the increased metabolic rate results in increased oxygen demand. Thus, an elevated body temperature compounds susceptibility to soft tissue necrosis in any person subjected to periods of sustained pressure. Turning schedules should be altered for the febrile patient and close attention directed to skin checks.

Edema Edema interferes with cell nutrition because the rate of diffusion of oxygen and metabolites from capillary to cell decreases in proportion to the distance between capillary and cell (Kosiak, 1961). Skin elasticity and resiliency are decreased in the presence of edema resulting in increased susceptibility to tissue necrosis and injury (Schell and Wolcott, 1966). Since edema of the lower extremities commonly occurs in the presence of circulatory disturbances and paralysis, positioning, exercise to control edema, and protective techniques are significant nursing strategies for patients with these deficits.

Some clinicians have considered decreased *vascular tone* as significant in pressure sore development. This could be a factor for the person with spinal cord injury during the stage of spinal shock.

Physical Factors

Sensory Deficit This is a prominent factor in the etiology of pressure sores because patients do not feel the early discomfort which indicates that they should relieve pressure. Anesthetic skin causes a deficiency in the natural warning system and must be replaced with habits of skin care and routine pressure relief.

Decreased awareness as a result of brain damage and some medications will interfere with perception of discomfort, altough sensation may be intact. The result will be a decrease in bodily movements.

Mobility Impairment A major element in the development of pressure sores, mobility impairment is often the reason pressure is applied for too long. In a state of health and when able to move, the body is never immobile for long periods. Even in sleep, one moves frequently. One study on frequency of movements of the elderly during sleep revealed a relationship between decreased body movements and pressure sore development (Exton-Smith & Sherwin, 1961).

Dry Skin Skin which has been robbed of natural lubrication can crack and become a potential site for ulceration. Liberal use of soap can result in chapping and cracking of skin as well as in irritation. Alcohol applied to the skin also has a drying effect. These agents and others that could decrease the protective function of skin should be used with caution. Attention must be given to appropriate oiling and lubricating of skin.

Incontinence Incontinence and subsequent poor hygiene increases susceptibility to pressure sore formation. This is a problem that can usually be managed through bowel and bladder programs and scrupulous hygiene.

Muscle Atrophy This is considered by some as a causal factor because there is a decrease in mechanical padding over bone.

Psychosocial Factors

It is rare to find mention of other than physical and physiological/metabolic factors in the literature. Surprisingly little has been written about the relationship between psychosocial factors and pressure sores. This area has probably been underestimated in importance, especially in the postdischarge phase when health professionals are not available to assess early neglect in items such as self-care routines and nutrition. Youngsters, who so often cannot discipline themselves to follow regimens, can be considered a group at high risk; their follow-up program should consider this factor.

Depression and decreased will to live probably influence the ability to care about and for one's body. Whether the individual feels that control of his or her destiny (and health as part of that destiny) is within personal control or is the responsibility of another person surely influences the outcomes of all aspects of health. What influence does the presence or absence of social support systems have on health outcomes? Does maintenance of follow-up by familiar staff members favorably influence compliance with skin care regimens? Research is lacking in these areas, but all probably have a significant effect.

DEVICES TO ASSIST IN MANAGEMENT

Correct utilization of devices adds a significant dimension to management. Staff and patient education in proper use, as well as the understanding that these devices do not eliminate the pressure relief requirement, is essential. The multiplicity of surfaces available for the patient to lie or to sit upon could present a baffling puzzle for the nurse and other health team members. Only in recent years has attention been addressed to studying the advantages and disadvantages of various support systems and to determining the degree of pressure exerted over skin. Selection of support surfaces is dependent upon individual patient needs as previously outlined. Proper maintenance and staff education are essential, since devices can actually contribute to increased pressure, moisture, and other problems.

Systems and devices developed for the prevention and treatment of pressure sores can be classified as follows:

1. Devices that assist in turning the patient
2. Devices that minimize pressure
3. Devices that intermittently alter pressure

Table 16-2 lists the various surfaces and devices in each category. To be effective, support surfaces should mold to the patient to assist in uniformly distributing pressure, and they should allow for the passage of water vapor. The device should also be financially and practically suitable for home use. Pressure will be increased if the support system is inadequate or not maintained, that is, distorted foam cushions or mattresses, pressure from mattress springs, overfilling or underfilling water beds and mattresses, mechanical problems with alternating air mattresses. The effectiveness of the best system can be reduced unless thought is given to what is placed between the patient and the surface. Plastic mattress covers, coarse sheets, draw sheets, and plastic underpads may increase pressure, prevent evap-

Table 16-2

Devices Used for the Prevention and Treatment of Pressure Sores

DEVICES THAT ASSIST WITH TURNING	DEVICES THAT ALTER PRESSURE INTERMITTENTLY	DEVICES THAT MINIMIZE PRESSURE
Stryker frame	Keane Roto-Rest bed	Water beds/mattresses
Circ-o-lectric bed	Alternating pressure mattress	Water cushions
	Mechanical cushions	Air beds and cushions
		Gel pads
		Foam mattresses and cushions
		Foam water cushions and mattresses
		Air fluidized bed
		MUD bed
		Cutout cushion

oration of water vapor, and result in an increase in local skin temperature.

Devices Designed to Assist with Turning

Circ-o-lectric Beds and Stryker Frames These are systems that are purported to assist in preventing pressure sores or in treating existing sores. However, it should be noted that these beds have no attributes that reduce or change pressure. In some situations, they may simplify turning and positioning. For example, following plastic surgery, patients may be bridged prone on stryker frames so that they may eat, read, or converse with a fair degree of comfort. Routine use of such systems limits the positions to which a patient can be turned and thus results in more frequent intervals of pressure over supine and prone bony prominences. Since both beds require strapping the patient between frames, safety is a constant concern. Neither bed is appropriate for home use.

Devices Designed to Alter Pressure Intermittently

Alternating Pressure Alternating-pressure mattresses can reduce pressures but do *not* eliminate them; patients continue to need regular turning. These mattresses consist of a polyvinyl bladder with air cells arranged horizontally or vertically. The mattress is attached to an electric pump system that alternately inflates and deflates a series of cells every 3 to 5 s. The alternation in filling of the air cells alternates the areas where pressure is exerted on the patient's skin. To be effective, it is essential that the mattress be maintained by inspecting connections, checking for punctures, and ensuring that the motor is functioning at all times. Few studies have been done that demonstrate the effectiveness of the mattress.

Keane Roto-Rest Bed This device consists of a support surface with foam blocks to maintain patients in anatomic positions and prevent them from sliding as the bed oscillates from side to side. The patient is never in one position for more than a few minutes. Disadvantages are the limitations on activity and vision, difficulty in carrying out care procedures, and heat buildup at skin surfaces. Recent models have attempted to overcome the latter problem with the use of a blower. Advantages cited are prevention and healing of pressure sores, as well as prevention of urinary stasis and pulmonary complications associated with immobility (Keane, 1970).

Devices Designed to Equalize or Minimize Pressure

Polyurethane Foam Mattress A compressible surface that conforms to the body distributes pressure more evenly. Earlier, mention was made of studies indicating that foam surfaces placed on the support unit assist in reducing pressure, but not to levels below capillary pressure. In recent years, a polyurethane foam mattress has been developed that reportedly reduces pressure over bony prominences to 20 to 25 mmHg (Reswick and Rogers, 1976). This mattress can easily be used at home. Many individuals with a sensory or mobility deficit do not need expensive mattresses. A 2-in-thick foam mattress placed over a standard mattress is adequate in most situations, both for home and hospital.

Seat Cushions Four-inch-thick foam seat cushions are frequently used in an attempt to decrease pressure over ischial tuberosities. A number of studies have shown that pressures remain far in excess of safe limits with foam cushions as well as with other cushions currently on the market (Souther et al., 1974; Houle, 1969; Mooney et al., 1971; De Lateur et al., 1976). High pressures over the ischial tuberosities can be reduced through the use of individually designed cutout cushions, which allow weight to shift somewhat to other weight-bearing areas, such as the posterior thighs. This type of cushion requires exact measurements of the individual patient and is usually provided through pressure clinics. Foam cushions lose elasticity over time;

thus the cushion should be replaced at regular intervals.

Gel Pads When used on a mattress or wheelchair, gel pads will decrease pressures but will not eliminate them. These cushions are quite heavy, which is a disadvantage for some patients who must lift the cushion for car transfers.

Flotation Devices Various types of these devices are available. They consist of systems filled with water or air, foam impregnated with water, and combinations of air, water, and foam. These systems are based on Pascal's law, which states that the pressure exerted anywhere in a mass of fluid is transmitted equally in all directions. A disadvantage in applying this principle to support systems is that the covering of a fluid-filled device can interfere with the flotation. Investigators have noted that the surface tension of the enveloping membrane of fluid-filled cushions prevents even pressure distribution. When resting on these cushions, the body is supported by the hammocking effect of the covering rather than by the fluid (Mooney et al., 1971). Inconsistency in filling of cushions or mattresses can be a major problem. Overfilling can result in an excessively firm surface; underfilling results in ischial tuberosities or other bony prominences bottoming out. Leaking of the fluidized material is a potential problem with all flotation systems.

Fisher and associates' study of local skin temperatures using various cushions revealed lower temperatures with use of a water flotation cushion as compared to foam and gel cushions (Fisher et al., 1978). This could be an advantage, as elevated skin temperature is thought to contribute to the negative effects of pressure on soft tissue. Fluid-filled cushions are heavy and therefore not easily managed by the person with weak upper extremities. Water and air cushions tend to provide an unstable sitting surface for some patients, notably those with poor trunk control, and can make transfers more difficult.

Translation of the flotation principle into mattresses or beds has met with more success in providing even weight distribution than have cushions. The *air-fluidized* bed provides a surface with pressures of 10 mmHg (Harvin and Hargest, 1979). This bed consists of a system in which air is pumped through a bed of fine medical-grade optical glass spheres. Air is introduced through a bottom chamber by a blower unit and flows upward at 40 ft^3 per minute. A loose polyester sheet covers the beads. The constant airflow results in water vapor evaporation. Initial problems with overheating and blower noise have been reduced in more recent models. Evaporative water loss can potentially result in dehydration of the patient with extensive sores or burns. This is unlikely to be a problem with the alert patient who drinks adequate fluids, but it could be a hazard for comatose or lethargic patients. During an evaluation of the bed, psychiatric changes of hysterical response, confusion, and agitation were reported. The investigation indicated that these changes occurred in 3 of 24 patients studied and were related to preexisting psychiatric problems (Newsome et al., 1972). Newsome also reported that burn patients positioned with fresh donor sites in direct contact with the surface of the bed healed rapidly. The weight and expense of the unit, 2400 lb, prohibits its use at home except in rare situations. However, the air-fluidized bed could prove beneficial in a hospital setting for prevention of pressure sores in high-risk patients and for treatment when multiple ulcerations are present.

Another *air support system* developed in England has been found to be effective in prevention and treatment of pressure sores. Problems with temperature control and dehydration of patients have not been noted in several years of use. Pressures are reported to be below capillary pressure in all positions (Redfern et al., 1973). This unit consists of polyurethane air sacs inflated by air pumped from a separate unit. Air flow through the system is constant. Air sacs conform to body contours as body weight displaces surplus air in the sacs, resulting in even distribution of weight. Evaporation of perspiration occurs because the air sacs are made of microporous material (Scales et al., 1974). Although it is an expensive unit, this bed has been issued for home use.

A *dry flotation support system* is also available. This unit consists of interconnected air balloons and is made for bed and wheelchair use. The body is said to immerse in the balloons. Thus far, studies on pressure of this system have not been published. Problems of air leakage from puncture and overfilling or underfilling of the unit can occur, but when properly used, pressures can be reduced.

Water beds can effectively reduce pressure over certain bony prominences (Lilla et al., 1975; Siegal et al., 1973; Redfern et al., 1973). Shoulder, knee, heel, and trochanter are subjected to pressures above capillary pressure (25 mmHg) when resting on a water bed, and thus turning remains necessary. Position change is also required to allow evaporation of moisture because the membrane enclosing the fluid is not vapor permeable. Economic considerations have resulted in the use of water-filled camping mattresses as substitutes for water beds. While the mattresses are not as effective as the bed, some decrease in pressure does occur. Underfilling and overfilling these mattresses interferes with flotation and could result in high pressures over bony prominences. Although the bed system contains a heating element, the mattresses do not, and cooling of the mattress can create discomfort for the patient. Water mattresses can be recommended for home use, but the potential for improper filling and leaking must be considered when making this selection and when educating the patient.

The *Rancho flotation bed* (MUD bed) consists of a colloidal suspension of pulverized barite (40 percent) in water (50 percent) and bentonite (10 percent). A thin, oversized plastic sheet that reduces shear and hammocking effect is placed over the flotation material (Reswick and Rogers, 1976). Patients are able to rest in prone as well as in side-lying and supine positions. Position changes are usually scheduled every 4 h, but it is possible to maintain patients for 6 weeks in one position after plastic reconstructive surgery (Wilson, 1976).

Selection of the proper support system for a patient is determined by response to a trial on a particular support as well as by individual need. No patient should be provided with a device for home use without an evaluation in the hospital. Pressure distribution, cost, weight, and control of heat and humidity are factors to be considered. Many of the units limit the patient's ability to participate in activities of daily living. In addition, a unit may not be realistic for home use, even though it may be necessary at some time during hospital stay. As soon as possible, the individual is placed on a regular bed with the mattress to be used at home. Because staff and patients may perceive these devices as eliminating the need for regular pressure relief, continued need for pressure relief such as turning must be emphasized.

New support surfaces should not be accepted without controlled studies of effectiveness. Controlled studies will be encouraged when nurses request that manufacturers' claims be substantiated by valid and reliable data. If studies are not available, nurses should do them.

Cost is, of course, a consideration when purchasing devices. The most expensive and exotic equipment is not necessarily the best for a particular patient or nursing unit. However, all facilities that admit patients with multiple sores or that may receive patients at high risk of developing pressure sores should have beds available that effectively distribute weight. This includes the air-fluidized or low-air-loss bed and water and MUD beds.

EXAMPLES OF ASSESSMENT AND MANAGEMENT OF RISK FACTORS

Once the role of risk factors is understood, the nurse can alter the plan of care to reduce the potential for skin breakdown. The following situations reveal the role that predisposing factors can play in pressure sore development and the need for nursing assessment and intervention.

A 15-year-old boy diagnosed as quadriplegic was admitted to a rehabilitation unit. At the time of admission, he was very thin, that is, 6 ft tall and weighing 125 lb. Bridging was difficult because of his body structure, so he was positioned on a standard mattress with a 2-in egg-carton foam mattress on top. Turning every 2 h resulted in mild hyperemia over bony prominences which disappeared within 15 min. The young man developed a temperature of 101 to 103°F as the result of a urinary tract infection. While his appetite had been poor, it now worsened as the elevated temperature and infection lingered. His hemoglobin remained at 10 g. Serum protein levels were slightly reduced. Within a few days, staff reported prolonged hyperemia and reduced the turning interval to 1½ h with no improvement. A persistent erythemic indurated area noted on the left trochanter prevented turning to this position. He was then transferred to a water bed and tolerated turning every 2 to 3 h.

Nursing intervention prevented a Grade I pressure sore from developing into a more serious grade. Earlier intervention when the fever began could have prevented the Grade I sore.

The following case study illustrates the role of inadequately assessed and maintained equipment in contributing to pressure sores, as well as the necessity for nursing assessment of predisposing factors.

A 21-year-old man was readmitted to the rehabilitation facility for treatment of a Grade II ischial pressure sore. He had been rendered quadriplegic, C6 level, 5 years previously and had a history of a pressure sore over one malleolus 2 years previously. He had been working, living independently, and driving his own car for the past 2 years. No other complications had occurred. While reviewing with him the circumstances surrounding the development of this sore, the following was revealed:

1. He had been depressed over recent loss of his job.
2. A 30-lb weight loss occurred. Although he had been about 20 lb overweight, this loss was sudden. He attributed the weight loss to "not enough money." It may have also been related to the depression which he acknowledged.
3. He had recently received a new wheelchair. Inquiries to determine whether the wheelchair had been checked by a physical therapist or whether he himself had checked the foot plate adjustment revealed a negative response.
4. He had been using a wheelchair cushion that was grossly distorted, that is, there was some fluid loss and the foam was hard and flattened.
5. He usually checked his skin in the morning. The day previous to noting the ischial sore, he had sat up for 16 h. His typical day consisted of sitting for about 12 h continuously with weight shifts.

When the above facts are analyzed, it is not surprising that this young man developed a pressure sore. Reviewing the circumstance surrounding the development of a pressure sore is essential. In this situation, predisposing primary and secondary factors, as well as lack of essential knowledge on the part of the patient, were revealed. The nurse, along with the rest of the team, reviewed all aspects of skin care and was instrumental in helping him to reenter the community.

MANAGEMENT OF PRESSURE SORES

Through the years, a mystique appears to have developed around the treatment of pressure sores. Untold numbers of substances have been put into and over pressure sores, and yet the action of many of the agents is not documented and the rationale given for others raises numerous questions. Recent comprehensive reviews of the literature on management of pressure sores revealed a need for better controlled studies to compare and contrast effects of various agents (Berecek, 1975; Michocki & Lamy, 1976; Sather et al., 1977). Some of the topical agents used were thought to hold promise for aiding in more rapid healing, but larger samples and controls were suggested. At times, the seeking of a new method to speed healing may take precedence over common sense, and pressure may not be alleviated while exotic substances are packed into a wound. Difficulties in studying pressure sore healing are encountered when one patient is compared to another, as there are so many clinical factors that contribute to impeding healing. In examining the data from certain studies on pressure sore healing, it appears that the attention given to the subject coincident to the study is a major factor in healing. One author states, "Reported success with poultices and applications is readily appreciated when one realizes that every thing that is put into these ulcers must be cleaned out, thereby accomplishing the second objective of cleaning and debriding the wound" (Shea, 1975).

Specific treatment of pressure sores depends upon the extent of the sore and the stage of healing. Goals for nonsurgical management are threefold: (1) relief of pressure, (2) wound cleansing and debridement, and (3) promotion of healing (Shea, 1975).

PRESSURE RELIEF

Pressure relief is a primary goal; without it, the extent of the sore will increase and healing will not occur, no matter what other treatment is used. If a single Grade I sore is present, pressure relief, cleansing, and dressing the wound, if open, and maintaining nutrition are sufficient for healing. A special support system is not necessary, since bridging or eliminating turning or sitting on the site is effective. In this way, erythemic areas can be eliminated within 48 to 72 h. if epidermal necrosis has occurred, 10 to 14 days are required for epithelial tissue growth (Enis and Sarmiento, 1973). Deeper sores can require months to heal. Multiple sores of any grade demand a program of bridging or the use of a bed that will evenly distribute pressure. The air-fluidized, MUD, or water bed can be used in these situations. When using the water bed, the nurse must remember that sitting and side lying markedly increase pressure. Turning continues to be necessary to prevent complications of immobility and, with the exception of the air bed, to allow moisture evaporation. The patient with ischial or posterior trochanteric ulcers must avoid sitting until healing is complete. If a sacral sore is present, a cutout back support can be fabricated to allow sitting. Whenever a sacral cutout is used, it is essential to check for pressure manually and to inspect the sacral area for hyperemia upon the patient's return to bed. If hyperemia is present, the cushion is ineffective, and sitting should be discontinued. Dressing activities and independent transfers are abandoned if they result in pressure or stress to the affected region.

Patients who are unable to sit can be mobilized on a stretcher; this is practical in the hospital setting but usually not at home. Numerous difficulties are encountered in maintaining a pressure relief program out of the hospital. Management of domestic responsibilities, work, school, and social obligations demand mobility; therefore, a decision to eliminate sitting becomes a difficult one for the patient. The nurse's support in helping to solve the problem of how to continue activities and in obtaining community help such as homemakers, tutors, visiting nurse, and rental of carts (if the home will accommodate them) may ease the burden.

Sustained pressure relief is, of course, required whenever Grade II, III, or IV sores are present. The patient is immobilized initially while the lesion is cleaned and debrided and again following plastic surgery until healing occurs. When possible, these patients should be mobilized on a stretcher. The change of scenery and activity that stretcher mobility allows can relieve some of the depression inevitable with prolonged hospitalization.

One last caution about pressure relief: *Never* use "doughnut" devices in an attempt to relieve pressure. Rather than relieving pressure, these devices cause further ischemia to the involved area.

WOUND CLEANSING AND DEBRIDEMENT

Cleansing

Mechanical cleansing by scrubbing is necessary to reduce infection. The degree of cleansing action should be such that viable tissue is not injured, and yet drainage and detritus can be removed. Maintenance of aseptic procedures and appropriate use of isolation techniques are necessary to control the spread of infection. Surface bacterial contamination is not considered a grave matter; however, suppuration and invasive infection are grave and must be treated (Schell and Wolcott, 1966). Frequency of dressing change and correct application can be significant in promoting healing of the ulceration. Dressings should not be so tightly packed or applied over the surface of the wound as to increase pressure; change of dressing should be carried out as often as necessary to remove accumulated drainage. Hydrotherapy can be an effect adjunct in wound cleansing.

Adhesive tape is not routinely advised for adhering a dressing to any individual and is strictly contraindicated in persons with insensitive skin or those in a debilitated condition. If several wounds are present or if a wound is quite extensive, a wrap of Surgi-Fix or stockinette can be applied. Surgi-Fix has the advantage of allowing air to reach the wound.

Debridement

Wound debridement removes foreign materials and necrotic tissue that interfere with healing; it can be accomplished through surgical, mechanical, or chemical means. Since debridement of necrotic tissue is basic to healing, it should be started early. Early debridement is considered to be lifesaving in some instances, for example, in the elderly and the severely ill patient (Enis and Sarmiento, 1973; Coopwood, 1976).

Necrotic wounds require surgical debridement followed either by wet-to-dry dressings or by application of proteolytic enzymes such as Travase and collagenase. Recently, dextranomer has been found to be helpful in aiding debridement (DiMascio, 1979). Each technique has its advocates. Wet-to-dry dressings using physiologic saline has been in use for some time as an adjunct to surgical debridement (Bailey, 1967; Shea, 1975; Enis and Sarmiento, 1973). Sterile mesh gauze (in one piece) is soaked in saline solution, excess solution is wrung out, and the gauze is packed into the sore. The packing must come in contact with all necrotic tissue, including that in the undermined regions. Three to four hours later, the packing is removed. During this interval, the gauze will have dried, becoming partially adherent to devitalized tissue. A thin, dry dressing is applied over the packing. Treatments are continued throughout the entire 24-h period. The debridement process is continued until the wound is clean enough to allow surgical repair.

Chemical debridement agents are nontoxic and nonirritating proteolytic enzymes, and yet they hydrolyze collagen, thus facilitating debridement. The enzymes assist in severing collagen fibers that bind necrotic tissue to the wound surface. Most of these enzymes are of vegetable, animal, and bacterial precursors (Michocki and Lamy, 1976). Disadvantages associated with their use include local irritation and allergic reaction. However, recent studies on the use of some enzymes indicate that these reactions were uncommon (Coopwood, 1976; Kerstein, 1975; Rao et al., 1975). These investigators also indicate that debridement time was shortened. When using proteolytic enzymes, the wound is cleansed with physiologic saline solution because some germicidal agents interfere with the enzyme action. The enzyme is applied over the entire area of necrosis and covered with moist dressing; moisture is necessary to activate the enzyme. The entire procedure is repeated three to four times daily. Eschar, which impedes enzyme contact with wound tissue, is surgically debrided, following which the enzyme is applied.

PROMOTION OF HEALING

Up to 50 g of protein can be lost daily through an open, draining pressure sore. A diet high in protein, calories, and vitamins is necessary to restore nitrogen balance and to promote healing of the wound. Generally, 100 to 150 g of protein and a minimum of 2500 to 4000 cal are required (Bailey, 1967). Anorexia is not unusual, especially in the presence of Grade III and IV sores, which are usually infected. Ingenuity is necessary if the food is to be ingested and not merely returned uneaten. Food preferences can be provided if family, patient, nurse, and dietician work together. Approaches that can prove helpful include serving small meals frequently, serving home-cooked meals brought in by family and friends, serving food hot, having snacks readily available, and having spices available for those who prefer them. With throughtful planning, cultural and developmental preference can be integrated into the diet. Ambulatory care nurses or dieticians must include guidance in low-cost foods that are high in protein for those patients managing their sores at home. Additional suggestions to stimulate the appetite are vitamins and drinking wine before meals. Anabolic steroids have also been advocated to stimulate the appetite and to promote nitrogen balance (Bailey).

Wound healing is impeded by the presence of anemia, protein depletion, infection, and dehydration. Intravenous fluids with antibiotics are indicated to treat the septic, dehydrated patient. Anemia, if severe, must be corrected through blood transfusions or with supplementary oral or injectable iron (Sather et al., 1977). Blood transfusions are not used with the sole intent of accelerating healing.

Despite the fact that wound healing is not accelerated by local or systemic therapeutic agents, numerous agents have been applied to pressure sores in order to promote healing. Correction of impediments to healing such as infection, vitamin and protein deficiency, and anemia allow healing to occur at a normal rate (Fulgham, 1977; Bailey, 1967). It must be remembered that a pressure sore is similar to other wounds and has a similar tissue response.

Claims that products or procedures promote healing of pressure sores are often based on studies that are poorly controlled or have included a limited number of subjects. To date, no treatment has proved superior to others to the degree that it is widely accepted in clinical practice (Berecek, 1975; Page and Goult, 1975; Sather et al., 1977). Agents and procedures that have been used to stimulate healing through local application include sugar, gold leaf, karaya, Gelfoam, low-intensity direct current (electrotherapy), hyperbaric oxygen, honey, trypsin, balsam peru, heat lamps, ultrasound, and ultraviolet light. Whenever local agents are used to stimulate healing, they must be critically evaluated. A potential problem is the widespread use of a treatment based on outcomes noted in one or two patients (Berecek, 1975).

SURGICAL TREATMENT

Surgical repair of a pressure sore must be preceded by debridement of necrotic tissue, establishment of a clean wound, and reversal of hypoproteinemia and anemia. Serum protein levels should be 6 g/100 mL and the hemoglobin should be 12 g (Herceg and Harding, 1971). Spasticity, if present, must be controlled prior to surgery.

The surgical procedure varies according to the location and extent of ulceration. Split-thickness grafts, removal of bone with flap coverage, and occasionally direct closure are techniques utilized in surgical repair of pressure sores. Bony prominences are resected to varying degrees depending on the anatomic location. Trochanters can be extensively resected, while the sacrum is smoothed down (Constable and Pierce, 1977). Radical removal of the ischium is not generally performed, as urethral diverticulum has been reported following total ischiectomy (Enis and Sarmiento, 1973).

Regardless of the surgical procedure, it is essential that resumption of pressure over the area be gradual. Following ischial repair and healing, sitting can be resumed for no more than 30 min on the first day that the patient is allowed up in the wheelchair. Skin inspection must be done after each period of sitting; pressure relief is done every 15 min. Following surgical ischial repair with flap coverage, 2 to 3 weeks of gradual upgrading of tolerance may be required to attain a 5-h sitting tolerance.

Following surgical repair of pressure sores, the patient is immobilized while healing occurs; for example, after a sacral flap repair, the individual is bridged prone for 4 to 6 weeks (Enis and Sarmiento, 1973; Bailey, 1967). It is essential that the goals of treatment, the treatment itself, and the time element be understood by the patient prior to surgery if cooperation is to be achieved. Meticulous postoperative nursing care is critical to prevent shearing and pressure over the surgical site.

PREVENTION: REVIEW OF KEY FACTORS

PRESSURE CONTROL

Control of pressure is the single most important element in prevention of soft tissue necrosis. The most critical means of controlling pressure include decreasing the time at risk through regular turning and bridging, doing wheelchair push-ups, and increasing the weight-bearing surface area through the development and use of appropriate support surfaces (Bailey, 1967). Nurses must be advocates to convince administrators and third-party payers of the need for adequate staffing to turn patients, to provide nutrition, and to otherwise decrease risk of tissue necrosis.

Early detection of potential ulceration is vital. Some staff members and patients believe that the risk for tissue breakdown is reduced with time. This can result in laxity in regimens of wheelchair pressure relief, turning, and skin inspection. Skin does not toughen; unlimited sitting is not possible; a given turning or sitting tolerance cannot be taken for granted. Skin care habits are lifetime regimens and cannot be abandoned or reduced in intensity.

Pressure clinics have grown in popularity in recent years. In addition to providing wheelchair cushions based on pressure measurements over ischial tuberosities, regular rechecks of skin and equipment are provided along with continual reinforcement of skin care habits.

Unfortunately, there is a dearth of studies on predictors for success in the patient whose discharge is imminent. A recent retrospective study of a small population of individuals with spinal cord injury revealed that pressure sores occurred more often in paraplegic males than in females or quadriplegic patients (Maccauley and Weiss, 1978). These findings are in agreement with the author's clinical impressions.

The question arises of whether such findings are related to physiologic, emotional, or social factors or to any combination of the three. Only through research will precise answers be available to help nurses and other team members develop more prescriptive plans of care.

The general indicators of high risk include patients with poor social resources, those who are depressed or in denial at the time of discharge, those who demonstrate poor ability to integrate skin care habits into daily routines, those who feel that responsibility for care lies with someone else, those who have had previous sores, and those who are slow learners. These are in addition to the primary and secondary predisposing factors discussed previously. Until further research is done in this area, there are often more questions and suppositions than answers.

For those patients considered to be at high risk, special consideration should be given to simplify home care routines such as bowel and bladder care, medication regimens, and skin care programs. A predischarge home assessment is critical. A patient may be reluctant to reveal to staff members that the living room couch with a sprung cushion is going to serve as the "bed."

It becomes obvious that more precise identification of the patient who is at high risk for pressure sores would allow more appropriate use of procedures and devices. Resources could be better used in follow-up programs to prevent further disability and rehospitalization.

When a high-risk patient is discharged, an

early recheck date should be scheduled, a referral should be made to the community health nurse, and home visits and frequent telephone contacts should be conducted by the rehabilitation staff. This not only serves to monitor the patient's progress but also communicates the interest and commitment of the staff. When possible, these patients should be followed by the same personnel upon return for rechecks. This reinforces the commitment and provides continuity. Although all these strategies will not eliminate risk, they will reduce the liability.

PATIENT/FAMILY AND STAFF EDUCATION

To reach all patients, including those at high risk, nurses must know available teaching methods and evaluation techniques. From a rehabilitation perspective the ultimate responsibility for prevention of soft tissue necrosis lies with the patient. Until the patient realizes that prevention is within personal control, the possibility of pressure sores is great.

Adolescents may be unable to integrate the necessary degree of responsibility. Parents are an integral part of the education process and carry a share of the responsibility. However, the parent is not always with the youngster, such as at school or on a date, so ways need to be found to help the adolescent assume responsibility.

General skin care measures of cleanliness, foot care, control of edema, and skin lubrication add a significant dimension to prevention of tissue necrosis. Prevention of complications such as thermal lesions, rashes, and bruising should be integrated very early into the care plan.

All staff members who work with patients at risk to developing pressure sores must be aware of this possibility. In addition to verbal, audiovisual, individual, and group educational experiences, patient learning is enhanced when all staff members know the behaviors expected and participate in reinforcing these behaviors. For instance, do all staff members encourage patients to shift their weight when they are with them?

CONCLUSION

Prevention of pressure sores has long baffled health professionals. However, with the data currently available and the research being done, there is reason to believe that the majority of pressure sores can be prevented. It is the responsibility of health professionals, especially nurses, to use the data in planning and giving care and in educating patients, families, and staff. Further research on the significance of various risk factors has been mentioned as a major need if prognostication of risk is to occur. Potentially significant work is being done on patient monitoring in the United States and in England. Thermography studies continue, and recently, radiometry (small, portable units to measure heat) has been developed (Trandel and Lewis, 1975; Trandel et al., 1975; Verhonick et al., 1972; Brand, 1976; Barton, 1976). These studies may result in a means of definitively noting the time required for skin to return to normal temperature following pressure application. Thus, scientific guidelines would be available for safely upgrading skin tolerance and for recognizing dangerous levels of hyperemia and heat. The development of accurate assessment scales is needed; research in this area could build on that which has occurred in recent years.

Research on support systems should continue. Each new device that is developed should be subjected to controlled studies to determine such things as its potential to reduce pressure and moisture buildup.

Prevention of pressure sores remains a multidisciplinary problem. Fortunately, bioengineers have been added to the team, and they should be utilized as resources concerning what devices are available and in the scientific evaluation of devices.

Further knowledge in the area of assisting

patients to internalize responsibility for self-care is needed. Along with this knowledge, research on patient education methods and evaluation of teaching are necessary. Dissemination of knowledge on skin care and adequate staff to implement strategies should be priorities. Improvement in follow-up programs is necessary; basic to improved programs is prediction of individual needs. Nurses are of primary importance in the prevention of pressure sores, and they have a responsibility to lead in studying some of the unanswered questions related to this prevention.

BIBLIOGRAPHY

Adams, L. S., and S. M., Bluefarb: "How We Treat Decubitus Ulcers," *Postgrad Med* 44: 269–271, 1968.

Bailey, B. N.: *Bedsores,* Edward Arnold, London, 1967.

Barton, A. A.: "The Clinical and Thermographical Evaluation of Pressure Sores," in R. M. Kenedi, J. M. Cowden, and J. T. Scales (eds.): *Bedsore Biomechanics: Seminar Proceedings, University of Strathelyde,* University Park Press, Baltimore, 1976, pp. 55–62.

Berecek, K. H.: "Etiology of Decubitus Ulcers," *Nurs Clin North Am* 10:157–170, 1975.

Berecek, K. H.: "Treatment of Decubitus Ulcers," *Nurs Clin North Am* 10:171–210, 1975.

Brand, P. W.: "Patient Monitoring," in R. M. Kenedi, J. M. Cowden, and J. T. Scales (eds.): *Bedsore Biomechanics: Seminar Proceedings, University of Strathelyde,* University Park Press, Baltimore, 1976, pp. 185–188.

Brattgard, S. O., S. Carlsoo, and K. Severinsson: "Temperature and Humidity in the Sitting Area," in R. M. Kenedi, J. M. Cowden, and J. T. Scales (eds.): *Bedsore Biomechanics: Seminar Proceedings, University of Strathelyde,* University Park Press, Baltimore, 1976, pp. 185–188.

Brooks, B., and G., Duncan: "Effects of Pressure on Tissues," *Arch Surg* 40:696–709, 1940.

Constable, J. D., and D. S., Pierce: "Pressure Sores," in D. Pierce and V. H. Nickel (eds.): *The Total Care of Spinal Cord Injuries,* Little, Brown, Boston, 1977.

Coopwood, T. B.: "Evaluation of a Topical Enzymatic Debridement Agent: Sutilains Ointment: A Preliminary Report," *South Med J* 69:834–836, 1976.

Dawson, R. L.: "Treatment of Pressure Sores," *Nurs Times* 70:1108–1110, July, 18, 1974.

De Lateur, B. J., R. Berni, T. Hongladarom, and R. Giaconi: "Wheelchair Cushions Designed to Prevent Pressure Sores: An Evaluation," *Arch Phys Med Rehabil* 57:129–135, 1976.

Dinsdale, S. M.: "Decubitus Ulcers, Role of Pressure and Friction in Causation," *Arch Phys Med Rehabil* 55:147–152, 1974.

DiMascio, Suzanne: "Debrisan for Decubitus Ulcers," *Am J Nurs* 79:684–685, 1979.

Enis, J. E., and A. Sarmiento: "The Pathophysiology and Management of Pressure Sores," *Orthop Rev* 2:25–34, 1973.

Exton-Smith, A. N., and R. W. Sherwin,: "The Prevention of Pressure Sores: Significance of Spontaneous Bodily Movements," *Lancet* 2: 1124, 1961.

Fisher, M. V., T. E. Szymke, and M. Kosiak,: "Wheelchair Cushion Effects on Skin Temperature," *Arch Phys Med Rehabil* 59:68–72, 1978.

Fulgham, D. D.: "Ascorbic Acid Revisited," *Arch Dermatol* 113:91–92, 1977.

Gosnell, D.: "An Assessment Tool to Identify Pressure Sores," *Nurs Res* 22:55–59, 1973.

Groth, K. E.: "Clinical Observation and Experimental Studies of the Pathogenesis of Decubitus Ulcers," *Acta Chir Scand* 87 (suppl. 76), 1942.

Gruis, M., and B., Innes: "Assessment: Essential to Prevent Pressure Sores," *Am J Nurs* 16: 1762–1764, 1976.

Guthrie, R. H., and D. Goulian: "Decubitus Ulcers: Prevention and Treatment," *Geriatrics* 28: 67–71, 1973.

Guttmann, L.: "The Problem of Treatment of Pressure Sores in Patients with Spinal Paraplegia," *Br J Plast Surg* 8: 196, 1955.

Hargest, T. S.: "Problems of Patient Support: The Air-Fluidized Bed as a Solution," in R. M. Kenedi, J. M. Cowden, and J. T. Scales (eds.): *Bedsore Biomechanics: Seminar Proceedings, University of Strathelyde,* University Park Press, Baltimore, 1976, pp. 269–275.

Harvin, J., and T. Hargest: The Air-Fluidized Bed: A New Concept in Treatment of Decubitus Ulcers, *Nurs Clin North Am* 5:181–187, 1979.

Herceg, S. J., and R. L., Harding: "Surgical Treatment of Pressure Sore," *Pa Med* 74:45–52, 1971.

Houle, R. J.: "Evaluation of Seat Devices Designed to Prevent Ischemia Ulcers in Paraplegic Patients," *Arch Phys Med Rehabil* 50: 587–594, 1969.

Husain, T.: "An Experimental Study of Some Pressure Effects of Tissues with Reference to the Bed Sore Problem," *J Pathol Bacteriol* 66: 347–358, 1953.

Keane, F. X.: "Roto-Rest," *Paraplegia* 5: 254–258, 1970.

Kerstein, M. D.: "Management of Amputation-Stump Breakdown," *Am Surg* 41:581–583, 1975.

Kirk, J. E., and M. Chieffi: "Variation with Age in Elasticity of Skin and Subcutaneous Tissue in Humans," *J Gerontol* 17:373–380, 1962.

Knox, J. M.: "Aging Skin," *J Am Med Wom Assoc* 21:659–61, 1966.

Kosiak, M.: "Etiology and Pathology of Ischemic Ulcers," *Arch Phys Med Rehabil* 40: 62–69, 1959.

―――: "Etiology of Decubitus Ulcers," *Arch Phys Med Rehabil* 42:19–29, 1961.

―――: "A Mechanical Resting Surface: It's Effect on Pressure Distribution," *Arch Phys Med Rehabil* 57:481–484, 1976.

―――, W. Kubicek, M. Olson, J. Danz, and F. Kottke: "Evaluation of Pressure as a Factor in the Production of Ischial Ulcers," *Arch Phys Med Rehabil* 39:623–629, 1958.

Landis, E. M.: "Micro-injection Studies of Capillary Blood Pressure in Human Skin," *Heart* 15: 209–228, 1930.

Lewis, T., and R. T. Grant,: "Observations upon Reactive Hyperemia in Man," *Heart* 12: 73–120, 1925.

Lilla, J. A., R. R. Friedrichs, and L. M. Vistnes: "Floration Mattresses for Preventing and Treating Tissue Breakdown," *Geriatrics* 30: 71–75, 1975.

Lindan, O., et al.: "Pressure Distribution on the Surface of the Human Body," *Arch Phys Med Rehabil* 46:378–385, 1965.

Maccauley, C., and L. Weiss: "Spinal Cord Injury in an Inner City Hospital," *Arch Phys Med Rehabil* 59: 76–79, 1978.

Malament, I. R., M. E. Dunn, and R. Davis: "Pressure Sores: An Operant Conditioning Approach to Prevention," *Arch Phys Med Rehabil* 56: 161–164, 1975.

Merlino, A.: "Decubitus Ulcers: Cause, Prevention and Treatment," *Geriatrics* 24:119–124, 1969.

Michocki, R. J., and P. P. Lamy: "The Care of Decubitus Ulcer Pressure Sores," *J Am Geriatr Soc* 24:217–224, May 1976.

Mooney, V., M. J. Einbund, J. E. Rogers, and E. S. Stauffer: "Comparison of Pressure Distribution Qualities in Seat Cushions," *Bull Prosthet Res* 10:129–143, Spring 1971.

Mulholland, J. H., C. Tui, A. M. Wright, V. Vinci, and B. Shafiroff: "Protein Metabolism and Bed Sores," *Ann Surg* 118:1015–1023, 1943.

Newsome, T. W., L. A. Johns, and B. A. Pruitt: "Use of an Air-Fluidized Bed in the Care of Patients with Extensive Burns," *Am J Surg,* 124:52–56, 1972.

Norton, D.: "Research and the Problem of Pressure Sores," *Nurs Mirror* 140:65–67, 1975.

Page, C. F., and W. R. Goult: "Managing Ischemic Skin Ulcers," *Am Fam Physician* 11: 108–114, 1975.

Putnam, T., L. Calenoff, H. Betts, and J. Rosen: "Sinography in the Management of Decubitus Ulcers," Unpublished paper presented at the 54th Annual Session of the American Congress of Rehabilitation Medicine, October 1977.

Rao, D. B.: "Management of Dermal and Decubitus Ulcers," *Drug Ther,* October 1976, pp. 8–16.

———, P. G. Sane, and E. L. Georgies,: "Collagenase in the Treatment of Dermal and Decubitus Ulcers," *J Am Geriatr Soc* 23:22–30, 1975.

Redfern, S. J., P. A. Jeneid, M. E. Gillingham, and H. F. Lunn: "Local Pressure with Ten Types of Patient-Support Systems," *Lancet* 2:277–280, 1973.

Reichel, S.: "Shearing Force as a Factor in Decubitus Ulcer in Paraplegia," *JAMA* 166:762–763, 1958.

Reswick, J. B., and J. Rogers: "Experience at Rancho Los Amigos Hospital with Devices and Techniques to Prevent Pressure Sores," in R. M. Kenedi, J. M. Cowden, and J. T. Scales (eds.): *Bedsore Biomechanics: Seminar Proceedings, University of Strathclyde,* University Park Press, Baltimore, 1976, pp. 301–310.

Roach, Lora B.: "Skin Changes in Dark Skins," *Nursing '72* 2:19–22, 1972.

Sather, M. R., C. E. Weber, and J. George: "Pressure Sores and the Spinal Cord Injury Patient," *Drug Intell Clin Pharm* 11:154–168, 1977.

Scales, J. T., H. F. Lunn, P. A. Jeneio, M. E. Gillingham, and S. J. Redfern: "The Prevention and Treatment of Pressure Sores Using Air-Support Systems," *Paraplegia* 12:118–131, 1974.

Schell, V., and L. Wolcott: "The Etiology, Prevention and Management of Decubitus Ulcers," *J Mo State Med Assoc* 63:109–112, 1966.

Shea, J. D.: "Pressure Sores: Classification and Management," *Clin Orthop* 112:89–100, 1975.

Siegel, R. J., L. M. Vistnes, and D. R. Laub: "Use of the Water Bed for Prevention of Pressure Sores," *Plast, Reconstr Surg* 51:31–37, 1973.

Souther, S. G., S. D. Carr, and L. M. Vistnes: "Wheelchair Cushions to Reduce Pressure under Bony Prominences," *Arch Phys Med Rehabil* 55:460–464, 1974.

Stewart, P., and G. W. Wharton: "Bridging: An Effective and Practical Method of Preventive Skin Care for the Immobilized Person," *South Med J* 69:1469–1473, 1976.

Trandel, R. S., and D. W. Lewis,: "A Small Pliable Humidity Sensor, with Specific Reference to the Prevention of Decubitus Ulcers," *J Am Geriatr Soc* 23:322–326, 1975.

Trandel, R. S., D. W. Lewis, and P. J. Verhonick,: "Thermographical Investigation of Decubitus Ulcers," *Bull Prosthet Res* 10:137–155, Fall 1975.

Trumble, H. C.: "The Skin Tolerance for Pressure and Pressure Sores," *Med J Aust* 2:724–726, 1930.

Unger, G. H.: "The Care of the Skin in Paraplegia," *Practitioner* 206: 507, 1971.

Vasile, J., and H. Chaitin,: "Prognostic Factors in Decubitus Ulcers of the Aged," *Geriatrics* 27:126–129, 1972.

Verhonick, P. J., D. W. Lewis and H. O. Goller: "Thermography in the Study of Decubitus Ulcers: Preliminary Report," *Nurs Res* 21:233–237, 1972.

Wildnauer, R. H., J. W. Bothwell, and A. B. Douglass: "Stratum Corneum Biomechanical Properties," *J Invest Dermatol* 56:72–77, 1971.

Williams, A.: "A Study of Factors Contributing to Skin Breakdown," *Nurs Res* 21:238–243, 1972.

Wilson, R.: "The MUD Bed and Its Implications for Nursing Care," *Nurs Clin North Am* 11:725–730, 1976.

17
frederick j. schneider

physical therapy assessment

INTRODUCTION

The nurse who functions in a rehabilitation setting interacts with and processes information from a wide variety of health professionals. Awareness and understanding of the information gathered by these colleagues on any patient enhances the rehabilitation nurse's ability to function effectively and efficiently. This chapter presents an overview of the most common evaluation procedures used by physical therapists. It will also try to provide the nurse with strategies and suggestions on how best to make use of this information. No attempt will be made to instruct nurses in the performance of any of these procedures, although it is acknowledged that professional spheres overlap and the nurse may well be proficient in some of these tasks.

Before discussing specific assessments and their relations to various clinical pictures, it will be useful to examine how assessment fits into the overall picture of patient care in a physical therapy setting. The physical therapists' primary goal in performing any assessment procedure is to gain as much insight as possible into a patient's functional level. This facilitates ongoing planning and implementation of a comprehensive treatment program and subsequently assists in ascertaining the effectiveness of that program.

The process of patient management within a physical therapy setting can best be understood by examining the conceptual drawing shown in Fig. 17-1.

The process of evaluation by gathering information from many sources, planning and implementing treatment, and assessing the outcomes of that treatment is analogous to the models of intervention with patients by most health-care practitioners. Characteristically, however, the physical therapist, at least in many instances, is one of those professionals who treats through a "laying on of hands." Ongoing assessments can be further broken down into two categories. One is the formal administration of periodic testing procedures to establish a (summative) evaluation of the functional outcomes of treatment; the other is the ongoing monitoring of the patient's performance during treatment and assessing whether the response being obtained is oriented toward its established goal. This sequential and constant monitoring of the patient's physiological and psychological status during treatment is a key component of a successful outcome. The sharpening of observational skills is inherent in the clinical education of a therapist and a hallmark of a competent practitioner. An example of this would be a therapist assisting a neurologically involved patient in the performance of therapeutic exercises with the patient lying on an exercise mat. By detailed attention to positioning of the therapist and patient (including manual contacts with the patient), recognition of the presence or absence of certain reflexes, and awareness of the responses of the patient, functional and controlled movement may be developed.

Evaluation procedures will be discussed in three sections based on the three primary physical systems dealt with in a physical therapy setting, neurological, musculoskeletal, and cardiopulmonary. A number of procedures will show considerable overlap between sections. For example, the evaluation of the motion present at a joint or the strength present in a muscle or extremity is common to most clinical physical therapy situations but is categorized by systems for clarity of discussion.

It must also be mentioned that a number of the procedures are identical with the examinations performed by physicians during the process of differential diagnosis. The therapist may be assisting the physician in further delineating the diagnosis (Fig. 17-1), but in most cases a therapist learns most by interpreting an evaluation that he or she has performed.

MUSCULOSKELETAL ASSESSMENT

The physical therapist's primary objective in performing any evaluation is to assess the functional state of the patient. Goal setting and treatment planning with the patient who is faced with a disturbance of physical mobility is geared toward

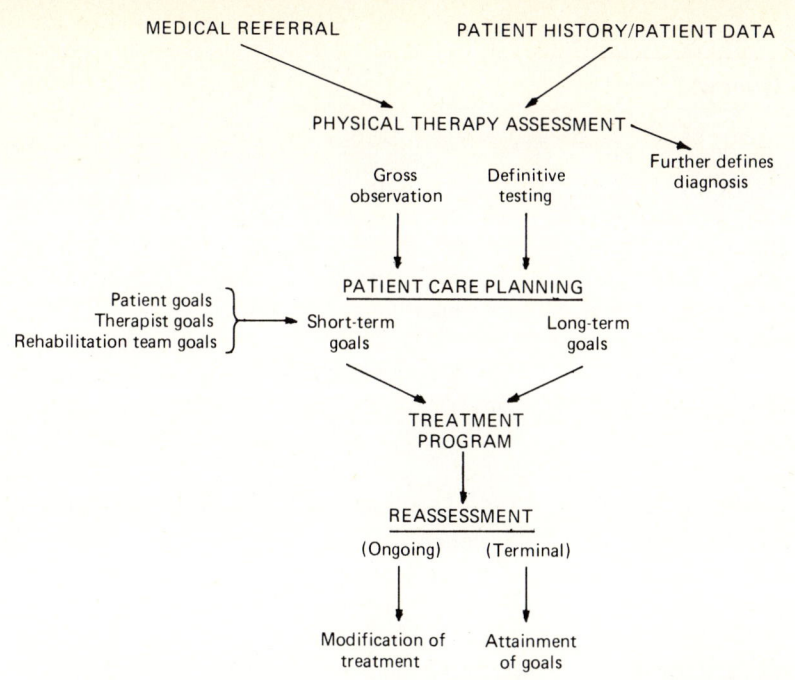

Figure 17-1
Conceptual model for the process of patient management within a physical therapy setting.

the attainment of functional controlled movement. The loss of physical mobility within one's environment is usually a result of involvement of the musculoskeletal or neurological systems or both. In this section we discuss assessment of muscular and skeletal function. The next section will deal with evaluation of those parts of the neurological system which, when affected, result in loss of mobility. It must be emphasized that the separation of systems in this presentation is for clarity and organization and that the two systems are rarely looked at separately in clinical situations.

MUSCLE ASSESSMENT

The evaluation of muscle function has for many years been the commonest of the testing procedures done by physical therapists. Muscle function can be examined by monitoring the types of electrical activity present or absent in the muscle-nerve complex. This monitoring procedure is called *electromyography*. Electromyography can provide accurate and objective data useful in the diagnosis of various disorders of the neuromuscular systems, but it cannot record the degree of weakness and subsequent loss or return of function in a muscle. This has to be done by manually isolating a muscle's function as much as possible and then grading the degree of weakness or strength present. This is referred to as *manual muscle testing,* and it can, when performed by a skilled therapist, provide an accurate picture of a muscle's clinical state. Reliable serial manual muscle testing can document the progression or regression of a patient's function. A number of factors can lead to muscle weakness: nerve involvement, lack of use, overstretching either through trauma or as a result of postural stretch weakness acquired over a long period of time, pain, and fatigue. Weakness of muscles may also be indirectly due to sensory deficits such as loss of proprioception or tactile sensation in a limb.

271 PHYSICAL THERAPY ASSESSMENT

Table 17-1

Manual Muscle Testing Grading Systems*

Normal	5	N	Complete range of motion against gravity with full resistance
Good	4	G	Complete range of motion against gravity with some resistance
Fair	3	F	Complete range of motion against gravity
Poor	2	P	Complete range of motion, gravity eliminated
Trace	1	T	Evidence of slight contractility, no joint motion
Zero	0	0	No evidence of contractility

* Both numerical and letter grades are presented; one *or* the other system should be used for a complete test.

Manual testing of muscle strength is valid with disorders involving (1) the muscle tissue (examples: muscular dystrophy, myopathies), (2) the neuromuscular junction (example: myasthenia gravis), and (3) the lower motor neuron, including the anterior horn cells (examples: peripheral nerve lesions and neuropathies, poliomyelitis). Disorders of the central nervous system involving levels higher than the anterior horn cells *cannot* be validly evaluated by the use of manual muscle testing, because central nervous system lesions bring into play reflex activity and altered states of muscle tone which vary with body position. In assessing loss of functional movement as a result of altered reflexive and tonal states, it is best to examine patterns of movement. This is discussed in the following section on neurological assessment.

To perform the manual muscle test, the examiner fixates and stabilizes a body segment in order to isolate a given muscle's action from others with similar function. The patient is then asked to perform an active contraction of that muscle; resistance is applied (when feasible) after the contraction, and the degree of strength is graded according to an established scale. It must be mentioned that there are only a few examples of a muscle being able to achieve a truly isolated movement of a joint (example: the flexor digitorum profundus, which alone flexes the distal phalanges of the fingers). However, the relative degree of individual muscle function can be tested by accurate knowledge of the muscle's origin and insertion, adequate fixation of the body segment, and clear commands to the patient.

Examples of grading scales and the systems used to assign grades are shown in Table 17-1. An example of the muscle examination form which the nurse is most likely to encounter on a patient's chart is shown in Fig. 17-2.

In addition to showing the clinical state of a muscle or muscle group, the manual muscle test can serve as a means of diagnosing various neuromuscular conditions. Most common is the detection of partial or complete involvement of peripheral nerves and nerve roots. For example, weakness of the deltoid, biceps, and brachioradialis muscles may be indicative of a nerve root impingement at the C5 and C6 level. An example of a form which relates peripheral nerve levels to muscle function is shown in Fig. 17-3.

The information given on a muscle strength evaluation can prove helpful to the rehabilitation nurse, offering insight into what can be expected of a patient functionally. For example, a patient whose lower-extremity muscle grades are all in the poor to fair range cannot be expected to perform a standing pivot transfer from bed to wheelchair.

SKELETAL ASSESSMENT

Skilled functional and pain-free motion cannot often take place where there is joint limitation of motion, joint capsular laxity, or joint pain. This section focuses on assessment of motion at individual joints and then examines the manner in which malalignment at multiple joints leads to postural dysfunction.

Joint Motion

In examining the motion present at any joint, two factors need attention: (1) What is the total range through which that joint can both actively and passively move a body segment and (2) what is the degree of stability present within the joint structure itself during movement? The first test is referred to as a *joint range-of-motion* (ROM) test and the second as a *joint play* examination.

Joint ROM Test Measurements of the mobility present at a joint can provide the patient and the rehabilitation team with reliable and objective feedback on progress in overcoming problems of joint range. The means of measurement most widely accepted is an instrument called a **goniometer.** This is essentially a protractor with two movable arms attached. By aligning the two arms along the long axes of two body segments attached to the joint and aligning the axis of the goniometer with the axis or fulcrum of joint motion, the active and passive motion of the joint can be measured in degrees. An example is elbow flexion and extension. Here one arm of the goniometer is aligned with the long axis of the humerus and the other with the long axis of the forearm, with both arms usually maintained in place during active and passive motion. The exception is that in some joints the anatomic axis shifts during motion of the body segment; therefore, the goniometer alignment is also shifted by the examiner. The alignment of the arms of the goniometer takes considerable skill for some joints, and most therapists utilize bony landmarks to aid accuracy of measurement. There are many sizes and types of goniometers; selection depends on the joint to be measured. Considerable difficulty arises in spinal measurement, and the only truly accurate measurement of a scoliosis curve, for example, is made by drawing the two axes of the spinal curve on an x-ray and measuring the degrees of curvature with a protractor. Even then, many scoliotic curves incorporate a degree of rotation around the long axis of the spine, and the two-dimensional radiologic measurement cannot assess the progress of this factor.

The skeletal system has hundreds of joints, and only a few are measured to ascertain functional loss. For example, the shoulder girdle complex contains seven joints, which all move to produce motion of the upper extremity on the trunk. Only two of them, however—the glenohumeral and the scapulothoracic (also called **scapulocostal**) joints—need be considered in order to assess movement in the shoulder's three planes of motion: flexion-extension, abduction-adduction, and internal rotation-external rotation.

Joint motion must always be measured in both passive movement (the examiner moving the joint) and active movement (the patient using his or her own muscles to complete the joint range of motion). It is important for the nurse reading a ROM report to know whether the measurement was done with active or passive movement. It is possible, for example, for a patient with quadriplegia to have full passive motion at the shoulder and, because of muscle weakness, to have considerable loss of active shoulder function.

It is also helpful for the nurse to know the cause(s) of the limitation of motion. In viewing the results of a definitive joint range-of-motion analysis, the nurse has to keep in mind that many factors contribute to limitation of joint motion; some of these promote a "static" limitation (bony intraarticular blockages, muscle-joint capsule contractures), while others relate to a limitation of a changing nature. An example of the latter would be limitation induced by spasticity of the muscles controlling a joint. Since the degree of spasticity can change with changes in the position of the patient, the nurse can make use of this information in patient care activities. A patient with limitation of motion caused by severe spasticity of the lower extremities may

Patient's Name ______________________ Ric No. ____________

Date of Birth ______________________ Date of Onset ____________

Diagnosis:

LEFT							RIGHT			
					Examiner's Initials					
					Date					
				NECK	Flexors	Sternocleidomastoid				
					Extensor group					
				TRUNK	Flexors	Rectus abdominis				
					Rt. ext. obl. } Rotators	{ Lt. ext. obl.				
					Lt. int. obl. }	{ Rt. int. obl.				
					Extensors	{ Thoracic group				
						{ Lumbar group				
					Pelvic elev.	Quadratus lumb.				
				HIP	Flexors	Iliopsoas				
					Extensors	Gluteus maximus				
					Abductors	Gluteus medius				
					Adductor group					
					External rotator group					
					Internal rotator group					
					Sartorius					
					Tensor fasciae latae					
				KNEE	Flexors	{ Biceps femoris				
						{ Inner hamstrings				
					Extensors	Quadriceps				
				ANKLE	Plantar flexors	{ Gastrocnemius				
						{ Soleus				
				FOOT	Invertors	{ Tibialis anterior				
						{ Tibialis posterior				
					Evertors	{ Peroneus brevis				
						{ Peroneus longus				
				TOES	M. P. flexors	Lumbricales				
					I. P. flexors (1st)	Flex. digit. br.				
					I. P. flexors (2nd)	Flex. digit. l.				
					M. P. extensors	{ Ext. digit. l.				
						{ Ext. digit. br.				
				HALLUX	M. P. flexor	Flex. hall. br.				
					I. P. flexor	Flex. hall. l.				
					M. P. extensor	Ext. hall. br.				
					I. P. extensor	Ext. hall. l.				

Measurements - Remarks:

KEY

5 N Normal — Complete range of motion against gravity with full resistance.
4 G Good* — Complete range of motion against gravity with some resistance.
3 F Fair* — Complete range of motion against gravity.
2 P Poor* — Complete range of motion with gravity eliminated.
1 T Trace — Evidence of slight contractility. No joint motion.
0 0 Zero — No evidence of contractility.

S or SS — Spasm or severe spasm.
C or CC — Contracture or severe contracture.

* Muscle spasm or contracture may limit range of motion. A question mark should be placed after the grading of a movement that is incomplete from this cause.

Figure 17-2
Sample muscle examination form. *(Courtesy of the National Foundation for Infantile Paralysis.)*

LEFT								RIGHT			
					Examiner's Initials						
					Date						
				SCAPULA	Abductor	Serratus anterior					
					Elevator	Upper trapezius					
					Depressor	Lower trapezius					
					Adductors	{ Middle trapezius / Rhomboids					
				SHOULDER	Flexor	Anterior deltoid					
					Extensors	{ Latissimus dorsi / Teres major					
					Abductor	Middle deltoid					
					Horiz. abd.	Posterior deltoid					
					Horiz. add.	Pectoralis major					
					External rotator group						
					Internal rotator group						
				ELBOW	Flexors	{ Biceps brachii / Brachioradialis					
					Extensor	Triceps					
				FOREARM	Supinator group						
					Pronator group						
				WRIST	Flexors	{ Flex. carpi rad. / Flex. carpi uln.					
					Extensors	{ Ext. carpi rad. l. & br. / Ext. carpi uln.					
				FINGERS	M. P. flexors	Lumbricales					
					I. P. flexors (1st)	Flex. digit. sub.					
					I. P. flexors (2nd)	Flex. digit. prof.					
					M. P. extensor	Ext. digit. com.					
					Adductors	Palmar interossei					
					Abductors	Dorsal interossei					
					Abductor digiti quinti						
					Opponens digiti quinti						
				THUMB	M. P. flexor	Flex. poll. br.					
					I. P. flexor	Flex. poll. l.					
					M. P. extensor	Ext. poll. br.					
					I. P. extensor	Ext. poll. l.					
					Abductors	{ Abd. poll. br. / Abd. poll. l.					
					Adductor pollicis						
					Opponens pollicis						

| CLINICAL RECORD | MUSCLE AND/OR NERVE EVALUATION—MANUAL AND ELECTRICAL: UPPER EXTREMITY |

DIAGNOSIS AND BRIEF CLINICAL HISTORY

LEFT		RIGHT
	← (Insert type of test given) →	
	EXAMINER'S INITIALS	
	DATE	
	SPINAL ACCESSORY NERVE	
	Sternocleido- —Stern. C2–3	
	mastoid —Clav. C2–3	
	Trapezius—Upper C2–4	
	—Middle C2–4	
	—Lower C2–4	
	DORSAL SCAPULAR NERVE	
	Rhomboids C4–5	
	LONG THORACIC NERVE	
	Serratus Anterior C5–7	
	THORACO DORSAL NERVE	
	Latissimus Dorsi C6–8	
	UPPER SUBSCAPULAR NERVE	
	Subscapularis C5–6	
	LOWER SUBSCAPULAR NERVE	
	Teres Major C5–7	
	ANT. THORACIC NERVE	
	Pect. Maj.—Clav. C5–7	
	—Stern. C6–8, T1	
	SUPRASCAPULAR NERVE	
	Supraspinatus C4–6	
	Infraspinatus C4–6	
	AXILLARY NERVE	
	Deltoid—Ant. C5–6	
	—Middle C5–6	
	—Post. C5–6	
	Teres Minor C5–6	
	MUSCULOCUTANEOUS NERVE	
	Biceps Brachii C5–6	
	Coracobrachialis C5–6	
	Brachialis C5–6	
	RADIAL NERVE	
	Triceps C6–8, T1	
	Brachioradialis C5–6	
	Supinator C6	
	Ext. Carp. Rad. C6–7	
	Ext. Carp. Uln. C7	
	Ext. Dig. Quinti C7	
	Ext. Ind. Prop. C7	

PATIENT'S LAST NAME—FIRST NAME—MIDDLE NAME   REGISTER NO.   WARD NO.

16—61553-2

MUSCLE AND/OR NERVE EVALUATION—
MANUAL AND ELECTRICAL:
UPPER EXTREMITY
Standard Form 528

(NAME OF HOSPITAL OR OTHER MEDICAL FACILITY)

Figure 17-3
Clinical form for relation of peripheral nerve levels to muscle function.

LEFT		RIGHT
	← (Insert type of test given) →	
	EXAMINER'S INITIALS	
	DATE	
	Ext. Dig. Com.—1 C6	
	—2	
	—3	
	—4	
	Ext. Pol. Long. C7	
	Ext. Pol. Brev. C7	
	Abd. Pol. Long. C7	
	MEDIAN NERVE	
	Pronator Teres C6	
	Palmaris Long. C6–8, T1	
	Flex. Carpi Rad. C6	
	Flex. Dig. Sub.—1 C7–8, T1	
	—2	
	—3	
	—4	
	Flex. Dig. Prof.—1 C8, T1	
	—2	
	Flex. Pol. Long. C8, T1	
	Flex. Pol. Brev. C6–8	
	Abd. Pol. Brev. C6–7	
	Opp. Pollicis C6–8, T1	
	Lumbricales—1 C7–8	
	—2	
	ULNAR NERVE	
	Flex. Carpi Uln. C8	
	Flex. Dig. Prof.—3 C8, T1	
	—4	
	Add. Pollicis C8	
	Abd. Dig. Quinti C8, T1	
	Opp. Dig. Quinti C8, T1	
	Flex. Dig. Quinti C8, T1	
	Interossei (dor.)—1 C8	
	—2	
	—3	
	—4	
	(palm.)—1	
	—2	
	—3	
	Lumbricales—3 C8	
	—4	

Key to Manual Muscle Evaluation:

100%	5	N	Normal	: Complete range of motion against gravity with full resistance
75%	4	G	Good	: Complete range of motion against gravity with some resistance
50%	3	F	Fair	: Complete range of motion against gravity
25%	2	P	Poor	: Complete range of motion with gravity eliminated
10%	1	T	Trace	: Evidence of contractility but no joint motion
0	0	0	Zero	: No evidence of contractility
		S	Spasm	} If spasm or contracture exists place S or C after the
		C	Contracture	grade of a movement incomplete for this reason

Key to Electrical Evaluation:
(Insert key used locally)

SIGNATURE OF THERAPIST   DATE

277   PHYSICAL THERAPY ASSESSMENT

CLINICAL RECORD	MUSCLE and/or NERVE EVALUATION—MANUAL and ELECTRICAL: TRUNK, LOWER EXTREMITY, FACE

DIAGNOSIS AND BRIEF CLINICAL HISTORY

LEFT		RIGHT
	(Insert type of test given)	
	EXAMINER'S INITIALS	
	DATE	
	INF. GLUTEAL NERVE	
	Gluteus Max. L5, S1, 2	
	SUP. GLUTEAL NERVE	
	Glut. Med. L4, 5, S1	
	Tens. Fas. Lat. L4, 5, S1	
	FEMORAL NERVE	
	Sartorius L2–4	
	Rect. Fem. L2–4	
	Vast. Med. L2–4	
	Vast. Lat. L2–4	
	Vast. Intermed. L2–4	
	OBTURATOR NERVE	
	Adductors L2–4	
	Gracilis L2–4	
	SCIATIC NERVE	
	Biceps Fem. L5, S1–3	
	Semiten. L4–5, S1–2	
	Semimem. L4–5, S1–2	
	POST. TIBIAL NERVE	
	Gastrocnemius S1–2	
	Soleus L5, S1–2	
	Tib. Post. L4–5, S1–2	
	Flex. Dig. Long. L5, S1–2	
	Flex. Dig. Brev. L5, S1	
	Flex. Hal. Long. L5, S1–2	
	Flex. Hal. Brev. L5, S1	
	Interossei S1–3	
	Lumbricales L5, S1–2	
	COM. PERONEAL NERVE	
	Tibialis Ant. L4–5, S1	
	Ext. Dig. Long. L4–5, S1–2	
	Ext. Dig. Brev. L4–5, S1–2	
	Ext. Hal. Long. L4–5, S1	
	Peroneus Long. L4–5, S1	
	Peroneus Brev. L4–5, S1	
	Peroneus Tert. L4–5, S1	

PATIENT'S LAST NAME—FIRST NAME—MIDDLE NAME   REGISTER NO.   WARD NO.

(NAME OF HOSPITAL OR OTHER MEDICAL FACILITY)

16—61537-2

MUSCLE AND/OR NERVE EVALUATION—
MANUAL AND ELECTRICAL:
Trunk, Lower Extremity, Face
Standard Form 529

pose a considerable problem with dressing and hygiene in the supine position, but in another position (side lying, for example) the activity may be accomplished with comparative ease.

Unfortunately, there are a number of different systems for expressing range of motion. The one most commonly used by physical therapists and endorsed by the American Academy of Ortho-

LEFT		RIGHT
	(Insert type of test given)	
	EXAMINER'S INITIALS	
	DATE	
	Diaphragm C3–5	
	Ext. Intercostals T1–11	
	Int. Intercostals T1–11	
	Sacrospinalis-Thor. T1–S3	
	Sacrospinalis-Lumb. T1–S3	
	Quad. Lumborum T12, L1–3	
	Rectus Abd. T5–12	
	Obl. Ext. Abd. T5–12	
	Obl. Int. Abd. T7–12	
	Iliopsoas L1–4	

Key to Manual Muscle Evaluation—Lower Extremity and Trunk:
- 100% 5 N Normal: Complete range of motion against gravity with full resistance.
- 75% 4 G Good: Complete range of motion against gravity with some resistance.
- 50% 3 F Fair: Complete range of motion against gravity.
- 25% 2 P Poor: Complete range of motion with gravity eliminated.
- 10% 1 T Trace: Evidence of contractility with no joint motion.
- 0   0 0 Zero: No evidence of contractility.
- S   Spasm   ⎤ If spasm or contracture limit range of motion, place S or C after
- C   Contracture ⎦ the grade of a movement incomplete for this reason.

KEY TO ELECTRICAL MUSCLE EVALUATION (*Insert key used locally as applicable to test*):

	MUSCLES OF FACE	
	Frontal is CR7	
	Corrugator CR7	
	Orb. Oculi CR7	
	Procerus CR7	
	Quad. Lab. Sup. CR7	
	Risorius CR7	
	Zygomaticus CR7	
	Orb. Oris CR7	
	Mentalis CR7	
	Quad. Lab. Inf. CR7	
	Triangularis CR7	
	Platysma CR7	
	Buccinator CR7	
	Temporalis CR5	
	Masseter CR5	
	HYPOGLOSSAL NERVE	

Key for Evaluation of Facial Muscles: N: Normal   SN: Subnormal   T: Trace   0: Zero

SIGNATURE OF THERAPIST   DATE

paedic Surgeons utilizes the erect anatomic position as the starting position (0°) for joint movement. Shoulder flexion then progresses from 0° to full range at 180°. It is important that nurses interested in utilizing this test information be familiar with the system of measurement and recording utilized within their institution.

The last factor that needs to be discussed in

279   PHYSICAL THERAPY ASSESSMENT

Name _____ RIC No. _____
Diagnosis _____ Onset _____
Anatomical position is considered zero and is the starting position.

LEFT				EXAMINER'S INITIALS		RIGHT			
				DATE					
			HIP	Flexion 0-125°	HIP				
				Extension 0-10°					
				Adduction 0-20°					
				Abduction 0-45°					
				Internal rotation 0-45°					
				External rotation 0-45°					
			KNEE	ROM 0-140°	KNEE				
			ANKLE	Plantar flexion 0-45°	ANKLE				
				Dorsi flexion 0-20°					
			FOOT	Inversion 0-40°	FOOT				
				Eversion 0-20°					
			SHOULDER JOINT	Abduction 0-120°	SHOULDER JOINT				
				Internal rotation 0-90°					
				External rotation 0-90°					
			SHOULDER COMPLEX	Extension 0-45°	SHOULDER COMPLEX				
				Flexion 0-180°					
				Abduction 0-180°					
			ELBOW	ROM 0-145°	ELBOW				
			FOREARM	Supination 0-90°	FOREARM				
				Pronation 0-90°					
			WRIST COMPLEX	Flexion 0-80°	WRIST COMPLEX				
				Extension 0-70°					
				Ulnar deviation 0-45°					
				Radial deviation 0-20°					
			THUMB	MP 0-70°	THUMB				
				IP 0-90°					
			INDEX	MP 0-70°	INDEX				
				PIP 0-120°					
				DIP 0-80°					
			MIDDLE	MP 0-90°	MIDDLE				
				PIP 0-120°					
				DIP 0-80°					
			RING	MP 0-90°	RING				
				PIP 0-120°					
				DIP 0-80°					
			LITTLE	MP 0-90°	LITTLE				
				PIP 0-120°					
				DIP 0-80°					

WEB SPACE (Distance thumb MP to index MP with thumb abducted to fullest range) _____
OPPOSITION (Finger reached) _____
REMARKS:

Figure 17-4
Range-of-motion measurement chart. *(Courtesy of the Rehabilitation Institute of Chicago.)*

measuring joint range is reliability. Serial measurements should be performed by the same therapist. Most studies and authorities agree that an experienced and well-trained therapist can consistently attain accuracy between measurements to within 5°. Joint motion recorded in intervals smaller than 5° therefore has little clinical meaning.

An example of a commonly used range-of-motion form is shown in Fig. 17-4.

Joint Play The ability to examine the integrity of a joint in both the extremities and the spinal column is critical to planning a successful treatment regimen for the patient suffering joint and joint-referred pain. Pain can be caused by hyper- or hypomobility of various joint structures, and the physical therapist treating painful orthopedic disorders can become highly proficient in the art of palpation of skeletal structures. This type of test is useful to assist the team in differentiating pain within a joint from pain referred to or around a joint from other organs and structures.

Postural Assessment

Postural malalignment can result in painful disabling conditions. Faulty body alignment may be caused by muscle imbalances in the form of either weakness or tightness. Three primary factors cause these imbalances: inheritance (body type), disease, and habit. Developmental and environmental factors play an important role in the formation of postural faults; therefore, it is essential that the cause or causes of the condition be established and that all members of the treatment team make a concerted treatment and teaching effort to alleviate the factor(s).

The process of postural assessment is based on two essential observational skills of the therapist: (1) the understanding of what constitutes good posture and body alignment and (2) the ability to recognize deviations from what is considered normal.

The assessment of faulty body alignment consists first of observation of the patient while standing, sitting, and walking (gait analysis). After observational assessment, the problem is further delineated through joint range-of-motion and muscle-strength testing. Only then can appropriate treatment programs be established. Little equipment is needed by a therapist in performing a postural assessment, although such items as a mirror, plumb line, and tape measure can prove valuable. Figures 17-5 and 17-6 are examples of forms used to record and communicate postural and gait-analysis findings.

In addition to definitive treatment, inappropriate habits of posture need to be detected and corrected. This is where the rehabilitation nurse can play an important role. Effective correction of poor postural habits needs a concerted and continuous effort by both patient and staff. On an inpatient unit—a low-back pain unit, for example—the nurse is most often in contact with the patient during activities of daily living and can therefore serve as a prime factor in modifying the patient's postural behavior.

NEUROLOGICAL ASSESSMENT

The patient suffering from dysfunction of any part of the nervous system, whether a peripheral nerve lesion or trauma to the brain, can pose one of the most complex and unpredictable clinical problems facing a rehabilitation team. While most diseases and injuries to the body run a fairly predictable course to recovery, injury or disease of the nervous system offers few well-defined clues to prognosis. Experienced clinicians who have dealt with a compression or neurapraxia of a peripheral nerve, the unpredictable remissions and exacerbations of multiple sclerosis, or the individualized complex reactions of the head trauma patient know well that there is no easy answer to patients' or families' question "Where do we go from here?" To deal with dysfunction of such a complex system, one would hope for highly accurate and objective assessment procedures to facilitate planning a course of treatment. Unfortunately, these are not available for problems of the central nervous system.

| Name _____ RIC No. _____ Birth Date _____ |
| Diagnosis _____ Onset _____ |

Date and Initials	Admission		Interim		Discharge	
	R	L	R	L	R	L
GAIN DEVIATIONS (✓)						
SWING PHASE						
Trunk: Lean backward						
Lean involved side						
Lean uninvolved side						
Pelvis: Lacks rotation						
Hip: Inadequate flexion						
Circumducts						
Hikes						
Scissors						
Internally rotates						
Externally rotates						
Knee: Inadequate flexion						
Inadequate extension						
Ankle: Equinus						
Varus						
Toes: Clawing						
Uneven arm swing						
Unequal length steps						
Uneven timing						
Other:						
STANCE PHASE						
Trunk: No lateral shift						
Forward at hip						
Weight behind knee						
Pelvis: Extreme rotation						
Drops other side						
Hip: Extreme adduction						
Internally rotates						
Externally rotates						
Knee: Hyperextension						
Excessive flexion						
Wobbles						
Ankle: In varus						
No dorsiflexion range						
No heelstrike						
Tacks push-off						
Toes: Clawing						
Other:						

Please list all equipment used at each evaluation:

Figure 17-5
Gait-deviation measurement form. *(Courtesy of the Rehabiliation Institute of Chicago.)*

Name.. Cl. No................ Doctor..
Diagnosis.. Date—1st Ex.:..............................
Onset... Date—2nd Ex.:............................
Occupation.. Height................ Weight.......................................
Handedness................................ Age................ Leg Length: Left................ Right................

PLUMB ALIGNMENT

Side View: Lt.. Rt..

Back View: Deviated Lt.. Deviated Rt.............................

SEGMENTAL ALIGNMENT

		Hammer Toes	Hallux Valgus	Low Ant. Arch		Ant. Foot Varus
	Feet	Pronated >	Supinated	Flat Long. Arch		Pigeon Toes
		Int. Rot. >	Ext. Rot.	Knock-Knees		
	Knees	Hyperext. >	Flexed	Bow-Legs		Tibial Torsion
	Pelvis	Leg in Postural Add.	Rotation	Tilt		Deviation
	Low Back	Lordosis	Flat	Kyphosis		Operation
	Up. Back	Kyphosis	Flat	Scap. Abducted		Scap. Elevated
	Thorax	Depressed Chest	Elevated Chest	Rotation		Deviation
	Spine	Total Curve	Lumbar	Dorsal		Cervical
	Abdomen	Protruding	Scars			
	Shoulder	Low	High	Forward		Int. Rotated
	Head	Forward	Torticollis			

TESTS FOR FLEXIBILITY AND MUSCLE LENGTH

Forward Bending .... Bk........ H. S........... G. S.........
Arm Overhead Elevation: Lt.................... Rt....................
Hip Flexors: Lt.................... Rt....................
Tensor Fas. Lata.: Lt.................... Rt....................
Trunk Extension:....................
Trunk Lat. Flex.: To Lt.................... To Rt....................

TREATMENT

Infra-red:........................
Massage:........................
Moist Heat:........................
Paraffin Bath:........................
Diathermy:........................
Exercises:
  F. L.: Pelvic Tilt
  B. L.: Pel. Tilt and Breath.
         Pel. Tilt and Leg Sl.
         Head and Sh. Raising
         Pectoral Stretch
         Straight Leg-Raise
         Hip Flex. Stretch
  Sd. L.: Stretch.................... tensor....................
  Sit.: Forward Bending
         To Stretch Low Bk.
         To Stretch H. S.
         Wall-sitting
           Middle Trapezius
           Lower Trapezius
  St.: Foot and Knee Ex.
         Wall-standing
Other Exercises:....................

MUSCLE STRENGTH TESTS

L		R
	Mid. Trapezius	
	Low. Trapezius	
	Back Extensors	
	Glut. Medius	
	Glut. Maximus	
	Hamstrings	
	Hip Flexors	
	Tib. Posticus	
	Toe Flexors	

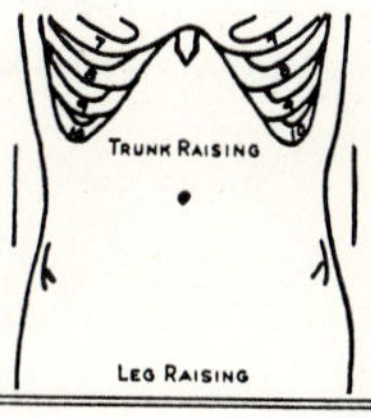

(Trunk Raising / Leg Raising diagram)

SHOE CORRECTION

Left		Right
	(Wide Heel) Inner Wedge (Narrow Heel)	
	Level Heel Raise	
	Metatarsal Support	
	Longitudinal Support	

NOTES: ....

Support:..

Figure 17-6
Postural examination chart. *(Used with permission of Florence P. Kendall, P. T., Baltimore, Md.)*

Every patient with central nervous system dysfunction presents a unique clinical picture, one that can change from moment to moment. The rehabilitation team is therefore faced with assessment techniques which are observational, subjective, and sometimes unreliable from one day to the next. For the physical therapist it is most important and helpful to separate program planning (prognostic) assessment from the continuous assessment of treatment (Fig. 17-1). The therapist must carry out carefully planned and ongoing evaluations of treatment in order to achieve success at goals attainment.

In this section neurological assessment is divided into two parts, involving (1) the peripheral nervous system (PNS) and (2) the central nervous system (CNS). The physical therapy evaluation of the CNS system is presented as a whole, not by diagnosis; whether the diagnosis is cerebral palsy, cerebral vascular accident, brain tumor, or spinal cord injury, the therapist is primarily concerned with determining how sensorimotor and perceptual dysfunction affect skilled and functional movement.

PERIPHERAL NERVOUS SYSTEM

Injury to or disease of the lower motor neuron (which includes all structures from the anterior horn cells to the neuromuscular junction and muscle tissue) results primarily in weakness, pain, and other sensory loss, with possible secondary limitation of joint motion. (Evaluations of muscle strength and joint motion were discussed in the preceding section on musculoskeletal assessment.) The evaluations discussed in this section are commonly performed by physical therapists treating PNS dysfunction.

Sensory Testing

Superficial and deep types of sensation are controlled by higher CNS centers such as the thalamus and cortex. It must be appreciated that complete or partial lesions of the lower motor neuron systems can be affected indirectly by higher thalamic and cortical centers. In addition, accurate sensory testing depends upon an alert, objective, and cooperative patient. Testing for sensory loss aids in locating the area of the nervous system that is affected. It also alerts the patient and team to areas of the body that might require careful monitoring during positioning, bracing, casting, transfers, and ambulation. Loss of proprioception or kinesthetic awareness poses an added problem for the therapist in training the patient in functional activities.

Superficial Sensation Superficial sensation testing includes assessing the patient's ability to perceive tactile or light-touch stimuli, differences in temperature, and superficial and deep pain. The areas of involvement are usually drawn on a body chart, with dermatomes outlined and classified as intact, impaired, or lacking sensation. Another common test of skin sensation is the two-point discrimination test, which requires the patient to distinguish two distinct areas stimulated simultaneously and records how close the stimuli can be to each other before the patient interprets them as one. Superficial and deep pain evaluations often include having the patient draw areas of pain on a body outline and then write a description of the pain. The therapist can utilize serial drawings to evaluate the effects of treatment and, if the drawings are inconsistent, to alert the patient and team to possible psychological manifestations of the pain.

Deep Sensation Deep sensation testing includes proprioception and vibratory sensation as well as deep pain sensations. Proprioception or joint-position sense is tested distally in the toes and fingers by having patients sense the passive movement of a digit while their vision is obscured. Vibratory testing utilizes a vibrating tuning fork or mechanical vibrator to stimulate both bony points and muscle bellies. The loss of either proprioception or vibratory sense provides valuable information to the physician in localizing a lesion between and within the peripheral and central nervous systems. For example, loss of proprioception with intact vibratory sense favors a lesion above the thalamic level. Proprioceptive loss leads to a disturbance of body image and must be taken into consideration in treatment planning and goal setting. *Stereognosis* is the ability to recognize objects nonvisually through feeling and manipulation. When hand sensation and motor function are intact, impairment of this ability tells the team that there is probably cortical dysfunction.

Reflex Testing

The evaluation of deep tendon stretch reflexes enables the therapist to identify neurological levels in relation to possible nerve root damage caused by herniated disks, osteoarthritis, or other pathologic processes. Reflex responses are reported as normal, increased, or decreased, and the evaluation is usually done bilaterally to compare one side with the other, since reflex activity varies among individuals.

Electrical Testing

Two simple tests of the excitability of the muscle-nerve complex offer valuable diagnostic and prognostic data for examining peripheral nerve injuries.

Strength-Duration Curve By stimulating the affected muscle tissue with an electric current which varies in duration, a curve can be plotted which compares the intensity of current, measured in milliamperes, that is needed to obtain a minimally visible contraction with varying current impulse durations, measured in milliseconds. Since nerve tissue is much more excitable than muscle tissue, the intensity and duration of current impulse needed for contraction rises with progressive denervation and falls with reinnervation. Serial strength-duration curves can plot patient progress.

Chronaxie Studies A time-saving procedure is to plot the changes occurring at one point on the strength-duration curve. The chronaxie is a factor of stimulus duration and is measured in milliseconds (ms). The chronaxie is normally less than 0.1 ms; it rises above 1 ms with partial and complete denervation.

Nerve Conduction and Electromyographic Studies

These studies can provide additional objective data on lower motor neuron status that can assist the physician in diagnosing impairment of the lower motor neuron system. They can be performed by therapists with advanced training.

CENTRAL NERVOUS SYSTEM

Disorders involving upper motor neuron dysfunction display a wide variety of clinical pictures depending on the area of the brain and spinal cord involved, the extent of involvement, and the stage of recovery. In assessing and treating CNS problems, the physical therapist is mostly concerned with sensorimotor loss that results in decreased function. This loss can have many labels, such as flaccidity, spasticity, rigidity, hypotonia, ataxia, athetosis, tremor, chorea, all of which are used to describe states of muscle tone as abnormal patterns of movement. Damage to this system also results in altered postural tone, abnormal reflex activity, and impaired balance reactions. The outcome is a decrease in the quality of functional and controlled movement.

The assessment of function or dysfunction in the CNS can have many parameters. With adults, the focus is often on describing the altered total movement patterns, or synergies, and charting recovery in stages related to the appearance or disappearance of these abnormal synergistic motor patterns. With children, movement dysfunction is related to the sequence of normal motor development.

Besides sensorimotor dysfunction, the physical therapist needs to be aware of other aspects of CNS disorders. Depending on the setting and the sophistication of the therapist, the assessment of these aspects may be carried out by the therapist or by other professionals. Assessments include the patient's levels of cognition, speech and language, bulbar and oral-motor function, body-image awareness, perceptual-spatial states, visual field and visuo-spatial orientation, hearing, and general affect. To plan a safe, efficient, and effective program of treatment, the physical therapist also needs to know the premorbid health status (for a noncongenital condition) and the present overall health status, along with pertinent socioeconomic information.

In assessing function with the CNS-involved patient, the therapist can make use of any of the applicable tests mentioned in other sections of this chapter. Some are more pertinent to this type of patient than others. Superficial and deep sensory testing and analysis of joint motion and gait will provide useful information with a large segment of this population. Cardiac and respiratory testing will be used when dysfunctions of these systems affect the rehabilitation program.

One test that is *not* applicable with upper motor neuron problems is manual muscle testing. Considerable confusion still exists among health professionals over the issue of strength as a primary goal in CNS rehabilitation and the limitations of manual muscle testing in evaluating motor function in these patients. Although these patients suffer from weakness, either as a primary problem (hypotonia) or as secondary disuse atrophy, the grading of muscle strength as outlined in manual muscle testing with lower motor neuron and musculoskeletal problems is not applicable. A number of factors present with CNS movement disorders contribute to this: (1) movement with CNS dysfunction most often takes place as mass patterns of movement involving whole muscle groups and body segments; (2) the effect of abnormal reflex activity present with upper motor neuron involvement can alter the tone in these mass patterns of movement; and (3) changes in limb position and total body posture can affect the quality and quantity of movement in a body segment. In essence, the primary goal becomes function through the *quality* of controlled movement and not the *quantity* or strength of movement.

What factors and tests, then, are important to the assessment of movement in the CNS patient?

Assessment of Muscle Tone

Assessment of abnormal muscle tone is observational, descriptive, and somewhat subjective in nature. The therapist's primary focus is on how tonal changes affect functional movements, balance, and posture in various positions.

Hypertonicity Hypertonic movement patterns are referred to as CNS *spasticity* or *rigidity*. Spasticity is defined as an abnormal increase in spinal stretch reflex activity, consisting of a sustained state of contraction of opposing muscle groups, which, at rest, most often results in a posture of increased flexion of body segments. Resistance to passive movement of the segment is a cardinal sign of hypertonia. Spasticity brings a sustained resistance, while other forms of hypertonia involve altered passive responses. Rigidity, for example, as found in Parkinsonism, presents a "cogwheel" effect or rhythmic give to passive movement and is indicative of thalamic dysfunction. Spasticity varies with the speed and direction of the passive movement, while the various forms of rigidity vary to a lesser extent with the speed of movement and are more symmetrical in terms of sustained contractions of both flexors and extensors. Hypertonicity is caused by an excitatory state present in the extrapyramidal system which excessively influences the anterior horn cell–lower motor neuron system, i.e., the hyperactive stretch reflex.

Hypotonicity Hypotonia is a level of tone which is less than that normally present in the body's antigravity muscles during rest. It is a state which demonstrates a decrease in stretch and normal postural reflex activity. Unlike spasticity and rigidity, there is a lack of mass patterns of movement, and stability or fixation of posture may be lost. This dysfunction of the CNS may be caused by the cerebellum and/or the extrapyramidal system by way of their decreased level of excitatory influence on the anterior horn cells and gamma efferent system. Hypotonus with CNS disorder is also called *flaccidity*. Hypotonicity may also be caused by damage in the peripheral nervous system to the proprioceptive or motor innervation of the muscle. Disuse atrophy of the muscles may also be considered hypotonia.

Parameters of Assessment The extent to which hyper- or hypotonicity affects function can be documented as slight, moderate, or severe. The assessment process for muscle tone focuses on the following five parameters.

Response to passive movement Hypotonic or flail body segments will allow passive movement to occur with no resistance, except in some rare instances where rapid movements into the end of joint range elicit a stretch reflex response. Hypertonic muscles, as discussed earlier, will demonstrate varied types of resistance to slow and fast passive movements against the pattern of hypertonicity; e.g., extensor spasms of the lower extremity will show resistance to passive flexion and assistance to passive extension.

Palpation The hypotonic muscle is soft and pliable to palpation, and its lack of resilience does not change with changes in the patient's body position. Hypertonic muscles are in an excitable state of often sustained contraction, especially if put on a stretch. They will feel firm on palpation, and tendons may stand out. Tapping of a hypertonic muscle belly may result in increased firmness or slight contraction through stretch reflex reactions.

Observation of posture Lack of postural tone (hypotonia) results in gravity becoming the primary force that determines a usually unstable posture. Flaccid limbs show no active controlled movement on changes in posture. Normal postural reflex activity is usually absent. With hypertonus, the extremities tend to assume a static posture, in either extension or flexion. Postural antigravity muscles determine the most common fixed posture—flexion in the upper extremity and extension in the lower. With severe spasticity or rigidity concurrent with massive CNS dysfunction, as in decerebrate states, total extensor postural states can exist in all four extremities, as well as the trunk, head, and neck.

Testing of reflex responses Because abnormal tone states are indicative of varying states of excitability of the stretch reflex, many clinicians evaluate tone by the elicitation and grading of this reflex. The activity of the stretch reflex is controlled by the balance of excitatory and inhibiting impulses reaching it from higher centers. Therefore, when the pyramidal system's inhibiting effect on this reflex arc is removed, hyperactivity of the arc, in the forms of spasticity and rigidity, results. Conversely, disruption of messages from the cerebellum and brainstem channeled through the extrapyramidal system decreases that system's excitatory effect on the stretch reflex arc, and hypotonia occurs.

The training of the therapist, physician, or nurse in the use of the percussion reflex hammer in eliciting the reflexes in various muscles provides a valuable tool for assessing tone. The quality and quantity of reflex activity in a muscle is usually graded +, ++, +++, or ++++ or as Grades 1 to 4 to signify degrees of excitability. Interpretation of the activity grade is based on the force and speed of contraction and relaxation of the muscle.

Many factors can affect the reliability and validity of reflex testing, which is subjective and must be correlated with other aspects of neurological assessment to provide accurate indications of function. For example, the degree of reflex excitability varies among normal subjects, so comparison of activity in the involved limb with that in the uninvolved limb is essential. Reflex activity also varies with changes in body position, so consistency must be maintained during and between testing sessions.

Effect of body movement and position on tone Changes in body position, especially head and neck movements, can significantly alter tonal states as a result of CNS damage causing the relaxation of certain inhibiting controls on primitive reflexes. For example, a patient with spastic left hemiplegia may have a strong asymmetrical tonic neck reflex. When the head is passively or actively turned to the left side, the extensor tone in the left arm may increase; turning the head toward the uninvolved right side may cause an increase in left-arm flexor tone. Another example is the labyrinthine reflexes, or midbrain righting responses, which may produce changes in extensor tone when, for example, the patient is turned from a supine to a prone position.

An understanding of these primitive reflexes and their inhibitory and facilitative postural effects on tone can greatly assist the nurse and therapist in planning the care and treatment of the patient with a CNS disorder.

Summary Tone can hinder or assist the rehabilitation team in helping a patient recover functional movement. It must be mentioned that many stimuli external to the patient can affect the degree of tone present. Loud noises, vibration, or sudden touches or movements can cause a significant increase in tone and may be counterproductive to treatment. The patient's emotional state is also an important factor to be considered in evaluating tone.

Assessment of Movement Patterns

CNS dysfunction often brings with it abnormal patterns of movement, which the physical therapist can classify and use to describe a patient's present state and process of recovery.

Many patients with a sudden onset of CNS dysfunction, as in cerebral vascular accident with resultant hemiplegia, will initially demonstrate a total lack of movement or tone called *flaccidity*. After the acute stage, movement or spasticity most often replaces the flaccidity.

When movement occurs in the presence of residual CNS damage, it has some common characteristics. The extremities, head, neck, and trunk lose the ability to perform skilled and controlled isolated movements of any body segment. These are replaced by mass or gross patterns of movement in which, for example, all segments of the arm move in a total flexion or total extension response. The patient is not able, for example, to extend the wrist and fingers while flexing the elbow and shoulder. Another example is the patient's attempt to roll from supine to prone in total extension, instead of breaking up the activity into isolated movements led initially by rotation and extension of the head and neck, as in normal rolling.

The neurophysiologic basis for these mass movement patterns is the central nervous system's provision of too much motor unit stimulation through a decrease in cortical inhibitory control activity. Normally, by the process of reciprocal inhibition, the agonist muscle groups at a joint (flexors, for example) relax when the antagonists (extensors) contract. This action is replaced by an excessive degree of co-contraction, or simultaneous contraction of agonist and antagonist muscle groups at the joint. The rotational component is also lost with these patterns of movement. These movement patterns can also be pure involuntary reflex responses. Brunnstrom (1970) labeled these stereotyped patterns of movements in hemiplegic patients *synergies*.

Factors which need to be observed in assessing the effects of these synergistic motor patterns on functional movement are:

- The effect of primitive reflex activity on movement patterns
- The symmetry of static and phasic motor behavior in various positions: supine, prone, quadrupedal, sitting, kneeling, half-kneeling, standing
- The rate at which the movement patterns occur
- The quality of the movement pattern in terms of the patient's ability to assume a posture or position, maintain the posture (stability), and then move while maintaining the posture (mobility)
- Whether the movement patterns are flexor- or extensor-dominated in various positions
- The effect of normal automatic balance reactions and protective responses on the patterns

Observation of synergistic movement patterns and of the ways they and other factors affect functional movement forms the foundation for an organized method of classifying the movement patterns of patients with hemiplegia. This method was developed by the physical therapist Signe Brunnstrom. Through her observations of large numbers of hemiplegics, Brunnstrom described four basic limb synergies. She also observed that hemiplegic patients progressed through similar sequences of recovery, and she classified these into six stages. These synergies and stages of recovery were incorporated into an *evaluation system* which has become widely accepted among rehabilitation centers and professionals and is, to this author's knowledge, the only form and procedure for assessing any type of CNS dysfunction that is widely used by physical therapists.

Because this type of evaluation is the one most often incorporated into the assessment of hemiplegic function, it is discussed here. The rehabilitation nurse will often hear in conferences that the patient is "in Stage 4" or "is coming out of synergy." The definitions of the four basic synergies and the six stages of recovery follow, and a version of the evaluation form is shown in Fig. 17-7.

The Basic Limb Synergies The following synergies are based on complete joint range with all components having developed. Wrist, finger, and toe responses are inconsistent with synergistic movements and are therefore not included in the observation of synergistic movements for assessment.

Upper-extremity flexion synergy When the sitting patient (elbow extended at side of trunk) is asked to lift the arm as high as possible, the result is retraction and/or elevation of the shoulder girdle, shoulder abduction or extension, elbow flexion, and forearm supination.

Upper-extremity extension synergy When the sitting patient (arm actively placed or supported in pain-free range of shoulder abduction, external rotation, and elbow flexion with forearm supination) is asked to straighten the elbow, the result is fixation of the shoulder in a somewhat protracted position, internal rotation of the shoulder, adduction of the arm in front of the body, full elbow extension, and forearm pronation.

Lower-extremity flexion synergy The patient can be tested supine, sitting, or standing, depending on recovery stage. When the patient is asked to bring the knee back toward the chest (with or without assistance), the result is hip flexion, abduction, external rotation, knee flexion, ankle dorsiflexion, and inversion, with possible extension of the great toe.

Lower-extremity extension synergy As with lower-extremity flexion synergy, this can be tested with the patient in any position. The lower extremity is supported in the end range of the flexion synergy and the patient is asked to straighten the leg. The result, which will occur with or without support of the lower extremity, is hip extension with possible adduction, knee extension, and ankle plantar flexion with inversion.

The Stages of Recovery The stages of recovery from a sudden onset of hemiplegia range from the initial flaccidity through reflex-dominated mass movements to voluntary controlled movement at isolated joints:

Stage 1   Flaccidity
Stage 2   Weak voluntary movements in synergy with spasticity predominating
Stage 3   Full synergy movements with spasticity still marked
Stage 4   Active movement deviating from the mass synergy pattern, spasticity decreasing
Stage 5   Movement mostly independent of synergy, spasticity minimal
Stage 6   Isolated joint movement with full voluntary control

Stage 6 is not considered normal movement as the patient knew it prior to the onset of hemiplegia. Some spasticity may linger, but the key aspect is full functional movement. Hand function may be assessed in six stages based on a progression from flaccidity through mass grasp to development of full prehensal control. These stages are listed on the form in Fig. 17-7.

The form shown is an adaptation of the longer one developed by Brunnstrom and fulfills the needs of one institution. Not shown here is the seven-page procedure guide which accompanies this form and helps to ensure its reliability and validity. The key to the development of this type of CNS assessment form is that the nurse,

PHYSICAL THERAPY ASSESSMENT

Name		Age		RIC No.		
Diagnosis				Onset		

1. Recovery stages (Brunnstrom)

	Admission	Discharge	Date and Initials	Admission	Discharge
Upper extremity			2. Motor control		
1. Flaccid			(Nonfunctional, assistive, functional)		
2. Spasticity					
3. Synergy initiated			Upper extremity		
4. Movements deviating from synergy			Trunk		
a) Hand to sacral region			Lower extremity		
b) Arm forward-horizontal			3. ROM (passive)		
c) Pro-sup elbow 90°					
5. Movements independent of synergy—raise arm:					
a) Side-horizontal					
b) Forward and overhead					
c) Pro-sup elbow 180°					
6. Isolated joint movements					
Hand			4. Sensory (severe, slight, N)		
1. Flaccid			Shoulder (Proprioception)		
2. Little or no active finger flexion			Elbow		
3. Mass grasp, no release			Wrist		
4. a) Lateral prehension			Hand		
b) Semi-vol finger extension			Hip		
5. a) Palmer prehension			Knee		
b) Cylindrical and spherical grasp			Ankle		
c) Vol. mass ext. digits			Toes		
6. All prehensal control			LE-Gait		
Lower Extremity			Upper arm (Tactile)		
1. Flaccid			Forearm		
2. Minimal voluntary movement in synergy			Hand		
			Thigh		
3. Hip-knee-ankle flexion sitting and standing			Leg		
			Foot		
4. Sitting-deviating from synergy			Body image		
			Visual field		
a) Flex knee beyond 90°			5. Other evaluation forms used		
b) Vol. dorsi-flexion (heel on floor)			ADL		
5. Standing-independent of synergy			Gait Deviations		
a) Knee flex with hip extension			ROM		
b) Dorsi-flex with knee extension			MMT		
6. Voluntary control					

Comments:

Figure 17-7
Hemiplegic evaluation form. *(Courtesy of the Rehabilitation Institute of Chicago.)*

therapist, and all other members of the team within an institution or system be cognizant of the forms, definitions, and procedures.

Assessment of Coordination and Balance

The cerebellum coordinates equilibrium, posture, and voluntary movement on the basis of input received from the gamma motor, sensory, vestibular, visual, and auditory systems and functions through brainstem centers and connections to control:

1. Balance reactions and tilting responses in all positions
2. The automatic protective reactions involved with equilibrium
3. The coordination of timed sequencing of skilled voluntary movement

Damage to areas of the peripheral and central nervous systems can affect cerebellar coordination of movement.

By an understanding of normal balance and other automatic protective reactions, the physical therapist can assess dysfunction of these through comparison with the normal. No formal tests are used to evaluate coordination and balance. During initial and ongoing reassessment, movement is observed in terms of rate, range, direction, and force and is related to its effect on function.

Assessment of Motor Development

The development of normal motor abilities in the baby, from early primitive reflex movements to purposeful controlled actions, serves as an index for the assessment of CNS dysfunction. The sequence of postural events in the baby—rolling, propping on elbows, sitting, propping on all four extremities, crawling, kneeling, and finally standing—is the sequence often followed also by adults regaining function after CNS disorders.

Developmental abnormalities in the baby and child, from slight developmental delay through severe forms of cerebral dysfunction, are assessed by comparison with normal motor development. Numerous standardized tests are available to evaluate dysfunction at various ages and levels of disability. Depending on clinical interests and amount of advanced training, physical therapists are capable of administering most or all of the pediatric assessments of sensorimotor disability. No attempt will be made here to discuss specific tests, but essentially, most developmental assessment tools focus on observing spontaneous and controlled behavior in various positions and recording these observations in relation to indices of normal development. The effect of reflexes on movement is noted. Specific reactions are evoked by tilting and moving the child in different planes and by the use of visual and auditory stimuli. More advanced tests for older children attempt to evaluate and correlate cognitive with motor abilities.

CARDIOPULMONARY ASSESSMENT

CARDIAC ASSESSMENT

When planning and monitoring activity for any patient involved in a rehabilitation process, it is vital to assess certain functions which individualize the activity according to the patient's tolerance or endurance. Endurance is related to many factors, among them the patient's age, motivation, and cardiopulmonary status, as well as the effects of the patient's current diagnosis and medications.

In the acute care setting it is the nurse and physical therapist who are often responsible for monitoring the initial activities of a patient recovering from surgery or acute illness. Even with the supervision and guidance of the best physician, this process is often risky, because the monitoring of the activity is usually subjective and observational in nature. Whether the activity is the patient's initial trial of sitting up at bedside or the ambulation of the patient with a walker, the nurse has little more by which to judge a safe activity level than gross monitoring of the patient's pulse, color, and respiration and verbal feedback. In order to decrease this risk, the nurse and physical therapist must work together to establish an organized and progressively increasing level of activity that has continuity throughout the day. This same approach of controlled and documented increases in activity can be carried over into the rehabilitation phase, when the team approach can bring increased monitoring and objectivity. The key to success is cooperation between all members of the team.

Definitive testing of cardiovascular function is usually limited to those patients who have dysfunction of the cardiac system. The physical therapist who specializes in cardiac rehabilitation has advanced training, either on the job or in formal postgraduate education, to perform most of the assessment procedures common to this area of medicine. The rehabilitation nurse should expect competence in these procedures only from a therapist who has special interest and training in this area.

The physical therapist, in many instances, is an important member of the team which plans and implements the rehabilitation program of the post-myocardial infarction patient. Determining the patient's levels of activity, ability to return to a previous life-style, and work capacity are important decisions for the patient and the physician. This evaluation process begins early, in the intensive care unit.

During the acute phase, when the patient is medically stable, electrocardiographic (ECG) monitoring is used to assess the patient's gradual increases in activity. The team of physician, nurse, and therapist plans a program of bedside exercises, increased sitting tolerance, and progressive ambulation. The ECG monitoring starts at bedside and continues during supervised ambulation. This early monitoring of activities assists the team in relating arrhythmias, angina, and other heart irregularities to the patient's level of activity and also provides the physician with information on which to base decisions regarding drug and other therapy.

After the acute phase, patients without complications or significant residual problems may become candidates for a more formal program of cardiac rehabilitation. Prior to any quantitative cardiovascular functional testing, the team needs to consider certain critical functions which will provide adjunct information on which to formulate a truly individualized rehabilitation program. Besides the patient's previous levels of physical exertion, the team needs information on the patient's preinfarction life-style; i.e., the emotional, cognitive, and environmental demands, especially in regard to occupation. The overall goal of any cardiac rehabilitation program is to return the patient to his or her previous life-style with, it is hoped, a change in the preinfarction factors, such as stress, tobacco consumption, and diet, which may have led to the onset of coronary disease.

Exercise Tests

The initial steps in formulating a cardiac rehabilitation program are a series of formal exercise tests, usually performed 2 to 3 months after the patient's discharge from the hospital. The trend is toward instituting this testing earlier, and some facilities are now beginning low-level testing prior to hospital discharge. The primary goal of testing is to establish a safe and appropriate baseline level of activity from which to start progressively increasing activities and also to serve as a guideline for recreational and occupational endeavors. Ongoing exercise testing will also provide feedback on the effect of therapy.

Exercise testing assists in ascertaining (1) the patient's functional abilities, (2) the relation of arrhythmias to activity level, (3) the threshold of activity at which myocardial ischemia occurs, and (4) the response of the patient's blood pressure. The therapist, under the supervision of a physician who is usually a cardiologist, can use a variety of methods to carry out this exercise or stress testing. An example of a long-used and basic test is the step test, in which the therapist or physician monitors the patient's reactions to going up and down one step; the quantifying factors in judging the patient's progress are the number of steps and the rate of activity.

Recent tests make use of bicycle ergometers

and, more commonly, treadmills. With these devices the level of activity can be more accurately controlled. The primary means of monitoring activity is the ECG. Abnormalities experienced may include dyspnea, chest pain, lightheadedness, and exertional hypotension (a decrease of 10 mmHg or more during exertion).

In addition to measuring the patient's overall response to activity, the therapist needs to evaluate the patient's activity level in different positions and with different types of exercise. Positional changes in relation to a static activity level may indicate orthostatic hypotensive problems which could alter the patient's occupational outlook and life-style. The patient also is usually evaluated against two types of exercise: isotonic and isometric. *Isotonic exercise* (movement against changing or accommodating resistance) is that offered by the treadmill, bicycle, etc. *Isometric exercise* (movement against a static form of resistance) determines the patient's reaction to static exertional activities such as pushing or lifting over a prolonged time. With isometric testing the Valsalva phenomenon can be brought into play. The *Valsalva phenomenon* is a change in cardiovascular response brought on by the increased intrathoracic pressures caused by straining with a fixed glottis against resistance. This can also cause marked elevation of blood pressure and can have serious implications for patients whose anticipated life-styles involve, for example, such activities as prolonged lifting or playing a wind instrument. Proper teaching on how to breathe while exerting can help to alleviate this threat. Depending on the patient's projected life-style or occupation, the therapist may want to evaluate the patient's response to activity in different environments (temperature, humidity) and different clothing and to evaluate the effects of drugs on activity. Stress testing can also be combined with pulmonary evaluations of blood gases, lung function, etc. This form of testing can provide a myriad of more sophisticated parameters of cardiac function which can be used in patient management and research and which are beyond the scope of this discussion.

The results of the exercise test provide the cardiac rehabilitation team with a *target heart rate,* which forms the baseline for the rehabilitation program. Most centers and authorities will allow activities which produce a heart rate of 20 beats per minute less than that at which abnormalities occur. The resulting program of activity is structured according to four variables, the intensity, duration, frequency, and type of activity. Periodic activity reassessment, along with psychological and dietary guidance, are important for achieving a successful outcome.

PULMONARY ASSESSMENT

Patients with pulmonary involvement, whether acute or chronic, often find themselves interacting with a physical therapist during the recovery stages. The physical therapist who specializes in the treatment of pulmonary dysfunction, often referred to as a *chest physical therapist,* is part of the pulmonary rehabilitation team along with the respiratory therapist, nurse, and physician. In intervening with the patient coping with the effects of various chronic lung diseases, such as chronic bronchitis, emphysema, asthma, or cystic fibrosis, it is particularly important that the patient also constitute a vital and active part of this team. The pulmonary rehabilitation team intervenes not only with patients suffering from primary lung disease but also with those who have decreased pulmonary function secondary to neuromuscular and other disease entities and with certain postoperative patients. A new area is the chest physical therapist's intervention with the high-risk neonate, in whom maintenance of adequate respiration by the use of chest physical therapy techniques is a vital adjunct to mechanical support systems.

The therapist's goal in assessment of pulmonary function is to assist in the diagnostic process or to plan a program of treatment. A complete evaluation by the therapist includes not only an assessment of pulmonary function but also an examination of the secondary musculoskeletal effects of the problem.

Medical History

The first area the therapist should address is the patient's medical history. A thorough examination of the patient's records and a discussion with the patient can provide the information needed to establish effective and realistic goals and a plan of therapy. Such factors as type and degree of previous treatment, previous and current lifestyle (tobacco consumption, allergies, levels of emotional stress, for example), and past and present environmental exposures pertinent to the disease, together with a general "feel" for the patient's and family's level of interest and motivation, are important for all members of the team. In addition, the results of pertinent radiographic studies should be noted by the nurse and therapist.

Definitive Testing

Observation of Breathing The nurse and therapist should observe the patient's breathing patterns, both at rest and when the patient is performing activities and is unaware of being observed. Specific findings that will assist the team in establishing goals of treatment might include (1) symmetry of breathing, (2) whether the thorax is maintained in an overinflated posture, (3) speech patterns, (4) overuse of the musculature considered accessory to normal breathing, (5) frequency and severity of cough, (6) color of skin and fingernail beds, and (7) pain and its relation to the patient's resting and movement postures. In regard to cough production, it is important to note the color, viscosity, and quantity of sputum produced.

Assessment of Breath Sounds In order to localize problem areas within the pulmonary system, the therapist and nurse need to be proficient in examining the quality and quantity of sounds heard or felt within the thorax and its connecting airways. The following three techniques can be used.

Palpation By feeling the chest wall with the fingers on the palm of the hand, areas of abnormalities can be found during breathing and coughing. Pleural effusion or fluid collecting in various areas within and outside the lungs can be felt. Bronchial airway obstruction and blockage cause vibrations. In addition, areas of the lungs not receiving ventilation can often be delineated by palpation.

Percussion Percussion of the patient's chest with the fingers is a technique that, if learned well, can differentiate air and fluid accumulations within selected lung and pleural cavity segments.

Auscultation The use of the stethoscope allows for monitoring of normal and abnormal breath sounds in the trachea, bronchi, and individual lobes of the lungs. Abnormal sounds that may be heard include:

- *Rales*—sounds produced by obstruction, broken down into many types depending on (1) whether the obstruction is "wet," i.e., secretions, or "dry," i.e., pleural thickening, and (2) the location within the trachea, bronchial airways, or lungs at which the obstruction occurs. Loud rales in the trachea and upper bronchi are referred to as *rhonchi.*
- *Wheezing*—high-pitched sounds more prevalent on expiration, indicative of bronchial narrowing and usually associated with asthma.
- *Friction rub*—a coarser sound found in pleural diseases such as pulmonary embolism, caused by thickening within the pleural cavity.

Assessment of Lung Function The pulmonary rehabilitation team uses various devices which record objectively the functioning of the lungs. Lung function tests are usually performed by the respiratory therapist but can be carried out by a trained chest physical therapist or nurse. Essentially, these tests assess the ability of the lungs to transport air during inspiration and expiration. Serial measurements provide data on the patient's response to therapy. By comparing test results with established norms based on age and body size, the team is able to quantify the progression of a pulmonary disease. These results also provide information establishing a more definitive diagnosis. Pulmonary diseases are usually categorized according to whether air transport is decreased by obstruction of the airways (asthma, chronic bronchitis) or by restricted ability of the rib cages, pleura, and lungs to contract during breathing (emphysema, pleural and pulmonary fibrosis).

Common test devices include flowmeters and spirometers. The following are examples of parameters which these devices measure.

Vital capacity The sum of the inspiratory capacity and the expiratory reserve volume. It is measured by having the patient perform the deepest possible inspiration, followed by a maximum expiration into a spirometer. Normal values vary greatly, depending on body size, with a range of 3.5 to 6 L.

Tidal volume This is the amount of air that is transported into the lungs on each inspiration and expired during quiet breathing.

Forced expiratory volume This is the amount of air that can be forcibly exhaled at the end of a normal breath. It can also be limited by time; that is, the amount exhaled in 1 s can be recorded as FEV_1. This gives an objective measurement of the degree of airway obstruction.

More sophisticated devices can provide measurements of the relative percentages of oxygen and carbon dioxide present during ventilation—useful, for example, for patients with emphysema, who have higher CO_2 levels because their damaged and overextended lung tissues cause increased dead air space and resultant decreased oxygen transport abilities. The team also makes use of radiographic chest and lung studies, blood gas analysis, and bacteriologic analysis of the patient's sputum in planning and reevaluating a therapy program.

Assessment of Posture The chronic pulmonary patient will present adaptions in posture which are a secondary cause of decreased pulmonary function. The physical therapist should perform an evaluation of the motion and mobility of the rib cage, the cervical, thoracic, and lumbar spine, and the shoulder-girdle complex. Common postural problem areas include (1) hypertrophy and tightness of the muscles considered accessory to breathing (anterior cervical and shoulder elevators), (2) cervical lordosis, (3) kyphosis and kyphoscoliosis, and (4) decreased chest expansion, including asymmetries of chest contour. Chest expansion is usually measured during inspiration and expiration with a tape at the axilla or the level of the fourth rib or in the epigastric area at the level of the ninth costal cartilage. Shoulder motion usually demonstrates tightness to shoulder internal rotation and scapula protraction.

In addition, the therapist and nurse need to be aware of the patient's overall level of tension, so that, if indicated, a program of relaxation exercises can be implemented.

The nurse and therapist need to coordinate their efforts in guiding and teaching the patient in an individualized program of positioning during all daily activities, breathing exercises, and in the mobilization of postural defects. Patient education over time is critical to maintaining a functional life-style.

OTHER ASSESSMENTS

Rehabilitation facilities and therapists use many other evaluation procedures and tests to assess the functioning of the patient or of assistive equipment used by the patient such as a prosthesis or orthosis. An example is the activities of daily living form shown in Fig. 17-8.

Functional evaluations of a patient's abilities have an important limitation. They assess the *quantity* of function present but not the *quality* of the movements involved in the performance of any function. For example, the fact that a patient can independently transfer in and out of a wheelchair does not tell the therapist and rehabilitation team whether the quality of that activity is such that the patient could benefit from therapy to upgrade this activity. If the goal of assessment is to evaluate the quality of the improvement noted in a patient, then the func-

Name	RIC No.	Birth Date
Diagnosis		Onset

METHOD OF GRADING
   0 — Activity cannot be performed
   1 — Activity can be performed with physical assistance of another person
   2 — Activity can be performed with supervision or verbal cues
   3 — Activity can be performed safely, independently and within reasonable time
   NA—Not applicable   NT—Not tested

Date and Initials	Admission	Interim	Discharge
APPARATUS			
Put on — remove braces			
Lock — unlock braces			
Put on — remove corset			
Put on — remove splints			
LOCOMOTION AND TRANSFER			
Wheelchair independence indoors			
Wheelchair independence outdoors			
In and out of bed			
In and out of wheelchair			
In and out of armchair			
In and out of armless chair			
In and out of bath and shower			
Toilet independence			
In and out of car			
Down and up from floor			
Move on floor, not in upright position			
Manage doors			
Standing balance			
Walk forward 30 ft			
Walk backward 5 ft			
Walk sideways 5 ft (to R, to L)			
Walk up and down ramp			
Walk up and down curb			
Walk outdoors			
Cross street with safety			
Up and down 6-in risers with rails			
Up and down 6-in risers without rails			
Public transportation			
Drive car			
FUNCTIONAL ABILITY			
Assume standing position			
Bed: Roll to right			
Roll to left			
Roll from prone to supine			
Roll from supine to prone			
Move on bed, not in upright position			
Sits up and maintains balance			
Sitting balance (head and trunk control)			
With support of UE			
Without support of UE			
Assume four-point position			
Assume kneeling position			
Knee walking			
Creeping (reciprocal, hands & knees)			
Crawling			

List all equipment used at each evaluation:

Figure 17-8
Activities of daily living form. (Courtesy of the Rehabilitation Institute of Chicago.)

tional evaluation is of secondary importance and does not provide adequate or complete assistance in treatment planning.

CONCLUSION

Any of the systems assessments may be combined to form an evaluation tool based on a given diagnosis or clinical picture, as shown by the hemiplegic evaluation form in Fig. 17-7. It is also, at times, helpful to combine the evaluations done by different professions into one form. In this manner, the specific factors that a facility or system deems necessary may be incorporated concisely and efficiently. An assessment procedure should not only be useful to the person performing it but should be understandable and available to any health professional intervening with the patient.

BIBLIOGRAPHY

Bobath, B.: *Adult Hemiplegia: Evaluation and Treatment,* 2d ed., William Heinemann, London, 1978.

Brunnstrom, S.: *Movement Therapy in Hemiplegia: A Neurophysiological Approach,* Harper & Row, New York, 1970.

Cash, J.: *Neurology for Physiotherapists,* 2d ed., Lippincott, Philadelphia, 1977.

Cyriax, J.: *Textbook of Orthopaedic Medicine, Vol. I: Diagnosis of Soft Tissue Lesions,* 6th ed., Williams & Wilkins, Baltimore, 1975.

Daniels, L., and C. Worthingham: *Muscle Testing: Techniques of Manual Examination,* 3d ed., Saunders, Philadelphia, 1972.

——— and ———: *Therapeutic Exercise for Body Alignment and Function,* 2d ed., Saunders, Philadelphia, 1977.

Frownfelter, D. L. (ed.): *Chest Physical Therapy and Pulmonary Rehabilitation,* Year Book, Chicago, 1978, chaps. 6 and 7.

Hoppenfeld, S., *Orthopaedic Neurology: A Diagnostic Guide To Neurologic Levels,* J. B. Lippincott Co., Philadelphia, 1977.

———: *Physical Examination of the Spine and Extremities,* Appleton-Century-Crofts, New York, 1976.

Johnstone, M.: *Restoration of Motor Function in the Stroke Patient,* Churchill Livingstone, New York, 1978.

Kendall, H. O., F. P. Kendall, and G. E. Wadsworth: *Muscles: Testing and Function,* 2d ed., Williams & Wilkins, Baltimore, 1971.

———, ———, and D. A. Boynton: *Posture and Pain,* Robert E. Krieger, Huntington, NY, 1975.

Mayo Clinic, *Clinical Examinations In Neurology,* 4th ed., Saunders, Philadelphia, 1976.

Moore, J. L.: "Clinical Assessment of Joint Motion," in John V. Basmajian (ed.), *Therapeutic Exercise,* 3d ed., Williams & Wilkins, Baltimore, 1978.

Pearson, P. H., and C. E. Williams, (eds.): *Physical Therapy Services in the Developmental Disabilities,* Charles C Thomas, Springfield, Ill., 1972.

Wenger, N. K. and H. K. Hellerstein, (eds.): *Rehabilitation of the Coronary Patient,* Wiley, New York, 1978.

18

beverly j. ritt
janie j. mccoley

functional
living skills

INTRODUCTION

APPROACHING THE PATIENT

The achievement of independent performance in functional living skills is one of the most important measures of a patient's rehabilitation. Physicians, nurses, and all allied health professionals look to these levels of performance in helping the patient define goals for the future. The patient's ability to reestablish a daily routine often determines his or her ability to reenter society. Occupational therapy (OT) assists the physically disabled person in this process.

In activities of daily living (ADL), the therapist asks the patient to perform routine daily tasks. These tasks become a self-test for the patient to gauge what can and cannot be done and how severe the disability may be. In addition, the process of adjusting to the disability will be reflected in these tasks. Thus, in approaching functional skills training, two factors are involved: the therapist's ability to understand the emotional status of the patient and the patient's readiness to learn.

Stages of grief and loss following a disability are described in other chapters of this book. These stages affect a person's ability to relearn functional living skills.

"I don't have any problems with dressing." **Denial** is the first reaction to the shock of traumatic injury. The patient does not believe that he or she will be unable to carry out self-care. The patient believes the situation is not permanent and that the therapist's time is being wasted.

The therapist must emphasize the here and now and verbalize the team's concern for the patient's ability to carry out self-care. The sessions are guided to provide tasks which will be initially successful; e.g., a hemiplegic is first asked to remove the shoe and stocking or sock from the uninvolved leg, initial training sessions are kept short, and time and tasks are increased as the patient's physical and emotional tolerance allows.

"I'm not stupid. I've dressed myself for 50 years." **Anger and hostility** at the therapist occur when the patient realizes he or she has a disability. In ADL training this patient will have little patience and will feel that the tasks are unimportant.

This is an attempt to avoid the task because of the recognition of disability; the patient fears failure. The therapist must verbally acknowledge the patient's anger and share with the patient the similar reactions of others; e.g., "You seem upset that you have to put on your shirt using only one arm. Most people I've worked with feel the same way." After acknowledging the emotion, the therapist provides shortened training periods and structured tasks to allow success. This encourages the patient to try more of the tasks that have been avoided.

"I can't do this, I'm crippled." **Depression** results when a patient begins to realize that the disability has changed his or her life-style. It can never be what it was, and it is not possible to visualize what it will be in the future. The focus is on the loss, to avoid planning for the future.

Depression interrupts ADL training. The patient has little motivation, and the emotional focus is turned inward, becoming self-pity. The patient feels no sense of worth and consequently has no desire to carry out self-care. Forcing the patient to perform at this time is not successful, and the therapist's approach should be supportive. If good patient rapport has been established, one can acknowledge depression and help the patient express what is being experienced. It is worthwhile to talk about depression because it is an expected occurrence. If inactivity continues for a prolonged period, however, an objective decision must be made regarding candidacy for a rehabilitation program. Lack of progress in self-care goals will be questioned by utilization review and third-party payers.

"I'll dress myself as soon as you make my arm better." **Bargaining** occurs when the patient is willing to work hard to regain normal physical function. The patient is aware of present

FUNCTIONAL LIVING SKILLS

inabilities but views them as temporary. The focus now is on the future and what may be regained with therapy.

The therapist's approach is to bargain in return by offering to do part of the task if the patient will complete it; e.g., "I'll start your trousers over your feet if you pull them up and fasten them." Another approach is to orient the task to meet the patient's goals. For example, "You'll be exercising your arm by putting on your shirt like this."

"I'll do whatever you say. If you want me to dress, I'll do it for you." This is an example of an *overcompliant* patient who may be experiencing a combination of reactions: anger, depression, or denial. Such patients will complete the task for the wrong reasons; they lack the motivation to learn the new skill for their own benefit.

The therapist can use this compliance to initiate practice of ADL skills. However, one must recognize the motivation behind the behavior. The motivation and behavior must be altered before successful outcomes of the training will occur. Rarely does a patient become independent in performing ADL if they are done only for someone else.

"I want to do as much for myself as I can." In the final stage, *acceptance,* the patient makes the most progress in functional skills training and begins to use his or her own problem-solving abilities. The therapist facilitates this by giving support and allowing the patient time to practice. Knowing how long to let the patient struggle is important. Frustration tolerance is higher at this stage because the patient wants to succeed. Giving assistance too early will interfere with problem solving; thus, the chief role now is to "sit on one's hands."

In addition to the patient's emotional readiness, other factors directly influence the success of ADL training: bed mobility, transfers, sitting and standing balance, upper extremity function and sensation, orientation to environment, vision and hearing, sensory and motor integration and learning ability, previous life-style and how it will alter, stress of the activity, and medical precautions. These factors have been evaluated in previous chapters; some of them will be mentioned throughout this chapter as they relate to ADL performance.

FORMAT

The format of this chapter provides a quick reference for the rehabilitation nurse. The problems of self-care are emphasized. Techniques for the hemiplegic and spinal cord–injured patient are presented in each problem area. Other disabilities that decrease coordination are discussed only when the techniques differ significantly from those used in these two conditions. Such disabilities could be multiple sclerosis, muscular dystrophy, or ataxia following brain trauma. All discussion of amputation in this chapter refers to upper extremity only. In each area, guidelines are given for the nurse and the occupational therapist, the available adaptive equipment is described, and the average time needed for each activity is estimated.

Our purpose is to provide information to enhance communication between the occupational therapy and nursing departments and, more importantly, benefit each patient in the rehabilitation program. The specific techniques and equipment can be easily referred to in this chapter. Self-care problems are discussed in an order similar to the sequence the therapist uses in treatment, with initial emphasis on feeding and hygiene, progressing to the more complex physical skills of dressing and bathing. Each skill is then subdivided by major diagnoses.

The format emphasizes the problem-solving approach in teaching self-care. Only basic methods are presented. Therapists, nurses, and patients must be flexible and adapt these basic techniques to meet patients' needs. The long-range plan is to develop patients' problem-solving ability, because the process of self-care adaptation continues after they leave the rehabilitation program.

SELF-CARE AREAS

POSITIONING

Correct positioning of the patient, both at rest and during activity, influences the success of self-care training. Nurses are concerned with proper positioning to prevent skin breakdown and contractures. Occupational therapy is able to provide orthotic and adaptive equipment to maintain functional positioning in the presence of spasticity, muscle atrophy, edema, pain, or joint destruction. It is the therapist's responsibility to instruct nursing personnel, the patient, and the family in the proper use and care of this equipment.

Hemiplegia

Night Positioning The resting position of the involved extremities will affect the patient's ability to perform therapeutic activities. The involved shoulder must be supported by pillows or a foam wedge, with the arm and hand elevated. This will reduce subluxation, edema, and spasticity and the pain and stiffness caused by retraction of the scapulohumeral complex. The patient will be more willing to attempt self-care if passive movement is pain-free. Use of wrist-hand ortheses (WHO) for night wear is a controversial issue.

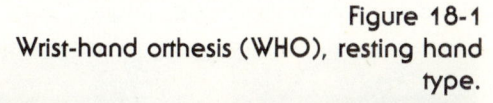

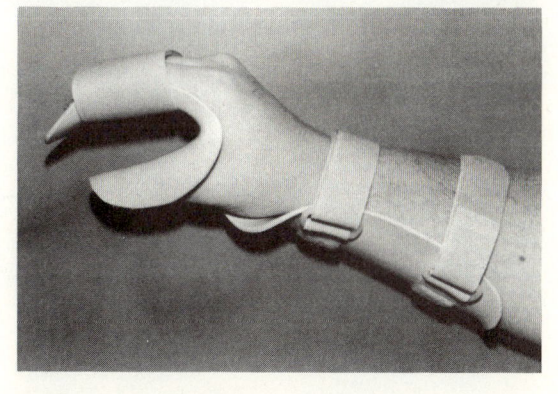

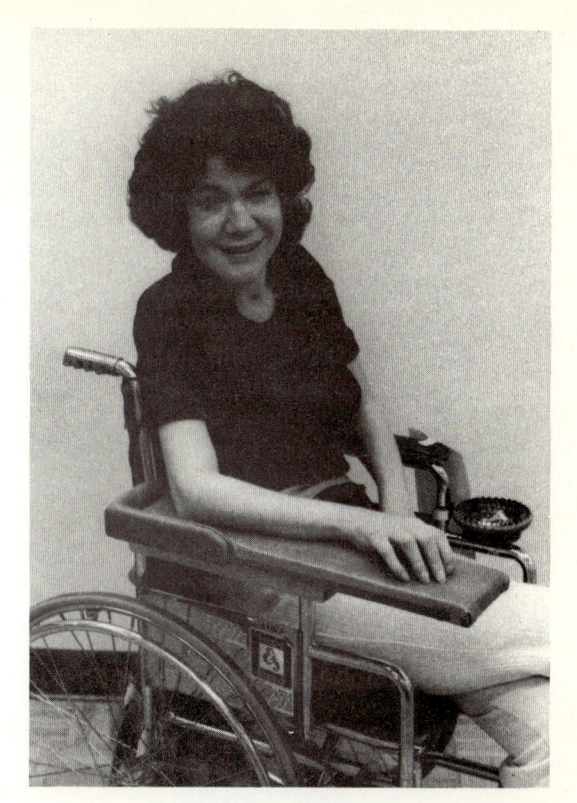

Figure 18-1 Wrist-hand orthesis (WHO), resting hand type.

Figure 18-2 Wheelchair armrest.

Traditionally, the resting-hand WHO was used (Fig. 18-1). More recent theories maintain that this type of rigid positioning may cause an increase in flexion spasticity (Bobath, 1978). The current emphasis is on preventing deformity through active treatment rather than application of an orthesis. Rehabilitation centers have various guidelines for orthesis use.

Day Positioning The purpose of daytime positioning is to provide safety for an extremity with impaired sensation, facilitate motor recovery, prevent abnormal posture, and control edema.

Patients sitting in wheelchairs may be provided with armrests (flat or elevated), lapboards, or overhead slings. The armrest provides static positioning of the extremity outside the flexion synergy pattern (Fig. 18-2). Lapboards or over-

301 FUNCTIONAL LIVING SKILLS

head slings encourage bilateral integration through active or passive mobility of the affected extremity. This body awareness is necessary in performing certain ADL skills discussed later in the chapter.

During prolonged standing or ambulation, a sling may be needed to support the involved extremity. Styles vary, each having positive and negative implications in the total treatment program. Indications for a sling would be subluxation, shoulder pain, or edema of the wrist and hand. Other slings or hand orthoses may be used more specifically by a therapist in muscle reeducation techniques. Slings that encourage mobility of the arm and decrease the flexion synergy pattern are the shoulder saddle sling and abductor roll sling as described by Bobath. Both

Figure 18-3
Shoulder saddle sling.

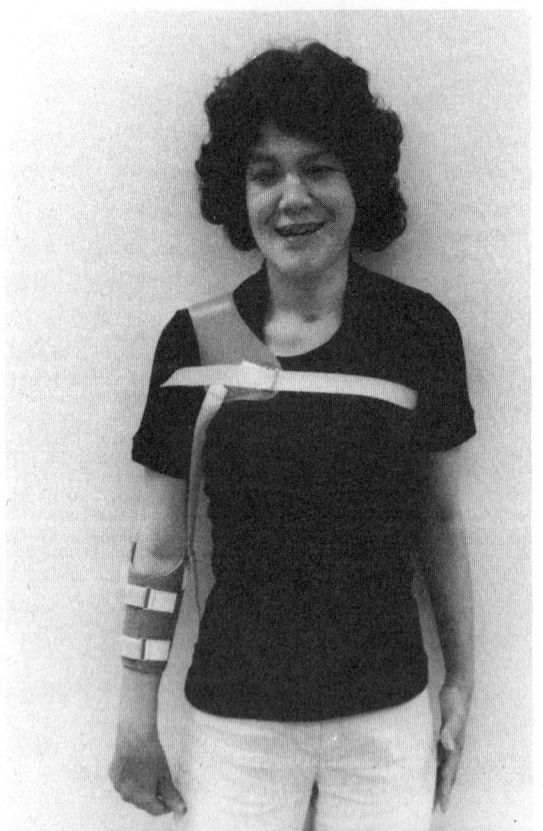

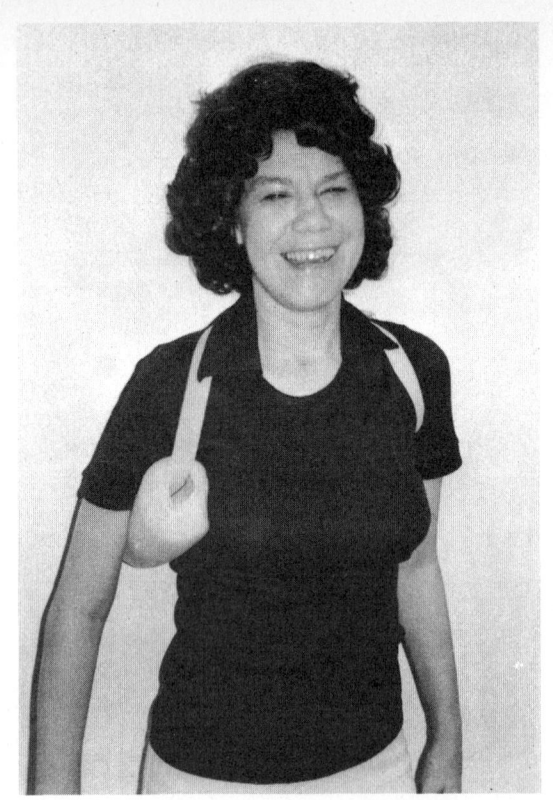

Figure 18-4
Abductor roll sling.

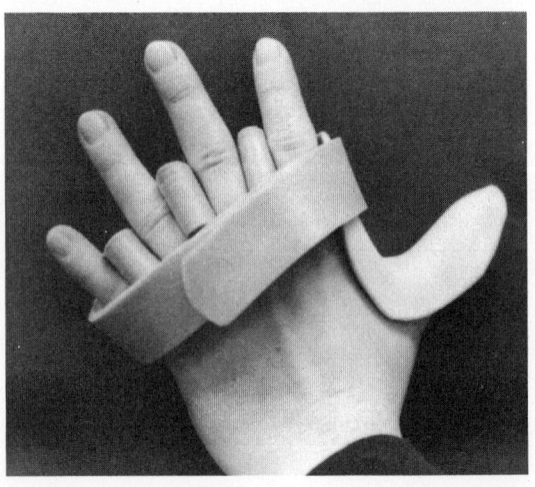

Figure 18-5
Hand orthesis that provides finger abduction.

provide support to the shoulder and hold the extremity in elbow extension (Figs. 18-3, 18-4). Another hand orthesis provides finger abduction to relax flexion spasticity (Fig. 18-5). Immediate application of such an orthesis in acute hospital settings helps to prevent deforming spasticity patterns.

The involved extremity should not remain statically positioned in an armrest or sling throughout the day. The patient is encouraged to passively position the extremity during activities; e.g., arm on the table top to stabilize paper while writing. This encourages the reintegration of all body parts necessary for independent self-care.

Spinal Cord Injury (SCI)

Night Positioning The patient who has lost upper-extremity muscle function requires equipment to prevent deformity from imbalanced muscle forces. Static types of WHO are indicated to maintain a functional hand position of 15° to 30° wrist extension, thumb abduction-opposition, 40° metacarpal (MP) flexion, and 15° proximal interphalangeal joint (PIP) and distal interphalangeal joint (DIP) flexion. Resting-type ortheses (Fig. 18-1) have been traditionally used for night wear. Use of a WHO with MP extension stop and thumb abduction/extension stop (long opponens with lumbrical bar, C bar, and thumb-post) is a more current practice (Fig. 18-6). This allows for some tightness to develop in the long finger flexors, which is an advantage for using a natural tenodesis pattern or other dynamic WHO. Night positioning is also necessary to maintain palmar arches to prevent a flat-hand deformity secondary to the loss of intrinsic musculature.

The therapist depends on nursing to remphasize to the patient the importance of using this equipment and to contact the therapist if problems result from pressure or interference with bed mobility.

Day Positioning The successful use of upper extremities for self-care depends upon trunk stability. High cervical injuries may require application of lateral trunk supports (Fig. 18-7) and

Figure 18-6
WHO with metacarpal (MP) extension stop and thumb adduction and extension stop.

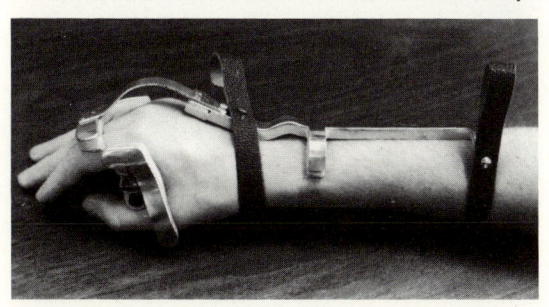

Figure 18-7
Lateral trunk support.

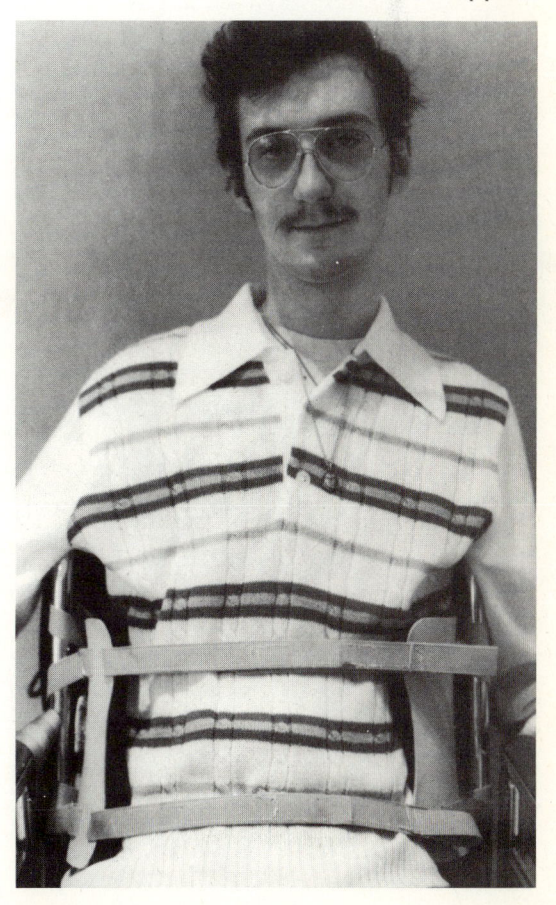

sion slings, are used to provide antigravity support when shoulder musculature lacks strength or endurance for prolonged arm placement in self-care activity. A functional WHO is used with the SEWHO according to patient need, to provide wrist extension for stabilization of the hand, thumb position for lateral prehension, or increased tenodesis action for three-point prehension. Specific orthoses for self-care are discussed in a later section of this chapter.

These examples demonstrate that rehabilitation involves the use of highly specialized adaptive equipment. The patient's ability to accept the use of equipment depends on two things: its positive introduction into treatment by the therapist and understanding and support for its benefit to the patient on the part of other team members. Gadget tolerance will vary with each patient and must be monitored by all team members, who must be in close communication whenever new equipment is introduced into the treatment program.

Other Disabilities That Decrease Coordination

It is especially frustrating to a patient to have motion available but lack the control to make it useful in self-care. The goal is to teach the patient positions that provide stability or control of motion. One of these positions is to keep the arms as close to the body as possible. Another is placing elbows and forearms on a table and pressing downward to inhibit unwanted motion. A raised table surface will decrease the amount of movement needed for activities of feeding and hygiene. Using two hands together will give increased control in a task. The application of these principles is discussed in subsequent sections of this chapter.

Arthritis

Proper positioning at rest and during activity helps to reduce deformities caused by the disease process. In arthritic patients, maintenance of independent self-care depends on adequate range of motion, preservation of joint function,

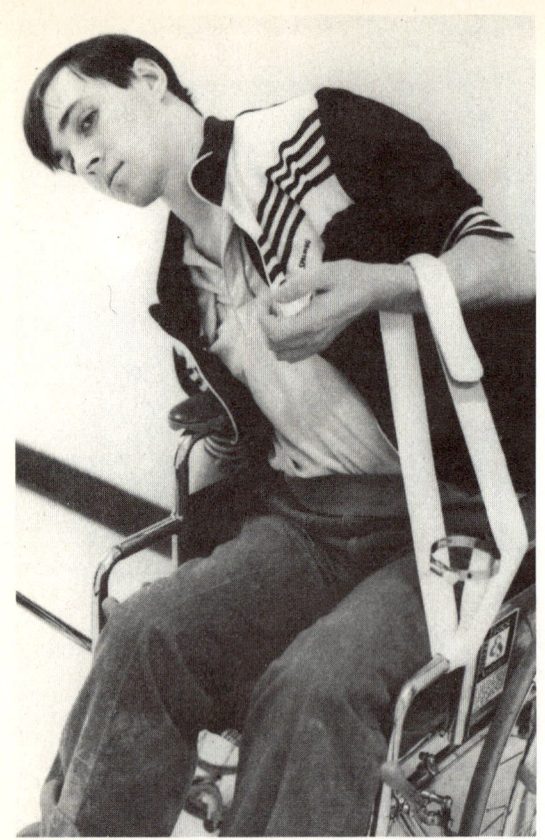

Figure 18-8 McCormick loop.

seat belts to prevent falling from the wheelchair. Leg separators may be used by persons injured at any spinal cord level to avoid adductor tightness, which would interfere with lower-extremity dressing, hygiene, and urinary care.

Patients with injury at or below C5 may use a McCormick loop to relieve pressure on the buttocks and maintain skin integrity. This is used by putting one arm through the loop and leaning in the opposite direction to raise the buttock from the wheelchair. Elbow flexion is then used to pull the trunk upright (Fig. 18-8).

Once trunk position and stability are achieved, the upper arm and hand may require additional equipment for function. Shoulder-elbow-wrist-hand orthoses (SEWHO), commonly called *balanced forearm orthoses* (Fig. 18-9), or suspen-

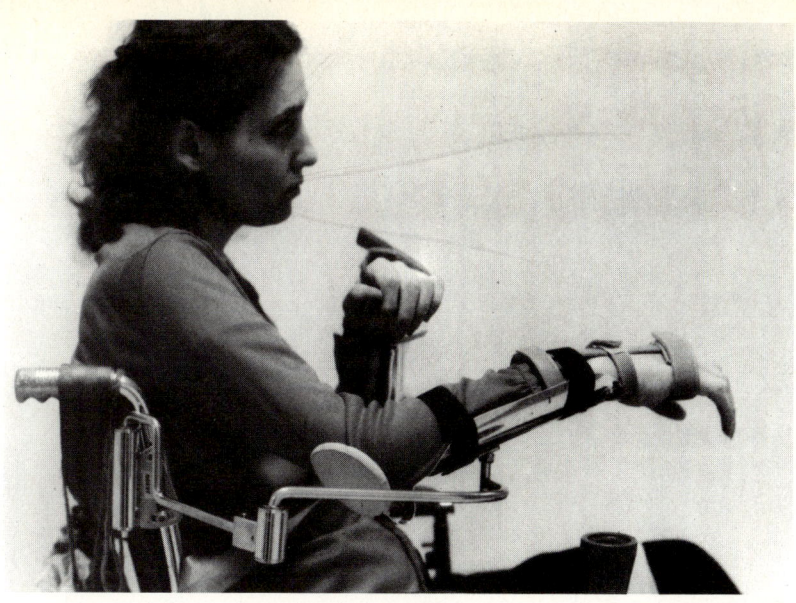

Figure 18-9
Balanced forearm orthesis/mobile arm support.

and, to the degree possible, avoidance of flexion contracture.

Night Positioning   A WHO (resting hand type) is commonly used to prevent pressure or stress on the joints, to prevent further deformity, and to reduce pain.

Day Positioning   Wrist-hand ortheses may also be used during activities by rheumatoid arthritic patients. If the disease process is active, an ortheses giving rest and support to all joints should be supplied. Tasks causing stress to joints should be stopped or at least reduced to a minimum. If the disease process is not active, ortheses may be used to provide support to the wrist or MP joints while allowing movement for functional living tasks (Fig. 18-10).

In addition to ortheses, the patient's ability to position the hands in approaching a task can decrease deformity and pain. The general guideline is to put the least possible stress on wrists and smaller joints of the hands. These joint-protection techniques can be applied to all tasks of daily living and are described in later sections of this chapter.

Amputation

Previous discussion on positioning has emphasized the application or use of ortheses and equipment. Positioning for the amputee emphasizes a different concept. A prosthesis replaces one or more limbs. Control of this device for function requires the patient to have a good understanding of body position and the muscles used to operate the mechanical components. Before manipulating an object the patient must determine three things: the standing or sitting posture, the angle at which the elbow must lock if the amputation is above the elbow (AE) or higher, and the correct position of the terminal device (TD) to give maximum surface contact with the object.

In subsequent sections of this chapter, the approaches to functional life tasks for the patient with amputation are displayed in chart form. The task is presented and guidelines are given by level of amputation, both unilateral and

305   FUNCTIONAL LIVING SKILLS

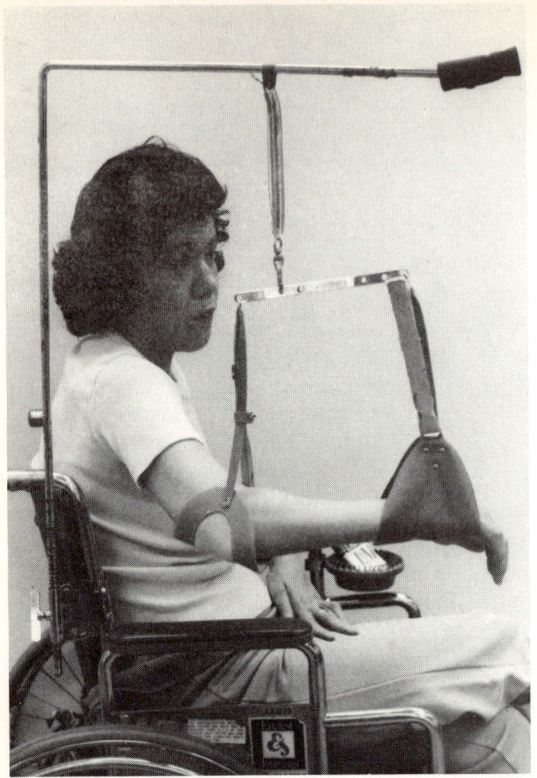

Figure 18-10
Overhead suspension sling.

bilateral. These guidelines will vary according to the patient's motivation and ability to solve problems.

FEEDING

In normal development, self-feeding is the first learned functional life skill. Likewise, feeding is approached early in a patient's rehabilitation program. The patient who is dependent on this skill must be fed three times daily by nurses, aides, or volunteers.

Hemiplegia

One-handed feeding techniques are used by the patient with hemiplegia. Training the nondominant extremity may be necessary. For the patient this is clumsy at first but achievable with practice and support from staff. Bilateral feeding activities such as cutting meat and opening containers are more difficult. Meat cutting is achieved by using a rocker knife (Fig. 18-11), which incorporates a rocking motion rather than sawing and eliminates stabilization with a fork. Containers such as milk cartons may be held between the knees and opened one-handed.

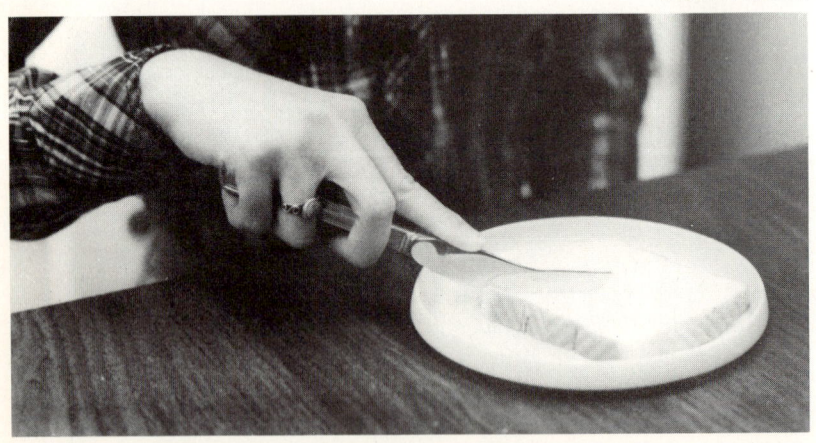

Figure 18-11
Rocker knife.

CHAPTER 18   306

Loss of sensation or movement in oral and facial muscles will affect feeding. Specific facilitation techniques may be applied and are explained in other chapters. Communication among team members is essential for carry-over of these techniques at mealtime.

Visual and perceptual deficits may also interfere. These problems are identified by the occupational therapist, who provides necessary remediation or compensatory training. Such deficits as hemianopsia may cause the patient to be unaware of one-half of the food tray. Until the patient learns compensation skills of scanning from left to right, the food tray should be set more to the unaffected side. As skill improves, this same activity (feeding) may be used to reinforce therapy by moving the tray more to the affected side. Emphasis again is on communication between the nurse and the therapist to ensure continuity in approaching the patient.

The time required for a hemiplegic patient to eat independently is 30 to 45 min, depending on the severity of visual-perceptual problems.

Spinal Cord Injury

Table 18-1 describes various functional levels of SCI patients and their feeding ability. The approach to feeding training depends on the

Table 18-1

Spinal Cord Injury: Feeding

PHYSICAL FUNCTION	UPPER-EXTREMITY ORTHESIS	ADAPTIVE EQUIPMENT	NONEQUIPMENT METHOD	TIME AND EXPECTED OUTCOME
Quadriplegia: Head and neck control, no arm placement	NA for feeding	Eating Aid	Dependent on human assistance (fed by another person)	1 h—partial assistance
Partial arm placement	Radial arm support or BFO—long opponens WHO with utensil cuff, or shoulder-driven tenodesis ratchet, or myoelectric WHO	Friction surface (Dycem), plate guard, long straw with holder, bent swivel or extended utensils, sandwich holder	NA	1 h—independent with equipment setup
Arm placement, wrist extension, no hand function	Tenodesis WHO	Lightweight glass, regular or built-up utensils, adapted knife	Palms used together to grasp cup or glass; regular utensil interlaced in fingers	30–45 min—independent
Arm placement, wrist extension, partial hand function	Tenodesis WHO as interim training device	Built-up utensils, adapted knife	Same as above	30–45 min—independent
Paraplegia: Full arm placement, full hand function	NA	NA	Independent	20–30 min—independent

Source: Adapted from material by Sharon Groch.

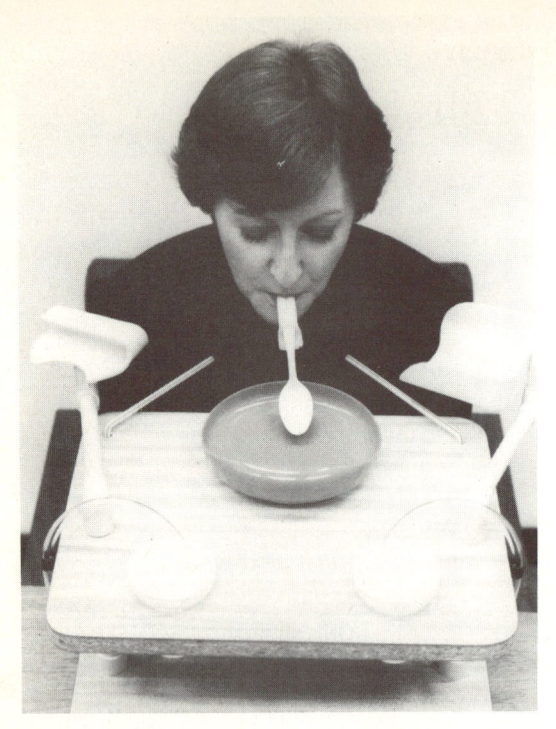

Figure 18-12
Eating Aid. (Used with permission of the Northwestern University Rehabilitation Engineering Program.)

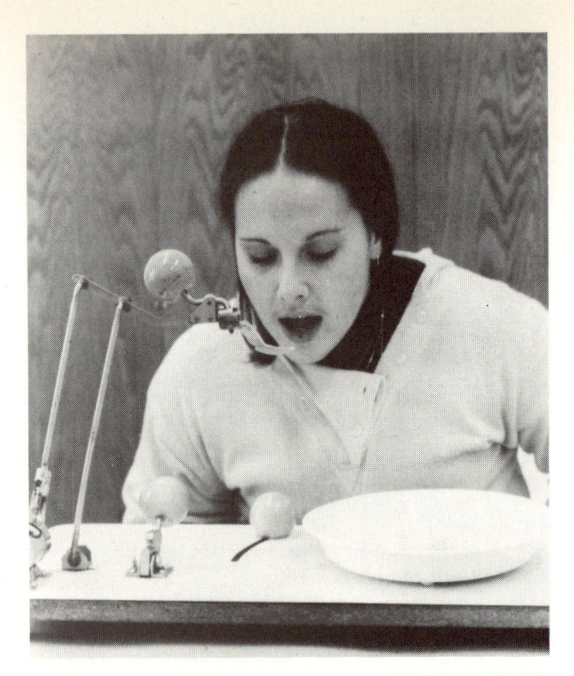

Figure 18-13
Cerebral palsy (CP) feeder. Eating set up for patient with partial arm placement and head and neck control.

Figure 18-14
Tenodesis-type WHO.

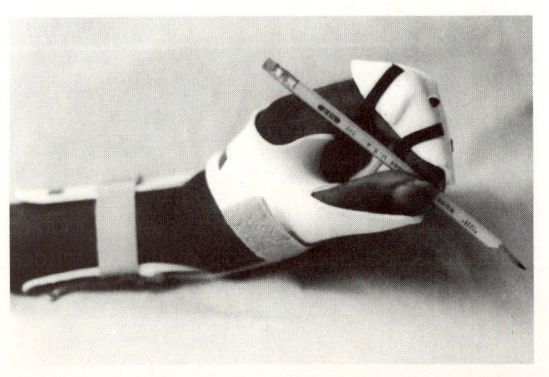

therapist's personal philosophy as well as the patient's tolerance of equipment. It is important for the therapist to provide patients with all possible alternatives and allow them to decide what works best.

The patient who has head and neck control but no arm placement will be partially independent in feeding with the use of highly sophisticated equipment. The Eating Aid, (Fig. 18-12) developed by the Northwestern University Rehabilitation Engineering Program, operates on a single pivot, allowing the patient to use lateral head movement to reach a specific food item. Note: the device is placed close to the patient so that no forward trunk motion is required.

Patients with quadriplegia who have head and neck control as well as partial arm placement have more available options for feeding. One common setup is shown in Fig. 18-13. A balanced forearm orthosis (BFO) or radial arm support allows antigravity motion in horizontal, vertical, and oblique planes. This orthosis requires a combination of fine adjustments made by the therapist according to the patient's available muscle power. Other adjustments should not be

CHAPTER 18   308

made unless the therapist has given specific instructions. A long opponens WHO with a built-in utensil cuff provides the necessary wrist support and a means to stabilize the eating utensil. The place must be stabilized on a friction surface with a plate guard attached. Utensil handles may need to be extended and bent in such a way as to compensate for unavailable motion and prevent dragging the hand in the food. A long plastic straw is used rather than picking up the glass.

Patients who have full arm placement with wrist extension require less equipment to be independent in feeding. A tenodesis WHO may be used to enhance patients' grasp and three-point pinch (Fig. 18-14). It may be necessary to provide a plate setup similar to that described above, e.g., plate guard and friction surface. Such patients, however, will be able to pick up lightweight glasses and use built-in handled utensils or possibly regular utensils. Unlike patients who do not have wrist extension, these patients may not require permanent use of equipment. Orthoses may be used as interim training devices to strengthen wrist extensors or encourage new patterning in hand function. Thus the patients may ultimately have a functional tenodesis pattern providing lateral pinch without an orthosis. Surgical procedures may be used to strengthen lateral pinch and decrease the need for an orthosis (Moberg, 1975). Surgery would be considered later in a rehabilitation program. Without an orthesis or surgery, alternative methods for feeding include placing the palms together to hold a glass, holding regular utensils interlaced between the fingers, and use of a utensil cuff (Fig. 18-15). An adapted knife will allow independence in meat cutting (Fig. 18-16).

Figure 18-15
Utensil cuff.

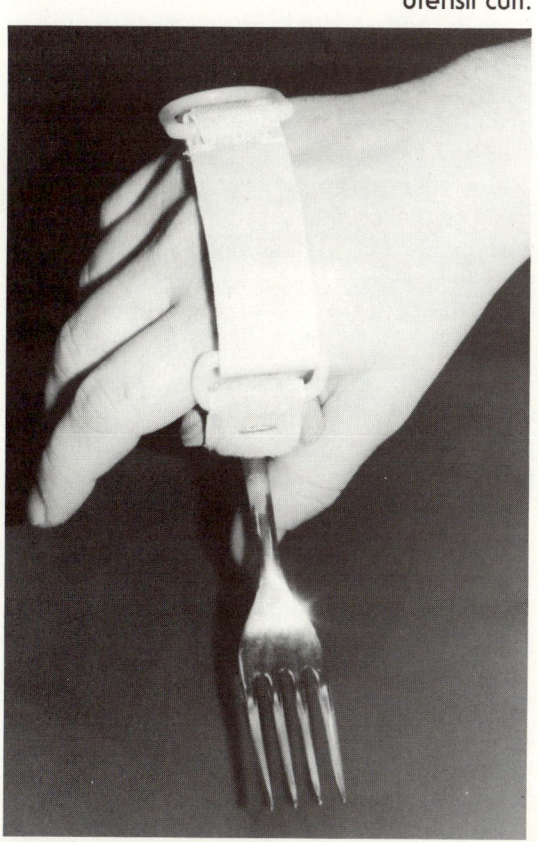

Figure 18-16
Adapted knife.

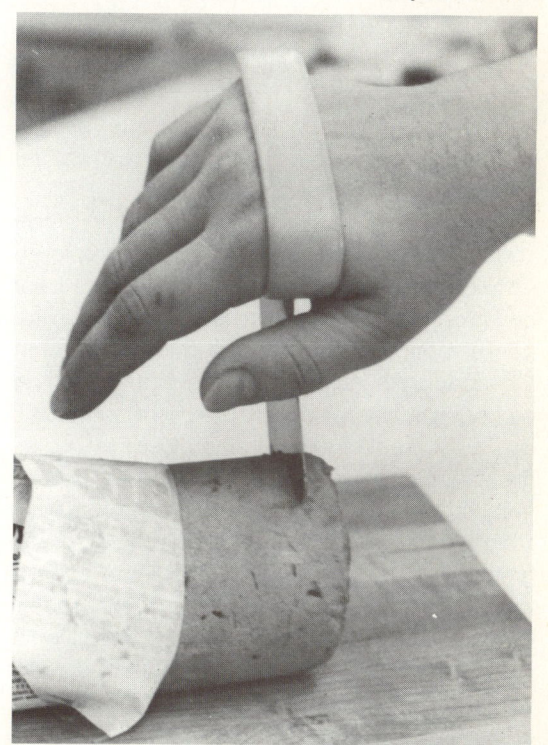

309 FUNCTIONAL LIVING SKILLS

Spinal cord–injured patients with full arm placement, wrist extension, and partial hand function will use a tenodesis WHO mainly for training purposes, e.g., to strengthen wrist extensors and correctly pattern remaining hand musculature. Without an orthesis, built-up handled utensils or combinations of techniques described earlier, such as using the joined palms or interlacing utensils in the fingers, may be used according to patient choice.

Again, emphasis is on providing the patient with all available options and allowing choice of the most comfortable equipment or technique. Team communication provides the necessary support to give each option an adequate trial prior to making this decision. If the patient chooses not to use an orthesis for feeding, this should *not* be considered an indication that the orthesis is no longer useful. As will be seen in the discussion of other functional living skills, an orthesis may serve as the sole means of independence in one task, i.e., writing. The usefulness of an orthesis must be judged by what it is used for, not by how often it is worn.

Other Disabilities That Decrease Coordination

For the patient who lacks coordination, feeding is a long and potentially frustrating activity, requiring 1 to 1½ h for completion.

Positioning principles discussed earlier in this chapter should be applied first for maximum stabilization. Having the patient's elbows bear down on the table helps to decrease the extraneous motion of the forearm and hand. Using the nondominant hand for the actual feeding process has been found to be more successful. Raising table heights eliminates some movement. Application of certain inhibition techniques such as joint compression and rhythmic stabilization prior to feeding will give the patient greater motor control. These techniques can be taught to nursing personnel and family members by the therapist so that carry-over is effective.

Only when the patient is positioned with maximum stability will adaptive equipment be of assistance. Trial and error are required to find the best combination of equipment. The patient must be made aware of this at the outset to avoid frustration. A friction BFO may be used with some success if the positioning techniques do not minimize upper arm motion. Plate stabilization is achieved by use of suction cups under the plate. Plate guards, of metal or plastic, stop the patient from pushing food off the plate. Utensils with weighted handles may be used, as well as long, reusable plastic straws, which allow the patient to drink while maintaining a stable body position.

Arthritis

The treatment emphasis with arthritic patients is to place as little stress as possible on the wrists and small hand joints. Utensils with built-up handles allow for larger, less straining grasp. Use of knives for chopping and cutting should be kept to a minimum. Meat may be cut by holding a rocker knife between the palms of the hands. Small or medium-size plastic glasses are used to reduce weight, thus requiring less grip strength. Using both hands to hold the glass is best. Cups should have large enough handles to allow all the fingers to fit through.

Severely involved arthritis patients who have minimal use of fingers may use a utensil cuff incorporated into a wrist-supporting WHO to hold feeding utensils.

Amputation

Feeding training with a prosthesis requires the use of basic principles of positioning and approach, realistic goal setting, and problem solving by the therapist and patient.

As mentioned previously, prepositioning of the prosthesis before beginning a task is the major factor leading to success. In cases of unilateral amputation, the prosthesis is most often used as the nondominant stabilizing assist to the intact extremity. If the intact extremity was not dominant premorbidly, training will be needed to switch dominance. In cases of bilateral amputation at the same level, dominance is maintained as it was premorbidly. In uneven bilateral amputation, the extremity with the lower level

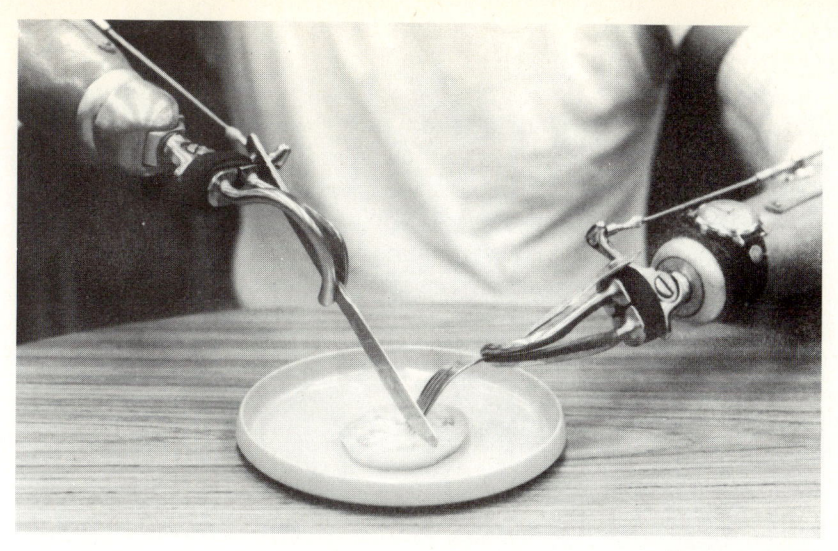

Figure 18-17
Position of bilateral prosthesis for cutting food.

amputation most often becomes the dominant extremity. With these guidelines in mind, the approach to training is to use the nondominant prosthesis as a stabilizer and the dominant prosthesis as the manipulator or mover in a bilateral activity. Thus, in accomplishing such bilateral feeding tasks as meat cutting, the fork is placed in the nondominant prosthesis and the knife in the dominant prosthesis (or hand, in unilateral cases). In Fig. 18-17, notice the varied position of the two terminal devices. This positioning is required in order to provide maximum surface contact between the flat edges of the object (utensil) and the neoprene lining of the TD.

Table 18-2 is a guideline for expected level of independence according to level of amputation. In addition to AE (above elbow), upper-extremity amputations are classified as BE (below elbow) and SD (shoulder disarticulation). Special equipment and techniques may be used in other ways than those cited, which are presented only as guidelines to determine initial expectations. The

Table 18-2

Amputation: Feeding

UNILATERAL BE	BILATERAL BE	UNILATERAL BE	BILATERAL AE	UNILATERAL SD	BILATERAL SD
Independent: intact extremity used with prosthesis assist, optional use of rocker knife	Independent: dominant prosthesis used with nondominant prosthesis assist	Independent: intact extremity used with prosthesis assist, optional use of rocker knife	Independent*: with difficulty: dominant prosthesis used; meat cutting independent	Independent: intact extremity used with possible prosthesis assist; meat cutting difficult; use of rocker knife	Independent with difficulty: dominant prosthesis used; meat cutting dependent; two-step feeder used

* May be possible with feet, especially if congenital amputee.

311 FUNCTIONAL LIVING SKILLS

actual outcome will depend on the patient's emotional status, acceptance of the disability, mechanical ability to control the prosthesis, creativity, and motivation to be independent.

HYGIENE

Oral and facial hygiene is approached early in a patient's rehabilitation for several reasons. The physical motions required to perform these skills coincide with the motions required for feeding, thus it is appropriate for training to occur in both areas simultaneously. Another important factor is the personal nature of these skills and the self-esteem involved in performing them independently. If a patient is dependent in hygiene, nursing personnel find themselves performing these tasks at least twice daily, in time which could be used more dynamically if the patient were independent. OT is available to provide the equipment and training, and with the support of nursing for carry-over, the patient will become independent in one more functional living skill.

Hemiplegia

As in feeding, the patient with hemiplegia will use one-handed techniques to perform oral and facial hygiene. The amount of practice needed will increase if the nondominant extremity is being used. If gross motion is available in the involved extremity, the patient will be trained to use that motion to assist with the task as well as to therapeutically upgrade the function of the involved extremity. Time required for face washing, care of the teeth, and shaving or applying makeup is 30 to 40 min.

Washing Face and Hands If the patient's involved extremity is flaccid, one-handed techniques are used, including passively cleaning the involved hand. A wash mitt may be used if the patient desires. If gross motion is available, the wash mitt is applied to the involved hand and the activity performed bilaterally.

Care of Teeth The toothpaste cap is removed by using a one-handed technique of grasping the tube close to the top and removing the cap with the thumb and index finger. Other options are holding the tube in the involved hand, if some grasp is present, or holding the tube between the knees. The toothbrush is placed on the counter to apply paste or is stabilized by use of the involved extremity. Actual brushing and rinsing is carried out in normal fashion. If the patient has sensory or muscle loss in the mouth, treatment will emphasize compensatory and facilitation techniques in brushing and holding water in the mouth for rinsing. Dentures may be cared for by using a suction hand brush attached to the side of the washbasin.

Hair Care Shorter hair styles are recommended for both sexes. Use of a mirror provides feedback while the patient practices using only one hand to comb the sides and back. Patients with perceptual problems or hemianopsia must be carefully trained to compensate so as not to miss combing some parts of the hair. Many women prefer to have their hair professionally styled. If this is not feasible, a hand-held dryer and curling iron can be used one-handed with patience and practice.

Shaving Electric razors are recommended for safety, particularly if the patient has loss of sensation on the involved side. Safety blade razors may be used if closely supervised initially. Therapists and nursing staff must be aware of the differences between patients with right- and left-sided hemiplegia. Such things as judgment, impulsiveness, and observance of safety precautions will help determine which technique is used and how much supervision is required. The presence of perceptual or visual deficits necessitates training the patient to compensate so as not to miss part of the face. Facial shaving takes 5 to 15 min, depending on the coordination of the extremity being used and the influence of perceptual-visual deficits. Leg shaving requires postural control and may have to be approached later in the program.

Nail Care Cleaning the nails of the involved hand is similar to premorbid care except that

CHAPTER 18 312

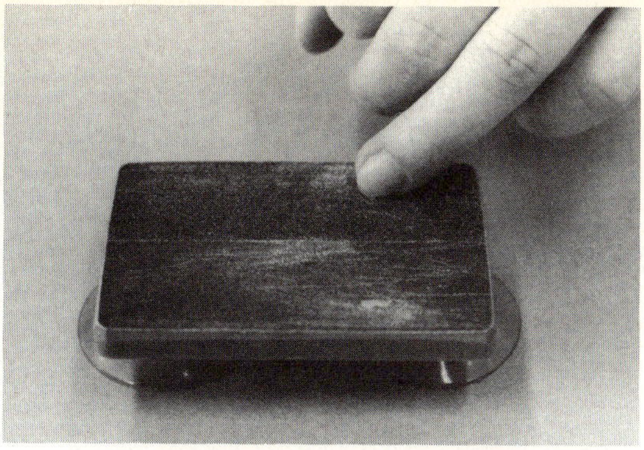

Figure 18-18
Adapted nail file.

the involved hand must be stabilized on a table or against one leg to prevent sliding. Nails on the unaffected hand may be washed by using a suction hand brush. An adapted file is recommended for managing length (Fig. 18-18). Adapted clippers are successful if gross motion is available on the affected side.

Deodorant Deodorant, whether it is a spray or roll-on type, is applied with the unaffected hand. An extremely flaccid or spastic extremity requires training in techniques for positioning the upper extremity away from the body for application. This may be done by lying supine and raising the affected arm above the head or by sitting and positioning the involved extremity forward on a table surface.

Makeup This activity is peculiar to each patient. Specialized adaptations are usually required according to types of makeup used. Containers may be opened one-handed as described for toothpaste or may require an adapted base to allow the container to remain upright while open. Much practice may be necessary, especially if the nondominant extremity is used. Sensory loss or perceptual deficits greatly influence the success of this skill. Using a mirror may only add to the problem initially, because of incorrect visual feedback. Sensory stimulation, facilitation, and other treatment techniques should be applied to ameliorate these problems as much as possible before this skill is practiced. Makeup was created to accent the positive; if misused, however, it will create a negative reaction. Therapists and nurses alike must give support and *honest* feedback as to whether makeup is positive or negative, helping the patient realize the practice necessary to achieve the desired effect.

Spinal Cord Injury

Oral and facial hygiene skills at different SCI functional levels are presented in Table 18-3. The equipment or method necessary and the expected level of independence are correlated with the physical function.

Spinal cord–injured patients with head and neck control but no arm placement are dependent in all areas of oral and facial hygiene with the exception of shaving, which may be done with the setup shown in Fig. 18-19. An electric razor on a gooseneck base may be attached to a table edge level with the patient's face. Head and neck motion is used to perform the task. Assistance is required in starting and stopping the razor and in applying lotions used before and after.

Partial arm placement allows an increase in the SCI patient's participation in oral and facial hygiene tasks. The use of antigravity equipment, such as BFO or radial arm support, may be approached in two ways. If available muscle power is limited, such equipment will be a permanent part of the patient's setup. The same equipment may be used on a short-term or interim basis while a patient is regaining full muscle potential. On this basis the gain is twofold: muscle strengthening occurs as a result of activity, and the patient's self-esteem improves with increasing ability to perform some basic self-care tasks. In either situation, trunk stability is achieved with lateral trunk supports or partial reclining of the wheelchair back. The BFO or radial arm support may be used either unilaterally or bilaterally, depending on the patient's ability and need. A long opponens WHO (dorsal-fitted WHO with wrist and flexion extension stop) gives wrist stabilization. A utensil cuff may be incorporated within the WHO for such hygiene activities, e.g., holding a toothbrush or a comb or brush with elongated adjustable handles. An electric toothbrush with an adapted handle which encircles the palm and back of the hand may be preferred because the additional brush motion provides more thorough cleaning. An electric razor with a similarly adapted handle is suggested for safety reasons.

As indicated in Table 18-3, application of deodorant or makeup is not an independent skill when a BFO is used, because of the placement required for reaching the underarms and the fine motor control required in applying makeup.

Patients with partial arm placement require approximately 30 to 45 min for oral and facial hygiene, with intermittent assistance for setups.

Independence in all six areas mentioned can be achieved by patients who have full arm placement and wrist extension. All hygiene items must be placed within reach, thus counter space must be adequate around the washbasin. With the increased scope of motion, the patient has more freedom to choose preferred equipment or methods for performing a hygiene task.

A tenodesis WHO providing three-point pinch

Table 18-3

Oral/Facial Hygiene Skills by Level of Spinal Cord Injury

PHYSICAL FUNCTION	FUNCTIONAL LIVING SKILL	EQUIPMENT AND METHOD	APPROXIMATE TIME AND EXPECTED OUTCOME
Quadriplegia: Head and neck control, no arm placement	Washing face and hands Teeth Hair combing Shaving Deodorant Makeup	NA NA NA Possible use of electric razor stabilized on gooseneck extension NA NA	Dependent—20–25 min by attendant Dependent—20–25 min by attendant Dependent—20–25 min by attendant Assistance with setup—15 min Dependent—20–25 min by attendant Dependent—20–25 min by attendant
Partial arm placement	Washing face and hands Teeth Hair combing Shaving Deodorant Makeup	In bed: wash mitt, and basin setup over bed; in bathroom: close to sink, wash mitt, octopus BFO-long opponens WHO with utensil cuff or BFO-long opponens WHO with adapted electric toothbrush As above with elongated handles on comb and brush As with no arm placement or BFO with WHO and adapted electric razor NA NA	Assistance—10 min Assistance—10 min Assistance—5 min Assistance—15 min Dependent—5–15 min by attendant Dependent—5–15 min by attendant

CHAPTER 18

Table 18-3 (continued)

Oral/Facial Hygiene Skills by Level of Spinal Cord Injury

PHYSICAL FUNCTION	FUNCTIONAL LIVING SKILL	EQUIPMENT AND METHOD	APPROXIMATE TIME AND EXPECTED OUTCOME
Arm placement, wrist extension, no hand function	Washing face and hands Teeth Hair combing Shaving Deodorant Makeup	Wash mitt or regular washcloth, octopus Adapted electric toothbrush, regular brush with utensil cuff or tenodesis WHO or two palms Adapted handles on comb and brush or tenodesis WHO Tenodesis WHO or two palms (possible use of adapted safety razor) Adapted container Special adaptation	Independent—15–30 min to complete all areas
Arm placement, wrist extension, partial hand function	Same as above	Equipment and method with no hand function; use of tenodesis WHO for initial training only; fewer adaptations necessary	Independent—15–20 min
Paraplegia: Full arm placement, full hand function	Same as above	NA	Independent—15–20 min

Source: Adapted from material by Sharon Groch.

may be used to remove a toothpaste cap or hold a toothbrush, comb, hairbrush, roll-on deodorant bottle, safety or electric razor, and a variety of makeup articles such as eyebrow pencils, mascara, and powder brushes.

Individually adapted equipment may be used instead of a tenodesis WHO. A utensil cuff will hold a toothbrush or safety razor. Adapted handles can be attached to a comb or brush, an electric toothbrush, or an electric razor. Spray-type deodorant containers may be adapted with wider levers or plastic spirals over the button (Fig. 18-20) so they can be depressed with the palm of the hand.

As mentioned in the feeding section, patients may eventually choose to use neither ortheses nor elaborate adaptations. This option is most successful when a stronger natural tenodesis pattern has been developed through wrist-extensor strengthening and some tightening of the long finger flexors. A surgical tenodesis of the extensor pollicis longus may also strengthen lateral pinch for increased performance in these tasks (Moberg, 1975). The two palms together may be used to hold a toothbrush and a safety or electric razor. The toothbrush handle may be interlaced in the fingers for stability. Toothpaste caps may be removed by stabilizing the cap between the teeth and rotating the tube with the palms. A tenodesis action resulting in a strong lateral pinch will serve to stabilize all items needed for oral and facial hygiene, including most makeup applicators.

Patients who have full arm placement, wrist

stability in performing the task. Thus the approach is to gain trunk stability, then peripheral stability of the extremities, coupled with any additional stabilization of the object itself.

As previously mentioned, raised work surfaces decrease undesired trunk movement by allowing the patient to remain in a more vertical position and decreasing excursion between the work surface and the face. The extremities should be held as close to the body as possible, therefore objects to be used should be placed close to the washbasin or immediate working surface. Two hands together should be used where possible to increase the stability of the object used in the task.

In washing the face, two hands are used to manage the washcloth, with the basin slightly raised and close to the body. Other tasks such as

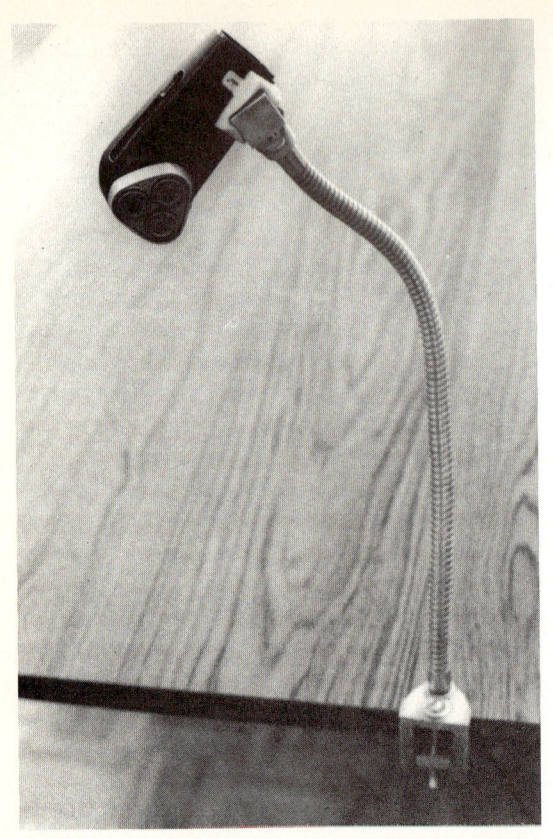

Figure 18-19
Shaving setup for patient with head and neck control.

Figure 18-20
Adapted spray deodorant container.

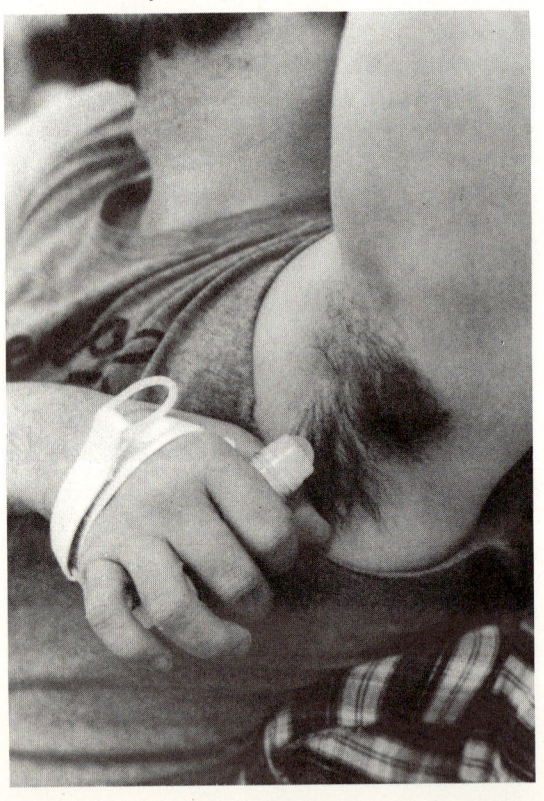

extension, and partial hand function may use, for training purposes, a tenodesis WHO or equipment adaptations and the methods described in Table 18-3 for those with similar arm and wrist function but no hand function. However, after the initial period, many hygiene adaptations are discontinued by patients with this degree of motion. On occasion a patient will continue to use a tenodesis WHO for one or two specific skills to achieve *total* independence.

Other Disabilities That Decrease Coordination

Independent performance of oral and facial hygiene skills will depend on the severity of the incoordination. The treatment goal is to achieve

CHAPTER 18   316

hair combing and brushing the teeth are performed with two hands to increase the control. Many small hygiene articles such as toothbrush, soap, makeup items, combs, and brushes may be placed on specifically adapted holders beside the basin to decrease the amount of manipulation needed to retrieve them for use.

The most important factor in this area of training is patient safety. Electric razors are preferred; nail care may be more safely achieved by having a manicure; and contact lenses may need to be replaced by regular glasses.

The time required to perform these tasks is directly related to the degree of coordination. Treatment emphasizes the patient's understanding of the concepts of increasing stability and application of these to individual skills. Thus the time to perform a task is also related to the problem-solving ability of the therapist and patient.

Arthritis

As mentioned previously, built-up handles are incorporated when possible; e.g., toothbrush, comb or brush, nail file. Fine, individual finger movements are avoided by loosening caps on toothpaste or adding an extended lever to push-button cans. Ortheses designed to provide wrist position and MP support during activities should be used during training. Oral and facial hygiene activities may also be performed while sitting; this in itself will help to conserve energy and reduce joint stress in other parts of the body.

Occupational therapy is responsible for communicating to nursing personnel the patient's level of independence and the equipment necessary for hygiene tasks, and the support and encouragement needed to carry over these skills are provided on the patient unit. This is a major link between the patient's initial training and independent performance in a home environment.

Amputation

Oral and facial hygiene skills require use of the basic positioning concepts referred to in previous sections. One major complication in hygiene is that conventional prostheses cannot be submerged in water, because the mechanical joints will lose their efficiency and become inoperative. Therefore the prosthesis must be used at a safe distance from water faucets.

Unilateral amputation allows the patient to perform most tasks using one-handed techniques, incorporating the prosthesis as an assist. This assistive use requires that the patient be fitted as early as possible, to avoid loss of spontaneous bilateral coordination; a temporary prosthesis is fitted as soon as major healing of the residual limb has occurred.

Independent performance by a bilateral amputee is dependent on the level of amputation. The basic principles to consider are which prosthesis will be dominant and in what position the terminal device will have the most surface contact with the object to be used.

Table 18-4 provides guidelines for the expected performance level and adaptive equipment necessary for the completion of oral and facial hygiene tasks. You are again reminded that these are merely guidelines, which may vary according to the creativity and problem-solving ability of both therapist and patient. It is important to note that the information provided throughout an amputation is based largely on the use of conventional-type cable-driven prostheses. The development of myoelectrically controlled prostheses may allow a wider range of possibilities in independent function. Myoelectric prostheses allow arm placement at more than 90 percent of shoulder flexion and at floor level while bending at the waist. These two activities are limited in cable-driven prostheses because of the length of the cable and the direction of pull. As in other evolutionary processes, however, the greater the sophistication the greater the chance for equipment breakdown and thus dependence during repair. Patients must be carefully educated in both the positive and negative aspects before deciding which type of prosthesis is best suited to their life-style. For example, if their vocation requires stressful labor, a myoelectric prosthesis may not be the best choice.

Table 18-4

Amputation: Oral/Facial Hygiene

HYGIENE SKILL	UNILATERAL BE, AE, SD	BILATERAL BE	BILATERAL AE	BILATERAL SD
Face washing	Independent—one-handed technique	Independent—soap stabilized on octopus, soft face brush with extended handle	Independence possible as in bilateral BE, but assistance often preferred	Assistance generally required
Care of teeth	Independent—one-handed technique; prosthesis may be used to stabilize paste tube to remove cap or hold brush to apply	Independent—paste cap remains loosened; may prefer putting paste in mouth rather than on brush	Independence possible as in bilateral BE; head motion used for brushing	Assistance generally required
Deodorant application	Independent—one-handed technique	Independent—spray or pump type placed on table and pressed, roll-on in small, round container	Independence possible with highly specialized adaptations, but assistance may be preferred	NA
Shaving	Independent—one-handed technique, electric or safety razor	Independent—safety razor, brush to apply cream; electric razor requires special adaptation for stability	Independent—electric razor with adaptation to hold in TD or place on table stand	Independent—razor placed on table stand (assistance often preferred)
Hair care	Independent—daily brushing, one-handed; wash and dry, one handed with prosthesis as assist; hand-held blow dryer, curling iron recommended	Independent—daily brushing Dependent—washing* Independent—drying with adapted hand-held blow dryer	Independent—daily care with adapted extensions Dependent—washing* Assistance preferred for drying	Dependent—cannot work above head, no cable excursion
Nail care	Independent—suction hand brush to clean and large-handled nail file recommended	Hand care—NA Foot care—independence possible, assistance usually preferred	Hand care—NA Foot care—assistance required, cable excursion very limited	Hand care—NA Foot care—dependent
Makeup	Independent—one-handed technique, prosthesis used to stabilize containers while removing lids or in use	Independent—individual adaptations to assist removal of caps, hold applicators stable	Independence possible as in bilateral BE, but assistance may be preferred	Assistance required for such fine motor activity so close to body

*Prosthesis should not be wet.

DRESSING AND UNDRESSING

Patients who are unable to dress themselves require assistance from nursing personnel. Occupational therapy can provide training and equipment to increase the patient's independent performance. A close working relationship between OT and nursing is effective. Just as nursing directly observes the success or progress of the OT training program, OT quickly discovers how well the self-care program is carried over in the nursing unit. Feedback from nursing that a patient is not performing as indicated by OT may mean that further training or adaptation is necessary. Likewise, if OT sees that skills are not being carried over on the nursing unit, perhaps reeducation of the aides, modification of the patient's schedule, or a different approach to the patient may be indicated.

OT generally teaches dressing in the morning on the nursing unit or during the day in the OT clinic. Information concerning the patient's *current* status must be effectively communicated by a means acceptable to both departments. Methods used and equipment needed may be communicated to nursing via 3 x 5 cards, care-plan kardex, or rounds when nursing and OT meet to discuss the patient's self-care status.

Additional benefits from dressing practice are increased muscle strength, general endurance, range of motion, balance, mobility, and stability in various developmental positions as well as self-esteem. The most common dressing techniques for shirt, trousers, underwear, and shoes and socks are described. Numerous variations may exist, however, according to specific patient needs. Application of other garments, such as tie, slip, dress, and outerwear, can be discussed with the patient's therapist.

Many severely involved patients will practice dressing to find their maximum level of performance before deciding whether to incorporate this activity into their daily life. Some persons choose attendant care to conserve energy and time for other activities such as a job or hobby. Others prefer to spend an hour a day dressing to maintain strength and range of motion while decreasing the burden of care on another family member. Nurses and therapists should work together to encourage patients to find their limits and be open to the available alternatives.

Hemiplegia

Underwear Underpants or shorts are put on while sitting.
Dressing:

1 Cross affected leg over unaffected leg.
2 Grasp front waistband in the middle.
3 Pull pants over affected leg up to knee.
4 Uncross legs.
5 Insert nonaffected leg into pants.
6 Pull pants onto both thighs.
7 Stand to pull pants over hips.
8 Sit to fasten.

If balance is not adequate to stand safely, the patient may sit in a straight armchair secured against the wall or in a locked wheelchair. Hips are elevated by leaning back against the back of the chair and pushing down with the unaffected leg. As the hips are raised, the pants are pulled up.

Undressing: Start in a standing position to remove pants from the hips. Return to a sitting position and remove the unaffected leg from clothing first. The affected leg is then crossed over the unaffected leg to complete the removal.

Bra Certain bra styles are recommended for a one-handed approach. Bras with elastic shoulder straps, all-elastic bras with no closure, or front-opening bras are easier to manage. Bras without these features can be adapted by adding elastic or Velcro.
Dressing:

1 Place bra on lap, inside facing up.
2 Hook opposite shoulder strap on affected thumb.
3 Push bra under affected arm and around waist.
4 Pull bra across back and bring to front.

5. Position involved arm close to body and hook bra in front at waist level (With large breasts it may be easier to fasten the bra above the breasts.)
6. Remove affected thumb from shoulder strap.
7. Turn bra so cups are in front, slightly off center toward uninvolved side.
8. Put affected arm in shoulder strap.
9. Move bra to center position and place uninvolved arm through straps.

Undressing: Take unaffected arm out first, then affected arm. Turn bra around so opening is in front and unfasten.

Shirt The method for putting on a pullover shirt can be used for any garment that goes over the head, such as a T-shirt, slip, or dress.

Dressing:
1. Place shirt face down on lap, head opening at the knees.
2. Separate bottom edges of shirt and place affected hand between them (Fig. 18-21).
3. Put affected hand in armhole and pull sleeve onto arm, above elbow.
4. Insert unaffected arm into other sleeve.
5. Gather shirt to the collar, lean head forward, and lift over head.
6. Push shirt back over both shoulders.
7. Pull shirt down in back and line up front sections.
8. Start buttoning at bottom to ensure alignment.

One-handed buttoning is facilitated by pushing the button against a firm surface, e.g., chest or arm. Initially buttoning is difficult, especially when using the nondominant hand. A buttonhook (Fig. 18-22) may be needed temporarily or for persons with incoordination.

Undressing: Unbutton shirt. Lean forward, grasp shirt at back of neck, and pull forward over head. Remove shirt from unaffected arm first, then from affected arm.

A second method begins with holding the shirt at the collar on the affected side:

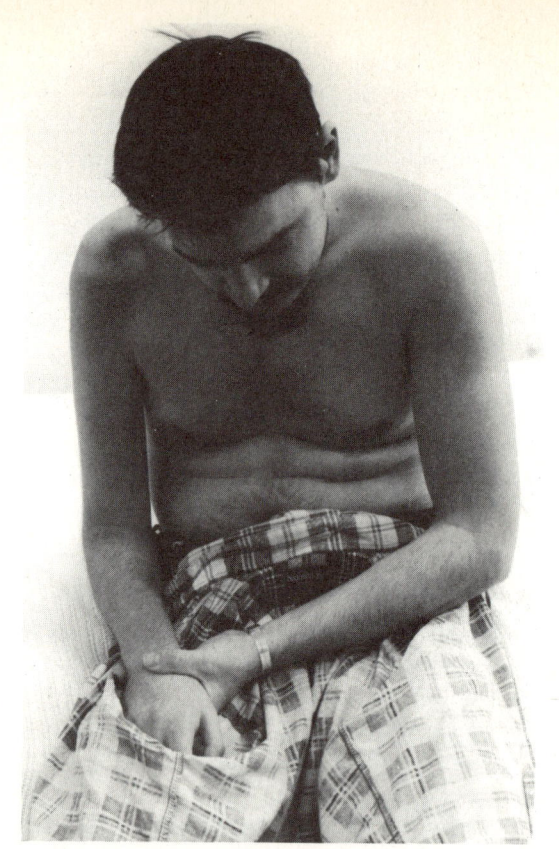

Figure 18-21
Positioning shirt for dressing.

1. Maneuver shirt sleeve over affected hand.
2. Pull sleeve up affected arm onto shoulder.
3. Pull shirt across back and insert other arm.
4. Line up shirt fronts for buttoning.

Undressing: Unbutton shirt. Push shirt off shoulders and shake unaffected arm out of sleeve. Remove shirt from back and affected arm.

Trousers Putting on trousers in a sitting position is the same as the procedure described for putting on underpants or shorts. A reminder: always thread the belt through the belt loops before putting on trousers; this requires less energy, and the process is easier to see.

For the patient with poor balance, putting on trousers in bed is safer:

CHAPTER 18   320

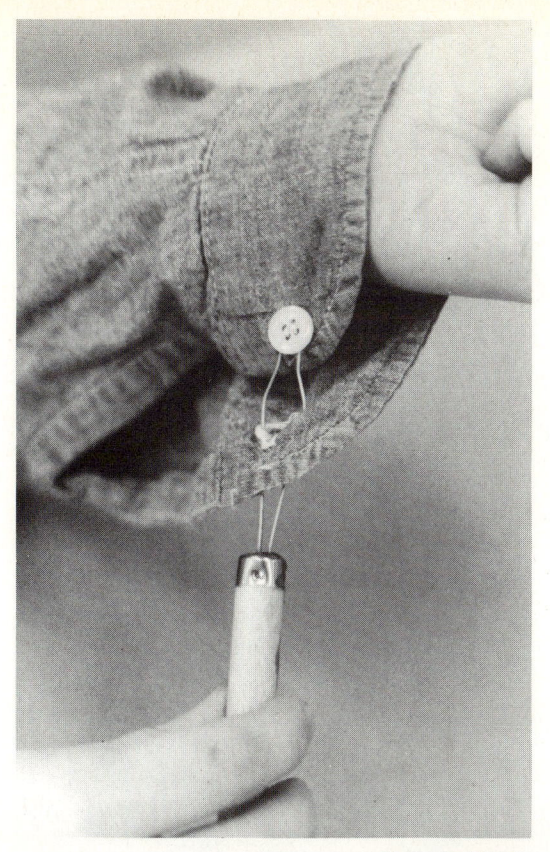

Figure 18-22 Buttonhook.

1. Lying supine, cross affected leg over unaffected leg, keeping unaffected knee bent to maintain position.
2. Hold trousers at zipper, place over affected foot, and pull up to knee (Fig. 18-23).
3. Uncross leg and insert unaffected leg into pants.
4. Pull pants onto thighs.
5. Bridge or roll from side to side to draw pants over hips and tuck shirt in.
6. Lower hips and fasten.

One-handed zipping is performed by separating the hand into two parts: (1) the thumb and forefinger and (2) the last three fingers. The function of the first part is to pull the zipper tab. The function of the last three fingers is to push the material tight against the body.

Removing trousers lying down: Unfasten pants. Bridge to elevate hips, and push trousers down from hips. Remove the unaffected leg first, then cross the affected leg over the unaffected leg and pull trousers off leg and foot.

Socks The main problem in putting on socks one-handed is to get them over the toes. First cross leg so that the foot is off the floor. To hold the sock open, insert the unaffected hand up to

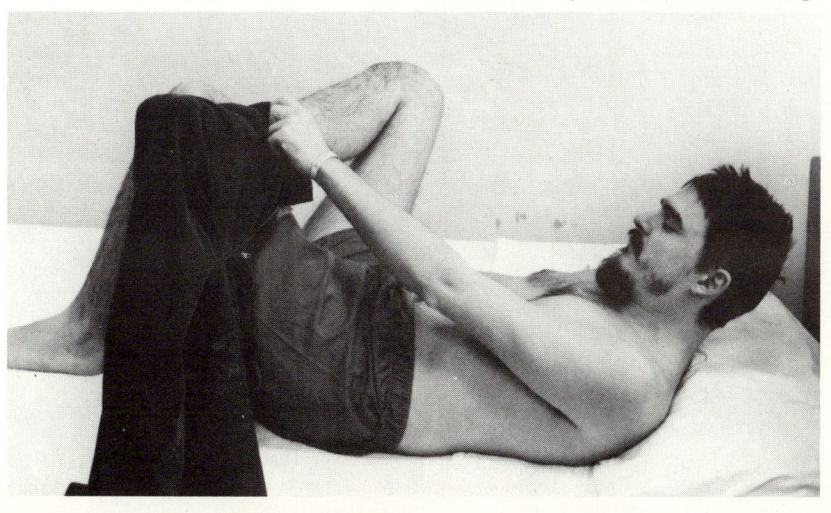

Figure 18-23 Positioning trousers for dressing.

321 **FUNCTIONAL LIVING SKILLS**

the knuckles in the top of the sock. Then spread fingers and thumb to create opening under palm. Slip sock over toes and slide hand out. Work sock over foot by adjusting material on one side and then the other. To remove sock, cross leg and push sock off the foot.

Panty hose are recommended for women to eliminate fastening garters one-handed and the struggle of pulling up a tight girdle.

Shoe and Ankle-Foot Orthesis Shoes that slip on without fastening are easiest to manage. When more support is needed from a tie shoe and laces are a problem, a variety of shoe fasteners can be substituted. Flex-a-lace elastic laces, Kno-bows, and Velcro straps are commonly used. Flex-a-lace elastic laces are laced in the shoe and left tied. The elastic gives as the foot is inserted and removed. Kno-bows is a plastic slide that grips the laces securely, sliding up and down the regular laces to allow removal of the foot. Velcro straps are attached by the therapist or orthotist. Shoelaces can also be tied with one hand, but this is time-consuming and requires patience and dexterity.

Putting shoe on unaffected foot: Place shoe on the floor and insert foot. Use a shoehorn if necessary to get heel in shoe.

Putting ankle-foot orthesis (AFO) on affected foot in a sitting position:

1 Cross affected leg over unaffected leg.
2 Hold orthesis by top bar and turn shoe so toes enter shoe at a slight angle (Fig. 18-24).
3 Pull shoe on foot as far as possible.
4 Uncross leg and insert shoehorn.
5 Place ankle directly under knee and press down on affected knee until heel slides into shoe.
6 Remove shoehorn and fasten.

Shoe aids (Fig. 18-25)—thermoplastic pieces shaped to fit the back of the shoe—can be used instead of shoehorns. These are put on the shoe before it is donned.

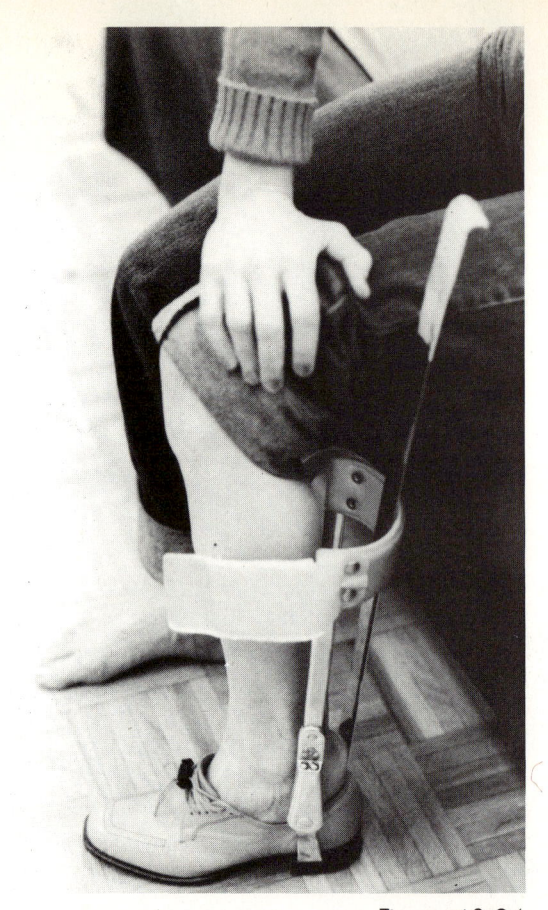

Figure 18-24
Positioning ankle-foot orthesis (AFO).

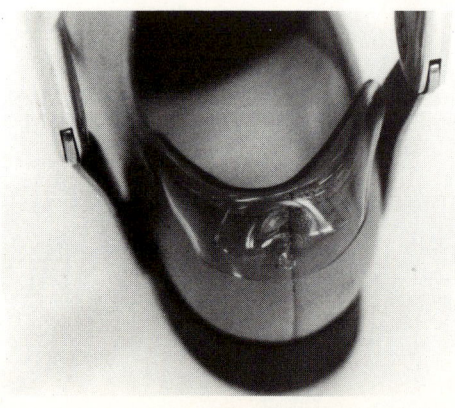

Figure 18-25
Shoe aid.

Removing shoe and AFO: Unfasten shoe and remove from unaffected foot first, using hand or front of other shoe. To remove AFO, cross the affected leg over the unaffected leg. Unfasten strap and push down on brace upright until shoe is off foot.

Time Initially it may take 1 h or more for a hemiplegic person to dress. An average time is 30 min. The possible range is 10 to 45 min.

Spinal Cord Injury

Dressing ability has been classified according to spinal cord injury levels. For example, C5 SCI patients can dress upper extremities (UE), C7 SCI patients can dress lower extremities (LE) and UE (Long and Lawton, 1975). The authors believe that this classification is misleading. Few SCI patients have complete cord injuries at one specific level. Diagnoses of C5–6 or C6–7 are common. Also, there have been several exceptions to the classification system; e.g., a C5 SCI patient who is independent in UE and LE dressing and a C7–8 patient who is dependent in LE because of poor range of motion in hip flexion and poor balance in a long sitting position. (The long sitting position is one in which the patient's knees are extended as contrasted to the short sitting position in which the patient's knees are flexed, such as occurs when sitting in a wheelchair.) Therefore basic techniques for UE and LE dressing are presented, with physical criteria for each task. Patient motivation is a critical factor, particularly in LE dressing, where maximum cooperation is needed. Also, head and neck ortheses necessary for spinal cord healing interfere with dressing training, since they limit head, neck, and trunk mobility. Often intensive dressing training cannot begin until the orthesis is removed or a soft collar can be worn.

Loose-fitting clothes with front fasteners are recommended in early training. V-neck T-shirts, pullover shirts with partial front zippers, trousers with elastic waistbands, slip-on shoes, and bras with elastic straps are some examples.

Loose-knit cotton underpants are recommended for some to protect against skin irritation and abrasions and to absorb perspiration. Jockey shorts do not wrinkle or bunch in the crotch as boxer shorts do; they also hold catheter equipment in position. Other patients prefer not to wear underpants, to save time in dressing. They may need trousers made of softer material than denim jeans.

Upper-extremity Dressing and Undressing SCI patients will be able to dress the upper extremities if they have fair to good bilateral arm placement, minimum half-hour sitting tolerance, and the ability to maintain balance using one UE or the back of the wheelchair for support. The wheelchair provides better support and is preferred to a bed for training.

Donning a bra begins by positioning the bra in the lap with top toward waist and outside facing up.

1. Hook thumb or fingers of one hand into strap on same side and lean forward.
2. Hook other hand and forearm on wheelchair to maintain balance.
3. Push bra around back as far as possible and let go.
4. Switch arms and lean forward again, reaching behind the back for released strap. (When sensation is absent in the hand, movement may be observed in the part of the bra remaining on the lap, or a reacher can be used.)
5. Fasten with loops sewn on ends (Velcro may replace hooks and eyes).
6. Insert thumbs into loops and bring together for fastening.
7. Turn bra to front by pulling and pushing on shoulder straps.
8. Hold one strap by opposite thumb and insert one arm. Repeat with other arm.
9. Push straps onto shoulders. (A dressing stick may be necessary for this.)

To remove the bra, hook thumb into strap and push out and down. Slip forearm and hand out of strap. Remove other strap. Turn bra by straps and unfasten.

The pullover shirt method is preferred for putting on open-front shirts, jackets, blouses, and dresses. To don a shirt, begin by positioning shirt on lap or table, collar at knees and label facing down. Put hands under shirt back and move toward armholes. Work shirt over arms and past elbows by shaking arm, pushing one arm against the other, and holding sleeve with teeth while pushing arm through sleeve. Using wrist extension or WHO, hook thumbs under shirt back, gather up material, and pass shirt over head. Shirt is worked into place by (1) shrugging shoulders to get material down across shoulders, (2) hooking wrists into armholes to pull free at axilla, (3) leaning forward, and (4) reaching back to slide hand against material. Line up shirt fronts for buttoning, using a buttonhook.

To remove front-opening shirt, use buttonhook to unbutton. Push shirt off one shoulder at a time. Rotate trunk and shrug shoulders to slide garment down arms as far as possible. Use thumbs in armholes to push sleeves down arms. With thumb hooked in armhole, flex elbow to pull arm out of sleeve. Repeat for other arm.

To remove pullover shirt, insert hand under shirt front and pull armhole down to slip it over flexed elbow. Pull arm out of sleeve. Repeat for other arm. Pull shirt over head by holding shirt between hands and pulling up and forward.

Lower-extremity Dressing and Undressing

Bed mobility is important for lower-extremity dressing independence. A person must be able to roll from side to side, assume and maintain a long sitting position, and reach the feet in a long sitting or side-lying position. Bed mobility aids are available to assist in these tasks, such as a trapeze, loops on an overhead Balkan frame, raised back support, side rails, and ladders or series of webbing loops attached to the foot of the bed.

Trousers can be donned and doffed in many different ways. One commonly used method is as follows:

To put on trousers, assume a long sitting position in bed.

1. Maintain balance in long sitting position, using one arm for support or leaning against back of bed.
2. Throw pants out so they lie straight on bed.
3. Slide arm under thigh and lift leg to chest.
4. Cross leg by putting wrist under calf.
5. Work pants over foot.
6. Uncross leg.
7. Push leg through trousers with one hand while holding pants with other hand in pocket or belt loop.
8. Repeat steps 3 to 7 with other leg.
9. Pull pants up with trouser loops, wrist against crotch area, or pressure of moistened palm.
10. Pull pants over hips by rolling from side to side.
11. Fasten.

A quadriplegic zipper pull (Fig. 18-26) or a metal ring attached to the zipper will facilitate zipping. Velcro, buttonhook, or a large hook and eye may be needed for waistband fastener. Elastic waistbands eliminate fastening.

To remove trousers, unfasten fasteners. Lying on the side, place thumb in pocket or waistband and push trousers down over hips. (If unable to extend elbow, hold arm in partial extension and pull body toward head of bed with opposite arm.) To push trousers down legs, either lie on side or long sit, place wrist under thigh, and flex leg. One arm holds the knee in flexion while the other works the pants off leg. A patient unable to lift the knee can use a dressing stick to push pants off over the feet.

Shoes and socks can be put on in bed or in the wheelchair. Positioning is important. The heel must be free and the body stabilized to permit both hands to work. Shoes and socks can be donned with one hand, but two are preferred. Zippers with rings, elastic shoelaces, Velcro straps, and slip-on shoes are the most common adaptations. If a shoe aid is used over the heel, it will

Shoes may be put on in bed, in the same way as socks, or in wheelchair. To put on shoes in a chair:

1 Place shoe on footrest.
2 Place wrist under knee and lift leg.
3 Lower leg until toe slips into shoe.
4 Push calf forward with wrist until heel of shoe catches on footrest.
5 Press down on knee to slide foot into shoe.

To remove shoe, cross leg and push shoe off heel, or use front of footrest to catch heel of shoe. Then lift leg up under knee until shoe slides off.

Time Initially, upper-extremity dressing for the quadriplegic person can take 30 min or more;

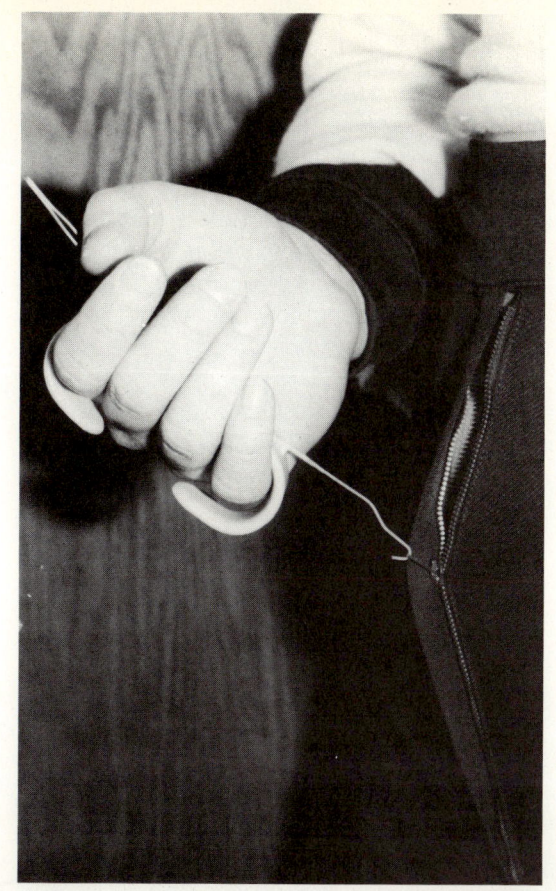

Figure 18-26
Quadriplegic zipper pull.

Figure 18-27
Sock donner.

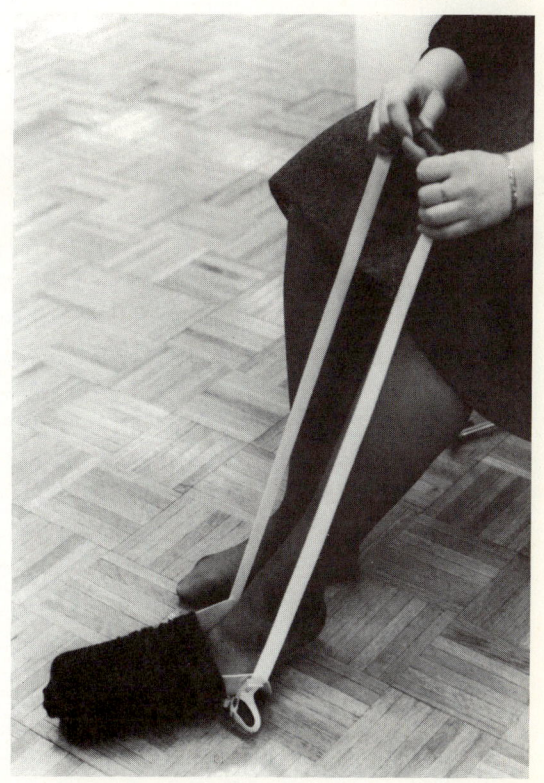

need a loop to facilitate removal after foot is in shoe.

To don socks, first cross leg over opposite knee, leaving heel free. Loops can be sewn on the sock, or a sock donner (Fig. 18-27)—a cone-shaped piece of thermoplastic with a loop attached to the back to aid in pulling—may be used. The sock is placed on the donner, using both hands and teeth if necessary. Then the donner is slipped out and the sock is adjusted with thumbs or damp palms.

To remove socks, push them off with thumb or fingers, providing heel is free. Dressing stick may be used.

325 FUNCTIONAL LIVING SKILLS

the average time range is 20 to 30 min, depending on undergarments and fasteners. The paraplegic in a stable sitting position can dress upper extremities in the same manner as an able-bodied person.

Lower-extremity dressing can initially take over an hour; the average time range is 20 to 30 min. Normal hand function allows the paraplegic person to perform lower-extremity dressing in less time with fewer adaptations or devices.

Other Disorders That Decrease Coordination

The previously mentioned postures of stability are also applicable in these disorders. For example, it may be safer for an ataxic patient to dress lower extremities in bed, where more surface contact is available for stability when pulling up pants. Upper-extremity dressing is more safely accomplished in a straight-back chair or wheelchair rather than sitting on the edge of the bed. If tremors interfere with fastening closures, adapted Velcro closures, zippers that are permanently closed at the bottom, buttonhooks, elastic waistbands, pullover shorts and bras, and slip-on shoes are recommended.

Arthritis

The ability to dress independently varies with the severity of the arthritis. Specific dressing methods and equipment are recommended to compensate for limited range of motion and prevent deformity or pain. Dressing sticks or reachers extend the reach for pulling on trousers, positioning shoes, and pushing shirts over the head (Fig. 18-28). A sock donner with a long loop can be used for sock application when hip flexion is limited or pain is present in the lower back. Built-up handled buttonhooks may be recommended to prevent deforming stress to the hands from fine manipulation, and Velcro adaptations may be used on bra, trousers, and shoes.

Time Average dressing time for a moderately severe arthritic patient is 30 to 40 min.

Amputation

Independence in dressing for the amputee depends on the level of amputation (Table 18-5). As in all functional living skills, it is important for nursing to focus on the use of the prosthesis as early as possible. Closures present the major coordination problem because of the rigid po-

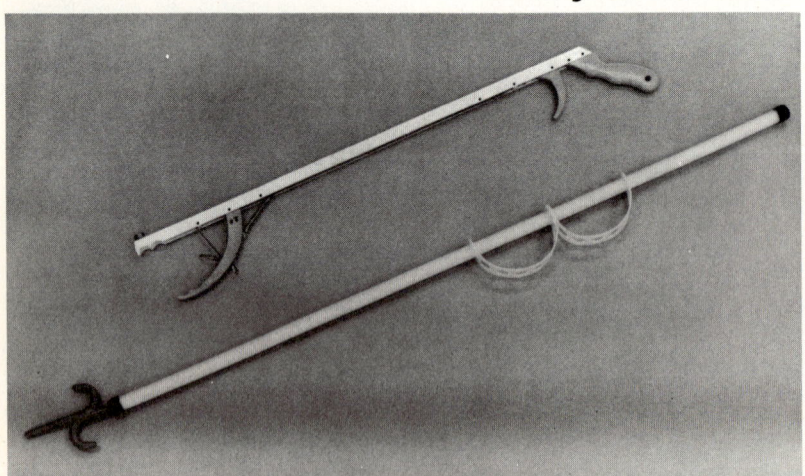

Figure 18-28
Dressing stick and reacher.

TABLE 18-5

Amputation: Dressing

DRESSING SKILL	UNILATERAL BE, AE, SD	BILATERAL BE	BILATERAL AE	BILATERAL SD
Putting on and removing:				
Prosthesis	No problem	Possible—teeth and one arm used to put on other arm sock	Possible—T-shirt with sleeves sewn closed used for arm socks	Difficult—hard to fasten harness—may need help
Shirt	One-handed technique (prosthesis inserted first)	Without prosthesis: pullover method; with prosthesis: either pullover or front-opening method	Without prosthesis: pullover method for T-shirt; with prosthesis: front-opening method, wall-hook assistance	Help needed with T-shirt, front-opening shirt possible
Bra	Prosthesis used to help fasten in front, then finished with one-handed technique	Bra omitted or front-opening bra used; strapless bra may be fastened in front and turned around, or bra may be fastened first and pulled on (BE and AE only)		
Trousers	One-handed technique using prosthesis to hold pants while fastening	Prosthesis used; elastic waistband eliminates need to fasten; hook or Velcro closure, ring or zipper tab		
Socks	One-handed technique or prosthesis used to stretch sock over toes	Feet or prosthesis used		
Shoes	Slip-on shoes used or prosthesis used to help tie (takes much practice)	Slip-on shoes		
Buttoning:				
Shirt	One-handed technique faster; prosthesis may be used to stabilize shirt bottom	Buttonhook and mirror used for top button		Buttonhook used, may need assistance
Cuff	Buttonhook used for cuff on uninvolved arm	With hook TD, cuffs buttoned before putting on shirt (cuff will slip over TD); with hand TD, buttonhook used (this is difficult)		

sition of the TD and lack of sensation. The problem can be avoided by the use of nonfastening clothes such as pullover shirts and slip-on shoes. If fasteners are desired, a wrist-flexion unit is necessary to make possible TD positioning close to the midline of the body (Fig. 18-29).

Time Unilateral amputees require 10 to 15 min, bilateral BE 15 to 20 min, and bilateral AE 30 to 40 min to dress independently. Bilateral SD patients usually opt not to dress themselves because of the great difficulty they experience and the time involved.

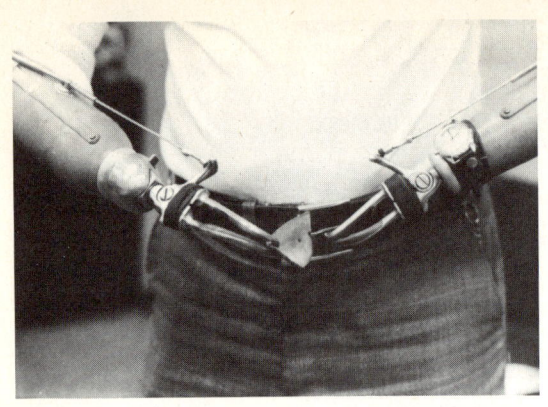

Figure 18-29 Wrist flexion unit used in midline activities.

BATHING

The nurse provides the patient with regular showers or baths at the rehabilitation center. The occupational therapist provides teaching and equipment to enable the patient to be independent in bathing at home. Nursing may also provide the patient with practice time to reinforce independent bathing methods and use of adaptive equipment. For occupational therapists and nurses to work together, three prerequisites are needed:

1. A bathing facility similar to the one in home environment, i.e., regular size tub or shower
2. Safety and adaptivie equipment: grab bars, benches, nonskid floor in tub or shower, flexible shower hose
3. Staff time for adequate supervision of the patient

Bathing is one activity during which the nurse or the therapist must strictly observe the patient. Potential for accidents is high because of slippery surfaces from soap and water on bare skin, sensory deficits which impair the ability to judge or feel the temperature of the water, and complex transfers from wheelchair into tub. Dry skin increases friction and resistance in transfers, while wet skin facilitates sliding. The patient's balance is altered from lack of supportive braces and from increased body tone caused by heightened sensory stimulation. The activity of bathing, like dressing, can be exhausting. The humidity and warmth can lower the patient's fatigue level and determine whether the patient has enough strength and coordination to maintain balance during transfer from the shower or tub.

Hemiplegia

Transfers When hemiplegic patients have fair to good sitting balance, they are ready to begin tub or shower bathing. Assistance and supervision are needed initially, but with repetition and increased confidence less help will be required. Methods for transferring a hemiplegic patient vary according to the patient's ambulation status. A patient who has good standing balance and walks with a cane may not need adaptive equipment. If standing balance is fair and the patient has difficulty rising up from sitting in the tub, a grab bar and low stool are used. The patient who can only stand and pivot will need a grab bar and bath bench. The standing pivot transfer is described here, as it is most commonly used in early stages of training.

1. Place wheelchair or straight chair parallel to tub.
2. Place bath bench (or chair with cane tips on legs) in tub.
3. Place one leg in tub. If this is the affected leg, assist with hand if necessary.
4. Hold grab bar, stand, and sit on bench.
5. Lift other leg into tub.

Make sure the bath bench is positioned close to faucets to allow reach without losing balance. Also position soap, washcloth, back brush, and shampoo within easy reach. An octopus (Fig. 18-30) to stabilize the soap is helpful.

Washing and Drying The unaffected arm is washed by placing the cloth over the unaffected leg, holding the cloth edge between the knees, and sliding the arm against the cloth. The axillary region is cleansed by holding the cloth in the

CHAPTER 18 328

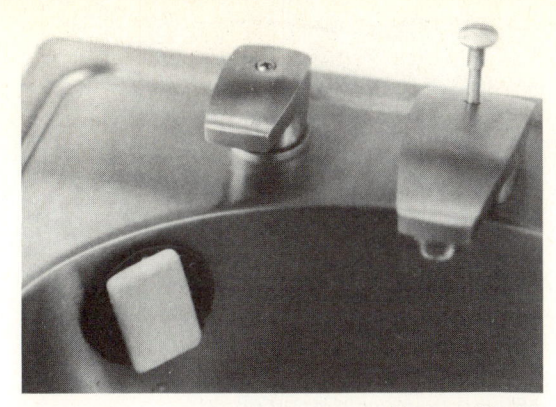

Figure 18-30
Octopus for soap stabilization.

unaffected hand and reaching under the arm. Weight is shifted from side to side to cleanse the buttocks. Precautions must be taken if poor sitting balance interferes with reaching the lower legs and feet. A long-handled bath brush may be used for this, as well as for reaching the back.

The unaffected arm is dried the same way as it is washed. The patient places the towel across the lap and rubs the arm against it. The axilla is dried by holding the towel in the unaffected hand and reaching under the arm. The back is dried by placing the towel on the back and pulling forward slowly, over first one shoulder and then the other.

Time From 45 min to 1 h.

Spinal Cord Injury

A person injured at C5–6 level or below can be expected to perform independently. Two functions are required before bathing training begins: (1) ability to reach all body parts with one hand or bath brush (patient uses other hand to maintain balance); (2) ability to transfer with supervision or minimal assist. Bathing transfers are similar to other SCI transfers which use a sliding board. A Lumex bath bench is used instead of a sliding board; it has legs that extend outside the tub, bringing the edge of the bench close to the wheelchair, and a deep seat for more support (Fig. 18-31). The bench should be positioned at the same height as the wheelchair. Other equipment needed might include a grab bar or a shower chair with cutout bottom to facilitate washing the buttocks. Shower curtains are easier to manage than a sliding door; a flexible shower hose may need adaptation for weak hand grasp. A paraplegic patient needs minimal adaptation; e.g., a grab bar for transfers to the floor of the tub. The procedure for washing and drying is as follows:

A wash mitt or cloth held between two hands is used for washing. Soap on a rope around the neck allows easy soaping of the cloth. The pressure of two hands is greater than one and is often preferred if balance can be maintained. A long-handled bath brush with adapted handle

Figure 18-31
Bath bench.

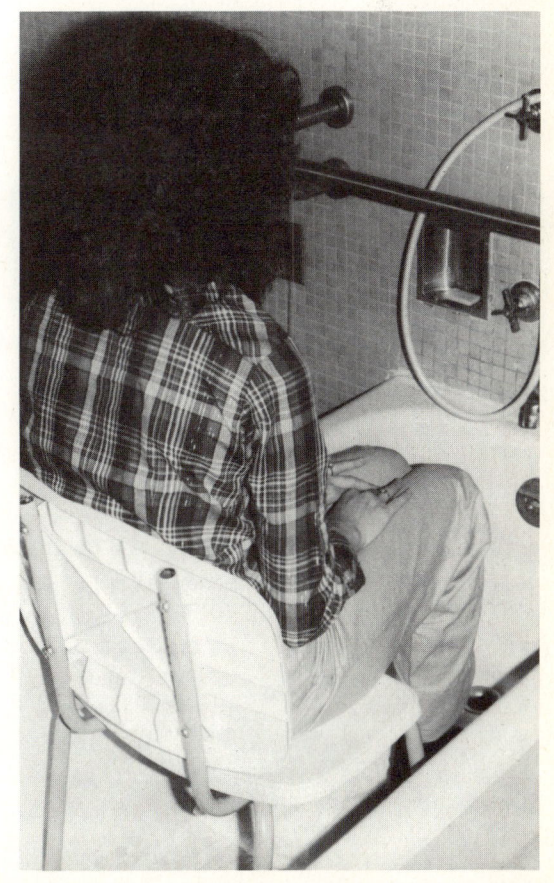

329 FUNCTIONAL LIVING SKILLS

can be used to reach the back and lower legs. For hair washing, shampoo is applied to the forearm or wrist, then to the hair. Tube shampoo is recommended for easier handling. Shampoo is rubbed into the hair by using pressure of the forearm and wrist or a brush that slips over the fingers. For rinsing an adapted flexible shower hose is used.

The hair and front of the body are towel-dried while in the tub. The towel is then placed on the seat and back of the wheelchair, and the patient transfers into the wheelchair to dry the back and buttocks. Other options are wearing a terry-cloth robe or adapting a towel with loops to dry the back.

Time   From 1 to 1½ h.

Arthritis

Techniques and equipment used for SCI and hemiplegic patients may be helpful for the arthritic patient as well. Range of motion and presence of deformity or pain define the approach, equipment needed, and level of independence. The time for the activity varies accordingly. Long-handled sponges and reachers are most commonly used when limited range of motion is present. The therapeutic benefit of soaking painful joints in warm water conflicts with the inabilty to stand up from the bottom of the tub. Solutions range from soaking only hands and feet to using a hydraulic bath seat to lower and raise oneself in the tub.

Amputation

The major problem in bathing with an amputation is that protheses must not get wet, as water disrupts the function of the mechanical joints. Ingenuity is important in this activity. Other body parts can be used, such as the head or feet, or a plastic cuff can be constructed by the occupational therapist to stabilize a sponge or bath brush. Other equipment may include wash mitt, bath sponge, sponge surface mounted on wall, adapted towel, or terry-cloth robe. See Table 18-6 for techniques and equipment used for different levels of amputation.

Time   From 30 to 60 minutes.

TOILETING

Nursing has the primary responsibility for toileting patients. An occupational therapist is trained to teach toilet transfers to patients and also provide training and equipment for clothing management, cleaning, menstrual care, and catheter care.

Hemiplegia

Unfastening closures with one hand is not difficult. Buttons and snaps come apart easily. Zippers may require more practice but usually slide down smoothly. If zippers stick, the patient must use the last three fingers as a second hand, i.e., holding the last three fingers close together, push

Table 18-6

Amputation: Bathing (Bath or Shower)

UNILATERAL BE, AE, SD	BILATERAL		
	BE	AE	SD
One-handed techniques and equipment as in hemiplegia	Adapted Magic soaper and wash mitt	Feet, wall-mounted sponges, adapted wash mitt, magic soaper, or terry-cloth chair covers; may need help setting up equipment	

CHAPTER 18   330

trousers against the body to stabilize the material and use the index finger and thumb to manipulate the zipper tab more effectively.

Unfastened trousers are slipped down over the hips in one of three ways, depending on the patient's balance and ability to transfer. The patient can push the pants down to knees (1) in the wheelchair prior to a pivot transfer, (2) while standing in front of a toilet before sitting, or (3) after sitting on the toilet. When assisting or supervising a patient in this skill, two factors must be recognized to ensure safety: the unaffected hand generally used for support is now used to get trousers up and down, and weight may be shifted from leg to leg during clothing management. Either one of these changes in postural support will alter the balance and create the potential for a fall. In addition, patient anxiety may increase because of the desire to avoid accidents. Anxiety plus a full bladder tend to increase spasticity, which adversely affects a patient's balance. The type of transfer will vary according to the patient's balance and strength. Communication with the patient's therapist provides information on the technique and the assistance or supervision necessary.

Cleaning the anal area is no problem if the patient can shift weight forward or toward the involved side without losing balance. Otherwise the patient must approach cleaning from the back and front separately.

The clothing can be managed after toileting while standing or while sitting in the wheelchair. If standing, the patient may lean the noninvolved side against the wall for more support (Fig. 18-32). If seated, the patient can rock from side to side or bridge to pull trousers over hips. One-handed fastening techniques have been described earlier, in the section on dressing.

Managing supplies for menstrual care may require practice in opening packages with one hand. Insertion of a tampon is normally a one-handed activity. Positioning and balance on the toilet are the main emphases. For those who use sanitary napkins, brands with self-adhesive backing are recommended.

Catheter use for a hemiplegic patient is usually

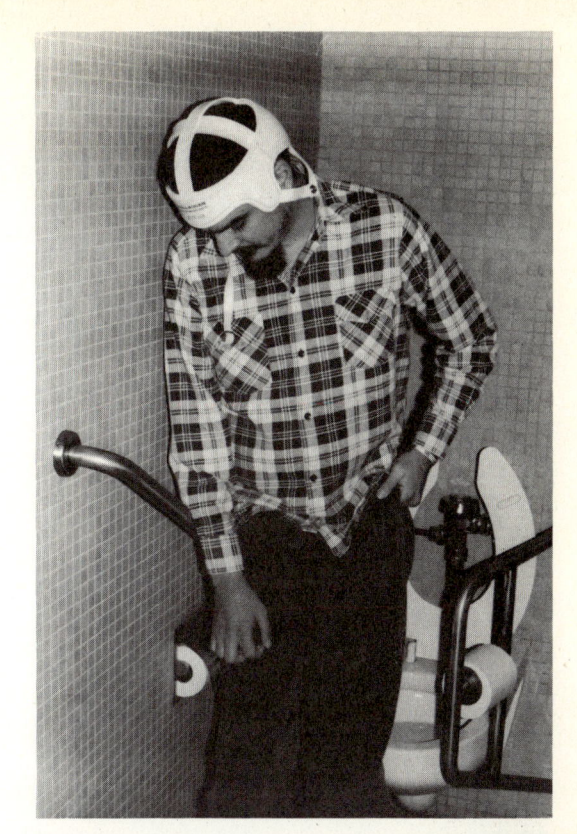

Figure 18-32
Managing clothing after toileting.

temporary and short-term. If it is permanent, the patient will probably be severely involved and unable to carry out independent catheter care. One-handed catheter techniques are discussed in the following section.

Spinal Cord Injury

Urinary management for quadriplegic patients has been presented in other chapters. Adaptive equipment and alternative methods to increase independence in urinary management are discussed in this section. Paraplegic patients have no problem with regular equipment. A reusable catheter for self-catheterization has been developed that allows simple, economical, and sterile catheterization (Wu, 1978).

331 FUNCTIONAL LIVING SKILLS

The role of the nurse and occupational therapist were well defined by a Midwest rehabilitation center (Groch, 1977). Nursing was responsible for:

1 Monitoring method of urinary management
2 Instructing primary care given in urinary management
3 Initiating urinary precautions
4 Contacting occupational therapist regarding problem areas in use of urinary equipment

The responsibilities of occupational therapy included:

1 Suggesting, fabricating, and instructing patient and family in use of adaptive clothing and equipment for increasing independence in catheter care
2 Providing work simplification techniques and safety precautions by giving alternatives in positioning and equipment handling
3 Providing resources for commercially and noncommercially available adaptive equipment
4 Maintaining communication with patient's nurse regarding current status in management of adaptive equipment

Managing Catheter and Leg Bag Patients with spinal cord injury at C5 level or below are ready to begin training in this skill if they are able to reach their feet and return to a sitting position independently. One of the first tasks to be mastered is emptying the leg bag. Adapted clamps are available to allow independent performance (Fig. 18-33). If the patient is unable to reach the feet, a Velcro or zippered opening is made in long trousers below the knee. The patient is able then to pull the catheter tubing out and into position on the toilet. If the toilet is not accessible, the SCI patient must learn to empty the catheter into a commode or urinal or other plastic container (e.g., detergent bottle) placed on the wheelchair.

Attaching the leg bag to the leg is the second skill commonly learned. The patient usually at-

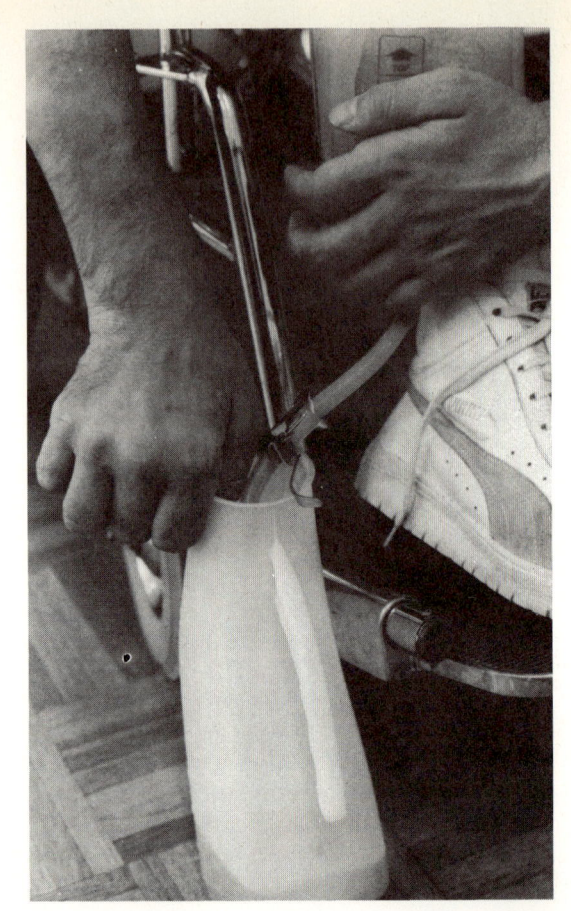

Figure 18-33
Adapted leg bag clamp.

taches the leg bag while in a long sitting position in bed. Straps are adapted with thumb loops and Velcro closures (Fig. 18-34). Positioning of the lower extremities increases independence, e.g., crossing the leg over the opposite knee to attach leg bag.

Connecting catheter tubing to the leg bag and changing the leg bag to a night drainage bag are done by using ortheses, natural tenodesis action, or pressure of palms together. Cone-shaped connectors must be used.

Usually independent bowel care and external catheter application are achieved next. For independent bowel care, suppository inserters and digital stimulators have been designed for use

CHAPTER 18   332

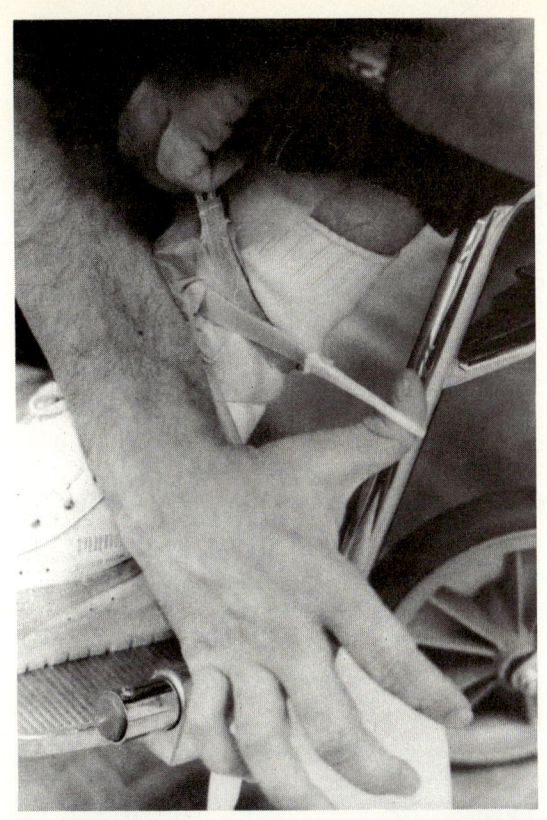

Figure 18-34
Adapted leg bag straps.

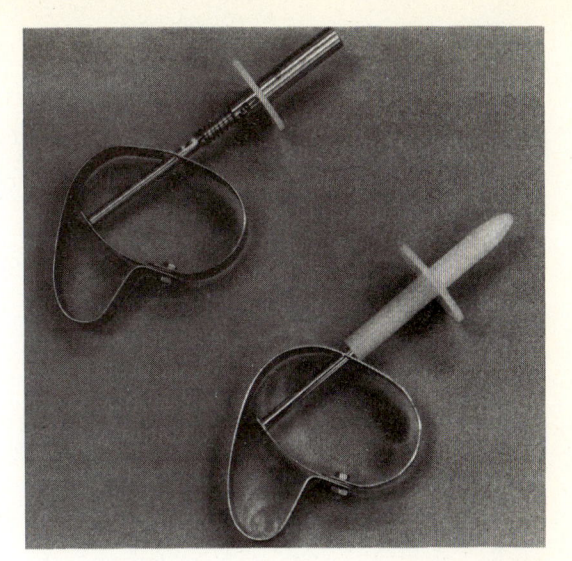

Figure 18-35
Suppository inserter, digital stimulator.

by persons with little hand function (Fig. 18-35). Both these devices require wrist extensor strength or wrist stabilization by an orthosis to apply adequate pressure. Patients must be able to assume and maintain a side-lying position or support themselves on a commode or raised toilet seat. Arm placement must be adequate to reach rectal area.

External catheter application is an independent skill with the aid of an adapted glue dispenser and posey strap. A patient may need to use an adapted vibrator to stimulate an erection prior to applying the condom.

Inserting an internal catheter for intermittent catheterization requires more dexterity in hand function. Spinal cord–injured patients may prefer either to have the sterile technique carried out by a primary care giver or to use the clean technique. The clean technique is done while in a wheelchair. Clothing is adapted to give access to the groin area. It is successful for females if an adapted mirror or knee spreader is used. This technique is preferred for independent function because of the inability of the high-level SCI patient to use sterile gloves. Patients may choose to use an orthosis or natural tenodesis for manipulation of equipment.

Sterilization for irrigation is one of the final steps learned in independent urinary management. All equipment must be adapted—cup holders, notched emesis basin, and a plastic thumb loop for the syringe. This activity requires much practice and individualized adaptation. Most spinal cord–injured patients who achieve independence in sterilization have an injury at C7–8 or lower. Table 18-7 summarizes the adaptive equipment used by SCI patients with quadriplegia.

Arthritis

Arthritis problems of limited range of motion, pain, and weak grasp are similar to those of spinal cord–injured and hemiplegic patients.

333 FUNCTIONAL LIVING SKILLS

Table 18-7

Spinal Cord Injury: Toileting

ADAPTIVE EQUIPMENT TO FACILITATE INDEPENDENCE

EMPTYING CATHETER	APPLYING LEG BAG	CONNECTING TUBING	APPLYING EXTERNALLY	INSERTING INTERNALLY
Deluxe catheter clamp Estebrook clamp Double-loop clamp Single-loop clamp Pants with Velcro or zippered opening on side of pant leg	Velcro straps or combination of cloth and Velcro or elastic and Velcro or loops on rubber straps	Uri-drain bag[a] Cone shaped connectors	Glue dispenser Posey strap[b] Vibrator	Adapted mirror Diamed catheter kit[c]

IRRIGATING OR STERILIZING	TOILETING	BOWEL CARE	WIPING
Cupholder Pyrex syringe Emesis bowl with notch Tongs	Male and female urinals[d] Commode Raised toilet seat Footstool Backrest Grab bar Overhead strap	Suppository insert[e] Digital stimulator[f]	Toilet tissue holder Wash mitt Adapted powder puff

a—Cheesebrough-Ponds, Greenwich, Conn.
b—Aamed, Forest Park, Ill.
c—Diamed, Elk Grove, Ill.
d—Maddack, inc., Pequannock, N.J.
e, f—BEOK Catalog Brookfield, Ill.
Source: Adapted from material by Sharon Groch.

Equipment needs and adaptations vary with the severity of disability. Raised toilet seats facilitate transfers and rising to a standing position. Seats may be padded to decrease pain and avoid unnecessary pressure on joints. Toilet armrests can be attached to fixtures to ensure safety during transfers. Extended toilet tongs allow positioning of toilet tissue when arm placement is limited (Fig. 18-36). These tongs can be built up or adapted with Velcro cuffs for patients with weak grasp. Other adaptive devices for menstrual and bowel care are the same as those used by hemiplegic or spinal cord–injured patients.

Amputation

Toileting procedures for patients with amputation are presented in Table 18-8 by level of amputation. Unilateral amputees (AE or BE) will use the prosthesis primarily as a stabilizer to (1) hold pants while fastening and unfastening, (2) position clothing, and (3) hold toilet tissue while tearing off a portion. Bilateral amputees have difficulty if the amputation is high, because the prosthesis cannot be positioned to provide adequate motion and pressure for wiping. Bidets are often recommended. Another option is to build in a rotation unit in the humeral section of an AE prosthesis which allows internal rotation.

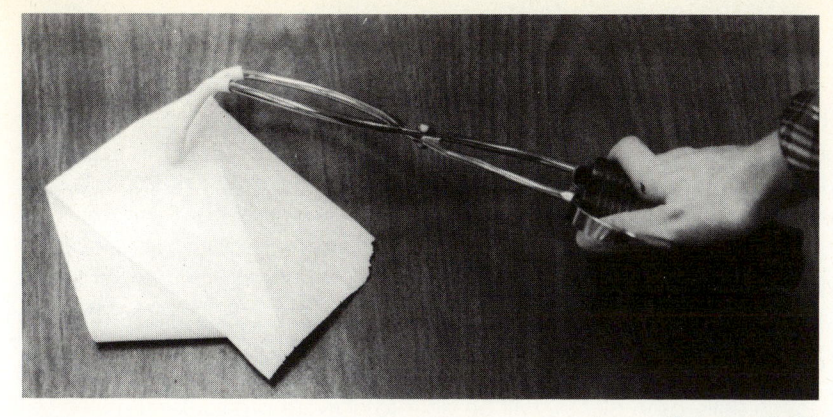

Figure 18-36
Extended toilet tongs.

COMMUNICATION

After serious injury, patients are naturally fearful because of the life-threatening nature of the situation. The fear is magnified if they are unable to communicate their fears and needs.

The nurse's role is of primary importance initially because of the dependence of the patient. In responding to a call light, nurses may find themselves doing a variety of communication tasks for the patient. These may include making phone calls, assisting in filling out and signing forms, adjusting a television or radio, or simply answering questions to comfort the patient. Occupational therapists can assist by providing adaptive equipment or positioning to allow the patient to perform many of these tasks independently.

Hemiplegia

Two major areas of communication must be attended to in this population: (1) the cognitive ability to understand and express verbal and written communication and (2) the motor ability to perform communication tasks. This phase of treatment is closely coordinated with the speech pathologist. Communication used in OT sessions and on the nursing unit should coincide with the level of treatment given in speech therapy.

Perceptual and visual deficits may interfere with the hemiplegic patient's performance of communication tasks. Perceptual retraining or compensation techniques will be emphasized in OT to gain independence in tasks such as dialing a telephone, writing, finding the call light, and operating television, radio, or typewriter.

It may be necessary to switch dominance to

Table 18-8

Amputation: Toileting

UNILATERAL BE, AE, SD	BILATERAL		
	BE	AE	SD
Other extremity used in one-handed techniques as in hemiplegia	Prosthesis used	Difficult with prosthesis; heel use or special devices such as Rimjet rotation unit	

335 FUNCTIONAL LIVING SKILLS

the uninvolved extremity to achieve the coordinated motor function necessary for writing. This process is enhanced by the need for the patient to perform other functional living skills with the unaffected nondominant extremity. Such tasks as feeding, hygiene, and dressing allow practice in coordinating grosser motions. Tasks demanding increased coordination and strength will be practiced in occupational therapy in preparation for writing training.

Spinal Cord Injury

Independence in communication skills, as in all functional skills, is related to the level of injury and remaining physical function. Table 18-9 provides a guideline for the equipment or technique used by spinal cord–injured patients at various levels.

Call lights are a major means of communication for patients immobilized in bed. Patients with only head and neck control have an immediate need for establishment of this method of communication. Advances in technology have provided electronic controls operated by the sucking in or blowing out of the breath. This "sip and puff" control can be quickly set up and the patient trained in minutes to operate a call light. Highly sensitive switches may also be strategically placed to be activated by chin pressure or head pressure. Patients with partial arm placement will be able to activate a pressure-sensitive pad fastened flat to the bed, close to the body.

Radio, television, and tape recorders may also be operated by the "sip and puff" method. Patients with some arm placement may be able to manipulate adapted extensions with an an-

Table 18-9

Spinal Cord Injury: Communication

PHYSICAL FUNCTION	CALL LIGHTS	RADIO/TELEVISION/TAPE RECORDER	TELEPHONE	WRITING
Head and neck control, no arm placement	Sip and puff, chin switch, or head switch	Sip and puff	Sip and puff or sparr telephone arm with mouth stick	PMV or other system or mouth stick to type
Partial arm placement	Sip and puff or gross arm placement used for lights fastened flat to bed	Sip and puff, BFO with WHO, or special adapted extensions on knob or switch	Sip and puff, shoulder-rest with typing stick or pencil to dial, BFO with WHO, or utensil cuff with pencil	PMV or other system, BFO with WHO to type (possibly), utensil cuff, or writing adaptations
Arm placement, wrist extension, no hand function	Side of hand used for lights flat on bed beside body	Adapted switches, WHO (tenodesis type), or lateral pinch (if good strength	WHO (tenodesis type) with pencil to dial, utensil cuff with pencil to dial, two hands to manage receiver, or residual hand function	WHO (tenodesis type), writing adaptations or typing sticks, or residual hand function to type or write
Arm placement, wrist extension, partial hand function	Placed within reach	Minor adaptations on knobs or switches or residual hand function	Residual hand function	Writing adaptations or residual hand function

Source: Adapted from material by Sharon Groch.

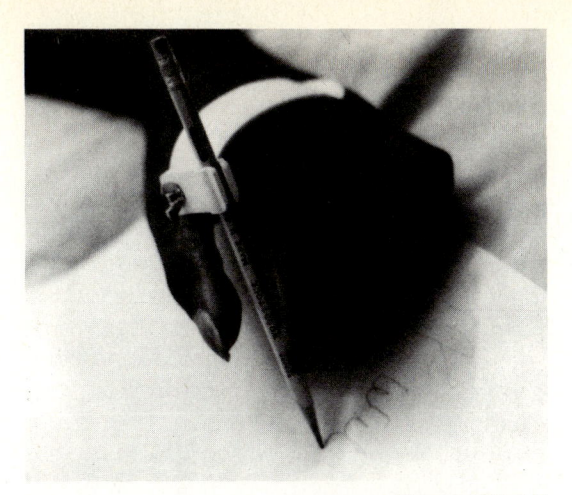

Figure 18-37
Adaptation for writing.

tigravity orthesis (BFO) and WHO. Patients having wrist extension with or without partial hand function may use a WHO (tenodesis type) to manipulate adapted switches or may choose to use residual hand function (natural tenodesis and lateral pinch).

A telephone may be managed by high-level SCI patients in one of two ways: (1) the "sip and puff" method or (2) use of a Sparr telephone arm to hold the receiver and a mouth stick to dial. Patients with more upper-extremity function will use a shoulder rest to hold the receiver in place and a typing stick or pencil in their orthesis for dialing. If wrist extension is available, the options are (1) use of a WHO (tenodesis type), (2) use of two hands together to manipulate receiver, (3) use of utensil cuff with a pencil for dialing, or (4) use of residual hand function.

Writing is one of the most important areas of communication to be dealt with for spinal cord–injured patients. Often this is a younger population who may be more actively pursuing educational and vocational goals. Scientific advances have given us specialized systems which allow patients with little function a means of typewritten communication. Spinal cord–injured patients with more arm placement may use a BFO with a WHO and typing sticks or pencils to type. Good arm placement and wrist extension allow use of a WHO (tenodesis type) and pencil, special writing adaptations (Fig. 18-37), or residual lateral prehension from a well-trained natural tenodesis.

The functional living skill of communication has been discussed for hemiplegic and spinal cord–injured patients to present the major approaches and equipment available to achieve independence. Other diagnostic categories are of no less importance and are frequently seen by both nurses and occupational therapists. This skill requires the use of the basic principles of object manipulation that have been presented. For example, incoordination requires achievement of maximum stability and positioning of the total body and the object to be manipulated prior to performing the activity. For typing, use of a typewriter keyguard at a table of proper height

Figure 18-38
Typewriter keyguard.

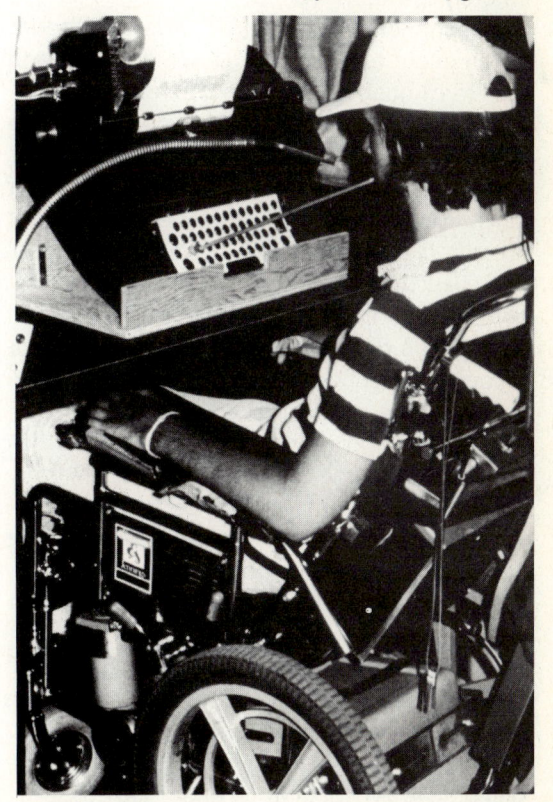

337   FUNCTIONAL LIVING SKILLS

increases the patient's success. The keyguard, a plexiglass plate that fits across the keys, prevents hitting unwanted keys (Fig. 18-38).

A patient's level of independent communication can make the difference in the ability to return productively to society. The cooperative efforts of speech therapy, occupational therapy, work evaluation, and nursing personnel will fulfill this goal in the rehabilitation of physically disabled persons.

PROGRESSIVE DISEASE

Self-care training for the person with a progressive disorder demands a different approach. A traumatic injury or disease process that can be stabilized allows independent function to be achieved and maintained. Progressive disease, however, is an inconstant process resulting in a continual decrease of physical function and ultimately loss of independent performance. The uncertainty of such a disease process impedes both patient and therapist in setting long- and short-term goals. There is no assurance that the level of performance achieved one day will be achieved the next day. In fact, little or no progress is expected because of the inevitable loss of function. As the disease progresses, the patient is confronted with the grief of each additional loss. Physical symptoms of pain and fatigue limit performance from day to day. Thus a varied approach is required, emphasizing self-care as an activity to enhance self-esteem and to allow patients some control in their lives.

In teaching patients how to perform with their current abilities, the therapist must prepare them for the next lower level of performance. For example, a patient with cancer of the spine is experiencing increased pain on a particular day that leaves her unable to dress her lower extremities and gives the therapist an opportunity to introduce adaptive equipment such as a leg lifter or dressing stick. Frequently this stimulates a discussion of the reality of having good and bad days. It also exposes the patient to the alternatives available as function decreases.

When patients are given alternatives for performance in all areas of self-care, they can give priority to activities for a given day according to available energy. An example of this would be a patient with amyotrophic lateral sclerosis who is independent only in feeding and in oral and facial hygiene and wakes feeling very weak but knowing that he has planned to take his family to a movie that evening. He must then determine how to use his energy throughout the day. He knows the importance of rest to avoid fatigue and has learned to select activities and use alternative methods. His decision may include having his wife assist in oral and facial hygiene and using a BFO for feeding. Instead of working on a string-art piece, he chooses a less fatiguing activity such as reading. His afternoon rest period is lengthened. By conserving energy throughout the day, he will enjoy the movie and still feel that he has maintained control of his day.

Simplifying activities to conserve energy is called **work simplification**. It may include sitting rather than standing, preplanning to eliminate tasks, and delegating tasks to others. While these seem to be simple concepts, patients unaccustomed to approaching tasks in this way may feel threatened by this needed change in life-style. Occupational therapy provides the environment to perform activities, with or without modification, which enables the patient to receive the supportive direction needed to alter daily routine. The patient's ability to adjust to this constantly changing life-style becomes the measure of progress in the treatment program.

CONCLUSION

The therapist is able to provide equipment and individual treatment sessions to determine the patient's level of independence. A maintained level of independence, however, comes in the carry-over of the designated routine. The therapist is responsible for communicating to nursing and families the routines to be followed and for giving instruction for special equipment. Therapy is successful only if the patient is given support and time to practice with others around. Nursing personnel are instrumental in monitoring consistent and proper use of equipment. Therapists also depend on nursing to help avoid loss of equipment and to communicate maintenance problems. It is only with this coordination of effort that a newly learned skill will become part of the patient's independent daily routine.

In this chapter you have learned that functional living skills are not easily taught to the patient. We have familiarized you with basic techniques and equipment used in self-care training. Not all techniques were presented, however, because of the variations in patients' individual needs. Each situation presents a new problem-solving opportunity for patient, nurse, and therapist. Certain questions must be answered to initiate effective training: Is the patient ready emotionally? Is the patient ready physically? What are the patient's goals? What techniques and equipment are available? How will the patient and staff handle failure or setback?

The timeliness of intervention depends on the nurse and therapist answering these questions together. Nurses need to be aware of this evaluation process and to give input to the occupational therapists as to the patient's treatment potential. Nurses need to know equipment and techniques to be able to give the patient support and to facilitate carry-over of the training. This is critical to the success of the training, since nurses often have more daily contact with a patient than the therapist does. Our effort has been to provide you with this information to enhance communication between OT and nursing and, more importantly, to benefit patients in their rehabilitation.

BIBLIOGRAPHY

American Academy of Orthopedic Surgeons: *Atlas of Orthotics: Biomechanical Principles and Application,* Mosby, St. Louis, 1975.

Bobath, Bertha: *Adult Hemiplegia Evaluation and Treatment,* 2d ed., Heinemann, London, 1978.

Ford, Jack R., and B. Duckworth: *Physical Management for the Quadriplegic Patient,* Davis, Philadelphia, 1974.

Harris, E. E.: "A New Orthotics Terminology: A Guide to Its Use for Prescription and Fee Schedules," *Orthotics Prosthetics* 27(2), June 1973.

Hopkins, H. L., and Helen D. Smith: *Willard and Spackman's Occupational Therapy,* 5th ed., Lippincott, Philadelphia, 1978.

Long, Charles, and Edith Lawton: "Functional Significance of Spinal Cord Lesion Level," *Arch Phys Med Rehabil* 36:250, 1975.

MacDonald, E. M., G. MacCaul, L. Mirrey, and E. M. Morrison: *Occupational Therapy in Rehabilitation,* Williams & Wilkins, Baltimore, 1976.

McKenzie, Mary, et al.: *Occupational Therapy Treatment Guide: Spinal Cord Injuries,* Rancho Los Amigos Hospital Occupational Therapy Department, Downey, Calif.

Moberg, Erik: "Surgical Treatment for Absent Single-Hand Grip and Elbow Extension in Quadriplegia," *J Bone Joint Surg* Vol. 57-A, No. 2, March 1975.

Pierce, Donald S., and Vernon H. Nickel: *The Total Care of Spinal Cord Injuries,* Little, Brown, Boston, 1977.

Self Care Activities of the Hemiplegic Patient, Division of Health, Department of Health and Social Services, Madison, Wis. (Pamphlet.)

Trombley, C. A., and A. D. Scott: *Occupational Therapy for Physical Dysfunction,* Williams & Wilkins, Baltimore, 1977.

Upper Extremity Prosthetics and Orthotics for Physicians, Surgeons, and Therapists, Prosthetic-Orthotic Center, Northwestern University Medical School, Chicago, August 1979.

Wu, Y., et al.: "Reusable Catheter for Sterile Intermittent Self Catheterization," *Arch Phys Med Rehabil* 59:557, 1978.

19
anita s. halper
deborah lynn korkos

acquired speech and language disorders in children

INTRODUCTION

The development of a child socially, emotionally, and cognitively depends upon language as the foundation. Imagine, if you can, the effect of a communication impairment during a child's formative years of development if language is perceived "as . . . a tool or mechanism by which the human organism is able to achieve its potential" (Rees, 1978). Interruption in the normal acquisition of these skills interferes not only with existing functions, but with future learning.

The purpose of this chapter is threefold: first, to describe the speech and language problems associated with traumatic head injuries in children under 10 years of age who are presumed to have had normal language and speech skills premorbidly; second, to describe the assessment procedures and general principles of therapy utilized by the speech-language pathologist; and third, to describe management techniques that can be employed by the nursing staff and taught to family members. The impact of these disorders on development and learning will be addressed.

NORMAL LANGUAGE DEVELOPMENT

Language develops in a series of predictable stages, each dependent upon the previous steps. These sequences are generally the same for all children and parallel biologic stages of readiness during the first 3 years of life.

Language development is often described in terms of receptive and expressive modalities. *Reception* refers to the decoding or understanding of oral language, while *expression* entails the encoding of meaning into verbal responses for interpersonal communication (Bzoch and League, 1978). The two processes are interdependent and are ongoing from the time of the child's birth (Muma, 1978).

During the first year of life, the child's receptive growth begins with auditory awareness and recognition of speech intonation patterns. This development progresses to the recognition of some words in context and the understanding of some simple statements and questions. Before the age of 1, the child does not truly comprehend isolated words or units, but rather responds to phrases with specific intonations in certain functional settings.

During the second year, the child begins to understand some simple requests supplemented by gesture, with a gradual increase in recognition of names heard in conversation. After the age of 3, the child has a receptive repertoire of nouns, verbs, and adjectives that seems to expand daily. In addition to the greater number of words and forms recognized, the child displays greater comprehension of syntactical structure.

Expressively, the infant begins to use oral language as a means of conveying needs and feelings of pleasure. The child moves from undifferentiated crying to selective emotional responses (including oral sounds) that are easily identified by a mother. In the 2 to 6-month period, as awareness of sounds made by the self increases, the child begins to babble or repeat sounds, often vocalizing in self-initiated sound play. This babbling or tuning of the child's vocal apparatus continues in various forms and stages until about 6 months. In the 8- to 10-month range, corresponding to increased understanding of certain symbolic gestures, intonation, words, and simple phrases, the child enters a period of *jargon* speech. In this period, the child "talks" to people and objects by chaining a series of syllables together with the intonation pattern of meaningful sentences. This stage appears to provide the child with early practice in the connected speech patterns to be later developed (Bzoch and League).

The child's first word often emerges around the first birthday, beginning with the names of favorite people, toys, foods, or actions. Use of jargon gradually decreases and the child relies on one- to two-word combinations to communicate. After about age 18 months, a rapid growth in expressive vocabulary becomes evident, as the child's growth in expressive vocabulary becomes evident, and the child's understanding of interpersonal communication increases. Simple two- to three-word phrases and sentences are produced to direct and interpret the environment. By the end of the second year, the child's vocabulary may have increased to 250 or more words. From this point, the expressive repertoire continues to expand and longer sentences of more complex form are generated. From 4 to 5 years of age, the child uses intelligible speech for social purposes, to communicate ideas, to acquire information, and to relate happenings. By the fifth and sixth years, the emphasis shifts to the interactional content and the child makes significant perceptual developments that form the basis of reading readiness. By age 6 to 7, the child is ready to acquire a visual language system and learns to read and write.

DESCRIPTION OF POPULATION

There are many discussions of acquired speech and language disorders in children, but no generally accepted diagnostic classification system currently exists. In order to correlate neurologic findings with observable clinical speech and language behaviors, and to facilitate communication among professionals, the classification system presented below was formulated and is utilized at the Rehabilitation Institute of Chicago. It is presented here to provide a framework from which to view this population.

Acquired Aphasia

Acquired aphasia is a language disorder that typically impairs functioning in all language modalities. (For more specific definitions of aphasia, refer to Chapter 12.) It results from left-sided brain injury, e.g., trauma, tumor, CVA (cerebrovascular accident), in the same areas that produce aphasia in adults. Chase (1972) indicates that damage to the frontal lobe results in motor disturbances of speech and frequently an accompanying right hemiplegia. On the other hand, he states that deficits occur in auditory comprehension and production of speech when the lesion is more posterior in the temporoparietal regions. However, the consequences of such damage ". . . do not produce the differential effects on speech production as a function of location that one observes in adult patients" (Chase). The acquired aphasia most often seen in children is the nonfluent type with restricted verbal output as the most clinically significant characteristic (Alajouanine and Lhermitte, 1965). Speech is generally sparse or telegraphic in nature with the more severely aphasic child having no functional oral expression skills. Word-finding difficulties, apraxia of speech, and agrammaticism (refer to Chap. 12 for definitions) are the major contributing factors to these problems. Auditory comprehension skills, although usually impaired, are often superior to oral expression skills. The prereading and prewriting skills of visual perception/conception and visual-motor skills in the child under 6 years of age and the reading and writing skills in the older child are also involved.

Right Brain Damage

The child who suffers damage to the right side of the brain usually does not present the true symbolic deficits seen in the child with acquired aphasia. Rather than specific symbolic dysfunction, problems lie in the inability to consistently utilize language skills because of inadequate attention, retention, perception, and memory skills.

Typically, the most common symptoms include reduced and fleeting attention and distractibility from internal and external cues. These are manifested in the child's inability to concentrate on a specific activity (e.g., conversation, television, eating) for more than a few seconds before attention shifts to another stimulus. Consequently, the child who appears to have problems understanding language may in actuality be prevented by variable attention and impulsivity from responding to and integrating the entire message.

Memory deficits for recent events further confuse the child regarding surroundings and ADL (activities of daily living). The child may not recall whether or not lunch has been eaten or whether therapies have been received. In an attempt to fill these memory gaps, the child may confabulate, using speech that is excessive, inappropriate, disorganized or irrelevant to the situation. This limited awareness and inability to monitor speech output makes the child difficult to control. Disorientation to time, place, and persons distorts the child's perceptions of where he or she is and why, often resulting in an inappropriate response. Visual-perceptual problems may coexist, affecting the child's perception of the environment as well as certain linguistic skills. Interruption in visual-perceptual functioning often precludes the development of reading and writing.

Thus, as in the adult, this disorder is one in which behavioral, cognitive, and perceptual deficits reduce the child's efficiency in utilizing language skills and deter the child's further development.

Generalized Language Deficits

Generalized language deficits are characterized by speech, language, and cognitive skills that are all reduced to a similar level. This reduction occurs as a result of bilateral brain damage sustained secondary to trauma, encephalitis, exposure to certain toxins or drugs, or pervasive brain tumors. It has been the authors' clinical experience that this type of language disorder occurs more frequently in children than does an isolated aphasia or dysarthria, possibly because of the smaller size of the child's head and the incomplete localization of function relative to the child's age. Characteristics associated with generalized language deficits include significant deficiency in all language and cognitive areas, particularly in dealing with abstract language concepts, reduced memory skills, and a delayed or latent response pattern. The child's level of performance in auditory comprehension and oral expression skills is typically stable; that is, there is not the variability or inconsistency often seen in the right brain-damaged child.

Dysarthria

Dysarthria is a speech disorder that affects the process involved in the production of speech, respiration, phonation, articulation, resonation, and prosody due to central or peripheral nervous system damage. As a result of this damage, muscles controlled by the affected nerves may evidence slow, weak, or incoordinated movement which often impairs the intelligibility of speech, as well as chewing and swallowing. (For a more detailed definition and classification of dysarthrias relative to neurological damage, refer to Chap. 12.)

In general, the problems are similar to those seen in adults; however, the effect of such damage on development of speech and feeding skills in the younger child is significant. For example, if the child has insufficient muscular control over lips and tongue, normal babbling and sound play may be impaired or absent. Consequently, the child will be unable to produce words and sentences necessary to develop language.

Multiple Speech and Language Disorders

Aphasia, dysarthria, and symptoms of right brain damage may coexist in children who have sustained multiple lesions. Generalized language deficits may also occur in the presence of a dysarthria, but concurrently occurring aphasia or symptoms of right brain damage are less common and are difficult to differentiate when present.

ASSESSMENT PROCEDURES

The evaluation of the traumatically brain-damaged child includes diagnosis of specific language disorders, identification of problem areas, measurement of the child's developmental level in each modality relative to chronologic age, and establishment of goals and priorities for the treatment program.

In evaluating the child, the speech-language pathologist typically assesses auditory comprehension, oral and gestural expression, visual perceptual/conceptual skills, and, when appropriate, reading or writing. An attempt is made to observe the child in both clinical and functional settings, that is, use of these skills in a test performance versus use in natural language situations. In addition, an examination of the peripheral speech mechanism for both vegetative (chewing and swallowing) and voluntary functioning is performed. A determination of hearing acuity is also an integral part of the evaluation.

Whenever possible, formal test measures should be utilized. Such tools provide objective and quantifiable data and allow for interdisciplinary communication. Often formal assessment is not feasible with this population because of the severity of impairment, inconsistency of performance, and the child's age. In such cases, informal measures including developmental scales and behavioral observations are employed. This information compares the child's level of functioning to selected scales of normal child development in each area.

A variety of commercially produced tests are available for assessment of the traumatically brain-damaged child. Test selection is often based on the speech-language pathologist's theoretical viewpoint of language. The more commonly used formal tests in the various modalities are described below.

Auditory Comprehension

Test for Auditory Comprehension of Language This test was developed by Dr. Elizabeth Carrow after several revisions and was published in 1973. It measures vocabulary and grammatical aspects of auditory comprehension without requiring a verbal response. Norms are provided from ages 3 years to 6 years, 11 months.

Assessment of Children's Language Comprehension This test was developed by Rochano Foster, Jane L. Giddan, and Joel Stark in 1972. The authors intended this tool ". . . to determine how many word classes in different combinations of length and complexity a child would be able to understand" (Foster, Glidden and Stark, 1972). A comparison of the percentage of items correct relative to the child's chronological age can be made.

Oral Expression

Developmental Sentence Analysis This two-part procedure was developed by Laura Lee in 1974. A language sample is analyzed according to the developmental order of sentence types and language acquisition (e.g., pronouns, verbs, conjunctions, etc.). Norms are provided for ages 2 years to 6 years, 11 months.

The Fisher-Logemann Test of Articulation Competence This articulation test was developed by Drs. Hilda Fisher and Jerilyn A. Logemann in 1971. It identifies faulty sound production through a picture-naming task. An analysis of articulatory errors is made.

Visual Perception/Conception

Developmental Test of Visual-Motor Integration The Developmental Test of Visual-Motor Integration was developed by Dr. Keith E. Beery in 1967. This test consists of copying 24 increasingly difficult geometric forms. Norms are available from 2 years, 10 months to 15 years, 11 months. Information regarding the child's overall level of visual-perceptual and prewriting skills, including such functions as the relationship of one object to another (spatial relationships), the location of those objects in space (position in space), and coordination of eye-hand movements (visual-motor coordination), is obtained.

Motor-Free Visual Perception Test The Motor-Free Visual Perception Test was developed by Drs. Ronald P. Colarusso and Donald D. Hammill in 1972. The authors indicate that the test measures five areas of visual perception—spatial relationships, figure-ground, visual closure, visual memory, and visual discrimination—and requires no graphic response. Norms are available from ages 4 through 9.

Reading Comprehension

Gates-MacGinitie Reading Tests This series of reading tests from kindergarten through grade 12 was developed by Drs. Arthur Gates and Walter MacGinitie. They measure reading readiness, vocabulary, comprehension, speed, and accuracy.

Written Expression

Picture Story Language Test The Picture Story Language Test was developed by Dr. Helmer R. Myklebust in 1965. It is a measure of spontaneous narrative-writing ability from a picture stimulus. An analysis of this sample yields age equivalents from 7 to 17 years for each of the following areas: length, syntax, and content.

Multimodal

Illinois Test of Psycholinguistic Abilities The Illinois Test of Psycholinguistic Abilities was developed by Samuel Kirk, James McCarthy, and Winifred Kirk, and the revised edition currently in use was published in 1968. This test evaluates auditory, visual, verbal, and motor functioning and determines discrepancies in growth among these skills. A composite psycholinguistic age, as well as individual age levels for each area tested, is provided. Norms range from the 2-year level to the 10-year, 11-month level depending on the subtest.

Peabody Individual Achievement Test The Peabody Individual Achievement Test was developed by Drs. Lloyd M. Dunn and Frederick C. Markwardt, Jr. in 1970. The authors designed this test to screen achievement in mathematics, reading, spelling, and general information. Norms for grade equivalents below first grade up to 12.9 grade level and age equivalents from the 5-year, 4-month level to the 18-year, 1-month level are provided.

PROGNOSIS

Prognosis for speech and language recovery and continued development depends upon certain variables. Significant prognostic factors include:

1. Site and extent of lesion: The literature supports the concept that the site and extent of the lesion will affect language recovery. Chase indicates that frontal lesions usually show more rapid recovery than temporal lesions. Van Dongen and Loonen (1977) cite two French works by Collegnon, Hécaen, and Angelergues (1968) and by Gloning and Heft (1970) regarding the effect of the extent of the lesion on recovery. They report that severe bilateral lesions are a negative prognostic indicator. In describing the course of recovery in acquired aphasia, Alajouanine and Lhermitte state "the recovery of speech—its speed and extent in particular—depends upon the situation, the extent and the reversibility of the cerebral lesion."

2. Duration of coma: There is little information available regarding the relationship between length of coma and recovery from the different speech and language disorders discussed in this chapter. Hécaen (1976) in his article on acquired aphasia states that "there is no clear relationship between the occurrence and duration of a period of coma and the persistence and severity of deficit." Those children who remain comatose for more than a 2-week period show poor intellectual achievement as measured by school performance (Heiskanen and Kaste, 1974). One can infer that this does affect overall language functioning.

3. Age at onset: A belief commonly held by many health professionals is that the younger the child is at the time of injury, the better the prognosis for speech and language recovery. However, the literature is inconclusive regarding this relationship. Lenneberg (1967) postulates that in children with unilateral lesions sustained before the age of 9, there

will be return of language. On the other hand, Oelschaeger et al. cite the case of acquired aphasia in a 10-year-old girl whose language abilities remained significantly impaired 1 year after onset, indicating both incomplete recovery and questionable prognosis. In other words, it is difficult to state at what age recovery will be complete and when residual problems will persist.

4. Time between onset and initiation of therapy: Therapy should be initiated as soon as the child is medically stable. Early intervention capitalizes on spontaneous physiologic recovery and facilitates the ongoing speech and language of development.
5. Severity of language deficit: Perhaps one of the most important prognostic indicators is the severity of impairment in the various language modalities, particularly auditory comprehension. Understanding speech is fundamental to the development of language.

In general, the authors' clinical experience reveals that prognosis for language improvement is better for aphasic, dysarthric, and right brain-damaged children than in those children with diffuse or multiple defects. It is clear from this discussion of prognostic indicators that further research is needed in this area.

INTERVENTION TECHNIQUES

Acquired Aphasia

Although there are a variety of approaches to language therapy, in all cases, treatment must begin at the child's developmental level of functioning in each modality. Goals must be set to move the child in an orderly sequence to facilitate reacquisition of previously established skills as well as stimulation of new learning.

At the onset of treatment, the primary focus is on auditory comprehension, which forms the foundation for all language learning. Therapy begins with vocabulary building, including a variety of grammatical forms such as nouns, verbs, and adjectives. Once the child's receptive repertoire has been significantly expanded, these words are used in simple commands of increasing length and complexity. As greater understanding of these terms is demonstrated, the child is taught to employ them verbally. In those children where apraxia of speech limits verbal output, therapy is directed toward imitation of oral movements, sound and word repetition, naming, and, finally, simple sentence production. Word-recall activities are an integral part of the treatment program in oral expression and include sentence completion tasks, categorical naming, and word-association activities. Visual training is employed simultaneously through the use of pictures and printed words to strengthen auditory and expressive associations. The development of prereading, reading, or writing skills is added when the child has mastered nonsymbolic visual activities.

Right Brain Damage

While rehabilitation for the aphasic child emphasizes language development, the primary foci of treatment for the right brain-damaged child are to increase auditory and visual attention spans, to orient the child to time, place, and person, and to improve visual-perceptual skills, including left-sided awareness. Further, all of these tasks are manipulated so as to facilitate the child's memory of recent events.

Therapy begins in a very structured environment where auditory and visual distractions are minimized; for example, the child faces a blank wall, the door is closed, and therapy materials are concealed. The child then performs relatively simple and unfrustrating tasks, generally starting with nonlinguistic activities and progressing to linguistic materials of increasing length and complexity. Visual rather than auditory input is stressed because the former serves to limit the child's excessive verbalizations. When the child is able to attend to a task for a 3- to 5-min period, therapy shifts to organization and sequencing of verbal output. For example, if the child has difficulty describing the steps involved in toothbrushing, the speech-language pathologist introduces picture-sequence cards depicting this. The child is then asked to order the pictures and describe the series of events sequentially.

As in the adult, therapy programs for the right brain-damaged child serve to improve the effectiveness and efficiency of language functioning. In addition, successful learning in the other therapies is facilitated as a result of increased task orientation, attention span, and memory.

Generalized Language Deficits

Therapy for the child with generalized language deficits is related to developmental status in each modality. Unlike treatment of the aphasic child, however, the focus of therapy is on stimulation of all language areas rather than the development of specific problem areas (e.g., word-finding skills) or compensatory techniques (e.g., association cues).

Treatment is centered around a core vocabulary of nouns, verbs, prepositions, and modifiers consistent with the child's developmental level. Ideally, this vocabulary includes meaningful and functional terms that can be reinforced in the other disciplines, e.g., body-part naming in physical therapy (PT), and clothing names in occupational therapy (OT). Stimulation is multiexperiential and emphasizes development in auditory comprehension, verbal expression, and visual perception. As with the mentally retarded child, attempts are made to establish terminal representational behaviors by constructing one part of the whole and adding to it systematically until the goal is achieved (Flahive et al.). For example, individual body parts are taught before integration into activities of daily living.

Dysarthria

The ultimate goal of dysarthria therapy is to increase the overall intelligibility of functional speech. While the basic principles for improvement of respiration, phonation, articulation, prosody, and resonance are the same as in adults (see Chap. 12), the procedures utilized with children must be different. For example, a 5-year-old child who needs to improve synchronization of inhalation and exhalation of the airstream would have difficulty understanding the process underlying this function and its role in speech production. Rather, the approach might be to teach the child to monitor air flow utilizing visual feedback (e.g., blowing water in a bottle to a certain level). Similarly, consonant and vowel production can be improved through reducing the rate of speech and overarticulating syllables rather than drilling on the production of individual phonemes.

An alternate means of communication must be considered for those children where the development of functional speech is not a realistic goal. The use of such systems is necessary not only to permit expression of needs and ideas, but is essential to the continued development of the child's conceptual language skills.

Multiple Speech and Language Disorders

In treating children with multiple speech and language disorders, the speech-language pathologist must ascertain those problems which interfere most significantly with auditory comprehension and oral expressive skills. For example, if a child has a moderate generalized language deficit and a severe flaccid dysarthria resulting in unintelligible functional speech, therapy for the dysarthria takes precedence. Thus, the immediate establishment of a means of communication is the first goal.

NURSING MANAGEMENT

Management of the child with a language disorder requires an understanding of the nature of the problems and their effect on the child's functioning in the environment. Carry-over by the nursing staff is an integral part of the therapeutic process.

Acquired Aphasia

For the aphasic child with limited comprehension, single words or short simple phrases supplemented by gestures may facilitate understanding. It is also helpful to limit background noise and the number of people speaking to the child at any given time. Comprehension is often improved by presenting one idea at a time, then slowly repeating or rephrasing if the child seems confused. Although the speech-language pathologist will provide specific information regarding the child's expressive ability, the nurse may also use experience in clinical observations to anticipate the type of response a child can produce. For example, for the nonverbal child with no functional speech, the nurse may use yes and no questions that allow a child to respond by a shake of the head rather than by struggling to produce a verbal response. Similarly, the nurse may ask the child to point or gesture needs whenever possible.

The nurse can also facilitate the aphasic child into conveying needs and wants while concurrently promoting carry-over of therapy goals. For the child who is experiencing word-finding difficulties, techniques similar to those used with adults may be employed. These may include having the child describe the function or characteristics of the word, write the word, or tell with what letter it begins. Some children require a longer time to formulate a verbal response. To encourage continuing communication efforts, it is critical that the child be given additional response time, that errors be accepted, and that there be no interruption. Above all, it is important not to anticipate what is going to be said and say it for the child.

Right Brain Damage

The key to effectively communicating with the right brain-damaged child is to elicit the child's attention and to structure the environment so as to limit distractions. Once this is achieved, the same principles for facilitating the aphasic child's understanding can be applied. To assist the child with recall of directions that have been given, the nurse asks the child to repeat them. Similarly, having the child describe daily activities and events sequentially will foster verbal organization and sequencing skills and will simultaneously increase orientation to the environment. Inappropriate or excessive verbalizations are best handled by ignoring and thus extinguishing these responses.

Generalized Language Deficits

Communicating with the child with generalized language deficits is relatively uncomplicated. The principal consideration is the use of simple, concrete language presented in brief verbal units. As with the right brain-damaged child, it is important to review instructions to ensure comprehension. In addition, the child may require extra time to respond.

Dysarthria

To promote the dysarthric child's continuing attempts to communicate verbally, the nurse must be supportive of the child's efforts without pretending to understand. This involves allowing the child adequate response time, repeating unclear words, and guessing the message, when necessary. In addition, the nurse should remind the child to reduce the speech rate, overarticulate words, and repeat when necessary. For the child whose speech is virtually unintelligible, the nurse may need to prepare a simple communication board containing pictures to convey basic needs (e.g., hunger, pain, or fatigue).

FAMILY COUNSELING AND EDUCATION

The role of counseling and education of the child's family is an integrated component of the total rehabilitation process. The speech-language pathologist will describe the nature of the language disorder, the child's level of functioning in each language area, and the goals, expected outcome, and duration of therapy. Family members are encouraged to observe the child in therapy to promote better understanding of the disability and the techniques that can be used to facilitate carry-over. As with the adult, if the services of a speech-language pathologist are not available, the nurse can direct the family to the American Speech-Language-Hearing Association or to a state speech and hearing professional association. Later in the therapeutic process, it may also be necessary to discuss appropriate school placement for the child.

CONCLUSION

The interdisciplinary management of the child with acquired communication problems is essential to effective language rehabilitation. The natural language situations which the nursing unit affords maximize the child's clinical success in therapy. Although each hospital varies in its differential diagnosis and management principles for the brain-damaged child, the underlying concepts outlined in this chapter can be adapted in many settings.

BIBLIOGRAPHY

Alajouanine, Th., and Francois Lhermitte: "Acquired Aphasia in Children," *Brain* 88:653, 1965.

Beery, Keith E.: *Developmental Test of Visual-Motor Integration,* Follett, Chicago, 1967.

Berry, Mildred Freburg: *Language Disorders of Children: The Bases and Diagnosis,* Appleton-Century-Crofts, New York, 1969.

Bzoch, Kenneth R., and Richard League: *Assessing Language Skills in Infancy,* Univeristy Park Press, Baltimore, 1978.

Carrow, Elizabeth: *Test for Auditory Comprehension of Language,* Urban Research Group, Austin, Texas, 1973.

Chase, Richard A.: "Neurological Aspects of Language Disorders in Children," in John V. Irvin and Michael Marge (eds.), *Principles of Childhood Language Disabilities,* Appleton-Century-Crofts, New York, 1972.

Colarusso, Ronald P., and Donald D. Hammill: *Motor-Free Visual Perception Test,* Academic Therapy Pub., San Rafael, California, 1972.

Darley, Frederick L., Arnold E. Aronson, and Joseph R. Brown: *Motor Speech Disorders,* Saunders, Philadelphia, 1975.

Dunn, Lloyd M., and Frederick C. Markwardt, Jr.: *Peabody Individual Achievement Test,* American Guidance Service, St. Paul, Minn., 1970.

Fisher, Hilda B., and Jerilyn A. Logemann: *The Fisher-Logemann Test of Articulation Competence,* Houghton Mifflin, Boston, 1971.

Flahive, Michael J., Joseph J. Auffrey, Robert L. Bancroft, Gregory Loeser, William L. Reed, and Julie Stoy: *Language Development—Perceptual Motor Training Program,* 2d ed., Muskegon Regional Mental Retardation Center, Muskegon, Mich.

Foster, Rochana, Jane Giddan, and Joel Stark: *Assessment of Children's Language Comprehension,* Consulting Psychologists Press, Palo Alto, Calif., 1972.

Fuld, Paula Altman, and Phyllis Fisher: "Recovery of Intellectual Ability After Closed Head Injury," *Dev Med Child Neurol* 19:495, 1977.

Gates, Arthur L., and Walter H. MacGinitie: *Gates MacGinitie Reading Tests,* Teachers College Press, Columbia Univ., New York, 1965.

Hécaen, Henri: "Acquired Aphasia in Children and the Ontogenesis of Hemispheric Functional Specialization," *Brain and Language* 3:114, 1976.

Heiskanen, O., and M. Kaste: "Late Prognosis of Severe Brain Injury in Children," *Dev Med Child Neurol* 16:11, 1974.

Irwin, John V., and Michael Marge (eds.): *Principles of Childhood Language Disabilities,* Appleton-Century-Crofts, New York, 1972.

Kirk, Samuel A., James J. McCarthy, and Winifred Kirk: *Illinois Test of Psycholinguistic Abilities,* Western Psychological Services, Los Angeles, 1968.

Lee, Laura L.: *Developmental Sentence Analysis,* Northwestern Univ. Press, Evanston, Ill., 1974.

Lenneberg, Eric H.: *Biological Foundations of Language,* Wiley, 1967.

Lezak, Muriel Deutsch: *Neuropsychological Assessment,* Oxford Univ. Press, New York, 1976.

Morehead, Donald M., and Ann E. Morehead (eds.): *Normal and Deficient Child Language,* University Park Press, Baltimore, 1976.

Muma, John R.: *Language Handbook: Concepts, Assessment, Intervention,* Prentice-Hall, Englewood Cliffs, N.J., 1978.

Myklebust, Helmer R.: *Auditory Disorders in Children: A Manual for Differential Diagnosis,* Grune & Stratton, New York, 1954.

———: *Development and Disorders of Written Language, vol. 1, Picture Story Language Test,* Grune & Stratton, New York, 1965.

Oelschaeger, Mary Lee, and John Scarborough: "Traumatic Aphasia in Children: A Case Study," *J Commun Dis* 9:281, 1976.

Rees, Norman S.: "Pragmatics of Language: Applications to Normal and Disordered Language," in Richard L. Schiefelbusch (ed.), *Bases of Language Interaction,* University Park Press, Baltimore, 1978.

Schain, Richard L.: *Neurology of Childhood Learning Disorders,* Williams & Wilkins, Baltimore, 1977.

Schiefelbusch, Richard L.(ed.): *Bases of Language Interaction,* University Park Press, Baltimore, 1978.

Stover, Samuel L., and Evan Zeiger, Jr.: "Head Injury in Children and Teenagers: Functional Recovery Correlated with the Duration of Coma," *Arch Phys Med Rehabil* 57:201, 1976.

Van Dongen, H.R., and M.C.B. Loonen: "Factors Related to Prognosis in Children," *Cortex* 13:131, 1977.

Worster-Drought, C.: "An Unusual Form of Acquired Aphasia in Children," *Dev Med Child Neurol* 13:563, 1971.

PART THREE

NURSING MANAGEMENT OF SELECTED PHYSICAL IMPAIRMENTS

20
jennifer mccarthy

brain damage
from stroke

INTRODUCTION

When circulation of the blood to the brain is disrupted, the nerve cells in the involved area die or are damaged. This interruption of blood flow is commonly called *stroke;* it is given this name because of the suddenness of onset. Since the nerve cells of the brain control motor activity, coordination, sensation, perception, speech, and thought, all or some of these may be temporarily or permanently impaired.

CAUSES

"Nearly all strokes originate in one of two ways. Either there is a closing off (occlusion) of one of the brain (cerebral) arteries or of one of the arteries in the neck which leads to the brain or there is bleeding (hemorrhage) of a diseased cerebral artery" (Howell, 1978). In occlusion, the artery can be blocked either by a thrombus or by an embolus.

Hemorrhage is the rupture of a weak or diseased artery; therefore, nerve cells that receive nourishment from this artery are abruptly cut off. In addition, the pressure exerted by the blood that flows from this artery can cause further cell death to brain cells in the area.

CONTRIBUTING FACTORS

Howell notes that "the cerebrovascular disease process tends to occur along with some other disease processes which may or may not be causal factors. For example, three-fourths of stroke victims have been diagnosed as having hypertension. Arteriosclerosis (hardening of the arteries) and especially atherosclerosis (narrowing of the arteries due to fat deposits) are usually found in the stroke victim. Cardiac disease, high cholesterol levels, overweight, heavy smoking and diabetes are known to be contributing factors" (Howell).

INCIDENCE

In the United States, 600,000 people per year have a stroke; approximately 200,000 of those die from it. Stroke occurs at all ages, but the average age of onset is 60. Strokes afflict all races, both sexes, and all socioeconomic levels, although not with equal frequency in each grouping. Medical researchers are currently looking at a variety of factors, such as stress on the job, dietary habits, exercise habits, and rest habits, to determine if these may be causative.

PREVENTION

Nurses, whenever or wherever they deliver care for patients, are involved in health assessment and teaching. This teaching should include information to help prevent strokes, with particular emphasis on the importance of regular medical checkups, where blood pressure can be checked and any other possible contributing factors, such as diabetes, can be monitored and controlled. The nurse may be involved in instructing patients regarding proper diet either for weight loss or to reduce cholesterol levels; in teaching methods to avoid or handle stress; or in counseling diabetics on diet, self-medication, and the importance of monitoring urine sugar/acetone levels. All patients should be encouraged to stop or dramatically reduce smoking. Finally, nurses can instruct patients with cardiac diseases or clotting abnormalities about the administration and side effects of any medication they may be receiving.

This chapter focuses on the nurse's role in the rehabilitation of the stroke patient. While it is hoped that this information will prove helpful to the nurse in acute health care agencies, in community-based nursing, and in nursing home facilities, nursing care unique to these situations will not be discussed. The reader is urged to utilize additional sources pertinent to each area.

REHABILITATION TEAM

The essential ingredient of a successful stroke rehabilitation program is the constant and active teamwork of properly trained personnel. "Experience has shown that a coordinated team effort leads to effective utilization of time and facilities, encourages rehabilitation to be practiced throughout the hospital, and allows all persons, including the attending physician, house staff, nursing personnel, rehabilitation specialists, family, and patient to cooperate effectively on formulation and executing an integrated rehabilitation plan suited to the individual needs of each patient" (Bureau of Health Planning and Resources, 1976).

The team generally consists of physicians, including a primary care physician, a neurologist, a psychiatrist, and house staff physicians; nurses, including general nursing staff and rehabilitation nurses; physical, occupational, speech, and vocational therapists; a social worker; a psychologist; and, of course, the patients and their families. Additional team members may include a recreational therapist, a nutritionist, a chaplain, and other specialists such as cardiologists.

NURSE'S ROLE

Where does the nurse fit into this large team? Many of the disciplines are directed at clearly defined areas in the patient's program. The nurse's role is to take what may be very complex medical, social, and psychological problems and deal exhaustively with each need without ever losing sight of the patient as an individual—that is, as a whole. As a result, the nurse assumes major responsibility for facilitating the integration of therapy programs into the patient's daily activities and for ensuring that family members and significant others receive instruction in and are involved in providing daily care to the patient. All activities are carried out with the goal of restoring maximum function of the affected area or areas.

ACTIVITIES OF THE NURSE

The nurse accomplishes this task by employing the tools of assessment, engaging in mutual goal setting with the patient and family, delivering direct care and teaching care to the patient and family, and gradually shifting care delivery to them. In addition, discharge planning and referral to community agencies are done. Unique roles the nurse assumes in rehabilitation with the stroke patient include providing a safe environment for the patient, preventing deformity and complications caused by immobility, reinforcing newly learned skills from other disciplines, and evaluating the patient's compliance with newly learned material. This last role is necessary to determine whether new learning is being retained. Vital to success is the nurse's constant observation and feedback to all members of the rehabilitation team.

All too frequently in hospitals nurses become overly protective of their patients. They often feel that their patients "belong" to the nursing staff. Although this attitude is not without some benefit, nurses can be quite perplexed by the all too obvious fact that the patients are not theirs alone. To begin with, patients do not "belong" to anyone. Moreover, it is often quite a shock when nurses realize that the patients are as valuable to the occupational therapist and the social service worker (and vice versa) as they are to the nursing staff (Martin, 1975).

ASSESSMENT

Whether the patient is entering a rehabilitation facility or beginning an active rehabilitation program within the acute care facility, the nurse should make a thorough assessment of the patient. "Obtaining pertinent data early is the only way goal-directed patient programs can begin early. The initial baseline not only indicates the areas in which the patient needs teaching and assistance, but serves as a means of measuring his progress. Data required for all disability and allergies, family and other social information" (Martin). Table 20-1 offers an example of a basic format that may be used in assessing the patient with completed stroke.

MILDLY VERSUS SEVERELY DISABLED

Should every stroke patient receive a rehabilitation program? Patients with the following characteristics may be considered to be mildly dis-

---

Table 20-1

Assessment Tool for the Patient with Completed Stroke

1. *Communication.* Does the patient:
   a. Use verbal means of expression?
   b. Follow direction on verbal command?
   c. Monitor his or her verbal expression?
   d. Use gestures?
   e. Follow direction given by gestures?
   f. Demonstrate a reliable yes/no response?
2. *Mental Ability.* Does the patient:
   a. Follow directions?
   b. Demonstrate recent and remote memory?
   c. Retain instructions?
   d. Demonstrate carry-over from one situation to another?
   e. Demonstrate good judgment?
   f. Control impulsiveness?
   g. Demonstrate the ability to be alone safely and for what period of time?
   h. Demonstrate lability?
3. *Self-care Activities.* Does the patient manage:
   a. Shirt/blouse?
   b. Undershirt/bra?
   c. Trousers/shorts?
   d. Dress?
   e. Fastenings, hooks, zippers, buttons, snaps?
   f. Socks?
   g. Shoes?
   h. Facial hygiene?
   i. Combing hair?
   j. Shaving?
   k. Applying cosmetics?
   l. Applying deodorant?
   m. Applying splint, brace, sling?
4. *Body and Environmental Awareness.* Does the patient:
   a. Protect involved extremities?
   b. Shave both sides of face?
   c. Remove food pocket from involved side of face?
   d. Dress involved extremities?
   e. Bump into objects in front?
5. *Diet and Fluids.* Does the patient:
   a. Need assistance in opening containers and cutting food?

Table 20-1 (continued)

Assessment Tool for the Patient with Completed Stroke

    b. Have the ability to feed self?
    c. Have chewing problems?
    d. Choke on liquids?
    e. Choke on solids?
    f. Drink from a cup, glass?
    g. Drink with a straw?
    h. Require frequent offerings of foods and fluid?
    i. Eat food from all parts of the tray?
6. *Skin.* Does the patient:
    a. Have sensation of touch in all parts of the body?
    b. Have sensation of hot and cold?
    c. Have areas of breakdown?
    d. Have areas of potential skin breakdown?
    e. Have edema of an extremity or extremities?
7. *Control of Bowels.* Does the patient:
    a. Indicate verbally or with gestures the need for evacuation?
    b. Eat appropriate diet?
    c. Drink sufficient fluids?
    d. Maintain established program, that is, daily, every other day?
    e. Do toilet hygiene?
    f. Use toilet or commode?
    g. Avoid accidents?
8. *Control of Urination* (in absence of catheter). Does the patient:
    a. Indicate verbally or with gestures the need for urination?
    b. Drink sufficient fluid?
    c. Use toilet or commode (female)?
    d. Use urinal (male)?
    e. Tolerate external urinary collecting device (male)?
    f. Do toilet hygiene?
    g. Avoid accidents?
9. *Mobility.* Does the patient:
    a. Have potential for contractures or subluxation?
    b. Come to a sitting position from lying position?
    c. Lift involved lower extremity into and out of bed?
    d. Come to a standing position?
    e. Tolerate wheelchair?
    f. Propel wheelchair?
    g. Ambulate?
10. *Wheelchair Transfers.* Does the patient:
    a. Position wheelchair safely prior to transfer?
    b. Lock brakes prior to transfer?
    c. Place involved foot firmly on floor during transfers?
    d. Do pivot transfer?
    e. Protect involved upper extremity during transfer?

Source: Nancy Martin, "Nursing in Rehabilitation," in I. Beland and J. Y. Passos (eds.): *Clinical Nursing,* Macmillan, New York, 1975, pp. 1012–1013.

abled and therefore in need of less sophisticated rehabilitation techniques:

1. Early partial recovery of dorsiflexion of the paretic foot, even though the ipsilateral arm may remain functionless.
2. Intact sensation or only partial loss of sensory modalities.
3. Minimal or no speech impairment.
4. Preservation of intellect. (Joint Committee for Stroke Rehabilitation, 1972)

The more disabled patient will require a greater number of specialists who are thoroughly familiar with stroke rehabilitation. In particular, the following groups will need specialized attention:

1. The hemiplegic child.
2. The young adult who has suffered a stroke.
3. The patient with bilateral cerebral or cerebellar involvement.
4. The patient with extreme spasticity or prolonged flaccidity.
5. The patient for whom special efforts seem justified, e.g., vocational reasons.
6. The patient for whom formal speech therapy is indicated. (Joint Committee for Stroke Rehabilitation, 1972)

All patients, no matter how severe their physical disability, have had their lives dramatically disrupted, and members of the rehabilitation team must be mindful that each patient is experiencing tremendous loss.

REHABILITATION POTENTIAL

Numerous studies have been done to determine what set of characteristics following stroke indicates good rehabilitation potential and when rehabilitation programs are best initiated. One study using "predictors including a pool of medical data, the age of the patient, psychological tests and the patient's educational level" indicated that

none of these predictor items showed a correlation with outcomes high enough to allow precise prediction of individual outcome....

Since a prediction on an individual basis was not possible, it was concluded that even the most severely involved patient should be provided with a therapeutic rehabilitation trial. There was no correlation between severity of the functional impairment at admission and the gains obtained in the rehabilitation program. The same predictors were used to predict whether the patient went home or to an institution. It was found that family income and involvement in support of the patient predicted this outcome, whereas medical data did not. (Lehmann, 1975)

GOAL SETTING

At the beginning of the active rehabilitation phase, the nurse should discuss goals with the patient. If they are able to communicate verbally, patients most often reply, "to walk and use my arm" or "to be 'normal' again" or "to go home and walk again." Patients with expressive aphasia may point at their paralyzed arm and leg or pick up the extremity, drop it, and then point to it. In addition, this group of patients will often point to the mouth. Family members often express similar goals. The nurse must assist the patient and family in breaking down general goals into individual, short-term, accessible goals. This enables the patient and family to have something concrete to work on and toward; for example, an initial goal might be for the patient to sit at the side of the bed unsupported, then learn to eat independently once the tray has been set up, and finally to cut meat independently. This creates a situation in which the patient can see progress, experience success, and receive positive reinforcement. All efforts are vital if the patient is to remain motivated in a sometimes lengthy rehabilitation program. The nurse must therefore look at each task the patient must relearn and break it down into graduated skill components.

For a newly admitted patient with neither sitting nor standing balance, dressing is an area that seems to offer no goals. In this situation, however, the goal might be assisting with removing trousers/skirt by rolling from side to side in the bed. Rolling for a hemiplegic patient is a major goal, as is attempting to manage the zipper with one hand by pressing the zipper against the body while pulling upward.

RIGHT BRAIN VERSUS LEFT BRAIN

Since nerve fibers cross in the brain stem, the right hemisphere controls the left side of the body and vice versa. The large hemispheres of the cerebrum are commonly known as the *left brain* and the *right brain* because each is specialized in its functions. They communicate with each other through a thick bundle of transverse fibers called the *corpus callosum,* the largest fiber system in the brain (Sperry, 1975).

The left brain, that which remains intact for the left hemiplegic or that which the right hemiplegic may lose, "is highly verbal and mathematical, performing with analytic, symbolic, computer like, sequential logic." The right brain, that which remains intact for the right hemiplegic or that damaged for the left hemiplegic, "by contrast, is spatial and mute, performing with a synthetic spatio-perceptual and mechanical kind of information processing that cannot yet be simulated by computers" (Sperry).

The relationship between language and thought continues to perplex neuropsychologists.

> Unquestionably, certain cognitive and intellectual abilities depend quite heavily on linguistic intactness: the ability to reason about abstract issues, the capacity to solve scientific problems, and, in most areas, skill at mathematics. (Just try to think about a comparison between socialism and communism without resorting to words.) However, an equally impressive list details reasoning powers that may be well preserved despite a severe aphasia: the ability to solve spatial problems, sensitivity to fine differences in patterns or configurations, and alertness to the emotional contours of a situation. (Just try to describe a spiral staircase using only two words.) (Gardner, 1975)

Finally, it is good to keep in mind that our commonsense notions of the relationships among mental abilities may be invalid. Pure alexia without agraphia is an example of this, in that these patients cannot read and yet they are able to write. "The same patients often can read numbers such as 'DIX' as '509' while proving incapable of reading it as 'diks.' They are able to name objects but are frequently unable to name samples of colors shown to them" (Gardner, 1975).

RIGHT HEMIPLEGIA

Patients with right hemiplegia have difficulty with speech and language. Speech/language disorders are described briefly in the following sections, after which care adaptations for the right hemiplegic are discussed. (For a detailed discussion of language disorders, refer to Chaps. 12 and 19.)

The following distinction can be made between language and speech: in speech disorders, verbal output is impaired because of weakness or incoordination of the muscles of articulation; in language disorders, verbal output is linguistically incorrect.

Broca's Aphasia

Aphasia is a term used to describe the language disorders resulting from brain damage. Broca's aphasia characteristically produces little speech, which is slowly emitted. This patient can say single, isolated words but cannot produce complete sentences. For example, if asked about the weather, the patient may say "raining." When asked what day it is, the patient may say "Monday." If urged to produce a sentence, the patient might produce "Today . . . Monday." These patients are unable to repeat a complete sentence given to them, such as "today is Monday" or "the weather is rainy" (Geschwind, 1970).

The relationship between linguistic and musical skills is complex. Some aphasic musicians are able to compose and perform, while others lose their abilities entirely. Gardner indicates that musical capacities may be organized in idiosyncratic ways across individuals (possibly related to how one learned music: by playing an instrument, singing songs, etc.) (Gardner, 1975). The patient with Broca's aphasia can often sing a melody correctly (Geschwind, 1970). Some speech therapy programs may thus attempt to utilize melodic chanting as a means of communication for these patients.

Wernicke's Aphasia

Generally, patients with Wernicke's aphasia have no paralysis of speech musculature of the opposite side. Speech is often rapid, effortless, and as rhythmic as normal speech, but it is without substance, conveying little information. There may be errors in word usage, for example, "spoot" for "spoon" or "fork" for "spoon." Geschwind (1970) describes an example of Wernicke speech as, " 'I was over in the other one, and then after they had been in the department, I was in this one.' " Thus the skeleton of grammar remains, but meaningful words are lacking. Patients with Wernicke's aphasia can write; however, here too, substantive words are lacking. They have severe receptive problems, that is, understanding both spoken and written language without any visual or hearing deficits (Geschwind).

Left Cerebral Dominance

The left side of the cerebrum is dominant for speech. This *left cerebral dominance* occurs, scientists believe, in no other mammal but humans. Geschwind and Levitsky (1968) demonstrated that differences do exist between the two hemispheres, with the left side being larger in 65 percent of brains, while the right is larger in only 11 percent. These differences have been found by Wade to be present at birth.

In adapting care for right hemiplegic patients the nurse should not assume that because the patient cannot speak or respond appropriately to speech, he or she is unable to communicate.

Yes–No Reliability

It should be established as early as feasible in the patient's stay whether the patient's "yes" and "no" responses are reliable and appropriate.

This can only be done by asking the patient simple questions. Using questions that relate to orientation, such as the day, time of day, place, or current president, are often inappropriate, since the patient has not had recent access to this information. Instead, you might ask the patient whose spouse is present, "Is this your wife/husband?," or the patient who has just completed breakfast, "Did you eat breakfast?" These questions should first be asked simply avoiding your own automatic gesture of pointing to the person or tray. Give the patient time to respond, and be alert to the patient's gesturing responses, such as head shaking. For example, Mrs. B. may only shake her head, or she may shake her head "yes" but say "no," or she may say 'no . . . no,no,no," pause then finally say "yes!"

Reliability of "yes" and "no" responses cannot usually be determined with one or two questions. However, bombarding the patient with many questions at one session may reveal that yes–no accuracy declines as the patient tires during the session. Thus, repeated attempts to establish yes–no reliability should be made during the patient's first week of rehabilitation stay and frequently thereafter to assess improvement. Although nurses must attempt to establish an early baseline, the first day of admission and even the first week may yield false data, since the patient may be unable to concentrate fully while coping with the awesome "change" a transfer to a rehabilitation hospital can present.

The nurse must also attempt to ascertain if the patient is accurate in "yes" and "no" responses for recent versus remote memory function. For example, Mr. G. only responds correctly to questions such as "Is this your daughter?" or "Do you live in Philadelphia?" but never to "Did you attend physical therapy?" or "Have you taken your medicine this morning?" Short-term memory losses are common and will be discussed later in this section.

If the patient fails to respond to questions appropriately, try adding gestures. For example, in addition to the simple spoken words of "Did you eat breakfast?," point to the tray. Finally, if this does not elicit an appropriate response, try using *only* gestures, such as pointing at the tray and imitating putting food in your mouth. Fordyce and Fowler (1972) note that aphasic patients sometimes become so adept at understanding nonverbal communication that we overestimate their ability to understand what is said to them. The aphasic patient may only be guessing what has been said by watching the speaker's facial expression or responding to the general tone of voice. They also note that talking while gesturing may only "jam" the circuits, so both methods should be tried.

Aphasic patients are commonly treated as if they are hard of hearing. One logical reason people speak loudly is because they find that it works. This is because when one shouts instructions are usually given in simple words, for example, "Stand up!" or "Turn over." Thus the input is significantly simplified (Fordyce and Fowler).

Since older patients do experience hearing problems more often, an accurate history of auditory testing may be necessary. To further complicate things, the hemiplegic with facial paralysis may be suffering from a hearing deficit on the affected side caused by collapse of the eustachian tube.

If the aphasic patient is bilingual, he or she is apt to lose all ability to communicate in the secondary language while retaining some abilities in the primary language, which may not be English. In addition, knowing the educational background of the patient is important before assessing reading or writing ability. McKenzie Buck (1970) notes that a vast number of our patients have little need for recreational reading once they leave public school. Patients may come to us with poor ability to read materials in sentence and paragraph form, and they may have little need to do so. Functional reading of labels, signs, and headlines may be an adequate goal. Remember that patients with Wernicke's aphasia who have problems with auditory receptive aphasia generally have equally as much trouble reading and writing.

Before attempting to assess reading ability, make sure that if the patient's history indicates the use of eyeglasses, these glasses are worn when the patient is awake. (A discussion of hemianopsia is given later in this chapter.) The patient who wears dentures should have them in while awake, since teeth are necessary to formulate sounds correctly.

Finally, the nurse should assess the patient for dysarthria, facial paralysis, mouth droop, ptosis of the eye, or drooling when placed in a sitting position. Ask the patient to stick out the tongue and move it up and down from side to side. Can the patient chew food of the same consistency as prior to the stroke? (Facial muscle paralysis can be present with or without aphasia.)

Dysarthria

Formal speech therapy by trained therapists is needed for aphasic patients. Nurses reinforce the therapy program by engaging patients in communication attempts and by placing patients in situations that allow them to interact with others. Room selection and roommate selection can play an important role in whether the aphasic patient makes attempts at social speech. Management of personal needs will cause the aphasic patient great distress if failure (i.e., incontinence) occurs because of missed communication. Thus, these areas of meeting the patient's needs should be worked out early in the program. Attempts made by staff members to establish a method of communication for the patient often work in practice sessions but not in real situations. For example, the patient may be supplied with a communication board containing words and pictures indicating yes, no, toilet, eat, pain, toothbrush, and the like. When asked to point to the toilet or point to the pain, the patient may quickly perform the task but be unable to use the board when in pain or when needing to use the toilet. The nurse should seek guidance from speech therapists when necessary and try as many tools as possible, taking care to introduce new materials slowly and to provide an adequate trial period. Nurses must be willing to discard the unsuccessful tool and try alternative methods.

Dysarthria is present in both the right and left hemiplegic. Care must be taken immediately to protect the sclera from drying if ptosis is severe. Taping the eye closed or patching it at night may be indicated along with frequent instillation of "artificial tears."

The distortion of facial expression caused by facial paralysis is at times severe. It may make family, staff, social friends, and especially the patient very anxious. This distortion, especially when coupled with drooling, probably contributes most to erroneous stereotyping of the patient as crazy, dumb, retarded, inhuman, and so on. It also may be the greatest deterrent for resuming social activity; that is, if you drool at the dinner table, you do not get many dinner invitations.

The importance of self-image and to future interpersonal relationships of assisting the dysarthric patient to attain at least a premorbid level of hygiene and to learn compensatory techniques to manage drooling cannot be overemphasized. Some patients have found it beneficial to practice eating in front of a mirror, which allows them to rehearse placing the utensil in the mouth and wiping the mouth frequently.

LEFT HEMIPLEGIA

Patients with left hemiplegia generally will not exhibit aphasia but instead will exhibit spatial-perceptual problems. These have to do with one's ability to judge position, distance, rate of movement, form, and the relationship of the body or its parts to surrounding objects. Patients with spatial-perceptual problems sometimes confuse up and down, inside and outside, right and left. They often walk or move into objects in their path, finding even the widest doorway too narrow to get through. Inability to read occurs, not because they cannot understand the words, but because they lose their place on the page.

Spatial-perceptual problems are more difficult to notice than speech problems, which often leads to overstimulation of the patient's abilities to accomplish tasks such as eating or dressing or safely transferring from, say, bed to chair. There is evidence to suggest that patients with severe spatial-perceptual deficits are less likely to learn independent self-care than are patients with severe aphasia problems (Fordyce & Fowler, 1972).

Behavior

The following phrases characterize behaviors often seen with left hemiplegia: talks incessantly; exhibits poor judgment; is unable to complete a task without errors; is frequently unaware of errors made; can do arithmetic, dial a phone, or use money appropriately; displays a very short attention span; is prone to confabulate, especially about still being engaged in activities that were common prior to the stroke; becomes easily lost; reads aloud fluently without comprehension; displays problems with concepts of time and space; ignores the left side of the body.

Anosognosia

Anosognosia is the inability to recognize or acknowledge hemiplegia by the patient. This is particularly found in patients with left hemiplegia. Patients may deny that the affected extremity belongs to them; for example, a patient may awaken at night and tell the nurse that there is someone else in bed or claim that he or she has been put in bed with a dead person. It is not uncommon for these patients to name their extremities, for example, "Charlie" or "Joe" or "the baby." Although this type of behavior appears bizarre and delusional, it is very important to understand the behavior and correctly interpret it to family and friends, who may believe it to be of a psychotic rather than an organic nature.

First, the sensation of the limb is different; imagine how your own limb feels when it "falls asleep." Second, as Ullman explains, the left hemiplegic "has difficulty in abstract thought. . . ." That is, "thinking becomes concrete. By this we mean that the actual or sensory quality of whatever it is the individual is experiencing determines his response rather than the meaning or abstract interpretation of the stimulus. The individual is bound to his actual experience and lacks the ability to step aside from it, reflect on it, and make reasoned judgements concerning appropriate courses of action" (Ullman, 1961). Thus, if the patient's arm feels "dead," the patient believes it is "dead."

The patient with anosognosia needs gentle, persistent reality orientation from staff and family members, such as saying, "I know it feels as if it's not your arm, but it really is." Unfortunately, interventions of this type produce only temporary results. However, the problem of anosognosia may improve as sensorium clears.

BEHAVIORAL CHANGES

The right hemiplegic patient approaches tasks with anxiety, fear of failure, and frustration. The left hemiplegic, by contrast, plunges ahead, totally self-confident and unaware of safety dimensions.

The right hemiplegic patient will need cueing and feedback on each step of a task, since this may be very stimulating. Simple gestures, such as a head shake or a pat of approval, often prove most effective. Again, it must be emphasized that the task should be broken down into step-by-step components, for example, wheelchair transfer to bed, locking the wheels, removing footrest, and placing feet flat on the floor. In addition, the steps of each operation should be known and rigidly adhered to by all assisting the patient.

The left hemiplegic patient will respond best to verbal directives without visual demonstrations or pantomime. Suggestions to slow down and reminders to follow each step in sequence, as well as positive reinforcement, will be necessary. Emphasis on giving single commands when directing this patient in self-care is imperative if maximal function is to occur; for example, if directed to stand up and turn around, the left hemiplegic may attempt to turn around without first standing up.

NEUROLOGIC CHANGES

The following discussion of neurologic changes pertains to both the right and the left hemiplegic.

HEMIANOPSIA

Hemianopsia, or blindness in one-half of the visual field, may be unilateral or bilateral. The majority of patients with hemianopsia have unilateral blindness or homologous hemianopsia. For the right hemiplegic, it feels as if the right half of each eye has been taped over, with the right visual field cut. The reverse is true for the left hemiplegic. Bilateral hemianopsia usually cuts vision in both outer halves of the visual field, leaving the patient with tunnel vision.

In assessing the patient for hemianopsia, the nurse can check peripheral vision by asking the patient to look straight ahead and then slowly bring an object into the patient's visual field, that is, starting the object on a plane slightly behind the ear of the patient and arm's length distance from the patient and bringing the object forward in an arc.

Functional tests or observations often prove easier to do. For example, when given a food tray, the patient with homologous hemianopsia will see only half the tray and therefore will eat from only half of the food on the tray. If asked to reproduce a simple "stick" drawing of an object, say a house, this patient will draw only half of a house. The patient's head will often be turned to the unaffected side, or the patient may not respond when spoken to if the input is coming from an area in which vision is blocked, but when you enter the patient's visual field, the response is as if you just entered the room. These patients frequently are unable to locate their rooms because they see only one side of it when leaving the room and being wheeled down a corridor; when returning to the room, they see only the other side. For these patients, the corridor is two different corridors.

Some patients who have experienced hemianopsia describe it as being able to see only half of an object, while other patients say they see half of the object clearly, with the second half appearing to be covered with a white drape.

One might wonder why these patients do not just turn their head and see the whole object. Some do; others learn to do this with the assistance of frequent reminders; still others, especially the left hemiplegic with anosognosia problems, will completely neglect one side of the body and environment. (Remember the left hemiplegic's thinking has become more concrete.)

Anosognosia and hemianopsia are different problems, and together they compound each other. These patients present safety problems, since they allow their affected arm to dangle and become caught in wheelchair spokes, or they may roll over on their arm, at times injuring it. Frequent patient checks can prevent many injuries, and utilizing adaptive equipment such as an arm rest that secures the patient's arm in a safe position is extremely helpful.

Bed placement and arrangement of the environment are of top priority for patients with hemianopsia. The bed should always be placed so that the patient's unaffected side is nearest the entrance to the room or that area in which the "action" is, no matter what view the patient is missing out the window. This enables patients to be aware of the area of the room in which most activities occur, since few staff members will squeeze themselves around a patient's bed by the windows to administer simple care or relate simple messages. Proper bed placement also allows the patient in a multibed room to see the other patients, witness social interaction, and hopefully attempt to socialize.

The patient's paraphernalia, such as get well cards, family photographs, body lotion, combs, brushes, and the like should be displayed or stored on the patient's unaffected side. Orientation aides such as calendars, clocks, or wristwatches should be on the patient's unaffected side or within the visual field. Most importantly, the patient's call light must be within easy reach on the patient's unaffected side and in the patient's line of sight.

MEMORY

Memory problems accompany almost all brain injuries. Comparatively little is known about how the brain stores material. There does seem to be two types of memory. Short-term memory refers to those facts that stay with us only a few minutes to a few weeks; for example, when you stay at a hotel, you remember the room number for the duration of your visit and forget it as soon as you leave. Long-term memory, on the other hand, is the retention of experiences for a long period of time. If you spent your honeymoon in a particular hotel, it is likely that you will remember your stay quite clearly (Buys, 1976). You may remember conversations that occurred, or you may be able to close your eyes and visualize the ocean view.

Memory seems to be a function across the brain; that is, it is not confined to one or two segments or localized only in one hemisphere. Researchers are beginning to study memory as a chemical function rather than as electrical activity. Moving from one stage—short-term memory—into another stage—long-term memory—requires a chemical step to fix the impression.

The chemicals currently under research are the hormones ACTH and vasopressin. (A Dutch pharmacologist, Dr. David DeWied, is credited with these discoveries.) "ACTH will prevent rats from forgetting a new skill for some time, vasopressin appears to engrave it in their memories forever. . . . Even though the amino acids from which the hormones are made can be found in common food stuffs, an active pituitary or hypothalamus is required to make them" (Pines, 1975).

Since ACTH is released naturally in the body during stressful or highly emotional situations, this may account for individuals having more vivid memories of events during times of anxiety, fear, hunger, pleasure, and anger.

Many people demonstrate difficulty "fixing" memory as they get older. The patient with cerebrovascular accident (CVA) exhibits particular difficulty in this area. The patient may demonstrate tremendous accuracy with remote memory or memory of old learning but have short retention of recent memory or new learning. For example, the CVA patient may be able to tell you in detail the events of a daughter's birth but be unable to remember your name, the day of the week, or what step is next in transferring to the bed from the wheelchair.

Generalizing or applying what is learned in one situation to another situation is another problem area related to memory function. Previously, we discussed the patient who is unable to use the communication board in a functional setting but is very accurate in a therapy session. Such patients may be able to transfer safely from bed to wheelchair in the physical therapy department but be unable to transfer in their hospital room or at home. The more closely the practice setting can resemble the actual setting, the more likely that the patient will be able to transfer the skill. Teaching the family members how to assist the individual and providing practice sessions in the patient's home via day or overnight passes are essential to success at discharge.

Since patients with generalization problems tend to become more disorganized in their thinking with any alterations of their schedule (i.e., changing therapy times around) or physical environment (i.e., changing rooms or roommates), they need consistent and rigid schedules, with any alterations being made slowly. The same personnel, a schedule of activities posted in the patient's room, and established routines for activities such as dressing or arranging the patient's tray are examples of this (Fordyce and Fowler, 1972).

Other aids for patients with generalization problems who can read include listing appointments or the steps involved in transferring and dressing on cards that the patients carry with them in a notebook. Staff members then focus on reinforcing the use of the notebook. If a patient is unable to read, pictures of the task in sequence form may prove helpful.

Fordyce and Fowler (1972) suggest using old memory aids to help patients negotiate in their environment. Examples of this include taping a family picture to the patient's bed, thus enabling the patient to find the bed; tacking a familiar object such as a hat or scarf to the door of the room thereby helping the patient identify the correct room. In addition, they suggest using old associations in teaching new tasks. An example of this might be the patient who calls his urinal a duck. Staff members should call it a duck when giving the patient directions to evaluate if the urinal is better managed in this way (Fordyce & Fowler, 1972).

How does one teach this patient? It should be reemphasized that each patient is going to be different: each had different mental abilities premorbidly, and damage to the brain occurs in different degrees and affects each individual differently. The approach is therefore geared to the individual patient. Speech therapy assessments, psychological testing, and the nurse's own observations will determine the approach. It is important that the therapeutic disciplines communicate with each other, that an approach is decided upon and given an adequate trial before modifications occur, and that such modifications be made slowly.

Social interaction and socially accepted behavior control seem to be very high-level skills. They are learned at more advanced ages than, say, speech and are usually continuously improved upon throughout life, though often not mastered. This is the ability to evaluate and correct one's own behavior for appropriateness. For example, you do not swear at your boss, you do not steal some item you admire, you comb your hair or put on makeup when going out, you leave a situation that makes you angry rather than pouring your drink on someone's head, and you leave food you do not like on your plate rather than throwing it on the floor.

Patients with brain damage can and do have problems with quality control. They may therefore respond to their environment in unacceptable ways. Nonpunitive, clear feedback about social errors should be given to the patient along with encouragement to correct the behavior. Feedback should occur immediately after an incident, since elasped time may block the patient's memory of the behavior in question.

ORGANIC AFFECTIVE LABILITY

Organic affective lability or emotional lability occurs when there is a loss of control over emotional expressions as a result of brain damage. The behavior manifested is rapid, unpredictable shifts from tears to laughter or to anger.

Patients with inappropriate emotional responses usually receive feedback or interactions from others appropriate to the behavior they are expressing but inappropriate to their feelings. For example, when he is anxious, Mr. S. laughs uncontrollably. He has a Broca's aphasia, and so he has difficulty quickly responding to requests made of him, and almost all social interactions make him anxious. The other patients in his room gradually stopped socializing with him, as he literally "laughed in their faces" when they approached him to eat dinner with them, to watch a game on television, to play cards, and to meet their families. Mr. S. was embarrassed about his behavior and desirous of participating in activities with his roommates. In this case, his behavior could be interrupted by telling him sharply to stop. And if given simplified directive statements, such as "television . . . (point at television), football game . . . yes?," Mr. S. could often communicate without laughter.

Most patients with organic affective lability have problems with uncontrollable crying. It is very easy to misinterpret this for depression on casual observance. Two differences are that affective lability crying has little or no relationship to the activity that was occurring when it started (i.e., nothing precipitates it) and that the behavior is easily interrupted by diverting the patient's attention. Snapping the fingers, clapping the hands, saying the patient's name authoritatively, directing the patient to look out the window, or just telling the patient to stop may interrupt the behavior.

PHYSICAL RESTORATION

The dangers resulting from prolonged immobility have been extensively described (Thompson, 1967; the reader should refer to this issue of the *American Journal of Nursing* for detailed discussion). Following a stroke, as soon as there is medical stability, the patient should begin an activity program including sitting up in a chair or wheelchair and/or ambulating. If sitting balance is poor, support can be given to the patient by utilizing chest straps and pillows and blankets to correct positioning. These activities are begun slowly, and the length of time of the activity is gradually increased as endurance improves. The following sections describe activities that nurses and physical and occupational therapists will participate in prior to getting the patient out of bed and throughout active rehabilitation. They will gradually teach the patient and family to assume these activities.

CONTRACTURES

A *contracture* is shortening of the muscle, which produces limitation of movement of a joint. Contractures in the stroke patient "occur most frequently in the shoulder adductors and rotators, the wrist and finger flexors, the hip flexors and external rotators; the knee flexor and foot plantar flexors" on the affected side. Correct bed positioning and range of motion activities are essential to prevention. Since the stroke patient, especially soon after onset, often does not actively use the unaffected side, positioning and range of motion activities apply to that side as well (Bureau of Health Planning, 1976).

POSITIONING IN BED

The patient should be positioned in bed horizontally, either in supine, side-lying, or prone position, except for activities such as eating. This is done to minimize flexion at the knee and hip joints, which frequently occurs as the patient slides down in the bed. Using the knee gatch of the bed or placing pillows under the knees may prevent the patient from sliding down in bed, but it will also contribute to hip flexion and knee flexion contractures.

Supine

In the supine position the unsupported patient will have extension at the ankles and external rotation of the legs with slight knee flexion. Therefore, the patient is brought down to the end of the bed so that the feet are flat against a footboard. The patient's heels are free from pressure when they rest over the open space between the mattress and the footboard. Trochanter rolls, when placed starting just above the hips along the thigh and just below the knee, will prevent external rotation and knee flexion. A trochanter roll made of a bath blanket or a towel and sheet is placed under the patient and rolled firmly under itself toward the extremity. Hip flexion is avoided because the bed is flat. The patient's head and shoulders are kept in proper alignment by using a flat pillow or no pillow.

Upper extremity positioning should be changed frequently, alternating the following three positions. First, the arms should be placed beside the body, with a small pillow or towel in the axilla of the affected extremity to maintain slight abduction of the shoulder and a pillow under the affected arm to provide elevation and minimize edema. The wrist should be supported with an additional towel to avoid flexion. The hand should be placed in either an open neutral position or around a hard cone or towel roll. Use of the towel or cone should be discussed with the physician and therapist (in some settings the occupational therapist and in others the physical therapist), since it is believed that use of these may sometimes increase synergies of flexion. If the patient has had special resting splints made to keep the wrist in neutral position, to allow for thumb opposition, and to minimize synergy of flexion, the splint should be applied.

The second position of the upper extremity is full extension to the side. This allows for maximal abduction of the shoulder and extension of the elbow. The arm is again elevated slightly on pillows to minimize edema, and the wrist is supported and the hand positioned as previously described. The arm may be pronated, the hand down or supinated and opened up toward the ceiling.

The third upper extremity position resembles a "Statue of Liberty" pose. The shoulder remains fully abducted, the elbow is flexed at a 90° angle, with the hand pointed toward the head of the bed. This may also be reversed, with the hand pronated or pointed down toward the foot of the bed. The nurse should change the arm position as frequently as possible and at least every hour.

Side Lying

For side lying on the unaffected side, the patient is again moved toward the foot of the bed, the unaffected leg is straight so that the foot is placed again against the footboard. The outer malleolus of this ankle is bridged in the space between the mattress and the foot of the bed. The hips and shoulders are placed in good alignment, that is, one directly below the other to maintain the natural S curve of the spine. The affected lower extremity is flexed at the hip and knee and brought in front of the lower leg. Pillows are used to support the entire length of the leg to avoid hip abduction. If the patient's hips are properly aligned, a pillow at the back is not necessary. The upper arm is supported on pillows in front of the patient's chest to avoid shoulder adduction, and the wrist and hand positions are maintained as previously described. Finally, a small pillow is placed under the head.

Many patients dislike this position, since the only parts of their bodies they can use are pinned against the bed. If hemianopia is present, the patient may be completely cut off from the environment. Patients naturally fight to correct this position by turning onto their back. Piling pillows up behind the patient's back generally only results in the patient's being "lost in a sea of pillows" as the patient tries to correct the position.

Having patients lie on their side when a family member is present to reassure them may be helpful. The best rule of thumb is to plan on positioning and repositioning this patient frequently. Side lying on the affected extremity is not recommended owing to risk of injury because of the often severe impairment in sensation. It also contributes to edema of the affected arm and hand. Patients will usually do more than enough side lying on their affected side as they struggle to reposition from the supine position. This naturally occurs because the affected arm and leg are swung across the body as the patient tries to turn, the side rail is grasped, and the patient rolls onto the affected side.

Prone

The prone position is excellent to prevent hip flexion and knee flexion contractures. The patient is again brought down to the foot of the bed so that the feet hang over the end of the mattress. Pillows placed under the thighs and below the knees alleviate pressure on the knees. Another pillow is placed under the abdomen to prevent hip hyperextension. If the patient is male and has a Foley catheter, this will facilitate drainage and free the scrotal area. If the patient is female, more pillows under the abdomen may be needed to avoid pressure on the breast.

Pads of towels or bath blankets are used under the shoulders to encourage adduction of the scapula and provide greater chest expansion. The arms are placed in one of three positions: along the sides of the body, out at the side, or by the patient's head. Finally, a small pillow is placed under the patient's head, and it should be turned toward the unaffected side to allow for maximal visual field. This position is also very frightening for the patient, since, again, the patient is virtually trapped against the bed. Staying with the patient or having family members stay with the patient is often very helpful. The patient's tolerance for abdominal lying can often be increased gradually by 5- or 10-min increments.

RANGE OF MOTION

Passively moving each joint of the affected extremity through a full range three times at least once a day and preferably twice is essential in preventing contractures (Bureau of Health Planning, 1976). One of the easiest ways to incorporate range of motion exercises into the patient's daily routine is during bathing. It is also an activity that family members can become involved in early in the patient's hospitalization and often assume responsibility for at least once a day. Passive ranging should always be done by providing gentle support over the joint; that is, an extremity must not be picked up or held in the middle of a long bone, since this can result in a fracture. The joint is ranged only to the point of pain; going beyond this point should be done only with a physician's order and is generally done by trained physical therapists. Physical therapists may utilize other therapy modalities such as heat or water to augment the activity.

Lower extremity range of motion "includes bending and straightening of the hip, knee and ankle" and should be given to both lower extremities for even mildly involved patients. This also helps prevent venous stasis in the lower extremities. Range of motion of the lower extremities can generally be discontinued as soon as the patient is actively walking (Bureau of Health Planning, 1976). "Conversely, full flexion of the shoulder, extension of the elbow, pronation-supination of the forearm, dorsiflexion of the wrist, and straightening and bending of the thumb and fingers are a routine which must be followed faithfully for a prolonged period" (Joint Committee for Stroke, 1972).

As soon as possible, patients are taught to do range of motion exercises themselves. This provides for active exercise of the unaffected extremity and actively involves the patient in rehabilitation, often before more strenuous therapy can be attempted. Patients with severe "spasticity have a tendency to substitute hyperextension of the lumbar spine for full flexion of the paretic shoulder." The patient may need assistance to avoid this. To avoid wrist injury, the patient should be taught to grasp the distal forearm rather than the hand when doing pronation-supination exercises. To stretch finger flexors, the palms of both hands are opposed and the uninvolved hand is slid distally, which causes the involved hand to dorsiflex at the wrist and fingers. The thumb should be extended and abducted separately. Finally, the fingers of the uninvolved hand should be interwoven with the fingers of the involved hand (Bureau of Health Planning, 1976).

The patient may receive specific aids for range of motion exercises for full adduction of the shoulder and extension of the arm, such as a door pulley attachment that the patient can use while sitting up in the wheelchair. These are usually prescribed by the physical or occupational therapist under the supervision of a physician. The patient should be supervised in these activities until staff members are certain that the aids can be safely used by the patient to avoid shoulder injury.

A material similar to "silly putty" may be used by the patient with some hand function to increase strength in finger flexion and extension. This is generally supplied by the occupational therapist.

PREVENTION OF PRESSURE SORES

Patients develop pressure sores from prolonged pressure over a bony prominence. This compression of tissue over a bone cuts off circulation to the tissue, and thus oxygen and food supplies are stopped and cell death occurs. (See Chap. 16.)

The patient should be turned every 2 h to avoid pressure sores. The heels, sacrum, scapula, and occiput are checked for redness after the patient is in the supine position. Following the side-lying position, the outer malleolus, trochanter, and shoulder are checked. Finally, after prone lying, the toes, knees, anterior tibial crests, and iliac crests are checked for redness. If redness occurs and has not completely resolved in 20 min, the patient should not be placed in this position again until complete resolution has occurred, and the subsequent length of time in that position should be reduced.

This population of patients, in contrast to the generally younger spinal cord patient population, may have concurrent medical problems, such as peripheral vascular insufficiency or diabetes, that compound the problem of pressure. Frequent turning, even hourly, may be needed.

A physician's order for antiembolus stockings should be secured for all patients, and the hose should be worn in bed, since venous stasis also decreases the flow of oxygen and nutrients to tissue.

In struggling to find a position of comfort, the stroke patient often uses the unaffected lower extremity as a lever. This rubbing of the foot against bed linens, even when antiembolus hose are worn, can produce enough friction and heat to cause redness and inflammation of the unaffected heel. Inflamed tissue is more prone to breakdown, and therefore it must be reemphasized that the nurse check bony prominences on the unaffected extremities as well. Use of sheepskin or foam under the heels or wearing boots of sheepskin can be helpful. However, removing pressure entirely is the only absolute prevention.

When the stroke patient is mobilized to the wheelchair level, the ischial tuberosities should be checked after sitting. Stroke patients generally do not have the endurance initially to sit for prolonged periods of time, but even if they do, the sitting tolerance of their skin should be carefully evaluated and slowly upgraded.

The problem of obesity that many stroke patients have makes repositioning themselves in a chair nearly impossible, even though they may have sensations of discomfort. Assisted weight shifts should be done every 20 min while the patient is sitting until the patient is able to assume this activity independently.

MOBILIZATION

Activities progressing from sitting to wheelchair mobility to walking are begun as soon as there are no medical contraindications. A patient who has had an intracranial hemorrhage generally will need to be kept flat in bed longer than a patient who has had a stroke from thrombosis or embolism. A patient with existing cardiovascular disease or one who has had a recent myocardial infarction will need a more gradual endurance-building program with close monitoring than will the patient with uncomplicated stroke. Patients with diabetes mellitus will need to have diet and insulin regulations evaluated and altered as their activity increases.

POSTURAL HYPOTENSION

When beginning sitting activities, the blood pressure should be monitored closely by the nurse, since orthostatic hypotension following cerebral infarction may further compromise the brain's collateral circulation, aggravating the ischemic injury already present. The patient should wear antiembolus hose. In addition, the head of the bed should be raised slowly, a few degrees at a time, and a blood pressure determination made at each new level.

BED ACTIVITIES

Sitting and coming to a sitting position are practiced once postural hypotension is overcome. Since the patient should use and practice techniques applicable to the home situation, a trapeze generally is not used on the bed. Patients often use the side rail, attempting to drag the body into a sitting position. This is difficult to do because when the hand is released from the side rail as the patient attempts to reach forward for a new grasp, nothing is supporting the patient, and usually gravity pulls the patient back to the reclining position. In addition, if the patient will not have side rails at home, learning to depend on them will be a handicap after discharge.

The nurse can begin teaching the patient to move the affected lower extremity using the unaffected leg prior to working on sitting activities. When the patient can do this, he or she should be taught to practice turning onto the unaffected hip, about a half-turn to the unaffected side, with the affected lower extremity crossed over the unaffected lower extremity. In this position, the patient can practice extending the unaffected arm to raise the torso off the bed; flexing the trunk at the same time should, with practice, bring the patient to a sitting position. The principle involved in this maneuver is to place the center of gravity of the body over the supporting base provided by the unaffected side, hand, hip and finally buttocks. Although this is difficult for all patients to do, the difficulty increases for an obese patient, since the weight that must be lifted is greater.

Special precautions may need to be taken for the patient with cardiovascular disease, since there is a natural tendency toward a Valsalva maneuver. Patients with serious cardiovascular disease may need to have a hospital bed at home after discharge so that the head of the bed can be raised, or they may be candidates for a trapeze. The physician should be consulted to determine activity restrictions in such cases.

As discussed previously, the right hemiplegic patient will do best with gestures and frequent feedback, while the left hemiplegic patient should be given short single-step directive statements, positive feedback, and support to slow down. Both will benefit from following the same procedure each time.

To sit at the side of the bed with feet dangling, the patient must be able to move the affected leg off the bed using the unaffected extremity. Until the patient can do this independently, the nurse assists, being careful to follow the steps the patient is to learn.

When the patient can come to a sitting position with the legs in bed and is able to move the lower extremity in the bed using the unaffected lower extremity, practice should begin on doing these activities simultaneously.

The hemiplegic patient tends to lean toward

the involved side, and therefore the patient should practice overcorrection toward the opposite side. The nurse must always stand by the patient who is sitting at the side of the bed until the patient can either transfer independently or is ambulatory.

STANDING TRANSFERS

The assisted transfer to the wheelchair from the bed is done following the same steps that the patient will eventually employ to transfer independently. The wheelchair is brought to the bed and placed facing either the head or the foot of the bed so that the patient's unaffected extremities will be closest to the chair. The footrest is removed or moved out of the way, and the chair is locked. The patient, after assuming a sitting position at the side of the bed, is brought to the edge of the bed so that both feet are flat against the floor. When doing any transfer, the patient should be wearing flat supportive shoes with nonslip soles. Inexpensive tennis shoes can be supplied by the family if the patient has no other appropriate shoes, since future shoe purchases may need to be a prescribed oxford, possibly worn with a short leg brace. The patient is then directed to or assisted to lean forward, flexing at the waist, followed by pushing up from the bed with the unaffected arm. This brings the patient's body weight forward and over the feet. It is important to remember to direct the patient to lean forward, since this seems to be a step frequently forgotten, especially by the left hemiplegic. For example, Mrs. G., a left hemiplegic patient, sitting at the side of the bed ready for transfer, is told "Now stand up." Instead of standing up, Mrs. G. straightens her legs, which results in her falling back across the bed.

The nurse should be positioned either directly in front of the patient, placing one hand under each axilla for support, or on the patient's affected side, supporting the dressed patient by holding onto the trouser or slacks top in back of the patient. The affected arm is not grasped, since injury to the shoulder might result. Whichever position is assumed, the nurse should stand so that one foot is blocking the patient's affected foot, which keeps the foot from sliding; in addition, flexing of the nurse's knee will block the patient's knee on the affected leg. This not only prevents the affected leg from buckling but also enables the nurse to assist the patient in fully extending the leg.

Once the patient has leaned forward, pushed up from the bed, and is standing straight with the nurse supporting the affected side, the patient can be assisted to turn, or pivot, on the unaffected leg. The patient should then be told to reach for the wheelchair arm rest for support and be assisted to a sitting position in the chair.

When doing the transfer, many patients will automatically reach up to the nurse's shoulder or lock the unaffected arm around the nurse's back in an attempt to gain greater support. This can injure both the nurse, who is now carrying most of the patient's weight, and the patient, since the nurse in this position cannot safely lower the patient into the chair. Therefore, patients should be discouraged from holding onto the nurse. Often, this is best done by giving the patient short, clear directions of what to do next; if the problem persists, a second person should assist with the transfer until the patient is more secure in the procedure.

Once the patient is in the wheelchair, the footrest on the involved side is repositioned; the patient is assisted to use the unaffected leg to lift the involved lower extremity onto the footrest. A safety belt is applied to prevent falling forward or to the side before the patient is assisted to unlock the brakes on both sides of the chair. Remember, the patient with hemianopia may forget that there is a brake to unlock if it falls outside the visual field, and the patient may not be able to include it in the visual field even when turning the head for scanning. Finally, the patient's position in the wheelchair is corrected so that the involved upper extremity is supported either with pillows (the shoulder abducted, forearm up on a pillow, wrist and hand supported) or with an adaptive arm rest that abducts the shoulder and elevates the arm and hand while supporting the wrist.

To transfer from the wheelchair back into the bed, the steps are essentially reversed. The wheelchair is placed so that the unaffected extremity is closest to the bed, the brakes are locked, the involved foot is taken off the footrest, and the footrest is removed or swung out of the way. The safety belt is removed, and the affected arm is taken off the adapted arm rest or the pillows are removed. The patient is then directed and assisted to lean forward while pushing up against the arm rest, straighten the legs, pivot on the unaffected leg, and lower to a sitting position while reaching for the bed with the unaffected hand. The affected leg is swung into bed using the unaffected leg, and the side rail is raised.

Transfers are gradually upgraded from the assisted one-person pivot, to standby assistance, and finally to independent transfers. Some patients may always need to be assisted because of lack of strength or inability to transfer safely because of balance or memory problems. However, if the patient can actively participate and follow cues or directions, it will facilitate those caring for the patient by increasing the patient's mobility.

Commode and Toilet Transfers

Transferring to the commode from the bed is done just like a wheelchair transfer. It is important to use a very stable commode chair with adequate brakes or to have a second staff member stabilize the chair.

Transferring to the toilet from the wheelchair for the fully dressed patient is more difficult. Clothing must be either removed or reapplied. The patient must stand on one leg, using the only functional hand to manipulate the clothes, thus leaving no hands to hold onto the grab bar.

Most patients, unless they are ambulatory, will be assisted in toilet transfers. If there are properly placed grab bars, the patient is directed to hold onto the bar for balance once the standing position is assumed, and the nurse will unbutton or unzip trousers and slacks or hold up dresses and pull down underclothing. When transferring back to the wheelchair, if the patient is wearing trousers or slacks, the nurse should pull these items up at least over the knee and hold onto them before the patient stands so that when the patient is assisted to stand, the slacks or trousers do not end up around the ankles. The underclothes and the outer garments are repositioned, but fastening is usually delayed until the patient is back in the wheelchair.

How do patients ever accomplish this independently? Some of the following shortcuts may help: Men can void while sitting in the wheelchair and may develop bowel habits that enable them to evacuate early in the morning or late in the evening, when street clothes are removed. Female patients, since they must use the toilet for voiding, will be doing more transfers. Many wear loose-fitting dresses and underclothes to make management easier. Some patients may decide to go without undergarments all or some of the time. If the patient wears slacks, elasticized waistbands are easier to manage. They may be pulled down to hip level while in the wheelchair before transferring, and they do not usually fall to the floor if left above knee level. Further, buttons, hooks, or zippers will not be a problem. The patient will need to have good standing balance. If the bathroom is constructed so that the unaffected side can be placed next to a wall, some patients are able to support themselves by leaning against the wall with the shoulder.

Physical therapists are actively involved in determining the easiest and safest method of transferring. They may make a home visit to evaluate the layout of the bathroom the patient will most frequently be using or request the family members to draw the bathroom layout and measure dimensions of the room. Adaptive equipment such as grab bars is recommended by the physical therapist. The family is taught to assist in transfers either by the nursing staff or the physical therapist. Family members will need to be taught the steps of the transfers and good body mechanics; their participation should be supervised until they are comfortable with the procedure.

WHEELCHAIRS

The wheelchair used should be the standard type with backrest and seat made of fabric or synthetic plastic. The leg rests should be detachable and made so that they can be moved out of the way. Brakes are located in front to be accessible to the uninvolved hand and are of the lever type. A safety belt similar to an automobile seat belt is used when the patient is independent with transfers or if the patient demonstrates no impulsiveness. A seat belt that fastens behind the patient or out of reach of the patient is appropriate for patients who attempt impulsive transfers in order to minimize the risk of falling. This seat belt is not applied tightly or restrictively but rather is utilized to serve as a reminder feedback tool for the patient to call either a member of the nursing staff or the physical therapist for assistance with transfers.

To self-propel the wheelchair, the footrest is removed on the unaffected side of the chair. The patient is then taught to use the uninvolved hand on the handrim while using floor contact with the normal foot in order to maneuver the chair effectively.

Wheelchairs should not be purchased by the patient or family, since many stroke patients will be ambulatory at discharge. If it is necessary to purchase a wheelchair, specific modifications of the standard chair can be obtained, such as elevated leg rests, swinging leg rests, detachable arms, desk-type arms, or extra-wide chairs for obese patients. If there is no physical therapist skilled in ordering wheelchairs in your facility, the wheelchair company representative should be consulted for specific directions on measuring the patient for a chair.

Although one-arm-drive wheelchairs are available, they are difficult to operate, more expensive, and often too wide for doorways. In general, they are used only for triplegic patients or patients with lower extremity amputation on the uninvolved side—in both cases, the patient must be capable of conceptually knowing which rim to propel.

Wheelchair Weight Shift

To correct position in the wheelchair or to relieve pressure, the patient is taught to lock the brakes, lean forward at the waist, and push up with the normal arm and leg, lifting the buttocks a few inches off the chair. Hemiplegic patients who have a tendency to slide down in the wheelchair should be reminded to flex at the waist, since attempting to move the buttocks back in the wheelchair by only extending the leg results in the chair tipping backward and/or the buttocks moving more toward the front edge of the wheelchair.

AMBULATION

Ambulation training is begun by the physical therapist when there has been moderate recovery of voluntary motor activity in the lower extremity. The patient should wear broad, low-heeled shoes. Exercises that require shifting the body weight alternately from one leg to the other are done to improve balance. Even when doing these, the patient is taught always to lean toward the unaffected side. If there is minimal impairment, ambulation may be relearned without special equipment; otherwise, training begins with the parallel bars. Once the patient has developed a gait with persistent leaning toward the unaffected side and slightly forward, training begins outside the parallel bars with a wide-based quad cane (Joint Committee for Stroke, 1972).

Once the patient is safely ambulating outside the parallel bars in physical therapy with supervised assistance, ambulation should be done on the patient unit. The nurse should be positioned on the paralyzed side because of the tendency to fall in that direction. If assistance with walking is necessary, the nurse should hold on to the back of a belt placed around the patient's waist. It should be emphasized again that the paretic arm is never grasped. The nurse should pay particular attention to the "swing" phase of walking, encouraging the patient to bend the knee and dorsiflex the foot.

A cane on the side opposite the involved lower extremity not only bears some weight but also provides proprioceptive input during the "stance" phase on the involved lower extremity. A broad-based quad cane is used for greater stability. A single-ended cane may be used as ambulation improves. Lightweight aluminum canes do not provide as much proprioceptive input as do heavy wooden canes, and therefore the latter are recommended, especially if there is proprioceptive loss in the involved leg. Finally, some patients, particularly older persons, may need thick-handled canes because of a weak hand grasp (Joint Committee for Stroke, 1972).

Stair climbing is taught to the ambulatory hemiplegic patient who has good strength and balance. Patients with minimal involvement may learn the normally used "step-over-step" method. More severely involved patients will be taught one step at a time. Ascending the stairs, the normal leg leads, and the paretic leg is pulled up after it. Descending, the paretic leg is advanced to the lower stair by bending the normal leg. Since a handrail on the uninvolved side is needed for both activities, handrails will be needed on both sides of the stairs in the home.

BRACES

If the patient is unable to dorsiflex the foot during the "swing" phase or has spasticity (of the talipes equinovarus) that presents difficulties in controlling the foot in a dorsiflexed position, a short leg brace may be needed. When a brace is prescribed, shoes may also be prescribed. After receiving a brace the nurse should teach the patient to inspect the paretic lower extremity for any pressure areas.

BEGINNING ACTIVITIES OF DAILY LIVING AND VARIOUS REACTIONS OF PATIENT AND FAMILY

Early involvement of the patient in activities such as moving in bed, washing the face, and brushing teeth is important in establishing the patient's active participation in self-care. Patients arrive at the hospital and/or rehabilitation facility with a set of expectations that often include "getting well" and "returning to normal." They often feel that "being cared for" or "ministered to" will result in their returning to premorbid levels of functions. Sometimes they and/or their families turn to religious beliefs, with the expectation that God will make them well. They may respond to their stroke and disability by denying that it has occurred and, more frequently, by denying that they will be left with any permanent limitations.

Social and cultural influences may diminish the patient's self-expectations to participate in care. These include the patient's or family's expectation of caring for the "afflicted" individual, as well as the patient's or family's expectations of how one lives and is cared for at advanced ages or after a stroke.

Mr. C., for example, was a successful businessman, president of his own company, who, while in the hospital for a fractured hip, suffered a left cerebrovascular accident. His resultant right hemiparesis and moderately severe Wernicke's aphasia left him with what appeared on admission to be potentially good ability to be independent with self-care. Mr. C. indicated he had planned to retire so that his son could assume management of the company, and he therefore proceeded to retire in a few months. In the weeks that followed, Mr. C. made brief attempts at activities of daily living (ADL) but quickly became frustrated, often saying "You help me" or "I'm paying for services here" or "This is your job." Finally, Mr. C. became very angry at the staff's insistence that he do or attempt self-care and insisted on private nurses. At discharge, Mr. C. had not learned self-care and was discharged with private duty nursing assistance. Interestingly, he and his wife did remain socially active. Although there were many dynamics at work in this situation, the conclusion drawn by nurses, therapists, psychologist, and social service personnel was that this "assisted, cared for" life was in fact what Mr. C. felt was his "due" on retirement and that being able to care for himself independently held less value for this particular patient than being able to afford attendants.

Although this is an extreme example, it illustrates one of the conflicts that can occur between the professional staff member's goals for independence and the patient's or family's goals. It should be reemphasized that on admission and frequently thereafter, the patient's goals should be discussed and that the nurse should assist the patient in setting short-term, reachable goals in order to gain the patient's full participation.

EATING

Eating is one of the first activities in which the patient can be involved. If there are no swallowing difficulties and if the patient can handle utensils, the assistance needed may be just to prepare the tray, cut up food into bite-size proportions, and open milk or juice cartons. Plate guards are useful for many patients to facilitate getting the food onto utensils. A combination fork-spoon may also be useful when eating foods in sauces or hard-to-"spear" foods, such as peas. If the patient was right-handed and is a right hemiplegic, there will be greater difficulty in managing eating with the left hand, and vice versa.

Patients with paralysis or paresis of facial musculature will have more difficulty managing chewing and swallowing. Because they may be unable to feel food in one side of the mouth, they fail to use the tongue to move the food back toward the throat where it can be swallowed. Instead, the food pockets in the side of the mouth, often between the gums and cheek, or it may fall out of the affected side of the mouth during chewing. Unable to detect the food pocket, these patients often continue eating, which results in overfilling the oral cavity, leaving the patient unable to swallow or chew. Patients with these types of problems benefit from eating in a quiet setting, such as their own room. If hemianopsia is present, they should be positioned in their room with their affected side toward the door. This is done because it cuts the patient off from confusion in the corridor area, thus minimizing interruption. A single food item at a time is given to the patient instead of the multicourse food tray. A staff member stays with the patient, giving either simple verbal cues or gestures to "take a bite," "chew," "swallow," and "check for food pockets." If the patient has difficulty swallowing food, all meals should be eaten while sitting erect, and the nurse should give reminders or assistance to flex the neck slightly, since it is easier to swallow in this position and aspiration is less likely.

Speech therapists are often involved in eating training if there is severe facial muscle paralysis. They may use techniques of stimulating facial musculature with a hand placed along the affected side of the jaw. In severe cases, techniques of icing (using an ice-cold spoon with a little ice water in the mouth) may be used. In situations such as these, the nurse will learn the particular care program to be used with the patient. Suction equipment should be at hand, and assessing the patient for aspiration is imperative.

NUTRITION

In some patients who have problems with quality control, it is necessary to give food items in the order they should be eaten. If presented with the entire tray, this patient usually eats the most desired foods first, dessert in most cases, and may never eat more nutritionally important items such as vegetables.

Finally, a calorie count may need to be implemented for patients with chewing and swallowing problems, for diabetics, for those who are easily distracted, or for those with poor appetite. The dietician is frequently involved in planning appetizing and nutritionally sound diets for these patients. Family members may be requested to provide favorite dishes to improve dietary intake in extreme cases.

DRESSING

Dressing using only one hand is a very difficult task and may be further complicated by hemianopsia, anosognosia, and perceptual impairments. When the patient is able to sit up in the wheelchair or chair, even if active physical therapy classes have not begun, the patient should be dressed in street clothes during the daytime. Since this will most likely occur before the patient has mastered sitting balance at the side of the bed, the nurse will utilize in-bed dressing procedures for the lower extremities.

Antiembolus hose will be applied by the nurse, and undergarments and slacks or trousers, if worn, will be started over the feet and pulled up on the lower extremities to mid-thigh, where the patient can reach them. The patient is then instructed to or assisted to roll from side to side, and when in the side-lying position, the clothing is pulled up to the waist.

Zippers can be closed with one hand by pressing in against the body while pulling the zipper up. The patient may be able to put on shoes once in a sitting position in bed; if not, assistance with the lower extremities may be necessary.

Once the patient has transferred to the wheelchair, the upper extremities are dressed. Bras will often have to be fastened by the nurse until the patient becomes more adept at one-handed techniques or until front closing or adapted bras with Velcro are available. The shirt or blouse that buttons up the front is placed on the patient's lap, unbuttoned, with the neckline or collar toward the patient's knees. With the unaffected hand, the patient reaches in through the affected extremity sleeve, grasps the affected hand, and pulls it through the sleeve to the armhole opening. Once the hand is through the sleeve, the fabric is slid up the affected extremity as close to the shoulder as possible. The patient then grasps the shirt collar and brings the shirt around the back. Finally, the unaffected extremity is placed through the appropriate sleeve. Remember, left hemiplegic patients may have difficulty with distinguishing up and down and inside and outside. Sewing brightly colored thread to the neckline may help such patients remember where the shirt should be placed when beginning the procedure.

After the shirt or blouse is on both arms, it is adjusted on the back and shoulders and then buttoned. Many patients are able to learn one-handed buttoning techniques. This task is difficult and frustrating for most patients at first. The nurse can facilitate buttoning by starting one button at the shirt neckline; this aligns the other buttons with the buttonholes. Short-sleeved, loose-fitting blouses and shirts will be easier to use when first learning.

Since buttoning the cuff on a long-sleeved shirt on the unaffected arm remains impossible unless fine finger control returns in the affected extremity, the patient can be taught to button this cuff before applying the shirt. The pullover shirt or dress is applied by placing the garment face down on the lap, with the neckline again toward the knees. The affected arm is placed through the armhole in a similar fashion as the button shirt. The shirt is brought over the head, and then the unaffected extremity is put through the armhole. Some patients place both arms through the armhole openings before pulling the garment over the head. Because the procedures do differ, it is generally less confusing for the patient to learn only one procedure to begin with.

Once the patient has good sitting balance, dressing the lower extremities will be done while sitting on the side of the bed. The occupational therapist will be involved in teaching dressing and undressing techniques. The nurse should be cognizant of the procedure each patient is using and follow it religiously. As with all activities, remember to give the right hemiplegic patient nonverbal cues and frequent feedback; the left hemiplegic will need short verbal directions and reminders to slow down.

Finally, adaptations for shoe closures, such as elastic laces, or learning one-handed tying or utilizing long-handled shoe horns will generally be made and taught by the occupational therapist. Many hemiplegic patients will wear only loafer-type shoes. As with all activities, the family should be taught the procedures as soon as possible and be involved in them whenever visiting.

HYGIENE

Hygiene is an activity in which at least partial participation can occur early. The goal the nurse should keep in mind is restoring the patient to at least the premorbid level of hygiene. That is, if a patient used to bathe only twice a week with partial or sponge baths in between, it will probably be unrealistic to expect the patient to shift to daily showering or tub baths. Of course, if the patient had poor hygiene habits, the nurse should encourage upgrading, but keep in mind that this may mean asking the patient to change a lifelong routine, which may be met with strong resistance.

Oral Hygiene

Oral hygiene in the stroke patient is extremely important, since, as noted earlier, there is a tendency for food to remain pocketed in the oral cavity. When this problem exists, the patient should be told to check for food pockets with the index fingers after eating. Patients should be reminded to brush their teeth at least twice daily and to rinse the mouth with clear water after each meal. Placing the patient in front of a mirror while brushing the teeth will help remind the patient to brush on both sides. The toothpaste usually can be squeezed onto the toothbrush with one hand; however, applying and removing caps may be difficult. The recommended flossing of the teeth is unfortunately a two-handed procedure; some patients may benefit from using a Water Pik to dislodge small food particles between the teeth and near the gums. All patients, unless they have recently been seen by a dentist, should do so during the hospitalization period.

If a patient wears dentures, they should be in, since, as noted earlier, they promote clearer speech as well as aiding eating and improving appearance. Following a stroke, particularly if facial musculature paralysis is present, dentures may no longer fit well. Many patients with full denture plates will therefore need to see the dentist. Cleaning of dentures with one hand can be accomplished using a brush attached by a suction cup to a flat surface or to the bottom of a bowl.

Facial Hygiene

Facial hygiene is another activity that can be done by the patient even in bed. A properly positioned mirror facilitates this. Male patients who must shave often can do this more safely with an electric razor. If the patient insists on using a blade razor, supervision is necessary until the activity has been done safely on at least three consecutive days. Patients with severe hemianopsia may be unable to shave one side of the face, since turning the head to include that side of the face in the visual field only turns the face out of view in the mirror.

Female patients should be encouraged to resume wearing makeup if this was their habit. Although it may be difficult to apply with one hand, practice usually improves results.

The patient can usually assist with partial baths in bed but will need help washing the strong upper extremity and under the arm. Tub bathing can be done once sitting balance is good.

The patient will need to have all necessary items on hand when bathing. This may be facilitated by having a simple list for the patient to refer to if the patient can read, or a picture list may prove useful when reading is a problem.

Transfer for Hygiene

Rehabilitation facilities may have showers that accommodate wheelchairs or into which the patient can walk and then sit in a chair. Although this does provide ease for managing bathing while in the hospital, it unfortunately misrepresents the problems the patient will face in bathing once the transfer has been taught at home. Tub transfers usually are taught by the physical therapist, but the nursing staff must plan to provide practice for the patient in tub transfers and bathing.

A tub bench is placed in the tub, and the patient transfers to it much the same as to a chair. The legs are swung into the tub while holding onto a properly placed grab bar. A hand-held shower will provide greater independence. Soap, washcloths, and towels should be placed within reach prior to beginning the activity. To bathe in this fashion, the patient will need to have excellent sitting balance.

HOMEMAKING

Homemaking activities such as cooking, cleaning, and laundering are usually taught by occupational therapists. If finances are no object, there are many aids and devices available to make chores more manageable; they include regular labor-saving devices such as sink garbage disposals, electric knives, microwave ovens, self-cleaning ovens, food processors, automatic defrost refrigerators, and front-loading washers and dishwashers for wheelchair-bound patients. Less expensive kitchen aids include mixing bowls with suction cups, one-handed egg beaters, handheld electric mixers, long tongs for reaching, and one-handed can openers. Meals can be simplified by using convenience foods or one-pot meals.

Clothing that requires minimal care should be selected to reduce the need for ironing. Floors can be cleaned with lightweight vacuum cleaners or by using a broom and a long-handled dustpan. Beds can be made from a sitting position.

Whenever possible, the patient should be given the opportunity to practice homemaking activities while in the hospital. Day and weekend passes also provide opportunities to practice. Prior to discharge, it is often helpful to have the occupational therapist make a home visit to evaluate needed equipment, rearrangement of existing supplies, and the accessibility of the home in general.

For information on infant care, see Patricia Galbreaith's book *What You Can Do for Yourself* (1974). It is filled with practical, simplifying steps to ease infant care.

BOWEL AND BLADDER

Nurses, either acting alone or in conjunction with physicians, assume major responsibility for bowel and bladder retraining programs.

BOWEL

When planning a bowel program at admission, it is important to have current data, including diet, fluid intake, medication, type of suppository if one is used, date of last evacuation, and the facility (i.e., toilet, commode, bedpan) used. The nurse will also need to know historical (premorbid) data, including usual evacuation pattern (i.e., daily, every other day, etc.), time of day evacuation occurs, whether evacuation occurs after coffee or with cigarettes, the usual stool consistency or frequency of diarrhea or constipation problems, and finally, if the patient has any history of hemorrhoids or bowel or intestinal disease. (See Chap. 15 for more detail on assessment.)

In this population of patients, the majority of whom are over 50 years old, the patients often have well-established habits that may include the frequent use of laxatives and even daily enemas. While it may be desirous to stop this practice and augment "normal" bowel evacuation by increasing bulk foods in the diet, increasing fluid intake, and using mild lubricating and mechanically stimulating suppositories, this may be impossible because of patient resistance to change or because of poor bowel response to the new program. In such cases, it may be advisable to continue the patient's own program and, if possible, gradually alter it. Most patients will not need chemically stimulating suppositories (i.e., diocytyl sodium or Dulcolax) and may find these very uncomfortable if abdominal cramping occurs.

Patients are probably unaccustomed to the lack of privacy that occurs when the nurse is in attendance for safety needs. This is not a time to engage these patients in interaction; instead, the nurse should stand quietly by, possibly physically supporting the patient to lean forward. If the patient seems too distressed by having someone in attendance, a stable commode chair equipped with safety straps could be utilized.

The majority of patients will not need to use suppositories after discharge. For this reason, teaching of suppository insertion is often delayed until the more finalized program near discharge is determined. There are some stroke patients who remain incontinent of stool, although these seem to be more the exception than the rule. Prolonged bowel incontinence and/or smearing of stool may be the most reliable indicators that the patient is a "poor rehabilitation candidate." Because of their inability to perform other self-care activities, these patients will often be discharged to nursing home facilities. The goal with such patients would be to establish a program that provides evacuation after a stimulus such as a suppository at nearly the same time every day or every two days to avoid incontinence.

BLADDER

Marks and Bahr (1977) explain the effects of brain damage on the bladder as follows:

> In certain types of brain damage, bladder function is disturbed. As urine collects in the bladder, the contractions usually occur with smaller volumes than normal because of a decrease in inhibition. This happens despite the patient's lack of desire to void. Often the patient does not even know he is emptying his bladder. At other times, the patient experiences the need to void only immediately before involuntary micturition. It is believed that brain damage at certain regions normally involved with bladder function prevent inhibition of the spinal reflex. Thus, frequently an uninhibited voiding occurs. That is why this abnormal bladder is referred to as an uninhibited neurogenic bladder.

Although frequency and incontinence are most common with the uninhibited bladder, some patients have brain lesions that cause urinary retention.

During the acute phase following a stroke, patients often will have an indwelling urinary catheter inserted if incontinence is present or retention is suspected. Often the catheter is not removed until just prior to or at the time of admission to a rehabilitation facility.

Since most patients will have urinary frequency and incontinence problems, the following procedure can be employed. Give fluids on a rigid schedule, at mealtimes or spaced hourly, and then keep an accurate record of output. Have the patient urinate every 2 h and note volumes. In addition, note all times of incontinence accurately, along with what the patient was doing when incontinent, that is, sleeping, laughing, tearful, or simply sitting quietly. This information gives the nurse an idea not only of how often the patient needs to be toileted but also of the times when the patient is least aware of the need to void. Be sure that recent urine cultures have been done and that sterile urine is present.

If the problem persists, male patients often make use of external catheters, of which there are a wide variety in a wide price range on the market. Since the male stroke patient may inconsistently be incontinent, (i.e., most of the time successfully using the urinal), the external catheter chosen should be inexpensive and easy to apply and remove with one hand. The patient will need to be taught how to avoid and check for pressure when applying the catheter. Female patients can use incontinence panties with disposable liners. As the skin will be in contact with urine, these patients should change the liner of the panty at least every 4 h, thoroughly wash the area, and allow some time to expose skin to air at least daily. Skin rashes will usually occur less often if the patient maintains an adequate fluid intake, keeping the urine dilute. Maintaining adequate fluid intake, especially with female patients, is a problem, since if they are incontinent, they prefer to avoid wetness, and if continent, they may wish to avoid difficult toilet transfers. Both male and female patients may tend to forget that they are supposed to drink fluids and they must therefore be monitored continuously to ensure adequate fluid intake.

PSYCHOLOGICAL RESPONSES

How a patient responds and eventually adapts to a stroke will generally be characteristic of that individual's coping abilities. The severity of the stroke, the resultant physical disability, the support or lack of it provided by family and friends, and the patient's perception of what has happened will all be major factors in the patient's response. Finally, what is lost and the significance of the loss to the patient directly affect the patient's sense of intactness, body image, and feelings of worth.

Strokes, for example, may precipitate or cause the loss of friends, a spouse, or a significant other. The patient may lose a life role such as breadwinner or homemaker or be unable to perform a specific skill or trade. Pleasurable pursuits such as singing, dancing, or reading may be impossible to pursue. Basic bodily functions, bowel and bladder control, sitting balance, and ambulation are frequently interrupted, if not permanently lost. Some psychiatrists believe that these last-mentioned losses are the most severe, since they are abilities mastered at such an early age (1 and 2 years old) that the individual has never known or defined "self" without them.

Generalizing, stroke patients respond to what has happened to them in the well-described grief pattern, which includes anger, denial, bargaining, and acceptance. However, stroke patients are different in that the behaviors exhibited by the patient responding to the stroke may be confused with behaviors manifested by brain damage. For example, Mr. L. is repeatedly found in his room alone, staring at a blank wall. Repeated efforts to encourage him to participate in conversations, dining with others, playing cards, and watching television have failed. Why? Is he depressed, anxious, or embarrassed about his speaking difficulties; fearful of failing at cards, which he once played well; uninterested in the options given; or overstimulated, causing him to seek out a quiet, less confusing place? Or consider Miss B., a right hemiplegic with severe aphasia, who strikes out at the nurse who is attempting to teach her and cries when being bathed and during range of motion exercises. Is she angry and frustrated at her new limitations; is she afraid that these "strangers" will harm her and, in fact, cause pain; or is she demonstrating emotional lability?

To determine what is making a stroke patient behave in a particular fashion, the nurse must repeatedly observe the patient, look for patterns, consult others on the rehabilitation team, talk to family members, and often by a process of elimination, determine the psychological status of the patient. The nurse should, of course, talk to the patient and offer verbal and physical (touching) support.

SOCIALIZATION

The self-image of the stroke patient, like all individuals, is determined by relationships to others and the ability to perform social roles. It seems logical, therefore, that positive interactions and relationships and successful performances of roles, such as host or hostess, bowler, or card player, will promote a positive self-image. Because of this, it is critical that stroke patients reestablish themselves as social beings, reassuming old roles or exchanging old for new activities when necessary. A great deal of the nurse's role here will simply be to encourage the patient and family to try things, to experiment. The nurse should caution the patient not to expect immediate perfection, and any and all efforts should be reinforced positively.

Many rehabilitation facilities will have therapeutic recreation departments that schedule a wide variety of activities, such as wheelchair bowling, attending movies, plays, ballets, and operas, visiting museums and zoos, and shopping in department stores. These activities serve to reinforce the abilities of the patient. They also allow the patient to go out, be seen in a wheelchair, and perceive the reactions of the able-bodied to them.

Finally, many communities have or are developing stroke clubs. These may serve functions such as offering an opportunity for patients after discharge to share common problems, express feelings, and participate in recreational activities.

SEXUALITY

Some stroke patients and their partners may find that the stroke disrupts their sexual lives very little; these are probably the exceptional few. Stroke patients who experience quality control problems may chase their partner around the bedroom or make inappropriate sexual overtures to the partner or acquaintances. The right hemiplegic who is very anxious when attempting any task is likely to be anxious about attempting sexual activities and will need much reassurance. Some partners may be "turned off" by the stroke patient's appearance or inability to do previously meaningful activities. Many patients and partners are fearful that sexual activities could cause still another stroke. And there are an unfortunate few patients who experienced the onset of their stroke while engaged in sexual activity.

The biggest obstacle to helping patients and partners solve problems is presenting the subject. For this reason, it is generally recommended that the nurse introduce the subject soon after admission, on the first day in many cases. While it would be the rare patient who sets this as first priority to discuss when worried about walking, talking, and using the hand again, it is a method of giving the patient and partner permission to approach the nurse later on the subject. For example, the nurse might simply say, "Before you go home, we will discuss any questions you or your partner have about sex."

If the patient does not raise the subject again, the nurse should. In all cases, it is important to find out from the physician if there are any contraindications and to inform the patient accordingly. This can be a perfect lead into further discussion.

If patients are going home on overnight passes, it is likely that if they shared a bed with someone prior to the stroke, they will do so during the overnight stay. The nurse might suggest to the patient or partner or both that the bed be placed against the wall to minimize the risk of falling out of bed and that the partner sleep on the patient's unaffected side. After the patient returns, the nurse should check on how things went. Just getting the conversation "into the bedroom" may open the discussion up.

Remember, nurses are not sexual therapists; they should merely try to assure that discussion is promoted between the partners, that practical solutions to often encountered problems are given, and that proper referrals are made.

PREPARING FOR PASSES

Throughout this chapter, there has been reference to weekend or overnight passes. They are very important to patient morale during a long hospitalization and help to isolate trouble spots prior to discharge.

Before the patient goes on pass, the individual assisting the patient with care will need to know dressing techniques, transferring, bowel and bladder programs, hygiene routines, and dietary considerations (as previously discussed). The following areas must also be taught: medications, (i.e., types, times, and side effects), seizure precautions and management of seizures, and safety/supervision needs for the patient.

MEDICATIONS

Medications are given to the patient on pass by family members or friends unless the patient has demonstrated the ability to self-medicate safely. To "safely" take medication, the patient must demonstrate, preferably for several days, the ability to know when medications are due, what medications are taken, and how to pour medication out of the bottle. A nurse at one rehabilitation hospital helped patients learn how to identify medication by making up medication cards on which the pills were glued in correct dosage next to the times they were to be taken. Teaching the patient about any side effects is desirable; however, if this is not possible, a family member should be so taught.

SEIZURES

Seizures can occur following any type of cerebrovascular lesion. Since they may occur as late sequelae, the nurse may encounter seizures infrequently. The following are nursing actions to be taken in the event of a seizure, and they are identical to the actions that family members should be taught to take. First, a plastic airway should be available for all patients known to have seizures. If the patient's teeth are clenched, however, do not pry them open. If a seizure occurs, the patient should be placed in a recumbent position. The patient's clothing should be loosened if it is restrictive. The extremities should be protected from injury but not restrained from moving. The airway can be improved by retracting the mandible while extending the neck. The nurse or family should be prepared to turn the patient quickly to the side if any emesis occurs. Finally, the family is taught to observe—to note the character, duration, and pattern of the attack and to note the patient's strength and motor ability following the attack. In most instances, the family is directed to call an ambulance and have the patient seen immediately in an emergency room, where evaluation and treatment can be promptly administered.

SAFETY

Safety and the amount or degree of supervision a patient must have is one of the most important concepts the nurse must convey to those who will assist the patient at home. The following are examples of safety considerations: If the patient is ambulatory, are the floors slick or are numerous throw rugs present? Can the patient be left alone? If alone, can the patient get out of the house or apartment in the event of fire? Is there anyone the patient can call for help? Can the patient use the telephone? Have grab bars been installed in the bathroom? Is the patient able to operate the stove safely? If alone, can the patient make a lunch or dinner?

DISCHARGE PLANNING

When planning for discharge, the nurse again verifies that all necessary teaching has occurred and that good understanding of care components has been demonstrated by the responsible party, that is, the patient, a family member, or a friend. Discussion of problems that have occurred on visits home and assistance with problem solving help to diminish the major problems the patient will encounter on the first few days at home.

The nurse should then give particular attention to the needs of the individual who will be assisting with care. Can the patient be left alone while this individual shops, goes to work or to school, and so forth? If not, arrangements should be made for someone to assist this person by spending a few hours a day in the home. The social worker is often the team member primarily involved in securing homemaking assistance or nursing assistance from community-based agencies.

The nurse will make referral to visiting nurse associations for patients who have an existing medical condition that must be monitored, such as hypertension, diabetes, or cardiovascular disease; for those patients who have been cared for only on a few occasions by the significant other or where techniques should be supervised at intervals to assure compliance and accuracy; or for those situations where reteaching is likely to be necessary. The patient or family may need the assistance of other health professionals (via future referrals) for optimal adjustment in returning to the community.

In addition, the nurse verifies with the physician when the patient will be seen again for a recheck and may recommend to the physician, to an outpatient-based social worker, or to an outpatient-based nurse that an early recheck occur if the nurse believes the patient to be at risk. Briefly, the patient at risk is one who has medical, social, or psychological problems that may endanger the patient should they become worse and who the nurse doubts will secure the appropriate assistance.

It is often necessary to wait until near the time of discharge before beginning vocational therapy and/or driver education. This is done to allow maximal clearing to occur, which in turn provides the patient, family, and therapists with a more accurate picture of future potentials. Outpatient therapy in vocational rehabilitation for the patient may be arranged after discharge in some cases.

CONCLUSION

Nurses have no more challenging patient than the stroke patient. Each is an individual, and each has been individually affected by the stroke. The author has often heard nurses disdain caring for "yet another stroke patient," with the phrase "they are all alike." This is a grossly inaccurate statement, and one can only feel that it is said out of ignorance or inability to observe. Nursing has a great deal of work to do in the future to establish better methods of assessment and care planning for the stroke patient and to improve the knowledge of the laity and health professionals regarding the affects of stroke.

With an ever more vigilant society casting a critical eye at health care in conjunction with a tidal wave of "baby boom" children fast approaching the "stroke" age, nursing will need to move quickly and decisively if we are to have the answers and the tools to meet the demands in stroke rehabilitation nursing in the future.

BIBLIOGRAPHY

Anderson, E., et al.: "Stroke Rehabilitation: Maintenance of Achieved Goals," *Arch Phys Med Rehabil* 58:345–352, 1977.

Beverly, E.: "Nursing Homes: Matching the Facility to the Patients Needs," *Geriatrics* 31: 100–110, 1976.

Bobath, B.: *Adult Hemiplegia: Evaluation and Treatment,* Heinemann, London, 1970.

Bourestrom, N. C.: "Predictors of Long-term Recovery in Cerebrovascular Disease," *Arch Phys Med Rehabil* 48:415–419, 1967.

Brett, G.: "Dressing Techniques for the Severely Involved Hemiplegic Patient," *Am J Occup Ther* 14:262–264, 1960.

Buck, McKenzie: "Dysphasia: The Patient, His Family, and the Nurse," *Cardiovasc Nurs* 6:51–56, 1970.

Buckley, J., et al.: "Feeding Patients with Dysphagia," *Nurs Forum* 15:69–85, 1976.

Bureau of Health Planning and Resources, Health Resources Administration: "Guidelines for Stroke Care," Department of Health, Education and Welfare, Publication No. (HRA) 76-14017, 1976.

Burnside, I. M.: "Clocks and Calendars," *Am J Nurs* 70:117–119, 1970.

Burt, M. M.: "Perceptual Deficits in Hemiplegia," *Am J Nurs* 70:1026–1029, 1970.

Buys, Donna: "Memory: Why We Remember . . . Why We Forget," *Family Health /Today's Health,* June 1976, pp. 38–40.

Carini, E., and G. Owen: *Neurological and Neurosurgical Nursing,* Mosby, St. Louis, 1974.

Carnevali, P., and S. Brueckner: "Immobilization: Reassessment of a Concept," *Am J Nurs* 70:1502–1507, 1970.

Chusid, J.: *Correlative Neuroanatomy and Functional Neurology,* Lange, Los Altos, Calif. 1976.

Dayhoff, N.: "Soft or Hard Devices to Position Hands," *Am J Nurs* 75:1142–1144, 1975.

Delehanty, L., and V. Stravino: "Achieving Bladder Control," *Am J Nurs* 70:312–316, 1970.

Diamond, Milton: "Sexuality and the Handicapped," *Rehabil Lit* February 1974.

Dolan, M.: "Autumn Months, Autumn Years," *Am J Nurs* 75:1145–1147, 1975.

Dzau, R.: "Stroke Rehabilitation: A Family Teaching Educational Program," *Arch Phys Med Rehabil* 59:236–239, 1978.

Edmond, R.: "The Hazards of Immobility: Effect on Motor Function," *Am J Nurs* 67:788–790, 1967.

Eliasson, S., et al.: *Neurological Pathophysiology,* Oxford, New York, 1978.

Ellis, R.: "After Stroke: Sitting Problems," *Am J Nurs* 73:1898–1899, 1973.

Feigenson, J., et al.: "Factors Influencing Outcome and Length of Stay in a Stroke Rehabilitation Unit," *Stroke* 8:351–356, 1977.

Fields, W.: *Neurological and Sensory Disorders in the Elderly,* Stratton, New York, 1975.

Fordyce, W. E., and R. S. Fowler: "Adapting Care for the Brain Damaged Patient," *Am J Nurs* 72:1832–1835, 72:2056–2059, 1972.

Galbreaith, Patricia: *What You Can Do For Yourself,* Drake, New York, 1974.

Gardner, Howard: *The Shattered Mind,* Knopf, New York, 1975.

———: "Brain Damage: A Window on the Mind," *Saturday Review,* August 9, 1975, pp. 26–29.

Geschwind, Norman: "The Organization of Language and the Brain," *Science* 170:940–944, 1970.

———, and W. Levitsky: "Human Brain: Left-Right Asymmetry in Temporal Speech Region," *Science* 161:186–187, 1968.

Gilbert, Arlene: *You Can Do It from a Wheelchair,* Arlington House, New Rochelle, N. Y., 1974.

Goffman, E.: *Stigma,* Prentice-Hall, Englewood Cliffs, N. J., 1963.

Goldenson, Robert M.: "Independent Living Ways and Means," in R. Goldenson (ed.): *Disability and Rehabilitation Handbook,* McGraw-Hill, New York, 1978.

Goodglass, H., and E. Kaplan: *The Assessment of Aphasia and Related Disorders.* Lea & Febiger, Philadelphia, 1972.

Griffin, K., et al.: "Teaching the Dysphagic Patient to Swallow," *RN* 37:60–63, 1974.

Haerer, A.: "Visual Field Defects and the Prognosis of Stroke Patients," *Stroke* 4:163–168, 1978.

Hart, Leslie A.: *How the Brain Works,* Basic Books, New York, 1975.

Hirschberg, G.: "Ambulation and Self-care Are Goals of Rehabilitation After Stroke," *Geriatrics* 31:61–65, 1976.

———, et al.: *Rehabilitation: A Manual for the Care of the Disabled and Elderly,* Lippincott, New York, 1976.

Hodgkins, Eric: *Episode: A Report on the Accident Inside My Skull,* Atheneum, New York, 1968.

Howell, Linda: "Stroke," in R. M. Goldenson (ed.): *Disability and Rehabilitation Handbook,* McGraw-Hill, New York, 1978.

Hurwitz, L. J.: "Helping the Asphasic to Communicate Again," *Geriatrics,* May 1973, pp. 102–106.

Huston, J.: "Overcoming the Learning Disabilities of Stroke," *Nursing '75* 5:66–68, 1975.

Joint Committee for Stroke: "Stroke Rehabilitation," *Stroke* 3:373–407, 1972.

Jones, Michael A.: *Accessibility Standards, Illustrated,* Capital Development Board, State of Illinois, 1978.

Kavchak-Keyes, Mary Anne: "Comeback from Disaster: Helping the Stroke Patient Learn to Help Himself," *Nursing '79* 9:32–35, 1979.

Klinger, Judith L., et al.: *Mealtime Manual for the Aged and Handicapped,* Simon & Schuster, New York, 1970.

Large, H., et al.: "In the First Stroke Intensive Care Unit," *Am J Nurs* 69:76–80, 1969.

Larsen, G.: "After Stroke: Optokinetic Nystagmus," *Am J Nurs* 73:1897–1899, 1973.

Lehman, J. F., B. J. DeLateur, R. S. Fowler, et al.: "Stroke Rehabilitation Outcome and Prediction," *Arch Phys Med Rehabil* 56:383–389, 1975.

———, ———, ———: "Stroke: Does Rehabilitation Affect Outcome?," *Arch Phys Med Rehabil* 56:375–382, 1975.

Librach, G., et al.: "Stroke Incidence and Risk Factors," *Geriatrics,* April 1977, pp. 85–96.

Lowman, Edward, and Judith L. Klinger: *Aids to Independent Living: Self-Help for the Handicapped and Elderly,* McGraw-Hill, New York, 1969.

Maney, J.: "A Behavioral Therapy Approach to Bladder Retraining," *Nurs Clin North Am* 11:179–188, 1976.

Marks, Robert L., and George A. Bahr: "How to Manage Neurogenic Bladder after Stroke," *Geriatrics,* December 1977, pp. 50–54.

Martin, Nancy: "Nursing in Rehabilitation," in I. Beland, and J. Y. Passos (eds.): *Clinical Nursing,* Macmillan, New York, 1975, pp. 989–1018.

May, Elizabeth E., Neva R. Waggoner, and Eleanor B. Hotte: *Independent Living for the Handicapped and Elderly,* Houghton Mifflin, Boston, 1974.

McCarthy, J.: "Hazards of Immobility: Effects on Gastrointestinal Function," *Am J Nurs* 67:785–787, 1967.

Olson, E.: "The Hazards of Immobility," *Am J Nurs* 67:780–797, 1967.

Penfeld, Wilder: *The Mystery of the Mind: A Critical Study of Consciousness and the Human Brain,* Princeton, Princeton, N. J., 1975.

Pfaudler, M.: "After Stroke: Motor Skills Rehabilitation for Hemiplegic Patients," *Am J Nurs* 73:1892–1896, 1973.

Pines, Maya: *The Brain Changers: Scientists and the New Mind Control,* Harcourt Brace, Jovanovich, New York, 1973.

———: "Speak, Memory: The Riddle of Recall and Forgetfulness," *Saturday Review,* August 1975, pp. 16–20.

Sarno, John E., and M. T. Sarno: *Stroke: The Condition and the Patient,* McGraw-Hill, New York, 1969.

Schroeder, L.: "Hazards of Immobility: Effects on Urinary Function," *Am J Nurs* 67:790–792, 1967.

Schultz, C.: "Nursing Care of the Stroke Patient: Rehabilitation Aspects," *Nurs Clin North Am* 8:633–664, 1973.

Schwartzman, S.: "Anxiety and Depression in the Stroke Patient: A Nursing Challenge," *J Psychiatr Nurs,* 14:13–18, 1976.

Shapiro, M., et al,: "Community Health Services for Stroke," *Stroke* 5:115–133, 1974.

Skelly, M.: "Rethinking Stroke: Aphasic Patients Talk Back," *Am J Nurs* 75:1140–1147, 1975.

Smith, G.: *Care of the Patient with a Stroke,* Springer, New York, 1976.

Sperry, Roger W.: "Left-Brain, Right-Brain," *Saturday Review,* August 1975, pp. 30–33.

Thompson, L.: "Hazards of Immobility: Effects on Respiratory Function," *Am J Nurs* 67:783–784, 1967.

Ullman, Montague: "Disorders of Body Image after Stroke," *Am J Nurs* 64:925–934, 1964.

Wade, M.: "Hazards of Immobility: Effects on Metabolic Equilibrium," *Am J Nurs* 67:793–794, 1967.

Washam, Veronica: *The One-Hander's Book: A Basic Guide,* Day, New York, 1973.

21
betsy schnek

brain damage
from trauma

INTRODUCTION

The rehabilitation of a patient who has suffered brain injury as a result of trauma is a problem of some magnitude. Each year in the United States more than 50 million persons are injured. Of these, about 3 million suffer injuries to the head (U.S. Dept. of Health, Education, and Welfare, 1969). A large proportion of these 3 million head injuries are caused by motor vehicles, especially automobiles. It has been estimated that more than two-thirds of the victims of automobile accidents sustain head injuries.

Another growing source of head injuries is motorcycle accidents. Far too often, serious head injuries are incurred by those riding motorcycles and involved in accidents because the riders are relatively unprotected. Helmets give some measure of protection, but some states are currently eliminating their laws requiring cyclists to wear helmets. Ohio, for example, no longer requires a cyclist to wear a helmet if the cyclist is over 18 and not a novice (first-year license). Snowmobile riders are also exempt in some states from wearing helmets. It will be interesting to see what this trend does to mortality and morbidity statistics.

Other causes of cerebral trauma include occupational injuries, falls, and gunshot wounds. Victims of violent crimes may experience head injuries as a consequence of beatings or blows.

The rehabilitation of the patient with cerebral trauma is difficult in many cases because of the multiple injuries that often accompany head injuries. Fractures of the extremities, chest injuries, and amputations are complications that are common.

Cerebral trauma occurs in all age groups and in both sexes, but the highest incidence occurs in relatively young men. Two-thirds of the 4 million persons injured annually in motor vehicle accidents are between the ages of 17 and 44. The incidence of death is also higher in young men; 30 percent of all motor vehicle accident victims who die are men between the ages of 15 and 24 (Feiring, 1974).

CLASSIFICATIONS OF HEAD INJURY

Trauma to the brain can be classified according to the nature of the head injury. The two main classifications used here are closed head injury and open head injury.

Closed head injuries are those in which there is no injury to the skull or which are limited to a simple undisplaced fracture. They may be considered mild, moderate, or severe. The mild head injury involves brief loss of consciousness without neurological changes. Moderate head injuries involve longer periods of unconsciousness, with abnormal neurological signs. Severe head injuries are characterized by prolonged periods of unconsciousness and abnormal neurological signs. The damage in a closed head injury results from movement of the brain against the skull. The movement of one surface against the other produces what is commonly called *shearing forces* (Fig. 21-1).

Open head injuries include compound fractures of the skull, scalp lacerations, and various amounts of cerebral destruction. If there is fragmentation of the skull, damage to the brain may be extensive.

FRACTURES

Fractures of the skull may be simple or compound. Linear fractures are simple breaks or breaks in the continuity of the skull without disruption of the bone (Fig. 21-2). The comminuted fracture is a fragmented interruption of the skull from multiple linear fractures. The third type of fracture, the depressed fracture, is a displacement of comminuted bone fragments.

CONCUSSION

Concussion has been described as a "jostling" of the brain's soft substance without contusion (Swift, 1974). Many authors equate concussion with mild head injury. Concussion is usually manifested by a loss of consciousness, sometimes for

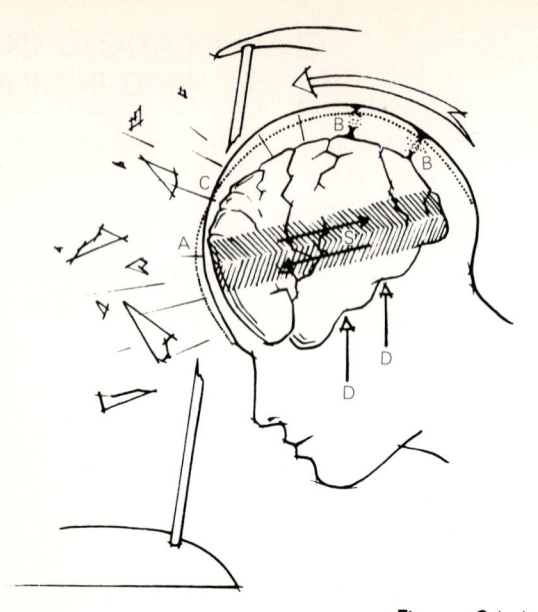

Figure 21-1
Closed blunt injury. Skull molding occurs at the site of impact. (A) Stippled line, preinjury contour; (C) solid line, contour movements after impact with inbending at vertex. (B) Subdural veins torn as brain rotates forward. (S) Shearing strains throughout the brain. (D) Direct trauma to inferior temporal and frontal lobes over floors of middle and anterior fossae. *(Adapted from Sven Eliasson et al., Neurological Pathophysiology, Oxford University Press, New York, 1978. Used by permission of the publisher.)*

just a few seconds, and loss of memory or traumatic amnesia. For most patients who suffer concussions, recovery is complete and fairly rapid, and there are no complications.

CONTUSION

A contusion involves multiple bruising of the brain and usually presents a more serious situation than concussion. The patient usually loses consciousness but may present with stupor and confusion. Contusions occur as a result of two different types of injury. The first is called coup and contrecoup. This injury involves bruising of the brain just beneath the site of the injury (coup) and directly contralateral to the impact site (contrecoup). The injury is caused by the rebounding of the brain against the surface opposite that to which the injury occurred. The second type of injury is caused by deceleration or acceleration. In deceleration the head in motion comes in contact with a stationary, unyielding object that brings it to an abrupt stop. An example of this occurs in automobile accidents, when the head hits the windshield. Acceleration, on the other hand, occurs when a moving object strikes the relatively immobile head, causing it to be set in motion. As a result of either type of injury, the head is compressed, and possible skull fracture occurs.

LACERATIONS

Brain lacerations involve a tear in the substance of the brain, usually at the point of application of force to the head or directly opposite the force site. Laceration of the brain may occur with almost no damage to the skull. Lacerations

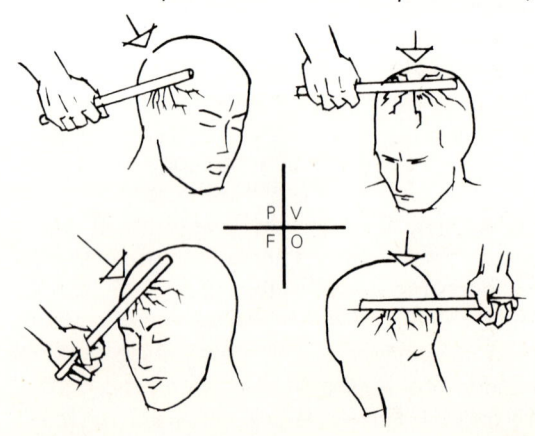

Figure 21-2
Linear fracture lines. *(Adapted from Sven Eliasson et al., Neurological Pathophysiology, Oxford University Press, New York, 1978. Used by permission of the publisher.)*

CHAPTER 21   388

Figure 21-3
Bullet wounds of the head. (A) Soft, low velocity bullets cause compound (open) penetrating wounds of the skull and dura and local laceration of the brain. (B) A high velocity bullet causes a compound penetrating wound of the skull and dura with severe laceration of the brain in its path. Expansion effects are transmitted throughout the brain. *(Adapted from Sven Eliasson et al., Neurological Pathophysiology, Oxford University Press, New York, 1978. Used by permission of the publisher.)*

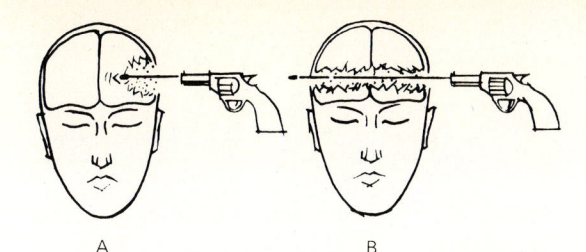

involving the base of the skull usually cause death within a short period of time.

GUNSHOT WOUNDS

Gunshot wounds cause a number of injuries, in part determined by the location of the entry and exit sites, the velocity and mass of the bullet, and whether the bullet changed shape after penetrating the skull. Not only does a bullet entering the head destroy the structures it passes through, but also expansion waves occur throughout the brain (Fig. 21-3).

SPACE-OCCUPYING HEMATOMAS

One of the complications of head injuries is space-occupying hematomas. These include epidural hematomas, subdural hematomas, and intracerebral hematomas. The blood clots act as masses in the brain, compressing vital structures.

EPIDURAL HEMATOMAS

Epidural hematomas occur between the dura mater and the skull. They are rare, but when they do occur, they constitute a surgical emergency. The middle meningeal artery is the vessel usually damaged. The hematoma usually expands rapidly, causing pressure and displacement of the brain, with death occurring rapidly unless there is surgical intervention.

SUBDURAL HEMATOMAS

Subdural hematomas are caused by bleeding into the subdural space, between the dura mater and the arachnoid. These clots can be classified as acute, subacute, or chronic, depending on the time of onset of symptoms in relation to the actual time of injury. Subdural hematomas may not present immediate danger to the patient but may be dormant for weeks or months. Such hematomas sometimes follow what seems to be an insignificant injury to the head. They, too, can often be effectively treated with surgery to remove the clot and allow the brain tissue to free itself from compression.

INTRACEREBRAL HEMATOMAS

These hematomas occur within the brain itself. They occur most frequently in the frontal and temporal lobes, usually near the site of the injury. Such hematomas arise as a result of damage to a deeply placed cerebral vessel and may be more difficult to diagnose than the other types of hematomas.

PROGNOSTIC FACTORS IN RECOVERY FROM HEAD INJURY

The ability of a patient to recover from head injury is determined to a great extent by the severity of the head injury and the amount of damage to the brain. Another important factor, however, is the skill of the health team in recognizing complications before they become well advanced and in treating the complications at an early stage. The nurse plays an invaluable role in safeguarding the patient from complications because the nurse is the one with the patient at all times. Still another significant factor in determining whether the patient survives the acute injury period is the skill of the health team in treating the multiple problems that a victim of head injury often suffers.

Attempts have been made to define objective indicators that would give some clues about a patient's potential recovery from serious head injury. Laboratory data and other diagnostic procedures have been found to be of little value (Feiring). The most reliable indicator is the depth and duration of unresponsiveness or altered consciousness. However, even this indicator is not without exception. There are many documented cases of patients, comatose and unresponsive for months, who have made a reasonable recovery against all medical odds.

IMPORTANCE OF REHABILITATION PHILOSOPHY

It is extremely important for the patient with cranial injury to be cared for by individuals who maintain and believe in a philosophy of rehabilitation. The patient should be approached with the notion that recovery will occur and therefore bodily structures and functions should be maintained. The rehabilitation of the patient will be greatly delayed if, initially, the nursing staff allows contractures to develop and decubitus ulcers to form. Rehabilitation does not take place only in formal facilities designed for that purpose. Some of the best rehabilitation nurses this author has known have been nurses in acute facilities who believe that any patient can benefit from some type of rehabilitation, and the sooner the better. Even in the intensive care unit, attention should be given to maintaining joint function and intact skin and to preventing other complications. The nurse serves as an advocate for the patient to ensure that preventable complications do not occur.

ADAPTATION OF NURSING PROCESS

The nurse utilizes the nursing process to plan for the care of the patient with cerebral trauma. Adaptations are made in accordance with the data presented by the patient; each victim of head injury presents a unique picture. Because many patients remain comatose for some time following injury, the nurse must rely on physical assessment skills and not on subjective data. The plan of care may be determined in part by the age of the patient and the other injuries suffered at the time of the head trauma.

CARE OF THE PATIENT WITH ACUTE HEAD INJURY

Many patients with head injuries are admitted to an intensive care unit, especially if the head injury has produced unconsciousness. The patient should be turned every 2 h to prevent reddening and breakdown of the skin, and should be kept on either side with the head slightly elevated to prevent aspiration and airway obstruction. Seizure precautions should be taken, and eye and mouth care should be instituted. Other signs that need to be assessed at intervals include:

1. Size and equality of pupils and reaction to light.
2. Level of consciousness and reaction to stimuli.
3. Pulse rate, blood pressure, and temperature (rectal temperatures should be taken).
4. Any movement of extremities and extremity strengths.
5. Drainage from orifices.
6. Any headache—site and character.
7. Incontinence, distention of bowel and bladder.
8. Seizure activity or unusual behavior.

COMMON COMPLICATIONS

Four common complications of acute cerebral trauma are respiratory difficulties, shock, increased intracranial pressure, and hyperthermia.

Respiratory Difficulties Severe respiratory distress indicates that the patient should be placed on a respirator and may require a tracheostomy. In patients with cerebral trauma, respiratory insufficiency produces negative effects by increasing the intracranial pressure and by inducing hypoxia.

Shock One of the most severe complications in a patient with cranial injury is shock. Irreversible shock causes 50 percent of the deaths following head injury. Symptoms of shock are pallor or slight cyanosis, cold moist skin, rapid pulse with thready characteristics, rapid shallow respirations, restlessness and anxiety, thirst, subnormal temperature, and low or falling blood pressure. Fluid replacement, without increasing intracranial pressure, is of primary importance.

Increased Intracranial Pressure Increased intracranial pressure must always be watched for by those working with persons who have sustained cranial injuries. Symptoms include slowly falling respiration, restlessness, irregular pupils, falling pulse rate, slowly rising blood pressure, increased headache with or without vomiting, diminished alertness and changes in level of consciousness, papilledema and visual disturbances, seizures, and increased cerebrospinal pressure. The probable causes of increased intracranial pressure are hemorrhage, cerebral edema, hematomas, or meningitis.

Hyperthermia Hyperthermia in the acute injury period is usually an indicator of injury to the heat-controlling mechanisms of the hypothalamus or of damage to the brainstem. Marked dehydration or infection may also be a cause. Treatment is symptomatic unless a treatable cause for the increased temperature is found.

COMMON PROBLEMS ENCOUNTERED DURING THE REHABILITATION PROCESS

Whether the residual brain damage is mild, moderate, or severe, the trauma can only be perceived as devastating to the family and significant others. The perception of the patient concerning his or her present state will, of course, vary according to the degree of awareness of what has really occurred.

For the most part, during the acute hospitalization, the patient will have been essentially sedentary. This may have masked the severity of brain damage, which will become apparent as activities of daily living are evaluated and increased. Even if the brain damage is minimal, staff members will be challenged to help the patient and, more particularly, significant others understand the meaning of the residual damage when the patient may be functioning well in so many areas. The motor ramifications of hemiplegia or hemiparesis are often easier to interpret than is lack of judgment in the absence of aphasia.

In any event, the rehabilitation staff must assess and address the residual damage. As nurses working with the unconscious patient during the acute phase must assume there is a reason to prevent complications, so, too, must nurses in the rehabilitation setting believe there is reason to determine the ways the patient can be helped to assume care and control of his or her life. The degree of recovery following severe head trauma can be absolutely astounding. It has happened, for example, that a young patient, admitted demonstrating uncontrolled and at times animalistic behavior, has eventually returned to college, successfully.

Rehabilitation workers, therefore, need to pace the physical upgrading program with a full understanding that mental clearing can occur. Most certainly it must be remembered that an unexpected and devastating event has happened to the patient and those significant to him or her.

The nurse who works with the cerebral trauma patient in the rehabilitation setting encounters a variety of physical and psychological problems, depending upon the area of the brain that was damaged.

RESPIRATORY PROBLEMS

It is not uncommon for the patient who has suffered acute trauma which required the use of a tracheostomy tube to continue with this tube after transfer to the rehabilitation facility. However, every effort should be made to wean the patient from the use of oxygen and eventually to remove the tube. While this is being done, caregivers must be aware of how the patient manifests hypoxia. Base line values of arterial blood gases should be obtained for purposes of comparison.

Short periods of time with decreasing oxygen concentrations and then room air are attempted until the patient is able to tolerate the lack of oxygen for longer and longer periods. When the patient is able to tolerate room air without a significant drop in arterial blood gas levels, the goal is then to attempt removal of the tracheostomy tube. Before the tube can be removed, the patient must be able to breathe efficiently without it. Most often, plugging of the tracheostomy tube for short periods of time is initiated, with continued checks of arterial blood gases. Gradually the period of time that the tracheostomy tube is plugged is increased until the span exceeds 24 h. After the tube is removed, the stoma usually spontaneously closes relatively quickly. In the event that it does not, surgical closure of the stoma may be deemed necessary.

Even after the patient has been weaned from all mechanical respiratory supports, it may be necessary to teach the patient, if he or she is alert enough, to perform exercises in order to strengthen the primary and accessory muscles of respiration.

PHYSICAL DISFIGUREMENT OF THE HEAD FOLLOWING CRANIAL SURGERY

Patients with traumatic head lesions may have had surgery to remove bone fragments, or to evacuate hematomas. Trauma to the skull at times is so extensive as to require removal of part of the bony skull, or this may be done to decrease further damage by confining the edematous brain in the skull's shell. Both procedures affect the appearance of the patient who may present with a shaved head encircled with scars, or a head that is misshapen from bony removal. Staff often unknowingly react to the appearance of these patients by facial expressions, staring, not looking at the patient when talking, or by avoiding the patient. All negative interactions can take away from the patient's sense of wholeness and worth. Finally, the patient may be frightened or disgusted by the reflection in the mirror.

For example, one female refused to leave her room for any activity and would cry and struggle if attempts were made to coax or force her from the room. Since she was aphasic and could not explain her feelings, but could indicate reliably "yes" and "no" with a headshake and hand gestures, the staff began an elaborate guessing game to find the cause. After several attempts without success, one staff member who had left the room said, "I don't blame her; I wouldn't want to leave the room either—looking like that." That, of course, was the problem. The solution, from then on, was the use of scarfs attractively tied over the head and, later, of expensive wigs when good healing of suture lines had occurred.

Loss of bony portions of the head is a more difficult problem, which requires that the primary goal be avoidance of further trauma to the brain. These patients must wear protective helmets at all times, while sleeping, and especially when mobile, whether in wheelchair or ambulatory. Recent surgical advances have made it possible for these patients to undergo corrective surgery with the use of skull prostheses, but these procedures cannot usually be done until the chance of edema has decreased. The time interval is usually 6 to 9 months following the initial surgery.

ACTIVITIES OF DAILY LIVING

The patient with head trauma who is undergoing rehabilitation will undoubtedly need assistance with activities of daily living such as dressing, hygiene, communication, and mobility. Approaches and techniques for these activities are considered in Part Two of this book.

Emotional Problems

It is common for the patient who has suffered brain injury to have some residual emotional problems. The emotional disturbance may be secondary to the actual physical damage or may occur because of emotional trauma. If the frontal lobes of the brain have been damaged or diffuse damage has occurred, any of the following may be manifested:

1. Loss of memory.
2. Euphoria.
3. Regression to an earlier level of adjustment.
4. Untidiness.
5. Impaired moral and ethical judgment.
6. Generalized apathy.
7. Uncooperativeness, irritability, antagonism, hostility, aggression and assaultiveness (Carini, 1974).

CONTROLLING THE ENVIRONMENT

More often than with any other brain-damaged population, the traumatic head-lesion patients display dramatic disorganization and impulsivity. When these patients enter a rehabilitation facility, they are bombarded by the change. The very stimulating environment in which the patient is expected to go to and through demanding and diverse therapy sessions and to establish and renew social abilities often produces regression, increased disorientation, and impulsiveness. Take the following example:

Mr. S., a single 25-year-old, enters a rehabilitation facility via ambulance accompanied by his sister and a friend. He had sustained a head injury in an automobile accident, minor facial lacerations, and multiple fractures on the left side of his body. He was unconscious for a short time and then, because of complications, spent several weeks in an intensive care unit (ICU). His sister explained he had been terribly upset in the ICU, often hallucinating and demonstrating combative behavior. The first day in a rehabilitation facility he was examined by a resident physician, then by his attending physician, and by a nurse. A parade of well-wishing visitors followed, often making cheerful comments like, "Now you're on your way." "You'll be good as new soon." "We'll take you home for a Christmas celebration with the whole family next week."

During the admission interview, the nurse found Mr. S. to be frequently tearful; he repeatedly expressed a desire to leave, demonstrated unreliability as a historian, and showed a tendency to confabulate. Later in the day, the patient was found asleep while visitors sat chatting around him in the room.

Mr. S. was unable to selectively receive and integrate stimulation. His difficulty became more obvious the next day.

Mr. S.'s day started quietly. He was awakened and dressed by a staff member, assisted into a wheelchair, and was able to feed himself breakfast in his room. He was then taken to an elevator where a new assistant took him to physical therapy where he waited in a vestibule crowded with other chatting patients. His therapy took place in a large brightly lit room with 50 other patients, 20 therapists, and the unfamiliar weights, pulleys, mats, bars, tilt tables, and exercycles. After this therapy, Mr. S. passed again through a crowded area to await his occupational therapy, where he again faced unfamiliar faces, equipment, tasks, and sounds. Mr. S.'s occupational therapist noted he seemed very "wide-eyed," anxious, and distractible. He was unable to follow simple directives, and after 20 min fell asleep. Shortly after, Mr. S. was returned to the nursing unit and was placed in a common area to await lunch. In this position he was visible from the nurses' station; however, in his line of sight were staff scurrying to and from the nursing station, and he was subjected to hearing call bells ringing, being answered, and to multiple pages. Mr. S. soon became tearful and began making repeated attempts to get up from his wheelchair.

This situation illustrates Mr. S.'s rapid decline in ability to maintain control and to appropriately respond to his environment when overstimulated. Note his attempts to escape the stimulation by falling asleep. In other instances, patients may return to their rooms and stare at a blank wall; some seem to relax best by listening to quiet music; still others seem to strike back at any nuance of stimulation.

The following measures were taken to maximize Mr. S.'s therapy regimes while minimizing the regression. Visitors were limtied to two per night for 1 h for the first week. Therapies were administered in Mr. S.'s room and the therapy schedule was adjusted to allow a 1 h rest break between each program. Since Mr. S. was in a semiprivate room with a quiet roommate, no room change was necessary. Meal trays were ordered to the unit and Mr. S. ate in his room. As much as possible, the same nursing staff was assigned to Mr. S., and an hourly schedule was written out in marking pencil, including all the day's activities, which was hung in Mr. S.'s room for reference.

These measures were strictly adhered to for 1 week. At that point Mr. S. seemed to be coping well with the program so one activity was upgraded. Mr. S. was escorted to physical therapy by familiar nursing personnel to be treated there in a quiet area.

Planning a rigid, stimulation-controlled program for the patient by gradual upgrading is believed to facilitate the traumatic brain-injured patient's ability to maximize treatment regimes.

This same population of patients, especially young people, often experience dramatic clearing and recovery. Families need to be given an overview of what to expect. They are often disheartened when the patient becomes worse; they have trouble understanding that their good intentions may be causative, and they have great difficulty with the term "brain damaged." In Mr. S.'s case, his family felt he was "going crazy." Obviously, care must be taken when explaining brain damage to families in order to verify their understanding.

SEXUAL ISSUES

Traumatic brain-injured patients often display a loss of inhibition, verbally swear, and abuse anyone around when frustrated. They also may make overt sexual overtures to staff working closely with them and to other patients or family. The primary intervention is consistent limit setting.

Because of the age of many of the patients with head injury, it is not uncommon for sexual matters to be high on their list of concerns. The patient may just be leaving adolescence, when sexual orientations become increasingly established. With the disability now also a concern, the patient may feel sexually unattractive and may feel the need to test how people perceive him or her. For patients with residual emotional difficulties, sexual urges and drives may be confusing. Lack of inhibition regarding sexual desires may also be present. Masturbation may occur, as well as sexual advances to others.

The approach to managing any inappropriate sexual behavior the patient demonstrates should be discussed by the rehabilitation staff in as objective a way as the approach to any other manifestation of inappropriate behavior. While the patient's sexual behavior may prove to be a high anxiety area for those in contact with the patient, it should nevertheless be addressed as early as it is noticed. Any nurse who discusses these issues with the patient must feel comfortable with the topic, or further embarrassment may result. The patient with a steady partner should be assured the opportunity to be alone at times with the partner in a private place. It will be the rare partner who will not need some counseling regarding sexual activity. Counseling should be given by whichever member of the rehabilitation team is designated for this responsibility, based on relationship with the patient and on comfort with the topic.

In all cases, the patient should be helped to be as physically presentable as possible. Such things as being cleanshaven, having makeup applied, and being dressed in clean, properly fitting clothing are essential in helping patients regain a positive image of themselves.

MAINTAINING A SAFE, THERAPEUTIC ENVIRONMENT

The nurse who works with a brain-damaged person may need to plan to compensate for the patient's poor judgment and impulsiveness. Supervision is a must. The patient may not be able to realize that some behavior is unsafe; therefore, reasoning with the patient may not help. Some patients regress to a childlike level.

Every effort should be made to assist the patient to develop mental and emotional control. Acceptable social behavior, as well as the ability to reason and cooperate, must be taught and developed. The nursing staff should think in terms of reality orientation—not only working with the patients about where they are and who they are but also about what behavior is appropriate. No one should talk "down" to the patient. Every effort should be made to increase gradually the scope of patients' socialization and to help patients maintain contacts and friends they had prior to the injury.

It is often difficult for the family and friends of the brain-damaged person to accept the behavior of the patient. They may continue to expect that the person will function as before the trauma. They may react as if the patient should be in constant control of feelings and actions. The patient who is unsuccessful in tasks or interactions may become further agitated. It is usually necessary for the nursing staff to control the environment to allow for the highest level of functioning by the patient. While this is true when the patient is attempting physical activities, it also holds for beginning social interaction. Interaction should increase but at a pace and in such a way as to be positive for all concerned. As friends begin to visit, they may be helped by knowing, before seeing the patient, what they will observe. The length of visits as well as the setting should be monitored. Everything possible should be done so that the patient will not fail during interactions.

SEIZURES

The incidence of seizures following trauma to the brain depends on the type of injury and the extent of brain damage. The first convulsion usually occurs within 6 months to a year after the trauma among 50 percent of those with severe head injuries (Carini). Convulsions are generally caused by scar tissue that exerts a pull on the brain. It has been found that seizure activity in patients may recede and cease with or without medications within a 3- to 4-year period.

The seizures experienced by patients who have brain damage may be grand mal, petit mal, psychomotor, or Jacksonian. The nurse has a responsibility to protect the patient from injury during the seizure. Clothing should be loosened if it restricts movement or breathing. If it is possible to insert a padded tongue blade or rubber wedge before the teeth are already clenched, this should be done. If the teeth are already clenched, however, no effort should be made because the chance of breaking a tooth or causing trauma to the patient or to the nurse is great. The patient's extremities should not be restrained, but should be protected from injury.

The nurse should also observe the pattern of the seizure, its duration, and its characteristics, i.e., which extremities are involved and whether the seizure activity is clonic or tonic. After the seizure, the patient should be turned on the side to prevent aspiration of secretions. As the pre-seizure level of activity is regained, the patient needs to be reassured.

Patients who have sustained cerebral trauma are usually maintained on anticonvulsant medication for at least several years after the injury.

The patient and the family must be taught about the medication regimen, the side effects, the desired action, and the importance of continuing to take the medication even though the patient remains seizure-free for long periods of time. This latter problem can be very real. Many patients, because they have been seizure-free for a period of time, feel they no longer need the medication.

BOWEL AND BLADDER PROBLEMS

The patient who has experienced a brain injury may experience bowel and bladder problems, especially after prolonged periods of unconsciousness. Diarrhea can be a critical problem with both conscious and unconscious patients if they must be maintained on tube feedings. Different commercial preparations or homemade varieties may need to be tried before one is found that satisfied nutritional requirements and at the same time does not cause diarrhea. Adequate fluid intake is essential for efficient bowel and bladder programs. Brain-damaged persons may forget that they are to drink specified amounts of liquid. Staff must watch for this and, when necessary, be physically present to ensure that the patient does drink. Additional information about establishing bowel and bladder programs may be found in Chapters 14 and 15 of this book.

NUTRITIONAL PROBLEMS

Nutritional problems may occur in patients who have suffered a cranial injury. Initial nutritional needs of the patients are met by intravenous fluids. These, however, do not provide adequate calories or nutrients if used for periods longer than a week or so. Long-term nourishment of the unconscious patient is usually accomplished with tube feedings. Several commercial preparations are available for liquid tube feedings, or tube feedings may be prepared at home in a blender. Usually 2500 or 3000 mL of a high protein, high vitamin preparation is given in 24 h; the caloric count is about equal to the fluid amount.

Nasogastric tubes can cause many problems. A nasal tube left in a nostril for an extended period of time without periodic cleansing and lubrication can result in crust formation or actual erosion of the nostril. (This author has actually seen an example of this erosion.) To avoid this problem, as well as to prevent discomfort and possible embarrassment to the patient, many physicians prefer to insert a gastrostomy tube in a person who needs tube feedings for an extended period of time. Changing the nasogastric tube from nostril to nostril every 3 days may also be done.

With either type of feeding tube, it is important to follow the feeding with at least 30 mL of water to prevent clogging of the tube. Residuals should be checked before each feeding, and the feeding should be reduced or held if the amount of the residual is significant. Patients should receive feedings while in high Fowler's position and should remain in this position for at least an hour after the feedings to prevent aspiration.

Once a patient regains consciousness, there may still be swallowing difficulties, most likely secondary to damage to the glossopharyngeal and vagus nerves. The first attempt at oral feeding should be made carefully with water to test for any dysphagia as evidenced by the patient's inability to swallow without regurgitation or choking, increased drooling of saliva, or decreased gag and swallow reflex. For patients with dysphagia, sitting straight up with support to the back and arms is helpful. The neck should not be hyperextended during feeding. Giving small amounts of food and coaching the patient to swallow are helpful also. Starting the patient with liquids, working up to semisolids, and then solids is usually possible with diligence. Most patients are better able to handle thicker liquids, such as milk shakes, than water or tea. Before any feeding is done, however, the nurse should test the gag and swallow reflexes to get a baseline on which to plan care.

The involvement of the family in problems of

feeding can be extremely helpful. Family members are usually more than willing to help the patient eat and to work slowly with the feeding process. Experience has shown that often patients will eat for a parent or spouse but not for the nursing staff. The nurse should supervise the family members until it is evident that they can safely feed the patient.

MOTOR PROBLEMS

Patients with cranial injuries may suffer a number of motor problems. These may include paresis or paralysis of one extremity (monoparesis or monoplegia), hemiparesis or hemiplegia, and paresis or paralysis of the muscles of the eye and those needed in chewing, swallowing, or talking. If any of these problems are present, the nurse and other therapists work to assist the patient to compensate for them and to prevent deformities. When in bed, the patient is positioned to maintain neutral alignment of all joints.

Range-of-motion exercises are given to all joints at least two to three times daily. Many head injury patients have a problem with spasticity, with resulting flexion contractures. If this tends to occur, braces or splints may be helpful to prevent foot drop, wrist drop, or other contractures. Slings should be used for flaccid, paralyzed arms when the patient is up in a chair or ambulating. A footboard should be used when the patient is in bed. If spasticity becomes a problem that interferes with functioning, a drug regime may be tried to decrease the spasticity. Extreme or prolonged spasticity may require surgical intervention.

Incoordination may present a difficult problem for the patient recovering from cerebral trauma. Although physical and occupational therapy may assist the patient in overcoming this, the nurse can help the patient undertake tasks slowly to minimize the incoordination.

COMMUNICATION PROBLEMS

Communication problems may be present in the patient with cerebral injury. The muscles used in talking may be involved so that clear verbal expression may not be possible. The patient may also be suffering from expressive aphasia, receptive aphasia, or global aphasia. For further discussion of these problems refer to Chapters 11 and 12.

No matter what the cause of the communication difficulty, the nurse must use the utmost patience in assisting the patient to express needs. Caregivers must try to anticipate the needs of the patient, yet at the same time not take away initiative by providing for all needs before the patient can ask about them.

Speech therapy can prove extremely helpful in the diagnosis of a speech problem and in working toward a solution. The nurse must be aware of any plan made by the speech pathologist so that the plan can be reinforced on the unit.

VOCATIONAL AND EDUCATIONAL COUNSELING

Because many of the patients who suffer head injuries are of working or school age, vocational and educational redirection and counseling may be necessary. Some patients may be able to return to previous jobs or educational programs, but many cannot. For those patients with residual motor deficits, training in more sedentary occupations may be required. Persons with residual intellectual deficits will need to be evaluated vocationally to see if they are able to function in a work setting and if so, for what type of work they are best suited. Factors such as safety, control of environmental stimuli, one- versus two-handed activities, transportation to and from work, and physical endurance must all be considered. Most often, vocational testing and subsequent counseling do not begin immediately upon the patient's entry into the rehabilitation facility but may continue after discharge on an outpatient basis. Most communities have access to vocational guidance services and rehabilitation services, which should be made use of by those patients who require them.

FAMILY INVOLVEMENT

The involvement of family or significant others is important from time of admission. By caring for the patient in any way possible, these people become involved in a real way and, in fact, gain firsthand knowledge regarding the totality of residual damage. Further, if the patient is to return home with them, they must become comfortable with the care involved before the patient is discharged. If, for instance, the patient has seizures, caregivers need to know the proper interventions.

Selected passes or leaves of absence play an important role in assisting the family to prepare for the patient's discharge. Usually the program begins with day passes and then progresses to overnight passes. Family members have an opportunity to care for the patient but know that they can return the patient to the hospital at any time. Family members should also be assured that they can call the hospital if they need advice.

A home evaluation should be made to assess the patient's living situation, and environmental changes to facilitate care of the patient should be suggested.

As the patient progresses in the rehabilitation program, family and significant others should have periodic, scheduled appointments regarding the patient's progress. They need tremendous amounts of support in their continued adjustment to what has happened. It is necessary to remember again that brain damage from head trauma tends to affect the late adolescent, and the concomitant alterations in life plans can be great. The more the family members understand about the patient's abilities and potential for success, the better equipped they will be for future planning and adjustments. For example, it is not unusual for a patient to regress and become increasingly depressed even when making significant improvements in all areas. As the patient clears mentally and increases independent activities, the patient also increasingly is aware of the tragedy that has occurred. Regression and depression are understandable, even appropriate. Rehabilitation workers know and accept this; families cannot be expected to.

DISCHARGE PLANNING

Many of the patients who have suffered cerebral trauma are able to return to their own homes. Some, however, remain unconscious or have residual motor or emotional problems that preclude their independent functioning. As a result, realistic planning must be undertaken to determine the best option for discharge care. Sometimes, home care is not in the best interest of either the patient or the family. Many families feel guilty for even considering other placement options than home care. The nurse should work with the families to help them choose the best alternative for the family as well as for the patient. When nursing-home placement is necessary, families should be assisted to find a facility that can meet the patient's needs.

For patients who do return home, plans should be made with their families or caregivers for visiting nurse involvement and for home health aides where needed. If not arranged beforehand, any financial referrals should be made. Follow-up care should be arranged before the patient is discharged. The family or patient should know the source of follow-up care, as well as the time and location of the appointment.

This young population of patients has a particular problem after discharge; they have little or nothing to do, and they suffer boredom and depression. Discharge planning with the family and patient should include scheduling in-home activities and out-of-home recreation. This is a difficult task since many of the patient's favorite hobbies and pastimes may be beyond physical abilities at the time of discharge.

Mr. M., a 24-year-old patient, suffered a skull fracture with brain trauma in a motorcycle accident. Mr. M. was a bartender at a local singles bar, had attended college for 3 years, but had quit to become a carpenter. For recreation he enjoyed jogging, skiing, and coaching the bar's female softball team. Mr. M. had several girlfriends, mostly casual acquaintances, and he lived alone. At discharge Mr. M. was ambulatory and able to do simple ADL (activities of daily living); however, his homemaking skills were limited, he was easily fatigued, and he still needed environmental controls on stimulation. He was discharged to live with his mother, 30 miles from his own apartment. Mr. M. could not return to work, or even visit the bar, since the noise and activity made him very anxious and fearful. He could not participate in his former recreational pursuits and since most of his friends lived at a distance and were casual relationships, he had few visitors. On recheck, 6 weeks postdischarge, he was severely depressed.

Preplanning an activity program, early rechecks, and visiting nurse referrals could have at least to some degree, short-circuited this problem.

CONCLUSION

Head trauma with residual permanent damage, no matter how mild, is a disastrous event. It is unexpected, and it is quick. Permanent damage is irreversible, although absolutely amazing recovery can occur. For this reason, optimism must prevail, but objective realism is also needed. The patient, family, and significant others need the utmost rehabilitation workers can offer.

BIBLIOGRAPHY

Adams, J.: "Patients Who Talk and Die After a Non-Missile Head Injury," *Nurs Mirror* 142:17, 1976.

Berkovsky, D.: "Physiological Effects of Closed Head Injury," *J Neurosurg Nurs* 4:125, 1972.

Blackwood, W., and J. Corsellis: *Greenfield's Neuro-Pathology,* Edward Arnold, Chicago, 1976.

Carini, E., and G. Owen: *Neurological and Neurosurgical Nursing,* Mosby, St. Louis, 1974.

Chaffee, E., and E. Greisheimer: *Basic Physiology and Anatomy,* Lippincott, Philadelphia, 1964.

Chusid, J.: *Correlative Neuroanatomy and Functional Neurology,* Lange, Los Altos, Calif., 1976.

Cross, A.: "Nursing Care of Patients with Head Injury," *Nurs Mirror* 145:15, 1977.

Eliasson, S. et al.: *Neurological Pathophysiology,* Oxford Univ. Press, New York, 1978.

Feiring, E.: *Brock's Injuries of the Brain and Spinal Cord,* Springer, New York, 1974.

Glass, S.: "Nursing Care of the Neurosurgery Patient," *J Neurosurg Nurs* 5:49, 1973.

Johnson, M.: "Emergency Management of Head and Spinal Injuries," *Nurs Clin North Am* 8:389, 1973.

Jolly, F.: "The Management of Head Injuries in Adults," *South Med J* 63:989, 1970.

Kaplan, H.: *The New Sex Therapy,* Brunner/Mazel, New York, 1974.

Knight, P.: "Rehabilitation of Head Injuries," *Nurs Mirror* 136:14, 1973.

Lucas, B.: "Nursing Care Study: Pregnant Car-Crash Victim," *Nurs Times* 70:451, 1976.

Nahum, A.: *Early Management of Acute Trauma,* Mosby, St. Louis, 1966.

Parsons, L.: "Respiratory Changes in Head Injury," *J Am Nurs* 71:2187, 1971.

Proctor, H.: "Management of Head Injuries," *Nurs Mirror* 145:19, 1977.

Quesenbury, J., and P. Lembright: "Observations and Care of Patients with Head Injury," *Nurs Clin North Am* 4:237, 1969.

Swift, N.: "Head Injuries: Essentials of Excellent Care," *Nursing '74* 4:26, 1974.

U.S. Department of Health, Education, and Welfare: *Types of Injuries, Incidence and Associated Disability. U.S. July 1965-June 1967,* Public Health Services Publication no. 1000, series 10, no. 57, 1969.

Willie, R. et al.: "Emergency Care of the Neurosurgery Patient in a Community Hospital," *J Neurosurg Nurs* 8:11, 1976.

Young, J.: "Recognition, Significance and Recording of the Signs of Increased Intracranial Pressure," *Nurs Clin North Am* 4:223, 1969.

22
dorothy l. gordon

multiple sclerosis

INTRODUCTION

The person who experiences multiple sclerosis is faced with a dilemma of certainty and uncertainty. The certainty is the reality of living with a usually progressive disabling disease; the uncertainty is how the disease will manifest itself in that person and what impact it will have on the life of the individual and significant others. This puzzling illness is a major crippler of young adults, male and female, usually appearing between ages 20 and 40. Although onset before age 18 and after 45 is known, it is uncommon. In the prime of life, the person who acquires multiple sclerosis is stressed with a neurological disease of unknown cause, unpredictable course, and no known cure.

The pathological accounts of the disease were initially given in the early nineteenth century. The French neurologist Jean Martin Charcot described the clinical manifestations in 1868 and made the first correlation of symptomatology with pathologic alterations. His work brought multiple sclerosis to the attention of the medical world, which today still seeks the elusive etiology of the disease. The search is reflected in the numerous etiologies postulated over the years: toxins, antecedent acute illness, vascular thrombosis and vasospasm, vexation, exposure to cold, and "constitutional peculiarity," among others. Current research efforts into etiology are concentrated in the fields of virology and immunology, with the interaction of the two an important consideration. There is emphasis on finding the cause of multiple sclerosis; once that mystery is solved, steps in prevention and treatment can be definitive. At present, prevention is not possible and treatment is symptomatic.

The certainties and uncertainties surrounding multiple sclerosis also affect health professionals. Since the disease does not lend itself neatly to criteria for diagnosis and cure, the feelings of success from the medical viewpoint are diminished. Distinguishing multiple sclerosis from other neurological diseases is made difficult since no specific diagnostic tests are available. Sometimes, a conclusive diagnosis cannot be made, yet the patient and physician are faced with a persistent and assorted array of signs and symptoms. Once a medical diagnosis is made, efforts to interrupt the progress of the disease are unrewarded, and the feelings of helplessness attributed to patients may also be experienced by the professionals charged with providing care. Nurses and others should be vigilant to prevent such feelings from turning into withdrawal from and abandonment of the patient. The plan of care for the person with multiple sclerosis requires discussion between the professionals involved about how to be realistic with patients who face an uncertain future, and at the same time not destroy their grounds for hope. A sensitivity to this dilemma provides no specific solutions but affords patients and professionals an opportunity to make the process a shared concern.

THE DISEASE

Knowledge of the pathology of multiple sclerosis is essential to understanding the fact that different clinical pictures of patients emerge. Although there are symptoms that appear more frequently than others, in any given patient the specific progression of the disease, and therefore its signs and symptoms, is uncertain.

Multiple sclerosis is a disease of the central nervous system. Upon autopsy, plaques or "scarring" can be found in such locations as the spinal cord, brainstem, cerebrum, cerebellum, and optic nerves; in general, peripheral nerves are spared. The pathological process involves the formation of these sclerotic "plaques." In these circumscribed lesions, the myelin sheaths and, to a lesser extent, the axis cylinders of the nerves are destroyed. Since nerves are insulated through the myelin sheaths, it is postulated that destruction of the latter results in the interruption of nerve impulse conduction. In early stages of the disease, the axis cylinder may be spared and

---

The author acknowledges the comments on and contributions to this chapter by Patricia B. O'Donnell, R.N., M.S., Clinical Nurse Specialist, Multiple Sclerosis Comprehensive Care Program, Johns Hopkins University.

there is a probable reversibility of the lesions; this may account for complete or partial recovery from symptoms.

The pattern of remission and exacerbation is a striking characteristic of multiple sclerosis. It is generally felt that over time there is a gradual increase in the severity of lesions and less recovery of function following exacerbation (DeJong, 1970).

The geographical distribution of multiple sclerosis reveals that it is more prevalent in the northern hemisphere; in the United States the incidence rate is five to ten times higher in Northern compared to Southern states. Rates of distribution among the sexes vary somewhat with the source reporting the figures, but the National Multiple Sclerosis Society says that the incidence rate is higher in women than men.

For approximately 500,000 Americans suffering from the disease, research into its etiology is a basis of hope. Since the epidemiological, clinical, and pathological features of the disease are consistent with a viral infection, a viral theory has received attention. Concurrently, immunological studies are being pursued as there is some evidence that certain histocompatability antigens are more prevalent in persons with multiple sclerosis. The interplay between viral and immunological phenomena is an area of investigation that is receiving concentrated attention as the search for knowledge about multiple sclerosis continues.

In summary, the factors known about the disease itself are the morbid anatomy (plaques seen on autopsy), some pathologic neurophysiology, certain epidemiological findings, and the revealing course of exacerbation and remission. Unknown factors are precise etiology, premorbid features, individual prognosis, and specific diagnostic tests and therapy (DeJong, 1970).

DIAGNOSIS AND CLINICAL MANIFESTATIONS

The medical diagnostic process itself is a period of uncertainty for both patient and physician. The patient may first approach the physician because of a single symptom that becomes particularly troublesome, or the patient may have a series of persistent signs that something is wrong. Upon careful inquiry, the person may recall less severe and transient problems which were attributable to something else and dismissed as trivial. Weakness of a muscle group is a common early sign; visual symptoms and sensory changes may also be initial complaints of note. Table 22-1 shows the first symptoms reported by 100 consecutive multiple sclerosis patients.

Signs and symptoms come and go; in any given individual there is no predictable course of events. One may experience the early symptoms and enter a prolonged remission with little problem in exacerbation. In others, periods of exacerbation and remission of symptoms occur more frequently. Occasionally a steady progressive course is exhibited. Traumatic events and emotional stress are generally cited as precipitators of both the disease and its exacerbations. Surgery, pregnancy, physical injury, and infections have all been implicated, but specific evidence is not conclusive and the mode in which such stressors operate is not understood. Particularly in the early stages of multiple sclerosis, the patient's subjective symptoms can be confused with hysteria, even after a careful clinical neurological examination.

Since no disease-specific test is available, the diagnostician relies heavily on history, neurological examination, and differentiation from other nervous system disorders. Demonstration that the lesions have disseminated both in time and place is a major criterion of note in differential diagnosis. The complexity of the problem of diagnosing multiple sclerosis is reflected in the medical literature where it is not uncommon for physicians to discuss what they tell patients and when. Generally, caution is advocated until there is confidence in the diagnosis.

Some helpful diagnostic tests reflect the areas of research into the etiology of the disease. Spinal-tap findings show that patients with multiple sclerosis have an elevated proportion of

Table 22-1

First Symptom Noticed in 100 Consecutive Patients with Multiple Sclerosis

WEAKNESS OR LOSS OF CONTROL OVER LIMBS	NUMBER
Involving both lower limbs	18
Involving one lower limb	14
Involving one upper limb	9
Involving one upper and one lower limb	7
Involving all four limbs	2
	50
VISUAL SYMPTOMS	
Blindness in one eye	16
Double vision	8
"Dimness" of vision	4
Homonymous field defect	1
	29
SENSORY SYMPTOMS	
Numbness and other painless paresthesias	11
MISCELLANEOUS SYMPTOMS	
Vertigo	2
Tremor	2
Multiple symptoms	2
Prosis	1
Loss of taste	1
Epilepsy	1
Impotence	1
	10

Source: Adapted with permission from John N. Walton: *Brain's Disease of the Nervous System*, 8th ed., Oxford Univ. Press, Oxford, 1977, p. 549.

gamma globulin to total protein in the cerebrospinal fluid and distinct bands of immunoglobulin G; however, this also may be found in other neurological diseases. Work related to histocompatability antigens reveals that some are found more frequently in persons with multiple sclerosis than in others (Paty, 1977b). Increased levels of measles antibodies in the serum of multiple sclerosis patients have been found, but elevated antibody levels for other viruses also have been demonstrated (Walton, 1977).

Electroencephalograms and electromyelograms contribute information in the diagnostic process; reports on the usefulness of computerized transaxial tomography in diffenential diagnosis have just begun to appear. Myelograms and pneumograms have a role in ruling out brain and spinal cord tumors.

The time between the person's seeking medical attention and the actual diagnosis may be prolonged. This period of uncertainty has been described by patients as a time of great difficulty and stress accompanied by feelings of helplessness. Lack of both information and reassurance creates a sense of aloneness and isolation for the person awaiting answers to questions. Indeed, some persons report having received the diagnosis with relief, even though it triggered other anxieties (Hartings). The nurse attending patients during this period can be caught between the physician's problem of making a definite diagnosis and the patient's desire to have an answer. Support can be offered by providing the patient with an opportunity to express concern and by helping make sure the person receives pertinent information during the period that diagnostic data are being gathered.

MEDICAL MANAGEMENT

With no known etiology of multiple sclerosis, options for medical management of the patient are limited. In addition, the unpredictability of the pattern of the disease makes evaluation of the effectiveness of therapies a difficult problem. For example, it is difficult to determine whether remission is a result of therapy or part of the natural course of the disease. The frequency, severity, and duration of exacerbations may be a guide but are not necessarily a valid or reliable measure of the success of medical therapy. In studies of the effectiveness of treatment regimens on multiple sclerosis, it is not uncommon to use scales or scores of disability (Kurtzke, 1965; Schumacher). Such measurement methods are also used during the rehabilitation process when a person's ability to function, in terms of mobility and activities of daily living, is commonly used as an assessment of response to a total program of treatment. A general review of considerations in conducting clinical studies on multiple sclerosis has been published by an ad hoc committee of the National Multiple Sclerosis Society (Brown, 1979).

Numerous pharmacologic agents including antimetabolites and immunosuppressives have been utilized in treating the person with multiple sclerosis, but their value has not been substantiated. Corticosteroids and/or adrenocorticotropic hormone (ACTH) have been useful in alleviating the severity of relapses, but long-term administration is not usually advocated. Other drug therapy in the treatment of the multiple sclerosis patient is in response to symptoms and complications. Diazepam (Valium), baclofen (Lioresal), and muscle relaxants may be used for relief of the discomfort and pain of spasticity, and medications such as propanolol or diazepam may be prescribed for tremor. Some patients reported relief of spasticity while using marijuana, and beginning research results have been reported (Check, 1979). Over a period of time, different medications may be utilized, reflecting both the ongoing studies in treatment and the lack of specific successful drug therapy in multiple sclerosis. Drug therapy for bladder and bowel problems is individualized, as is the possible use of tranquilizers and antidepressants.

Although results are inconclusive, the use of linoleic acid in the form of sunflower seed oil may hold some promise in alleviating the severity of relapses, and there are continuing studies in this area. Low fat diets are prescribed in some instances.

As part of medical management, a rehabilitative medicine program is generally begun at some stage as the disease progresses. The physical medicine and rehabilitation personnel are called upon to assess whether or not the patient is utilizing maximum functional potential, and whether or not active intervention is of value. There is no evidence that indicates a rehabilitation program influences the pathologic process of the disease in any way. However, in many cases, an individualized activity program can be helpful in preventing complications that arise from disuse, and such a program may facilitate mobility. The goal is to help the patient lead a useful and functional life.

There are differing opinions regarding the value of exercise programs and the use of rest. Some people recommend complete bed rest during exacerbation (Schumacher, 1970; Russell, 1976); others claim it does nothing to influence the course of illness and has negative qualities, such as contributing to depression (Tourtellotte, 1977; Rusk, 1977). The latter view recommends activity programs that can be realized within the patient's limitations (Rusk).

Rehabilitative medicine measures may include passive, active, and/or resistive exercise, use of braces, canes, or walkers, provision of adaptive devices, and training in activities of daily living. Specific therapies are utilized according to the particular presenting problem or problems experienced by the patient. Since an increase in body temperature is thought to bring on a temporary exacerbation of symptoms, the use of heat in physical therapy is generally avoided.

In severe cases of multiple sclerosis, surgical intervention may be employed to relieve the deforming spasticity and permit positioning of the extremities. Alcohol and phenol blocks are also sometimes of help.

Euphoria is a state of mind frequently attributed to the person with multiple sclerosis, although situational depression is not unexpected or uncommon. Intellectual functioning may sometimes be diminished, but emotional changes seem to be more common (Walton). Counseling in individual or group sessions may be indicated to assist the person in coping; if emotional problems become profound, psychologic or psychiatric consultations may be recommended and put into effect.

Wonder Cures

Since conclusive treatment for multiple sclerosis is not yet within the armamentarium of the medical world, those with the disease are potentially vulnerable to charlatans and "wonder" cures. Certainly the phenomenon of remission lends fertile ground to claims of success in alleviating the disease. Providing as much objective information as possible, teaching the patient and significant others about the disease, and maintaining an open communication link with professionals may help prevent someone from taking advantage of multiple sclerosis patients and their families. Understanding the desperation which leads patients to seek magic answers is important. An open communication line provides the nurse with the opportunity to counsel the patient about unsafe wonder cures; the patient, however, eventually decides the course to be pursued.

NURSING MANAGEMENT

Nurses will encounter persons with multiple sclerosis in the hospital, the home, the work scene, nursing homes, or rehabilitation centers. Since the average life expectancy after the first symptoms appear is over 25 years (DeJong), a nurse's contact with any one patient could be over a lengthy time span. On the other hand, the nurse may have only a brief exposure to a patient. Since a general objective is to keep the multiple sclerosis patient out of an institution, it may be that hospital nurses see patients only during diagnostic periods or relapses when manifestations of their symptoms are acute. Nurses in rehabilitation centers may see them when an active program is considered to have potential benefit for functional performance. In industry or clinics, nurses may be in touch with those continuing their life's work with some minor adjustments, while nurses in nursing homes see the severely disabled who require maximum care. Assessment of persons with multiple sclerosis at their particular time and place in the course of the disease is the basis for an individualized plan of care. Although general goals are consistent throughout patient care, priorities and methods of intervention are tailored to the individual's status whenever and wherever the nurse and patient meet.

PREVENTION OF EXACERBATION AND COMPLICATIONS

Since relapses or exacerbations are acute problems, and since complications may be life threatening, nursing intervention designed to put the person at less risk is an important part of care.

Good health is a person's best defense against illness and should be maintained whenever possible in the person with a chronic disease, such as multiple sclerosis. Consequently, patient education is aimed at preventing complications and is a major activity in nursing management. The person with multiple sclerosis is faced with a large number of problems as a result of changes affecting the body, and the energy required to cope with these problems may place great strain on the patient. Therefore, in assessing whether the person has complied with teaching, it should be kept in mind that this disease often is typified by a lack of energy.

It is generally accepted that stress can provoke an exacerbation or, at the least, can aggravate some symptoms. Therefore, counseling and teaching the patient about the avoidance of both physical and psychologic stress is a nursing activity. It is unrealistic to expect that all stressful events can be avoided, but awareness of them can be of value; when they are unavoidable, perhaps their effect can be diminished.

Fatigue

Fatigue is a common problem faced by the person with multiple sclerosis. Assessment of the person's daily schedule and life-style by the nurse and patient can serve as a basis for planning a rest and activity schedule to avoid severe tiring. For example, judicious scheduling of a nap during the daytime may help the individual to complete the day's activities at work or home. Sitting periods of rest are considered by some to be more valuable than lying down, and a good night's sleep aids the ability to tolerate an activity-filled schedule.

Fatigue in the person with multiple sclerosis seems to decrease motor power to a greater degree and extent than other conditions. This lessened power, or weakness, is attributable to the pathologic process and consequently is not reversible by exercise or other modalities. However, there also exists the probability that some weakness from disuse can be present, as well as fatigue from improper use of muscle groups. Activity to counteract this phenomenon may be of help in promoting the individual's potential to remain mobile. An important part of the nurse's role is to coordinate activity programs with the patient and other professionals. For example, if the patient is on a physical therapy schedule, this is considered in planning the patient's pattern of living. If the person is in a working environment, the nurse may arrange the person's schedule to accommodate a rest period. The effort by patients to remain active may be overwhelming in some cases; as a result, they may respond by refusing to participate in any activity. It is important to keep this in mind and to help the person understand differences between the disease problem and the disuse problem. This difficulty is underscored by personal accounts of patients; one described his major problem in coping with multiple sclerosis to be how to avoid overtiredness and yet not "opt out" (Burnfield).

An increase in body temperature due to fever, use of thermal modalities, and exposure to sun is associated with exaggerated symptoms in multiple sclerosis. In cases of fever accompanied by fluctuation in symptoms, treatment of the underlying cause by the physician is indicated. Generally, the worsening of symptoms in response to heat is not considered an exacerbation since a return of the body temperature to normal relieves symptom severity (Schumacher). Consequently, persons with multiple sclerosis should be made aware of the wisdom of staying out of situations associated with excessive heat, such as hot cars in the summer or sports events in the midday sun. In general, the increased symptoms may recede when the person returns to air conditioning. Activities should be planned for early morning or late evening; for those with a heat intolerance to exercise, a swimming program where heat dissipation can take place may be a useful alternative.

Nutrition

Part of maintaining general strength and health is adequate nutrition; therefore, the general nutrition of the patient with multiple sclerosis is of concern to the nurse, and teaching the patient about nutrition is in order. On general principles, a well-balanced diet is often recommended. The nature of the disease makes the multiple sclerosis patient susceptible to fad diets which claim to be instrumental in relieving symptoms. Patients should be instructed to contact their primary nurse or physician regarding any dietary claims from nonmedical personnel. This is of particular importance in the person with multiple sclerosis because certain diets have been used in medical management. Gluten-free, low fat, and the Evers-Root diets have been medically prescribed, as has the supplemental use of linoleic acid in the form of sunflower seed oil; no conclusive results from these dietary interventions have been reported, however. A misinformed patient should be cautioned not to try to combine these diets all at once and consequently suffer from poor nutrition.

If the patient has incoordination or visual complications, the mechanics of feeding may become a problem in nutrition. If this is so, the nurse may help the patient acquire adaptive tools and can help plan the patient's eating routine. Arranging plates, cups, and saucers consistently and within reach of the person may be helpful. Plate guards, adaptive drinking cups, and weighted utensils can be used as self-help devices to facilitate feeding. Use of napkins or bibs will protect clothes from possible spillage; the latter should be used sparingly as a consideration in relation to the person's self-image.

Some persons may have difficulty with chewing and swallowing. To help ease this difficulty, eating time should be unhurried and the atmosphere made as pleasant as possible. Semisolid or soft foods may be easier to manage, and the person should use small mouthfuls and chew slowly. Sensory losses in part of the facial area may require the person to chew and swallow on the unaffected side. Dysphagia is an uncommon problem but may be present. If feeding difficulties progress, consultation with an occupational or speech therapist may be helpful in planning care. In severe cases, tube feeding may be the recourse.

Good oral hygiene following meals helps remove remaining food particles and prevents dental problems which could lead to infection. Toothbrushes with soft bristles help prevent possible damage to tissue, particularly if sensory loss is present. Built-up handles on toothbrushes may facilitate closer brushing by making the brush easier to grip by persons with weakness. Regular dental checkups and care are part of the health maintenance of patients with multiple sclerosis.

Emotional Stress

Helping patients avoid or handle emotional stress can be approached by reviewing with them their areas of concern. An assessment of situations the patient perceives as stressful can be used to assist in recognizing such situations and, if feasible, to eliminate or avoid them. The nurse can explore this subject while taking the patient's health history and gathering information to devise a plan of care. The family also can contribute useful information. The nurse can be important in making the patient's contact with the health-care system less stressful; this includes helping to arrange appropriate schedules at clinics or within an institution, assuring that the person receives courteous treatment, providing information, and tendering direct assistance. Stress imposed on the patient by duplicated efforts, inadequate communication between team members, and inconsideration of the patient's individual situation can be reduced by the coordinating activities of the nurse.

In relation to stressful situations in the patient's life-style, cooperation of family and significant others is valuable. The patient who is slow in bathing and grooming may tie up the bathroom as the family starts a busy morning schedule, or the patient can remain socially active only if a family member is regularly available to provide transportation. These may not seem major problems to some people, but the presence of such situations, daily, may serve as sources of irritation stress. Sometimes the stress can be prevented or alleviated through help in planning and coordinating a family's daily schedule. Referral to an appropriate agency may be needed to help solve problems which patients and families cannot manage alone.

Physical Stress

As indicated earlier, pregnancy and surgery are events that are thought by some to induce relapses; however, in the case of surgery, physicians seem to think that when surgery is clearly indicated on its own merits, it should not be avoided (Tourtellotte). Pregnancy appears to carry a calculated risk for the mother in relation to exacerbation, and this subject merits serious consideration in a population of patients in the childbearing age. Not only the fact of pregnancy itself, but consideration of day-to-day child care and family life in relation to disability are matters for patients and spouses to discuss and decide. For example, persons who become moderately or severely disabled may have physical difficulty in carrying out child-rearing tasks. The nurse can facilitate a conference where the patient and significant others will receive medical advice and counseling regarding the case. Once a decision is made, the nurse may be a continued support.

Since infections and fever can be deleterious to the person with multiple sclerosis, efforts should be exerted to prevent their occurrence. If the person by necessity must have an indwelling catheter, then meticulous catheter technique is necessary; both the patient and significant others should be taught appropriate care.

Skin Care

The person with multiple sclerosis also needs to give attention to the integrity of the skin. Not infrequently there may be sensory loss which renders the individual insensitive to pain, temperature, and pressure changes; this insensitivity could lead to tissue damage and subsequent infection. The nurse, therefore, should help the person become aware of this possibility and should give instructions concerning safety. Caution about bath or shower temperature, as well as such concerns as cigarette burns of the finger, should be included. If the person with multiple sclerosis must spend time in bed or a wheelchair, then efforts to prevent pressure sores must be employed. High-risk sites are bony prominences and areas with sensory loss. If the person is in a stage of the disease where spasticity and flexion contractures give difficulty in positioning and skin care, flotation pads and water beds may be used.

In efforts to avoid, reduce, or alleviate psychologic and physical stress, the goals set by the nurse and patient are to be considered. Achievable goals can offer the person the opportunity to acquire a sense of accomplishment and to reduce the stress of failure. In goal setting, the person's abilities rather than disabilities should set the tone for planning and implementing care.

MAINTENANCE OF MOBILITY

A goal in the care of the person with multiple sclerosis is the maintenance of mobility as long as possible. During early stages of the disease, problems of imbalance and coordination may be the major sources of concern. Varying patterns of motor dysfunction can arise in the progress of the disease. For example, some people manifest hemiplegia; others have paraplegia and/or quadriplegia. The particular intervention, of course, is suited to the difficulty being experienced.

Range-of-motion exercises to both affected and unaffected extremities are given. The exercises may be active, in which case the patient is able to move all joints through the range of motion without help; if the person cannot accomplish this alone, then assistance can be provided by family, after teaching by the nurse or therapist. Patients who are depressed or who have unrealistic goals of ambulation may stop their range-of-motion exercises when unable to achieve their objective. This highlights the importance of continuing encouragement from the nurse so that the person will persist in the exercise program.

In some cases, a wheelchair may become a necessity. A wheelchair should be chosen carefully and should include features of convenience and assistance to the individual. The prescription of a chair is made by the physician or therapist after assessment of the person's needs and the environment in which the person will function. For example, desk arms on the wheelchair may make it possible for the person to work at a desk or table, and swinging footrests and removable arms make transfers easier.

Efforts are made to keep patients from becoming bedridden. If the person does spend a great period of time in bed, then basic measures to combat problems of immobility are used by the nurse. Positioning can be attended to by using pillows and linen rolls, the goal being body alignment. Positions are changed on a regular-routine basis, and when possible the person can be taught to turn alone or with assistance. Devices such as a pull rope on the bottom of the bed or a trapeze bar can help the bedridden person move about in bed. Sturdy side rails facilitate this and also act as a safety device to prevent falling. Not only are the physical problems of immobility important, but attention must be directed to the potential psychologic and social isolation of the bedridden person. Bedridden persons cannot go to others or to places others go. Consequently, they are dependent on caregivers, family, and friends for contact, conversation, and diversion. The lack of such personal contact and stimulation can contribute to behavioral changes (Stryker, 1977).

For the person with incoordination in the lower extremities, gait training may be of use. An assessment and planned program by a physical therapist can be incorporated into a total plan of care. Using a widened base of support and employing weighted canes or walkers are techniques to improve stability. Braces are used occassionally but not extensively for the person with multiple sclerosis.

If the person becomes homebound, clearing obstacles out of common traffic pattern areas will make ambulation easier. Loose rugs should be avoided and, if possible, ramps should be constructed over stairs. These precautions facilitate mobility but also entail safety measures to prevent falls or injuries. It would be anticipated that multiple sclerosis patients with motor and visual problems would have more accidents, but experience does not bear this out. Perhaps the person's concentration and attention to getting about compensate for the instability, or perhaps they restrict their activities.

Some persons can remain mobile with careful planning of activity patterns. For example, shopping routes can be studied and pathways mapped out which are barrier-free and also permit places for the person to sit and rest.

In instances where spasticity becomes a severe problem in maintaining motion, mild stretching may be of some value. A preventive daily program may forestall complications of progressive shortening of muscles. Cold packs to reduce spasticity have been utilized; packing the joints in cold towels for 15 min before range-of-motion exercise may help alleviate some of the tightness from spasticity. If spasticity becomes severe to the point of deformity and if it interferes with the ability to provide care, surgical intervention or the use of drugs or blocking agents may be medical treatments. These symptomatic treatments may or may not be of value.

Although pain does not seem to be a major difficulty for most patients with multiple sclerosis, it may be present in the form of backaches, muscle cramps, and spasms. It is thought the backache is secondary to an abnormal gait or posture. This pain and the other discomforts are generally relieved with mild analgesics or muscle relaxants. Spinothalamic tract pain, experienced as a burning sensation, also may be a discomfort for the person with multiple sclerosis. As in other chronic illnesses, narcotics and potentially addictive pain relievers are generally avoided.

Other sensory changes in the form of paresthesias may be experienced by patients with multiple sclerosis; there is actually no treatment for these and they are not incapacitating. Lhermitte's sign may be present, a sensation of electric shock shooting into the extremities upon flexion of the neck.

Vision

Among the cranial nerves affected by multiple sclerosis are those involving vision. Visual impairment hinders the person's interaction with the environment and can be a major difficulty in mobility. In multiple sclerosis, such changes may manifest themselves in any number of ways since the optic and oculomotor tracts can be the target of attacks. Common disturbances are diplopia, blurred vision, and loss of visual acuity.

Diplopia can be alleviated by the use of an eye patch or frosted lens over one eye; the covered eye may be alternated. The nurse should remind the person that using an eye patch will result in lack of depth image; although this may cause difficulty in ambulatory activities and therapies, it is generally superior to the confusion which can result from constant viewing of double images.

Glare from the sun, bright lights, and television may disturb the patient but can be reduced with sunglasses.

If diminished vision occurs, bright color contrasts may be of help to a person in identifying certain items. In some cases, magnifiers may be useful. When the person is in the home, environmental changes should be kept at a minimum and family should be instructed to tell the patient about any changes which occur.

Partial to complete blindness also may be experienced by the person with multiple sclerosis; if indicated, the nurse may refer the person and family to a local society for the blind or to another resource. If blindness is present, it is important to identify oneself to the patient, using sound or touch as a substitute for visual cues. Many libraries have books available in large print, and services such as "talking books" can be obtained. Some patients who have visual symptoms and who also need to rest at certain periods of the day use the talking book services during rest and state that they "read" more than previously.

MAINTAINING INDEPENDENCE IN ACTIVITIES OF DAILY LIVING AND SELF-CARE

Maintenance of the ability to care for oneself in day-to-day activities contributes much to the patient's feeling of self-worth. The problems of incoordination and tremor may make the routine handling of many items a distressing act. Sometimes, teaching the person to reach with both hands or to rest the elbow on a surface as a fulcrum will be helpful. Adaptive devices with weights and special handles have been mentioned as tools for eating. Consultation with an occupational therapist can help the nurse and the patient identify self-help devices that will assist the person in maintaining independence in activities for daily living.

In the home, adjustments to common areas of usage can facilitate daily activities. In the bathroom, grab bars securely and strategically placed should be available. Raised commode seats may help the person to maintain independence in care of the bowels. Showers instead of bathtubs may help the person remain independent in bathing; a tub seat makes it possible to sit while showering or bathing. If bathtub bathing is the only means available in the patient's home, then the nurse must teach transfer techniques. Strategic placement of furniture throughout the house helps many people maintain independence and mobility. Being able to "furniture walk" (using appropriately placed pieces of furniture as support items) may help to keep the person mobile around the home. Tools and devices around sinks, such as suction cups to hold soap and long-handled brushes, are useful in some cases.

There are myriad adaptive devices available which may make independent function achievable. The nurse should become familiar with these and their use in order to be a resource for the patient and family. In many instances, the nurse may be the one to suggest modifications and to do the teaching and training. However, in other circumstances, the expertise of the occupational and physical therapists is drawn upon for specific recommendations and training.

Personal care and appearance are important elements of independence and self-worth. In addition to bathing activities, grooming and dressing may be troublesome because of incoordination, spasticity, and visual problems.

Modification in clothing and adaptive tools can help some persons maintain self-care in dressing; for example, Velcro for fastening of openings can be used in place of a zipper, which may be unmanageable. A long-handled shoehorn can make putting on shoes easier. Training in dressing techniques may enable a person to perform that activity independently also. There are numerous strategies and illustrative sources available for donning clothes; the technique employed reflects the difficulty experienced by the individual. For the person with multiple sclerosis manifested as hemiplegia, the approaches used may be different from those for the person with quadriparesis; consequently, an individual assessment and plan for dressing can be facilitated by the nurse.

Hair care, makeup, shaving, and other grooming efforts are to be supported and encouraged. These may be time-consuming activities for the disabled individual, and depressed or discouraged patients may find it easier to neglect them than to expend the energy required; however, they are valuable because they contribute to a sense of well-being and achievement when accomplished.

MAINTENANCE OF URINARY AND BOWEL FUNCTION

Although not all persons with multiple sclerosis experience urinary problems, they are a frequent occurrence. The particular pattern is unpredictable. Difficulties may appear early or at any time in the disease course. In concert with other symptoms, the type of bladder function problem which manifests itself is related to the location of the involvement in the neural pathways.

A hyperactive reflex neurogenic bladder is one common syndrome, indicating a lesion above the actual urinary reflex arc. Urgency and frequency are manifestations that can be troublesome to the person, both from a discomfort and a social point of view. These symptoms are sometimes treated successfully with belladonna-type preparations. Patients who find that changes in temperature, a change in position from sitting to standing, excitement, or anxiety brings on urgency can anticipate it. If nocturia is present, the nurse may suggest the patient restrict fluid intake for several hours before bedtime. In more severe cases, there may be urgency accompanied by incontinence, in which case the problem is more difficult. The nurse can encourage attention to keeping the perineal area clean and dry. If the patient is mobile, a regular and frequent emptying of the bladder may be tried; if the patient is bedridden, the nurse or family can offer the bedpan regularly.

A nonreflexive bladder may be present if a plaque occurs in the urinary reflex center of the sacral spinal cord. Since somatic and parasympathetic centers are close to each other, this condition usually is accompanied by a flaccid external sphincter (Tarabulcy, 1970). There is usually some loss of urinary control, ranging from stress incontinence to constant dribbling. The nurse may instruct the patient and family in use of Crede's method (suprapubic manual pressure) as a means of intervention which may be of help. The use of sanitary napkins as padding can be suggested for social occasions. Special rubber pants are available through surgical supply houses. For males, the external catheter can be used. For bedfast persons, diapering is sometimes recommended; the demeaning effect this may have on the person should be of concern to the nurse who is considering this intervention.

The person with multiple sclerosis may experience retention of urine similar to that seen in patients with spinal shock bladder. This retention can be frightening for the patient, and it is not unusual for a person with multiple sclerosis to appear in a local hospital emergency room seeking help. The nurse can teach the patient and family to try proper positioning, the sound of running water, and pressure over the suprapubic area to relieve retention; they also can be taught catheterization techniques. The patient can be instructed in self-catheterization. If incoordination or other problems make this unfeasible, family members can be prepared to perform catheterization if required.

Where appropriate, the use of intermittent catheterization is preferred over indwelling catheters (Tarabulcy). If an indwelling catheter is employed, general teaching concerning adequate fluid intake, maintenance of acid urine, and careful catheter technique constitutes a basic nursing measure. Prevention of infection and renal complications is of major importance. In severe urinary problems that are unresponsive to symptomatic treatments, surgical interventions such as ilial conduits may be performed.

In relation to bowel function, constipation can be a complaint of the person with multiple sclerosis. General weakness and decreased activity contribute to the problem. A bowel movement every day or every other day is not generally necessary, and the nurse can help the patient to understand this.

Adequate fluid intake and a diet with appropriate bulk may be all that is needed. The nurse can help the person establish a regular routine, such as scheduling a visit to the bathroom 20 to 30 min after breakfast (or other meals) to take advantage of the gastrocolic reflex. Mild laxatives or suppositories can be used for the occasional problem. A regularly scheduled bowel regimen generally helps solve the difficulty, and a bowel training program is one approach that may be employed. If, in extreme cases, fecal impaction occurs, oil retention enema or manual removal can be utilized. A full bowel's pressure on the bladder may contribute to frequency and urgency.

Fecal incontinence is rare but can occur. A bowel training regime can be taught or directed by the nurse; a regularly evacuated bowel will prevent both the physical and social disturbance of an unexpected stool. Should diarrhea be present, other causes must be ruled out.

PROMOTION OF PSYCHOSOCIAL FUNCTION

Facing the uncertainty of a chronic illness with an unpredictable course imposes great stress on the person with multiple sclerosis. Anxiety and depression can be frequent manifestations of this stress, as can frustration, anger, and hopelessness. The behavioral response of the person with multipe sclerosis involves closely interrelated factors, including organic, psychologic, and social involvement. A person's premorbid personality, the site and extent of brain involvement, functional loss from the disease, and the response of others in the social milieu contribute to the pattern of response and adaptation.

Unlike someone who experiences a sudden and defined permanent change in physical and functional ability, the person with multiple sclerosis usually contends with a fluctuating situation; consequently, the psychologic response also may fluctuate. The pathway of adapting to life with chronic disability generally involves transition and acceptance; since there is no "constant" factor around which the person with multiple sclerosis can organize and marshal resources, this pathway is most difficult.

One group of professionals have identified three categories of issues requiring particular adaptive behavior by the multiple sclerosis population (Hartings, Pavlov, Davis, 1976). The first is "ambiguity of health status," mainly reflecting the uncertainty encountered during the diagnostic period. "Marginality" refers to the fine line many persons experience between illness and health. For example, many persons with a minimal degree of visible physical disability are functionally limited in their capacity to meet all the requirements of daily living. The third issue is described as "uncertainty of the future status" and relates to the problem in predicting what the pathway and outcome will be. As these issues reemphasize, even though the disability experienced by any one person may not be severe, the course of multiple sclerosis can constantly produce stress. This is important for the nurse and others to remember since their contact with the person may come at varying times of the person's illness experience. On an individual basis, the nurse should provide an empathic ear and allow for expression of anxieties, frustrations, and fears. Reflective listening may assist the person to marshal and direct the resources for coping.

As in response to any stress, the person adopts any number of coping strategies. One behavior reported to be seen quite frequently early in the disease experience is denial (Weinstein, 1970).

In general, the nurse and other team members support such coping strategies, recognizing the need for a sense of control by the individual. If denial becomes obstructive to necessary care, however, it may become a target for intervention; in such instances, it should be approached with consideration, in consultation with other members of the health team and the family. Denial is a valuable mechanism to the person working toward emotional coping with reality, and in the course of events it can resolve to acceptance. Some persons may, however, never completely give it up. It is important for the nurse to recognize denial when it occurs rather than be caught up in it. Concealing symptoms, refusing assistance, persistently seeking someone to deny the diagnosis may all be indicative of denial (Matson and Brooks, 1977).

Another behavioral manifestation frequently attributed to multiple sclerosis patients is euphoria; in fact, in the past it was described as a cardinal symptom. Generally speaking, euphoria is a term used to describe the elevation of mood and exaggerated sense of well-being and happiness seen in persons with multiple sclerosis, even in the presence of severe disability. Some professionals now doubt that euphoria is prevalent in these patients; they contend that some observers may not be able to fathom the degree of adjustment possible in persons with severe deficits (Matson and Brooks). An awareness that some persons with multiple sclerosis manifest exaggerated emotional behavior is helpful information to the nurse who encounters sudden laughter and/or tears with little or no apparent stimulus. Calm acceptance and understanding are of service to the person, who also may not understand why the behavior occurred. In rehabilitative efforts, changes in behavior may interfere with a person's ability to participate fully in a program of activities; psychologic or psychiatric counseling may be indicated. However small the number, the nurse should be aware that there are some persons with multiple sclerosis who do experience emotional disturbances; psychoses and dementia are reported to appear infrequently, usually in those with severe involvement in later stages.

The disabling effect of multiple sclerosis often places the person in a position of dependency; as a consequence, the individual may need to rely on others for help. This can range from dependency regarding such things as transportation to dependency for total personal care. Such needs can be a source of conflict within the person and within the family and social group. The dependency also may effect changes in roles within the family. Again, since the course of events is unpredictable, the process of change in roles for the person and significant others encompasses a particularly stressful pathway to adaptation.

Strategies to assist the person to maintain as much independence as possible are important nursing interventions. The person is involved in decision making related to care; this is an ongoing consideration throughout the course of any experience with multiple sclerosis. The level of decision making should be considered. For example, if situations are complex and frustrating to the point of interfering with care, incremental decision making can be used; the alternatives for a choice may be presented to the person for a decision, rather than asking the person to identify the alternatives. Similarly a decision can be structured to require a simple yes or no answer. The nurse can facilitate situations in which the patient can experience a sense of autonomy; drawing on the individual's interests and abilities is a useful strategy. The nurse also may be of help to the family as they experience the illness of a loved one. Assisting them to understand that they, too, are experiencing a change can be helpful. They can be assisted to understand that, at times, frustration and anger with the ill person are not abnormal responses. The patient and family can be encouraged to focus on determining and capitalizing on strengths and abilities rather than on limitations.

The nurse may facilitate or participate in group sessions with patients and families or refer to existing groups. The rationale for such groups is that persons who share a similar difficulty find a source of strength in that sharing. Group efforts may take several directions and encompass several purposes at once. They can be educational, with sharing and discussion, or they can be social function–oriented. Professional guidance can direct the group toward a positive working experience rather than serving as a forum for dwelling on symptoms and negative concerns.

The nurse and other health team members may be the targets of the frustration and anger experienced by patients and families, and they need to be aware of and to accept this fact. Indeed, staff may themselves need an outlet for honest sharing of their frustrations. Care must be exercised not to reject patients for their anger, for such rejection contributes to the further experiencing of aloneness or alienation described by these people.

Body Image and Sexuality

Another area of psychosocial concern in the person with multiple sclerosis relates to body image. Persons undergoing such things as changes in walking, changes in talking, and changes in excretory function experience an assault on their body image. As such alterations occur in oneself, perception of relationships with others can change. Indeed, whether one perceives oneself to have changed or not, it may be found that others respond differently when they learn the person has multiple sclerosis; this is a stressful situation for all involved. Persons with multiple sclerosis are no different from anyone else in that they are concerned with their appeal to others as valued persons. Persons with multiple sclerosis have reported feeling the withdrawal of others; this holds true not only in day-to-day living but with health personnel (Davis). The nurse can be a catalyst to prevent this within the health-care setting.

Interacting with the concept of body image is that of sexuality. Although physical sexual performance is a component, this concept includes the total sexual identity, behavior, and tendencies of individuals. Davis' (1973) descriptions illustrate the impact multiple sclerosis had on a patient's ability to function in a familial role, such as mother and/or wife. This concept extends to such things as expectations regarding the maintenance of friendships that were unfulfilled for the person with multiple sclerosis.

Since there can be both motor and sensory neurologic involvement in multiple sclerosis, some difficulties with physical sexual activities may indeed occur. Because the manifestations of the disease are not identical in given persons, however, this may or may not be a problem. Concern about such problems may translate into fear of an inability to function as a sexual partner. Davis interviewed some men who reported feeling guilty for not being able to sustain a sexual relationship with their wives; some women claimed they were abandoned by their husbands shortly after the diagnosis was made, on the grounds of being found not sexually attractive.

Although there has been increasing interest in sexuality and sexual needs of disabled persons, many health-care workers remain uneasy with this topic. In a comprehensive rehabilitation program, one would expect sexuality to be an acknowledged subject of concern, with appropriate resources available to help patients with their problems. However, persons with multiple sclerosis are not necessarily found in such locations. Therefore, the nurse and other team members again should be alert to this legitimate area of concern for the person with multiple sclerosis. If they cannot provide the information or help the person needs, health personnel should make an appropriate referral. Again, there should be careful assessment to determine the specific problems. Sexual difficulty may or may not be attributable to the disease; an underlying problem could be the cause. For example, vaginal yeast infections are not uncommon in females with or without multiple sclerosis, and they can be a source of dyspareunia. The nurse may be the person to whom the patient confides about sexual difficulties; depending on ability and skill in assessment, the nurse can provide information, counsel the patients and significant others, refer to a gynecologist or urologist, and may refer persons to social workers or others to help with their adjustment.

Social Needs

Social interaction and activity may decrease if the person becomes more physically limited; a major objective in intervention is to prevent social isolation. One study demonstrated that social needs increased as disability increased but were less likely to be met as disability increased (Braham et al.). Talking, one means by which people interact socially, can be a problem for the person with multiple sclerosis. The problem of dysarthria is not uncommon in these persons and may be more severe when they are excited or fatigued. A frequent symptom and complaint is known as "scanning" speech, an interruption between syllables and words. Changes in tone of voice and slurring may also occur. All these may cause difficulty in communicating, in person as well as on the phone, and can add to the individual's sense of isolation. An assessment and consultation with a speech pathologist can aid the nurse and the patient in a program to alleviate some of the problems of speaking. Resistive exercise for muscles used in phonation may be of some value. Problems with speech volume and pronunciation appear to be more responsive to a treatment program than do difficulties of rhythm and rate (Block and Kester, 1970). In severe cases, complications with speech, visual, and motor problems present a true challenge to health personnel in communicating with the patient.

As mentioned earlier, some of the social needs of the person with multiple sclerosis may be met through group activity. Bowling groups, fishing groups, travel groups, etc. are available in many locations; if they are not organized in a given community, the nurse can be instrumental in instigating them. Today, persons with disability are freer to travel than formerly, and pamphlets on accommodations are available from the airlines and government. Architectural barriers exist, but inroads are being made in accessibility to those with disabilities. Church groups, "friendly visitors," and other volunteer community organizations may be drawn upon to help meet social needs of persons with multiple sclerosis.

A valuable resource for both the nurse and patient is the National Multiple Sclerosis Society. This organization, with local chapters, supports research, programs for people with multiple sclerosis, and education of the public.

Another resource to assist in meeting social and vocational needs is the vocational rehabilitation program available in all states. In some instances, job retraining may be available to allow the person to function productively; in others, adaptive devices may be provided which assist the person to continue to work.

One problem which exists for multiple sclerosis patients and families, as well as others, is the assortment and fragmentation of resources which may be available; it is difficult to gain information or access to them. One study of persons with multiple sclerosis and their families pointed out that just because one agency is helping a person is no guarantee that this person does not need help from others (Braham et al., 1975). The nurse, in the role of coordinator, can work with the social worker and others to assist the patient and family in gaining access to potential sources of assistance.

CONCLUSION

Multiple sclerosis presents a confounding situation for patients, significant others, professionals, and society. In spite of vast resources in the health-care armamentarium, no one has yet learned how to prevent or cure this disease. Compared to the prevalence of other disease groups, the number of people who suffer from multiple sclerosis may not be large; however, since its primary target is the young adult population and since it is a chronic illness, its effect is great. Persons with multiple sclerosis and their significant others continually cope with the uncertainty of the future. Physically, psychologically, and socially there may be changes, but these are unpredictable in any given situation; this lack of a constant around which to marshal resources is quite stressful. Nursing and other health-care workers must be attuned to a careful assessment of where the multiple sclerosis patient is, both in time and place. One of the areas which presents difficulty for patients and professionals is developing and maintaining a sense of hope, while at the same time confronting reality. Although no magical cures exist, there is hope through research and, in any given person, there is hope that remission will occur and remain.

The nurse may be the only person to see the patient and family in settings that range from an occupational site to a nursing home, from a clinic to a comprehensive rehabilitation center. The nurse, therefore, is in a position to assist, care for, teach, counsel, and refer the person experiencing multiple sclerosis.

The nurse also can participate in and may conduct research related to the person with multiple sclerosis. The element of fatigue in multiple sclerosis patients merits attention, particularly in relation to the value of rest and activity patterns. Spasticity also is a problem that continues to need study. The needs and concerns surrounding pregnancy and childbearing, the interaction of mobility and body image changes, and the adaptive behavior of families are areas for study. The pattern of remission and exacerbation with its implications for teaching and compliance is another fruitful area for investigation.

BIBLIOGRAPHY

Antel, J. P., et al.: "Suppressor Cell Function in Multiple Sclerosis: Correlation with Disease Activity," *Ann Neurol* 5(4):338–342, 1979.

Bates, D., et al.: "Trial of Polyunsaturated Fatty Acids in Non-Relapsing Multiple Sclerosis," *Brit Med J* 2:932, 1977.

Block, J. M., and N. C. Kester: "Role of Rehabilitation in Management of Multiple Sclerosis," *Mod Treat* 7(5):930, 1970.

Braham, Sara, et al.: "Evaluation of the Social Needs of Nonhospitalized Chronically Ill Persons," *J Chronic Dis* 28:401, 1975.

Brown, Joe R., et al.: "The Design of Clinical Studies to Assess Therapeutic Efficacy in Multiple Sclerosis," *Neurology* 29(9)(part 2):1–23, 1979.

Burnfield, Alexander: "Multiple Sclerosis: A Doctor's Personal Experience," *Brit Med J* 1:435–436, 1977.

Check, W. A.: "Marijauna May Lessen Spasticity of M.S.," *JAMA* 241(23), 1979.

Current Research in the Fight Against Multiple Sclerosis, National Multiple Sclerosis Society, New York, 1975.

Davis, Marcella Z: *Living with Multiple Sclerosis: A Social Psychological Analysis,* Charles C Thomas, Springfield, Ill., 1973.

DeJong, Russell: *Enemy of Young Adults,* National Multiple Sclerosis Society, New York, 1977.

———: "Multiple Sclerosis: History, Definition and General Considerations," in PJ Vinken, and GW Bruyn (eds.), *Multiple Sclerosis and Other Demyelinating Diseases, Handbook of Clinical Neurology,* vol. 9, American Elsevier, New York, pp. 45–62, 1970.

Detels, Roger: "Epidemiology of Multiple Sclerosis," *Adv Neurol* 19:459–473, 1978.

Dillon, Ann M.: "Nursing Care of the Patient with Multiple Sclerosis," *Nurs Clin North Am* 8:653, 1973.

Hartings, Michael, Marcia Pavlov, and Floyd Davis: "Group Counseling of M.S. Patients in a Program of Comprehensive Care," *J Chronic Dis* 29:65, 1976.

Herschberg, Gerald, Leon Lewis, and Patricia Vaughn: *Rehabilitation,* 2d ed., Lippincott, Philadelphia, 1976.

Jontz, Donna L.: "Prescription for Living with Multiple Sclerosis," *Am J Nurs* 73:817, 1973.

Kurtzke, J. F.: "Geography in Multiple Sclerosis," *J Neurology* 215:1, 1977.

———: "Further Notes on Disability Evaluation in Multiple Sclerosis," *Neurology* 15:654, 1965.

MacRae, Isabel, and Gloria Henderson: "Sexuality and Irreversible Health Limitations," *Nurs Clin North Am* 10:587, 1975.

Matson, Ronald R., and Nancy A. Brooks: "Adjusting to Multiple Sclerosis: An Exploratory Study," *Soc Sci Med* 11:245, 1977.

Matthews, W. B., et al.: "Effects of Raising Body Temperature on Visual and Somatosensory Evoked Potentials in Patients with Multiple Sclerosis," *J Neurol Neurosurg Psychiatry* 42(3):250–255, 1979.

Maugh, T. H.: "Multiple Sclerosis: Genetic Link Viruses Suspected," *Science* 195:667, 1977.

McAlpine, Douglas, Charles Lumsden, and E. D. Acheson: *Multiple Sclerosis—A Reappraisal,* 2d ed., Williams & Wilkins, Baltimore, 1972.

Mei-Tal, Varda, Sandord Meyerowitz, and George Engel: "The Role of Psychological Process in a Somatic Disorder—Multiple Sclerosis," *Psychosom Med* 32:67, 1970.

Multiple Sclerosis Indicative Abstracts, Federation of the American Societies for Experimental Biology, Bethesda, Md. Bimonthly abstracts.

O'Donnell, Patricia B: "Multiple Sclerosis: Disease Process and Nursing Implications," unpublished seminar paper, University of Maryland, 1976.

Paty, D. W. et al.: "HLA in Multiple Sclerosis: Relationship to Measles Antibody, Nitogen Responsiveness and Clinical Course," *J Neurol Sci* 32:371, 1977.

Paty, Donald W.: "Multiple Sclerosis: Recent Advances in Diagnosis, Clinical Immunology and Virology," *Can Med Assoc J* 117:113, 1977.

Paulley, J. W.: "Psychological Management of Multiple Sclerosis," *Psychother Psychosom* 27:26, 1976/1977.

Plummer, Elizabeth: "The M.S. Patient," *Am J Nurs* 68:2161, 1968.

Pulton, T. W.: "Multiple Sclerosis: A Social-Psychological Perspective," *Phys Ther* 57(2):170–173, 1977.

Rusk, Howard A.: *Rehabilitation Medicine,* 4th ed., Mosby, St. Louis, 1977.

Russell, W. R.: *Multiple Sclerosis: Control of the Disease,* Pergamon Press, Oxford, 1976.

Schumacher, George: "Multiple Sclerosis," reprint by National Multiple Sclerosis Society from H. F. Conn (ed.), *Current Therapy,* Saunders, Philadelphia, 1970.

Smith, Bernard H.: "Multiple Sclerosis and Sexual Dysfunction," *Med Aspects Hum Sexual* 10:103, 1976.

Stryker, Ruth: *Rehabilitative Aspects of Acute and Chronic Nursing Care,* 2d ed., Saunders, Philadelphia, 1977.

Sutherland, J. M.: "Etiology of Multiple Sclerosis," *Med J Aust* 1:237, 1977.

Tourtellotte, W. W.: "Therapeutics of Multiple Sclerosis," in H. L. Klawans, ed., *Clinical Neuropharmacology,* Rowen, New York, 2:179–199, 1977.

Tarabulcy, Edward: "Bladder Disturbances in Multiple Sclerosis and Their Management," *Mod Treat* 7:941, 1970.

Walton, John N.: *Brain's Disease of the Nervous System,* Oxford Univ. Press, Oxford, 1977.

Warocqurer, R. et al.: "Lymphocytes in Multiple Sclerosis," *Lancet* 958, 1977.

Weinstein, Edwin A.: "Behavioral Aspects of Multiple Sclerosis," *Mod Treat* 7:961, 1970.

Witte, Pamela G., and Lynn Baker: "Group Therapy with Multiple Sclerosis Couples," *Health Soc Work* 2:188, 1977.

23

dorothy l. gordon
margaret m. stevens

spinal cord injury: acute phase

INTRODUCTION

The description of a person paralyzed from spinal cord injury, found in the Edwin Smith Surgical Papyrus and written about 5000 years ago by an Egyptian physician, reflects the general attitude which prevailed regarding the prognosis for such individuals until the twentieth century:

> Thou shouldst'say concerning him; One having a dislocation in the vertebra of his neck while he is unconscious of his two legs, and his two arms, and he dribbles. An ailment not to be treated

During World War I, the life expectancy of people with spinal cord trauma was 6 to 12 months after injury. Although advances were made in medicine and surgery, it was not until World War II that hope was offered the individual for an extended life. Usually, however, this meant institutionalization and custodial care. Today, *given appropriate treatment in specialized centers,* life expectancy is not significantly shortened (National Spinal Cord Injury Model Systems Conference, 1978).

Although there were some early pioneers in a multidisciplinary approach to management of the spinal cord injured, the specialized care which requires expertise in both personnel and technology left it an area where generalized progress was slow. Today, however, advances are being made. The concept of a total treatment program focused on one specific diagnostic group may have done more to advance the prognosis for the cord-injured than any other factor. This concept, coupled with advances in surgery and rehabilitation, has offered the opportunity for many persons to live productive and meaningful lives. Essential to its success is the recognition that informed, coordinated, and expert care is required from the time of spinal cord injury through the individual's return to the community. The acute care portion of that process is the subject of this chapter.

INCIDENCE IN SOCIETY

It is estimated that there are 120,000 to 150,000 cord-injured persons in the United States, and each year 10,000 more persons are added. The majority of injuries are caused by vehicular incidents of some kind; penetrating wounds, sports, and falls also contribute a sizable number. Recent figures indicate that about 50 percent of the cord injuries are quadriplegic and 50 percent paraplegic (National Spinal Cord Injury Model Systems Conference). Although injuries are the major concern of this chapter, it should be remembered that persons may become paraplegic or quadriplegic from other conditions or diseases.

The spinal cord–injured population is in general young adult (average age 28 years) and male, reflecting the activities involved in the major causes. Females are represented in lesser numbers. The impact of this devastating injury on society is realized, therefore, not only in the severity of the physical loss to the individual but also in productivity, disrupted family lives, and health-care cost. As indicated earlier, the outcome for these people was considered hopeless previously, and the health-care philosophy was custodial; current management philosophy is rehabilitative in nature, offering improved physical and psychosocial benefits for the individual and economic benefits for society. Although it is difficult to compute the expense of such injuries, there is a growing body of data to demonstrate that the cost for persons treated and rehabilitated in a coordinated system is considerably less than for others. Accompanying the trend of improved prognosis and return to society is the growing visibility of persons with spinal cord injury. The nonhandicapped individual finds contact with a paraplegic or quadriplegic person a not uncommon occurrence; this is a great change from the time when the disabled were kept at home or institutionalized, in essence "out of sight, out of mind" to society. Testimony to this increasing visibility of all handicapped persons is seen in such phenomena as the removal of architectural barriers and the growing activism among the disabled.

SYSTEMS OF CARE

A major impetus to improved management of the spinal cord injured in this country has been the federal and professional commitment.

The National Institute of Neurological Disease and Stroke has supported major research and demonstration projects in neurologic injury. The Veterans Administration has spinal cord centers for such injuries acquired in connection with the services.

Eleven centers have been supported across the country since the early 1970s by the Rehabilitation Services Administration; three more were added in 1978. Training of ambulance technicians and hospital emergency room personnel in proper early immobilization and management of cord injury is a large part of the system. Protocols for care during both acute and rehabilitative phases are developed and implemented by multidisciplinary teams. Health maintenance and lifelong follow-up are considered essential ingredients to the programs, and a coordinated effort between hospitals, rehabilitation centers, emergency systems, and public health is required. The data accumulated from these systems, in turn, permit evaluation of the care and of impact on society. A commitment to this total care concept holds promise for continuing advances in patient management, health-care cost savings, and stimulation of research.

Regardless of the setting, a key professional in the continuum of care necessary for the spinal cord injured is the nurse. Nurses view patients from a holistic perspective, are taught to communicate effectively, and have coordinating abilities essential to the care of these people. They possess a knowledge base which is necessary for intelligent nursing care of these individuals. Such care is goal oriented and includes close collaboration with the plethora of health team members involved in complex management of the spinal cord injured. In the acute phase of care for the cord-injured, efforts are directed to saving life, stabilizing the patient's condition, and preventing further neurologic deficit. A transition period then occurs when medical and surgical refinements may be necessary preparatory to the person's participation in an active rehabilitation program. Throughout this early care, there is need for coordination and setting of priorities for efforts by the team so that maximum benefit may be available to the patient. Recovery from such an injury and preparation for an altered life-style consume vast quantities of energy on the patient's part; incoordination and discontinuity in the care system should not make additional demands on that energy store, and the nurse plays a key role in seeing this does not occur.

PHILOSOPHY OF CARE

The devastating effects that a spinal cord injury may have are readily apparent to the members of the health team; consequently, an element of personal threat may be involved when professionals are faced with their own human vulnerability. This needs to be acknowledged. Not to be forgotten are issues regarding quality of life and human worth. One outcome of improved early management of the cord-injured is that more persons with high level, cervical injuries are surviving, resulting in a growing number of quadriplegic persons in society. Since a person's attitudes and feelings influence the ability to deliver needed care, the nurse's personal response to such situations needs attention. The examination and development of a philosophy of care regarding the severely injured who will survive with permanent disabilities provides the health professional with the foundation necessary to make services available to the patient. Such inspection of values has particular application in the acute care of the person with high spinal cord injury, since personnel are well aware of what the residual impairment may be. Closely akin to this is "survivor's guilt," a reflection of the resentment the patient may have toward anyone not disabled. This can be more threatening to the health worker close in age and circumstances to the disabled person (Weller and Miller, 1977b). Another consideration is the health-care team's attitude toward the patient's response to injury. Cord transection is awesome to the affected person, regardless of the level at which it occurs. People respond to their trauma as individuals and do not necessarily follow a set pattern of behavior. The literature written by persons who have experienced cord injury often includes advice to professionals not to expect a single "acceptable" or "appropriate" response by all persons with disability.

SPINAL CORD INJURY AND ITS EFFECTS

ANATOMY REVIEWED

The central nervous system comprises the brain and spinal cord. The spinal cord is encased and protected within the bony vertebral column consisting of seven cervical, twelve thoracic, five lumbar, five sacral, and four fused coccygeal vertebra. Fibrocartilaginous disks lie between the vertebrae, and the bony spinal column is supported by ligaments and muscles.

The spinal cord does not run the full length of the vertebral column. It extends from the base of the skull at the foramen magnum to the lower edge of the first lumbar vertebra. Due to differing growth rates cord segments and vertebral segments are not together (Fig. 23-1).

The spinal cord consists of a central canal and an H-shaped mass of grey matter surrounded by white matter. Encasing it (moving outward) are the pia mater, cerebrospinal fluid, arachnoid mater, dura mater, a cushion of epidural fat, and vertebrae. Sensory fibers in the posterior portion of the cord ascend to the brain; motor impulses descend from the brain in the anterior portion of the cord.

Spinal nerves originate in the cord and emerge through the vertebral foramina; each has an anterior and posterior "root." These spinal nerves and the cranial nerves (plus the parts of them composing the autonomic nervous system) comprise the peripheral nervous system (Fig. 23-1). This system has both sensory (dorsal) and motor (ventral) fibers and connects the periphery and organs of the body to the spinal cord and brain.

TYPES OF INJURY

Considering the anatomy involved, it can be seen that injury to the spine may affect several types of structures, including vertebrae (bone), muscles and ligaments, the spinal cord, and nerve roots (neurological tissue).

Bone Injury It is possible for a person to have fractures of the bony spine without incurring neurological damage to the spinal cord itself. These people are observed and managed carefully to prevent further damage since they would be predisposed to cord injury if the fracture were to become dislocated or unstable. Vertebral injury can be grouped into three categories: subluxation, compression, and fracture dislocation. These result from directional forces on the bony column that occur at the time of injury. Flexion, extension, and rotation, as well as axial forces, can be exerted in an accident. The circumstances surrounding the incident in which the trauma occurred often help the physician determine the type of injury present and provide direction for appropriate medical and surgical management.

Neural Damage Damage to the spinal cord has dire consequences, for destroyed central nervous system tissue does not regenerate; the result can be permanent loss of motor and sensory functions below the level of injury or illness. The types of spinal cord damage which can accompany vertebral injury include concussion, contusion, laceration, compression, or hemorrhage into the substance of the cord. Spinal roots also may be damaged or destroyed. Neurologic deficit depends on the extent of damage to the spinal cord and the level at which it occurred. Complete disruption of the cord results in loss of all motor and sensory function below the site of injury; this is usually due to a "physiologic transection" and rarely to actual severance. If part of the cord is disrupted, the neurological deficit relates to the cord substance destroyed and is detected by neurological examination. Since the bony vertebral column and spinal cord levels do not totally correspond, it is important for physicians and others to specify whether the level of injury is being expressed as vertebral or cord.

SPINAL SHOCK

Two functional disorders occur when the spinal cord is *completely* disrupted. All *voluntary* motion below the level of injury is lost and all sensation from those parts is abolished. Spinal shock (spinal areflexia) also occurs. This is a transient condition in which there is decreased synaptic excitability of the neurons below the level of damage; the clinical manifestation is the absence of somatic reflex activity and a flaccid paralysis. Since the autonomic nervous system is involved, particularly in higher lesions, hypotension, bladder paralysis, and interference with defecation may occur. Spinal shock may last hours to weeks, and persons with incomplete lesions have a return of reflexes in a shorter period of time than those with complete lesions.

Recovery from spinal shock begins with the return of any reflex activity which previously was absent and which returns progressively over a period of time. A flexor activity pattern usually occurs first, when stimulation elicits twitching toes or a flexor withdrawal of foot, ankle, knee, and hip; in some instances, a mass flexor response takes place. Over a longer period of time, extensor activity becomes strong although flexor patterns usually are dominant. Along with the return of somatic reflex activity, a reflex bladder may appear. Sensations such as burning in the buttocks and lower abdomen may also accompany the recovery from spinal shock (Mountcastle, 1974).

Permanent Disruption of Function

Most patients who have spinal cord injury will display the minimal signs of damage immediately. There is continuing research into the etiology of *permanent* paralysis. Although ischemia results in cellular anoxia, the exact mechanism causing the neural tissue to be permanently destroyed is unclear (Yeo, 1976; Ruge, 1977a). Whether or not any given individual will show increasing neurologic deficit or improvement is unknown at the time of injury. It is perplexing that in the early stages after injury, it is difficult to distinguish those who will recover from those who will not. As Ruge states, "The unparalyzed may become paralyzed and the paralyzed may

Figure 23-1
Illustration of vertebral column, spinal cord segment, and schematic view of the spinal cord. (A) The vertebral column with the surface of the spinal cord exposed. Samples of CSF are usually taken in the lumbar region, where the meninges extend below the cord. (B) A spinal cord segment. (C) Schematic view of the spinal cord. Note that beginning in the thoracic region spinal nerves emerge from the vertebral column at points progressively lower than their origin. The spinal nerves below the spinal cord are collectively termed cauda equina. (From L. L. Langley et al., Dynamic Anatomy and Physiology, 4th ed., McGraw-Hill, New York, 1974. Used with permission.)

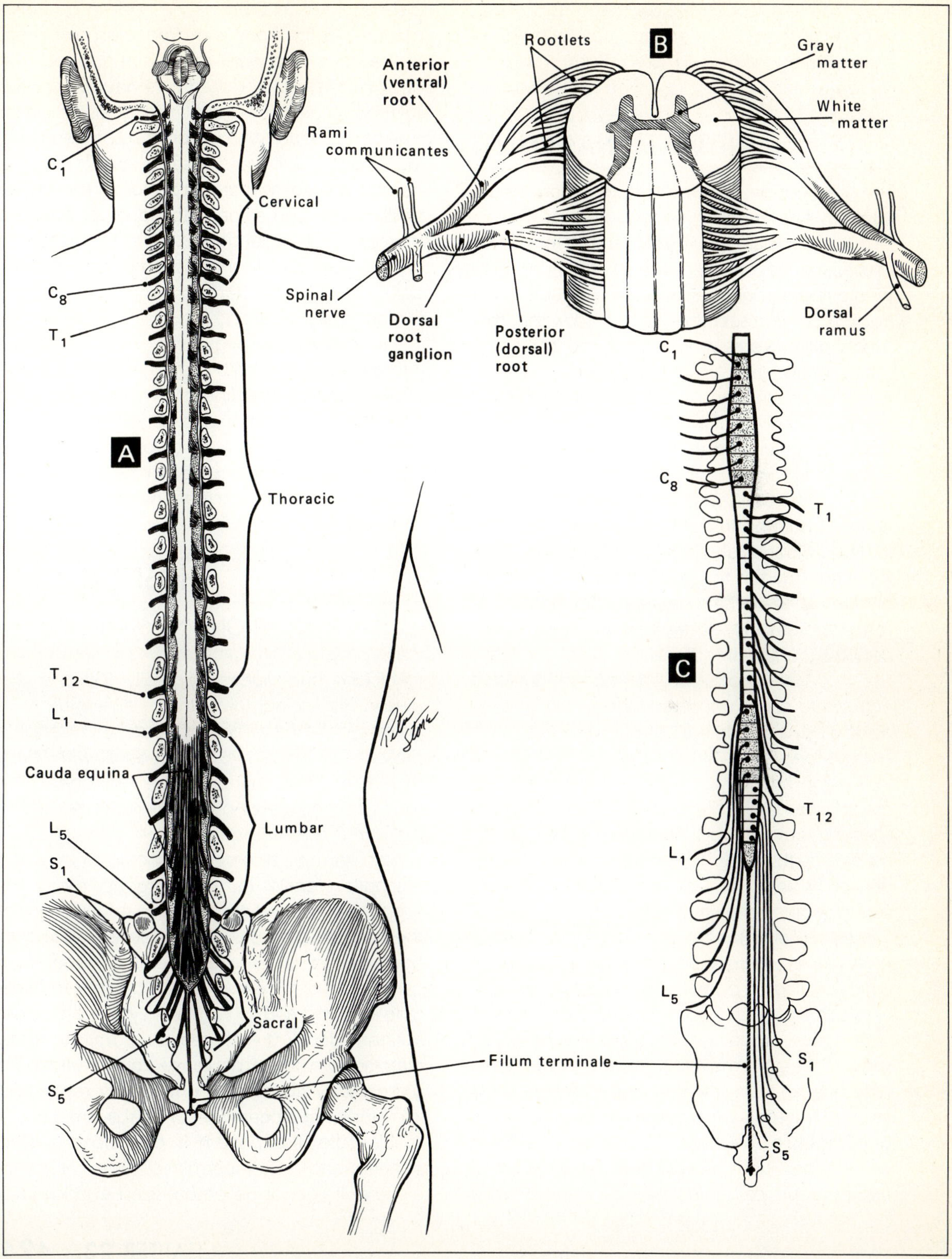

A
B
C
C1
Cervical
C8
T1
Thoracic
T12
L1
Cauda equina
Lumbar
L5
S1
Sacral
S5
Filum terminale
Rootlets
Gray matter
White matter
Anterior (ventral) root
Rami communicantes
Spinal nerve
Dorsal root ganglion
Posterior (dorsal) root
Dorsal ramus

improve even though experience of many supports that there is little hope for recovery in complete lesions one day old" (Ruge, 1977a).

INITIAL MANAGEMENT

The scene of an accident sets the stage for the initial assessment and management of the suspected spinal cord–injured victim. The fate of the injured patient often rests with the individual who arrives first on the scene. An unstable bone fracture can transect the spinal cord within moments after a person is moved improperly, resulting in quadriplegia or paraplegia.

Common sense and a few basic principles can guide the individual who assists at an accident where a spinal cord injury may have occurred. A spinal injury is suspected when a person is found in an unusual body position that under normal anatomic integrity would be impossible. If the individual is alert, one should ask questions regarding pain in the neck or back, numbness or tingling in the extremities, and inability to move or feel the extremities. An unconscious person should be treated as if a spinal injury has occurred, for a force on the head significant enough to cause unconsciousness may also be associated with additional trauma in the vertebrae of the neck.

The individuals generally most qualified to properly remove people from an accident are specially trained paramedics and emergency medical technicians. The majority of nurses and physicians have not received instruction in extricating people from wreckage or swimming pools without causing further damage. Unfortunately professional medical people sometimes find it difficult to admit a lack of knowledge or experience in this area.

A person suspected of having spine injury should not be removed from wreckage when only one rescuer is present unless the person's life is threatened by explosion, drowning, etc. If at all possible, the rescuer should wait for assistance. When help arrives, one should place a firm hard surface behind the victim's back while a second person supports the neck in a neutral position. As the body is moved, all major areas of the head and trunk must be supported. The neck must be maintained in a neutral position by the placement of two firm objects on either side of the head, such as sandbags, rolled clothing, or any readily accessible objects. Taping the head to the board also is acceptable. Immobility of the neck and spine is the goal. Specialized stretchers and spinal boards are often carried on ambulances and should be employed if available. (See Folsom, 1975, or similar publications for further elaboration.)

The receiving hospital facility will be aided by information gathered by personnel at the scene of the accident. Baseline information about the patient's initial motor and sensation levels as well as his or her level of awareness will assist the hospital personnel to determine whether the patient has improved or deteriorated since injury.

HOSPITAL CARE

RESUSCITATION AND STABILIZATION

Physicians and nurses generally first see the person with spinal injury in the emergency department. Whether or not neurologic deficit is present at admission, all persons with back injuries should continue to be managed as if they had fracture or dislocation until danger to the spinal cord is ruled out.

If an immobilizing device is not in place when the patient arrives in the emergency room, it is employed immediately. Initial stabilization of the cervical spine is usually achieved with sandbags placed at either side of the head, or a cervical collar. Several types of collars are available and the choice is made by the physician. Patients ideally are placed on a Stryker frame directly from the ambulance cart to eliminate unnecessary transfers to emergency room and x-ray tables. If placed directly on the emergency room table, the patient is put into a supine position and is not permitted to roll, turn, or elevate. It cannot be emphasized enough that these people should not be moved indiscriminately. For example, they *never* should be set up, twisted, and pulled to remove clothing, to have x-rays, or to be transferred. The emergency room staff needs to be aware of proper handling procedures themselves and to see to it that other departments involved during the admission process are well informed.

To transfer a patient with a back injury, principles of immobilization and alignment must be followed. The patient's body must be moved as a log, and such a maneuver may require four to six people so the spine is well supported.

It should be kept in mind that the patient may experience pain at the site of injury. Explanation prior to every step must also be given to help alleviate anxiety.

Although physiologic stability is of major concern during resuscitation, nurses and others should be attentive to the patient's emotional and psychological state. Patients have reported that they are not always clear what has happened to them and the period of admission has been found to be very stressful (McDaniel and Sexton, 1970). During initial management, the staff may be preoccupied with necessary tasks in resuscitating the patient, but they should not forget to give reassurance that everything possible is being taken care of and should provide explanations of what is taking place.

Emergency room resuscitation measures are directed at stabilizing the patient's physiologic status to permit definitive neurologic treatment. Vital signs are monitored frequently. Hypotension is not uncommon in the spinal cord injured, but the physician must determine whether or not the etiology is due to hypovolemia or spinal (neurogenic) shock. The latter usually results from loss of sympathetic vasomotor control, and bradycardia is one manifestation. Since these patients frequently have multiple injuries, differentiating between the two types of shock may be difficult. This poses a problem in management, and philosophies between physicians vary. One guideline used is to treat the low blood pressure if urinary output is below a specific number of milliliters per hour. The goal of treatment is to prevent spinal cord ischemia and possible extension of the neurological deficit. Based on physiological observations, either fluid replacement, plasma expansion, or vasopressor drugs may be prescribed by the physician to treat the hypotension.

Careful assessment of respiratory efficiency is performed to determine whether or not ventilatory support is needed. Arterial blood gases, vital capacity, and tidal volume are obtained. A person with a cord injury level at C4 and above can be expected to experience a compromised ability to maintain respiration. When necessary, therefore, oxygen, intubation, and ventilatory support may be initiated.

Depending on the extent of injury, the presence of other injuries, and the patient's condition, central venous pressure and arterial lines may be inserted during the resuscitation period for close monitoring of the patient's cardiorespiratory status.

Complete blood count, serum electrolytes, and urinalysis are obtained. An indwelling catheter generally is inserted during the initial management phase to closely monitor the output, composition, and specific gravity of urine. For the cervical-injured person with diaphragmatic breathing, the reduction of gastric dilatation is important. A nasogastric tube may be utilized to reduce potential for vomiting and aspiration. Care must be exercised during insertion of the nasogastric tube to prevent neck movements; this requires expertise of medical personnel and is generally attempted while the patient is awake and can cooperate by swallowing (Yashon, 1978).

When neurologic deficit is present, corticosteroid treatment is currently given in many centers since it is believed to decrease cellular edema from injury (National Spinal Cord Injury Model Systems Conference; Ruge, 1977a). Generally, the initial dose is given by "push" and a decreasing amount is administered every 6 h until discontinued. Mannitol also may be prescribed to decrease an edema secondary to the trauma.

During the early assessment of the patient's status, an abbreviated neurologic examination

Table 23-1

Neurologic Level and Key Muscle Function for an Abbreviated Neurologic Examination

NEUROLOGIC LEVEL	MUSCLE FUNCTION
C4	Diaphragmatic movement
C5	Lift elbows to shoulder height
C6	Flex elbow
C7	Extend elbow
	Extend wrist
C8/T1	Hand grip
L3	Lift leg or flex hip
L4, L5	Extend knee
L5	Plantar flexion of boot
S1	Dorsiflex foot

of the functional status of key groups of muscles can be checked. By systematically observing the patient's ability to perform certain functions, an estimate of the level of injury can be determined.

As can be seen, Table 23-1 indicates key movements that can be used in a *gross* assessment of the level of spinal cord lesion. The *absence* of the ability to perform these would lead one to suspect the level of damage was at the neurological level indicated. A bilateral assessment is needed, for the lesion may or may not be complete.

As soon as possible, a complete neurological examination is completed. The importance of a careful neurological examination during early acute care of the spinal cord injured cannot be overemphasized. It provides information locating the level of injury, the extent of cord injury (complete or incomplete), and the part of the cord most affected (anterior, posterior, central). Periodic neurological examinations can help determine whether there is increasing cord damage and will guide decisions for medical action.

It is important to reiterate that during early care of the person with quadriplegia, the function at C3 to C5 level is critical. It is here that the phrenic nerve arises and serves the diaphragm, the major muscle of respiration. Close observation of respiratory integrity of any person with quadriplegia is imperative, for an ascending injury level may result in respiratory incapacity and death; this is extremely important in the first 72 h after injury. Recognition of respiratory changes permits time for ventilatory support to be instigated.

One of the key prognosticators looked for by physicians in the neurological examination is the presence of perianal sensation (sacral sparing) and *voluntary* anal sphincter control. The presence of both gives favorable evidence for recovery of both motor and sensory functions. Absence of the perianal sensation is a serious sign that the damage may be irreversible; *reflex* anal contraction is considered evidence of a complete cord lesion (Meyer et al., 1975).

X-rays of the spine are taken to determine the presence and extent of bony injury. If the person must be sent to the x-ray department for this purpose, it is imperative that someone be present to assure that improper movement of the patient does not occur.

Lesions of the spinal cord may be complete or incomplete, progressive or stable, and the nerve roots may or may not be damaged. Because of the various forces that can occur in an injury, different neurological syndromes may be revealed upon examination. The reader is referred to a neurosurgical or neurological text for discussion of some of the classic syndromes which may occur, such as anterior cord syndrome, central cord syndrome, Brown-Séquard's syndrome and others. A review of Fig. 23-1, especially the cross section of the spinal cord, will elucidate the possiblity for the numerous findings on neurologic examination.

DEFINITIVE TREATMENT

When initial steps to immobilize the patient have taken place, and other resuscitative measures are under control, definitive management of the spinal injury itself remains. Principles underlying this are alignment of the spine, stabilization of the bony spine, and decompression (relief of compression) of the neurologic structures. Current management philosophy is that a person with spinal cord injury should be mobilized into the active rehabilitative process as soon as possible and this is reflected in the methods selected to achieve that goal (Pierce, Nickel, 1977). The trend today is for teams of neurosurgeons and orthopedic surgeons, with consultation from a physiatrist, to determine the optimum definitive treatment for the individual.

Regardless of the level of injury, closed or external alignment is generally attempted. For cervical injuries, this most often entails various types of skull tongs and traction to align the vertebral column and relieve pressure on neural tissue. The amount of traction is prescribed by the physician and generally is related to the level of injury. A halo device is one of the popular types of cervical traction now employed. It can be applied in the emergency room, affords stability of the cervical spine, and permits transfer of the patient for x-rays, myelogram, and surgery if necessary. Traction weights can also be applied. The device is a circular hoop which is secured to the skull by steel pins; in turn, it is attached to vertical rods rising from a vest or molded chest jacket on the patient. For thoracic or lumbar fractures, the patient may be placed on a frame where padding can be used to either flex or extend the spine as necessary. In some instances, positioning with rolls and pillows in a hospital bed may be employed (Pierce and Nickel).

There are different opinions regarding the use of myelography and surgery in early management of the person with a spine injury. Since myelograms are not without risk to the patient, their use depends on the physician's judgment of how valuable the information elicited will be in determining further treatment.

There was a time when laminectomies were performed on most persons with spinal injuries. However, many surgeons now think that immediate surgery is indicated only when there is neurologic deterioration that has not been halted with conservative means (Ruge, 1977a; Pierce and Nickel). Once it is determined that spinal surgery is indicated, the surgical approach must be determined. The surgeon may use an anterior approach if there is evidence of anterior bony pressure on the cord. If the symptoms indicate posterior pressures, then a posterior approach (or laminectomy) may be performed. Surgery for stabilization of the spine is generally desired at the same time the decompression procedures take place. Stabilization surgery provides a stable spine, protecting the spinal cord from further damage due to movement, and permits the patient to begin activities earlier. Harrington rods or spinal fusion are two methods used. When neurological changes are not urgent, orthopedic stabilization procedures are delayed until the patient's condition changes.

Following surgery, patients may remain in stabilizing traction, halo devices, or casts until bony healing has occurred. Their care generally continues on a Stryker wedge frame or on other types of special beds. In some instances where lower level injuries are involved, the patient may be placed in a regular bed with special positioning and handling prescribed (Pierce and Nickel). The general guideline for transferring the patient to a standard bed and beginning out-of-bed activities of daily living is the physician's determination that the spine is stable.

It should be remembered that persons with spinal damage often have other injuries that require early surgery. Therefore, the spectrum of care for the spinal injured person in the *acute stage* may range from a few days for those with no neurological damage and stable spines to several months for those with extensive neurological damage and accompanying injury.

Research Although surgical and stabilization methods have been improved, the ability to actually prevent permanent paralysis and sensory loss eludes the medical community. Since it is not known whether the ischemic deterioration of the cord is due to specific chemical, vascular, or other processes, interventions remain nonspecific. There is some work taking place experimentally in humans in which, it is hoped, cooling of the damaged cord within 8 h after injury may result in recovery of function. Although this effort appears somewhat successful in animals, the medicolegal aspects involved in experimentation have slowed study in humans. Hyperbaric oxygen has been used experimentally with animals, and some success has been demonstrated (Tator). Investigation on patients is just beginning (Bedbrook, 1978).

Rehabilitation Although a stable spine and a stable medical condition signal a person's ability to participate in an active rehabilitation program, appropriate handling and management of the person with an acute spinal cord lesion are part of that process. Prevention of neurological deterioration and other complications, as well as maintenance of the integrity of functioning systems, comprises a major component of the rehabilitation process during this phase. Not only is spinal cord injury a physical devastation, it imposes trauma on the psychologic system of the individual and significant others. Assisting the patient and family to cope with the changes dramatically imposed on their lives is a critical component of the care ministered during the acute-care period; when the time comes for an active encompassing rehabilitation program, psychological as well as physical stamina is required. Collaborative teamwork among those caring for the person acutely ill with a spinal cord injury also facilitates the overall progress to an active rehabilitation program. Early consultation from physical and occupational therapists, social workers, and physiatrists helps in efforts to capitalize on all aspects of care that eventually help the patient reach a productive and meaningful life.

NURSING GOALS AND MANAGEMENT

An acutely injured patient with spinal cord trauma presents a tremendous challenge to nursing. Every body system is ultimately affected by cord transection, especially when the injury occurs in the cervical spine area. Additional body trauma may be present, complicating the patient's condition. The nurse must be able to identify current patient problems as well as anticipate future ones. An individualized definitive plan of care is a necessity for each patient. Plans of care constantly require updating based on continuous nursing assessment. Throughout the acute stage, the underlying theme of care is maintaining body function at an optimum level to facilitate the rehabilitative course. Essentially, the rehabilitation process begins hand in hand with acute management.

The type and location of injury play a major role in determining the quantity and type of nursing care the patient needs. The quadriplegic person is potentially more dependent than the paraplegic person since there is greater loss of function with the greater injury. Nursing intervention is goal directed and coordinated with patient, family, and other nursing services.

GOAL: INTENSIVE MONITORING OF PHYSIOLOGICAL AND PSYCHOLOGICAL STATUS

Almost all body systems are dramatically affected by spinal injury, and during the acute-care stage these parameters must be carefully monitored. Early assessment of pertinent body response will serve as a baseline for comparison. The frequency of recurrent assessment depends upon the patient's condition and the system being evaluated. A predetermined assessment protocol guides the nurse and ensures that critical information is obtained. As the assessment is performed, an important point occurs when the nurse is able to analyze and synthesize the independent observations into a holistic view of the patient's overall condition.

The nursing neurologic examination should be done every hour. As the patient's condition stabilizes, it may be done less frequently; timing usually is determined by the physician. The components of this assessment include level of consciousness, sensation, motor function (quality, type of movement, and strength), pupillary signs, and reflexes. The patient is approached in a calm, reassuring manner. The nurse must observe signs of the patient's comprehension of the spoken word. A functional response may be exhibited if the patient looks to the examiner on stimulation or attempts to complete a command. If the patient is able to talk, the nurse decides whether the conversation seems appropriate to the environment and the patient's orientation to time and place. A concomitant head injury may affect the sensorium more directly, resulting in a sleepy or comatose state. Continuous observation is important for identifying trends in the level of the sensorium.

Motor movement is assessed by type and quality as well as strength. The patient is observed for spontaneous movement; this can be a reflex spastic muscle jerk or an intended purposeful act. Specific motions which the patient has intact are noted. For example, motion such as flexing or extending the elbow will give the nurse a good basis for assessing the level of injury (see Table 23-1).

Sensation can be assessed through the use of a dull-sharp object, namely a safety pin. The nurse begins the examination by starting with the toes and asking the patient to say when the pin is felt as it progresses toward the head. Care must be taken to avoid injuring the patient by breaking the first barrier of defense—the skin. The nurse may be given incorrect information by patients who want to feel and please. For instance, patients may state that they can feel the pin on the leg, but later during bathing, they cannot identify the touch. It also must be remembered that lesions of the cord can be incomplete and a patient may, indeed, have varying levels of muscle function and sensation. Marked changes in movement or sensation, particularly those indicative of a rising level of involvement, should be grounds for immediate notification of the physician.

Patients with complete transections experience loss of afferent stimulation below the site. During early stages the line between sensation and nonsensation is clear; however, this demarcation may become less distinct as compensatory overlap from other spinal segments occurs (Guttman, 1976). Phantom sensation may occur in the early periods but tends to resolve over time. Pain at the site of injury also may be present for a period of time.

Since it is not uncommon for spinal injuries to accompany head injury, an examination of the head and pupils is important. Particles of glass and dirt may be embedded in the scalp, or small areas of scalp laceration may be easily missed. The nurse may discover these when turning the patient. Bruising behind the ear can be indicative of basilar skull fracture.

Pupils should also be assessed to determine if light reaction is present and if the dilation or constriction of the irises is equal. Spontaneous patient blink can be observed when normal saline or artificial tears are dropped in the eye. In the unconscious patient, the presence of the blink indicates brainstem functioning. Corneal reflex is elicited by gently stroking cotton across the cornea and observing any closing of the lid. Corneal checks should be done only on deeply unconscious patients and, infrequently, to prevent corneal abrasion.

Respiratory assessment of a patient includes noting the presence and rate of respiration, breath sounds, ability to cough and mobilize secretions, and the color of skin. The depth and character of chest movement in the cord-injured is highly important. Persons with thoracic and cervical-level injury may have affected intercostal muscles; as noted before, cervical injury at C5 poses grave problems since the phrenic nerve is affected. Laboratory data such as arterial blood gases also provide information for assessment of the respiratory system.

The rate and rhythm of the pulse, blood pressure, presence of major body pulses, and presence or absence of edema contribute to evaluation of the cardiovascular status. In intensive care units, central venous and pulmonary artery pressure measurements provide tools for determining the cardiovascular stability. Regular blood pressure readings also are taken. Sinus bradycardia and low systolic blood pressure are frequent findings in the early stages of spinal cord injury due to the impact on the sympathetic nervous system. Because of the autonomic system response and general system instability,

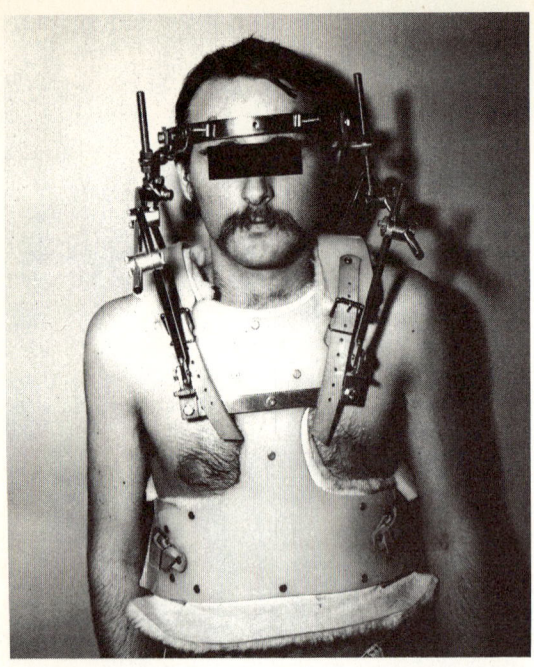

Figure 23-2
(*a*) Front view of halo traction with vest. Note fleece lining. (*b*) Side view of halo. (*c*) Posterior view of halo traction with vest. The halo ring can be utilized with weights to apply cervical traction during early management; later, the vertical stances are connected to a vest apparatus as shown.

particular attention must be given to signs of pulmonary edema and congestive heart failure when fluid replacement takes place. One should be aware that a major complication for these patients is venous thrombosis with possible embolus. Some centers place patients on heparin prophylactically (Casas et al., 1978).

Closely related to the cardiovascular system is renal functioning. Hourly urinary output checks generally are necessary to validate adequate perfusion of the kidneys during early stages of acute injury; such frequent output checks require the use of an indwelling catheter. Specific gravity, presence of sugar, ketones, and microscopic blood are additional aids in urinary assessment and should be done minimally every 8 h. Color, odor, and presence of sediment also are noted.

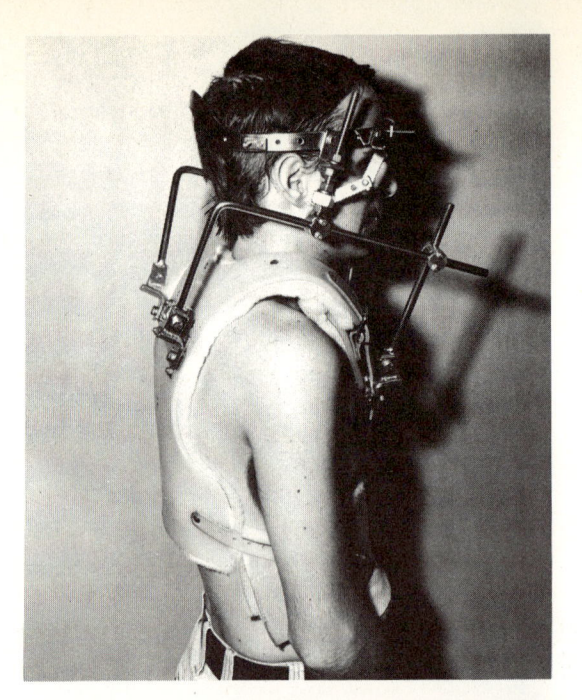

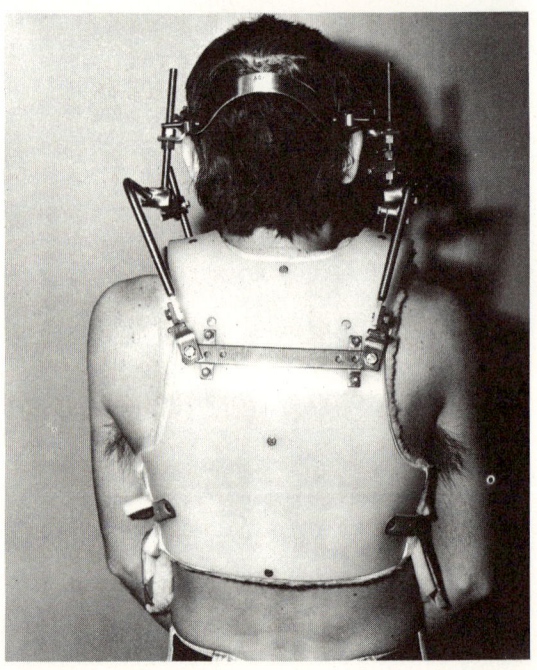

The current management preference for the cord-injured is to remove the indwelling catheters as soon as feasible and to institute intermittent catheterization (Pierce and Nickel; Guttman).

A major complication that may occur in the spinal cord–injured person is acute gastric ulceration and bleeding which may occur in the first week post injury and thereafter (Kewalramani, 1979). Monitoring of hematocrit, blood pressure, pulse as well as contents of emesis, gastric drainage and stool can serve to alert staff to changes indicative of gastrointestinal bleeding.

The laboratory data are an important adjunct to therapy for assessing the metabolic functioning of the spinal cord–injured patient, as well as others. Low values of hemoglobin and hematocrit indicate sufficient red cells for the transport of oxygen; potassium imbalance can result in arrhythmias; and dangerously low sodium levels can lead to unconsciousness. Leukocyte count helps assess the clinical picture of infection. It is important that the nurse be familiar with normal values and promptly report significant changes. Correlation of the clinical signs of the patient with laboratory trends should be done.

One enemy of the spinal cord patient is the pressure sore, and this remains true from time of injury thoughout life. The integrity of the skin must be assessed at each turning of the spinal cord–injured person. Bony prominences are especially prone to breakdown. Reddened areas should be made known to each person caring for the patient and addressed in the patient's care plan. Sites which do not return to normal color within 2 h of pressure relief are of major concern. An additional source of skin breakdown in the acutely ill patient is the area of invasive line insertion; with the administration of steroids, wound healing in cut-down sites often is poor.

The psychological assessment capitalizes on the nurse's awareness of response to crisis. With a basic understanding of the responses which may occur, the nurse can anticipate and effectively intervene. Since the acutely injured person may have a tracheostomy, the ability to verbally communicate distress is eliminated. Similarly, clues such as facial expressions may not be readily observed when the person is in a prone position or on a Stryker frame. Consequently, the nurse must intelligently use assessment skills.

Often, nurses tend to disregard infection as a variable requiring assessment. Invasive line sites, tracheostomy sites, open wounds, and incisions in the traumatized patient must be checked routinely for signs of redness, pus, odor, or any unusual appearance or drainage. Urine and tracheal secretions should be cultured routinely, and elevated temperatures should be reported immediately. Infection is a major enemy to the spinal cord–injured person and is never taken lightly.

The patient with cervical cord injury has a defective heat retention-release mechanism due to loss of sympathetic controls. They generally manifest ambient temperature. In attending these patients with lack of sensation, external applications of heat and cold must be used with meticulous caution to prevent injury. Whenever possible, sponging with tepid water is preferred to hypothermia blankets to reduce temperature. Blankets should be used in place of hot water bottles.

GOAL: TO PREVENT NEUROLOGICAL DEFICIT

Immobilization and stabilization of the spine are vitally important in the early management of the cord-injured. In the emergency room, immobilization is carried out in conjunction with activities related to restoration of circulation and support of the airway. The type of treatment is related to the level of injury.

Cervical Injury

The cervical spine is most easily treated with traction applied to the skull; this pulls neck vertebrae into alignment. As noted earlier, tongs are the most familiar form of cervical traction. There are several different types but the principle is to immobolize and align the spine. The halo traction is popular now because a patient in a halo ring can be connected to cervical traction initially, and later, with additional pieces added, the device allows the patient to be upright and mobile in a wheelchair (Fig. 23-2).

Collars are less effective in maintaining immobilization. Soft collars are the least acceptable method because the patient is able to move the neck too freely. A rigid two-piece collar is more effective and is an important adjunct to therapy when the x-ray films are not clear and cervical injury is not confirmed (Fig. 23-3). Two- and four-poster braces are other devices which can be used, especially after spinal fusion (Fig. 23-4).

Cervical traction requires a special nursing regime. All types have some form of skull pins, and the skin area surrounding them must be cleaned of crusts every 4 to 8 h. A bacteriostatic solution of ointment also may be used. Screws on the pins should be checked frequently for tightness. The prescribed pounds of weight should be known and checked; traction care includes measures to ensure that weights hang free.

Collars pose special problems because of skin irritation. Special skin care can be administered with **caution**. *With physician approval,* a cervical collar's anterior section can be removed if another person supports the chin while the neck is washed and dried thoroughly. Throughout any procedure, the patient should be informed of the plan of care and should be cautioned not to move the neck.

Thoracic and Lumbar Injury

Thoracic injuries do not require the use of traction. Immobilization is maintained by appropriate positioning and support, in some cases with the use of special beds.

If a general hospital bed is used, bed boards are placed beneath the mattress for firmness and added support. The patient is rolled side to side in a log position. A minimum of two personnel are necessary to turn small patients, a third or fourth person is needed for the larger patient.

Lumbar injuries are managed in essentially the same way as thoracic injuries.

Special Beds

The Stryker wedge frame is probably the most popular form of modified bed for the spinal patient. The patient must meet certain weight requirements in order to fit on the frame since anyone weighing more than 200 lb cannot be safely managed. The frame allows the individual

Figure 23-3
Illustration of rigid two-piece collar (after Stewart). This is one example of several types of rigid collars.

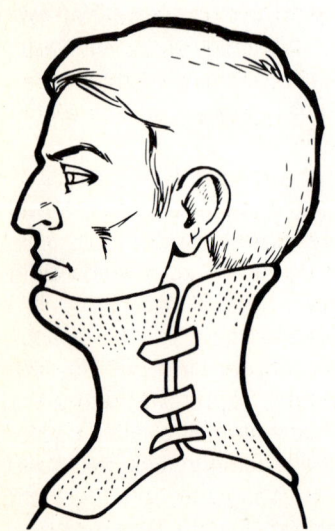

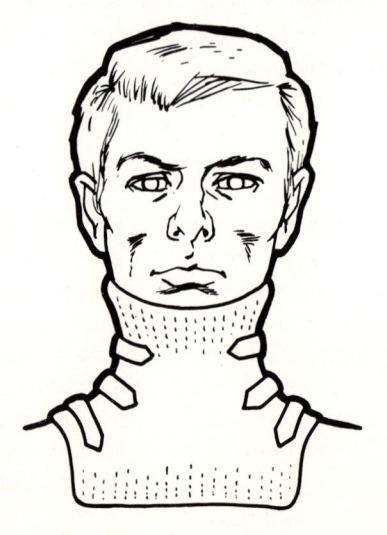

CHAPTER 23   432

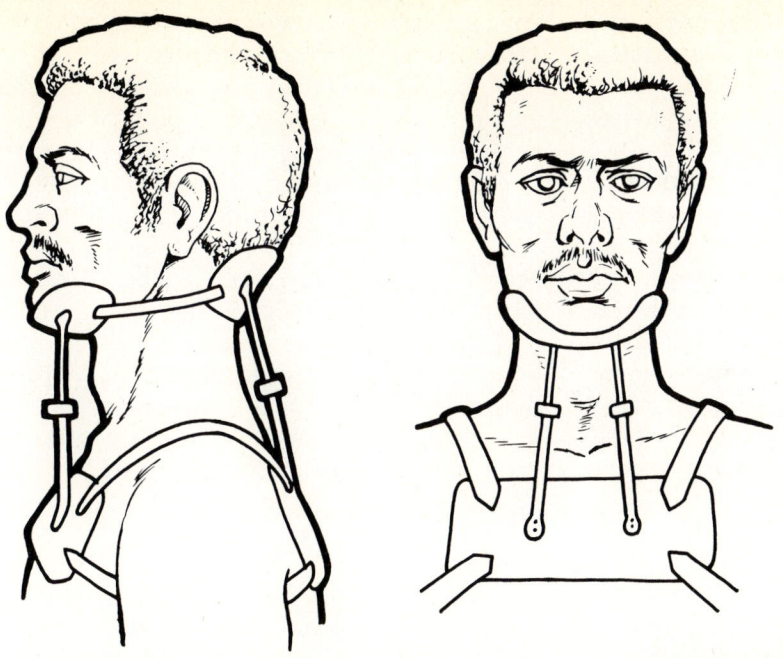

Figure 23-4
Illustration of four-poster brace. Four vertical supports hold chin and occiput pads to maintain position (after Stewart).

to be kept in alignment and turned frequently. It also permits the patient to be placed into Trendelenburg's position for chest physiotherapy, and into reverse Trendelenburg for preparation in developing sitting tolerance.

The disadvantage to the Stryker frame lies with the patient's inability to see the environment, except the floor, when on the abdomen, or except the ceiling while on the back. Prism glasses are very beneficial for refracting images for better visualization. Another common complaint is fitting of the face piece while the patient is lying on the abdomen. Facial edema occurs when the patient's condition necessitates frequent Trendelenburg positioning. This edema can be counteracted to some extent by reversing the tilt of the frame after the patient's blood pressure has stablized.

When turning a patient on the Stryker frame, some key points are important to remember. Cervical traction must be maintained at all times. Traction is lost when the weights rest on the floor or the knot on the traction rope rests against the pulley system, blocking the pull on the tongs or halo. To avoid this situation, the patient must be kept pulled down on the frame. Whenever moved up or down on the frame, the patient's body should be supported by two people on each side, another maintaining traction and supporting the neck. The movement should be one smooth action, all personnel using care not to flex or extend the body.

When ready to turn the Stryker, the patient's extremities should be secured onto the frame with straps. With decreased sensation in the hands, quadriplegic patients can have considerable soft tissue damage if the hands are caught in the turning ring. Additionally, a paralyzed arm left hanging loose can cause joint damage at the shoulder. The patient should be turned in one slow sustained movement to prevent sudden shifts in body position. A patient suffering from multiple trauma may have invasive tubes and lines that must be watched closely to prevent

433 SPINAL CORD INJURY: ACUTE PHASE

accidental removal. Although it seems impossible at first glance, a patient with chest tubes, intravenous lines, nasogastric tubes, Foley catheters, and intubation can, indeed, be turned when care is used (Fig. 23-5).

The patient who has experienced cardiopulmonary instability must be carefully observed during and after the turning period. The patient who is intubated should be suctioned well both tracheally and orally prior to turn, and care must be used to prevent occlusion of the tube once the patient is on the abdomen. For the respirator-supported patient who has the tubes disconnected for turning, only minimal delay (a few seconds) should be allowed to lapse prior to replacing the respirator.

If the patient experiences difficulties or physiologic instability when placed on the abdomen, the patient should be turned onto the back.

A behavioral response to turning may also occur. For anyone, healthy or ill, turning on a frame is a frightening experience. Careful explanation is required to help allay these fears. A gradually increasing time span may be necessary to assist the patient in adjusting to lying on the abdomen. The person should not be left longer than 2 h in either the prone or supine position.

For the obese patient, a regular hospital bed may be necessary for management. As with any spinal lesion, specific medical and nursing orders are needed to determine patient positioning and activities. A spinal fusion, followed by application of the halo jacket or hard collar, may be done sooner in the obese patient than in others to allow for more mobility.

Circ-o-lectric beds have not been found desirable by some physicians for use in the acute care of spinal cord–injured patients. There is risk of malalignment as the patient is turned and, in addition, a period of weight bearing is experienced as the bed turns. Other concerns include orthostatic hypotension which can occur as the patient becomes upright on the bed.

The Roto Rest and the Stoke-Mandeville-Egerton Turning Bed are examples of other special beds utilized in some spinal cord centers. Water, mud, and air beds also have been used for spinal cord injured, but these are useful in the later phase after danger of further damage to the cord is past. Regardless of the type of bed utilized, some essential points apply. When a cervical injury is present, the neck should never be flexed or extended. The patient is always turned as a whole, well-supported unit. The beds should be maintained in proper fuctioning condition. Improper techniques and equipment can result in further bone or nervous tissue damage to the patient. If a skull traction device becomes disconnected from the bone, immediately prevent the patient from turning the head by immobilizing the neck with sandbags, intravenous fluid bags, linen rolls, or similar devices on either side of the head. Have another person notify the physician as soon as possible.

Figure 23-5
Intensive care nurse with person on Stryker frame. Note endotracheal tube is in place connected by tubing to a mechanical respirator.

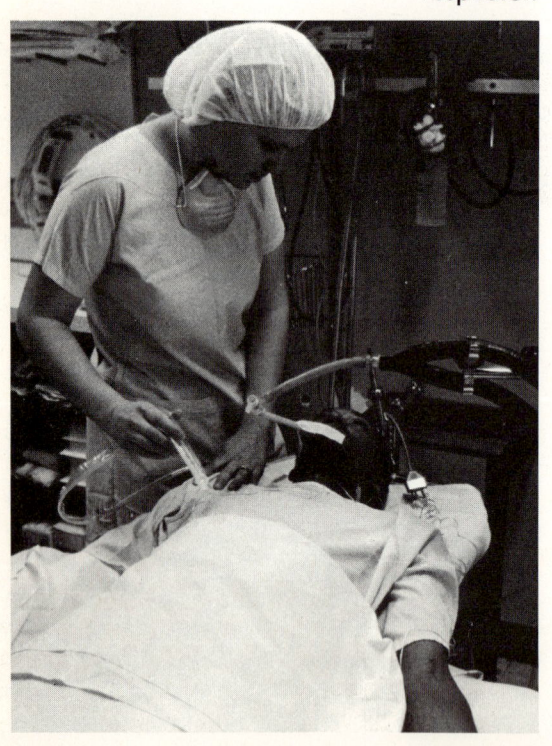

Orthostatic hypotension is a hazard of immobility for any patient. The person who has experienced high thoracic or cervical neck injuries is especially susceptible to the problem because of the loss of sympathetic control. The implications of orthostatic hypotension become apparent when the spinal cord–injured patient is raised to a sitting position after prolonged bedrest and promptly becomes markedly hypotensive. This phenomenon can be avoided by gradually elevating the patient over several days to weeks. The tilt table is often used in physical therapy to assist the patient in gradual sitting.

GOAL: TO PREVENT RESPIRATORY DISTRESS AND COMPLICATIONS

Respiratory distress is an ever-present treat to quadriplegic persons, especially those with injury at C5 and above. Loss of the phrenic nerve's innervation of the diaphragm and loss of intercostal muscles are life threatening. From the moment a patient enters the acute facility, a vigorous preventive therapy program is imperative to maintain respiration and combat pneumonia and atelectasis.

Many centers are utilizing tracheal intubation or tracheostomy as a means of administering optimal oxygenation and preventing collapse of lung segments during the acute spinal shock phase. This ensures that a patent airway is maintained, and the evacuation of retained secretions is made easier. Sterile technique is critical in suctioning to prevent infection. Cleansing around the tracheostomy stoma with acetic acid is effective in deodorizing foul-smelling anaerobic stoma secretions. Good tracheal toilet can be maintained by lavaging the trachea with sterile normal saline, suctioning, and inflating the lungs with an Ambu bag (in the adult). A mechanical respirator may be used to support acute respiratory insufficiency or may be necessary to sustain life.

Patients with midcervical lesions commonly have difficulty when the mechanical ventilation is stopped. A respirator with a "patient assist" may be used to gradually wean the patient from mechanical ventilation. Many intensive care units utilize specific respiratory criteria to determine the patient's ability to support respiratory functioning. Several days to weeks may be required on assistive breathing before the patient can maintain an adequate oxygenation level and clear the airway secretions.

Other respiratory measures may be instituted whether the patient has a tracheostomy or not. Assisted cough involves a coordinated effort between nurse and patient. The patient takes as deep a breath as possible, and the nurse assists the cough by pushing the abdomen inward and upward. This forces the diaphragm to rise and pushes secretions into the lower airways for easier removal. This procedure should not be done after the patient has eaten. Assisted cough and deep breathing should be done not less than every 2 h, slightly less frequently at night. A goal is to improve respiratory function so the patient can cough and mobilize secretions.

Postural drainage, clapping, and percussion are also important activities for clearing secretions from the lungs. The physician's assessment must be made to determine the degree to which the patient may be moved into position for postural draining. A patient's overall cardiovascular stability must be established prior to placing the patient in Trendelenburg's position for chest physiotherapy. Signs of cyanosis and decreased level of consciousness should be watched for, especially in the patient who has low arterial oxygen level. Arterial blood gases will show the results of aggressive chest management; these blood samples may be taken every 6 to 12 h to identify problems before they become unmanageable. Arterial catheter lines are very helpful for constantly monitoring the blood pressure as well as facilitating the drawing of blood samples. The nurse should know the hospital blood gas norms in order to identify problems.

Mobilization, either by turning or sitting (when allowed), also contributes to prevention and clearing secretions. For the patient who has been placed in a halo jacket, it is possible that the jacket will inhibit respiration. These patients must be checked frequently. For persons with potential respiratory emergency, endotracheal tubes or tracheostomy tubes should be readily accessible.

Every nurse and physician who comes in contact with the patient in a halo jacket should be aware of the technique for removing the front section of the jacket in the event of an emergency. Steps listing the procedure for removal and the precautions should be kept at the bedside; the special wrench needed for the bolts also must be kept close at hand for fast retrieval.

GOAL: TO MAINTAIN ALIGNMENT AND JOINT MOTION

Functional alignment and movement of joints through their range of motion are important activities in the care of the cord-injured person from time of injury. Utilizing pillows and linen rolls will help prevent internal and external rotation of legs. The heels must be kept off the bed, either by pillow supports under the calves or with special sheepskin protectors or booties. During back lying, a footboard is used to prevent foot drop. Some nurses favor using high-topped sneakers on patients for this purpose; however, fungal toe infections and heel breakdown can result if care is not taken.

To assist in preventing joint contractures, an early range-of-motion (ROM) program is important. Prior to beginning such a program, a specific doctor's order must be obtained so that all the individuals responsible for the person's care will be aware of any limitations. Full range of motion to hips is often contraindicated in the patient with postoperative Harrington rod insertion. ROM to the trapezius and rhomboidal muscles may not be allowed in the cervical-injured patient because of the muscles' insertion to the cervical spine. Several weeks may elapse before the physician will allow full range or resistive exercises to certain joints.

Every joint possible, however, should be moved through ROM four times a day. This is accomplished by passive or active exercise, depending on muscle strength. For example, if progressive exercises are in order, the nurse can have the patient lift intravenous bags (if available), starting with 500 mL size and progressing to 1000 mL size.

The patient may not always want to be turned or have ROM exercises and may seek to have the nurse eliminate them; the nurse, believing a favor is being done, may be contributing to complications.

During the first 24 to 48 h after admission, a consultation in physical therapy and occupational therapy is important. Early contact with these departments is needed to obtain a muscle evaluation and to facilitate a coordinated plan of care that begins to make maximum use of the patient's neuromuscular potential. Joint splints can be fashioned to support the paralyzed joints in a functional position. An example of the importance of this is the wrist in the person with cervical injury; potential must be maintained for eventual use of the hands. Patient participation in some activities of daily living may also be implemented according to the individual's ability.

GOAL: TO MAINTAIN URINARY OUTPUT, PREVENT INFECTION, AND FACILITATE BLADDER TRAINING

Attentive management of the urinary tract is crucial in preventing the complications of renal calculi and urinary tract infections. Infections by gram-negative organisms may result in septicemia and can cause death. From the moment of insertion of an indwelling catheter, sterile technique and subsequent frequent care of the catheter and the closed drainage system are extremely important. In the acutely injured patient who generally has a flaccid bladder as a result of spinal shock, the indwelling catheter provides the clinical means of evaluating kidney perfusion, general hydration, and of measuring urinary output. After the blood pressure and urinary flow have stabilized, the question of continuing the use of the indwelling catheter or removing it must be determined. When feasible, intermittent catheterization is the current method of choice although some controversy persists (Yashon; Pierce and Nickel).

The purposes of intermittent catheterization include minimization of urinary infection possibilities and provision of the opportunity for resumption of bladder functioning. The frequency of its use is directed to specifically determined residual urine. Consequently, if begun early, it is done more frequently, especially if the patient is on intravenous or increased fluid intake; care must be exercised to avoid overdistention of the bladder.

A systematic procedure is important to the eventual outcome, so a protocol related to fluid intake, residual urine, and frequency of catheterization should be utilized. Special catheter teams are organized for this purpose in some institutions.

During the acute stage, the patient who is able to tolerate liquids by mouth should try to reach an oral intake of 2500 to 3000 mL per day. This permits the kidneys to be perfused adequately and prevents infections by flushing bacteria and deposits out of the system. If intravenous fluids are necessary, the quantity of fluids also will be prescribed. Suggestions from the dietitian may be helpful in guiding the patient as to what fluids to drink to maintain acid urine. Acidic urine helps combat the formation of renal calculi, which are one complication due to immobilization. Cranberry juice is commonly given for this purpose and, in some areas, ascorbic acid is used (Pierce and Nickel).

Spontaneous voiding may sometimes occur. If the patient voids frequently, the bladder should be catheterized to check for residual urine. Some physicians prefer to use urinary antiseptics, such as Mandelamine, in conjunction with catheterizations to reduce infection.

GOAL: TO PREVENT GASTROINTESTINAL COMPLICATIONS AND FACILITATE BOWEL CONTROL

The person with an acute spinal cord injury may have food and fluid restrictions until the status of the gastrointestinal tract is determined. Generally there is distention and atonia; paralytic ileus also may occur, particularly accompanying lower thoracic and lumbar fractures. If the patient is to undergo surgery, vomiting and regurgitation could be hazardous. Nasogastric tubes may be employed either as treatment or prevention.

As soon as peristalsis returns, oral feeding can be started, progressing from liquids to solids. The nurse can facilitate adequate nutritional intake in several ways. Choosing foods for meals gives the patient some part in decision making. A patient on a turning frame may find it easier to eat while lying on the abdomen. Pitchers of liquids can be rigged on a platform, with a straw or hose connected within reach. Hand devices may be utilized early to allow the patient to self-feed. Care must be used not to overly frustrate the patient by making too many demands on the remaining functioning level.

For the patient who is unable to eat for a period of time, feeding via a gastrostomy or nasogastric tube may be necessary. Parenteral hyperalimentation may also be used to attempt to counteract massive muscle loss.

A well-balanced dietary regimen is vital to recovery and potential rehabilitation. A dietitian can be an important member of the team to help ensure that the patients receive adequate nutrition.

In response to injury, some patients develop stress ulcers. These most often appear within the first 4 weeks and can result in death from hemorrhage (Kewalramani, 1979). Emesis, gastric drainage, and stool must be checked for evidence of bleeding. Antacids may be used prophylactically when the patient is on steroid therapy.

The initial incontinent bowel movement of

the spinal cord–injured person may be large, followed by liquid stools until the intestinal tract is emptied. Bowel movements may then be absent for several days until the patient begins to eat. It is important to avoid fecal impaction; awareness of and recording of the bowel activity are an important part of care.

Whenever bowel sounds return, a bowel control program can be implemented. Complications of paralytic ileus and abdominal trauma may delay this.

A typical bowel program is generally done in the morning on an every-other-day basis. Dulcolox or glycerin suppositories are given after the rectum has been manually emptied. The number of suppositories is eventually reduced and, for some patients, only digital stimulation of the anus will be necessary. A carefully kept record of the results is important. The program may require modification when diarrhea occurs.

As the patient becomes ready to participate in self-care, it is time to begin teaching about the effects of diet and food on bowel movement.

The earlier bowel and bladder training occur, the easier it is for the rehabilitation facility to pursue the rehabilitative goals. Not every patient will be ready for bowel and bladder programs, but those who are will be closer to and more prepared for the rehabilitation therapy ahead. During the early stages, the nurse can be informally teaching the person about the changes that have occurred, relating the bowel and bladder regimens to the future. Excretory functions are private matters for most people, and it is not unusual for them to be uneasy or embarrassed about asking questions.

GOAL: TO PROMOTE SKIN INTEGRITY AND PREVENT FORMATION OF PRESSURE ULCERS

A major complication of care for any patient is disruption of skin integrity and the formation of pressure sores. Persons who have paralysis and loss of sensation from spinal cord injury are particularly susceptible to these ulcers. Once they are formed, they are a source of infection and a site of nutrient loss throughout their life-span. The lengthy time required for their healing interrupts the patient's recovery and ability to participate actively in rehabilitation. Later, these ulcers may cause a major disruption in living activities. Consequently, prevention of pressure areas is a prime nursing measure.

Essentially, these sores arise when there is prolonged tissue ischemia caused by a pressure exceeding tissue capillary pressure. Kosiak (Krusen, 1971) demonstrated that a pressure of 70 mmHg applied for 2 h resulted in microscopic muscle tissue changes. Particularly susceptible areas are those overlying bony prominences.

The person with spinal cord injury is especially prone to pressure sores because of vasomotor changes, paralysis, and lack of sensation. Since tissue integrity relies on delivery of oxygen and nutrients to cells via capillaries, interference with that process results in cellular damage and necrosis; lack of muscular movement and tissue edema can constitute that interference. The loss of sensation for pressure and pain that normally causes one unconsciously to shift position to remove pressure also interferes.

Additionally, parts of the skin below the lesion may become dry and scaly due to lack of sweating, and conversely, excessive sweating may occur in unaffected areas. Some of these patients may be acidotic or alkalotic during the early post injury phase; this also makes them risks for tissue problems. The nutritional status of the individual contributes to the potential for skin breakdown, and the acutely injured person will be suffering from metabolic changes that result in protein loss and other imbalances.

The major nursing intervention aimed at promoting tissue integrity and preventing the formation of decubitus ulcers is turning the patient to relieve pressure from major sites a *minimum* of every 2 h. Obviously, the patient's position will affect distribution of the areas most susceptible to breakdown (Table 23-2).

Before turning the patient, the nurse must pay special attention to these major sites by padding, ensuring dryness, and eliminating wrinkles. A

Table 23-2

Position Related to Sites Particularly Subject to Pressure

POSITION	PARTICULAR PRESSURE SITES
Prone	Forehead, cheekbones,* chin
	Shoulder
	Anterior iliac spine
	Knees
	Anterior tibial crest
	Dorsum of foot
Supine	Occiput
	Scapulae
	Elbows
	Sacrum
	Heels
Side	Ear
	Head of humerus
	Great trochanter
	Superior iliac spine
	Lateral and medial knee surfaces
	Lateral malleolus

* Particularly on sling of Stryker

turning regimen includes not only the relief of pressure but inspection of the skin sites and proper positioning. Location of a reddened site signals danger, and that site should be free of any pressure until the redness is gone.

Inspection of the skin of the acutely spinal cord injured also should include areas around dressings, tong (pin) sites, splints, cast edges, and intravenous and arterial lines. If elastic stockings are used, they should be removed every shift. Cervical collars and braces can be especially irritating to the skin as can the vest of a halo jacket; these cannot be removed without medical orders, but the area around their edges can be examined.

Teaching the patient and family the importance of skin care can be started early by demonstrating meticulous attention to regular inspection of the body surfaces and explaining relief of pressure as a reason for position change.

The nurse and others must be alert to possible injury to the senseless limbs of the cord patient during the admission and stabilization process. During the numerous activities surrounding early treatment and resuscitation, it should not be forgotten that the patient has descreased sensation to pain, touch, temperature, and location of the body parts. A carelessly handled paralyzed limb can be pinched or scraped unintentionally, but the beginnings of tissue breakdowns have already occurred. It should be remembered that if the acuteness of the patient's condition interferes with turning every 2 h, relief of highly susceptible pressure points should be attempted with massage and some padding. Doughnuts are contraindicated since they constrict vessels surrounding the pressure site.

Having the patient in a Stryker wedge frame or other special bed facilitates skin care and relief of pressure when the frame is turned and used properly. If the patient is cared for in a regular bed or is able to progress to a sitting position, then a nursing assessment should heed the location of greatest pressure points. Shearing forces also can contribute to occlusion of capillary supply, and this should be kept in mind, particularly for persons not sitting at a 90° angle.

In addition to pressure and shearing force, friction, tissue edema, moisture, and temperature are variables that can influence pressure-sore formation.

Friction can be avoided by positioning, careful placement, and removal of sheets or other padding under the skin. Sheepskin may be a help in reducing friction. Local heating and cooling devices such as hot water bottles should be avoided. Skin needs to be protected from excessive dryness or wetness. Excessive perspiration, drainage, urine, and feces contribute to the skin's susceptibility to breakdown. Wetness for 15 min or more can cause maceration. Skin should be washed with a mild soap and water and thoroughly dried. There are some antiseptic foam products available for use over potential breakdown areas that may be of some use. Gentle rubbing around potential sites can increase circulation. Heavy use of powders and oils is more detrimental than helpful.

If possible, intramuscular injections should be

avoided. The thighs, deltoids, and abdomen are sites of choice on a rotation basis if injections must be used. Frequently the acutely ill patient has intravenous lines in place which can be utilized for parenteral administration.

GOAL: TO PROVIDE AND MAINTAIN ADEQUATE NUTRITION

The nutritional status of the person with an injured spinal cord is highly important to progress during recuperation, rehabilitation, and throughout life. During the acute stage, these patients experience metabolic demands imposed by the body's response to trauma. In many cases, these demands are compounded by the additional stress of surgery. The problems of immobility are also present, complicated by actual pathophysiology. For example, in normal persons immobilized for periods of time, there is decreased muscle tone from inactivity; in the spinal cord–injured person, there are changes in muscle tone due to the interrupted nervous system.

Initially, then, the metabolism of the body is catabolic in nature as the body marshals its resources in response to the stresses incurred; in doing so, it draws upon body reserves. Since a general atony of the gastrointestinal tract occurs and oral intake is usually restricted, the normal intake source of nutrients is interrupted at a time when the body requires more. Consequently, the person must be given appropriate nutritional support to provide energy for healing and recuperation, as well as to prevent serious depletion of body reserves.

Fluid and electrolyte replacement is important and standard treatment in early postinjury care. If prolonged periods of restricted intake occur, then attention is given to other supplements. The protein stores of the body are the most fragile in response to trauma, and a decrease in skeletal muscle mass begins early following injury. The provision of adequate protein is a major consideration in nutritional care, and the ability to keep a person in positive nitrogen balance is a signal that catabolism is under control (Downey and Darling, 1971). Adequate calories must accompany any protein given to ensure its proper utilization.

If the patient's condition stabilizes after several days and oral feedings can begin, the nutritional status of the patient may come under control so that major nutritional intervention may not be necessary.

There is growing attention to the nutritional status of traumatized persons and the influence of nutrition on the individual's recuperation and general condition. Consequently a nutritional team, or most certainly a dietitian, should be consulted in early management. When the time comes for oral feedings, consideration of appetite and patient preference is important. Progression to solid foods is individualized according to the patient's condition and ability to tolerate a full diet. In prolonged periods of depleted intake, when the gastrointestinal tract is functional, supplemental feedings may be in order.

Not only are calorie intake and types of nutrient important; other nutritional considerations also are relative. Calcium balance is monitored because immobility, as well as steroid therapy, contributes to bone demineralization and possible kidney stone formation. Citric fruit juices are generally avoided; cranberry juice is utilized to promote acid urine, inhibiting calculi formation. Anemia may be present, and iron supplements may be given. For the proper functioning of the bowel, adequate fluid and bulk food are usually recommended.

Nursing considerations in feeding persons with acute spinal cord injury include the possibilities that these patients may be on special turning frames, may have partial body casts, or may wear halo vests. Patients who have been on ventilators may have some dysphagia, and care should be exercised to avoid aspiration. If the patient has a tracheostomy, there also may be discomfort on swallowing. One should also be alert to regurgitation around or through the trachea, which is indicative of a fistula. If the patient has the ability to do so, self-feeding should be encouraged. However, fatigue of very weak muscles is to be avoided. Patients with a cervical injury at C7 may be able to feed themselves and do some grooming while prone on a Stryker frame. Those with thoracic and lumbar injuries who are on a frame also may perform these activities in relation to feeding.

Once a patient is able to be elevated from lying flat, use of assistive devices may be helpful for those with some function in the arms. Planning a feeding and eating program with the nurse, dietitian, and occupational therapist can facilitate the patient's achieving and retaining optimum nutritional status.

Family members and significant others can help and be helped regarding the patient's nutritional needs. They can contribute a list of the patient's food preferences and can be encouraged to prepare some favorites to appeal to the patient's appetite.

GOAL: TO PROVIDE PSYCHOLOGIC AND EMOTIONAL SUPPORT FOR THE PATIENT AND FAMILY

The event of spinal cord injury has impact on the patient's personal and cognitive as well as physical being. The family and significant others in the patient's sphere of activities also are affected. The nurse, as the professional in most intimate contact with the patient during most of the acute-care period, is in the position to observe the patient's behavior closely and to interact effectively. Health team members are part of the patient's environment; accordingly, their behavior has an impact on the person's adaptation to the trauma. In the stress of the early intensive efforts dedicated to resuscitating and stabilizing the cord-injured patient, the staff's orderly noninteraction may be a defense mechanism to assist them to cope with the situation (Weller and Miller, 1977b). Although in some instances this is reassuring to the patient, carrying it to the extreme can isolate and make the patient more frightened. Reassurances and explanations are important parts of care for the psychological and emotional response of these patients.

Spinal cord–injured persons and others have described several stages in response to their situation. These stages often are described as shock/disbelief, denial, anger, depression, and acceptance. Although the framework is useful in identifying and understanding behavior and in planning intervention, a review of research in the field (Trieschmann, 1978) points out that there is no current evidence to support the belief that there are inevitable stages of adjustment. Further, there is no evidence of such a construct as *spinal cord personality* and, indeed, there is considerable reason to describe the spinal cord injured as a very heterogeneous group. That there is a strong psychological response to the event is not in question; the point to be made is that several types of response may be experienced by an individual, and the individual requires and expects intervention as needed.

One should keep in mind that the person who suddenly becomes paraplegic or quadriplegic has made a rapid transition from a socially valued, independent, whole person to a physically disabled, socially devalued person. In essence, there is an instantaneous change to "one of them," the group whom one previously felt sorry for. Although the stigma attached to the disabled population may be more of a problem to handle during rehabilitation in the community, the initial reality is that one is dependent on other persons. The paraplegic individual cannot move about in bed, cannot control bowel and bladder; for the person rendered quadriplegic, this means total dependence on people and on machines such as ventilators. The person is called upon to cope with the possible permanence of this state as well as to adapt to the physical trauma. Since the outcome in terms of paralysis is not conclusive initially, the patient often cannot be told right away what to expect. However, the physician sometimes may give a poor prognosis to the family and not to the patient, under the rationale that the information given to the latter so early may cause the patient to give up hope. Such game playing saps energy from both staff and families during communication with the patient (Roglitz, 1978). Some patients support such an approach on the basis that hope should not be removed since it is essential to being able to "carry on" (Roglitz; Caywood, 1974). Others indicate that there should be no undue delay (Kinash, 1978; Brookman et al., 1976) in being given information.

Whatever the belief about when and how to provide information to the patient, at some phase of care the spinal cord–injured person begins to seek answers to "Will I ever walk again?" The question may not be expressed in those words, but as time passes and there is little or no return of function, the reality of the situation becomes difficult to ignore. As opposed to persons with amputations, these people see all of their extremities present and intact, and the hope for returning function is difficult to relinquish.

It is not easy for the patient to ask questions concerning the ultimate outcome and it is not easy for the staff to supply the answers. Generally this information is given by the physician, but the bedside staff may be the ones who get the questions. The nurse can be alert to the questions that the patient needs to ask, explore those concerns, and see that the appropriate information reaches the patient. Patients have indicated that they many times "knew" the answer, but didn't want to ask the physician because they were not ready to accept the answer. In any individual case, the answer may, of course, vary; regardless of the answer, the staff can help the patient work with the current reality. For example, one can point out to the person that even if the outcome is unknown, the situation now (such as range of motion or eating) needs attention whether one is to walk or not.

Response to the Event The newly injured cord patient may indeed be in a state of shock or disbelief at the situation. The immobilizing devices, special beds or turning procedures, the loss of sensation, the presence of monitoring and ventilatory equipment all lend a sense of unreality. Patients have described this as a fearful period. They suffer fear of choking, fear of falling, fear that the staff may make an error. Constant reassurance that their needs will be cared for, that procedures will be explained, that instructions will be given about the routines employed will contribute to the patient's sense of trust and help decrease fear and anxiety. Stooping to make eye contact with the patient on a Stryker frame reassures the individual of importance and identity. Reassurance through touch is communicated by remembering to make the contact above the level of sensation loss.

In the consuming effort required by staff to meet the physical requirements of the acutely injured cord patient, attention to the psychological needs cannot be put aside. The often forgotten idea is that little things mean a lot.

Particularly during the earliest days postinjury, the patient may seem withdrawn from the situation. Although this may be attributed to the overwhelming nature of the episode taking place, the nurse and others should keep in mind that the effect may partially be contributed by sedation given for pain, by metabolic imbalance, or by lack of sleep due to the treatment regimen. Since alcohol and drug use may have been involved in the traumatic incident, withdrawal signs and symptoms from these substances may influence the patient's psychological and behavioral state.

The denying patient may be encountered during the acute phase of care. Denial is described as a defense by the normal ego to shield itself from the engulfing reality (Hohmann, 1975). The nursing staff and others should be gentle and understanding with the denying patients and should not try to enforce reality upon them. At the same time, the nurse must avoid being drawn into the denial. The cheerful and cooperative denier can cause consternation among the staff, but usually these persons do not make demands, and this may make it more comfortable for the staff to enter into the denial. The patient with the "wonderful spirit" may lend some of this bravado to the family, who need it at that time (Weller and Miller, 1977b). Hohmann says that the person will relinquish denial when there is sufficient experience with the disability to recognize positive and gratifying experiences which can occur despite the disability. When the facade of denial begins to be dropped by the patient, the nurse should recognize this as a sign of progress and help explain it as such to the family. Staff and families caught up in the denial may experience anxiety as *they* are faced with confronting the reality of the patient's condition.

Episodes of anger, depression, and anxiety may occur during the acute phase of care and need to be accepted with understanding; since this phase may last several days or several months, a spectrum of behaviors and responses may be anticipated. One should remember that a normal outlet for emotions is physical activity. The immobilized and paralyzed patient does not have this outlet. In the case of the person with a tracheostomy, even the verbal expression of emotion is hindered. Although the sensations are impaired in spinal cord injury, emotions are not. Strong emotional and psychological response to devastating injury is normal. When behaviors are extreme, the staff should consult the services of a psychiatrist. Talk of suicide in these persons is not exceptional; however, if characteristics of a plan for carrying it out appear, psychiatric intervention should be sought immediately.

Patients report that cheerful staff, friends, and relatives are a source of comfort to them, as are bathing, position changes, and touch (Kinash). Consistent, dependable care is important to convey a sense of worth and to allay apprehension. Fostering the patient's sense of control helps in the situation of dependence on others. Patients should be encouraged to participate in decisions, no matter how small. They also should be permitted to be as directive as possible. For example, following directions as to how the patient likes food prepared or the preferred sequence of bathing and grooming activities can be important.

If visiting is limited because of intensive care routines, provision for communication should be made. Telephone conversation for the immobilized person can be a source of pleasure and contact with others. The patient, with the aid of the nurse, can initiate as well as receive calls. Notes and mail are important communication links, as are such things as taped messages from friends and families.

Since sensory alteration is part of the situation, the patient should be oriented to time and place frequently. Temporal cues such as calendars and clocks should be made available and visible. Battery-operated radios, especially the patient's own, can be used in intensive care units; TV sets can be used in other areas. Prism glasses are an aid for reading or viewing television.

Family and Significant Others The family or significant others of the patient are initially under stress as a result of not knowing whether the patient will live or die and also because of the possibility that the person may be permanently disabled. Their need for information about and communication with the patient cannot be forgotten during the initial time-consuming patient care. Conferences with team members are important since they not only serve the family but also provide staff with information that enables them to deliver more individualized care to the patient.

During a time of crisis, there is a need to organize around some activity; families often are left with little activity except to wait. Contributing information to the care plan or bringing in personalized items for the patient are examples of useful activities. Even though clarifying insurance arrangements or trying to get assistance from referral agencies may be sources of irritation when people are concerned about a loved one, these activities do provide families with functions to accomplish which can be helpful to them in the sense of "doing something." Weller and Miller (1977b) observe that a family's response to spinal cord injury of a loved one often takes the form of panic; accompanying this may be one of two types of response, hovering or fleeing. Nurses see the former in the family constantly in attendance, overseeing, and anxiously asking questions about the patient's care. The latter are the family whom the nurse and social worker find very difficult to contact and who rarely appear at the patient's side. The staff may need to encourage families to make regular but limited visits to reassure the patient that he or she still is considered important. Since the families are a vital part of the patient's environment, their interaction with the patient needs to be assessed so that appropriate assistance to them can be offered as necessary.

Sexual Needs The impact of spinal cord trauma on sexual function has received much attention, but this aspect generally is focused upon during rehabilitation. Acutely injured patients may or may not raise questions concerning their physical sexual activity in the future. In males, reflex erections are not uncommon when spinal shock is subsiding, unless there is direct involvement at the S2-4 and cauda equina. Such erections occur spontaneously upon stimulation during catheterization or bathing. Since menstruation is not neurally controlled, females usually continue to menstruate as before (Claus-Walker et al.) and in postrecovery can conceive and deliver babies. There also have been cases where pregnant women have suffered cord injury and delivered normally.

The nurse caring for the spinal-injured person needs to be aware of the concerns patients have about sexual ability. When questions arise, they should be answered to the best of the nurse's knowledge concerning the individual circumstances. In reality, the physical capacity to peform the sexual act may not be known until later in the rehabilitation phase due to recovery from spinal shock. Since sex and sexuality have special intonations for individuals, satisfaction may be achieved in many ways; concerns may thus involve more than physical activity. Nurses are in daily contact with patients. They may be the ones who receive questions and, if they sense that the patient has a question but encounters difficulty asking it, they can make it known that it is a legitimate and appropriate subject for discussion. If uncomfortable in handling this, the nurse can make a referral, then follow through. Since this is generally a young population, spouses or significant others may be the ones with concerns and they, too, need assurance that this is an appropriate topic for discussion.

Sexual behavior is only part of a person's sexuality. The spinal cord–injured person, like any other, is concerned about appearance, self-concept and self-esteem. The ability to relate to a significant other has import for one's self-image, as does the capacity to perform in one's sexual role. The latter includes not just the role involved in sexual activity, but in "fathering" and "mothering," as well as being able to "provide" or "nurture." Concerns about these matters may indeed emerge in the early periods following injury, and the opportunity for expression of these concerns should be provided.

GOAL: TO FACILITATE CONTINUITY AND THE REHABILITATION PROCESS

It is almost a cliche to hear the phrase "rehabilitation begins at the time of admission to the hospital." In the case of the person with traumatic cord injury, the phrase should be restated, "rehabilitation begins from the time of injury." Since the desirable outcome for rehabilitation is functional ability, the more potential a person has to work with, the more function that can be achieved. Consequently, recognizing a possible spinal cord injury at the accident site, making appropriate transfer with immobilization to prevent further neurologic trauma, and employing stabilization techniques to permit early mobilization are important to the rehabilitation outcome. During the acute-care phase, the appropriate management of paralyzed limbs, the prevention of pressure ulcers, and the avoidance of urinary infections are extremely important to the person's eventual ability to participate in an active rehabilitation program. Time lost through infections, contracted joints, or failure to coordinate transfer to a rehabilitation facility are hindrances in the process.

The nurse can ensure the continuity of care by anticipating patient needs and planning to meet them. Depending on the type of acute-care facility the patient is in, a variety of resource team members may be present to collaborate.

CHAPTER 23   444

As many as possible of the professionals, non-professionals, and others involved in the patient's care should meet, set goals, and coordinate their activities for the patient's and family's benefit. The medical management alone may involve neurosurgeons, neurologists, orthopedists, urologists, and physiatrists. Physical therapists, occupational therapists, and social workers need to be involved with nursing staff early in patient management. Team conferences and team members' cooperation in the plan of care will aid in reducing unproductive and inconsistent efforts. They also will permit the patient to utilize more energy in overcoming the trauma. For example, the physical therapist and nurse can collaborate on the plan for maintaining range of motion, rather than having the patient subjected to regimens from both. Certain interventions can be planned for the time the patient is in a supine position, leaving prone time for sleeping. Planning discharge to an appropriate facility should begin as soon as possible. Coordinating such items as bladder and bowel training programs with the other institution can decrease the need for changes whenever transfer occurs.

As it becomes evident to patient and family that survival has been accomplished but the disability remains, they need to be introduced to the idea that a productive and meaningful life can be achieved, even though the process may be long and drawn out. At the time long-term goals are set, care must be taken to continue to establish short-term goals which can be achieved so the person has a renewed sense of accomplishment. A functional life in a wheelchair may be possible, but the patient needs to acquire the ability to sit before that can occur. Consequently, when elevation activities are begun, the goal to be set might be the ability to sit 15 min without dizziness or undue fatigue.

Teaching the patient and family what is being done and why contributes to their ability to care for these things when they are at home. There is one major transition in the process, over time, with which people may need some help. The patient has to be taught to perform, insofar as possible, without assistance. Just as it is difficult for staff not to "do everything" for the patient, it may be more difficult for the family. Patient, family, and team conferences can be helpful for learning as well as adjustment.

When the time comes for the patient to be transferred to a rehabilitation facility, this should be recognized as a significant moment. It offers hope for the future, but it also reinforces the reality of permanent disability. Additionally, the patient and staff face termination of a significant relationship; indeed, this time of transfer to another facility has been identified as one of stress for patients (McDaniel and Sexton). Patients have expressed a sense of fear at being transferred to the rehabilitation environment. In this essentially unknown situation, they may have been told they are going to learn how to live with their disability. They must, however, give up the security of being "cared for" in a familiar environment; at the same time, they have concerns about what they will or will not be able to accomplish.

Communication between the agencies involved is important, as is communication between staffs. The family can be encouraged to visit the rehabilitation facility ahead of time and to share their findings with the patient. Complete records are important for continuity, and liaison persons may prove invaluable.

Occasionally, the patient will be transferred to other acute facilities or to an intermediate care facility until the patient can take an active role in a full rehabilitation program. Continuity and planning are as important in these instances as they are in transfer to a rehabilitation facility.

Staff in acute-care facilities often do not have the benefit of seeing or knowing the long-term progress made by the patient with whom they have worked so diligently. Liaison and feedback are important for them also, since they can provide clues on improving care in relation to rehabilitation needs of patients. Such feedback also provides them with some sense of accomplishment in contributing to the process by which the patient eventually returns to home or community.

CONCLUSION

The person with spinal cord trauma requires expert and coordinated care from the time of injury through return to the community. During the acute phase of this episode, the emphasis is on stabilization of the patient's general condition as well as on management of the spine and cord trauma to prevent neurologic deterioration. When these tasks have been accomplished, the patient requires continuous attention to prevent any deterioration in physical or psychologic condition so that, when the time is right, participation in the rehabilitation process can take place to the fullest extent. These principles obtain whether one speaks of the person with paraplegia at the L4-5 level or quadriplegia at C5. The nurse is a key contributor in direct care and also maintains a vital coordinating function.

More persons than before are surviving spinal cord damage; they also have a greater chance of returning to the community as contributing and valued citizens. Although there have been strides in surgical management of spinal trauma, the actual prevention of permanent paralysis has been elusive. Research efforts toward regeneration of central nervous system tissue have contributed little that can yet be considered significant for the human who has lost both motor and sensory function. Research in these areas is essential to solving the problem of spinal cord trauma. Research into implantable devices to substitute for lost function has turned up help for selected persons, and investigations into tissue pressure and the prevention of pressure sores are ongoing areas of exploration.

Nurses can and have participated in such studies at various levels. Clinically, there are fruitful areas for nursing research in positioning as related to functional outcome, in prevention of pressure, in the problems which can be attributed to sensory alterations, and in effective teaching methods for patients and families.

Although the numbers of spinal cord–injured persons are not great when compared to other conditions such as stroke or heart attacks, the devastation that spinal cord injury imposes on the individual and those in the surrounding constellation is impossible to ignore. The majority of these persons are in the active, productive period of life when this major trauma occurs; failure to provide appropriate care from injury through rehabilitation would impose an immeasurable loss to them, and to society.

BIBLIOGRAPHY

Albrecht, Gary (ed.): *The Sociology of Physical Disability and Rehabilitation,* University of Pittsburgh Press, Pittsburgh, 1976.

Allen, Marshal B., et al.: *A Manual of Neurosurgery,* University Park Press, Baltimore, 1978.

Barry, Jeanie: *Emergency Nursing,* McGraw-Hill, New York, 1978.

Bedbrook, G.: "Spinal Injuries and Hyperbaric Oxygen," *Med J Aust* 2(14):618–619, 1978.

Bracken, M. B., et al.: "Classification of the Severity of Acute Spinal Cord Injury: Implications for Management," *Paraplegia* 15:39–326, 1978.

Bromley, Ida: *Tetraplegia and Paraplegia,* Churchill Livingstone, New York, 1976.

Brookman, R., et al.: "Information in the Early Stages After Spinal Cord Injury," *Paraplegia* 14:95–100, 1976.

Burke, David: "Pain in Paraplegia," *Paraplegia* 10:297–313, 1973.

Casas, E. R., et al.: "Prophylaxis of Venous Thrombosis and Pulmonary Embolism in Patients with Acute Traumatic Spinal Cord Lesions," *Paraplegia* 15:209–214, 1978.

Caywood, Tim: "A Quadriplegic Young Man Looks at Treatment," *J Rehabil* 40:22–24, 1974.

Claus-Walker, J., et al.: "Immediate Endocrine and Metabolic Consequences of Traumatic Quadriplegia in a Young Woman," *Paraplegia* 15:202–208, 1977–78.

Cornell, S. S., et al.: "Comparison of Three Bowel Management Programs," *Nurs Res* 22:321, 1973.

Downey, John A., and Robert C. Darling: *Phys-*

iological Bases of Rehabilitation Medicine, Saunders, Philadelphia, 1971.

Feustel, D.: "Autonomic Hyperflexia," *Am J Nurs* 76:228, 1976.

Folsom, Farnham: *Extrication and Casualty Handling Techniques,* Lippincott, Philadelphia, 1975.

Frost, Elizabeth: "Physiopathology of Respiration in Neurosurgical Patients," *J Neurosurg* 50:699–714, 1979.

Griffith, E. R., and R. B. Trieschmann: "Sexual Functioning in Women with Spinal Cord Injury," *Arch Phys Med Rehabil* 56:18, 1975.

Guttman, Ludwig: *Spinal Cord Injuries: Comprehensive Management and Research,* 2d ed., Lippincott, Philadelphia, 1976.

Heilporn, A., and G. Noel: "Reflections on the Consciousness of Disability and Somatognosis in Cases of Acute Spinal Injuries," *Paraplegia* 6:122–127, 1968.

Hohmann, George: "Psychological Aspects of Treatment and Rehabilitation of the Spinal Cord Injured Person," *Clin Orthop* 112:81–88, 1975.

Isaacs, Norma: "The Treatment of Acute Spinal Cord Injury Using Local Hypothermia," *J Neurosurg Nurs* 10:95–101, 1978.

Kewalramani, L. S.: "Neurogenic Gastroduodenal Ulceration and Bleeding Associated with Spinal Cord Injuries," *J Trauma* 19(4):259–265, 1979.

Kinash, Rose G.: "Experiences and Nursing Needs of Spinal Cord Injured Patients," *J Neurosurg Nurs* 10:29–32, 1978.

Krusen, F., et al.: *Handbook of Physical Medicine and Rehabilitation,* 2d ed., Saunders, Philadelphia, 1971.

Larrabee, J. H.: "The Person with a Spinal Cord Injury: Physical Care During Early Recovery," *Am J Nurs* 77:1320–29, 1977.

Lindh, Kathleen, and Gail Rickerson: "Spinal Cord Injury: You Can Make a Difference," *Nursing '74* February: 41–45, 1974.

Mack, E. W., and W. M. Dawson, Jr.: "Injury to the Spine and Spinal Cord," *Hosp Med* 12:23, 1976.

Maynard, F. M., and K. Imai: "Immobilization Hypercalcemia in Spinal Cord Injury," *Arch Phys Med Rehabil* 58:16, 1977.

McDaniel, James W., and Allan Sexton: "Psychoendocrine Studies of Patients with Spinal Cord Lesions," *J Abnorm Psychol* 76:117–122, 1970.

McFadden, J. T.: "Anterior Open Reduction of the Fractured Cervical Spine," in D. Ruge and L. Wiltse (eds.), *Spinal Disorder,* Lea & Febiger, Philadelphia, 1977, pp. 373–379.

Merritt, J. L.: "Urinary Tract Infections, Causes and Management with Particular Reference to the Patient with Spinal Cord Injury: A Review," *Arch Phys Med Rehabil* 57:365, 1976.

Messard, L., et al.: "Survival After Spinal Cord Trauma: A Life Table Analysis," *Arch Neurol* 35:78–83, 1978.

Meyer, Paul, et al.: "Fracture Dislocation: Cervical Spine Transportation, Assessment and Acute Management," Northwestern University, Chicago, Ill., unpublished paper, 1975.

Minckley, Barbara B.: "Emotional Aspects of Intensive Care," in L. E. Miltzer, F. G. Abdellah, and J. R. Kitchel (eds.), *Concepts and Practices of Intensive Care for Nurse Specialist,* 2d ed., Charles Press, Bowie, Md., 1976, pp. 371–385.

Mountcastle, Vernon B. (ed.): *Medical Physiology,* vol. 1, Mosby, St. Louis, 1974.

National Paraplegia Foundation: *Nursing Management of Spinal Cord Injuries,* Chicago, 1975.

National Spinal Cord Injury Model Systems Conference: *Proceedings,* National Spinal Cord Injury Data Research Center, Good Samaritan Hospital, Phoenix, Ariz., April 20–21, 1978.

Nursing Grand Rounds: "Caring for the Totally Dependent Patient," *Nursing '76* 6:38–43, 1976.

Nursing Grand Rounds: "Pitfalls of Emotional Involvement: Sympathetic Nursing Care of a Patient with Spine Injury," *Nursing '76* 6:42–47, 1976.

Osterholm, Jewell: "The Pathophysiological Response to Spinal Cord Injury: The Current

Status of Related Research," *J Neurosurg* 40:5–33, 1974.

Pepper, G. A.: "The Person with a Spinal Cord Injury: Psychological Care," *Am J Nurs* 77:1330–36, 1977.

Perine, G.: "Needs Met and Unmet," *Am J Nurs* 71:2128, 1971.

Pierce, Donald, and Vernon H. Nickel (eds.): *The Total Care of Spinal Cord Injuries,* Little, Brown, Boston, 1977.

Roglitz, Cathy: "Team Approach in the Acute Phase of Spinal Cord Injury," *J Neurosurg Nurs* 10:117–120, 1978.

Rosillo, Ronald, and Max Foge: "Emotional Support," *Psychosomatics* 11:194, 1970.

Rottkamp, B. C.: "An Experimental Nursing Study: A Behavior Modification Approach to Nursing Therapeutics in Body Positioning of Spinal Cord Injured Patients," *Nurs Res* 25:181–186, 1976.

Ruge, Daniel: "Spinal Cord Injuries," in D. Ruge and L. Wiltse (eds.), *Spinal Disorders,* Lea & Febiger, Philadelphia, 1977(a), pp. 357–367.

Ruge, Daniel, and Leon Wiltse: *Spinal Disorders: Diagnosis and Treatment,* Lea & Febiger, Philadelphia, 1977(b).

Shontz, Franklin: *The Psychological Aspects of Physical Illness and Disability,* Macmillan, New York, 1975.

Sorensen O., and A. Nachemson: "Early Mobilization of Patients with Unstable Fractures of the Thoracic and Lumbar Spine," *Scand Rehabil Med* 11:47–61, 1979.

Stewart, T. D.: "Spinal Cord Injury: A Role for the Psychiatrist," *Am J Psychiatry* 134:538, 1977.

Tator, Charles H.: "Acute Spinal Cord Injury: A Review of Recent Studies of Treatment and Pathophysiology," *Can M J* 107:143–149, 1972.

Trieschmann, Roberta B.: *The Psychological, Social and Vocational Adjustment in Spinal Cord Injury: A Strategy for Future Research,* Easter Seal Society for Crippled Children and Adults of Los Angeles County, April 30, 1978.

Trombly, Catherine Anne, and Anna D. Scott: *Occupational Therapy for Physical Dysfunction,* Williams & Wilkins, Boston, 1977.

Vandam, Leroy D., and Allan B. Rossier: "Circulatory, Respiratory and Ancillary Problems in Acute and Chronic Spinal Cord Injury," in S. G. Hershey (ed.), *Refresher Course in Anesthesiology,* vol. 3, Lippincott, Philadelphia, 1975, pp. 171–182.

Weller, D. J., and P. M. Miller: "Emotional Reactions of Patient, Family and Staff in Acute Care Period of Spinal Cord Injury: Part I," *Soc Work Health Care* 2:369–377, 1977 (a).

———, ———: "Emotional Reactions of Patient, Family and Staff in Acute Care Period of Spinal Cord Injury: Part 2," *Soc Work Health Care* 3:7–17, 1977(b).

Yashon, David: *Spinal Injury,* Appleton-Century-Crofts, New York, 1978.

Yeo, John D.: "A Review of Experimental Research in Spinal Cord Injury," *Paraplegia,* 14:1–11, 1976.

Young, John: "Development of Systems of Spinal Injury Management with a Correlation to the Development of other Esoteric Health Care Systems," *Ariz Med* 27:1, 1970.

24
marjorie a. boyink
susan m. strawn

spinal cord injury: postacute phase

INTRODUCTION

Providing nursing care to spinal cord–injured persons requires nurses to use all their basic skills. These patients require some nursing management of nutrition, fluid intake, elimination, respiration, mobility, health maintenance, and socialization. Nurses must have a knowledge of physiology in order to understand how spinal injury affects the body and how to develop a plan of care.

Highly skilled staff members are required to work with the spinal cord–injured patient. They must have the intellectual ability to provide and direct care and the emotional maturity to interpret and modify behaviors, as well as technical skills. Training programs provided for staff by the institution should be specific enough to cover all the physical and emotional care requirements of the spinal cord–injured person. It is really not possible for a spinal cord–injured person to work through the postinjury adjustment if staff members are inept.

The patient population being considered in this chapter is the late adolescent to middle-aged adult who has experienced trauma to the spinal cord with resultant limitations in motion and sensation. Persons who are very young or very old at the time they sustain spinal cord trauma have additional care needs, although the basic concepts apply to all age groups.

No differentiation is made between quadriplegics and paraplegics, as all patients must learn how to manage care. The needs of the two groups are similar, although their functional abilities vary. The quadriplegic patient must learn care in order to direct others; the paraplegic patient must learn self-care.

The problems of those patients with very high level lesions, who have virtually no voluntary motor function, are not addressed separately. These patients require close medical and nursing supervision. Most of them have respiratory complications that will keep them very close to, if not in, an institutional setting for the remainder of their lives. Unfortunately, they may have little more than the ability to breathe, think, and talk.

The preceding chapter considered the acute-care management of the person with spinal cord injury. This chapter addresses the care needs of the person once the medical condition has stabilized sufficiently to allow transfer to a rehabilitation facility. It also deals with preparations the person must make for reentry into the community.

The care of the spinal cord–injured person can be most rewarding for the nurse. In comparison with the length of time the patient will live with the disability, the amount of time the nurse spends with the patient is almost microscopic. In that very short period, the nurse must equip the patient with the skills necessary to survive, assist in moving the patient through the stages to acceptance of the disability, and still provide necessary physical care and surveillance. The nurse strives for improvement in physical abilities, prevention of disabling complications, and education of the person to function as a healthy, contributing member of society. Success can provide rewards unlike those in any other area of nursing.

CARING FOR THE PERSON WITH AN UNSTABLE SPINE

ADMISSION PROCESS

Transfer of the patient from an acute-care setting to a rehabilitation unit or center causes great anxiety for the patient and the family. The usual fears associated with moving into an unfamiliar environment, meeting new people, and having to learn new routines are coupled with the expectation that in this setting recovery will occur. Usually the patient has been given some explanation of the process of rehabilitation, perhaps no more than a remark that there will be more frequent physical therapy sessions. It is unlikely that the patient has been adequately prepared to cope with the impact of the new setting.

The extent of the dependence becomes more evident when the patient realizes that the injury affects the ability to move about or to obtain assistance. By reviewing material available from the transferring hospital, the nurse should be able to determine in advance if special equipment will be necessary and arrange to have it on hand before a patient arrives. For example, some patients cannot grasp and press the button on a call light or even call out to alert the staff to some need. The appropriate type of signal system should be available for immediate use by such patients. Almost all patients can effectively use a pressure or geriatric pad because it requires only slight pressure or movement to be activated. If the patient has no hand function, the pad can be placed close to the head and activated with a slight turn of the head.

At the time of admission, the patient and the family are told how the new environment is different and what the basic expectations are. The nurse offers simple information regarding daily routines, therapy sessions, other activities, how families can reach the patient by telephone, mealtimes, visiting hours, policies on drug and alcohol usage, laundry facilities, and a brief overview of the program. In this way, the nurse can help to allay some of the anxiety of the patient and the family.

Visiting hours in a rehabilitation setting often begin later than in an acute hospital so that the patient is not distracted from therapies. This change may create anxiety for the family member who has been at the patient's bedside all day in the general hospital. Allowing family members to visit other than at the scheduled time affords them the opportunity to become more familiar with staff members and helps to eliminate some of the fear that stems from not knowing what is happening. The presence of a familiar person can be a great comfort to a patient during this difficult transition period.

It should be explained that the patient has been transferred to this new setting in order to relearn self-care, but meanwhile the staff will provide care. Families need to know that in most instances the patient will be given day passes away from the setting after they learn how to care for the patient. Families also need to be told how and when they will learn what they need to know to provide the care.

INITIAL ASSESSMENT

A nursing interview and assessment based on the patient's physical, psychological, and social history provide the information necessary for development of the initial plan of care. Whenever possible, information is obtained from the patient so that the nurse can gain insight into how the patient perceives effects of the injury.

The following areas may serve as guidelines for the admitting nurse.

General Information What is the patient's account of the injury and course of treatment up to this point? Is the patient on any medications? What are they? How often are they taken? Is there a history of allergies? Has there been a recent infection? Are there other medical problems such as diabetes or respiratory or cardiovascular problems?

Skin Care What is the general condition of the skin surface, nails, and hair? Is there a bedsore? Are there limb contractures? What is the patient's current turning schedule? How is he or she positioned?

Bladder Care If there is an indwelling catheter, what is the size and when was it last changed? If intermittent catheterization is being used, how frequent are the catheterizations? What is the amount of urine obtained; what is the residual? Has the patient been receiving bladder irrigations? If so, how often and with what solution? Is the male patient wearing an external catheter? If so, what type is it? Has the patient experienced any problems with the bladder program? What is the character of the patient's urine?

Bowel Care What is the nature and frequency of the current program? What time of day is the program given? Has the patient had any problems with constipation, diarrhea, or hemorrhoids? When was the last bowel movement?

Respiratory Care Has the patient had any respiratory problems before or since the injury? Does the patient have a tracheostomy? Is assistance required to mobilize secretions, or can the patient cough? Has a respiratory program been established?

Functional Abilities Is the patient able to assist with dressing, feeding, hygiene? If so, does the patient require any special equipment to perform the activity? Has the patient been involved with bowel or bladder care?

Nutrition What is the current diet? Are there special food or fluid preferences? What is the amount of fluid intake? What is the patient's normal weight? Has there been a significant weight gain or loss? Are there any special eating problems? Does the patient wear dentures?

Sexual History Was the patient sexually active prior to the injury? When was the female patient's last menstrual period? Has she used contraceptives? If so, what kind? In the case of a preadolescent female, has menstruation begun? Has the male patient had an erection since the injury? Is there a history of penile discharge? Has anyone discussed sexual options with the patient?

Psychological History The psychological history includes a brief description of the behavior the patient exhibits at the time of admission. Because the admission process is for most persons a stressful experience, the observations made by the nurse may provide insight into how the patient will respond to stress in the future. Although the information is very difficult to elicit at admission, efforts should be made to learn about previous coping patterns.

Social History The social history includes the patient's family structure. If the patient is an adult, was he or she employed? What was the nature of the work? With a younger patient, it is important to obtain information about schooling. The nurse should also inquire about the patient's avocational interests.

Family Involvement The involvement of family members and friends is crucial to the rehabilitation process and should be encouraged. As the program progresses, it will be necessary to have one or two persons come in to attend therapy and learn physical care of the patient. Family members may become anxious about the amount of time that they will need to spend away from work or home. The nurse should try to reassure them that work and home responsibilities will be considered as much as possible when their involvement in the patient's program is planned. If family members cannot visit on a regular basis, the nurse can, at the time the patient is admitted, introduce family members to members of the team who are available. Also, the names of staff members and their phone numbers should be offered to the family.

DEVELOPING A PLAN OF CARE

As the nurse makes an initial assessment and introduces the patient and family to the setting, the nurse will begin to establish and implement an initial care plan.

Early Bowel Care

The majority of spinal cord–injured patients have no sensation of a full bowel and no ability to exert control over the anal sphincter. Therefore, a structured program is devised for the management of stool elimination and the control of incontinence.

In many institutions, management of bowel routines has been delegated by the physician to the professional nurse. The success of the patient's bowel program depends in large measure on the nursing plan, the patient's cooperation, and the nurse's subsequent surveillance and evaluation. It is possible to develop a plan for the patient with spinal cord injury that eliminates bowel accidents, can be managed in a reasonable time span, and is physiologically sound.

What may seem to be a relatively insignificant part of the total patient-care plan for other patient populations looms very large when the alternatives to a managed bowel program for the spinal cord injured are considered. Bowel accidents are tantamount to social disaster. Incontinence is associated with infants or with the old and the infirm.

The nurse's asssessment of the patient's stool elimination patterns must take into account previous bowel habits, life-style, eating habits, and present neurologic levels.

To develop a plan of action, the nurse first determines a consistent time interval for evacuations. Initially the patient is placed on a daily program that will assist in establishing a pattern. The nurse can then determine which position is best for the patient to have an evacuation. In the early stages of spinal cord injury, the lack of spinal stability is a consideration. The patient may have to have the bowel program in the recumbent position because of the lack of stability or because of poor sitting posture.

Bedpans are to be avoided at all costs; instead, incontinent pads should be used to contain the stool. Because the patient now has skin that is insensitive to pressure, the danger of developing sores is greatly increased. A quadriplegic patient who is transferred from a general hospital may have a perfect ring around the buttocks from sitting on a bedpan all night. Any reference to incontinent pads as diapers should be avoided by nursing staff and families. It is easy enough to infantilize the care required by a very dependent patient without labeling it that way.

It may be difficult to determine a suitable time for the bowel program. Demands on the patient's time are made for therapies, clinical appointments, visitors, and recreational trips. The great portion of nursing care, including management of bowel programs, is usually given in the evening to accommodate the demands of therapies.

This imporant aspect of the care of the patient with spinal cord injury requires consistency and sufficient time if the bowel program is to be successful. In many settings the nurse has the freedom to develop and carry out a plan but in others must consult with the physician before instituting any program. Generally, bowel programs for spinal cord–injured patients consist of bisacodyl suppositories administered against the wall of the rectum. The anal sphincter is gently stimulated by a gloved finger. Medications such as stool softeners or peristaltic stimulants may be required, although ideally the stool consistency will be managed by proper diet and fluids.

The effectiveness of the bowel program can be evaluated only if accurate records are kept. (See Fig. 24-1 for a sample of one type of bowel record sheet.) In evaluating the program, the nurse looks for an absence of bowel accidents and a minimum or absence of such problems as constipation, diarrhea, and fecal impaction. A plan to correct problems as they occur is implemented with the approval of the physician. Many of the problems can be managed with dietary changes or with different time intervals.

The records should be kept by the auxiliary nursing staff members who give the care but they should be supervised by the professional nurse. Unreported absences of evacuations can lead to severe impactions with the consequence for the patient of a series of cleansing enemas, missed therapies, soiled clothing, and general malaise. The plan for the patient's bowel routines is recorded on the nursing-care plan or bowel record, according to the policies of the institution.

Early Bladder Care

Urinary tract management is the single most important aspect of the care of the spinal cord–injured person. The greatest incidence of morbidity and mortality in the spinal cord population occurs because of diseases of the urinary tract (Pearman and England, 1973). It is of utmost importance that the nurse and the physician develop a plan of care to eliminate or minimize this health hazard and that they work closely with the patient to develop a long-range plan for preventive health maintenance.

In making the initial assessment, the nurse considers the neurological status, the present method of management, the patient's medication regimen, the patient's willingness and ability to take fluids, and the physical characteristics of the urine. The type of bladder management program used initially reflects the philosophies or practices of the institution.

A sound understanding of the anatomy and physiology of the urinary tract, as well as an understanding of the various methods that may be used to manage urinary tract care of the spinal cord–injured person, is essential. Insertion of an indwelling catheter for the spinal cord–injured person is perhaps the oldest, most widely used method of management in this country. In England, however, intermittent catheterization under strict aseptic technique has long been practiced by Guttman (Abramson, 1976). This method of draining the bladder has become more widespread in this country over the past decade. Modifications of the technique have included the clean technique developed by Lapides (1974) at the University of Michigan and the sterile no-touch technique used by Lindan (1975) in Ohio.

Attempts at developing or encouraging reflex-type voiding rarely succeed at first because of the areflexic or spinal shock state most patients are in at the time of injury. This areflexic state can be expected to subside within the first 3 months.

When the patient arrives at the rehabilitation facility, changes may be made in the management of urinary care. For example, an intermittent catheterization program may be used rather than an indwelling catheter. The patient needs to be reassured that the nurse and the physician will continue to monitor urinary tract care.

The patient's care plan focuses on maintenance of a healthy urinary tract. At this time, although there is the possibility of an infection, the urinary tract is probably healthy and intact except for the problems that exist because of motor and sensory losses (inability to recognize a full bladder and to control the sphincter).

Even though the patient may not have a total grasp of the problems, he or she should be included in the development of the care plan, especially those parts that require active involvement. The nurse finds out what fluids the patient likes, when to offer them, and how much to give at one time. The patient can learn to become aware of urine quantity and quality. Initially, quantity will be monitored by accurate intake and output. Recognition that certain urine characteristics, such as clarity and a lack of odor, are healthy should assist the patient in learning to make judgments when problems do occur.

Initial bladder management routines for male and female spinal cord–injured patients are the same. Alternative methods for the two sexes are covered in a later section.

Meticulous hygiene habits are essential to good health. Hands should be washed before and after each bladder procedure, including manipulation or emptying of collecting devices. The wearing of gloves may be necessary to control the spread of infections. Staff members and patients need to be taught how to handle urinary equipment to avoid contamination of those parts that are to remain sterile. Good perineal hygiene habits decrease the risk of ascending urinary tract infections. Female patients are especially prone to infections because of the short urethras and the closeness of the urethra to the vaginal and anal orifices.

Development of an evaluation tool is not as simple for urinary care as it is for bowel management. Periodic laboratory checks of urine

Figure 24-1
Bowel Program Record. *(Used with the permission of the Rehabilitation Institute of Chicago.)*

REHABILITATION INSTITUTE OF CHICAGO
BOWEL PROGRAM

Patient's Name Plate

MEDICATION _____

___ Prune Juice   ___ Digital Stim.
___ Dulcolax Supp.   ___ Toilet _____ Chux
___ Glycerine Supp.   ___ Spontaneous

DATE	PROGRAM		EVAC. TIME	FACILITY USED	STOOL TYPE			STOOL AMT.			SUP.AD.		REMARKS
	METHOD	TIME			L.	S.	H.	S.	M.	L.	S.	A.	

L=Liquid   S=Small   S=Self
S=Soft   M=Medium   A=Assist.
H=Hard   L=Large

BOWEL

455   SPINAL CORD INJURY: POSTACUTE PHASE

and renal function tests, such as blood urea nitrogen (BUN) and serum creatinines, are needed as well as radiologic studies. The nurse can monitor the urinary tract by observing urine quality and quantity.

One phenomenon related to urinary output, although it occurs infrequently, is worth discussing. Some patients may take their usual amount of fluids during the daytime but have very little daytime urinary output. They do not become edematous, nor do they seem to be in any distress. Diuresis often occurs after they have been put to bed. The cause is unknown at this time but possibly may be vasomotor instability. The condition may present problems such as nocturnal autonomic dysreflexia and unobserved nocturnal bladder distention.

Early Skin Care

At the time the spinal cord–injured person is admitted, the nurse designs a program that promotes and maintains skin integrity. The plan should be simple enough to be managed eventually by the patient and the family.

Because of impaired motion and sensation, the skin is vulnerable to many types of problems, including pressure sores, edema, burns, frostbite, and rashes. The most hazardous of these problems, pressure sores, do not just happen but are the result of prolonged pressure over one area.

Factors to be considered when a care plan is developed are the patient's present skin condition, limb contractures, general body type, age, and limitations in mobility. If a sore has already developed, the patient needs to be positioned in such a way as to avoid pressure on the area until it has healed. If the patient is experiencing pain or is very debilitated, it may be necessary to avoid certain positions or limit the time spent in them.

The initial plan should alert staff to the presence and management of existing skin problems as well as outline a turning and positioning regimen. For most patients, a schedule that requires changing positions every 2 h is advisable. After each turn, skin surfaces should be checked for any signs of redness. It is not uncommon for skin over the bony prominences to be somewhat pink; however, this should resolve within 30 min once pressure is relieved. If it does not, that position should be avoided until there is no further sign of redness. It is essential that good lighting be used when skin checks are performed. When redness persists, gentle massage around but not over the area of redness helps. Areas of unresolved redness must be checked frequently because they will develop into pressure sores if not managed correctly.

Many newly injured spinal cord patients wear an external spine-stabilizing device. For quadriplegic patients this is some type of cervical orthosis; for the paraplegic patient it is a trunk support. When skin inspections are made, the skin areas covered by these devices must not be neglected. On the patient unit, only a nurse, with the physician's permission, may remove a brace. If the patient is wearing a halo cast, it is generally possible to check the skin surfaces under the cast if a flashlight is used.

Developing a Turning Schedule The old cliche about individualizing care plans has merit once again as attempts are made to develop a plan for sitting, turning, and positioning. Daily activities, personal preferences, pain, and mobility orders should all be considered. With all positions, it is essential that spinal alignment be maintained. The patient may be allowed to be upright or may be restricted to lying flat. Early in the patient's program, the most common positions are side lying and back lying (see Fig. 24-2 and Fig. 24-3). Prone lying is generally medically contraindicated until the spine has stabilized.

Wheelchair Sitting Initially the patient's wheelchair time should be limited to 1 to 2 h. If the patient has very sensitive skin or is debilitated, a shorter period is advisable. If, after sitting, the patient has any ischial or sacral redness that does not resolve within 30 min, sitting should be discontinued until the redness disappears. Sitting is then resumed for a shorter period of time. Skin should be checked after each sitting. As the patient's condition stabilizes, it is necessary to

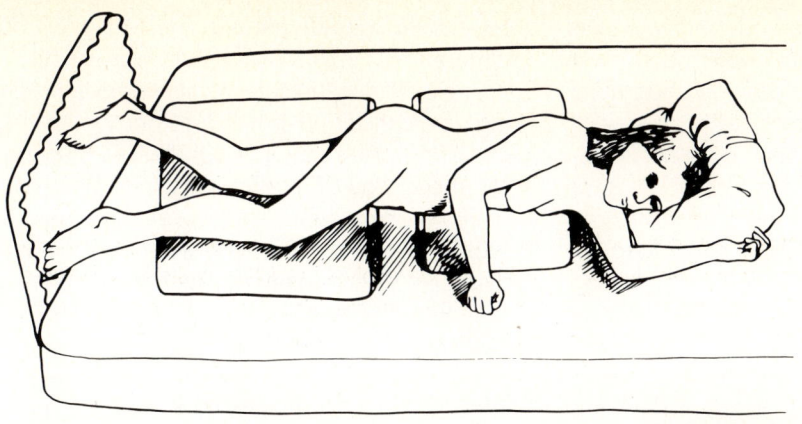

Figure 24-2
Positioning on side: bridging. *(Used with the permission of the Rehabilitation Institute of Chicago.)*

upgrade skin tolerance and adjust schedules according to the person's needs after discharge.

Early Respiratory Care

The development of a plan of care for managing the respiratory problems of the spinal cord–injured person relates directly to the level of injury and to the amount of injury to the respiratory tract. If the spinal cord lesion is above the C3 to C4 neurological level, there is an interruption in innervation to all of the musculature involved in respiration. Initial emergency needs will probably have already necessitated a tracheostomy and the implementation of some mechanical breathing device.

Persons with complete injuries to the cervical level above the third vertebra rarely survive. The need for ventilatory assistance at the scene of the accident is so acute, recognition of the problem so rare, and skilled personnel so infrequently available that most persons die almost immediately.

Patients with injuries at the third and fourth cervical level may have interruption to the innervation of the diaphragm via the phrenic nerve. At this point, innervation to all other respiratory musculature has been interrupted, so it is critical to maintain a patent airway and to prevent further trauma to the cord and the phrenic nerve by maintaining good alignment of the vertebral column. Respiratory involvement

Figure 24-3
Positioning on back: bridging. *(Used with the permission of the Rehabilitation Institute of Chicago.)*

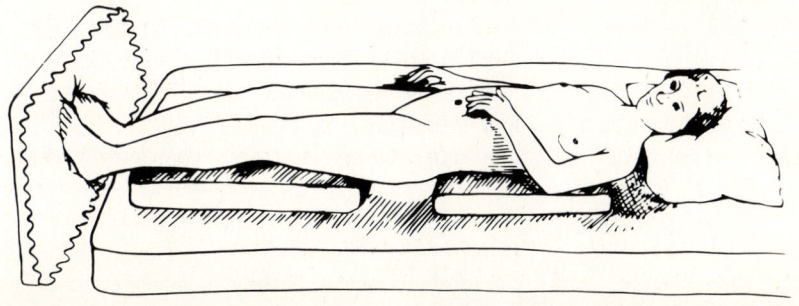

457   SPINAL CORD INJURY: POSTACUTE PHASE

from the C5 to C6 level and below occurs because of mild to moderate impairment of the musculature of the rib cage and the abdominal muscles. More severe respiratory embarrassment, with actual tracheal damage, may occur because of piercing injuries such as gunshot or stabbing wounds. Respiratory embarrassment may also occur as a result of severe spinal column misalignment or displacement, causing pressure against the trachea.

Respiratory involvement in patients with spinal cord injuries lower than the cervical area is more likely to be directly related to trauma to the chest cavity rather than to impaired innervation. Rib fractures, pneumothorax, or piercing injuries to the chest may make surgical procedures, drainage tubes, and nasopharyngeal suction necessary.

Frequently, patients are ready for physical upgrading or a rehabilitation program long before they are freed of respiratory problems. It is certainly best for the patient to attain some degree of respiratory stability before entering a rehabilitation program. A vital capacity below 500 mL does not allow for much active participation in a program of physical upgrading. The need for endotracheal suction more often than once an hour limits a patient's endurance and ability to participate in an aggressive program. The need for continuous oxygen therapy or for continous ventilatory support may or may not prevent a patient's admission into a rehabilitation program.

If a patient with respiratory problems is to be admitted, the facility must be able to provide adequate respiratory care, and staff should be able to articulate reasonable goals the patient might achieve. Provisions for maintenance of a patent airway, adequate gaseous exchange, and freedom from infectious organisms are essential.

If 24-h-a-day surveillance is required for maintenance of a patent airway, this must be provided. If the patient can call for help or clear secretions, this ability is built into the care plan.

Adequate gaseous exchange requires close monitoring of physical signs and blood gases, in addition to measurement of the respiratory parameters.

Guaranteeing an infection-free environment may be difficult. It must be remembered that one of a nurse's major responsibilities is controlling the spread of infectious disease. Meticulous respiratory hygiene techniques are mandatory to avoid cross-contamination between patients. Staff members with respiratory infections should not work with these patients.

Although in most larger clinical facilities respiratory therapy departments provide care, the nurse needs to gain skills in postural drainage and chest physiotherapy, including percussion, vibration, and cupping. Because sufficient bony healing may not have taken place and the rigors of aggressive postural drainage or chest physiotherapy can cause additional trauma to the spine, alternatives may have to be considered.

One technique to be learned by all persons who care for spinal cord–injured persons is that of assistive coughing. Effective coughing occurs because of increased pressure caused by contraction of abdominal muscles and subsequent elevation of the diaphragm. The nurse externally provides that pressure for the spinal cord patient. The nurse applies both hands with fingers spread wide to the anterior lower rib cage, then exerts pressure as the person coughs; this usually assists in mobilizing secretions (see Fig. 24-4). Pressure can also be applied over the abdomen to assist in coughing. Splints, binders, or pillows can be used against the diaphragm if these measures increase patient comfort.

Phrenic Nerve Stimulators

When persons with high cervical injuries C1 to C3 survive the acute phase of treatment, decisions must be made about long-term respiratory management. These patients, at least at first, are invariably dependent on some form of mechanical ventilation.

In a few centers, surgically implanted phrenic-nerve stimulators or pacemakers have been used with the high quadriplegic patient (Vander-Linden et al., 1974). Electrodes are implanted bilaterally over the phrenic-nerve innervation to

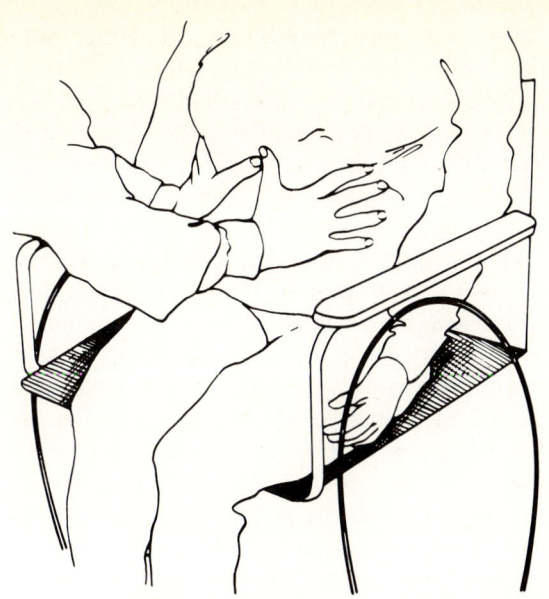

Figure 24-4
Assistive coughing. *(Used with the permission of the Rehabilitation Institute of Chicago.)*

the diaphragm. Following a period of healing, about 2 weeks, the electrodes and the phrenic nerve are stimulated by an external transmitter. Initially, the patient may not tolerate more than 5 min of diaphragmatic stimulation at a time. Ultimately, tolerance may be increased sufficiently for the patient to tolerate wearing the stimulator for 12 h on either side of the diaphragm. Removing the stimulator from one side and placing it on the other side of the diaphragm allows half of the diaphragm to rest.

Nursing care following the period of adjustment to the stimulator is relatively simple. Adequate oxygenation and maintenance of a patent airway are of critical importance. The transmitters consist of boxes that resemble transmitter radios. Attached to these transmitters are circular antennae that are taped over the area of the implanted electrodes. During the time each particular transmitter is turned off, skin surfaces under the antennae should be inspected daily for excoriation.

A regular schedule is maintained for switching the antennae from one side to the other. If the units are battery powered (usually by a 9-volt battery), a regular schedule for battery changes is set up. Education of all staff is critical. The nurse must be on the alert for faulty equipment and have a plan for replacement or repair. Nursing staff and therapists need to check the antennae to make certain they have not come loose after transfers and therapies. An Ambu bag with necessary adapters must be available at all times. Other aspects of the patient's care are no different from those for any other patient with chronic respiratory problems.

Phrenic-nerve stimulator implants allow considerable freedom. Patients may even gain mobility via a mouth- or tongue-controlled wheelchair. This is a rather remarkable degree of independence compared with the umbilicallike existence of a patient tied to a respirator. Although at this time only a small number of phrenic stimulators have been implanted, it is likely many more will be implanted in the future.

Early Supportive Emotional Care

Spinal cord injury is one of the most devastating physical insults a human can experience. The injury produces results that are immediate, are often irreversible, and affect all aspects of the person's life. Alterations in the ability to move about or to function within the family unit have a direct effect on emotional state. The need to depend on others for the simplest tasks of living can be profoundly depressing.

The professional staff should be open, honest, and realistic about the type of injury, yet never completely take away hope for recovery. How does one communicate to a patient that he or she will never walk again? A detailed neurological examination and/or surgical inspection of the cord allow the attending physician to form a prognosis. If the injury is permanent and irreversible, the patient is told that ambulation may never be possible. This provokes responses from the patient and the family that range from anger to profound disbelief. Yet it is important that they be given this information, and, in fact, they have a right to hear it.

Successful rehabilitation depends largely on the patient's ability to adjust psychologically. The efforts of the treatment team are meaningless if the spinal cord–injured patient is not able to regain the sense of being a worthwhile human being.

It is not possible to discuss fully in this chapter the complex psychological problems of the person with a spinal cord injury. However, some of the more critical periods during the initial process of rehabilitation will be discussed briefly.

The patient's first day of therapy can be overwhelming. Most likely this is the first time the patient has worn street clothes since the injury. Clothing may fit poorly if the patient has lost a great deal of weight. The patient may begin to realize that this is what life will be like when he or she is issued a wheelchair.

The patient is encouraged to participate actively in self-care as soon as general condition and physical abilities make this possible. Again, the patient is struck with how dependent he or she is. The eagerness to achieve may begin to fade. "Why should I bother to try to feed myself when it takes an hour and the food just gets colder?" "What difference does it make if I dress myself if it takes forever?"

The utmost patience is required of staff working with patients at this time. It may be difficult for staff members to stand by while the patient struggles to learn to hold a toothbrush or to pick up a piece of silverware or to do a wheelchair transfer, but their feelings cannot begin to compare with the frustration the patient experiences. Gentle encouragement is needed constantly. Never should the patient sense that staff members are impatient. It is necessary to reassure the patient that the job was done well and to remind the patient that it will take time to master these skills.

It is not uncommon for patients to become angry and depressed over their struggles. They may become belligerent and demand that staff provide the care, or they may become withdrawn and verbally abusive to those around. At this time, the nurse needs to help the ancillary staff working with the patient to realize that this type of response is not unusual in light of what the patient is experiencing. Without a basic understanding of the grieving process and help in gaining insight into the patient's behavior, staff members may begin to personalize the patient's responses and get into power struggles with the patient.

It is common for visiting patterns to change once the patient enters the rehabilitation setting. There may be a deluge of well-meaning friends who did not visit in the acute setting. The patient then must cope with griefstricken looks and awkward periods of silence from persons not seen since before the injury. Sometimes a patient feels abandoned by family and close friends who visited regularly in the acute-care hospital but now come less and less frequently.

The nurse needs to be aware of the effect these sessions have on the patient. Prolonged visits can be physically exhausting and anxiety-provoking if the patient is not comfortable with the visitors. It may be necessary for the nurse to suggest limiting the length of visits and the number of visitors. By observing the quality of interactions during visits and patient responses after visiting hours, the nurse gains insight into how the patient and the family may be coping with the disability. Is the patient an active participant in conversations? Do conversations merely take place around the patient because the patient is not able to put others at ease? Do family and friends spend more time away from the patient because they are uncomfortable?

The challenge to the professional staff working with these patients is an enormous one. The glib, empty phrase often found on nursing care plans, "Provide emotional support to patient and family," takes on special meaning when the professional considers the permanence of the injury. Patients and families need much gentle assistance to work through their feelings of loss and at the same time begin making necessary adjustments in life-styles.

Functional Abilities

Although a goal of the rehabilitation program is the achievement of maximal independence, it is not necessary to stress participation in functional activities, e.g., feeding, dressing and hygiene, in the initial nursing-care plan. Because the patient may not have a stabilized spine and because mobility and agility may be impaired by a cumbersome orthosis, upgrading of functional skills may need to be delayed until bony healing occurs.

Provided the patient has some degree of hand function, certain tasks can be done initially. Oral and facial hygiene and feeding require very little torque on the spine. However, dressing, transfers, and positioning activities are not advisable for the patient with a healing spine.

Even a person with little hand function can be allowed some measure of independence. The wise nurse recognizes the importance of teaching the person the components of care as soon as possible. Also, direction must be given to the persons providing care.

The nurse, on the basis of an assessment of physical capabilities and the neurologic lesion, will have determined the activities in which the patient may be able to participate, and will share that information with the patient. It is necessary to establish demands that are not overwhelming.

Family members must be involved in this part of the plan so they can be supportive of the patient's present goals. It may not be easy to communicate to families that initial unsuccessful attempts to develop some independent skills are ultimately in the patient's best interest. The tendency to mother or infantilize dependent patients is strong and perhaps develops out of pity at seeing a once-active person incapable of handling self-care. Families, visitors, and staff may all be tempted to do too much. However, the nurse must recognize that at times it is perfectly acceptable to give the care a patient can do independently. The skill comes in knowing when to stand back and when to provide the care.

Mobility

Until the physician writes wheelchair mobility orders, certain precautions are taken to ensure that further trauma does not occur to the spinal cord. If the institution does not have a policy for the immediate management of new patients, the following guidelines can apply until specific mobility orders have been written.

The patient is positioned supine in bed. When turning, the patient can be logrolled to one side or the other by three to four staff members. Strict attention is paid to maintaining alignment of the spinal column. A small pillow or folded bath blanket may be used to support the head. A spinal orthosis, if the patient is wearing one, is not to be removed.

Having basic guidelines that are applicable to all patients with a recent history of spinal cord trauma eliminates staff confusion and decreases the risk of further injury.

Lack of wheelchair mobility orders need not mean that the patient is confined to bed. The patient may be transferred, by a three- or four-person lift, to a cart to attend therapies or to visit outside the room. Most patients feel more secure if placed on a cart with side rails. However, a cart without rails suffices if staff members make certain that the patient does not fall by placing safety straps across the knee, waist, and chest areas.

Because of spinal instability, poor trunk balance, and the possibility of orthostatic hypotension, most patients begin sitting activities in a reclining wheelchair. Before transferring the patient into a reclining chair, staff must make certain that the wheelchair's angle-adjustment bolts are tightened securely so that the back of the chair does not drop when the patient is transferred. The paraplegic patient with a body cast or brace may not be able to tolerate sitting upright at 90° because of the pressure of the orthosis over the iliac crest and suprapubic areas. However, it may be possible to cut away the lower portion of a plaster body cast to allow the patient to sit upright.

As spinal stability increases and trunk balance improves, the patient becomes ready for a standard wheelchair. Certain patients, especially those with high cervical injuries, may need a high-backed chair for additional head and shoulders support. An electric reclining wheelchair permits the patient with minimal function to independently propel the chair and to alter position by changing the angle of sitting.

For patients with questionable judgment or poor trunk balance, a seat belt is needed to guarantee safety. Additional precautions such as lateral trunk supports and a chest strap may be necessary for those patients who have little or no trunk balance.

TEACHING PLAN

The development of a comprehensive teaching plan outlining those aspects of physical care that are to be learned or relearned is a basic nursing function. The purpose of a teaching plan is twofold: to prepare the patient and family for home passes and to prepare for the patient's discharge. For the plan to be effective, it must be tailored to the individual needs of each patient. The nurse actively involves the patient in the development of the plan. One nurse assumes responsibility for assessing the patient's needs, devising the plan, and teaching the patient. However, the nurse may delegate specific areas of teaching to another staff member. Current teaching goals are detailed in the patient's care plan. This information alerts staff members to the teaching method for the patient and tells them how to reinforce the patient's learning.

The first step in setting up a teaching plan is determining the patient's physical needs, that is, bowel, bladder, and skin. The need for specific teaching in other areas, such as respiratory, is dictated by the patient's level of injury. The nurse needs to know about the patient's functional abilities so as not to erroneously encourage a skill that the patient is unable to perform. Last, the nurse needs to have some idea of the patient's intellectual capabilities. The ultimate goal is for the patient to manage or direct care. However, it may be necessary to begin teaching a spouse or parent if the patient is unable or unwilling to learn.

When determining teaching needs, the nurse considers what the patient has already learned. If the patient has started self-bladder irrigations, that skill should be reinforced as soon as possible. Existing physical complications may suggest that teaching be started around a specific problem. If the patient has a bedsore, the nurse might begin by teaching skin care. If the patient is having respiratory difficulties, it may be appropriate to teach the patient and family coughing and deep-breathing exercises. A specific goal such as a day or an overnight pass also determines areas to be taught. Generally speaking, the simpler aspects of care should be taught first, and as the patient's knowledge increases and confidence is gained in abilities, more complex material can be introduced. When incorporating new skills into the plan, the nurse arranges time with the patient for return demonstrations.

Patients express readiness to learn in several ways, e.g., by asking questions about their condition and about procedures, or by intently watching care that is being given. Family members' behavior also can reflect a patient's interest in learning care. They may initiate involvement in simple aspects of care, such as feeding or hygiene. They may remain in the patient's room when care is provided to observe or participate. Conversely, they may visit infrequently without giving any reason, or they may break teaching appointments.

Most of the teaching is informal, on a one-to-one basis, with the nurse explaining why and how procedures are done and why the various aspects of care are important. When it becomes evident that the patient is ready to become more actively involved in the learning process, the nurse needs to plan the most effective presentation of the material to make it easily understandable.

Because of the number of things that must be learned by the person with a spinal cord injury, it is suggested that the nurse work with a general guideline that can be modified according to each patient's needs. Following is an outline of areas that should be considered when a patient's teaching plan is designed. The list is not meant to be all-inclusive. More attention will need to be paid to some aspects of care and less to others as the nurse formulates a plan for each patient.

1. Skin care
   a. Turning and positioning
      (1) Side
      (2) Prone
      (3) Supine
      (4) Bridging
   b. Wheelchair push-ups
   c. Skin checks
   d. Pressure sores
      (1) Cause
      (2) Prevention
      (3) Management
   e. Upgrading of skin tolerance
   f. Bathing
2. Bowel
   a. Suppository insertion
   b. Manual removal of stool
   c. Digital stimulation
   d. Signs of fecal impaction
3. Bladder
   a. Insertion of Foley or straight catheter
   b. Bladder irrigations
   c. Application of leg- and night-drainage bags
   d. Techniques to stimulate voiding
   e. Application of external catheter
   f. Symptoms and management of urinary tract infections
   g. Cleaning of urinary equipment
   h. Procurement of urinary equipment
4. Respiratory
   a. Deep-breathing exercises
   b. Assistive coughing
   c. Postural drainage
   d. Symptoms and management of chest congestion
   e. Care of respiratory equipment
5. General
   a. Symptoms and management of hypotension
   b. Symptoms and management of autonomic dysreflexia
   c. Taking temperatures
   d. Management of dependent edema
   e. Management of spasticity
   f. Application and care of antiembolic hose
   g. Range-of-motion exercises
   h. Care of special cushions or mattresses

If the patient is fearful about certain procedures, the nurse might consider first demonstrating on a mannequin. For the patient who does not appear to have a good understanding of how the body functions, it is helpful to use simple diagrams to explain basic anatomy and physiology. Before giving printed material to a patient, the nurse needs to have some idea of the patient's reading abilities. Group teaching is useful for presenting basic topics such as skin care and bowel and bladder function, although the nurse must still individualize teaching around the patient's specific needs. Audiovisual aids may also be helpful in teaching certain aspects of care. It is impossible to recommend any one approach because the needs of each patient are unique. What must be remembered is that the type of plan formulated by the nurse can enhance or inhibit the patient's learning.

The assessment of learning is an ongoing process. During teaching sessions, the nurse takes cues from the patient's facial expressions. Does the patient say he or she understands the material, yet look confused? Does the patient ask questions? Does the patient initiate follow-through with newly learned skills or need to be reminded? Is the patient able to remember material when questioned later?

It may be more difficult to evaluate the caregiving abilities of family members. Certainly the nurse can gather some information when the patient returns from a pass. If the patient's skin is in good condition, it may be assumed that turning and positioning routines were followed. If the skin is not in good condition, it is obvious that for some reason regimens were not followed. Even though family members actively participate in the patient's care during an occasional weekend, it is difficult to evaluate their ability to deliver care at home under a variety of circumstances. If expectations are not specified at the beginning of the program and reinforced throughout, family members may become passive observers rather than active participants.

Finally, the nurse must remember that not all patients and families are willing or able to learn all aspects of care. Occasionally, families are unwilling to learn cathererization. They may be fearful of harming the patient, or they may find the task distrasteful. A person may be helped to overcome these feelings; however, if this is not possible, other options must be considered. Most community nursing agencies can provide certain aspects of care for the patient. Before recommending such an agency, the nurse must be familiar with the particular service offered by various agencies. In time the patient and family may find it more practical to learn the care rather than to be dependent on someone else.

CARING FOR THE PERSON WHOSE SPINE HAS STABILIZED

INCREASED STABILIZATION AND MOBILITY

When the spine has stabilized, the patient needs to be weaned from the orthosis. This is done gradually in order to prevent undue strain on the muscles of the involved area.

For most patients the period following removal of the orthosis can be a traumatic one. Often the patient believes that, as the spine heals, function will return. Therefore, when stabilization occurs and the orthosis is removed, it is not unusual for the patient to become depressed or angry and for staff to see regressive behaviors. The patient may begin to miss therapies and want to stay in bed all day. Those aspects of care that the person could manage independently may be neglected. There may be physical acting out or verbal abuse.

The patient and family must be helped to understand that this reaction is not unusual. If the patient loses interest in care, the nursing staff must assume responsibility for care until the patient is once again able to manage independently. Forcing self-care is often more harmful than helpful and may result in a power struggle that neither the patient nor the staff can win.

Rather than being depressed when the orthosis is removed, some patients are excited with their new freedom. As a result, they may become overzealous with certain aspects of care, mobility, and living in general. If not supervised closely, these patients could accidentally harm themselves.

Another response to removal of the orthosis is fear of further injury now that movement is no longer restricted. The patient becomes reluctant to participate in more aggressive activities. With gentle encouragement from staff, this hesitation can be overcome rather quickly. The concern, however, should not be minimized.

Once the orthosis is removed, activities are possible that were previously prohibited because of spinal instability or the presence of a brace. Lower extremity dressing can be started. Transfer techniques may be taught. The patient can assume a more active role during turning and positioning. More aggressive recreational activities can be included in the program.

IMPROVED PHYSICAL STATUS

As healing of the spinal cord occurs and the accompanying cord edema diminishes, reflex activity below the level of the lesion becomes noticeable. The return of reflex activity means the patient is recovering from the state called *spinal shock*. The period of spinal shock varies (Pierce and Nickel). Both somatic and automatic reactions are depressed during this time. Some reflexes may return within hours, others not for several weeks or even months. Not surprisingly, the first signs of reflex activity that produce motion of an extremity are usually interpreted by the patient and family as a sign of returning function, even though there is no voluntary control of that motion.

Now that the patient shows signs of physical progress that is directly related to recovery and the return of some neurological function or reflex activity, work can begin toward the finalization of care routines that will be used at home.

BOWEL PROGRAMS

In addition to the increase in reflex activity, the increased mobility allowed by a healing spinal column permits a patient to develop more normal patterns of bowel and bladder elimination. For example, patients may assume the sitting position for bowel movements, and urination may occur because of a reflex stimulated by a full bladder.

The patient's bowel program until this time has probably consisted of a bisacodyl suppository administered by the nursing staff every day or every other day, and most likely evacuations are still occurring on incontinent pads. The patient has probably not played a very active role in the management of the program, other than to eat the foods recommended by the nurse and to take medications at the prescribed interval. If the patient has not been involved, now is the time for more active participation. Patients and families must learn all the components of bowel program management.

Sitting for a bowel evacuation is, of course, physiologically natural in that it allows gravity and abdominal pressure to be utilized in passing the stool. As soon as a sitting posture can be assumed at 90° and a sitting tolerance of 1 to 2 h has been achieved, the patient needs encouragement to plan activities to allow time for sitting on a commode. This may mean that some social activities have to be curtailed and that rest periods must be planned prior to the time of the bowel program.

The use of a commode chair is recommended since most patients, because of poor trunk balance, cannot sit safely on a regular toilet seat. Various types of commode chairs are available. Some commodes come equipped with padded seats, which are certainly advantageous for desensitized skin. Most have wheels or casters which help mobility but not stability. Some are equipped with a portion of the seat cut out along the side to allow for self-insertion of a suppository, manual removal of stool, and perineal care. Some commodes can be rolled over a toilet seat; these often double as shower chairs. The type of chair best suited for the patient can be determined by the patient, the nurse, and the physical therapist.

The time chosen for the bowel program takes into consideration the patient's life-style. Utilizing the gastrocolic reflex is helpful in reducing the amount of time required for an evacuation. It may be best to have the program in the evening if a patient is a full-time student or employee with early morning deadlines. It may be necessary, if the patient is dependent on others for this aspect of care, to plan the bowel program for a time when assistance is available.

An active sexual life may lose some of its spontaneity if a major portion of time is spent in physical care activities. Because bowel care is such an intimate, yet basic function, the patient may not want to have the sexual partner provide the care, or the partner may not want to provide the care. For this function, the plan should be to engage the help of someone else if assistance is needed.

The frequency of evacuation in a well-controlled program varies from patient to patient. Some patients require an every-day program, while others may have an evacuation as seldom as every 3 days. A major goal of any program is an absence of bowel accidents and such problems as fecal impaction, diarrhea, and bowel-related dysreflexia. This requires the patient's utmost cooperation during the time a bowel routine is established. An experimentation with medications, timing, and diet that can be done in the hospital provides for a more successfully managed bowel program after the patient is discharged.

Stimulation of the anal sphincter may be necessary to allow sphincter relaxation and subsequent evacuation. Administration of a suppository may provide sufficient digital stimulation. More likely it will be necessary to stimulate the anal sphincter by gently rotating a well-lubricated gloved finger or a commercial digital stimulator around the anal opening for about 30 s.

If a suppository is inserted, lubrication usually is not required. The suppository must be inserted high into the rectum and against the wall of the rectal mucosa. Some suggest manual removal of stool found low in the rectum to facilitate insertion of the suppository. The suppository must make contact with the rectal wall in order to be effective.

The use of strong cathartic-laxative medications should be avoided as much as possible. Very strong laxatives increase the unpredictability of evacuation. Every attempt should be made to utilize natural products including fruit and fruit juices, high fiber vegetables, such as carrots and celery and whole grain breads, and cereals such as bran, granola, or whole wheat. When constipation is a problem, a methylcellulose product such as Metamucil that helps supply required bulk may be considered. A number of such products are available. A medication such as casanthranol helps stimulate peristaltic action. Other medications are stool softeners that consist of sodium or potassium dioctyl sulfosuccinate. Some medications combine two or three of these substances in one capsule.

Different procedures may have to be used in patients with atonic or areflexic bowels or lower motor lesions. Patients with such bowels are those with lumbar, sacral, or cauda equina lesions or other lower motor neuron disorders such as poliomyelitis. They have considerable difficulty in establishing a bowel program. If bisacodyl suppositories are ineffective, carbon dioxide suppositories may work. It might be necessary to use low enemas or to manually remove the stool on a regular basis. The same dietary recommendations are made and the same medications are usually employed as for other spinal-injured patients.

Bowel Program Complications

Patients and families need to be taught the warning signs and management of bowel complications. Absence of stool following the usual mechanics of a bowel program may mean a high fecal impaction or severe constipation or both. The patient or caregiver should learn how to do a gentle rectal examination to determine if there is stool in the rectum. A small oil retention enema or other enema may be used, or it may only be necessary to remove the stool manually. Increasing fluid intake, perhaps including prune juice, and increasing the use of stool softeners are other options. The patient may need something a little stronger, such as bisacodyl orally, to initiate a bowel movement. The reasons for constipation should be explored. A new medication, a change in diet, a decrease in activity, or a febrile episode may have been contributing factors.

Autonomic dysreflexia, with its unpleasant symptoms, may result from a fecal impaction, inadequate evacuation, or simply stool in the rectum. This condition may also result from a distended bladder. The headaches, piloerection, anxious feelings, and slowed pulse are all indications of the very acute medical emergency that can affect the spinal cord–injured patient whose injury is above the level of T6.

Autonomic dysreflexia occurs when sensory transmitters ascend the spinal cord, signifying a full bladder or rectum, and reach the level of the lesion (Pearman and England). Because the message is interrupted at this point, impulses are transmitted to the autonomic nervous system, and an arteriolar spasm occurs in the skin and viscera. This sympathetic response is manifested by elevated blood pressure and profuse sweating. The elevated blood pressure is noted by receptors in the carotid sinus, which transmits impulses via the ninth and tenth cranial nerves to the vasomotor center in the brainstem, which in turn transmits impulses to the sinoatrial node on the heart. Bradycardia results. This is a compensatory mechanism meant to reduce the hypertension. However, as vasodilatation does not occur below the level of the lesion, the hypertension persists.

Any institution that is likely to treat patients with spinal cord injury needs to have a protocol indicating staff intervention in the event a patient experiences autonomic dysreflexia, as it is indeed a medical emergency. Often the nurse is the one who manages this emergency, as there may not be time to contact a physician. The symptoms must be immediately recognized and the cause explored.

The treatment for autonomic dysreflexia is simple; one merely eliminates the cause. A plugged catheter must be changed or a fecal impaction removed. Dysreflexia can occur when a leg bag is full, and, in turn, the bladder is distended. Whatever the cause, it must be corrected immediately. The patient will get some relief of the headache and hypertension if the head is elevated, although an analgesic may be required later. The hypertension and bradycardia normally subside when either the bladder or the rectum is emptied.

Patients and their families must receive a thorough explanation of autonomic dysreflexia and how to handle it. The patient may be encouraged to wear a Medic-Alert bracelet.[1] A written explanation of the phenomenon and its recommended treatment, carried by the patient in a wallet, is another option in the event the patient must enter an unfamiliar emergency room. Some families have been taught to take blood pressures and have been sent home with sphygmomanometers and stethoscopes, although this is probably not necessary. The other symptoms are so obvious that taking blood pressure may only delay treatment.

Most spinal cord–injured patients do not experience severe dysreflexia with normal bowel programs. The few who do may find that applying an anesthetic ointment such as dibucaine hydrochloride to the anal opening decreases the severity of the symptoms. However, the anesthetic ointment retards the action of the bisacodyl suppositories, thereby lengthening the time before evacuation. This method must be used only with physician approval. Severe, unrelenting dysreflexia may require management by other means, such as ganglionic blocking medication.

The presence of loose stools usually signifies one of two problems. Large, copious, loose stools probably mean diarrhea. Small, oozing stools often mean the presence of a fecal impaction. Again, the patient and family must be taught the importance of doing a rectal examination to help determine the cause, as obviously the treatment varies. Determining the cause of loose stools is important so the cause can be eliminated. Treatment for massive diarrhea requires some fluid, dietary, and possibly medication alterations.

Alternate Methods for Bowel Elimination

A few alternative methods can be employed in managing bowel routines. The regular use of enemas is not generally encouraged. One possibility is longer intervals between evacuations. Infrequently, one encounters a patient who has had a colostomy. This surgical procedure may have been done because of trauma to the colon at the time of the initial injury. In this case, the surgeons may later consider closure if there is minimal colonic injury.

The patient who has developed serious ischial or sacral-coccygeal pressure sores may have a temporary or permanent colostomy performed to eliminate contamination of the lower back, thereby promoting healing. At times patients prefer a colostomy because of ease in management. Occasionally, a colostomy is performed initially because someone has determined it will make life easier for the patient. Obviously, surgical intervention to achieve bowel control is a very drastic measure. It cannot be discounted because in rare situations it does have merit.

BLADDER MANAGEMENT PROGRAM

The type of long-term bladder management program a patient uses is jointly determined by the patient, the physician, and the nurse. Many factors are taken into consideration before the final plan is established. The health of the patient's urinary tract is determined before any decisions are made. Routine intravenous pyelogram and cystogram studies establish whether

---

[1] Interested staff and/or patients are encouraged to contact Medic-Alert Foundation International, Turlock, CA 95380, (209) 632-2371.

the structures of the urinary tract are disease-free; determination of serum creatinine and BUN levels also helps in the assessment of kidney function. A urinalysis and a test for culture and sensitivity determine whether any infection is present. Other factors that must be considered are the skills of the patient or the person who will be providing care, the availability of health-care facilities, and whether the patient is sufficiently reliable to maintain good techniques and follow-up regimes.

A 19-year-old paraplegic male was readmitted to a rehabilitation facility for general upgrading. During his stay the patient was placed on an intermittent catheterization program every 4 h. Initially the patient followed through well, catheterizing himself every 4 h and using sterile technique. Slowly the staff began noticing changes. The patient was not catheterizing himself every 4 h; often the time between catheterizations was 5 to 8 h, with an increased volume of urine output. Sterile technique gave way to whatever was convenient for the patient at the time.

When staff members talked with the patient, it became evident that he felt the program interfered too much with other activities. Discussions with the patient about the hazards of overdistending the bladder and the possibility of infection from sloppy technique made no difference. The patient, the physician, and the nurse together decided to reinsert an indwelling catheter until the patient felt he was ready to try intermittent catheterization again.

The economics of certain programs also need to be considered. For example, a patient on public assistance should not go home on an intermittent catheterization program using sterile disposable kits as, in all probability, public aid will not pay for the cost of disposable equipment.

Indwelling Urethral Catheters Long-term management with an indwelling catheter is probably best for those patients who are quadriplegic and must rely on others to provide care. Indwelling catheters decrease the probability of bouts of autonomic dysreflexia as well as providing continuous drainage and reducing the chance of pressure-induced reflux with subsequent hydronephrosis.

Until medical and nursing technology devises a suitable external collecting device for the female patient, the use of the indwelling catheter is the best option available. The need to transfer to a commode, in addition to managing clothing, makes reflex voiding for women too problematic to be practical in most cases. The use of long-term intermittent catheterization for female patients is rarely successful because of the awkwardness involved in positioning and the unsuitability of most female clothing for this technique.

Some women may elect, however, to be catheter-free. They manage leakage by using incontinent pads and waterproof panties. Even though their skin is continually wet, they can avoid maceration and excoriation by using petroleum-based skin preparations or any suitable waterproof barrier preparation.

An indwelling urethral catheter does present some management problems for the patient. The presence of a catheter provides a ready access to the bladder for bacteria; consequently, the urine is almost always infected. The anchoring balloon may be a precipitating factor in the formation of bladder calculi.

In males, the development of penile-scrotal fistulae is directly related to the use of an indwelling catheter. The fistulae can easily be prevented if the catheter is taped to the patient's abdomen, decreasing the urethral angle where this problem occurs. It is wise to tape the female patient's catheter to her thigh to lessen the chance of its accidentally pulling out, with the balloon then causing urethral damage.

Intermittent Catheterization Intermittent catheterization includes a variety of techniques that are being used quite widely as a means of emptying the bladder at regular intervals. Patients with areflexic bladders may remain on intermittent catheterization permanently. The method may be used effectively with patients who have dyssynergic bladders, which do not empty when full because of elevated sphincter pressure. Prior to the onset of reflex or spontaneous voiding, intermittent catheterization can be used to empty the bladder (Sperling, 1978; Perkash, 1978). As the methods and the objectives of intermittent catheterization vary from institution to institution and from patient to patient, the nurse must have a clear understanding of what the technique can or should achieve.

If intermittent catheterization is decided upon as the method of choice for long-term management, the nurse may wish to teach the patient the clean catheterization technique devised at the University of Michigan for home use (Lapides et al., 1974). Commercially available sterile catheter kits are really too expensive to be considered for long-term use.

Reflex Voiding When reflex voiding is the desired outcome, the physician closely monitors bladder pressure and sphincter-opening pressure. If the bladder pressure is considerably less than the sphincter pressure, bladder emptying is inadequate because of the excessive sphincter pressure. This causes residual urine to remain in the bladder. Residual urine is a good medium for bacterial growth and subsequent bladder infection. Various means are used to reduce the amount of residual urine. Medications such as bethanechol chloride, which provokes an autonomic response and may cause more complete bladder emptying, may be used. Diazepam may be prescribed if sphincter spasticity prevents the sphincter from relaxing and subsequent bladder emptying. Treating the bladder infection may reduce the amount of residual urine.

If all these interventions fail, the physician may recommend a surgical procedure called sphincterotomy. This procedure involves making one or more cuts in the internal sphincter. Some degree of sphincter pressure is reduced, thereby allowing more adequate emptying. The procedure does have some undesirable side effects. Most significantly, it may temporarily or permanently impair the male patient's ability to have an erection (Rosen, Nanninga, and O'Conor, 1973). Following the surgery, the patient wears an indwelling catheter. Some minimal bleeding can be expected. After a period of about 7 days, intermittent catheterization to reestablish the reflex voiding patterns is resumed.

External Urinary Collecting Devices Male patients whose bladder management program involves reflex voiding probably will prefer to use an external collecting device in order to decrease the possibility of urinary incontinence. Many different products are available. Disposable varieties are constructed of condoms or a similar rubber sheath. Adhesive or elastic tape can be used to hold the device in place. Because the use of elastic tape, or anything that encircles the penis, may have a tourniquet effect, the patient must apply the external catheter carefully so that circulation is not impaired. It is not uncommon for tapes to be applied so tightly that the penis becomes edematous and sores develop. In a few rare cases, gangrene has occurred, and the patients have had to undergo a partial amputation of the penis. By overlapping tape ends, the patient can eliminate this problem. All male patients must be instructed to check the skin of the penis daily to prevent the development of excoriations or sores.

Teaching the Patient Long-Term Bladder Management In developing a plan for long-term urinary tract management, the nurse must teach the patient to use the powers of observation. Normal, healthy urine is crystal clear, yellow, and free of unpleasant odor. Any variations should cause the patient to question why. Has fluid intake been adequate? Is there a possibility the urine is infected? If the patient has been instructed to maintain a certain urinary pH, he or she needs to be instructed to use a dipstick or Nitrazine paper to check the pH on a regular basis. Desirable pHs are thought to be in the acidic range, the rationale being that pathogenic bacteria do not grow in acidic media and calculi have less opportunity to form (Pierce and Nickel).

Grit in the indwelling catheter lumen or in the urine may indicate bladder calculi or the tendency to form them. The presence of mucous shreds probably indicates an infection. Urine that is pink-tinged or obviously bloody may be indicative of either calculi or infection. An unpleasant odor is often indicative of infection.

Although it is not necessary to maintain a strict, written record of intake and output, the patient must be able to determine if the amount of intake roughly equals that of the output, including insensible loss. This is especially important if the patient's catheter tends to plug or residual urine volumes are high.

The patient may be instructed by the physician to eat an acid ash diet in order to maintain an acid urine. This diet is high in protein and low in fruits except for cranberries and dried fruit. The eating of dairy products by the spinal cord patient is not so controversial as it once was (Hirschberg et al., 1976). At one point, dairy products were eliminated because they were believed to cause or contribute to the formation of bladder calculi by overloading the system with calcium. Now it is thought that a normal but not excessive amount of dairy products will not cause the patient to develop bladder calculi.

Maintenance urinary tract medications vary. Among the more common are those that increase urine acidity, such as ascorbic acid, methenamine mandelate, and hippuric acid. Acetic acid bladder irrigation also may be prescribed. Bactericides such as antibiotics or sulfonamides are used only in the presence of an infection.

A major part of health maintenance is follow-up care. The spinal cord–injured patient should have at least annual intravenous pyelograms and kidney function studies. It may be wise to have these studies done every 6 months for the first 2 years after injury. This is especially important for the patient who is catheter-free, as he or she may be experiencing some rather serious kidney problems but be completely asymptomatic (Nanninga, Rosen, 1976).

Alternative Methods of Bladder Management Some alternative methods of bladder management may be used for the spinal cord–injured patient. One relatively new method is the surgical implantation of electrodes in the sacral or voiding center of the spinal cord. When these electrodes are mechanically stimulated by the patient, voiding occurs. These implantations are still in the investigative stage.

Another method is a ureteroileostomy, also a surgical procedure. The ureters are implanted into a portion of the ileum that has been fashioned into a pouch and opens onto the abdomen. The urine is collected in an ostomy appliance. The indications for this procedure may be severe bladder-related autonomic dysreflexia or unmanageable urinary incontinence found in some female patients.

Suprapubic cystostomy may also be considered. Urinary drainage is managed by an indwelling catheter through the stoma. This catheter is usually of a larger diameter than a urethral catheter. The procedure is sometimes done as part of the treatment plan for penile-scrotal fistulae, when urinary drainage must be diverted from the urethra. It may also be used in female patients to avoid the use of a perineal catheter.

Autonomic Dysreflexia One of the most dramatic and bizarre problems related to spinal cord injury is the phenomenon known as autonomic dysreflexia or autonomic hyperreflexia. Autonomic dysreflexia occurs in those patients whose injury is at the T6 level or above. It is an autonomic reflex response to visceral distention (bowel or bladder) or stimulation of the skin. This phenomenon has been discussed in the section on bowel management but is mentioned again here because most often it is related to bladder distention or bladder instrumentation.

URINARY TRACT INFECTION

As was mentioned previously, the major cause of mortality in spinal cord injury patients is disease of the urinary tract (Pearman and England). Most of the disease processes either can be prevented or can be treated if caught early enough. Therefore, the nurse wants to be certain that the patient has a thorough understanding of potential urinary problems, how to prevent them, and the necessity for follow-up care. Because renal disease may be asymptomatic, it is an even greater hazard.

The most common urinary tract disease is infection. Although a bladder infection may not be life threatening, infections of the upper urinary tract can be. The body does have some defense mechanisms against urinary tract infections. The first defense is the mechanical washing of urine from the upper tract down. Urine is also thought to have some antibacterial qualities. The most important defense against upper tract infections is an intact vesicoureteral valve (Merritt, 1976). Damage to this valve, because of continued intravesicle pressure, high residual urines, or infrequent emptying of the bladder, and the presence of bacteria cause reflux of urine into the ureter. When this goes unchecked, the infection proceeds from ureteritis to hydroureter and hydronephrosis. Infections can be prevented or controlled by antibacterial medications, meticulous techniques during catheterizations or instrumentations, the giving and teaching of good perineal hygiene habits, the intake of adequate fluids, not allowing the bladder to overdistend, and maintenance of an acid urine.

RESPIRATORY PROGRAM

With increased mobility and improved vital capacity, the spinal cord–injured person is better able to handle secretions and is therefore less likely to develop severe respiratory problems. Because of partial or total paralysis of the respiratory muscles, patients with high cervical and thoracic lesions must learn new breathing techniques. For most patients this involves learning diaphragmatic and deep breathing as well as assistive coughing. Patients with high cervical lesions may need to be taught glossopharyngeal breathing to augment vital capacity. In addition, the caregiver of a person with known respiratory problems should be taught postural drainage, vibration, and percussion. All patients and their families should be cautioned to avoid persons with upper respiratory infections.

Although the physician directs the patient's respiratory program, the nurse needs to be familiar with exercises used for increasing vital capacity and mobilizing secretions. Once the patient has been taught, the nurse still is responsible for reinforcing these techniques daily on the patient unit. At the time of discharge, the patient and the family are instructed to continue with deep-breathing and assistive coughing exercises once or twice a day at home as a preventive measure.

The patient with a high cervical lesion is likely to require a tracheostomy. Depending on the level of the lesion, the patient may require part- or full-time ventilatory assistance. Respiratory care for the person with a tracheostomy includes suction to remove secretions, chest physical therapy and postural drainage to help loosen and mobilize secretions, intermittent positive pressure and deep-breathing exercises to expand the lungs, humidity to keep secretions moist, and oxygen therapy if hypoxia exists.

The feasibility of removing the tracheostomy tube is determined by the physician prior to discharge. As the respiratory status improves, switching to a fenestrated tube that allows use of the patient's own airway should be considered. The tracheostomy or a tracheal button may remain permanently if there is tracheal stenosis or if the patient cannot mobilize secretions adequately.

As the patient with a tracheostomy approaches discharge, the nurse assesses long-term manageability of the respiratory program. The nature and frequency of respiratory treatments need to be reviewed and attempts made to gradually wean the patient from treatments. If the patient is receiving intermittent positive pressure breathing treatments, consideration is given to decreasing frequency. If ultrasonic nebulization is being used, the patient may be tried on room humidity. Rarely is oxygen therapy needed at home. The pattern of suctioning should be evaluated. Would the patient be able to manage 6 to 8 h without suction during the night if aggressive chest therapy and suction were done just prior to bedtime? The time to experiment is when the patient is still in the hospital with trained personnel available to help if problems arise.

Respiratory Equipment

In addition to reviewing the program, the nurse determines what type of equipment is necessary for home use. For example, a suction machine may need to be ordered. Whenever possible, a portable machine should be obtained in addition to the regular unit. The portable unit can serve as a back-up in an emergency situation as well as allowing the patient the freedom to leave the house.

Suction catheters need to be ordered. The family needs to be taught how to clean the catheters because it is economically impractical to use a catheter only once. Equally important, but often overlooked, is how to clean and make minor repairs on the suction machine. Preferably the same type of equipment that is used for teaching will be ordered for the home. The family needs to know where to obtain extra supplies.

The ultimate goal for the patient is the prevention of respiratory complications. As awareness of breathing patterns increases, the patient is better able to recognize the signs of impending respiratory distress. With knowledge of respiratory techniques, the patient and the family can manage problems before they become critical. However, before weekend passes and ultimate discharge, options for emergency care must be discussed with the patient and the family.

SKIN AND HYGIENE

As mobility increases and endurance improves, the nurse begins to anticipate with the patient what the daily routines will be after discharge so that skin tolerance can be upgraded accordingly. Schedules have to be planned around the availability of the person who will care for the patient. Many patients can increase sitting tolerance sufficiently to allow for resumption of school or work schedules. Persons with sensitive skin may need to experiment with different types of equipment before a significant increase in sitting time becomes possible.

It is not possible to design a fixed schedule for repositioning. The patient's therapy schedule necessitates different positions for different programs, e.g., sitting up for activities of daily living and reclining in physical therapy for exercises. What is essential is that the family, the patient, the nursing staff, and the therapists know the position tolerance and that they share responsibility for seeing that the patient does not exceed the time in a certain position. If self-turns are possible, the staff must make certain that the patient actually does them. As the patient learns more about the program, staff members should encourage the individual to assume increased responsibility for alerting caregivers when it is time to change position.

Increasing Sitting Times The initial 2-h sitting schedule is increased in 30-min increments. If after several days there are no complications, the sitting time can be increased again. Although this approach may seem tedious, the patient is less likely to develop a pressure sore that would make sitting impossible. If at any time there is redness that does not resolve within 30 min, the patient should avoid sitting again until the skin is clear. Wheelchair push-ups and leaning from side to side are encouraged every 15 min as a means of relieving pressure (see Fig. 24-5 and Fig. 24-6).

The same plan can be used for upgrading the patient's turning schedule. It is unlikely that a turn every 2 h will be practical for the patient or family to manage over a long period. Therefore, the nurse and patient must work toward a schedule that will minimize the frequency of turns needed during the night. Certain positions can be maintained for longer periods of time if attempts are made to upgrade tolerance in those positions that are comfortable.

Prone Positioning Prone positioning may be tolerated by many patients for 6 to 8 h. Most patients are reluctant to assume the prone position because it limits their view of the surroundings and, for some, creates difficulties in signaling for help. When positioned properly, the patient may tolerate prone lying for longer periods of mine if the position can be tolerated. The patient needs to schedule rest periods according to evening activities. If at any point skin complications occur because of prolonged sitting, the nurse and the patient must revise the program. If it appears that the patient is willfully exceeding sitting tolerances, staff intervention is necessary to prevent serious complications. Patients can be encouraged to make independent decisions about sitting times when they are regularly checking their skin, indicating an understanding of pressure relief (see Fig. 24-8).

Special Hygienic Needs and Other Considerations Developing and implementing a turning and positioning schedule is only the first step in preventing potential skin problems. Ill-fitting clothing may bind or wrinkle and cause irritation, especially in the gluteal and perineal areas. Shoes must be checked frequently to make certain of proper fit. Old shoes may become too

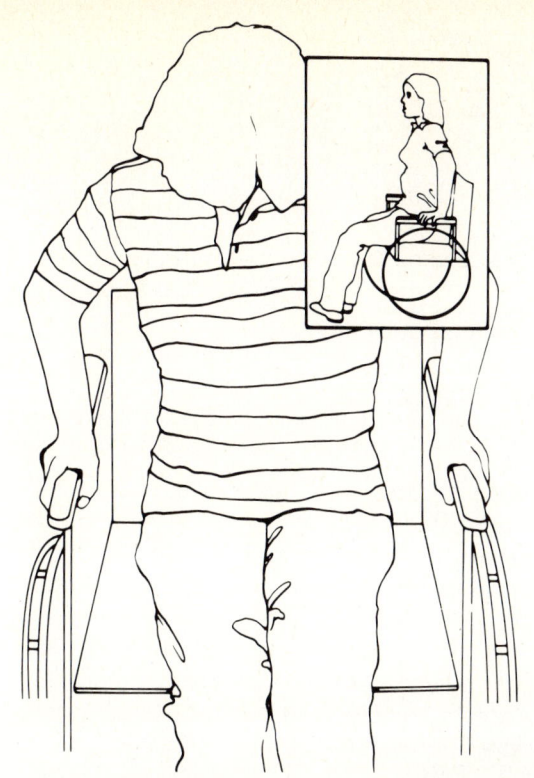

Figure 24-5
Wheelchair push-up. *(Used with the permission of the Rehabilitation Institute of Chicago.)*

Figure 24-6
Wheelchair pressure relief by leaning to one side. *(Used with the permission of the Rehabilitation Institute of Chicago.)*

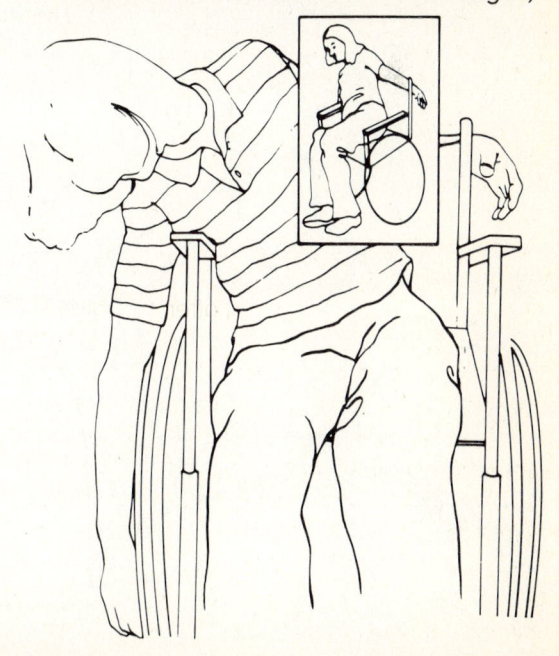

time than lying on the back or sides (see Fig. 24-7). To begin using this position, the patient may try it for brief periods during the daytime. The nurse uses pillows or pads to support the shoulders and protect the iliac crests, the patellae, and the tibial shafts and feet. As with all positioning, the patient needs to be told how long the position will be maintained, and a staff member should return to the patient at the designated time to change position.

Once skin tolerance has been upgraded, the schedule that is to be followed at home can be implemented while the patient is still in the hospital. For example, if the plan is for sitting 8 to 10 h while at work or in school, then the patient ultimately should be in the wheelchair for that length of time during the day to deter-

473 SPINAL CORD INJURY: POSTACUTE PHASE

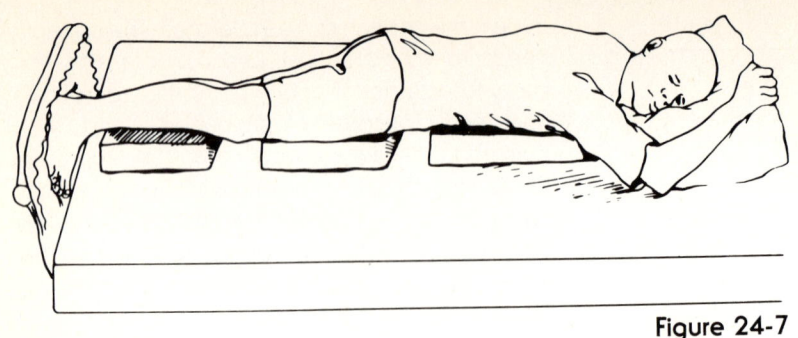

Figure 24-7
Prone positioning: bridging. *(Used with the permission of the Rehabilitation Institute of Chicago.)*

tight if the patient has developed dependent edema. New shoes may be too large or too small and cause blisters.

Because of impaired sensation, the patient may not be able to distinguish temperature extremes and, as a result, may suffer burns or frostbite. More than one patient has sustained burns because of not testing the bath water or shower temperature. Other patients have been burned because they held hot cups of coffee between their legs as they moved from the cafeteria line to the table. Burns can result from touching hot radiators or hot water pipes beneath sinks.

Wet clothing or perspiration can cause skin irritation. Perineal rashes resulting from moist skin surfaces rubbing together can be a persistent problem if meticulous hygiene is not used. The

Figure 24-8
Skin check. *(Used with the permission of the Rehabilitation Institute of Chicago.)*

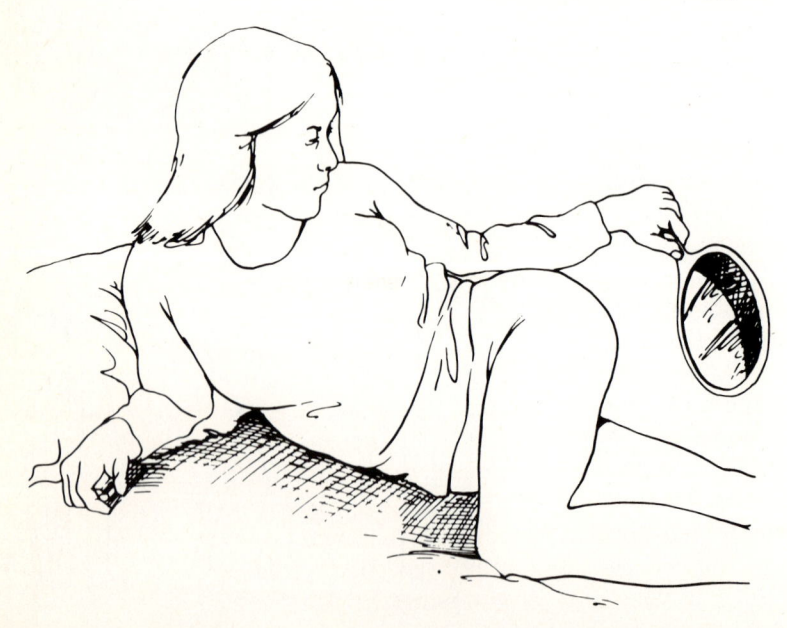

CHAPTER 24   474

patient who sweats excessively needs more frequent bathing and clothing changes to be dry and comfortable.

Basic to any skin care program is good hygiene. If a complete bath daily is not possible, at least facial, underarm, and perineal areas should be washed and teeth brushed. A shampoo usually can be given while the person is lying in bed, on a cart, or sitting in a wheelchair. Male patients should be offered a shave if they are unable to shave themselves. Women should be assisted with shaving legs and underarms. Attention should be paid to both fingernails and toenails.

When planning for hygiene needs, the nursing staff needs to allow time to help the patient with grooming. Helping fix the hair a certain way and putting on makeup, perfume, or after-shave lotion can help to restore a good self-image. Provisions can be made for laundry facilities so the patient's clothing is neat and clean. The use of strategically placed mirrors may also reinforce a positive self-image.

One aspect of hygiene that tends to be neglected with spinal cord–injured patients is dental care. If the patient cannot manage this independently, routine brushing may be neglected. If the nurse becomes aware of major dental problems, she might request a dental consultation. Plans should be made for dental care after discharge. A dentist who can and will work with the wheelchair-bound needs to be located.

EMOTIONAL READJUSTMENT

While spending time in an acute-care setting and then in a rehabilitation facility, the patient becomes aware of all the changes resulting from the injury. The most striking difference is limited mobility. In all probability, the patient cannot walk. If the spinal cord injury is in the high cervical area, the patient may not even be able to propel a wheelchair. The patient may not be able to meet bodily needs for breathing, eating, drinking, and eliminating wastes without being dependent, totally or in part, on someone else. The realization of these changes certainly affects the behavior of the patient and may at least temporarily affect participation in a rehabilitation program.

Changes in the family may occur as a result of the patient's disability. A great physical distance between the family and the rehabilitation facility may cause a change in relationships. Perhaps a role reversal will be needed between homemaker and breadwinner. An already strained family relationship may not be able to withstand the test of a catastrophic injury.

Despite all problems, sometimes the human spirit has remarkable resiliency. The struggle for survival and the will to live are very strong. Consider the following case history:

A male patient arrived at a rehabilitation facility with a diagnosis of paraplegia after a fall. The admitting sheet listed birthplace as unknown and no next of kin. The home address was a transient hotel. The patient was a junkman. During his rehabilitative stay, the patient experienced horrendous pressure sores, severe urinary tract problems that included renal involvement, severe spasticity, and what was interpreted as generally uncooperative behavior.

As of this writing, 8 years later, the man is still alive, residing in a transient hotel, periodically drunk but amazingly free of pressure sores and with very few urinary tract problems. Predicting success for this man 8 years ago was not even considered. Although his existence may seem marginal to some, it is apparently meeting his needs. For reasons obscure and astounding to most, this man chose to live.

There are various behavioral models that can be used to describe and interpret the behaviors exhibited by a person who has suffered a loss of function. The classic stages of mourning apply to the loss experienced by the spinal cord–injured person. Denial of the disability, anger that it happened, depression because of the overt changes brought on by the injury, and eventual acceptance, shown by adaptive coping behaviors, are the stages of emotional adjustment virtually all patients go through. No patient, however, moves into or through this or any other model in classic textbook fasion. Rather, there is a moving in and out of each stage, back and forth and around again.

One description of the process is proposed by Rigoni (Pierce, Nickel). He uses the terms *pre-shock* and *shock* phase to describe the very early stages when the patient is unaware of what has happened, even though perception of reality is clear. The second phase, *defensive retreat,* is the denial stage. Rigoni's third stage is the *acknowledgment,* or awareness-depression, phase. Last, he describes the *adaptation phase,* when the patient has some positive experiences because of rehabilitation efforts and realistic goal setting.

Pepper (1977) uses Erikson's model of psychosocial development, likening the process of adjustment to the first three developmental tasks of trust, autonomy, and initiative.

In the first stage, *trust,* the dependent infant's needs being met by the mother are likened to the needs of the very dependent spinal cord–injured person being met by the clinical personnel in the critical-care facility. The establishment of trusting relationships at this stage of recovery is essential to the development of healthy coping mechanisms later on.

The second stage, *autonomy,* is the period of development in which the child struggles to attain self-control. This, Pepper contends, is not unlike the struggle the patient experiences while attempting to gain some control over the body and its functioning, e.g., mobility and bowel and bladder control.

The third stage, *initiative,* is the struggle for sexual identity in the child, the development of a sense of awareness of moral responsibilities, and the satisfaction that comes from achievement of goals. The person who has experienced a change or loss of sexual function because of a spinal cord injury may see this as a failure of self. Redefining values and roles becomes a significant part of the total readjustment period.

Denial is exhibited by the spinal cord–injured patient in a variety of ways. The patient may work like a trouper in therapies or may refuse to learn care, deeming it unnecessary. Responses such as, "If I work hard in therapy, I shall get better," or "Why should I practice using a hand splint when I'm going to get well soon?" are not uncommon. It is likely that the prognosis, if known by the patient, has not yet been internalized. Another example of denial is that a patient or family may insist on renting equipment rather than buying it because the condition is only temporary.

Understanding staff members working wih the patient during this time do not take away hope but gently encourage the patient to focus on short-term rather than long-term goals.

Awareness of the disability is strikingly evident in some patients early in their hospital stay and obviously absent in others. Along with an increasing awareness of the problems of being disabled is a depression of varying depths. The nurse is alert for some of the more obvious signs of depression. Not attending therapies is frequently one sign. The beginning awareness that all the exercises in the world will not cause a return of motion and function only serves to increase the patient's frustration. If therapy does not work, what will?

One rather universal sign of depression is the sheet-over-the-head syndrome practiced by a great majority of cord-injured patients when they are in bed. If patients are physically unable to pull the sheets up, they frequently ask staff to do it for them, or they close their eyes and turn their heads. This phenomenon serves to visually block out the world immediately around them. The profoundly depressed patient frequently refuses to eat or drink. Experiencing depression is a very real part of the entire readjustment process for nearly all patients. In fact, the nurse might become more concerned about compliant persons who seem always to be cheerful than about those who are obviously depressed.

The efforts of staff members who work with depressed patients are directed at supporting the patients through the depression by providing the care they are unable to manage, and also accepting their current emotional state.

Most patients moving through the rehabilitation process experience feelings of anger. Sometimes the patients' anger may be rational and directed at the actual cause of the accident—another person, themselves, a situation that provoked the injury, or a violent act. Many times the anger is directed at the family, at the institution, or at the staff. Frequently the anger is diffuse, and the patients do nothing but voice complaints about everything. Nursing auxiliary staff members are particularly vulnerable to the patients' attacks because of the amount of time they spend with the patients. It is not unusual for staff members working with such patients to become frustrated because none of their efforts seems to relieve the patients' anger. If staff members are not helped to deal with their feelings, they may in turn become angry with the patients.

It takes a sophisticated staff to sort out the patients' feelings and redirect their energies toward achievement of positive goals. Staff members must feel comfortable in allowing patients to express anger and also must be comfortable when telling patients that some behaviors are less than acceptable. Being disabled does not give them license to be obnoxious.

Staff members must be able to recognize the patient in emotional distress, and to discuss the problem and the approaches to solving it in an intelligent and interdisciplinary manner. More sophisticated therapy such as psychiatric consultation and subsequent psychotherapy may be indicated. Structured group therapy is another option. On a simpler scale, well-chosen rooms, roommates, and staff members, plus a supportive family, may be all that are required to help a patient cope with the disability. Keeping family and friends involved in the process and keeping the communication lines open assist all involved in making the necessary adaptations.

Acceptance of the disability comes only with time and after the person experiences some positive rewards from the efforts of rehabilitation. Patients still need to maintain or develop close personal relationships but may feel that their ability to develop such relationships has been affected. Patients need to have meaningful experiences, such as positive rewards for academic achievement or employment, but achieving these rewards may now be more difficult. The physical upgrading and intellectual skills gained by the person going through a rehabilitative or adjustment process are the prerequisites needed for success in life outside the institution.

ISSUES OF SEXUALITY

Decreased sensation and lack of motor ability do not mean that an individual's sexuality need be diminished. A person with injury to the spinal cord is the same sexual being as before the injury. An individual who premorbidly had a strong sexual drive continues to have that drive. A person with shy, retiring ways or a limited sexual interest in all probability does not change. Flirtatious or provocative behavior may never change, in spite of a young female staff nurse's wishes that it might. An ongoing interest in personal appearance is not altered in those who value attractiveness.

Because of the nurse's frequent involvement in the patient's intimate physical care, the nurse is often the one first approached about sexual concerns. The patient wonders whether others will find him or her attractive and whether it will be possible to satisfy a partner. Specific questions about functional abilities or techniques may arise. The nurse's response to these concerns, if not handled in a sensitive manner, may reinforce the patient's doubts and make it appear that this is an unacceptable topic. If this occurs, the patient may be reluctant to bring up sexual concerns with anyone, for fear of the same response.

It is unrealistic to expect that all nurses can comfortably respond to the patient's questions; often discussions are avoided because the nurse feels inadequate. Although receiving accurate information is important, frequently it is more meaningful for the patient to have someone to listen, and to be able to express fears to a concerned person. When the nurse is unable to answer specific questions, the patient can be referred to someone on the rehabilitation team who can provide the answers.

In addition to helping the patient address feelings of sexuality, the nurse is sensitive to the needs of the person who was involved sexually with the patient before the injury. Will sexual relations be possible? Will there be a difference? The patient's partner needs to know that the patient will continue to have sexual urges and that sexual activity will still be possible, although it may be necessary to alter techniques.

As is the case with so many other aspects of spinal cord injury, the level of the lesion has much effect on the type of physiologic response the patient experiences. The sexual release normally experienced with orgasm will probably take on different dimensions. Some cord-injured patients have described the sexual act as a "head trip." The patient may or may not experience the same physical sensations as premorbidly.

Spinal cord injury has some effect on the motor ability necessary to perform the sexual act. Both the male and the female patient must make adaptations in positioning.

The most obvious physical changes affect the male patient. An interruption in transmission of messages along the spinal cord has some effect on the male's ability to produce or sustain an erection. The neurological pathways involved in producing an erection are parasympathetic fibers in the sacral spinal segments and sympathetic fibers of the hypogastric plexus. In the spinal cord–injured male, erections occur because of reflex activity when there is surface stimulation of the glans penis. This may occur when the patient is being catheterized or when an external urine-collecting device is being applied. It may also occur when clothing is being put on. The patient initially finds this unnerving, so it is wise to explain early that this erection is probably a reflex type and not psychogenic in origin.

Comarr alludes to the inability of most spinal cord–injured males to ejaculate (Comarr and Gunderson, 1975). According to some authorities, ejaculation may occur. However, when it does, it is frequently retrograde, or back into the bladder. David and Ohry report experimentation using a rectal electrostimulator, with resultant ejaculation in the 16 cases studied (David, Ohry, and Rozin, 1977). They also found severe disturbances in spermatogenesis and spermiogenesis thought to result from chronic infections or epididymitis. Obviously, ejaculation of healthy viable sperm is necessary for impregnation. Accurate data are not widely available on spinal cord–injured males' ability to impregnate. Comarr cites studies that indicate 3 percent of male patients sire progency (Comarr, and Gunderson, 1975).

The female who has been injured has different problems. It is not at all uncommon for the female patient past menarche to experience amenorrhea for the first few months after injury. The nurse might consider another cause of amenorrhea: the possibility of pregnancy at the time of injury. The authors remember at least two amenorrheic females who did not have periods until they delivered children some months later.

Unlike the male patient who has difficulty siring children, the female can conceive as soon as the ovulatory cycle has resumed. This is an important fact for the nurse to remember when giving counsel for out-of-the-hospital passes.

The female, like the male, must rely on receiving sexual gratification in other ways, for the sensation of orgasm requires neural pathways that are no longer intact. Unless there have been concurrent pelvic injuries, there is no physiologic reason that prohibits intercourse for the female patient.

One very elemental concern that certainly is the responsibility of the physician and the nurse is birth control or contraceptive advice. Because the male patient probably does not ejaculate, there may be no need for birth control measures. However, this should be determined by the physician, and the patient should be given appropriate advice.

In the case of the female patient, birth control becomes more complicated. The spinal cord injury has not affected her fertility, and therefore she should consider making preparations for contraception. The method used should be decided upon jointly by the patient, the gynecologist, and the attending physician. The physicians may wish to avoid using oral medication because of the serious side effects that are vascular in origin. Although no research has been done, the use of hormone-based birth control pills should probably be discouraged because of the susceptibility of spinal cord patients to the development of emboli (Shaul et al., 1978). One of the various ultrauterine devices (IUDs) may be selected if the patient can check to see if it is in place, although a lack of sensation may be a contraindication. Other mechanical agents such as vaginal diaphragms or spermicidal jellies may be preferable if the patient has the hand function to insert them. Although not as reliable as other means, the side effects of these agents are fewer. The patient may elect to have a tubal ligation as a means of birth control.

If pregnancy is desired, the female patient can be assured that it will be relatively uneventful. A vaginal delivery is possible, although the obstetrician may wish to admit the patient to the delivery corridor somewhat prior to the due date to decrease the possibility of a precipitate birth. Those patients with an injury at the level of T6 or above may have the added risk of autonomic dysreflexia when labor begins.

An obvious problem for patients confined to a hospital for an extended period of time is the lack of privacy. Most patients with spinal cord injuries are generally assigned to multiple-bed rooms that afford little privacy. If sexual retraining is to be an integral part of the program and not something that is left only to weekend passes, then space must be provided for the patient to experiment alone or with a partner.

Because of the physical problems, it may be necessary at first to plan for coitus rather than allowing it to be a spontaneous occurrence. The earlier discussion of how bowel programs may decrease spontaneity is pertinent here. What to do with indwelling catheters is certainly another issue. Removal of a catheter just prior to coitus, for males and females, is one way of managing. The patient can then proceed, being reasonably certain the bladder is empty of urine so that an accident is unlikely. The male patient may elect to fold the catheter back along the penis and put on a condom. This method will not hurt either the male or his partner. The female may choose to leave the catheter in but tape it up on her abdomen so that it is out of the way. The person using intermittent catheterization should empty the bladder prior to coitus to decrease the possibility of an accident.

The spinal-injured man and his partner should experiment with methods that will trigger and sustain an erection. Stimulation of the glans penis by the partner, using manual or oral means, will probably be sufficient. If the male is unable to satisfy his partner because of a flaccid penis, there are alternative methods that can be used. One simple method is "stuffing," which literally involves stuffing the flaccid penis into the woman's vagina. The use of dildos or vibrators is another option. At one time there was some discussion of silicone implantation to cause a permanent erection; this method, however, never received wide acclaim. The other options involve satisfying the female partner either manually or orally.

There may be motor problems because of the lack of control of extremities or because of an excess of spasticity that makes positioning experimentation necessary. Some positions may be next to impossible because of the increased lower extremity spasticity they provoke. For those patients with higher level injuries, the top or dominant position may no longer be feasible.

It is most important that the message be conveyed to the patient that, while there are many, many guidelines for sexual activities, there is no secret method that will work for all. The patient is responsible for experimenting with the partner and finding the method that is mutually satisfying. Experimentation while an inpatient at a rehabilitation facility allows the patient to discuss problems encountered with staff members who are qualified to assist.

One of the more important aspects of attempting to provide sexual information to the patient is to determine who shall do it. Years ago sex was an issue few persons discussed with patients. If anyone did, it was most likely the physician because this was one of the few topics that was relegated up the ladder of the medical hierarchy. Patients deserve to receive information from intelligent, competent clinicians. They should not have to obtain information from other patients or from well-meaning but essentially uninformed staff members. It is tragic if the patient receives no information whatsoever.

The clinical team is responsible for determining how sexual issues should be managed and who will provide the information. The physician or the nurse may provide information on the physical impairments and how to manage certain physical problems. The physical therapist may be the one to help with the positional problems. The psychologist or social worker may handle the emotional issues. Obviously these are traditional roles. Perhaps the social worker cannot discuss intimate feelings with a certain patient but a nurse can. Or maybe the physical therapist or the nurse can handle all the issues involved. If the nurse's comfort level with the information is limited, someone else should provide it. However, the nurse should be aware of who is conveying information.

Nursing, at times, may seem to ask the impossible of the younger members of the profession. Most staff nurses are young and female, and most spinal cord–injured patients are young and male. The message given to the staff nurse by professional superiors is not to become emotionally involved. Much of the physical care of the patients involves management of the most intimate parts and functions of the body. Because of similarities in age, and because the patient is not "ill," it is very possible that feelings other than nurse-patient can arise.

It is not reasonable to assume that nursing curricula will have included a course on how to attain a comfort level while providing sexual counseling to someone close to one's own age. In all probability, content on sexual dysfunction because of physiologic or neurologic impairment was never discussed, nor was how to handle a potentially romantic involvement with a patient. The nursing department, or perhaps the entire institution, becomes responsible for providing the educational opportunities and the emotional support needed by both the young nurse and the young patient.

Perhaps the following suggestions may be helpful. Off-premise fraternization with inpatients should be discouraged. Practically speaking, the nurse must remember that the patient needs both time and energy to devote to the rehabilitation process. There will be plenty of time after discharge to develop a relationship if that is what both nurse and patient want. The nurse may wish to examine personal motivations for developing a relationship and to make a careful determination that what is felt is more than sympathy. If this is done and the two continue over a period of time to be attracted to each other, the couple can certainly be encouraged to develop their relationship.

DRUG AND ALCOHOL ABUSE

A concern of many hospitals today is how to deal effectively with the problem of illicit drug and alcohol use among patients. For many reasons, the young spinal cord population is particularly vulnerable to the use of nonprescription drugs and alcohol. Such use was a way of life for some patients premorbidly. Drugs and alcohol may now provide an escape from the hard-core reality of being physically disabled. Perhaps the energy that once was expended in physical pursuits is now best released with use of mind-altering substances. Some patients, particularly early adolescents, may find it difficult to resist peer pressure.

Regardless of the reasons, the problem is one that cannot be ignored. There are no simple solutions. It is foolish to think that the problem is confined to patients who can open a bottle of beer or roll a "joint." Often the patient who is most physically disabled is the greatest offender. For the safety of all patients and staff, an institutional policy governing illicit drug and alcohol usage is needed. Included in the policy should be types of action that can be taken by the staff if a patient is found abusing the policy. Clear-cut rules on how many infractions constitute a reason for disciplinary action are essential. If it is to be effective, the policy must be supported by all staff members and known by all patients.

Nurses are confronted with drug and alcohol problems more than any other team members. Because most drug and alcohol use occurs during evening hours when the patient is not in therapy, the nurse is usually the one who witnesses the incident and must deal with the change in the patient's behavior.

If the nurse is to maintain any control, the policies must be enforced as much as possible. Repeated infractions that are not dealt with serve to frustrate and anger the staff and encourage the patient to continue using drugs.

Administrative discharges and other types of disciplinary actions offer only a temporary solution. If the problem is to be minimized, for it is unlikely that it will ever be resolved totally, institutions must address the factors that influence drug and alcohol usage. At times, known drug users will be admitted for treatment. In this situation it is most unlikely that established behaviors can be changed. If the patient is suspected of using drugs, it might be wise to consider asking personnel in a local drug abuse program for help in managing the problem.

Two factors, more than any other, influence the use of drugs and alcohol. The first, as mentioned previously, is a patient's inability to deal with the reality of being disabled. For this patient, drugs and alcohol help to blot out the injury. The second factor, particularly for the adolescent or young adult, is boredom. Many young persons have difficulty using unstructured time in sedentary activity. Premorbidly, free time was most likely spent with friends, going to movies or parties, and participating in sports. In the hospital setting there is limited opportunity to work off excess energy.

This problem is somewhat easier to manage if there is a recreational therapy department. Staff can be called upon to involve the patient more actively. Nursing staff can stimulate group games, parties, and other events that will help fill empty hours.

The problem of illicit drug use is inevitable when young persons are institutionalized. However, patients abusing drugs and alcohol cannot be ignored because there are potential hazards. Combining illicit drugs and alcohol with prescribed medications can have a lethal effect. Impaired judgment, brought on by mind-altering substances, can pose safety problems to patients and those around them. The problem of drug and alcohol abuse can be controlled somewhat with reasonable policies and with patient and staff cooperation.

WEEKEND PASSES

A part of the rehabilitation process that is as important as any other therapy is the weekend pass. The pass itself has many purposes. As an integral part of the resocialization process, passes are invaluable. The pass provides a short period at home when the family and patient can try to make the adaptations necessary for the care of the patient outside of the hospital. It is a good time to define problems and attempt to solve them before the patient is discharged. Passes also give the patient and family the opportunity to begin to reorder previously established routines and to adjust to the new changes in life-style.

The pass can be viewed as a small vacation for the patient, provided the problems encountered are minimal. Surprisingly, the therapeutic value of weekend passes is not always viewed that way by the third-party payers (insurance companies or public assistance departments). Views are changing, but some patients may still find that they are billed directly for time spent on pass. This is not a small problem. Patients should be aware of both institutional and third-party payer policies before leaving the hospital on the first pass.

Because most patients are eager to go home on pass as soon as possible, an early focus of the teaching plan should be to provide the essential information that will get everyone through those first 48 hours at home. The rudiments of skin, bowel, and bladder care should be covered, along with medication administration. Recognition of problems such as bladder distention and febrile episodes and what to do about these problems should be covered. Learning wheelchair-to-car transfer is essential.

Because passes away from the hospital setting tend to be stressful times, the nurse may attempt to ease the situation by excluding certain aspects of care. The patient may be sent home the first weekend with disposable urinary equipment. An overnight pass the first weekend that will not coincide with the night of the patient's bowel program may be in order. Possibly the patient can learn to sleep in the prone position, which will eliminate the number of turns needed during the night. Eventually, however, the patient and family must learn how to do all necessary care at home. The time to begin is during passes, not after discharge.

It may be wise to encourage the family not to plan a lot of entertaining during the first weekend pass. Fatigue and anxiety levels are usually high, and added stress is inadvisable. If the family appears extremely anxious about taking the patient home, the nurse might suggest a day or an overnight pass rather than a full weekend.

First weekend passes are usually approached with ambivalence by the patient. While eager to leave the confines of the hospital, the patient naturally fears what will be found outside. "Will I be able to get around in my wheelchair?" "Will I remember what I've been taught?" "How will friends and relatives react to me?" The patient's feelings and the family's anxiety make the first weekend pass a critical event in the rehabilitation process.

First weekend passes are more often than not traumatic for everyone involved. The physical care may actually overwhelm the family, particularly the person giving the care. The first attempt at sexual relations may be disastrous. The patient will experience for the first time being disabled in his or her own home and will quickly realize how inaccessible the bathroom and basement have become.

Architectural obstacles become noticeable. Carpeting, narrow doorways, and stairs limit mobility. The patient is burdened with the thought of renovating the home or moving to another location and the implications this will have for the family. Once again the patient is struck with the realization of dependence. Activities done at one time without thought now require the assistance of one or more persons. The first pass can leave the patient feeling depressed and defeated. Family members may wonder silently, "Will we ever manage?"

Following the pass, ideally there should be separate debriefing periods for both the patient and the family. Both may be reluctant to talk openly, fearing that future passes may be withheld or that they will be thought of as failures if the pass did not go well. The nurse needs to reassure the patient and family that this new experience is normally a difficult one and that staff members are available to help work through the problems encountered at home.

Because problem areas can be identified and possible solutions explored, the weekend pass can be viewed as a very important part of discharge planning.

ENCOURAGING RESPONSIBILITY FOR SELF-CARE

Being physically disabled and a temporary resident in an institution foster some degree of dependence. Initially, this dependence serves a useful protective purpose for the patient. Until the patient has an understanding of personal care requirements, staff members need to provide care.

Eventually the patient begins to assume responsibility for care; ideally this is while the patient is still hospitalized. Encouraging a dependent person to attempt a task, allowing the freedom to experiment and make errors, and providing the necessary supervision is no small job for the staff. Some staff members may tend to hover anxiously or attempt to do the task for the patient. Still others may simply withdraw and not provide either the physical or the emotional support the patient needs to succeed. Unfortunately, when a patient has become physically proficient in a task or is considered to be independent, staff members may think no more assistance is required. Yet this is frequently a time when a patient requires the most support.

The development of a separate independent living unit is ideal. Such a hospital situation often leads to informal group discussions of real problems that do not arise on routine patient units. When no living unit is available, the nurse can incorporate certain aspects of it on the regular ward. If the patients are functionally capable of independence, they should be able to do the following:

1. Obtain an alarm clock. The patients should set the clock for the time for them to get up in the morning. This places the responsibility for punctuality on the patients.
2. Care for genitourinary equipment. Patients should be responsible for all genitourinary care such as disinfecting leg bags and irrigation sets, and should follow the procedures of the institution.
3. Develop communication skills. Patients should be encouraged to discuss physical problems with the physician and change in therapy schedules with the therapist.
4. Administer medications. Patients should be responsible for going to the nursing station for medications and for pouring them under supervision. They should also learn the purpose of each medication, side effects, and possible synergistic reactions (e.g., what happens when diazepam and alcohol are mixed).
5. Make decisions. Patients should be allowed to make decisions; for example, about going on an outtrip or doing the bowel program or living with the consequences of doing the bowel program at midnight.
6. Recognize and manage problems. Patients should know what to do about reddened skin and how to report changes in urine quality or an elevated temperature.
7. Make plans. Patients must set the alarm clock early enough to awaken, bathe, dress, eat, and arrive at therapy in time for the first appointment. This planning requires having the wheelchair and clothing at the bedside the night before.
8. Assume an active role in the rehabilitation program. Being the key person on the rehabilitation team, each patient should attend interdisciplinary conferences and be an active participant in the discharge plan.

Although the foregoing list is not complete, it suggests how patients can have some control over the rehabilitation program and can have some experience managing daily activities.

One nurse on an independent unit recorded the following note in a patient's chart:

> Patient deals actively with problems he encounters (e.g., after recent problem over a weekend he spoke with his M.D. the next day). Patient initiates activities and activity passes in the evenings. Drinks a lot of beer but monitors this in accordance with medications and activities scheduled for the next day.

Functionally dependent patients must be able to give detailed directions on how to change catheters, when and how to change positions, and how to manage problems. These persons can learn to check their own skin if someone positions mirrors in such a way that ischial and sacral areas can be visualized. They might also be given short courses in assertiveness and interpersonal relations as they need both skills to be able to direct the necessary care.

To again be in control of even a portion of one's life helps improve one's self-esteem. To be able to exert some form of independence is a most important step in the recovery process. Not all patients attain this control within the first year after injury.

> One middle-aged male quadriplegic patient spent the first 2 years after injury at home alternately with his girlfriend and with his sister. He had resisted learning about his care, and family preparation for discharge was most inadequate. Many social and physical problems occurred, including massive pressure sores. Eventually he was placed in a nursing home.

With some intensive counsel from an outpatient nurse and a social worker, Mr. T. finally realized he would have to assume responsibility for his care and subsequently learned and directed it. He learned how to negotiate with personnel in the nursing home to obtain the necessary basic care such as frequent turns and adequate fluids. He also learned how to negotiate with public aid agencies and other health agencies to obtain care and supplies beyond those available in the nursing home. It has taken Mr. T. not months but years to regain control of his life. He is now able to live outside an institution in his sister's home and is cared for by an attendant. Those things important to him—his family, friends, baseball games on television, and several daily cans of beer—are again a real part of his life and, more important, his ability to be in control of his environment.

PROBLEMS RELATED TO SPINAL CORD INJURY

This section discusses some physical problems related specifically to spinal cord injury and some that occur because of the patient's immobilization. Not all of the problems affect every person with spinal cord injury. However, the nurse should know about the problems and help patients understand the problems, and learn how to manage them if they do occur.

SPASTICITY

Spasticity occurs in the spinal cord–injured person because of stimulation of an intact reflex arc below the level of the injury. Although it frequently presents problems in positioning and mobility, spasticity can benefit the patient by maintaining muscle mass and can be utilized by the patient in transferring into and out of a wheelchair, once the patient has learned how to trigger and control the spasm. Maintenance of muscle mass can decrease some of the problems related to change in body image because there is no impact of atrophy owing to muscle disuse.

Stauffer (Pierce and Nickel) describes spasticity as "an increased stretch reflex in a muscle motor unit below the level of the injury." He states that spasticity does not occur until about 3 months after injury, or after the areflexic, spinal shock stage. The first pattern to develop is that of flexor spasticity. After about 6 months, extensor spasticity appears. After about 1 year, spasticity reaches a plateau.

Severe, unrelenting spasticity or a sudden onset of it after 1 year usually is an indication of a physical problem. The nurse and the physician need to investigate the cause, which is usually not readily apparent. Among the more common causes are bladder infections or calculi, skin problems, ingrown toenails, and shoes that are too tight. If spasticity interferes with the patient's normal living, it can be managed medically with drugs such as diazepam and dantrolene sodium. Spasticity may require surgical or chemical intervention such as cordotomy, rhizotomy, or phenol blocks, but these destructive measures are used only as a last resort. Surgical or chemical elimination of spasticity increases muscle atrophy and eliminates the reflex arc utilized for sexual function and bowel and bladder elimination. Consequently, the patient may find it very difficult to accept this method of treatment.

REFLEX SWEATING

Because of interruptions in the spinal sympathetic pathways, spinal cord patients become vulnerable to aberrations in sweating patterns. Those with complete lesions do not experience thermoregulatory sweating below the level of the lesion. Patients with incomplete lesions experience some sweating below the level of the lesion. Most sweating experienced by patients with spinal cord injury is part of the mass reflex phenomenon that is related to spasticity and autonomic dysreflexia and occurs because of a stimulus below the level of the lesion. Reflex sweating does not occur in patients whose lesion is below T10 (Fast, 1977). When reflex sweating does occur, it may be indicative of a problem such as urinary tract infection, or stones, or fecal impactions.

While the cause is being investigated, management of sweating should be directed at patient comfort. Towels wrapped around the head and neck, change of clothing or bedding, and avoidance of chilling are of great help. The patient must replace fluid by drinking more liquids. Some physicians choose to use a medication such as Pro-Banthine to control excessive bouts of sweating, but a patient may find the side effects unpleasant.

THERMOREGULATION

Because the internal body temperature is controlled by centers within the hypothalamus, interruption of the neural pathways causes a major problem with thermoregulation in the quadriplegic patient. As vasodilatation and sweating do not occur in response to environmental heat and vasoconstriction and shivering do not occur in response to cold, temperature control must be achieved by external means. A spinal-injured person is well advised to avoid temperature extremes. Sun bathing or being outdoors in extremely hot weather can cause sunburn on desensitized skin and an elevation of the internal body temperature. It may be necessary to cool the person with a sponge bath. For a person living in an area where environmental temperatures go very high, an air conditioner may well be an important part of the survival equipment. Adapting to colder weather is usually not so difficult or inherently dangerous because one tends to put on adequate clothing and not remain in the cold for long periods of time.

Febrile episodes related to infections must be treated aggressively because of the cord-injured person's inability to normalize body temperatures. When the usual modalities of sponging and increased fluid intake do not seem to work, it may be necessary to consider the use of a hypothermia blanket, with care taken not to drop the body temperature too low. Temperature elevations to 105°F are not uncommon during febrile episodes.

PAIN MANAGEMENT

Decreased sensation does not mean the person does not experience pain. Pain below the level of cord injury is particularly difficult to treat as it does not always respond to conventional treatment methods. Davis (1975) categorized pain secondary to spinal cord trauma into three types.

The first is *pain at the site of trauma,* which does not last much more than 2 weeks to a month.

The second type is *pain referred from damaged nerve roots.* This pain is much more complicated and can become a chronic problem for the patient, who describes a burning, sometimes stinging sensation. In time, adhesive arachnoiditis may complicate this pain. Analgesics should be given on a regular schedule rather than on an as-needs basis. The physician may order diphenylhydantoin for pain relief. Decompression laminectomies, transcutaneous nerve stimulators, even dorsal column stimulator implants may be indicated. Treatment is for chronic pain. It is not a pain to be ignored, yet it is important that the patient not let it become the focus of life.

The third type is *pain below the injury.* This pain is also of a chronic nature and may be described as phantom pain, or a sensation rather than pain. It is apparently influenced by anxiety, fatigue, alcohol, marijuana, cigarettes, and exercise. Psychologic help may be indicated if there is no apparent pathology but the pain is immobilizing.

ORTHOSTATIC HYPOTENSION

Orthostatic hypotension, characterized by a drop in blood pressure when the patient assumes an upright position, occurs as a result of the spinal cord–injured patient's being immobilized in the recumbent position for a prolonged period of time. If care is not taken to initiate the patient to a sitting or standing position gradually, the patient can experience dizziness, hypotension, tachycardia, and fainting. In time, as the patient adapts to the upright position, postural hypotension no longer poses a problem.

To avoid orthostatic hypotension, the patient should not go directly from lying flat in bed to sitting upright at 90°. If a reclining wheelchair is available, the patient should begin sitting at 45°. The wheelchair angle should be increased 10 to 20° at a time, until the 90° position can be assumed without complications. If the patient has a straight-backed wheelchair, the position should be increased gradually in bed before transfer to the wheelchair. When the patient begins to feel dizzy, the wheelchair should be tilted back or the bed lowered. Once this is done, the patient recovers quickly. Sitting should then be resumed at a lesser angle. The physician may wish to prescribe ephedrine sulfate to be given 1/2 h prior to the patient's getting up.

An abdominal corset may be needed to help prevent pooling of blood in the abdomen. Antiembolic hose worn to help prevent stasis are also advisable.

Because the effects of hypotension can be very frightening, the patient may become reluctant to sit in the wheelchair or may want to avoid increasing the angle of sitting. The nurse should explain carefully the reason for the hypotension, and assure the patient that the position will be increased gradually and that the patient will not be left alone immediately after getting up.

THROMBOPHLEBITIS

Thrombophlebitis in the patient with a spinal cord injury may result from prolonged immobility and decreased circulation. The initial treatment plan, therefore, should include measures to help prevent venous thrombosis by increasing blood flow and decreasing stasis in the lower extremities. The nurse should do range-of-motion exercises regularly. Lower extremities should be elevated periodically throughout the day. Garments such as girdles, garters, and knee-high stockings that may restrict venous flow should not be worn. Thigh-high antiembolic hose, which help to increase venous flow through the use of a pressure gradient, should be considered.

Early signs of thrombophlebitis include muscle ache, stiffness, edema, and increased warmth in the lower extremity. Because of sensory impairment, the patient may not be aware of any soreness. Nursing staff must be alert to change in leg size or temperature. The physician must be notified immediately of any findings.

Doppler ultrasonic flow studies and impedance phlebography may be needed for conclusive diagnosis (Cudkowicz, and Sherry, 1978). If findings are positive, the physician determines whether anticoagulation therapy is needed. Initially the patient should be put on bed rest. The physician should give specific orders for positioning and exercising. Care should be taken to avoid massaging the extremity for fear of breaking up the clot. Calf and thigh measurements should be taken daily.

If anticoagulant therapy becomes necessary, the nurse will need to reconsider various aspects of the patient's program. It is best to avoid decatheterization programs during this time because repeated catheterizations may cause trauma to the urethra and result in bleeding. Vigorous digital stimulation should be avoided during bowel programs. Care must be taken to avoid trauma during wheelchair transfers.

OSTEOPOROSIS

One phenomenon directly related to immobility can potentially cause problems for the spinal cord–injured person. The phenomenon is the development of osteoporosis and the subsequent problems of calcium utilization or excretion.

The equilibrium or homeostasis that occurs during normal bony growth depends on mobility and weight bearing (Olson, 1967). The balance of calcium in the bony matrix is upset when mobility and weight bearing are eliminated. Bony growth ceases, and the supply of bony calcium becomes severely diminished. At the same time, there is further demineralization with the excretion of bony phosphorus and nitrogen. Demineralization, or osteoporosis, leaves bones in a somewhat weakened and brittle state.

Attempts to prevent osteoporosis over the years have never proved very successful. If calcium is increased in the diet, it is merely excreted in the urine and feces. No known medication is effective. Most effective in delaying or diminishing osteoporosis is the use of the tilt table or braces to allow the patient to stand, so that a weight-bearing situation is created.

According to Stauffer (Pierce and Nickel), it takes at least 1 year for sufficient osteoporosis to develop to cause pathologic fractures. Then the fractures occur exclusively in the long bones of the extremities, with very little torque or trauma to the limbs. Because the patient has no or decreased pain sensation, the initial sign that a fracture has occurred may be a snapping sound. The next sign may be swelling or discoloration at the site of the fracture. Diagnosis is confirmed on x-ray. Surgical pinning is possible, but this method is not the treatment of choice when osteoporosis is present. Traction tends to immobilize an already immobilized person even more.

Plaster casts are probably the most widely used method of treatment for fractures, yet the potential for development of pressure sores under the cast is very great. Often the cast is bivalved to allow for daily skin inspection and pressure relief. It is possible to use a posterior mold or splint and an Ace wrap in lieu of a cast if the extremity is flaccid. Another method of immobilization is using a pillow as a splint and wrapping it with an Ace wrap. This can also be used as an emergency measure. Further cast care, including petalling the tops and regularly checking circulation (pulses and blanching of nails), is most important for patients who have no sensation and therefore no warning that a skin problem may be developing.

Claus-Walker et al. (1972) studied calcium excretion in quadriplegia and found that early hypercalciuria resulted from changes in body fluid distribution, absence of sympathetic activity, and renal vasodilatation. They noted restoration of normal calcium levels within the first year after injury. A normalizing or homeostatic mechanism seems to operate following trauma.

ECTOPIC BONE

The etiology of a problem variously known as ectopic bone, heterotopic bone, myositis ossificans, and heterotopic ossificans is unknown, even though one might think it is related to the development of osteoporosis. This extra bony growth usually develops around the hip joints and sometimes at the knee. The nurse may be the first to note the formation of ectopic bone. A swelling is seen over the iliac crest, or lateral to it, which feels warm to the touch. Laboratory data probably reveal an elevated serum alkaline phosphatase.

The mass may or may not cause problems. The major problem is a decrease in range of motion. Surgery may be effective, but not until the bony mass has matured. Some physicians do not advise anything but conservative measures. Maintenance of range of motion should be encouraged and may even help alter the course of the disease.

Differential diagnosis is sometimes difficult. One quadriplegic patient had a bony mass diagnosed as an osteogenic sarcoma. On surgical removal, the mass was found to be ectopic bone. Heterotopic bone also may be confused with thrombophlebitis.

CONTRACTURES

The development of contractures is not uncommon with the spinal cord injured. The prevention and methods of treatment are so well documented elsewhere that there is no need for discussion here. However, spasticity is a major contributing cause to the development of contractures in the spinal cord injured. The use of medication to control spasticity may be indicated, or a surgical release of the contractures may be necessary. One of the more common contractures in the quadriplegic patient is the upper extremity flexion contracture caused by the active elbow flexors which are innervated at the C6 level. Because innervation to the extensors occurs at T1, contractures are likely to develop unless a range of motion is maintained and good positioning techniques are practiced.

SCOLIOSIS

Scoliosis is very likely to develop in the young child or adolescent who is injured. The use of corsets or orthoses to prevent this deformity has not been very effective. Encouraging the patient to sit upright to maintain good sitting posture and carefully monitoring this posture may help. Trunk-strengthening exercises also may be of benefit. While the child is growing, the nurse should frequently monitor the wheelchair to ascertain that the height of the chair back is adequate, the foot pedals are in good position, and the chair fits the child. Some, but not all, surgeons recommend surgical intervention (Griffiths, 1974) in young adolescents prior to the growth spurts of puberty to decrease incidence of spinal deformation.

ACUTE ABDOMEN

Because of decreased sensation and the elimination of the normal warning mechanisms, it is more difficult to diagnose acute abdomen in spinal-injured patients than in the general population. The clinical team working with spinal cord patients should be aware that acute abdominal problems can occur. Sudden anorexia and a temperature elevation may be clues to a problem. Some authors (Dollfus et al., 1974) have found that a rise in local skin temperature, as well as an abdominal x-ray, is helpful in the diagnosis of appendicitis.

ANTICIPATING DISCHARGE

The specific components of discharge planning have not been emphasized in this chapter. However, the purpose of all the nurse's care is to prepare the patient to live in the community. The goal of the nursing-care plan and the teaching plan is to maintain body integrity and prepare the patient and the family for the patient's eventual discharge and continued health maintenance.

The plan for physical care following discharge must include education for the person who will provide the care, whether it is an attendant, a family member, or the patient. Because of the nature of the physical disability, certain types of equipment are needed to help provide the care. Heavy equipment such as wheelchairs, hospital beds, and commodes must be ordered enough in advance of the actual discharge date to ensure arrival in time. The patient should have the name of either the vendor or the manufacturer, as servicing will be needed later on. Small expendable supplies and medications must be requested and a source of supply located in the community.

When at all possible, the nurse should determine which supplies may be reused in the home environment. In this age of disposable equipment, nurses may not always remember that continued use over a long period of time of sterile disposable catheter sets, irrigation sets, or tracheostomy care sets is prohibitively expensive. With the use of ingenuity and some sound nursing principles, patients and families can be taught methods for cleaning and reusing most items. Such methods should include careful washing with soap and water and the use of a bactericide such as dilute chlorine bleach or some readily available bactericidal agent. The patient will not be introduced to nearly as many pathogenic organisms in the home setting as in the hospital, which eliminates many of the hazards of cross-contamination.

Care after discharge should be closely monitored until the patient and the family have demonstrated the necessary skills and gained sufficient confidence to be able to give care independently.

Community health agencies or outpatient clinics can check patients; telephone follow-up is another method of monitoring. If distance is a factor, the patient must be referred to another health-care system. Final reports or discharge summaries are provided to those monitoring the care. These reports include descriptions of procedures and techniques that the patient and family have been taught.

The plan for spinal cord–injured patient follow-up provides for regular laboratory and x-ray studies of the urinary tract, including an intravenous pyelogram, BUN, and urine cultures. This health-maintenance program is to continue for the rest of the person's life. It may be necessary to alert health-care agencies in the community if the patient may possibly need emergency care. Not all emergency room personnel know how to recognize or manage autonomic dysreflexia. The local paramedic group may need to be alerted to a patient with potential respiratory problems.

The discharge plan must incorporate principles that help maintain the health of the individual. The plan should allow the individual to live as nearly normal a life as possible. All energies need not be directed toward maintaining health. Some ought to be reserved for gainful employment, education, and pleasure activities. Plans can be simplified to conserve energy. Using a hydraulic lift for transfer activities may be advisable. Upgrading skin tolerance and developing certain positions that allow for longer periods between turns are other considerations.

Patients can be advised to anticipate some minor problems after discharge. Keeping a change of clothing and a catheter set at work may save both time and energy. Keeping an adequate amount of supplies on hand in the event deliveries are not made on time is another good plan.

A person with spinal cord injury can make a successful adjustment to the community. This adjustment does not occur by accident. The person must have an adequate understanding of the disability. A reasonable plan should be devised that will enable the patient to maintain optimum health after the return to the community.

BIBLIOGRAPHY

Abramson, Arthur S.: "Management of Neurogenic Bladder in Perspective," *Arch Phys Med Rehabil* 57:5, 1976.

Babcock, James L.: "Spinal Injuries in Children," *Pediatr Clin North Am* 22:2, 1975.

Benvenuti, Christine: "Independence for the Quadriplegic: The Bantam Respirator," *Am J Nurs* 79:5, 1979.

Braakman, R., I. Orbann, and M. Blauw-Van-Dishoeck: "Information in the Early Stages after Spinal Cord Injury," *Paraplegia* 14:1, 1976.

Bregman, Sue, and Robert Hadley: "Sexual Adjustment and Feminine Attractiveness Among Spinal Cord Injured Women," *Arch Phys Med Rehabil* 57:9, 1976.

Bruck, Lilly: *Access,* Random House, New York, 1978.

Burke, David C., and D. Duncan Murray: *Handbook of Spinal Medicine,* Raven Press, New York, 1975.

─────, and T. S. Tiong: "Stability of the Cervical Spine after Conservative Treatment," *Paraplegia* 13:3, 1975.

Campbell, Joyce, and Charles Bonnett: "Spinal Cord Injury in Children," *Clin Orthop* 112, 1975.

Champion, Victoria L.: "Clean Technique for Intermittent Self-Catheterization," *Nurs Res* 25:1, 1976.

Christopherson, Victor A., Pearl P. Coulter, and Mary O. Wolanin: *Rehabilitation Nursing: Perspectives and Applications,* McGraw-Hill, New York, 1974.

Claus-Walker, J. R. Campos, R. E. Carter, C. Valbona, and H. S. Liscomb: "Calcium Excretion in Quadriplegia," *Arch Phys Med Rehabil* 53:1, 1972.

Comarr, A. Estin, and Bernice B. Gunderson: "Sexual Function in Traumatic Paraplegia and Quadriplegia," *Am J Nurs* 75:2, 1975.

Cornell, S. A., L. Campion, and S. Bacero: "Comparison of Three Bowel Management Programs," *Nurs Res* 22:4, 1973.

Cudkowicz, Leon, and Sol Sherry: "The Venous

System and the Lung," *Heart and Lung* 7: 1, 1978.

D'Agostino, Janet, and Patricia Welch: "The Phrenic Pacemaker: A Promise of a New Breath . . . and New Life . . . for Respiratory Patients," *Nursing 79* 9:5, 1979.

David, A., A. Ohry, and R. Rozin: "Spinal Cord Injuries: Male Infertility Aspects," *Paraplegia* 15:1, 1977.

Davis, Joan E., and Celestine B. Mason: *Neurological Critical Care,* Van Nostrand-Reinhold, New York, 1979.

Davis, R.: "Pain and Suffering Following Spinal Cord Injury," *Clin Orthop* 112, 1975.

Dollfus, P., F. Jurascheck, G. Adliand, and A. Chapius: "Impairment of Erection after External Sphincter Resection," *Paraplegia* 13: 4, 1976.

———, G. L. Holderbach, J. M. Husser, and D. Jacob-Chia: "Must Appendicitis Be Still Considered as a Rare Complication in Paraplegia?" *Paraplegia* 11:4, 1974.

Downey, John A., and Niels L. Low: *The Child With Disabling Illness,* Saunders, Philadelphia, 1974.

Fast, Avital: "Reflex Sweating in Patients with Spinal Cord Injury: A Review," *Arch Phys Med Rehabil* 58:10, 1977.

Feustal, Delycia: "Autonomic Hyperreflexia," *Am J Nurs* 76:2, 1976.

Griffiths, E. R.: "Growth Problems in Cervical Injuries," *Paraplegia* 11:4, 1974.

Gruis, Marcia, and Barbara Innes: "Assessment: Essential to Prevent Pressure Sores," *Am J Nurs* 11:76, 1976.

Habeeb, Marjorie, and M. D. Kallstrom: "Bowel Program for Institutionalized Adults," *Am J Nurs* 76:4, 1976.

Heslinga, K.: *Not Made of Stone,* Charles C Thomas, Springfield, Ill., 1974.

Hirschberg, Gerald G., Leon Lewis, and Patricia Vaughan: *Rehabilitation,* Lippincott, Philadelphia, 1976.

Kinash, Rose G.: "Experiences and Nursing Needs of Spinal Cord Injured Patients," *Neurosurg Nurs* 10:1, 1978.

Kovic, Ron: *Born on the Fourth of July,* McGraw-Hill, New York, 1976.

Kunin, C., and J. DeGroot: "Self-Screening for Significant Bacteriuria," *JAMA* 203, 1975.

Lapides, J., A. Diokno, B. Lowe, and M. Kalish: "Followup on Unsterile, Intermittent Self-Catheterization," *J Urol* February 1974.

Lawson, Norman: "Significant Events in the Rehabilitation Process: The Spinal Cord Patient's Point of View," *Arch Phys Med Rehabil* 59: 12, 1978.

Lindan, Rosemary, and Virginia Bellomy: "Effect of Delayed Intermittent Catheterization on Kidney Function in Spinal Cord Injured Patients," *Paraplegia* 13:1, 1975.

Mathews, Nancy C.: "Helping a Quadriplegia Veteran Decide to Live," *Am J Nurs* 76:3, 1976.

Merritt, John L.: "Urinary Tract Infections, Causes and Management with Particular Reference to Patients with Spinal Cord Injury: A Review," *Arch Phys Med Rehabil* 57:8, 1976.

Mooney, Thomas O., Theodore M. Cole, and Richard Chilgren: *Sexual Options for Paraplegics and Quadriplegics,* Little, Brown, Boston, 1975.

Ohry, A., M. Molho, and R. Rozin: "Alteration in Spinal Cord Injured Patients," *Paraplegia* 13:2, 1975.

Olson, Edith: "The Hazards of Immobility," *Am J Nurs* 67:4, 1967.

Paradowski, William: "Socialization Patterns and Sexual Problems of the Institutionalized Chronically Ill and Physically Disabled," *Arch Phys Med Rehabil* 58:2, 1977.

Pearman, John W., and Ernest J. England: *The Urological Management of the Patient Following Spinal Cord Injury,* Charles C Thomas, Springfield, Ill., 1973.

Peppee, G. A.: "The Person with Spinal Cord Injury: Psychological Care," *Am J Nurs* 77: 8, 1977.

Perkash, Indes: "Intermittent Catheterization Failure and an Approach to Bladder Rehabilitation in Spinal Cord Injury Patients," *Arch Phys Med Rehabil* 59:1, 1978.

Pierce, Donald S., and Vernon H. Nickel: *The Total Care of Spinal Cord Injuries,* Little, Brown, Boston, 1977.

Richards, B.: "The Social and Psychological Aspects of Sexuality," *Nurs Mirror Midwives J* February, 1976.

Rosen, Joel S., John Nanninga, and V. J. O'Conor: "Silent Hydronephrosis, A Hazard Revisited," *Paraplegia* 14:2, 1976.

Rozhoy, Melissa: "The Young Adult—Taking a Sexual History," *Am J Nurs* 76:8, 1976.

Ruge, Daniel: *Spinal Cord Injuries,* Charles C Thomas, Springfield, Ill., 1969.

Shapiro, Barry A., Ronald A. Harrison, and Carole A. Trout: *Clinical Application of Respiratory Care,* Yearbook Medical Pub., Chicago, 1975.

Shaul, S., J. Bogle, J. Hale-Harbaugh, and A. Norman: *Toward Intimacy,* Human Sciences Press, New York, 1978.

Shoenfeld, Y. et al.: "Orthostatic Hypotension in Amputees and Subjects with Spinal Cord Injury," *Arch Phys Med Rehabil* 59:3, 1978.

Smith, Dorothy: "Survivors of Serious Illness," *Am J Nurs* 79:3, 1979.

Smith, Jim, and Bonnie Bullough: "Sexuality and the Severely Disabled Person," *Am J Nurs* 75:12, 1975.

Smith, P. H., and J. B. Cook: "Micturition Patterns in Paraplegic Patients Following Spinal Cord Injury," *Paraplegia* 13:4, 1976.

Sperling, Keith: "Intermittent Catheterization to Obtain Catheter Free Bladder Function in Spinal Cord Injury," *Arch Phys Med Rehabil* 59:1, 1978.

Stover, Samuel L., Keith L. Lloyd, C. S. Nepomuceno, and Leslie L. Gale: "Intermittent Catheterization," *Paraplegia* 15:1, 1977.

Stover, Samuel, C. J. Hataway, and H. Zeiger: "Heterotopic Ossification in Spinal Cord Injured Patients," *Arch Phys Med Rehabil* 56: 5, 1975.

Stryker, Ruth: *Rehabilitative Aspects of Acute and Chronic Nursing Care,* Saunders, Philadelphia, 1977.

Teal, Jeffrey C., and Gary T. Athelstan: "Sexuality and Spinal Cord Injury: Some Psychosocial Considerations," *Arch Phys Med Rehabil* 56:6, 1975.

Thomas, D. G.: "The Effect of Trans-Urethral Surgery on Penile Erections in Spinal Cord Injury Patients," *Paraplegia* 13:4, 1976.

Trieschmann, Roberta B.: *The Psychological, Social and Vocational Adjustment in Spinal Cord Injury: A Strategy for Future Research,* Rehabilitation Services Administration, Department of Health, Education and Welfare, 1978.

VanderLinden, R. G., L. Gilpin, J. Harper, M. McClurkin, and D. Twilley: "Electrophenic Respiration in Quadriplegia," *Can Nurse* 70:1, 1974.

Wallace, Shirley G., and Albert D. Anderson: "Imprisonment of Patients in the Course of Rehabilitation," *Arch Phys Med Rehabil* 59:9, 1978.

Walsh, J. J.: "The Spinal Cord Disabled," *Nurs Mirror* February, 1976.

Warson, Norval: "Pattern of Spinal Cord Injury in the Elderly," *Paraplegia* 14:1, 1976.

Wehrmaher, Suzanne, and Joann Wintermute: *Case Studies in Neurological Nursing,* Little, Brown, Boston, 1978.

Wright, Beatrice A.: *Physical Disability: A Psychological Approach,* Harper & Row, New York, 1960.

25
hildegarde myers

upper extremity
amputation

INTRODUCTION

Until the 1950s, persons who underwent amputation were essentially neglected by medicine, nursing, limb manufacturers, and therapists. At that time, a few orthopedists, engineers, scientists, therapists, and some of the more knowledgeable limb manufacturers pooled their ideas for the betterment of both lower and upper extremity amputees. Suddenly the limb manufacturer became a prosthetist, and the artificial limb became a prosthesis. The Veterans Administration, faced with the large numbers of amputees injured during World War II, no doubt led the way in the significant changes in amputee management. New artificial joints, cables, systems of harnessing, improved socket shapes and sizes, and better methods of attaching the devices to the body were devised and became available. It was a fascinating era of scientific progress in providing provident care for the amputee. Influential people became involved, national committees were formed, government help was sought and obtained, and schools in prosthetics were initiated. For the first time in history, doctors, prosthetists, and therapists attended educational programs together, where each learned the overall objectives of amputee management as well as their own particular roles in the care and training of these patients. The physicians (usually orthopedists) learned that there was more to amputations than removal of an extremity.

THE TEAM APPROACH

In addition to the surge of interest in prosthetics new surgical techniques were developed, and far more importantly, the physician learned to work with others toward a common goal. As the leader of the group, the physician realized there must be input from prosthetists and other health professionals to complete the rehabilitation of the amputee. In this way, the "team approach," so common in the management of health care today, was born. This approach included regularly scheduled clinics in which all members of the team were present and where every patient was seen for initial evaluation, for written prosthetic prescription, and for checkouts when the prosthesis was ready. When there were problems and/or when prosthetic training was completed, routine follow-up clinic rechecks by the same team were scheduled. Gone were the days when the surgeon told amputee patients to get themselves an artificial limb by looking in the Yellow Pages of the telephone directory. Gone also were the days when the limb maker, after fabricating an artificial limb without medical advice and with little scientific background, gave the prosthesis to the patient with the only instruction being to "go home and learn to use it." Sometimes, much to the distress of the patient and family, the limb came by mail. Too often, the artificial limb was left to hang in the closet or was put away in the basement. Before 1950, particularly for the upper extremity amputee, the artificial limb was most inadequate and seldom functional. At times, the limb was worn as a passive device to fill a sleeve so that clothing would fit better.

Fortunately, there were and are many more lower extremity amputations than upper extremity amputations. The lower extremity prosthesis has always been more acceptable because it is not visible, the amputee needs it to get about, and it does not have to substitute for the many intricate and complex functions of the hand, wrist, and elbow. In spite of numerous improvements, there is no way present upper extremity prostheses can perform the involved grasping, pinching, and squeezing movements of the fingers against the thumb; the flexion and extension of both fingers and wrist; or the supination-pronation of the forearm, let alone replace the loss of sense of touch (McClinton, 1976). Therefore, the emotional and functional problems resulting from an upper extremity amputation are likely to be greater than those caused by the loss of a lower extremity. Lower extremity amputees may, for example, have such a smooth gait that they can "pass" as being able-bodied, something upper extremity amputees can never do. The upper extremity amputee clearly fits

Goffman's description of a discredited person and must therefore face stigma management (Goffman, 1963).

Proper selection and fitting of a prosthesis and training of the amputee in its use are aimed at replacing, as much as possible, the loss the patient has suffered. Hopefully, the prosthesis makes the patient feel less disabled, aids in daily activities and on the job, causes clothing to fit better, and is helpful in maintaining proper posture.

Nurses employed in hospitals have not been involved in the rehabilitation of the upper extremity amputee, in large part because of the amputee's brief hospitalization following surgery. Usually the unilateral upper extremity amputee requires little physical care, because surgical dressings are done by the surgeon and because the patient can be up and about at once to attend to daily needs. The patient may be discharged to outpatient care before the nurse recognizes and/or can address the patient's and family's anxieties and distress. The nurse can, however, supply the supportive role that these patients sorely need. The surgeon does provide this support, but often the patient may perceive the doctor's hurried manner as nonsupportive and therefore will be unable to gain any solace or information. The support needs to be a daily occurrence, repeated many times, and carried out with family members present. The nurse can assure the patient that there is a prosthetic device for every level of amputation, from hand to shoulder; that each person is prescribed with the device that best meets his or her needs; and that there will be referral to an amputee clinic team for prescription, training, and follow-up care. The amputee should be made aware that the doctors, prosthetists, and therapists on the clinic team are experts in the field so that the best that science has developed will be available. Every effort should be made during the initial hospitalization to acquaint amputees with the clinic team members who will work with them after discharge from the hospital. The amputee clinic team is usually composed of an orthopedist, a prosthetist, and physical and occupational therapists. Occupational health nurses, insurance nurses, school nurses, community nurses, and specialists in the fields of social work, psychology, and research become members as needed.

TYPES OF UPPER EXTREMITY AMPUTATIONS

Basically there are two types of acquired upper extremity amputation: unilateral and bilateral.

Unilateral   A unilateral amputation involves the loss of a portion or all of one extremity. This type of amputation leaves the patient with the remaining arm as the predominant side for two-handed activities and provides an opposite arm and shoulder for harnessing and operating the prosthesis. Regardless of whether the patient was right- or left-handed, the remaining extremity becomes the dominant side.

Bilateral   With a bilateral amputation, a portion or all of both upper extremities is lost. These people clearly have more than double the disability of unilateral amputees. For instance, with no sensation in either extremity, one must rely on sight to perform all activities such as finding a keyhole to unlock a door in the dark, taking an object such as coins out of a pocket, or finding lipstick in a purse.

ABOVE- AND BELOW-ELBOW AMPUTATIONS

In addition to the two basic types of upper extremity amputations, a major division of acquired amputations includes those that occur below the elbow (BE) and above the elbow (AE). This distinction is crucial to the fittings and functions of the prosthesis because of the complexities and limitations of the above-elbow prosthesis as compared to the below-elbow prosthesis. Correspondingly, the skills and work the above-elbow amputee is required to master are greater than those required of the below-elbow amputee.

Acquired shoulder amputation is any above-elbow amputation in which no above-elbow function remains, which means that the amputee must use the muscles of the back and opposite extremity to operate the prosthesis. Functional prosthetic use with this level of amputation is very limited.

TYPES OF PROSTHESES

Many devices have been made to replace partial loss of the hand. If the thumb is amputated, a device can be fabricated so that the fingers have something to oppose for grasping, and the same is true if the thumb is intact but the fingers are lost (Fig. 25-1). All of these devices are ugly and are usually not accepted by the amputee, except for laborers who must be able to grasp to do their job, and they usually wear the device only while working. Such amputees have the advantage of sensation, flexion-extension at the wrist, and pronation-supination of the forearm. Because of these advantages, the amputees frequently elect not to be fitted with any device, and they become particularly dexterous with the part of the hand that remains intact. For instance, they can grasp a fork between fingers if the thumb is missing and can develop surprising strength and adroitness in activities of daily living. If the thumb is intact, the second and third fingers can take the place of the index finger for opposition. The primary grasping parts of the hand are the thumb and the index finger. Loss of the other digits does not constitute much of a handicap except cosmetically.

The person with a wrist disarticulation can be fitted with a hook or a hand, but it is difficult to get a good cosmetic appearance because the terminal device will usually make that extremity longer than the remaining arm. Again, supination-pronation of the forearm is retained, which makes function with this device much smoother and more dexterous.

The below-elbow amputee is dependent on length of the below-elbow stump for function.

Figure 25-1
Partial hand prosthesis that provides thumb opposition. *(Used with permission of Northwestern University Prosthetic and Orthotic Center.)*

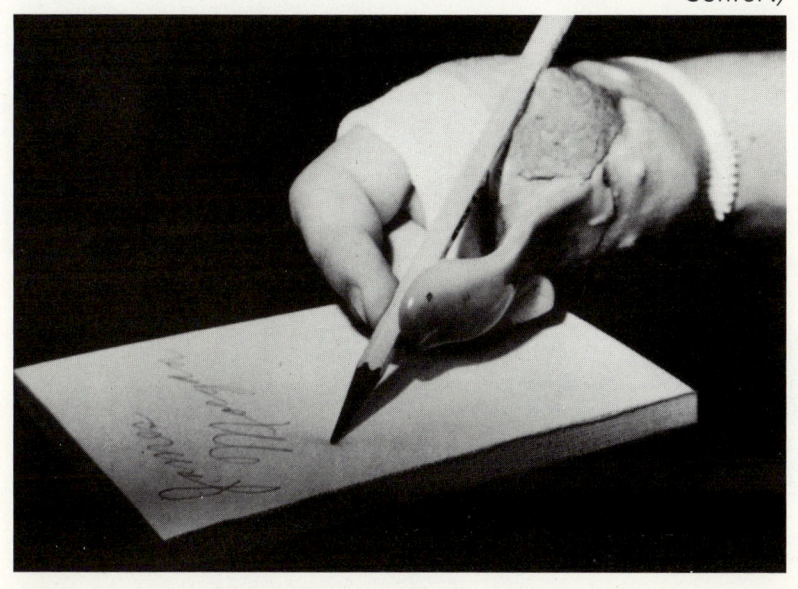

If the stump is long enough, the prosthetist can fit a socket whereby some supination-pronation function of the forearm is retained. If the stump is short, however, the terminal device will have to be manually prepositioned for forearm supination and pronation. Supination-pronation is so much a part of normal use of the upper extremities that its loss presents a frustrating situation in all activities. For instance, in eating, food is picked up with the forearm pronated, but in order to get the food to the mouth, the forearm must be at least partially supinated. In dressing, brushing the teeth, bathing, or using toilet paper, pronation-supination of the forearm is required. Therefore, the bilateral amputee is particularly frustrated and limited in self-care if the amputations are too high to have retained supination-pronation.

The above-elbow amputee has additional problems: the artificial elbow must be locked and unlocked. The elbow unit placed in the above-elbow prosthesis permits the forearm of the prosthesis to be flexed (Fig. 25-2). This procedure is managed by arm flexion, while positive locking and unlocking at any angle of the flexion is achieved by arm extension control acting on an alternator mechanism. This unit also has an adjustable friction turntable attached which provides manual prepositioning of arm rotation. In addition to the elbow-locking operation, there is loss of supination-pronation of the forearm, flexion and extension of the wrist, sensation, and intricate hand movements. The function of fittings for shoulder disarticulations and forequarter amputations is limited indeed, and the prosthesis is worn primarily as a holding device for the dominant side and for cosmesis.

When the amputee has more than one limb missing, problems are multiplied. An amputee with an arm amputation above the elbow and a leg amputation above the knee will usually need help in putting on the prosthesis. A few can manage to apply their own prostheses with special adaptations such as a pelvic belt instead of suction suspension. The less agile will need help. The above-elbow bilateral amputee will also usually need help. The older person who has also suffered a stroke will be advised to use a wheelchair instead of trying to get about with a prosthesis. One young woman who lost both

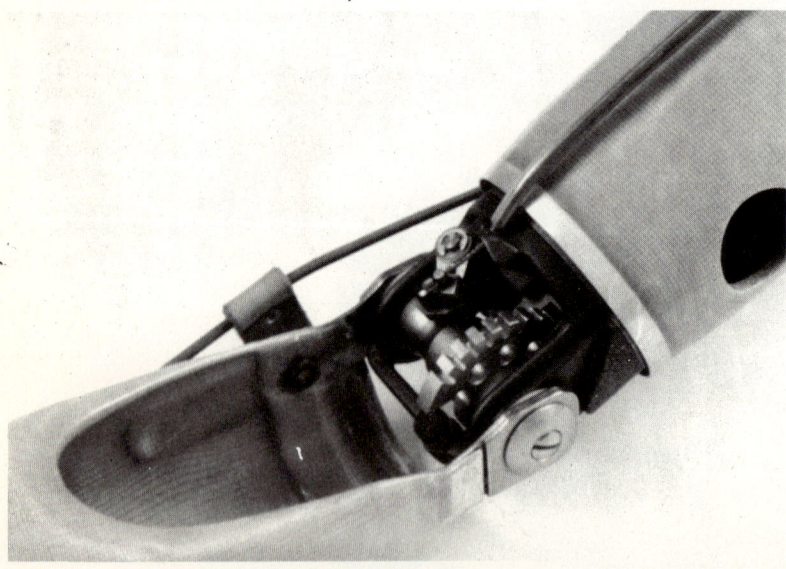

Figure 25-2
Upper-extremity prosthesis elbow unit. *(Used with permission of Northwestern University Prosthetic and Orthotic Center.)*

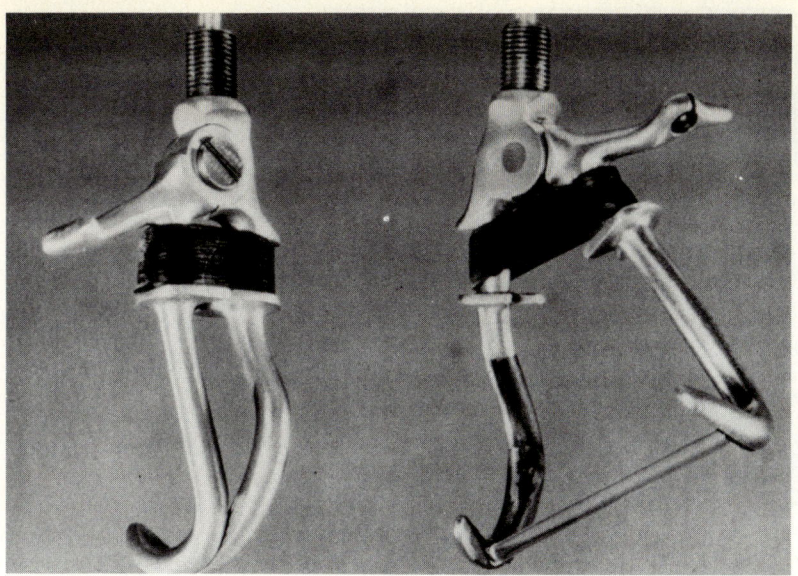

Figure 25-3
Voluntary opening two-fingered hook. *(Used with permission of Northwestern University Prosthetic and Orthotic Center.)*

lower extremities above the knee and one upper extremity above the elbow was not considered for lower extremity prostheses but was fitted with an above-elbow prosthesis and discharged in a one-arm-drive wheelchair. She became very skillful in maneuvering the wheelchair and returned to managing her own home. It is necessary to keep in mind that the human being can tolerate just so much gadgetry. Overzealous provision of unnecessary devices can frustrate the patient to the point of refusing to use necessary equipment.

TYPES OF TERMINAL DEVICES

Many terminal devices have been developed, and some are startling in their claims of usefulness. Although many of these have been discarded as inadequate, the two remaining basic types of mechanisms in terminal devices are those that permit voluntary opening and voluntary opening and closing. Each can be found in either hand or hook. The voluntary opening hook or hand is opened by the amputee by active use of the shoulder control and is closed by relaxation of the shoulder control. The voluntary opening and closing device is both opened and closed by the shoulder control. The terminal device found to be the most useful over the years, accepted by professionals and patients alike, is the voluntary opening two-fingered hook and the cosmetic hand (Figs. 25-3 and 25-4).

The hook most commonly seen is the voluntary opening, conventional, single-load hook. The grasp force is attained by the use of rubber bands. Thus the force can be increased or decreased by increasing or decreasing the number of rubber bands. One rubber band is equal to approximately 1 lb of fingertip grasp. The width of the grasp of these hooks is about 3 in, enough to grasp a can of beer. Occasionally, you will see one of these hooks with springs instead of rubber bands. The hooks can be manufactured from steel or aluminum alloy, depending on the workload for which they are to be used. The grasping surfaces can be plain metal or have a neoprene lining for better grasp and holding. Each hook has a projection near the wrist that is used to stabilize objects such as a knife when cutting meat.

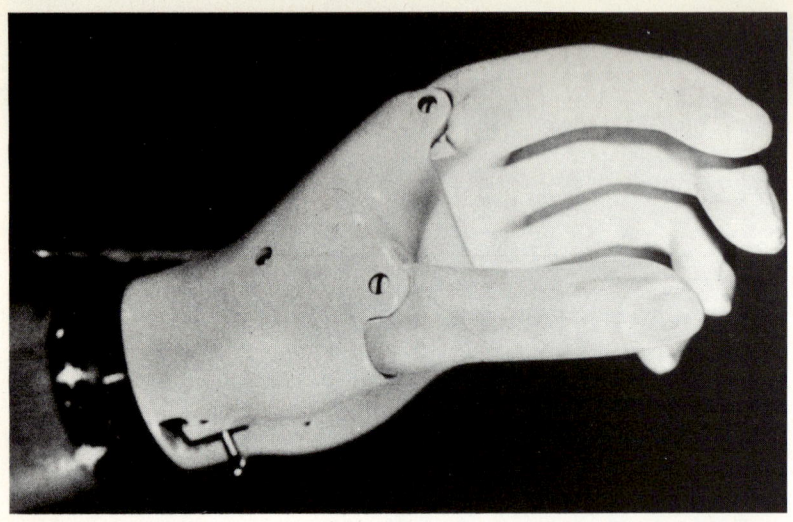

Figure 25-4
Cosmetic hand without glove. *(Used with permission of Northwestern University Prosthetic and Orthotic Center.)*

The voluntary opening and closing hooks and hands are also operated by the shoulder control. The amputee must open the device and close the device with shoulder action, because as the hook opens, it locks in the open position with relaxation of the shoulder control and stays locked until the amputee actively contracts the shoulder control to release the grasp and the fingers automatically return to the closed position. Thus the patient with a voluntary opening and closing terminal device must use a "double shuffle" action to operate the hook, which requires more energy to operate than the more simple voluntary opening hook. This terminal device does not hold up well to stresses and strains of heavy duty.

The prosthetic hand can be passive or active because the amputee will find that he or she has lost much of the dexterity that is present with the hook. The expected service life of a cosmetic glove is 3 to 4 months. Much depends on the amputee's ability to avoid staining from such things as ball-point pens, paints, and some fruits and vegetables, as these stains cannot be removed. Also, the glove covering changes color just from exposure.

The use of both hand and hook is easily accomplished with the same prosthesis because a wrist unit is built into the prosthesis so that the hook can be removed and the hand readily snapped into its place. The amputee is always trained initially with the hook because it is lighter in weight and much more functional. After skill has been gained in using the hook, the hand is often found to be too awkward and heavy for any practical use but will be worn for social functions.

REACTION TO AMPUTATION

Usually new amputees have never seen a stump before they see their own, and they are absolutely overwhelmed that a part of them is no longer there. For some, it is a tragedy that they cannot accept even though the limb is obviously missing. Adjusting to loss, altered body image, role reversal, concept of self, and vocational changes are all at issue (Pfefferbaum and Pasnau, 1976; Wright, 1964). In one case, a middle-aged man slipped and fell under a train and lost one arm above the elbow and one leg above the knee. He was an experienced electrician, and he could not accept the fact that he would be unable to do the climbing and the intricate handwork required on electrical jobs. However, with encouragement, good prosthetic care, and vocational counseling, he was able to return to the job as the supervisor and advisor to other, less experienced electricians.

Loss of an extremity is similar in many respects to the death of a family member (Parkes, 1975). The amputation affects not only the amputee but indeed all who are concerned with the welfare of the new amputee. In the case of the electrician, his wife was taught to bandage the stumps. Because bandaging was such an essential part of his preprosthetic care, it had to be done with a certain technique and had to be repeated at least three times a day to be effective. The wrapping procedure is usually too difficult for upper extremity amputees to do alone. Although his wife was eager to help, the sight of her husband's stumps made her so ill that at first she would have to interrupt the bandaging to vomit. Gradually, she controlled the vomiting, but she never got over her revulsion about the stumps.

There is something about seeing a stump that is very disturbing to most people; at times, the experience can be devastating. A new secretary hired for a physical therapy department had been chosen not only because she could type well and had a pleasant personality but also because she said disabled people did not bother her. (Only persons with severe physical disabilities were treated in this department, and all were visually apparent to everyone who worked in the department.) Everything was working well until amputee clinic day arrived, and the new secretary saw a stump or two. She was unable to sleep that night and handed in her resignation the next morning, saying she "couldn't take the chance of seeing another stump."

It is absolutely essential for all health workers—doctor, nurse, therapist—to consider and involve the family in the planning and rehabilitation of the amputee. If the family cannot accept the amputation and the prosthetic device, neither will the amputee. When, for example, a parent of a young amputee hangs the new prosthesis in a closet, it will be the rare child who takes the "new arm" out of the closet and struggles into it alone.

A young nursing student was in an accident in which she lost her right arm above the elbow. Much family support and encouragement were needed because this young woman not only had to face the complex cosmetic and social implications of amputation but also had her chosen career halted in midstream. After completing her prosthetic training and becoming skillful in the use of her prosthesis, she met a young man who was accepting and understanding about her disability. They were married, and she became a happy housewife and mother. Without the support of family plus an effective prosthetic program, she would have remained withdrawn, refusing prosthetic fitting and training.

When an amputee perceives that the immediate family does not want to look at or touch the stump, it is very likely they will not be asked to help with wrapping the stump, even though the amputee knows such wrapping is essential. Efforts should be made early to determine the ability of the family to participate in preprosthetic stump wrapping and care because of the significance of preparing the stump properly and quickly for prosthetic fitting. When such is not the case, the issue should be addressed directly and the patient referred to outpatient care. Significant others who can participate in the wrapping should be involved. If several months pass without a prosthetic device, the amputee will become one-handed in habits, and it is unlikely that the unilateral upper extremity amputee will seek or effectively make use of a prosthetic device.

PREPROSTHETIC CARE

Although the emotional needs of the amputee are often greater than the physical needs, one physical procedure is absolutely essential and should be started as soon as the stitches are removed, namely an effective wrapping program that will shape and shrink the stump (Fig. 25-5). The technique used is crucial so as not to injure the stump but to shrink and shape it before the patient is referred to a prosthetist for measurements for the prosthetic socket. If effective bandaging is not done prior to fitting of the socket, the stump will shrink with socket wear and use, and as a result, the socket will be too large. Sockets are expensive, and early replacement can be avoided with proper wrapping. Along with the wrapping program, stump exercises are needed to maintain range of motion and strength. The amputee, following the trauma of an amputation, is inclined to hold the remaining part tightly, with the shoulder high and the elbow flexed close to the body. An effective wrapping and exercise program will hasten rehabilitation because a properly shaped stump, plus adequate range and muscle strength, will be ready for fitting sooner, and there will be no contractures to stretch out or muscles that need to be strengthened before fitting can take place. If instructed, the amputee can carry out a routine exercise program that will be most effective.

PRESCRIPTION AND PROSTHETIC FITTING

The importance of the amputee clinic team cannot be overemphasized for the care and progression of all amputee patients. Invariably, an upper extremity amputee is soon transferred to outpatient care. Hospital care is no longer needed after the initial surgical procedures, and the amputee is quickly discharged to the home environment. Therefore, it is essential that he or she be followed by a progressive clinic team where an appropriate therapy program is established, to be done at home or on an outpatient basis, depending on the severity of the problem and the ability of the patient and family to cope with it.

When the stump is ready to be fitted, a prescription (Fig. 25-6) is written by the clinic team using the knowledge and expertise of all its members. The prosthesis is then fabricated per prescription by a prosthetist who has had special training in the techniques of limb manufacturing.

KINEPLASTY

Sometimes, in specially selected cases, the surgeon has suggested a kineplasty type of operation. This is a surgical procedure in which a tunnel is created in a muscle, and the tunneled muscle is then used to activate the terminal device. The ideal amputation for this type of procedure is a medium to long below-elbow stump, and the biceps muscle is used to form the tunnel. The biceps muscle is excised at its insertion at the elbow, and a tunnel is made in the freed end. The amputee uses this single muscle tunnel to operate the terminal device instead of using body motions with the conventional harnessing. By eliminating the across-the-shoulders harness, the amputee can be much

Figure 25-5
Stump wrapped above elbow. *(Used with permission of Northwestern University Prosthetic and Orthotic Center.)*

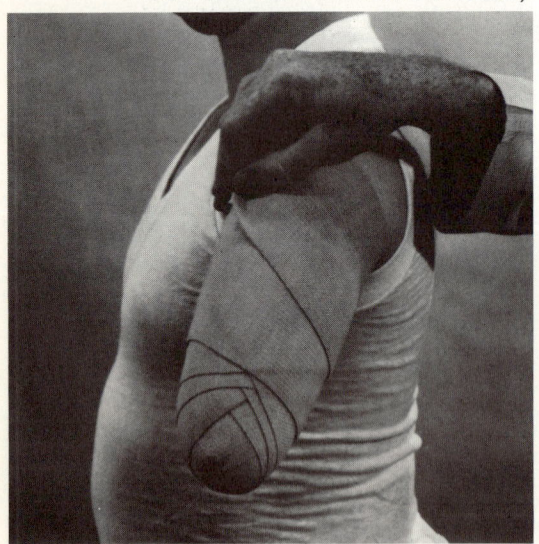

UPPER-EXTREMEITY AMPUTEE PROSTHETIC PRESCRIPTION

Name _____ RIC No. _____ Date _____

Age _____ Male _____ Female _____

Amputation type: Partial hand: L____ R____   Elbow disartic.: L____ R____
                  Wrist disartic.: L____ R____   A/E: L____ R____
                  B/E: L____ R____   Shoulder disartic.: L____ R____
                                                      Forequarter: L____ R____

I. TERMINAL DEVICE:
    Hook _____
        Voluntary opening _____
        Voluntary closing _____
    Hand _____
        Voluntary closing _____
        Voluntary opening _____
        Passive type _____
        Cosmetic glove _____

II. WRIST UNIT:
    Standard friction type _____
    Positive lock (quick disconnect) _____
    Flexion unit (specify R____ or L _____
        if bilateral _____)
    Oval unit _____
    Round unit _____

III. SOCKET (plastic laminate):
    Single wall _____
    Double wall _____
    B/E: Split (for step up hinge) _____
          Socket to fit around olecranon? ____
              yes_____ no_____
          Preflexed socket _____
    A/E: Socket to fit over acromion?
              yes_____ no_____
          Ant. & Post. wings _____
    S/D:

IV. ELBOW:
    B/E: Flexible dacron hinges _____
          Rigid single axis _____
          Rigid polycentric _____
          Step up _____
          Stump actuated lock _____
          Other _____
    A/E: Inside locking joint _____
     &   Outside locking joint _____
    S/D: Harness controlled lock _____
          Manual controlled lock _____
          Turn table _____
          Spring assist _____
          Electric elbow _____

V. CABLE SYSTEM:
    Bowden cable: _____
        Standard _____
        Heavy duty _____
        Nylined _____
    B/E: Forearm lift assist _____
    A/E: Dual control _____
     &   Triple control _____
    S/D: Excursion multipler _____

VI. HARNESSING:
    Width of webbing; ½"_____ 1"_____
    Figure of 8: Regular____ Ring_____
    B/E: Shoulder saddle _____
          Triceps cuff: leather____ plastic____
                       full____ half____
    A/E: Chest strap _____
     &   Opposite shoulder loop _____
    S/D: Perineal strap _____
          Belt strap _____
          Nudge control _____
          Shoulder joint _____
          Flex. - Ext. _____
          Abd. _____

VII. STUMP SOCKS:
    How many? _____
    Ply _____
    Wool _____
    Cotton _____

REMARKS:

LIMB SHOP: _____

PHYSICIAN: _____

Figure 25-6
Upper-extremity amputee prescription form. (Used with permission of the Rehabilitation Institute of Chicago.)

more facile in using the prosthesis over the head, behind the back, or, in fact, in almost any position. There are many pitfalls with the kineplasty. The tunnels must be kept scrupulously clean. There is a special technique in performing the surgery, and if the tunnel is not satisfactory, the amputee must resort to the conventional below-elbow prosthesis without the powerful biceps muscle as a flexor of the elbow, since there is no way to reattach the muscle at the elbow.

Bilateral amputees should not be considered for kineplasty prostheses, as they will have too much difficulty keeping the tunnels clean and applying the prostheses. Furthermore, preprosthetic strengthening and mobility programs are more extensive for the tunnel users, since the muscle must be reeducated functionally, its size, strength, and mobility must be developed, and the tunnel must be toughened to tolerate the pull of the pin in the tunnel. Therefore, the kineplasty patient will be off the job longer because the preprosthetic process is more prolonged. However, the kineplasty patient has better control and better sensory feedback, and the more complex voluntary closing terminal device is frequently of value.

ACTIVITIES OF DAILY LIVING

Amputees have been most ingenious in their efforts to live comfortably in spite of their problems with activities of daily living. For example, they change to loafer-type shoes to avoid the cumbersome task of tying shoelaces; they use elastic on the cuffs of their shirts or blouses in place of the traditional button and buttonhole so that they can get the garment on and off without buttoning and unbuttoning the sleeve; they cut all their meat at one time instead of the more socially acceptable cut-and-eat procedure; they do not carry coins in the pocket on the amputated side. The bilateral amputee will carry coins, house keys, and the like in a small purse attached with a chain to a belt of some type at the waist. There are many adaptations that amputees devise and use, depending on the level of amputation, the ability to tolerate gadgetry, and how adept they are in using the prosthesis.

TRAINING

Training starts the day the prosthesis is delivered to the clinic and has been accepted as satisfactory. Since the prescription was written as a team effort, the prosthesis fabricated by a member of the team, and the training done by the clinic therapists, a general feeling of responsibility exists so that errors are corrected, changes made, and revisions accomplished with a minimum of friction and difficulty. The training is usually initiated in the physical therapy department, with follow-up activities in the occupational therapy department to give the amputee experience in use. In training the amputee, a thorough checkout is done first, including evaluation of the efficiency of suspension and harnessing, comparison of the length and size with the remaining extremity, and assessment of comfort, workmanship, and cosmesis (Fig. 25-7).

**Figure 25-7
Above elbow prosthetic device with harnessing.** *(Used with permission of Northwestern University Prosthetic and Orthotic Center.)*

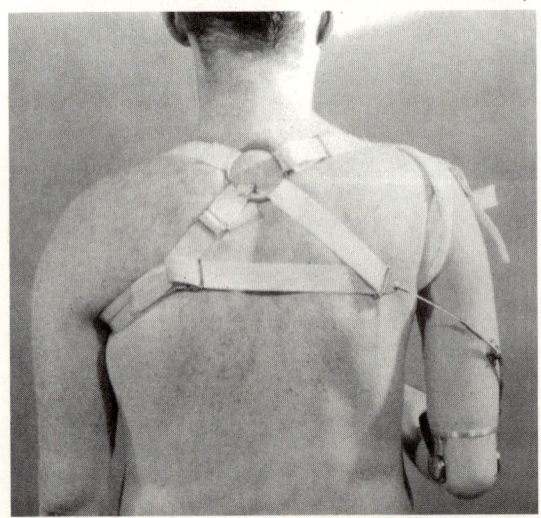

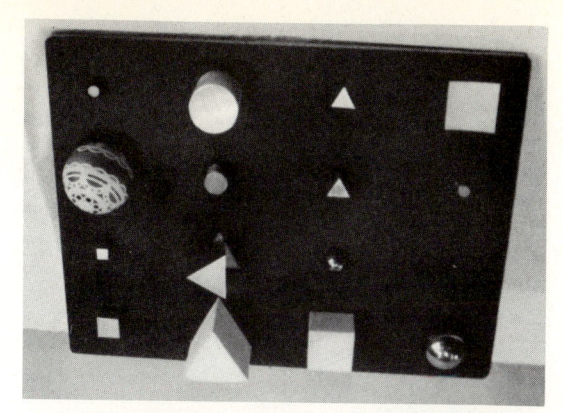

Figure 25-8
Amputee training board. *(Used with permission of Northwestern University Prosthetic and Orthotic Center.)*

When this checkout is satisfactory, training for all upper extremity amputees begins with instruction in putting on and taking off the prosthesis. Next, control of the terminal device is taught. This includes prepositioning for forearm pronation-supination activities and learning how to open and close the terminal device. In addition, the above-elbow amputees must learn to lock and unlock the elbow joint.

The amputee is taught how to grasp objects, control the amount of pinch to apply, and approach an object to pick it up through the use of a training board containing objects of various sizes, shapes, and consistency (Fig. 25-8). When these activities are mastered, the amputee is literally drilled in activities of daily living, such as putting on and taking off the prosthesis, buttoning buttons, tying a tie, wrapping a package, fastening a bra, using eating utensils, and picking up paper cups, glasses, and the like. It is always kept in mind that the prosthesis is used as an aid to the remaining extremity. The unilateral amputee should not be asked to do a one-handed activity with the prosthetic side. The prosthesis is used essentially as a holding device. For instance, in sharpening a pencil, the prosthetic side holds the pencil in place while the normal extremity performs the more complicated procedure of grasping and turning the handle. A good trainer of amputees will always demonstrate to the patient how an activity can be done, or how other amputees have been able to accomplish the act, before asking the patient to do an activity for the first time.

STUMP SOCKS AND PROSTHESIS CARE

Stump socks are used by most upper extremity amputees. The socks serve as a cushioning between the stump and the socket wall, absorb perspiration, and are a hedge against the development of blisters; in addition, the amputee generally feels more comfortable with them. The socks are usually made of cotton stockinette material, although other materials can be used if preferred. One grandmother knitted angora wool socks for her grandson's congenital below-elbow stump. A fresh sock should be worn at least daily and whenever needed. Socks should be washed after each wearing and rinsed thoroughly.

Also during training, the amputee is taught how to clean the prosthesis socket with soap and water, how to care for the hook, how to replace rubber bands as they become worn, how to care for and clean the cosmetic glove, and how to scrub the harness when necessary. The amputee should be encouraged to wear a cotton T shirt under the prosthesis.

During training, it is wise to have a family member present to see and appreciate progress so that the amputee will find encouragement and understanding at home. Amputees do not take the prosthesis home until they are proficient in its use. It is interesting to note that when an amputee becomes skillful in the use of the prosthesis, the prosthesis becomes less noticeable to others.

FOLLOW-UP PROGRAM

Regular checkup visits to the clinic are both supportive for the amputee and a means of keeping the prosthesis in good condition so as to avoid major repairs with loss of the prosthesis for several days. More than one prosthesis is not recommended, because the stump changes in shape and size over the years, making the standby prosthesis impractical; also, the development of new and improved parts will be desirable in future prostheses. Replacements depend on the adequacy of the initial fitting, how much it is used, financial arrangements, and quite often the desires and temperament of the patient. For the child amputee, of course, the replacements must correspond to the growth pattern, which usually means a new prosthesis every 3 years during the growing years. In the meantime, repairs and replacement of parts are performed as needed.

CONCLUSION

The upper extremity amputee needs the support of nurses employed in hospitals even though the patient will be under their care for only a brief time and will present few physical needs. While it is easily understood that the nurse caring for the amputee will rarely have any involvement during the prosthetic stage and beyond, timely, purposeful interaction with the patient and family immediately following surgery can assist immeasurably in positively preparing them for what will follow. The amputee is experiencing a painful but necessary mourning period and will need time and assistance to accept the amputation. In addition, referral to a competent amputee clinic team is of the utmost importance.

The need to include significant others in the patient's rehabilitation is absolutely essential, for their support and understanding are vital in helping the amputee cope with the continuous emotional episodes that will occur. Even when highly skilled in the use of their prostheses, amputees constantly face embarrassing situations in public. For example, people often shy away when they see a hook showing at the end of an amputee's sleeve. Furthermore, there is no way to avoid the frustration facing bilateral upper extremity amputees when cashiers drop change on the counter instead of handing it to them, and they must laboriously collect the coins or walk out without the change.

Although much has been accomplished in the way of scientific knowledge about prosthetics and about the need for team approach, much continued research is needed to improve the manufacture and the function of the product. Surgeons strive to preserve more and more of the extremity by using new and experimental surgical techniques. Research is being done in the application of electronics, but this is a costly endeavor. Above all, following any upper extremity amputation, we must accept the fact that some things cannot be replaced: loss of sensation, the many intricate functions of the hand, the change in appearance or cosmesis, and the need for sight to operate the terminal device effectively.

BIBLIOGRAPHY

Anderson, M., C. Bechtol, and R. Sollars: *Clinical Prosthetics for Physicians and Therapists,* Charles C Thomas, Springfield, 1959.

Chaiklin, H., and M. Warfield: "Stigma Management and Amputee Rehabilitation," in J. Stubbins (ed.): *Social and Psychological Aspects of Disability: A Handbook for Practitioners,* University Park, Baltimore, 1977, p. 605.

Goffman, I.: *Stigma: Notes on the Management of Spoiled Identity,* Prentice-Hall, Englewood Cliffs, N.J., 1963.

Halsled, L. S., et al.: "Sexual Attitudes, Behavior and Satisfaction for Able-Bodied and Disabled Participants Attending Workshops in Human Sexuality," *Arch Phys Med Rehabil* 59:497–501, 1978.

LaBorde, T., and R. Meier: "Amputations Resulting from Electrical Injury: A Review of 22 Cases," *Arch Phys Med Rehabil* 59(3):134–137, 1978.

McClinton, V.: "Nursing of the Upper Extremity Amputee and Preparation for Prosthetic

Training," *Nurs Clin North Am* 11:(4) 671–677, 1976.

Parkes, C. M.: "Psycho Social Transitions: Comparisons to Loss of Limb and Loss of Spouse," *Br J Psychiatry* 127:204–210, 1975.

Pasnau, R., and B. Pfefferbaum: "Psychologic Aspects of Post-amputation Pain," *Nurs Clin North Am* 11(4):679–685, 1976.

Pfefferbaum, B., and R. Pasnau: Post-amputation Grief, *Nurs Clin North Am* 11(4):687–690, 1976.

Wright, B.: *Physical Disability—A Psychological Approach,* Harper, New York, 1960.

———: "Spread in Adjustment to Disability," *Bull Menninger Clin,* 28:198–208, 1964.

26
betty quinn*

lower extremity
amputation

INTRODUCTION

The purpose of this chapter is to point out the tremendous need for all nurses to gain proficiency in the art of patient and family education and to learn to assist the patient and the family or significant others in establishing realistic goals. This should be done within the structure of a short-term program that leads to long-term acceptance of the situation. A great deal of consideration must be given to many facets so that each facet may be accepted or rejected as an appropriate short-term goal in the step-by-step attainment of the desired long-term results. If such a plan does not mirror the actual goals of the patient and others most closely involved, nothing will be gained.

All involved parties need to learn that some failure along the way does not mean that a particular plan should be abandoned. A failure at any given stage frequently enhances the coping mechanisms so that a more appropriate method may then bring success. Such success is achieved through the cooperation of the entire rehabilitation team. It must be explained in advance that although a suggested approach might not work, it is certainly worth a try.

EDUCATIONAL NEEDS OF PATIENT AND FAMILY OR SIGNIFICANT OTHERS

PREAMPUTATION

Diagnostic or surgical procedures (scheduled or anticipated) prior to amputation should be explained thoroughly. The explanation should cover the reason the procedure is being carried out, as well as the methods used (Jones et al., 1978). It is extremely helpful to patients to describe the sensations that they may encounter during and after the procedure. Knowing what to expect usually allays a patient's normal fear of the unknown. The patient will later recall the possible results and thus will be less shocked by these events. If a patient has been told that an arteriogram may feel like a wave of heat along a blood vessel, gaining in intensity until it feels like an explosion, the patient will be likely to remember this when the feeling actually occurs. This memory will relieve the mental anguish following the flash of thought that says "Dear God—this is it!"

A patient is usually quite aware of the nurses' show of concern, however unintentional, when they dash around following the patient's femoral-popliteal bypass, busily checking peripheral pulses. When a patient has been forewarned of the need for such action, it will seem merely like a routine check and will thus lessen any apprehension. Furthermore, if patients have been made aware that the bypass surgery may not be successful, they will gradually begin to cope with the inevitable and dreaded thought of possible amputation.

Traumatic injuries leave little time for explanation, but nurses should use the time before the surgical amputation to convey as much information as possible. They should concentrate on the affirmative results that are hoped for, such as removal of irreparably damaged tissues so that the circulatory system may be reunited to do its work in feeding the remaining viable tissues, prevention or lessening of infection, or alignment of all parts in order to have them in the proper anatomical relationship for the most functional usage.

POSTAMPUTATION

Residual Limb Care

Care of the stump will be a lifelong process for amputees, so it is imperative that they be taught the basic elements of this care as soon as possible. Great emphasis must be given to proper routines of skin care, positioning, exercise, and ways of shrinking and shaping the stump. If a rigid dressing, such as a plaster stump wrap, or an immediate postsurgical fitting (IPSF) has been applied in surgery, it will probably remain in

*Ms. Quinn is herself a bilateral lower extremity amputee.

place for a week or 10 days (Engstrand, 1976). Then the stitches will be removed, and a new dressing will be applied for a similar period of time. This method does not obviate the need for education on shrinking and shaping; it merely postpones it. Patients still need to know all the basic stump care procedures because the shrinkage will vary in relation to ambulation for a good many months. The rigid dressing is intended to lessen edema and pain, and the IPSF gives the added convenience of immediate ambulation (Fig. 26-1). The rigid dressing, with or without the immediate postsurgical fitting, will eventually be removed, and stump care will be necessary for the next step, the temporary prosthesis.

The skin must be kept clean and dry. But if the skin becomes too dry, it will scale, flake, and perhaps crack, thus delaying use of the prosthesis (Fig. 26-2). If the skin becomes too soft, it will be unable to tolerate the demands of the prosthesis, pressure sores will develop, and the rehabilitation process will be delayed.

Exercises will help the patient to build up muscle strength while gaining progressive ambulation. Isometrics can be advantageously used from the first postoperative day. Proper positioning and neutral body alignment help avoid contractures of hip flexors and in the popliteal area of below-knee amputees. Prone positioning several times a day is essential for avoiding such contractures. If the patient uses a wheelchair, a board must be placed to extend the below-knee

Figure 26-1
Below-knee amputation with rigid plaster dressing and immediate post surgical fitting (IPSF). *(Used with permission of Northwestern University Prosthetic and Orthotic Center.)*

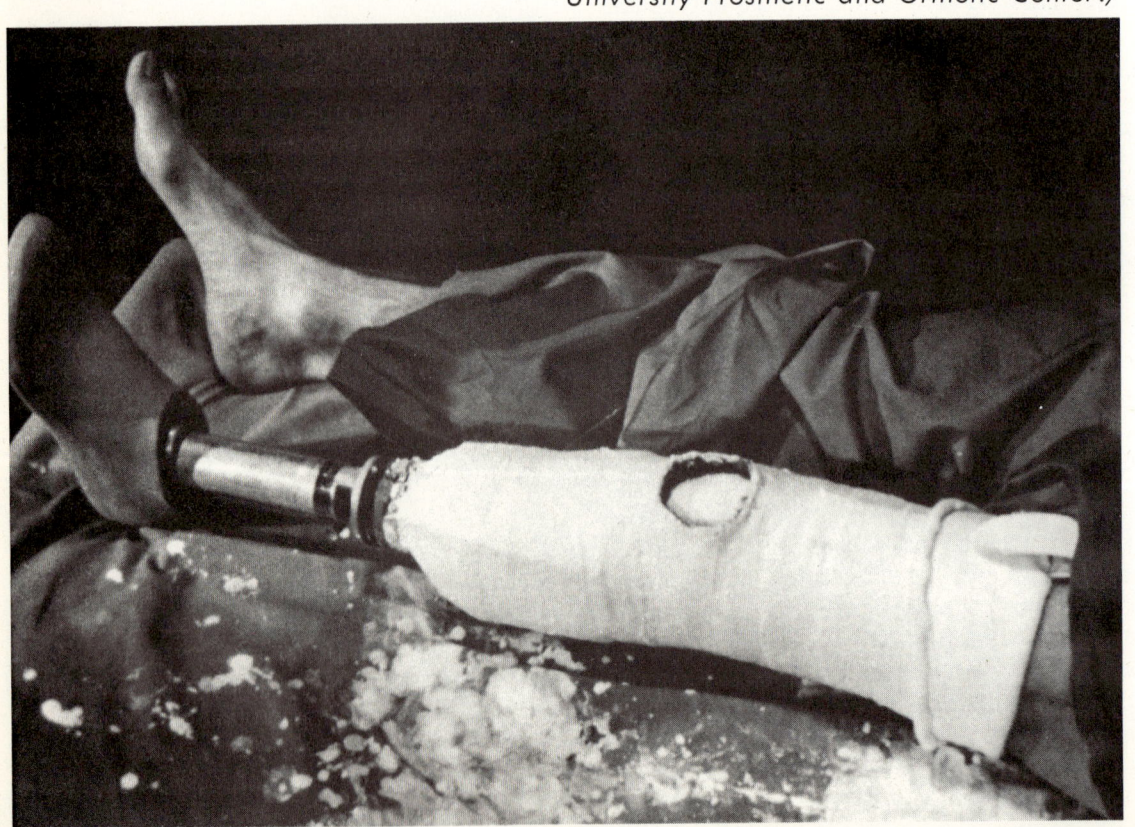

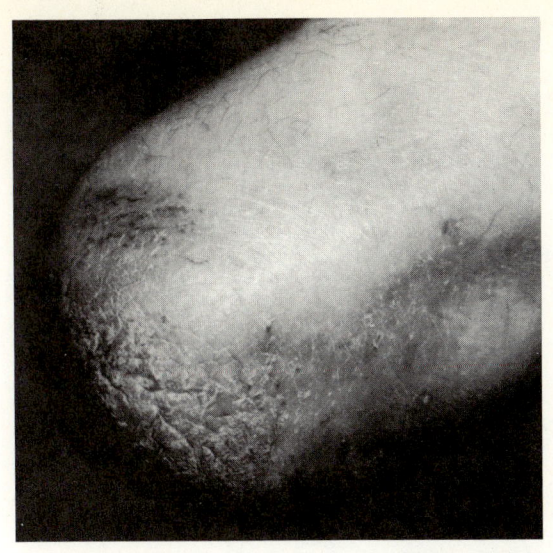

Figure 26-2
Lower extremity stump, cracked and too dry. *(Used with permission of Northwestern University Prosthetic and Orthotic Center.)*

stump. (Figures 26-3a,b, 26-4, 26-5, and 26-6 illustrate some of the exercises the amputee should do.)

Properly applied elastic bandages aid in shaping the stump, and patients must learn how to apply such bandages (Jones, 1978). If this is not possible, a family member or significant other must be instructed. The stump should be wrapped in spirals, not with circular turns, as the latter may constrict the circulation. Wrapping the distal end of the stump more firmly than the proximal discourages edema and produces a shape more conducive to a good prosthetic fit.

POSTOPERATIVE PAIN

Pain is a matter of semantics. What may be an annoying sensation to one person may well be severe pain to another. Nurses should endeavor to make nonjudgmental assessments. There are both advantages and disadvantages to discussing phantom pain and phantom sensation with the patient, although Solomon (1978) states it should be discussed. It is truly difficult for a new amputee to evaluate the difference between real and imagined pain (Lee, 1976). I kept telling myself that I could not be having pain in that foot because it simply was not there. How could it hurt? But it did. A few months later, I was readily aware of a phantom sensation when my missing big toe began to itch like mad. Nurses would do well to give credence to the patient's complaint by carefully comparing the subjective symptoms with the objective ones and then acting in accordance with good, basic nursing care. Perhaps if nurses think of it as referred pain, they might have a better perspective. Why should anyone have a headache simply because they have been constipated for several days? The area that hurts is not always where the problem lies.

Stump appearance is initially a real shock to patients, even if prior to amputation they have been told what to expect. They should be told how the stump will look but also that the amputation is only the beginning and that the results will be essentially of the patients' own making. This is not easy to get across to the amputee, since visualizing the loss of a limb is absolutely devastating. Family members and significant others are commonly initially frightened by seeing the stump and totally overwhelmed at the thought of having to touch or handle it for cleaning and wrapping. This apprehension can be reduced if the nurse actually guides the hands of the patient or significant other during beginning contact with the stump.

DIETARY AND FLUID NEEDS

Dietary needs are too often neglected. Because lower extremity amputees expend extra energy in ambulation, they need more calories. This is a prime concern for diabetics taking hypoglycemic medicine. Usually more carbohydrates will be necessary, but protein intake is equally vital to balance the diet and afford normal nutrition.

Most lower extremity amputees find that they perspire much more than they did prior to

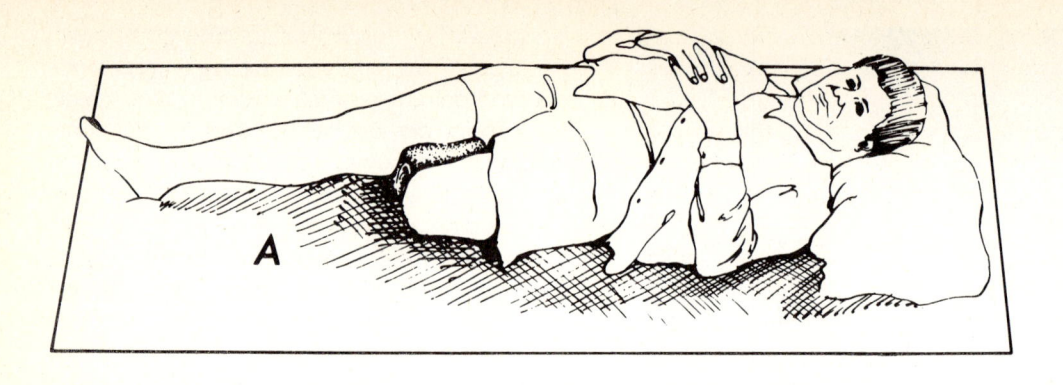

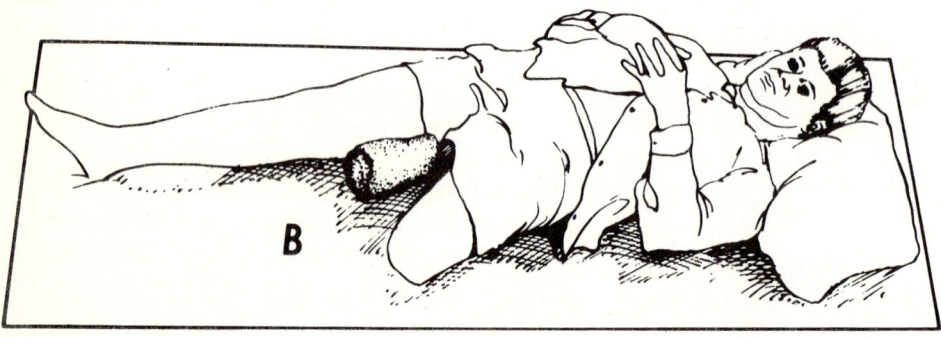

Figure 26-3A and B
Hip abduction-adduction. A small towel roll is placed between the thighs. The stump is moved laterally as far as possible, then moved in toward the other leg to squeeze the towel roll for 5 to 7 counts. The exercise should be repeated according to increasing tolerance and endurance. *(Used with the permission of the Rehabilitation Institute of Chicago.)*

amputation, but they fail to realize that this is the result of the new combination of additional energy expenditure, the loss of body surface for evaporation, and the limitation of air evaporation on the stump when it is encased in wool, acrylic material, and/or plastics used in the liner and prosthesis. The increased diaphoresis is not necessarily confined to the stump (it seems to be more predominant in the scalp). If there are no medical contraindications, additional salt may be needed to replace that lost in profuse diaphoresis. An adequate fluid intake must be encouraged to prevent dehydration and urinary tract problems. Urinary tract problems can develop because amputees have a tendency to allow the bladder to overload and to drink insufficient fluids because toilet facilities are frequently unavailable within a comfortable walking distance.

PREPARATION FOR MOBILITY

The amputee needs to use positive measures to strengthen the upper extremities and to achieve free-standing balance on one leg (like a stork). Extreme muscular strength is needed so that the patient can use both hands at the same time, without leaning on anything. Try to stand on one leg, not leaning on the bathroom sink, and use both hands for shaving or putting your hair up in curlers. For free-sitting balance, a different set of muscles needs strengthening.

There is no reason, except other medical problems, that a unilateral below-knee amputee cannot transfer to toilet, wheelchair, bed, or car independently. But nurses must be very much aware that these patients are frightened and insecure. They need encouragement within realistic limits.

Learning to transfer to a wheelchair without a prosthesis should begin in the acute hospital setting, thus starting the rehabilitation process. Even a bilateral lower extremity amputee should be taught immediately to transfer from bed to wheelchair to toilet and return, because all through life these actions will be necessary. Certainly, it is a great deal easier for the amputee to use the wheelchair to get out of bed to go to the toilet than it is to attach a prosthesis for this purpose.

Early ambulation with or without a prosthesis should be encouraged so that the amputee will become accustomed to the diminished weight without a prosthesis or what seems like additional weight with it. Whether a walker or crutches will work better depends on the individual. Crutches enable the amputee to utilize a more natural stride and require strengthening of trunk muscles used in balance. It is often difficult for the patient to achieve a rhythmic gait, but confidence and practice will overcome such problems. When a patient uses crutches to walk without a prosthesis, nurses should give frequent reminders about posture and neutral alignment of the stump. If this is not stressed, knee and hip flexion contractures may result. Amputees generally seem to flex the hip with an above-knee stump and to flex the knee with a below-knee stump.

Figure 26-4
Hip extension from Thomas position. Both legs are flexed toward the chest. The hands hold the nonamputated leg close to the chest. The stump is lowered forward and pushed down into the lying surface from 5 to 7 counts. The exercise should be repeated according to increasing tolerance and endurance. *(Used with the permission of the Rehabilitation Institute of Chicago.)*

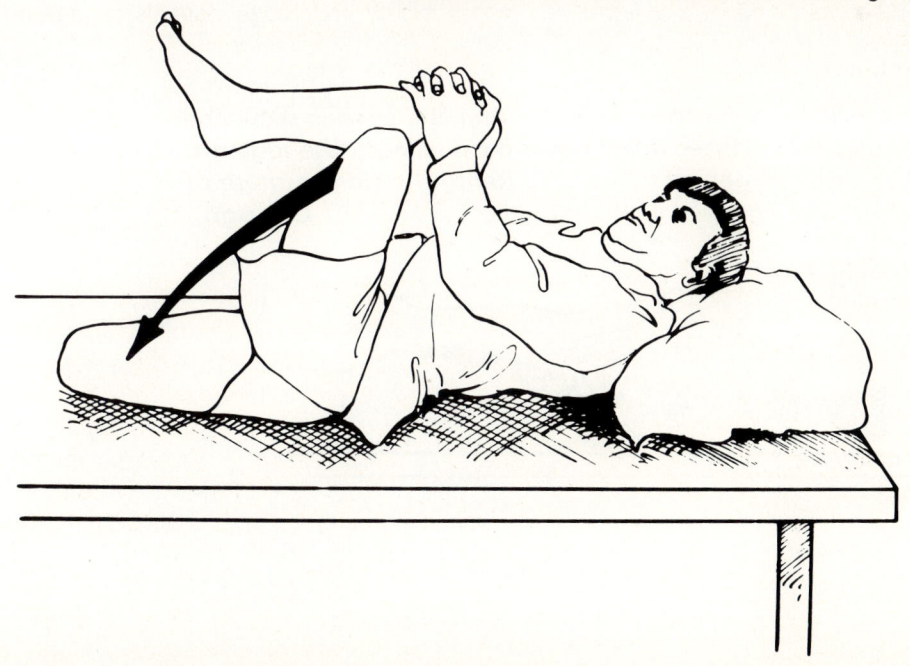

TEMPORARY AND PERMANENT PROSTHESES

Temporary pylons other than the previously mentioned IPSF or rigid dressings are usually worn by the amputee while the stump is still in the early shrinking process. The reasons for wearing the pylon need to be explained to patients. Pylons are frequently a cosmetic shock for which patients should be prepared. They can be told that a pylon is an artificial foot, the same size as the normal foot, with a piece of "pipe" between the foot and the plaster socket that fits around the stump, topped with straps on each side acting like garters that attach to a waist strap (Fig. 26-1). Patients should be made aware that it is not at all what the finished product will look like. The pylon can be made a bit more normal in appearance if the pipe is shaped with foam and dressed up with a stocking. The shoes worn with the temporary pylon need to be comfortable and yet sturdy enough that they will not cause a shuffle or uneasy gait.

At this point, a schedule is set up to test the patient's skin tolerance with the temporary prosthesis. This is often a progressive schedule of time on and time off, with no weight bearing at first. The length of time that the prosthesis is worn is gradually increased. When it is established that skin tolerance is sufficient, progressive ambulation begins. If the patient is ambulating in the physical therapy department, concurrent floor ambulation may not be advisable. Frequent skin checks are necessary during the progressive "on-off" period to establish tolerance. The stump should be wrapped when the temporary prosthesis is off.

Preplanning for the definitive prosthesis benefits patients. When, by trial of the temporary prosthesis, it has been determined that the amputee is a candidate for a permanent prosthesis, proper shoes should be available for the first appointment with the prosthetist. The comfort and support of the normal foot are of prime importance, as the prosthetist will need to order a foot of proper size. The height of the heel should be the one most comfortable to the amputee and one acceptable for the rest of the life of that prosthesis. As little as one-eighth of an inch can change the pitch that will be built into the prosthetic leg at the final adjustment. Changes in heel height after that time will produce aches and pains in muscles.

Nurses should encourage patients to discuss

Figure 26-5
Face lying should be done several times a day. This position should be assumed on a firm surface, with the hips flat and legs close together.
(Used with the permission of the Rehabilitation Institute of Chicago.)

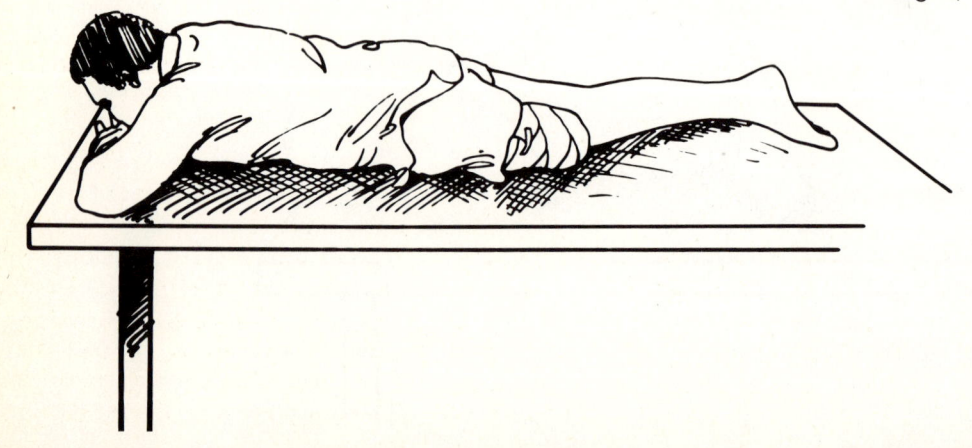

Figure 26-6
Isometric hip extension. A small towel roll is placed under the stump. The stump is pressed down into the towel until the buttocks are lifted off the lying surface. This position is held 5 to 7 counts and repeated according to tolerance and endurance. (*Used with the permission of the Rehabilitation Institute of Chicago.*)

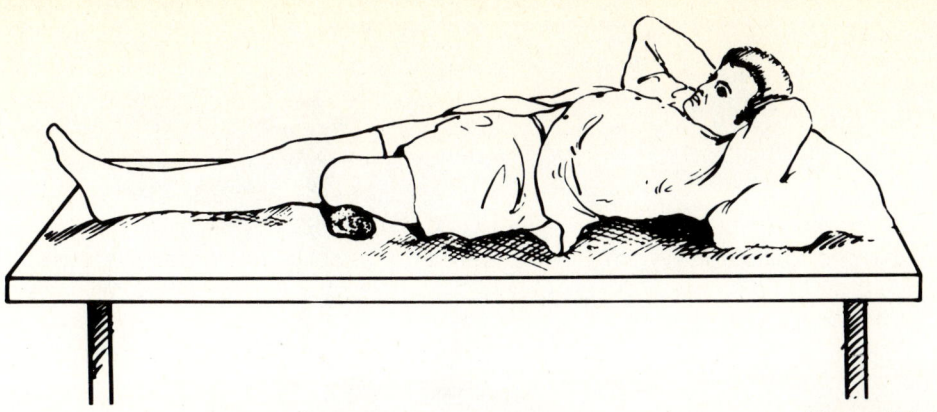

any problems of fit with the prosthetist, to ask questions, and to be candid about indicating where there is too much pressure or how the prosthesis feels. Language barriers can cause a problem if the prosthetist and amputee do not understand each other. At such times, an interpreter is needed to ascertain that the amputee does, in fact, understand what is being done to the prosthesis and how it is meant to be used.

At the first appointment, in preparation for making the initial mold, several things should be expected. The strong leg will be measured and outlined on heavy paper for duplication in the finished prosthesis. Proper foot size will be established, and the shoes will be left with the prosthetist. A thin plaster cast will be applied and molded to the stump, preferably with some weight bearing on the stump while it is drying. A mold made while the patient is only sitting cannot possibly fit the stump, as the pressure points will differ.

The prosthetist examines ambulation with the temporary pylon and can explain which type of foot would be most beneficial. The most popular is called the SACH (stable ankle, cushioned heel) foot (Fig. 26-7). For the below-knee amputee, rotators are sometimes suggested. They decrease the torque forces on the tissues within the socket but tend to make the leg about 1/2 lb heavier.

The patient needs to consider the initial cost of the prosthesis, the number of adjustments included in that cost, the approximate cost anticipated after initial adjustments have been made, and whether the prosthetist makes any guarantee of satisfaction. Were adequate measurements taken to assure that there would be no pelvic tilt? Is the foot angled properly for both walking and sitting? Does the skin tone match that of the normal foot? Is the foot the correct size for the shoe? (See Figs. 26-8 and 26-9.)

With professional guidance, the amputee should be able to assess the knowledge and ability of different prosthetists and choose the one who sounds sincere in interest and will work with the patient in attaining maximum comfort and utilization of the prosthesis. The criterion of choosing a prosthetist should not be initial convenience of location, even though temporary lack of mobility may make it difficult for the patient to shop around. Often, there will be a prosthetic clinic in the area. Patients can request suggestions about various prosthetists and then choose the one who would be best for them.

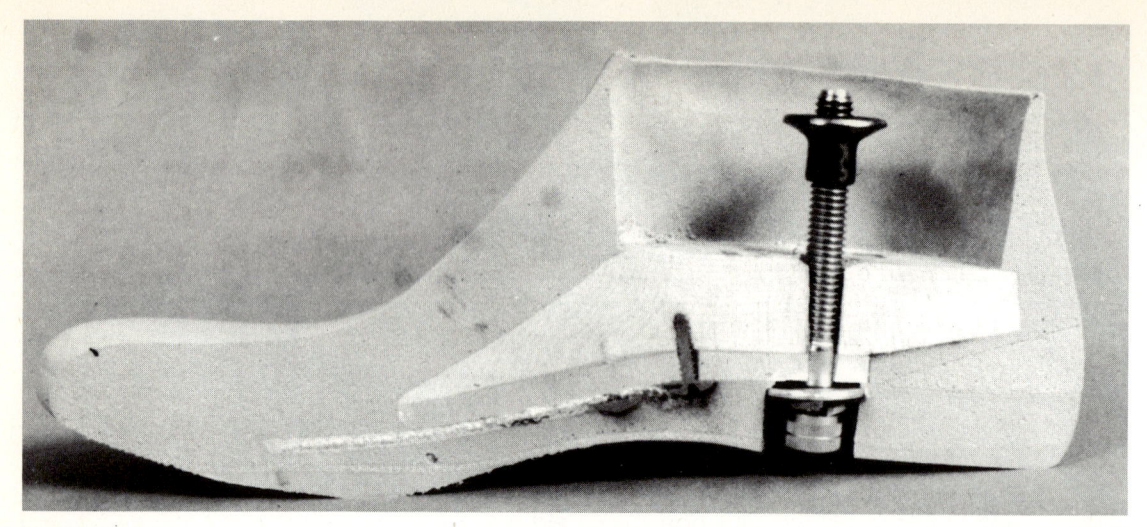

Figure 26-7
SACH (stable ankle, cushioned heel) foot. *(Used with permission of Northwestern University Prosthetic and Orthotic Center.)*

The greater the amount of remaining limb, the greater the rehabilitation potential, but that does not mean that an above-knee amputee cannot be as independent as a below-knee amputee, provided that the prosthesis fits properly, the patient is properly motivated and has good general health, and the training is pertinent to the additional limb loss. Usually even a bilateral above-knee amputee can get along with one cane, and those with two good below-knee stumps seldom need any assistive device.

Activities to be stressed include proper care of the prosthesis, the liner if one is used, and the stump socks. The new amputee may need to change stump socks several times a day to prevent skin irritation from perspiration. An adequate supply of socks of the proper size for the stump should be kept on hand. As time goes on and the stump shrinks more, the size will need to be changed. A combination of various thicknesses may be used. The socks should be washed as soon as they are removed because the perspiration deteriorates them. Acrylic socks may be machine washed and dried, but wool socks must be washed by hand as other wool products are. They take a long time to dry, as they should not be hung up or placed near heat. The liner should be wiped nightly with a soapy cloth and rinsed with a cloth wrung out in warm water.

As soon as any squeaks are heard in the foot, the prosthetist should be notified so that moving parts can be checked. Oiling may be all that is necessary, but amputees should not try to oil the parts themselves because proper machinery is needed to keep everything in alignment.

EXPECTED PROBLEMS WITH AMBULATION

Before patients are discharged from physical therapy, they must be taught how to fall and how to get up, because fall they will, sooner or later. The important thing is to plan the campaign and not get flustered. Usually patients are taught to lean to the strong side when falling and then to put the weight on the strong side while gradually getting onto the strong knee. Next they can use their arms to assume a "jackknife" position. Then, by placing one hand on the strong thigh, the amputee can pull the prosthetic leg up as the strong knee is extended and an erect posture is gained.

Ambulation in bad weather is something that must also be practiced, as it does make a difference in balance. In a strong wind, it is easier for the amputee to lead into it with the strong leg, as in going uphill, while taking smaller steps with the prosthesis. A bilateral lower extremity amputee will find a cane useful because it aids the balance. Walking on snow and ice, as well as on wet pavement, requires extra caution. Amputees should slow their gait and gradually place weight on the prosthetic side to secure a firm underfooting.

Balance is not much of a problem in a familiar terrain, indoors, or on a level surface. However, that balance is rather easily lost when the amputee walks on cobblestones or on open ground, where it cannot be assumed that the place the prosthetic leg is going next is nice and flat. A cat that is stalking very cautiously puts one paw ahead and "tests" the area for solidity before placing the weight on that foot. This is a good plan for amputees to follow lest they put the foot into an unexpected pothole, thus losing balance.

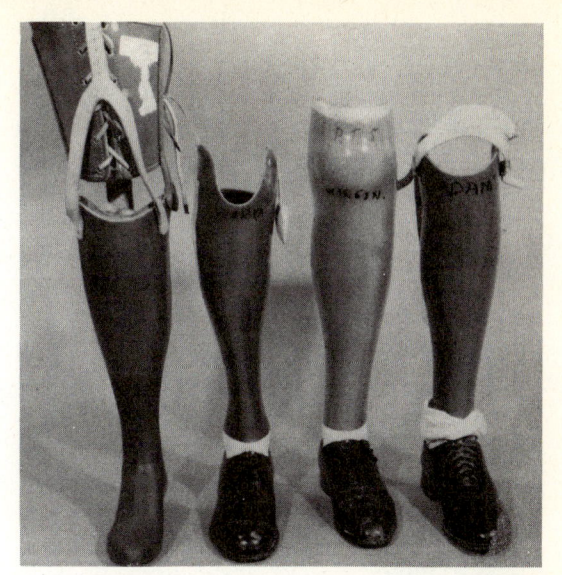

Figure 26-9
Types of below-knee prostheses. *(Used with permission of Northwestern University Prosthetic and Orthotic Center.)*

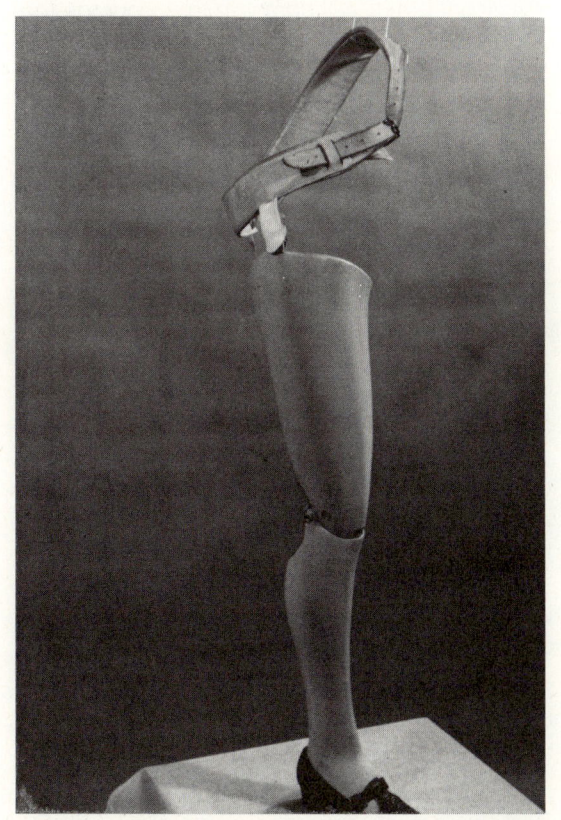

Figure 26-8
Above-knee prostheses with pelvic band. *(Used with permission of Northwestern University Prosthetic and Orthotic Center.)*

MOTIVATIONAL NEEDS OF THE PATIENT

ASSISTANCE IN SETTING REALISTIC GOALS

Much soul-searching is needed for the patient to achieve a realistic approach to life in the future. The amputee should be encouraged as soon as possible to start to plan what may well be a totally new way of life. A person who has been relatively inactive in the past cannot be expected suddenly to have cross-country skiing as a goal. It will suffice for most if they can return to their premorbid activities, even though one or two of the activities will be more difficult to perform or may be performed in a different way.

Some will have the determination to succeed in handling the prosthesis almost as well as the natural leg. Others will tend to give up and decide it is not worth the effort. This latter group must be given additional help in goal setting, as there will be numerous possibilities that they will not think about alone. For instance, would it not be better for them to be able to use a prosthesis, rather than a wheelchair, for getting around the house? It is meaningful to be able to feel "dressed" in the home, as opposed to feeling like an invalid in a wheelchair. If the amputee has driven a car and enjoyed it, it will be easier to get to the car with the prosthesis, even if it is necessary to take a wheelchair along for long shopping trips.

Patients should know that there are many differences in the fabrication of a prosthesis. A prosthesis can be made to withstand very heavy use or merely for light work. The amputee should be able to master the prosthesis and make it do the desired work rather than allowing the prosthesis to determine what can be accomplished.

ESTABLISHING MOTIVATION TO ATTAIN MAXIMUM POTENTIAL

Nurses should be absolutely truthful if they want patients to achieve realistic attitudes about their goals. If amputees are to achieve maximum potential, they will need help and encouragement over the many tough spots they will encounter. Many times, there will be a feeling of "I just can't do it." At those times nurses must push patients just a bit harder while telling them honestly that the weariness is understandable but that they must go on. If there is nothing available to lean on or sit on, patients must take the extra steps to a spot where they can lean or sit. After about 2 min, with weight off the prosthesis and a few isometric muscle contractions, amputees can be on the way again. But how will they know this unless they are told before it happens?

Common sense is the best ally in problem solving, and amputees will gain experience as they face calculated risks. Increasingly difficult goals should be set in a planned manner so that amputees will gain in self-confidence. It is no cause for shame when a bilateral lower extremity amputee freezes at the thought of going down a flight of stairs on crutches. This is normal, but as soon as it is done for the first time, it becomes a short- and a long-term goal because the patient knows the feat can be repeated.

As the amputee becomes more experienced in prosthetic ambulation, alternative methods of performing activities can be attempted. Even though the new method may not work, at least it has been tried. The support of the family or significant others will do much to encourage the taking of calculated risks. Such risks must be taken if the patient is not going to be wrapped in cotton wadding for a lifetime.

PSYCHOSOCIAL NEEDS OF THE PATIENT

REGAINING CONTROL OF THE LIFE SITUATION

Following an amputation, the patient needs to determine what type of life situation will be desirable, although at this point the individual may have lost almost total control of the situation. No option was offered concerning the amputation itself; the decision was a lifesaving one and unavoidable. Now, however, thought must be given to a choice of a prosthetist, what kind of work can be realistically attempted, what living plans should be made, and in general what can be done to brighten the years ahead. There is the question of body image and how best to cope with it, along with the fear of rejection by family, significant others, and society in general.

As amputees are trying to sort out all these things, it is obvious that nurses must somehow find a way to help them arrive at the most realistic solution. What that is will vary with each individual. They must find some spark that will give the needed motivation. It may take prolonged searching to come upon anything that will make the patient accept the fact that life must now be lived minus a normal appendage.

If nurses can get the amputee to realize that the use of a prosthesis can become as routine as shaving or brushing the teeth, it will help. As hard as it may be to believe, it is really true that there comes a time when an amputee forgets that a leg is artificial. It seems to "belong" if it is a properly fitted limb and is under the control of the amputee. As time passes and ambulation gait improves, there will come a nice surprise one day when a limp becomes apparent momentarily and someone says to the amputee, "Oh, what did you do to your foot? You're limping!"

VARIABLE FACTORS IN NEED OF CONSIDERATION

SCIENTIFIC RESEARCH

In recent years, scientific research has resulted in numerous, ever-improving types of lower extremity prostheses. The prosthetist has some range of choice in determining which one will be of the best functional use to the individual amputee. It is to be hoped that research will now produce a liner that can be adjusted by the wearer so that some pressure points can be eased without a trip to the prosthetist. Some below-knee amputees need to add socks to keep the stump from "bottoming out" in the socket, but the additional sock thickness over the knee joint itself causes too much pressure on the bony areas, so that it is not tolerable. Perhaps a liner could be developed with quilted surfaces between which air or water might be used at specific points to relieve pressure. If amputees could be taught to manage this, they could remain functional and comfortable at the same time. The mere addition of stump socks does not alleviate the situation because more padding may be needed at one point than at another.

AGE SPAN

While motivation will vary through any age group, it is more common to find the younger age group highly motivated. This can have a great effect on the setting of goals and acceptance of prosthetic training. An older person who has no family and therefore may be going into a nursing home will probably have far less motivation than a teenager who is eager to get back into action. Therefore, different goals are expected within various age groups and among various life situations. There are vast differences in energy available to be expended, and some individuals are more willing to work harder than others. Also, if other medical problems are involved, these will almost certainly hinder the total program.

ACCEPTANCE BY FAMILY OR SIGNIFICANT OTHERS

While there are varied ways of achieving acceptance, the most realistic way is to show the family or significant others what is possible for the amputee to accomplish. Then, it is hoped, the others involved will promote realistic independence, knowing that the amputee will ask for help whenever necessary. The family and others should allow the amputee to do alone whatever can be safely done, and they must be warned about being overprotective so that all involved may proceed to live normal lives.

If small children are involved, their natural curiosity will come out, and they will want to "see the leg." It will become rapidly evident when they are shown the prosthesis that it is the stump they want to see. When the amputee can handle such incidents honestly and accept the curiosity, there will be little further trouble about the acceptance of the whole neighborhood.

ADJUSTING TO THE UNEXPLAINED "WHY'S"

The lower extremity amputee uses a great deal more energy than normal and, for this reason, runs into a few additional problems. Levels of fatigue vary with each individual and at each progressive stage of rehabilitation (Fisher & Gullickson, 1978). It takes several weeks in a new situation or location for amputees to learn to pace their energy output adequately because they must do this by trial and error until achieving a pace acceptable to self, family, employer, and terrain. Once the locale has become familiar and a feeling of security has developed, amputees can change their pace as necessary to avoid total exhaustion.

SEXUAL BEHAVIOR

Accepted definitions of "body image" seem to vary, but one definition is simply "a description of one's body by the person." If "beauty is in the eyes of the beholder," then in a sexual relationship, two persons must make a decision about proper body image. As in any relationship, the persons involved must communicate in order to achieve the understanding necessary for mutual comfort.

Communication takes many forms, especially in sexual behavior. Nurses can give some ideas to patients about new ways of communicating after loss of a body part. Nurses are well aware that amputees are not about to "grow a new limb," but they must remember that the patients may not have accepted this fact at some given phase of rehabilitation.

What is sexuality, other than being sexual in whatever way best expresses a feeling? Amputees should be advised that they must take the initiative so as to answer the questions in the partner's mind. If the amputee goes into a shell or refuses to address the situation, it will be difficult for the partner to know what is desired. Inhibitions have even less place in the sexual behavior of a person with any handicap than they have in wholesome, natural, or "acceptable" behavior in general. Reinstein feels amputees should be encouraged to resume sexual activity as soon as their medical condition is stable (Reinstein et al., 1978).

Nurses must not judge what is "best" for the patient and partner in any sexual relationships. They are totally wrong, and therefore accountable, if they choose to impose their own moralities upon others. It is a fact that not all nurses are willing to counsel, or capable of it, in this facet of rehabilitation nursing, but the very least they can and must do is keep an open mind and give knowledgeable advice to patients as to whether they may need what is commonly called sex counseling or sex therapy.

CONCLUSION

Nurses should explain as much as possible about preoperative and postoperative experiences because the patient will be better able to adapt if these are known. Much assistance is needed for amputees to set realistic goals that are within their capabilities and the family's understanding and acceptance. The attainment of such goals will require numerous tactics on the nurses' part, of persuading, chiding, nudging, encouraging, and pushing, adding honest praise as each hurdle is overcome and each goal reached. The setting of progressively more difficult goals gives patients the opportunity to realize that they are making progress and that by working hard enough, they will probably be able to achieve the next goal. Many factors must be considered on an individual basis and discussed in depth with both patient and family or significant others so that parties involved understand the capabilities of the amputee. These capabilities must be encouraged even though there may be need to take some calculated risks. If there is an understanding that help will be requested when really needed, if only to conserve energy for more important tasks, then good understanding and mutual acceptance will have been reached. When nurses can say honestly that they have put the necessary time and effort into their teaching of these fundamentals and that their involvement has been deep and thorough with both patient and others involved, then they can lay claim to being rehabilitation nurses in the truest sense of the words.

BIBLIOGRAPHY

Alexander, J., and R. Goodrich: "Videotape Immediate Playback: A Tool in Rehabilitation of Persons with Amputations" *Arch Phys Med Rehabil* 59(3):141–144, 1978.

Buck, B., and A. Lee: "Amputation: Two Views," *Nurs Clin North Am* 11(4):641–657, 1976

Couch, N., J. David, N. Tilner, and C. Crane: "Natural History of the Leg Amputee," *Am J Surg* 133:469–473, 1977.

Engstrand, J.: "Rehabilitation of the Patient with a Lower Extremity Amputation," *Nurs Clin North Am* 11(4):659–669, 1976.

Fisher, S. V., and G. Gullickson: "'Energy Cost of Ambulation in Health and Disability: A Literature Review," *Arch Phys Med Rehabil* 59(3):124–233, 1978.

Hinterbuchner, C., P. Mondall, and J. Sakuma: "Rehabilitation of Patients with Dual Disability of Hemiplegia and Amputation," *Arch Phys Med Rehabil* 59(3):121–123, 1978.

Jones, D. A., C. F. Dunbar, and M. M. Jirovec: *Medical Surgical Nursing: A Conceptual Approach,* McGraw-Hill, New York, 1978.

Kegel, B., M. L. Carpenter, and E. M. Burgess: "Functional Capability of Lower Extremity Amputees," *Arch Phys Med Rehabil* 59(3): 109–120, 1978.

Nicholas, G., and W. Demuth: "Evaluation of the Use of Rigid Dressings," *Surg Gynecol Obstet* 143:398–400, 1976.

Pasnau, R., and B. Pfefferbaum: "Psychologic Aspects of Post Amputation Pain," *Nurs Clin North Am* 11(4):679–685, 1976.

Pfefferbaum, B., and R. Pasnau: "Post Amputation Grief," *Nurs Clin North Am* 11(4):687–690, 1976.

"Pre-Prosthetic Care for Above-Knee Amputees," Rehabilitation Institute of Chicago, Chicago, 1978.

"Pre-Prosthetic Care for Below-Knee Amputees," Rehabilitation Institute of Chicago. Chicago, 1978.

Quinn, L. B.: "It's Worth the Effort," *RN,* October 1976, pp. 57–68.

Reinstein, L., J. Ashley, and K. Miller: "Sexual Adjustment after Lower Extremity Amputation," *Arch Phys Med Rehabil* 59:501–504, 1978.

Roon, A., W. Moore, and J. Goldstone: "Below-Knee Amputation: A Modern Approach," *Am J Surg* 134:153–158, 1977.

Solomon, G., and M. Schmidt: "A Burning Issue: Phantom Limb Pain and Psychological Preparation of the Patient for Amputation," *Arch Surg* 113:185–86, 1978.

Stern, P., and P. Skudder: "Amputee Amputation I, Lower Limb Amputations, *NY State J Med* 77(9):1436–1440, 1977.

Wiley, L., et al.: "Battered Body: A Teenage Amputee Taught Us Four Tips for Better Long Term Management," *Nursing* 78(8):36–41, 1978.

Wilson, A. B.: *Limb Prosthetics,* 5th ed., Krieger, New York, 1976.

27

verna cain
janet a. marvin

third degree burns

INTRODUCTION

Nursing management of the severely burned patient is often difficult as a result of the patient's pain, emotional stress, and physical limitations. The person who has experienced deep dermal or full-thickness skin loss has suffered a significant injury that may produce tremendous physiological, as well as psychological, changes. These changes can be extremely debilitating, creating long-lasting and often permanent effects. Measures to maintain not only physical but also psychological function are imperative during the initial phase of care. Health disciplines must keep in mind that the extent of burn injury does not always correlate with the extent of disability. Rehabilitation can be influenced by many factors, requiring the cooperative efforts of all members of the burn team.

GENERAL PHYSIOLOGICAL RESPONSE TO BURN INJURIES

When the integrity of the human organism is threatened, the body's defense mechanisms are called into action. The response is generally related to the extent of the injury. In a severe burn injury, there is extensive destruction of skin, the body's first line of defense. Some of the normal functions of skin are to maintain fluid and electrolyte balance, regulate body temperature, and protect the body from invasion of foreign matter. As a result of skin loss, large amounts of fluids, electrolytes, proteins, and heat are lost. The open wound becomes a prime source for the development of infection. Besides skin loss, destruction of subcutaneous tissues, muscles, and bones may occur depending upon the temperature and the duration of exposure to the burning agent. Severe stress is placed on many vital organs as they attempt to reverse the process created by the injury. The response of these organ systems is briefly outlined in the following section.

CARDIOVASCULAR AND RENAL RESPONSE

A burn injury to the skin may produce capillary damage or destruction. Many of the superficial capillaries are destroyed. The endothelium of the remaining capillaries may be damaged by the release of vasoactive substances such as histamines, which cause an increase in capillary permeability. The normal exchange of fluids between the blood and the extracellular space is altered, causing a rapid shift of plasma from the intravascular to the extravascular space at the site of the burn. In patients with significant burns [i.e., those greater than 20 percent of the total body surface area (TBSA)], there is a generalized response allowing the loss of fluids and plasma proteins into interstitial tissues throughout the body. The lymphatic system, which normally carries away excess extravascular fluid, is rapidly overloaded and may well be damaged by the burn injury. The plasma loss may exceed several liters, creating a reduction in circulating blood volume. Although there may be some direct thermal injury to red blood cells in the peripheral circulation at the time of injury, this amount is insignificant, and red blood cell loss is not a problem during the first few days after injury. Continued red blood cell destruction has been described that may predispose the patient to anemia at 5 to 10 days following the burn (Loebl, 1974). The degree of red blood cell destruction varies with the extent of injury.

Although the body immediately initiates a protective measure to decrease the fluid loss through peripheral vasoconstriction, this is usually inadequate to maintain normal circulation. Cardiac output and blood flow are greatly reduced, thereby decreasing profusion of vital organs. Thus, vital organs begin to suffer from inadequate perfusion if the process is not immediately reversed. At this stage, the body's defense mechanisms will not function to correct these processes. Therefore, shock is imminent, and death will occur if intravascular volume is not replaced.

Splanchnic vasoconstriction may cause visceral blood flow to be greatly diminished. Obvious effects of this are seen in the kidneys. Poor renal blood flow causes damage to kidney cells that may result in oliguria or decreased urine output. Direct muscle damage and red blood cell destruction cause release of a heavy pigment load (myoglobin and hemoglobin) into the bloodstream to be filtered by the kidneys. Irreversible kidney damage will result if these pigments are allowed to accumulate in the kidney.

Burn Shock

The major cause of shock is hypovolemia, or the loss of circulating fluids. In severe burns, as much as 50 to 60 percent of the fluid loss may occur in the first few hours after injury. The first 24 to 48 h are considered the most crucial in the treatment of burn shock. Management during this period is directed primarily at adequate fluid resuscitation, which should provide the body with the substances that have been lost: primarily electrolytes, water, and plasma proteins. The restoration of fluid volume may be obtained by a number of formulas. One of the most popular is the crystalloid or Baxter formula, which is illustrated in Fig. 27-1. (Baxter, 1973). Monitoring fluids accurately is critical during this phase. The nurse should be alert to any deviations from normal in the signs and symptoms of adequate fluid resuscitation, as shown in Table 27-1. With early and meticulous attention to fluid resuscitation, even patients with greater than 90 percent burns may survive the shock phase.

Circulation to the Burn Wound

The burn injury causes immediate destruction of many vessels within the dermis and underlying subcutaneous tissue. The amount of destruction varies with the intensity of the heat produced by the burning agent and the great variation of the thickness of the dermis throughout the body. Furthermore, many vessels may not be destroyed initially, but as a result of progressive edema and reduced blood flow in the distal circulation, small vessels may become temporarily or permanently occluded. This progressive destruction occurs over a period of 48 to 72 h. With progressive destruction of the microcirculation to the dermis, increased tissue necrosis occurs. Therefore, the wound may increase in depth. Jackson, in schematically representing the progressive nature of the injury, developed the zonal concept (Jackson,

Figure 27-1
Baxter formula. Fluid administration 1st 24 h and 2d 24 h.

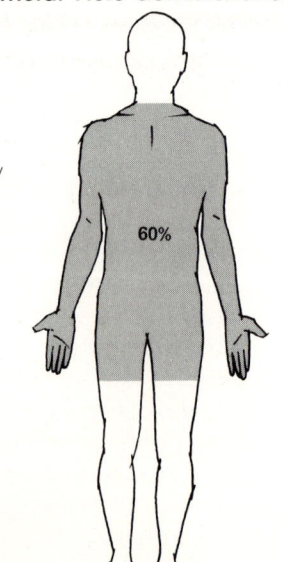

First 24 h:
  Lactated Ringer's
  4 mL/kg body weight/% body surface burn/24 h
  No plasma or plasma substitutes
  No dextrose containing solutions
  Administered:
  1/2 of 24° total — 1st 8 h
  1/4 of 24° total — 2d 8 h
  1/4 of 24° total — 3d 8 h

60%

Second 24 h:
  Dextrose in water sufficient to maintain the serum Na^+ < 140 meg/L
  KCl supplements to maintain serum K^+ within normal limits
  Plasma or plasma substitutes to return plasma volume to normal

Table 27-1

Signs of Adequate Resuscitation

1. Clear sensorium
2. Urine output:
   20–50 mL/h in children
   30–70 mL/h in adults
3. Slightly high normal pulse
   80–100 in adults
   100–120 in children
4. Central venous pressure below 12
5. Absence of ileus or nausea

1953). He depicts the full-thickness portion of the wound as the zone of coagulation. This zone is surrounded by an area of deep partial-thickness wound that he calls the zone of stasis. These two zones are surrounded by a zone of hyperemia, which is the zone of superficial partial-thickness injury. Studies have shown that the zone of stasis often progresses to a zone of coagulation during the first 72 h (Zawacki, 1974). The progressive coagulation is caused by a lack of oxygenation and nutrition of tissues owing to microvascular occlusion and poor perfusion.

In addition to the problem of microvascular occlusion, macrocirculation may also be impaired in a circumferential full-thickness wound of an extremity. The inelasticity of the full-thickness injury causes the eschar to act as a tourniquet in this case, and as swelling increases, circulation to the distal part of the extremity is impaired. This problem can be alleviated by making linear incisions through the eschar on the lateral and medial side of the extremity. These incisions, called escharotomies, are made only through full-thickness eschar down to viable subcutaneous fat. The incisions allow for decompression and improved blood flow.

PULMONARY RESPONSE

Pulmonary complications are among the leading causes of death in the severely burned patient. Thirty percent of major burns (greater than 20 percent TBSA) are complicated by smoke inhalation. The mortality of major burns with smoke inhalation ranges from 30 to 60 percent in most studies (Zawacki, 1977; Moylan, 1974; Kangarloo, 1977). Burn patients are also predisposed to other pulmonary complications such as pulmonary edema, pneumonia, atelectasis, and pulmonary emboli.

Respiratory Complications

Early pulmonary complications may be the result of inhalation of hot air and noxious gases. *Carbon monoxide intoxication* is frequently seen in patients exposed to smoke. This intoxication itself may lead to death. Actual thermal damage to the upper airway from exposure to hot air and noxious gases may lead to edema and **upper airway obstruction**. Edema of the upper airway and vocal cords may be detected by wheezing, hoarseness, and stridor, as well as rapid, labored respirations. Maintaining the airway and removing secretions may require the placement of an endotracheal tube or performance of a tracheostomy. Burns to the chest and abdomen cause pain and restrict movement of the respiratory muscle. Often an escharotomy must be performed to allow for better excursion in circumferential full-thickness burn of the chest. This procedure is usually performed along the lateral borders of the chest wall and across the diaphragm. Irritation of the tracheobronchial tree from noxious products and smoke may cause mucous membrane swelling and increased production of secretions in both the upper and lower airways. This irritation may result in sloughing of the mucosal lining, predisposing the patient to pneumonia. This process is frequently not evident in the first 48 to 72 h. The chemical pneumonitis caused by this injury is frequently associated with prolonged morbidity and high mortality.

Pulmonary edema may result from fluid overload during initial fluid replacement or from injury to the pulmonary vasculature. The pulmonary vasculature may be affected by the initial histamine response and increased capillary permeability. Fluid then collects in the interstitium of the lung. Decreased cardiac output prevents efficient emptying of the pulmonary artery. Continued congestion leads to pulmonary hypertension with resulting pulmonary edema.

Later complications may result from *aspiration,* *hypostatic* or *infectious pneumonia, pneumothorax, pulmonary embolus, atelectasis,* or *bronchiectasis.* The nurse should be observant for any signs indicating respiratory distress. Assisted ventilation is often required in these particular patients.

How Rehabilitation Might Be Affected by Respiratory Complications

The goal of rehabilitation is to maintain normal function and to increase function in restricted areas. This is best accomplished with the active participation of the patient, both psychologically and physically. Tremendous amounts of energy are required during activity and exercise periods. Complications that prolong bed rest, such as smoke inhalation, interfere with mobility. Prolonged bed rest may also create other problems, such as pressure sores, plantar flexion, contractures, or muscle atrophy, or may lead to respiratory conditions, such as atelectasis or pulmonary emboli. Respiratory complications increase the patient's need to conserve energy. The patient tires easily upon exertion as a result of the inability to maintain oxygenation. The nursing care priorities during this period are to provide adequate ventilation, appropriate antibiotics and other medications as ordered, nutrition, and rest. An active-assisted or gentle-passive range of motion exercises, splinting, and positioning are important to maintain joint function. At best, these supportive measures may not be totally adequate in preventing some loss of function in the severely ill patient. Nonetheless, it is important that every effort is made to maintain normal joint function.

IMMUNOLOGIC RESPONSE

Patients with severe burns appear to have increased susceptibility to infection owing to the breakdown of defense mechanisms, as well as to the loss of skin protection. In extensive burns, the generalized vascular response of fluid shifts into the extravascular space creates an initial overwhelming inflammatory response. White blood cell counts increase dramatically to between 10,000 and 20,000. Over a period of time, however, the phagocytic activity of white blood cells becomes suppressed as a result of the overall response (Alexander, 1971). The ability to remove foreign bodies, cellular debris, and organisms is inhibited. Abnormalities are also seen in the reticuloendothelial system, which is essential for normal phagocytosis and antibody formation (Munster, 1972). The lymphatic system which drains interstitial fluid is already stressed by the initial inflammatory response. Damage to the lymphatic system produces a decreased amount of circulating antibodies (immunoglobulins) in the blood (Muir, 1974). The body's natural defenses are no longer capable of protecting against invasion of large numbers of pathogenic organisms.

Another factor that adds to lower resistance to infection is age. Burned patients less than 2 years of age and those over 65 years have a higher incidence of sepsis and mortality related to sepsis than do others with similar burn injuries. In infants, the problem is usually related to poor antibody response. Older patients are generally undernourished and physically debilitated. Also, exacerbations of latent degenerative processes may be brought on by the stress of the injury. Thus, these patients often show a major deficit in host defense response.

The burned patient is in constant danger of contracting infection, not only from normal flora but also from exposure to personnel, other patients, and contaminated equipment. It is therefore necessary to provide an aseptic environment for protection of the burned patient. The degree of isolation will be dictated by the severity of the burn injury.

Septic Response

The burn wound is a perfect medium for the growth of disease-producing organisms. Invasion of bacteria is facilitated by the loss of the natural barrier, skin. Decreased circulation resulting from altered vascularity of the wound may delay the inflammatory response, allowing organisms to proliferate before phagocytes can reach the area. If the wound covers only a small area, the body's defenses may inhibit growth and eliminate the organisms. In extensive wounds, the organisms continue to multiply and invade local tissues in large numbers. The lymphatics normally remove these organisms, along with other debris, and transport them to the lymphatic ducts. Organisms not destroyed by the reticuloendothelial macrophages in the lymph nodes will be transported to the bloodstream, thus causing bacteremia. The patient will develop a generalized septic response to this invasion and may exhibit the signs and symptoms associated with sepsis in the burn patient, as seen in Table 27-2. As noted in this table, the nurse should be aware of the early signs of sepsis, which are increased pulse and respiration, confusion, either hypothermia or hyperthermia, ileus, and spilling of glucose in the urine. If the septic response is diagnosed early, therapeutic modalities can be initiated that may prevent further septicemia. Once organisms have continued to invade the bloodstream and overwhelm the defenses of the body, septicemia is certain to occur. Endotoxins released into the bloodstream by gram-negative organisms frequently cause a generalized response leading to septic shock. Once septic shock occurs, chances of survival are slim. Because of this, sepsis must be identified and treated immediately with appropriate therapy. This includes appropriate antibiotics, supportive care including fluid replacement, and ventilatory support, as well as excision or removal of infected tissues.

Effects of Infection on Wound Healing

Infection plays a major role in the prolongation of wound healing. A brief look at wound healing at the molecular level may help in understanding this phenomenon. Longacre (1972) classifies the stages of wound healing as the lag phase, the fibroblastic phase, and the phase of maturation. The lag phase is characterized by invasion of polymorphonuclear leukocytes, dilatation of blood vessels, and excessive edema. At the same time, the rudiments of healing begin with mitosis of endothelium to develop new capillaries and proliferation of epithelial cells from any remaining epidermal remnants. The fibroblastic phase is characterized by a decrease in polymorphonuclear leukocytes and an increase in fibroblasts (mononuclear cells). The spindle-shaped fibroblasts then stretch out along fibrin strands of the clot and along newly developing capillaries to form new granulation tissue. The granulation tissue is then replaced by scar tissue during the maturation phase. Scar tissue develops from the formation of collagen bundles. Winter (1974) has noted that there is usually a prolonged lag phase in the healing of the burn wound owing to the progressive vascular changes in the wound. These progressive changes lead to delayed localization of polymorphonuclear leukocytes, thus preventing the development of the normal host defense response to infection. Wound colonization at this point tends to prolong the lag phase further as a result of a more intense inflammatory process. The intense inflammatory response increases the number of polymorphonuclear leukocytes in the wound and thus delays the beginning of the second phase of healing.

Table 27-2

Signs of Septicemia in Burns

Early signs
1. Disorientation
2. Ileus
3. Hyperthermia or hypothermia
4. Tachycardia
5. Tachypnea
6. Glucose intolerance
7. Unexplained acidosis

Late Signs
1. Hypotension
2. Decreased urine output
3. White blood cells (< 5000)
4. Decreased platelet count

METABOLIC RESPONSE

Metabolism is the process by which the body produces energy required to sustain life. The metabolic process is regulated by various mechanisms throughout the body. The central nervous system and endocrine system, with their release of catecholamines and hormones along with enzyme systems and various feedback systems, function to maintain a constant metabolic balance. These mechanisms are largely dependent upon one another. Malfunction or abnormality in one area will create profound reactions from other areas in an attempt to maintain homeostasis.

Increased Metabolic Rate in the Burn Patient

Conditions that place added energy requirements on the body produce alterations in the metabolic response. A severe burn tremendously increases the energy needs of the body. The severe stress is created by loss of skin, body heat, fluids, and electrolytes, which stimulates the regulatory mechanisms to respond at an increased rate. The response is further augmented by cold exposure, pain, fear, and anxiety. All of these afferent stimuli increase the production of catecholamines, which interact with other hormones to exert direct cellular effects, thus altering normal function.

Factors that modify the metabolic response are preexisting disease, injuries to vital organs that create abnormal organ system function, preexisting nutritional and physical conditions, and age. The very young and the elderly are less tolerant of changes in metabolic rates.

The metabolic rate in a burned patient is directly related to the extent of injury, that is, total body surface area burned. In the patients with less extensive burns, the body's natural defenses are able to stand the stress produced by alterations in the metabolic rate. In burns greater than 30 percent TBSA in adults and greater than 20 percent TBSA in children, the metabolic rate shows a marked increase. An extensive effort should be made to meet these increased energy demands. Fluid therapy, as previously mentioned, is essential to maintain normal fluid and electrolyte balance. The prevention of cold stress, with its increased energy demands, may be accomplished by use of mechancial devices such as hypothermia blankets and heat shields. Analgesics, tranquilizers, and psychological support may be used to alleviate pain and enxiety.

Nutritional Needs of the Burned Patient

The severely burned patient generally requires twice as many calories as a normal person in order to meet these metabolic demands. A high-calorie, high-protein diet is required to maintain positive nitrogen balance and promote healing. Weight loss is a serious problem in these patients, since it represents to a large extent the loss of the lean muscle mass of the body.

The hypermetabolism of the burned patient is characterized by increased metabolic rate, weight loss, and negative nitrogen balance. Wilmore (1974) has related these changes to a reset of the hypothalamus, which causes an increase in catecholamine production. Hormonal changes occur as a result of the increased levels of catecholamines which favor the breakdown of proteins for energy utilization. The resulting hormonal imbalance gives rise to an increased ratio between glucagon and insulin, with glucagon production greatly increased over that of insulin. The normal relationship is for more insulin than glucagon to be produced. Glucagon favors the breakdown of protein by gluconeogenesis for the release of glucose for energy. Insulin has almost the opposite effect; it favors the storage of protein and the utilization of carbohydrates and fats for enery. Under this altered hormonal control, the protein of the lean muscle mass is used in deference to fat stores for energy production. Thus the picture of an increased basal metabolic rate, negative nitrogen balance, and weight loss is seen in those patients with inadequate nutritional support. If this process is allowed to continue without adequate caloric and protein support, the patient may die of the complications of malnutrition.

Effects of Metabolic Response on Rehabilitation

Preventing the loss of lean muscle mass of the body is of paramount importance to early ambulation and use of injured extremities. The loss of muscle strength through muscle wasting may increase the tendency toward contracture. Active exercise throughout the patient's initial course may reduce muscle wasting and actually help to increase the appetite of this anorexic patient. Thus the combination of adequate nutritional support and early exercise therapy may enhance the ability of the patient to prevent disability related to contracture formation.

PERMANENT CHANGES THAT MAY OCCUR IN THE INTEGUMENTARY, NEUROLOGICAL, MUSCULAR, AND SKELETAL SYSTEMS

The changes that occur in the integumentary system can often be devastating for the patient and family. Superficial skin loss usually results in minimal, if any, residual effects. However, deep dermal and full-thickness injuries generally leave telltale signs in the form of skin discoloration and hypertrophic scarring. The quality of regenerated or replaced skin is never the same as normal skin. This is in part due to the increased susceptibility to injury and the inelasticity of scar tissue. Also, scar tissue contracts as it matures. Even with early grafting of burn wounds, skin contracture may cause loss of function. Skin contracture eventually leads to muscle shortening. As the muscles become shortened, joints become immobile and may become ankylosed if not corrected.

How the Burn Wound Heals

Burn wounds, not unlike other wounds, heal by wound contracture, granulation, and epithelialization. Superficial second-degree burns heal primarily by epithelialization from epidermal appendages such as hair follicles and sweat glands (Fig. 27-2). These wounds generally heal within 10 to 14 days and result in minimal scarring. Deep dermal burns heal by wound contracture and epithelialization. This process may take several weeks, depending on the depth of injury and areas of the body injured. In the deep layers of the dermis, the epidermal appendages, primarily the sweat glands, are usually more distant from one another. This is in contrast to the hair follicles, which appear primarily in the upper layers of the dermis and generally are closer together (Fig. 27-2). As always, there are exceptions to every rule. For example, the hair follicles of the scalp extend deep into the dermis, while there are no hair follicles, only sweat glands, on the soles of feet and palm of the hands. Hypertrophic scarring is the hallmark of the deep dermal burn.

The full-thickness wound heals by wound contracture, development of granulation tissue at the base, and epithelialization from the wound edge with lysis of the eschar. This is obviously a lengthy process and ineffective in the closure of large full-thickness wounds. Studies have shown that epithelialization from the wound edges takes place at the rate of 0.25 mm per day (Erickson, 1972). In full-thickness burns, the eschar separates, leaving a base of granulation tissue. The fibrosis that develops in this area and in the deep dermis in deep partial-thickness burns is responsible for contracture and deformities seen in the burned patient.

The eschar that forms over the burn is both a protective mechanism and a potential hazard. It protects the wound and underlying structures from dessication and necrosis as the wound begins to granulate. At the same time, there is the ever-present hazard of proliferation of bacteria within this nonviable matrix, as well as the potential for invasive wound infection.

Debridement of Eschar

The removal of the devitalized tissue as soon as possible is essential to provide a recipient area for grafting, to decrease the danger of infection,

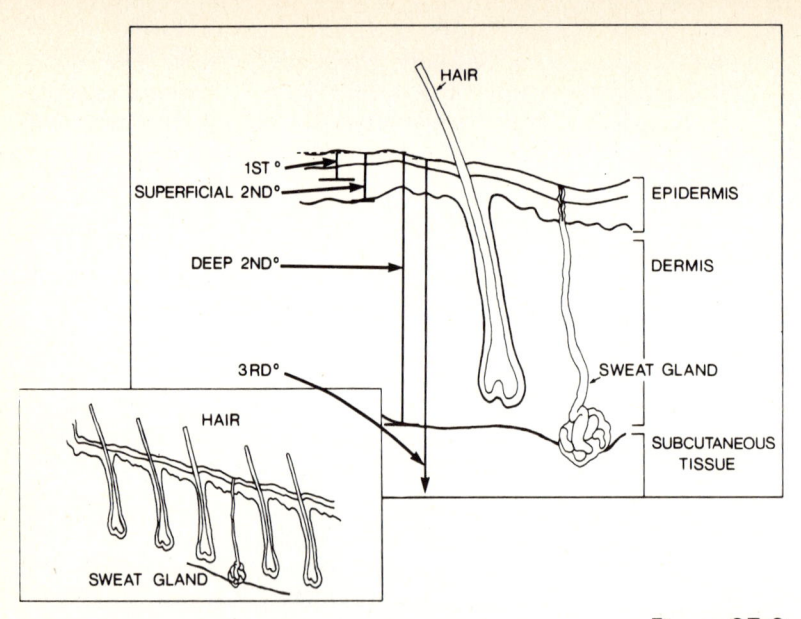

Figure 27-2

In this cross section of skin note the closeness and abundance of hair follicles appearing primarily in the upper dermal layer. In contrast, sweat glands are generally fewer in number and more distant from one another.

and to minimize deformity. Debridement may be performed by several methods.

Conventional mechanical debridement requires the persistent removal of loose, necrotic eschar as it separates from the burn wound. Within 7 to 10 days, bacterial growth causes a natural separation of the eschar from the wound, allowing it to be removed easily. This method is slow and painful for the patient, often requiring several weeks of daily debridement therapy. This method also allows the infected eschar to remain in contact with healthy underlying tissue, thus increasing the chance of sepsis.

Enzymatic debridement, although currently utilized less frequently than other methods, allows the eschar to be removed more rapidly than with conventional mechanical debridement. Bacterial enzymes placed directly on the wound dissolve the eschar, thus exposing the underlying tissue. This may be accomplished on a small wound in 3 to 5 days. The incidence of uncontrolled sepsis has rendered this method impractical in the moderate to severe burn injury (Hummel, 1974).

Surgical debridement may be indicated for several reasons in the deep dermal or full-thickness injury. In severe burns, survival may be threatened by the extent of the injury. Initial surgical debridement of the eschar, with subsequent placement of autograft or homograft, reduces the percentage of burn injury, thereby reducing the body's response to injury. Burke (1976) has reported a reduced mortality in children with this technique. The early removal of burned tissue may prevent infection and hasten wound healing even in small and moderate-sized burns, thereby reducing morbidity. Also, more normal appearance and function may be preserved by early excision and closure of the smaller wound, especially in areas such as the dorsum of the hands.

Several surgical procedures and special instrumentation have been developed to improve the surgical approach to the burn wound. The two

CHAPTER 27 528

most frequently used surgical procedures for removal of the burn wound are tangential excision and primary excision. *Tangential excision* refers to the sequential shaving of the dead tissue until a viable bleeding base is reached. This technique lends itself best to deep dermal and superficial full-thickness burn wounds. *Primary excision* is removal not only of the burn wound itself but also the underlying subcutaneous fat down to the fascial plane. This is done most often in large, deep burns where survival is the primary concern. With either procedure, immediate closure of the wound with autograft or homograft is imperative. The advent of special instrumentation such as improved dermatones and special surgical knives, as well as coagulation devices such as the CO_2 laser, the Argon laser, and electrocautery surgery, has improved the success of such excisional procedures.

Split-Thickness Skin Grafts

Skin grafts are used to cover open wounds that either will not heal or will require a lengthy period for healing. Grafting is accomplished by transferring skin from one area, the *donor site*, and placing it on the base of the excised burn wound or granulation tissue, the *recipient site*. Epidermis and a portion of the dermis are removed from the donor site at a depth of 0.012 to 0.018 in. The thickness of the graft is determined by the area to be grafted and by whether the donor area will need to be used a second or third time for grafting. The amount of donor graft is determined by the area to be covered and by the availability of donor sites. Sheet grafts are usually used for cosmetic areas such as the face and hands and over areas of function such as joints. Expanded graft techniques are utilized when there are limited donor sites and large areas to be covered. The mesh graft, one of the more common expansion techniques, is made by running a sheet of skin through a machine that produces a network of slits, thus allowing the skin to be stretched in a fishnet fashion so as to provide coverage of a larger area. Early debridement and early wound closure by skin grafting tend to produce less scarring than if primary healing is allowed to occur in deep dermal burns. Unfortunately, however, hypertrophic scarring continues to develop in grafted areas that are under constant tension and movement, such as over the volar aspect of most joints.

Scarring and Maturation

Deep dermal burns heal by a combination of contracture and epithelialization whereby the wound becomes smaller as a result of the force of the tension on the wound. After the burn heals, the scar maturation process continues for a period of up to 2 years. The exact mechanism of hypertrophic scarring is not clearly understood. Hypertrophic scars are thought to be created by an apparent inflammatory process in which there is abnormal formation of collagen fibers. Collagen bundles tend to form in whorls, centering around clusters of cells of small vessels (Baur, 1977). Some of the central cells are macrophages, while others are fibroblasts. It is theorized that tension along or across scars produces a response of increased collagen deposit and decreased collagen breakdown (Longacre, 1972). Tension produced by vigorous exercise over involved joints may lead to reinjury with subsequent inflammation, which increases the tendency of the scar to contract.

The scar appears raised, hard, and firm. It looks red and angry in people with fair skin and may appear reddish brown, gray, or even black in people of dark skin. Mature hypertrophic scars tend to decrease in size, becoming soft and pliable over a period of months to years. Hypertrophic scarring is often confused with *keloid* formation, which is seen most frequently in blacks, Orientals, and some dark European races. Young individuals of these races are more frequently affected than adults. Keloids are rarely found in the elderly. Keloids differ from the hypertrophic scar only in the amount of scar production. Keloids tend to increase in size, growing beyond the original wound to produce excess scarring in a mushroom shape. Small keloids may be treated with steroid injection to accelerate collagen breakdown. Treatment of large keloids is often discouraging, since excision requires skin grafting for closure, and the resulting wound may form similar lesions.

Physical Limitations as a Result of Wound Contraction

Wound contracture, generally seen in deep dermal and full-thickness burns, may present any number of problems, especially when joints are involved. As soon as scar tissue is formed, it begins to contract. It is this contraction of scar tissue that causes the deformity seen in severe burns. Bands in the form of scar tissue tend to pull joints down in the direction of least resistance. Thus, joint mobility becomes impaired. Limited joint mobility may severely hamper the rehabilitation of these patients.

Scar tissue has no elasticity, and therefore it does not grow at the same rate as normal skin. Children with severe burns are prone to deformities as growth spurts occur. Since the scar tissue may not grow as rapidly as the body structure, contractures and deformities increase. Deformity or limitation of joint function may require early surgical release to prevent irreversible damage. Unfortunately, early surgical procedures performed for contracture release often require additional surgery after the maturation process. When surgical procedures can be delayed for at least 12 to 18 months after final wound closure, reconstructive and cosmetic results are optimized.

Physical Limitations as a Result of Muscle Shortening and Loss of Muscle Tissue

Joint contractures commonly result from contracture of healing scar tissue while the patient lies in a flexed, abducted position, "the position of comfort." With disuse, muscles begin to atrophy. Muscle shortening and atrophy are the result of immobility, and long periods of exercise are required to improve function. If wound contracture and muscle atrophy are allowed to proceed, permanent loss of function may be the result. When the injury has resulted in loss of muscle tissue, as seen in electrical burns, function may not always be regained. Muscles must be strengthened, and often other muscles must be enlisted to take over the function of the lost tissue.

Physical Limitations as a Result of Loss or Damage of Nerves and Tendons

When the burn is deep enough to expose major nerves and tendons, immediate coverage with skin is indicated to prevent further damage resulting from dessication and necrosis with resultant loss in function. Tendons exposed to the air for any period of time necrose and die with loss of function of the involved joint. Nerve damage, especially to major nerves, will result in the loss of sensation or function in the involved area. These losses may be either temporary or permanent, depending upon the degree of nerve damage.

TREATMENT AND PREVENTION OF LONG-TERM DEFORMITY AND DISABILITY

Effective treatment and preventive therapy should be initiated immediately following the burn injury and followed throughout the hospitalization. Contracture deformities have long been a threat to the termally injured patient. Adequate positioning and exercise are difficult to manage and so are often overlooked during the initial resuscitation phase. By the time complications are noted, there may be loss of joint function that will be difficult to correct. Therefore, early intervention and preventative therapy are essential to enable the burned patient to return to a state of optimal function.

EARLY MANAGEMENT

Early management of the thermally injured patient requires the cooperation of the entire burn team. Therapy should include a comprehensive positioning, splinting, and exercise program regardless of the severity of the patient's condition; a nutritional program that meets and maintains the increased caloric requirements of the patient; and a consistent regime aimed at infection control.

Positioning and Splinting

The primary concern with burns involving joints is early positioning and splinting. Continuous evaluations should be made by the nurse and the therapist to monitor effective maintenance of joint function. Splints and conformers may be necessary to maintain adequate function and prevent contractures. An example of a typical neck splint is seen in Fig. 27-3. The use of neck conformers applied over the topical agent has been found to be successful in maintaining contour and decreasing muscle tightness and contracture in deep burns of the neck (Willis, 1973).

Figure 27-3
A typical neck conformer used to maintain the normal extension and angle of the neck.

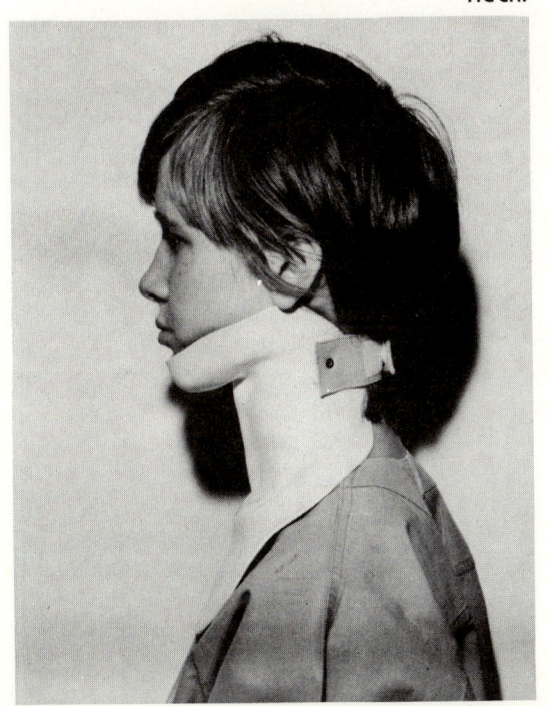

Pillows should be discouraged to avoid flexion of the neck. During the early phases of healing, neck conformers may not be well tolerated by some patients. Other methods of applying stretch and hyperextension may be necessary. The double mattress technique easily facilitates full extension with minimal discomfort to the patient. A supine position is assumed, with shoulders placed near the edge of the top mattress, thereby allowing the patient's head to rest on the lower mattress (Fig. 27-4). The head of the bed may be raised to a 45 to 50° angle without interfering with position.

Splinting should be considered whenever there is difficulty in maintaining range of motion in major joints. Particular attention should be given to the axilla, elbow, wrist, hand, knee, ankle, and foot. Early axillary and knee contractures can be prevented by proper positioning. Splints, as seen in Fig. 27-5 a–c, may be necessary to maintain hand, elbow, and ankle function. When splints are necessary, they are worn at night and whenever the patient is not exercising the involved area. Infants and small children usually require special individualized approaches for adequate positioning. Because of their size, they have the unique ability to wiggle and squirm out of the most elaborate conformer. Splints and conformers, particularly those being applied for the first time, should be evaluated frequently by the nurse or therapist for proper fit. Initially, splints should be removed and evaluated every 2 to 4 h for the first 24 h. The nurse should observe for signs of pressure, increased edema, or decreased sensation in the extremity. An improperly fitting splint or conformer should be readjusted before reapplying. After 24 h, the splints should be removed and reapplied at least every 8 h to ensure proper fit and positioning.

Exercise

Active or passive exercise is essential to maintain range of motion and muscle strength in the early phase of burn care. Active exercise should be encouraged as soon after admission as possible. Supervised physical therapy should be carried out at least twice a day. The patient should be

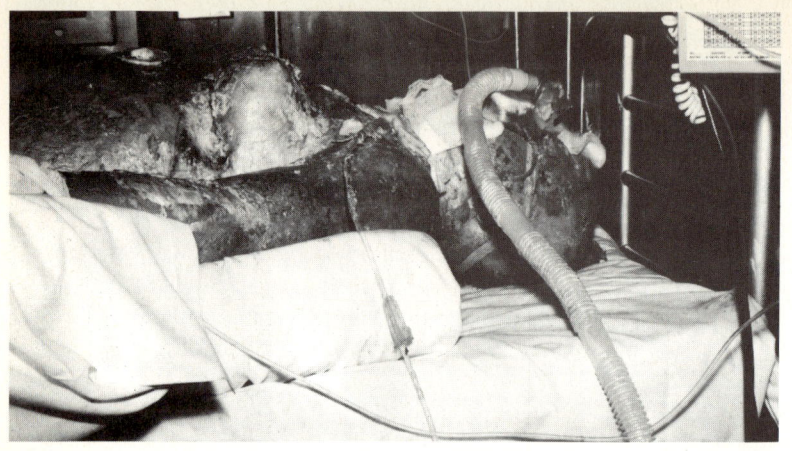

Figure 27-4
The split mattress technique helps to maintain the neck in extension when a conformer cannot be used.

instructed to carry out independent exercise periodically during the day. The extreme pain experienced by many patients may limit their ability to comply with therapy. Exercising in conjunction with hydrotherapy tends to enhance muscle relaxation and decrease pain. Analgesics or tranquilizers may be necessary to facilitate a more productive, less stressful exercise session. The nurse should encourage and assure the patient that exercise is an important part of treatment. When the patient is unable or unwilling to carry out active range of motion, the nurse or physical therapist should perform gentle passive range of motion.

Diet

Nutritional requirements are doubled in the severely burned person. Burned patients in general tend to have poor appetites and may be unable to consume the large quantities of food required. A diet high in protein and calories is essential during the period of wound repair. Liquid dietary supplements are often required to supply the caloric needs. Gastric hyperalimentation with continuous tube feeding is commonly initiated when oral intake is inadequate. Intravenous hyperalimentation may be required when the patient's clinical status does not permit gastric feedings.

Caloric needs should be evaluated on a daily basis during the acute phase of hospitalization. Calorie counts by the dietitian provide initial and periodic assessment of the patient's actual intake. Accurate measurements of daily weight and fluid balance are valuable tools for assessing the patient's metabolic state. Continuous reevaluation of caloric count, daily weight, and intake and output records allows the nurse to monitor the adequacy of the nutritional therapy.

Infection Control

As mentioned previously, infection is a constant threat in the thermally injured person. Sources of wound infection may be endogenous or exogenous. The most common endogenous source is the gastrointestinal tract; the most common exogenous source is cross-contamination. Staff members frequently carry organisms on their hands from one patient to another. Good handwashing techniques are essential to decrease the incidence of cross-contamination. Another frequent source of cross-contamination is equipment entering the patient area that may harbor organisms when not adequately cleaned. An *isolation protocol* should be developed that takes into account all the possible sources of contamination. This isolation program should be simple enough to ensure that it will be carried

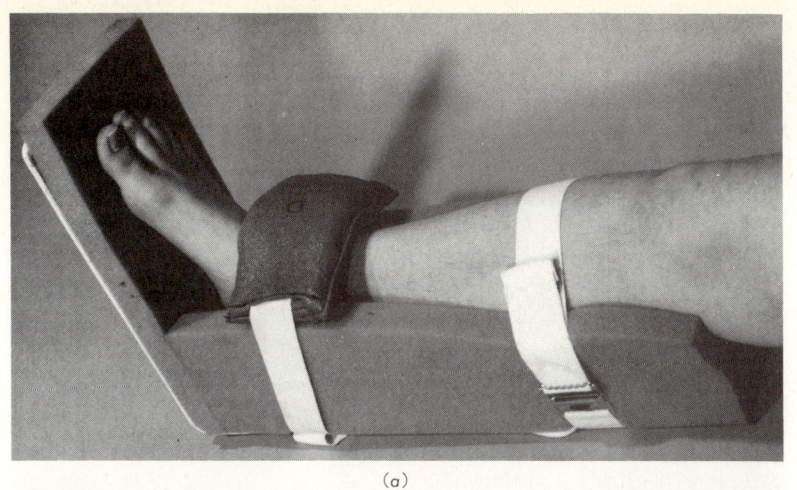

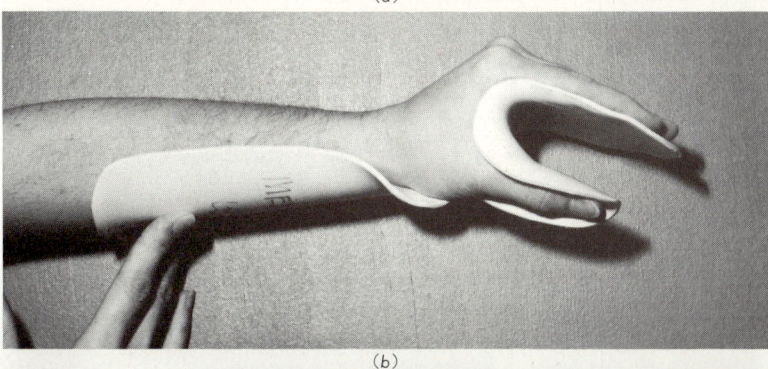

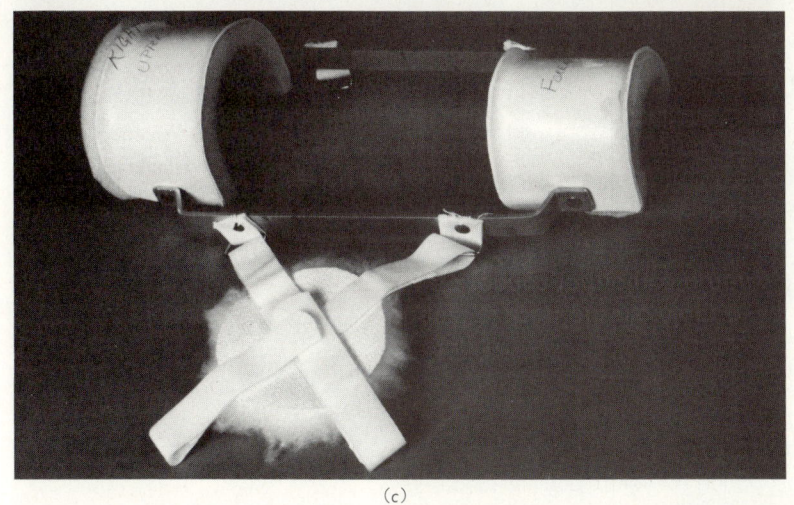

Figure 27-5

(a) A typical foot splint used to maintain the foot in a neutral position. (b) A hand splint used to maintain wrist extension, MP flexion, and PIP and DIP extension. (c) An elbow splint used to increase and maintain elbow extension.

out. The most elaborate isolation program can be ineffective if there is one break in technique.

Improved wound care techniques may contribute more to the control of infection than any other factor. The colonization of the wound may be effectively limited by topical application of antibacterial agents. The most commonly used topical agents are listed in Table 27-3 along with the bacterial spectrum for each agent. Topical therapy has been found to be most effective when used in combination with thorough washing and daily debridement. Unfortunately, with the continued use of these agents, strains of resistant organisms have begun to appear. It has become apparent over the last few years that topical agents are not the total answer to preventing colonization of the burn wound. Early removal and timely closure of the burn wound may prove to be the definitive answer.

Early Closure of Wounds

Great strides have been made in the treatment of burns as a result of early excision and coverage of the wound with autograft. Many physicians are now evaluating deep dermal and full-thickness injuries for excision soon after admission rather than allowing the eschar to separate naturally. Children and elderly persons frequently present difficulties in determining the depth of injury owing to the thinness of their skin. Initial injuries may appear shallow and seem to increase in depth within several days. When allowed to heal spontaneously, these injuries may produce severe scarring. Early excision and closure of wounds decreases the incidence of the severe deformities seen in deep dermal injuries. Once the wound is covered with skin, the incidence of infection is greatly reduced. The general response of the body to the injury is decreased when a significant portion of the burn wound is grafted.

Surgical excision is generally performed within the first 5 to 7 days after injury. After this period, the bacterial counts in the wound may be high enough that there is risk of introducing large numbers of organisms into the bloodstream. It must be remembered that the graft procedure is only effective if the graft adheres. Precautions must be taken to protect the graft until circulation is reestablished and it is adherent to the wound surface. The nurse should observe for blood or serum that may collect under the graft. Any fluid

Table 27-3

Topical Agents

AGENT	SPECTRUM
Silver nitrate	Effective against most staphylococci and *Pseudomonas*
	Not effective against *Enterobacter, Klebsiella,* or *Aerobacter*
Mafenide acetate (Sulfamylon)	Wide range of gram-positive and gram-negative organisms and most anaerobes
	Not effective against *Providencia stuartii* or *Serratia marcescens*
Silver sulfadiazine (Silvadene)	Wide range of gram-positive and gram-negative organisms, as well as *Candida albicans*
Polyvinylpyrrolidone and iodine (Betadine)	Wide range of gram-positive and gram-negative organisms, as well as some fungi

collecting under the graft will cause it to slough. Splinting, bulky dressings, or skeletal traction may be required to prevent movement and mechanical trauma with the consequent disruption of the graft. The graft is usually firmly adherent within 3 to 5 days. Activity and exercise may be resumed as soon as the graft is firmly adhered. Range of motion exercises are enhanced after grafting, since the pain associated with movement is diminished.

LATER MANAGEMENT

Prevention of joint contractures in the acutely burned patient by early proper positioning and splinting cannot be overemphasized. Aggressive early physical therapy facilitates later management of the severely burned person. If a vigorous program of splinting and physical therapy has been followed, muscle tightness and contractures may be avoided. If, however, contractures have been allowed to form, they may present difficult if not impossible problems to correct.

Positioning, exercise, and pressure should be continued following spontaneous healing and grafting of burns. Even though the skin may appear soft and smooth initially, contracture of the wound may initiate the formation of deformities within a few weeks to months. The patient may be impressed by the appearance of the healed burn and feel that positioning and exercise are less important at this time. The nurse and the therapist should be acutely aware of the complications that can occur following wound closure. This will allow them to instruct the patient properly in the need for continued therapy.

The newly healed burn often manifests a warm, red, firm tissue that continues to change actively until the scar matures. The scar tissue tends to pull and shorten over joints when there is no resistance, but it readily responds to constant stretch and pressure. Therefore, continued positioning, splinting, and pressure are imperative during this phase.

Conformers and Dynamic Splints

With the development of plastic splints and conformers, some measure of protection against scar contracture has been afforded the burned patient. These devices are made of plastic materials that are easily molded and modified as necessary. The plastics used can be molded at the patient's bedside or in the clinic by heating the material either with a heat gun or a water bath. This allows for continuous reevaluation and refitting of the splints.

Once the burn wound has healed or been grafted, a strict program of splinting is necessary to maintain stretch over the involved joints. Some areas present more difficulty than others; severe burns of the neck and axilla involve formidable management problems. Figure 27-6 shows examples of these typical burn deformities.

Neck contractures are characterized either by multiple narrow bands or by extensive scar tissue extending from chin to sternum with loss of the cleft. Prevention requires continuous splinting until the scar tissue is mature. Neck conformers may be flexible or rigid depending on the amount of pressure needed. The design is determined by the size of the burn area or skin graft. The neck conformer has two purposes: (1) to apply pressure to the scar to limit hypertrophy, and (2) to maintain the angle between the mandible and the sternum. The neck conformer should be evaluated frequently for proper fit to prevent undue pressure and skin breakdown.

Axillary contractures are very common and may involve either the anterior or the posterior axillary folds or the entire area. Burns of the axilla should be splinted in a position of 90 to 110° of abduction, with 10° of forward flexion to prevent bracheal plexus injuries. Constant pressure provided by large semicircular sponges placed in the axilla and secured with an elastic wrap has proved effective in preventing and correcting axillary contractures in children (Parks, 1977). Airplane splints, which allow the axilla to be abducted with the elbow either flexed or extended, have been used effectively in nonsurgical correction of contractures and following surgical releases (see Fig. 27-7). The airplane

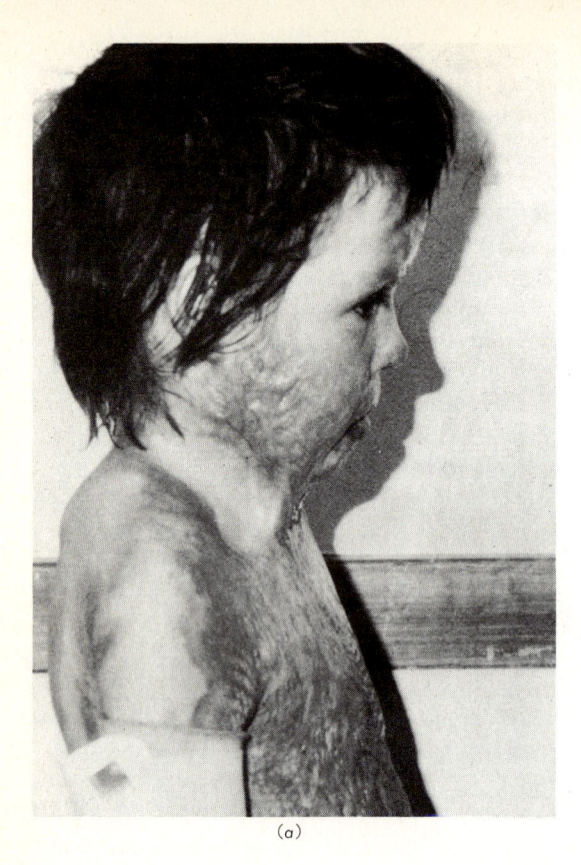

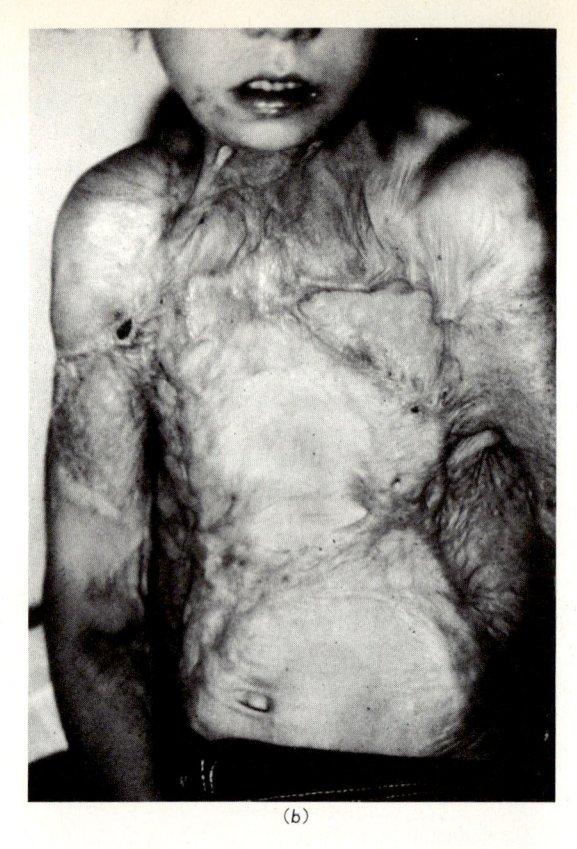

Figure 27-6
(*a*) Notice the loss of neck extension and angle in this typical burned neck contracture. (*b*) This shows both neck and axillary contractures after burn injury.

splint is anchored by a corset fitting snugly around the waist. Two adjustable metal rods are attached to the corset and angled up to suspend the arm at the elbow. The splint should be well padded and checked periodically for pressure sores. It is difficult to utilize the airplane splint when the burn involves the trunk because of irritation created by the corset.

The dorsum of the hand is most vulnerable to thermal injury. Although much of the initial damage to the hand may be irreversible, secondary deformities can often be prevented by early range of motion and splinting. The typical burned hand deformity presents with the characteristic pattern of hyperextension of the metacarpophalangeal joints and hyperflexion of the proximal and distal interphalangeal joints, flattening of the palmar arch, abduction of the thumb, and loss of wrist extension (see Fig. 27-8). Prevention of these deformities requires daily evaluation of position and splinting. Dynamic splints, which are capable of applying constant, even pressure and stretch to specific areas of the hand, may provide effective results. Dynamic splinting is a fairly simple method of solving a major problem. This may be accomplished with a volar splint, using rubber bands and hooks glued to the patient's fingernails to apply traction to the hand and fingers. Figure 27-9 shows a hand in a dynamic splint. Traction with this device may be continuous or only at night, depending on the patient's progress. Other types of dynamic hand splints are the hay rake and the banjo (Fig. 27-10 a and b). These splints are frequently used after early excision and grafting of the hand or in surgical reconstruction of the hand.

The nurse should continually evaluate splints and conformers for pressure areas and skin breakdown. Splints may be either padded with 1/2-in foam or applied over an appropriate dressing to avoid maceration or breakdown from pressure. They should never be applied directly over the wound, healed skin, or grafted area. Spontaneonsly healed skin and grafted skin are very sensitive, and any abrasion created by movement of the splint may create pressure necrosis of the skin. Patients being discharged with a splinting program should thoroughly understand the method of application and the importance of continued use.

Exercise

The most pronounced changes in range of motion caused by scarring usually occur during the first 2 to 3 months following spontaneous healing or grafting of burn wounds. Many patients lose range of motion after discharge from the hospital as a result of lack of supervision or motivation in carrying out appropriate exercises at home. The patient needs to understand the dynamic process that will continue until the scar tissue matures. The effectiveness of exercise therapy should be evaluated frequently and modified as necessary. This may require physical therapy sessions two to three times a week to maximize the effectiveness of the exercise program. Exercise therapy should be carried out in conjunction with a splinting and pressure regime to optimize the results.

Pressure Garments

Spontaneous healing of deep burn wounds results in the replacement of the normal integument with a highly active growing tissue lacking the normal skin characteristics. During the active healing phase, the use of pressure garments has been shown to be effective in controlling the proliferation of hypertrophic scars, thereby reducing contractures. Jobst custom-made elastic garments that provide constant controlled pressure to most anatomic areas are available (see Fig. 27-11). Detailed measurements are obtained

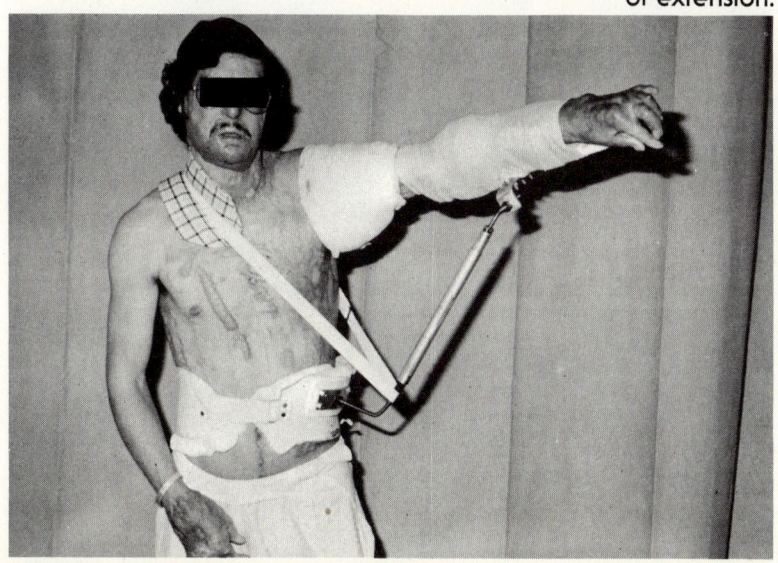

Figure 27-7
The airplane splint is used to maintain the axilla in 90°+ of extension.

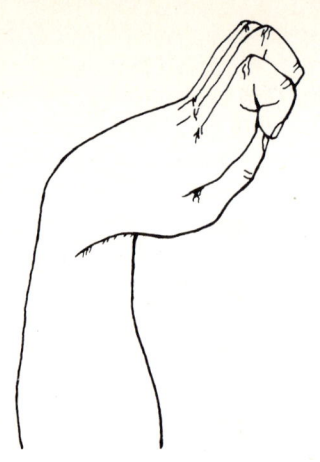

Figure 27-8 Diagram of the typical burned hand deformity.

for individualized custom fit (see Fig. 27-12). In order to be effective, pressure garments must be worn day and night. Noticeable changes in scar tissue and contracture formations have been demonstrated with interruption of pressure for only 8 h (Parks et al., 1977). Patients are provided with two sets of garments so that one set may be washed without interrupting pressure therapy. Areas of the body that are irregular in contour, such as the face, neck, and axilla, may require additional methods of producing pressure in conjunction with the elastic garment. The face presents difficulty in obtaining uniform pressure around the nose and eyes. Sponges inserted under the elastic face mask may be adequate, depending on the amount of pressure required. If additional pressure is needed, a plastic mask that is molded to the contour of the face may be necessary to obtain adequate pressure (see Fig. 27-13). The problems and methods involved in applying pressure to the neck and axilla have been discussed previously. The Jobst pressure garment, although effective, is expensive. They become very uncomfortable during the summer months, and many patients find it difficult to comply with therapy. A thorough evaluation should be made of the amount of pressure required and the ability of the patient to comply with the program. The patient should be instructed thoroughly and should understand the need for constant pressure. The nurse should explain the negative as well as the positive features of the garments.

Elastic woven wraps (Ace bandages) are a less expensive method of obtaining desired pressure in some areas such as upper and lower extremities. Elastic wraps should be applied in a figure-eight fashion to provide even pressure. The patient and a family member should be taught how to apply the bandage and alerted to the signs of inadequate circulation. The problem with this method is that it is difficult to achieve and maintain constant pressure. Pressure provided in this manner should be well supervised. All pressure garments should be evaluated frequently for adequate fit and refitted as necessary.

Figure 27-9 A volar splint with rubber bands may be used as a dynamic splint to improve joint function.

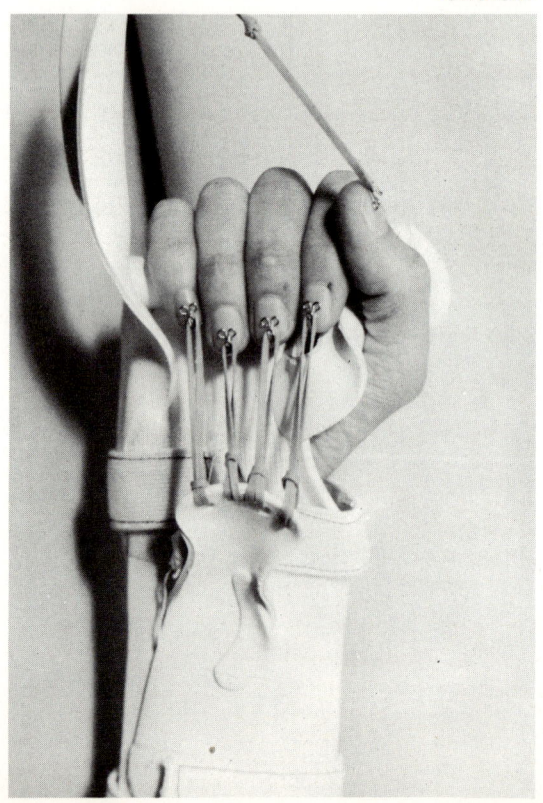

CHAPTER 27 538

Prosthesis

Some burned patients may actually experience the loss of an extremity as a result of the severity of the injury. This is especially true of the patient with electrical injury. These patients suffer not only the disfigurement of scarring but also the deformity of loss of a body part. Coping with the loss of a body part and learning to accept a prosthetic device may be an extremely difficult and highly discouraging process. Learning to use the prosthetic arm or leg will require hard work on the part of the patient. Examples of two types of prosthetic arms may be seen in Fig. 27-14 a and b. The nurse will need to give continued support and encouragement to prepare the patient and family for the difficult times ahead.

PSYCHOSOCIAL ADJUSTMENTS

The severely burned patient is suddenly faced with an extreme test of coping abilities. The time of transition from protective mechanisms to acceptance varies greatly from patient to patient. A variety of coping mechanisms are used in making the transition. The patient must accomplish several major tasks before transition can be completed. The feelings of inadequacy, hostility, guilt, denial, and personal rejection must in some measure be resolved or minimized. Close relationships that provide emotional support to the patient are extremely important during this period. Relationships that enable the patient to feel valued by significant others tend to enhance self-esteem and provide hope even in the face of permanent disfigurement or disability. Emotional support may be provided by family members, other patients, friends, or clergy.

Physical progress plays an important role in the patient's ability to improve emotionally. Progress can mean improvement in the function of a major joint or new skin covering an area that was once a large, open wound. The patient can begin to reassess the injury and set goals as progress continues. The human organism shows remarkable resilience in adapting to change. The severely burned person slowly comes to

Figure 27-10 (a) Hands may be maintained in the hay rake after grafting procedure for optimum joint function. (b) The banjo splint is another dynamic splint used to maintain position after grafting.

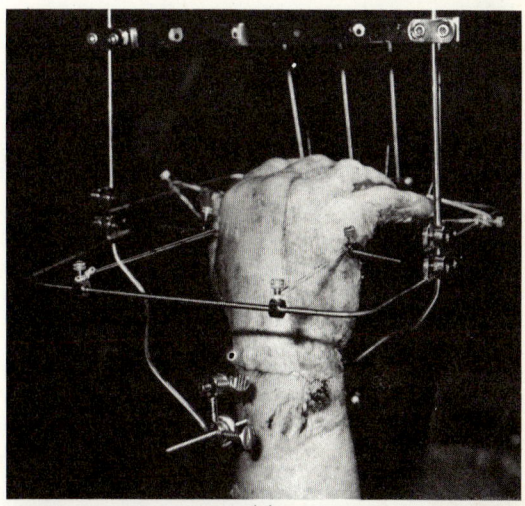

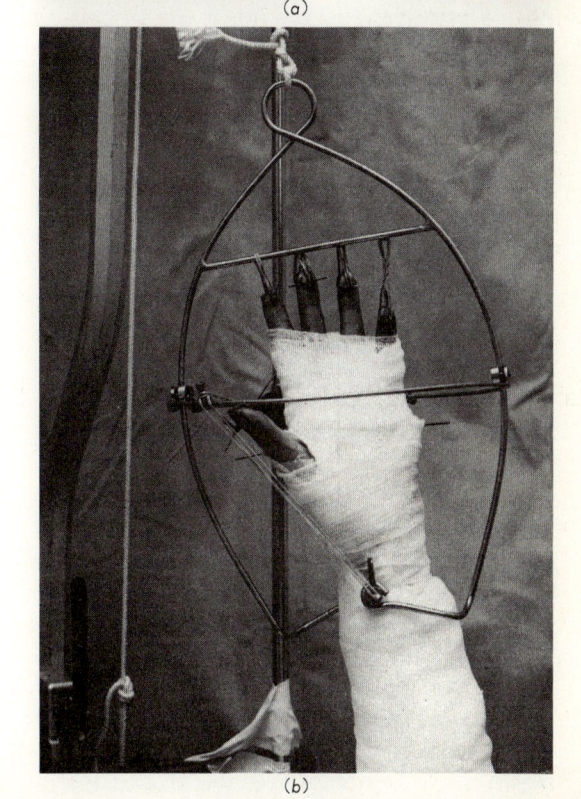

(a)

(b)

recognize the reality of physical limitations and disfigurement. As acceptance occurs, the patient begins to adapt to the new situation and seeks new sources of gratification, reliable relationships, and self-respect.

The majority of thermally injured patients are able to complete the transition without apparent long-term psychological complications (Hamburg, 1974). The significant few who are not able to adjust pose a major problem for the burn team. As the patient becomes aware of the changed body image, there may be a persistent refusal to acknowledge reality. Some patients may even avoid any recognition of the injury. The regressive childlike behavior of the patient may evoke anger from staff, friends, and family. Social interactions should be monitored for signs of rejection and hostility. Psychotherapeutic intervention focusing on the accident and its meaning to the patient will be most important at this point. Periodic psychotherapy sessions are often required after discharge from the hospital. It may be necessary to involve family members or significant others in the patient's therapy.

Does the Extent of the Burn Injury Dictate the Outcome of Rehabilitation?

The effect of disability on future plans is one of the most common sources of concern. One might assume that the severely injured patient would have more difficulty adjusting than the patient with a minor injury, but this is not necessarily true. There are many factors that may determine the patient's response to disability and the outcome of rehabilitation, and these factors vary from patient to patient. One factor is the patient's previous use of coping mechanisms. The extensively burned patient who was able to cope appropriately with prior stressful situations generally responds well to rehabilitation from the burn injury. Another factor is the length of time required for rehabilitation. Rehabilitation is a step-by-step process that allows the patient to gradually change the focus of future aspirations in the way of physical recovery. The patient with a severe injury who recovers over a period of months becomes able to accept

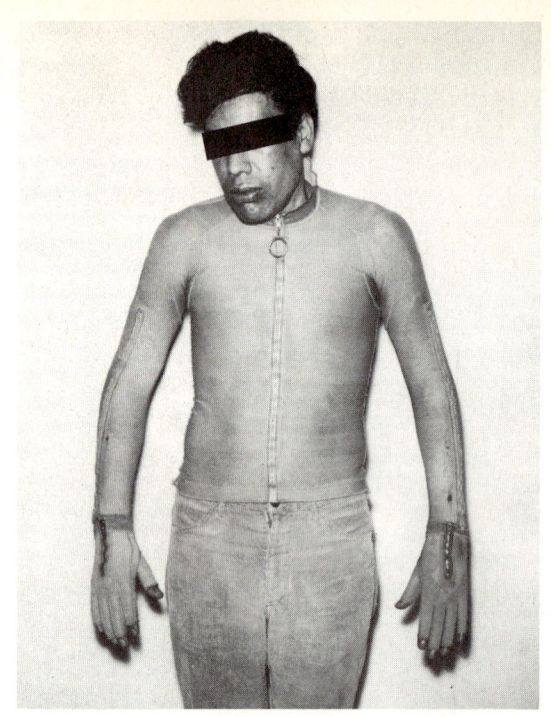

Figure 27-11
Jobst, an elasticized garment, is used to apply even pressure over areas of hypertrophic scarring.

disfigurement and disability and seeks gratification and self-esteem through new avenues. The patient who sustains what is erroneously termed "insignificant" burns may develop a very negative approach to rehabilitation. Often, this patient expects a short period of morbidity and is completely overwhelmed with the realization of the time required for scar maturation and the slow return of function. For example, a young athlete may become hostile and angry when a small burn on the lower leg requires 6 months or longer for complete recovery. Even superficial burns on the hands may be especially disturbing to the patient whose vocation requires fine dexterity or dealing directly with the public. Burns of the face are of concern to most patients but may have pronounced emotional effects on young people who are especially sensitive to appearance.

Society places great value on physical fitness

CHAPTER 27   540

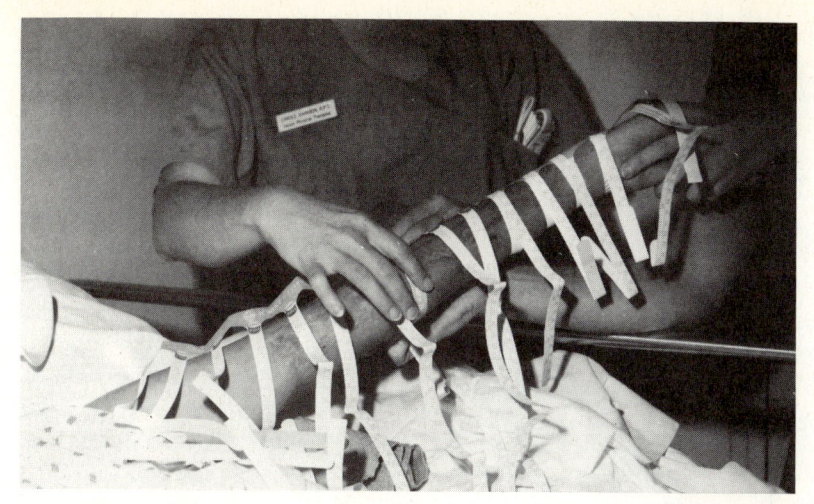

Figure 27-12
To ensure proper fit of the elastic garments, detailed measurements must be taken of each body part to be covered.

and appearance. Individuals place different values on different anatomical areas of the body. An insignificant injury to one patient may not be insignificant to another. The outcome of rehabilitation is generally determined by the patient's overall emotional response to the injury. Inevitably, there are physical limitations and disfiguring elements directly related to the severity of the burn injury, but how the individual perceives the disability or disfigurement is based on self-perception. Therefore, rehabilitation may be said to be effective when the patient perceives that successful reintegration into society has been completed.

Figure 27-13
The clear plastic mask shown here has been molded to fit the contour of the child's face. Adequate pressure is maintained by securing the mask with Velcro straps to a cap worn by the child. The diagram emphasizes the uniform pressure which is obtained around areas of the eyes, nose, mouth and chin.

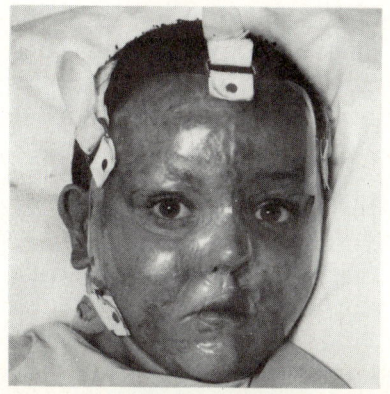

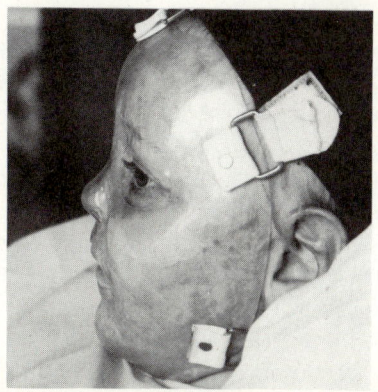

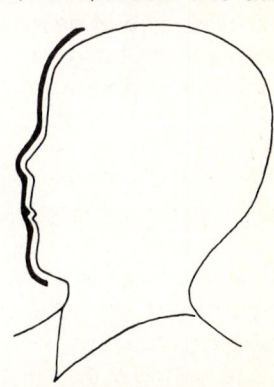

541   THIRD DEGREE BURNS

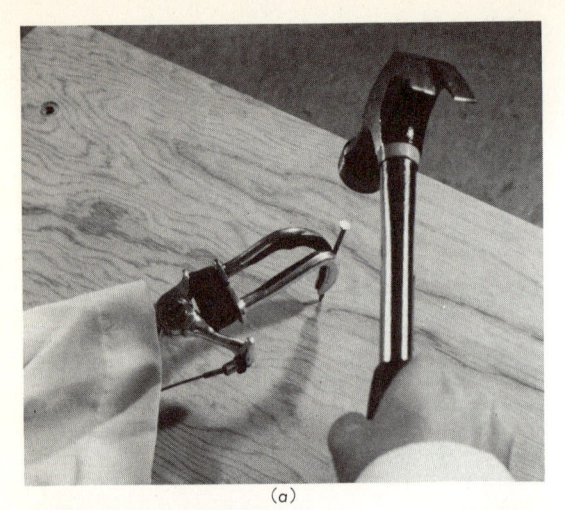

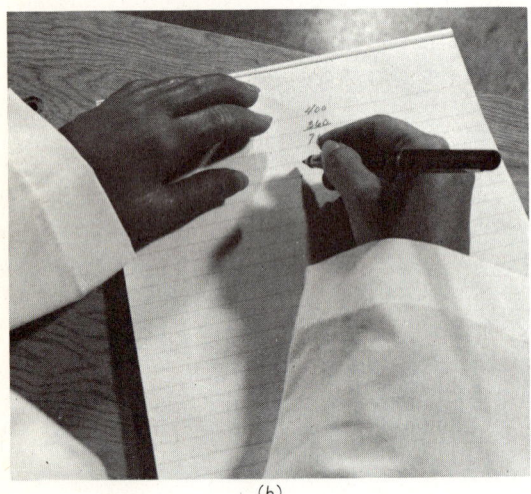

Figure 27-14
(*a*) The hook-type prosthesis may be useful in performing many jobs requiring a high degree of dexterity. (*b*) The cosmetic prosthetic hand may be used for a more normal appearance but is relatively useless when dexterity is required.

Looking at Each Patient as an Individual

An essential part of rehabilitation is a thorough evaluation of each patient to assess his or her needs adequately. Each patient's requirements will be different and should be based on an individual assessment. In the initial assessment, the nurse should attempt to obtain information concerning the patient's past experiences, cultural and ethnic background, relationships with significant others, and financial status.

Past Experiences The patient's hospital and rehabilitation course may be influenced either negatively or positively by past experiences. Information should be obtained regarding previous hospitalizations or serious illnesses of the patient, family members, or close friends. A bad experience from a prior hospitalization may be manifested by anger and hostility. The patient may be uncooperative with therapy and, in some instances, may attempt to interfere with treatment. Also, some patients may have known someone who either died or was badly scarred as a result of a burn injury. Many elderly patients frequently enter the hospital not expecting to survive. They have seen many of their friends grow old and die either in a hospital or in a convalescent center. Young children pose a different problem. Often, hospitalization represents a new experience, that of prolonged separation for parents and child. This in itself may give rise to stress and emotional problems. The inquisitive nurse may find that providing the child's favorite toy may reduce some of the fear of separation. The nurse should also seek information about previous personal or family crises and how the patient reacted to these experiences. This type of questioning often uncovers unresolved problems that may affect the patient's response to injury or hospitalization.

Cultural and Ethnic Background Cultural and ethnic differences, though not always a major problem, can present difficulties for staff members as well as for the patient. Cultural differences in dietary habits may be a factor in the nutritional management of the burned individual. Also, superstition or cultural beliefs about health and disease may interfere with the patient's cooperation with various treatments. Lack of communication can be a major stumbling block to treatment and understanding of the rehabilitation needs. Communication problems do not always involve a difference in the spoken language but often relate to understanding medical versus nonmedical terms.

The patient who speaks limited English is often more difficult to evaluate than the patient who speaks no English. Frequently, staff members erroneously assume that the patient understands when nonverbal positive gestures are used. For example, smiling and nodding, especially among Oriental and other Eastern cultures may only be a polite response when verbal communication is difficult. Some Eastern cultures see the hospital as a place to go only when very ill and survival is not anticipated. Many have never before required hospitalization and feel threatened by the lack of understanding and the unfamiliar surroundings. The hospital is an institution where the physician, nurse, therapist, and other health professionals provide all medical and physical needs of the ill. The patient may be willing and cooperative during supervised therapy, but a lack of understanding may limit the patient's ability to participate in an unsupervised program. The periodic use of a language interpreter may eliminate problems that could develop in such situations.

All too frequently, there may be lack of communication among groups of people who appear to be speaking the same language. Some cultural groups such as black Americans, American Indians, and chicanos learned to speak several languages: English and the "language of survival," or "street" language. Often the same words may not have the same meaning. Sentence structure may be different, with slang or native language interjected. It may often be difficult to understand the patient's motives, intentions, or goals. The young black patient who feels guilt associated with the injury and is apprehensive and suspicious of staff members may express anger and hostility, while the elderly black or the American Indian may exhibit withdrawal with quiet acceptance of the situation. A sincere attempt should be made to assess the individual's cultural values and attitudes in order to set realistic goals. It would certainly be of little value to initiate scar preventive therapy if the patient is a member of a culture or ethnic group that regards scarring as a symbol of beauty or disfigurement as a sign of accomplishment in reaching maturity.

Different cultural groups, as well as different age groups, may respond in a dissimilar manner to a similar situation. The role of the nurse is to establish an effective line of communication and understanding in this often difficult situation.

Family Support The patient's main source of emotional gratification during this highly stressful period will be provided by the family and close friends. It is important to ascertain who the patient considers to be the significant persons. Conflicts between the critically ill patient and family members or among family members may add to the stress of the injury. Family members should be told frequently of the patient's condition by one or two members of the burn team. Often confusion arises when too many staff members try to intervene with a particular family. Channeling family concerns and information through a limited number of team members will reduce the risk of double messages and will improve communication.

The family should be encouraged to participate in the patient's rehabilitation therapy. They should be helped to understand the patient's goals for rehabilitation and how and when they can assist the patient to accomplish them. Some families tend to be overprotective and not allow the patient to try to achieve the desired goals. Other families may have expectations far above the patient's abilities and thus inhibit progress by robbing the patient of a sense of accomplishment. The patient usually regains a sense of worth and self-esteem through the acceptance and encouragement of family members and close friends.

The nurse should assess the ability of family members to cope with the patient's physical limitations and disfigurement. Family conferences should be provided whenever necessary to assist the patient and family in reaching these goals. Clinical observations show that patients with poor support systems generally tend to be less motivated. Although they may cooperate during supervised therapy, rarely do they follow through without supervision. When a source of substantial emotional support can be provided these patients, they may respond more appropriately to therapy.

Financial Status The patient recovering from a burn injury may find it difficult to concentrate on physical therapy or other treatments if the family is experiencing financial difficulties. Thoughts of how to pay the hospital bill, prevent the accumulation of personal debts, or feed and shelter the family may preoccupy the patient's mind. Often these problems are exacerbated by loss of a family dwelling or other personal property. Efforts to continue therapy may be unsuccessful until the patient's anxieties are decreased. Social services may need to intervene in an attempt to obtain emergency funds. The patient and family may be eligible for temporary public assistance or long-term, low-cost loans to meet these financial obligations. Community resources may often be used to assist the family in this situation. When the patient no longer perceives finances as an immediate crisis, treatment usually becomes more productive.

Patient Reaction to Injury and Hospitalization The patient's response to injury will be dictated not only by past experiences but also by the nature of the injury itself. The patient's approach to the injury depends in large part on the nature of the accident, the self-image that results, and how the accident is viewed. Progress and treatment may be complicated if there are feelings of guilt associated with the injury. The patient who feels responsible for the accident or for someone's death as a result of the accident may feel that pain and disfigurement are deserved punishment and so will respond negatively to the treatment and therapy programs. If the injury was self-inflicted or the result of criminal activity, the patient may appear depressed, withdrawn, and fearful.

The child whose injury was the result of abuse or a self-induced accident may be withdrawn, feeling guilty and responsible for the injury. They often become attached to staff members and the hospital environment because they either fear further punishment upon returning home or feel the need to be punished for creating so much trouble. In such cases, the patient and family will need much support from the whole staff. It is essential that the staff remain objective and nonjudgmental toward the parents in a suspected child abuse case. The patient's guilt or nonguilt will need to be dealt with openly in a realistic manner if emotional improvement is to occur. Often, long-term psychological or psychiatric intervention may be necessary.

Anger, a common response during this period, may be directed at God for allowing the injury to occur or at the burn staff, who control and direct the care and limit activities. In other cases, anger may be self-directed when progress is slow or the patient feels responsible for the injury. Often, when complaints of pain and discomfort appear to be ignored and therapy is reinforced by family members, the patient may feel deserted and express anger toward certain members or the whole family. The nurse should be aware of the patient's need to express anger. The patient often needs help in expressing this anger in an acceptable manner. Some patients need a firm approach from the nurse to understand how to cope with their anger.

Fear and apprehension related to the unknown aspects of hospitalization, the injury, and disfigurement may create any number of problems. Much of this can be eliminated by careful explanations of treatment and progress. Finding motivation and positive reinforcement presents a challenge for the nurse, therapist, and entire burn team. Without a positive outlook, however, fear and apprehension may be difficult to overcome.

HOSPITAL DISCHARGE AND REENTRY INTO SOCIETY

Rehabilitation Fears

Once the burned patient no longer sees survival as a threat, other fears may come into focus.

The response to treatment will be determined by the patient's ability to cope with these fears and apprehensions as attention is directed toward going home. The person experiencing a severe burn injury often spends many weeks in the hospital, away from family members, close friends, and normal activities. The total environment is often one of loneliness and dependency. Personal contacts are limited to the burn unit staff, who are accepting the patient's disfigurement, and to brief visits from family members and close friends. The patient's new world is smaller, more comfortable, and more secure. For the patient, contemplating reentry into the real world may produce severe anxiety. Although the patient enters the hospital with a fear of the unknown, he or she now must think of leaving a familiar place, a place that accepts the patient's changed body image. Thus the patient may find anticipation of going home a fearful adventure. Returning to normal relationships with family members and friends may add to this fear. Thus, reentry into society may be one of the most difficult areas of recovery for the burned patient.

Feelings of inadequacy may produce fears of being a burden to the family when prior responsibilities cannot be resumed immediately. The patient, especially a child, may acutely perceive alterations within the family structure and no longer feel included as a member. Much understanding and assistance are needed at this time from both the nurse and the family members. The patient must learn to cope with, accept, and adapt to being different in order to function as a productive person within the family unit and the community.

As the patient prepares to go home, the primary concern may be the altered self-image created by the injury. Apprehension may be manifested by frequent complaints of pain. Although the patient may continue to experience pain associated with joint limitations and exercise therapy, the severe pain experienced with open wounds should be diminished. Pain at this point may generally be controlled with mild analgesics and muscle relaxants. The patient who suffers severe disfigurement may have extreme difficulty controlling these anxieties. Psychiatric therapy and drugs aimed at antianxiety and antidepressant therapy may be beneficial.

Society has not yet learned to accept the scarring and disfigurement of the burn victim. Physical appearance is highly valued, and those who do not measure up to the standard are often severely penalized. Thoughts of strangers staring and making shocked comments, as well as rejection by family and close friends, make the outside world seem less desirable. Special anxieties may arise in connection with particular problems such as sexual functions. If the injury affected the genitalia, the patient will be concerned about decreased masculinity or femininity.

The nurse should be aware of the possible concerns related to the injury and should attempt to elicit verbal confirmation by the patient. Daily discussion of these fears may alleviate seeming problems or help the patient adjust to real problems. The patient will need support from family members and close friends, as well as staff members, to cope with these problems. Psychiatric intervention may be necessary if anxieties cannot be resolved.

Future Orientation

The patient suffering a less severe injury or the patient who has sufficient coping mechanisms may have less difficulty with a positive approach to the future. Once the patient is able to progress toward accepting disfigurement and scarring, the business of planning for the future can get underway (Steiner & Clark, 1977). The nurse should be observant for nonverbal and encourage verbal cues that indicate the patient is ready to make future plans. Patients with adequate coping mechanisms may reach this phase earlier and with less stress than other, less motivated patients. As soon as the patient starts thinking of what lies beyond the immediate healing process, it is the time to begin planning for the future. The patient often looks to the nurse and other disciplines for direction and positive options regarding the future. As the family and close friends become actively involved with the patient in planning for the future, they will need to understand that a period of readjustment may be required. This period of readjustment will often require learning to perform many self-care activities. The patient often feels helpless and useless during this period. If the injury was severe, a transfer from the burn unit to a rehabilitation unit may be indicated. There, the patient will be able to concentrate on self-care and further develop plans for the future.

Discharge Planning

The patient and family should be alerted that discharge plans are underway, allowing time for emotional adjustment and for arrangements to be made for the homecoming. Although discharge planning is the responsibility of the whole burn unit team, the primary responsibility often rests with the nurse. Because nurses are involved in day-to-day patient care, assessment, and evaluation, they are often the ones best suited to facilitate comprehensive coordination of discharge planning.

Discharge planning should begin on the day of admission as the nurse fills out an initial "nursing history" of the patient. A nursing history that includes pertinent information regarding both the patient and significant family members enables the staff to develop an in-depth nursing care plan as well as an individualized discharge plan. Support systems need to be explored early to ascertain availability and reliability of resources for the patient during the rehabilitation and postdischarge period. Some patients may have poor support systems and require the assistance of community resources and referral agencies. It is essential to identify early which agencies are available to the individual patient and to make referrals prior to discharge. Cooperative input will be required from all disciplines associated with the patient's care. Upon identifying the needs of the patient and family, the various referral agencies should be contacted by the appropriate person. That person may be the nurse, the social worker, the physical or occupational therapist, or another member of the team.

Patient and family teaching should begin upon admission to the hospital or as soon thereafter as possible. Although teaching is carried out by all members of the burn team, the nurse is with the patient for the longest period of time and will provide most of the teaching and instruction on a day-to-day basis. Providing gradual teaching and information enables the patient and family to be less overwhelmed and better prepared as the time for discharge approaches.

Timing is an important factor; the patient and family will need to be ready for the impending discharge if plans are to be successful. The most elaborate plans may often fail if the patient or family is uncooperative as a result of emotional stress or is unable to comply because of lack of understanding or support systems. The discharge plan should be developed in keeping with the family's ability to carry out procedures in the home.

Individualized planning should be considered in methods of testing and instructions. Continual assessment and evaluation of the patient's emotional and physical progress are essential. Physical limitations may require special considerations in developing independence. The nurse will need to assist the patient in setting realistic goals that can be accomplished. Progress in gaining independence may be more effective in an environment where the patient is in contact with other patients who are working toward similar goals. The family must be taught not only about the patient's limitations but also the importance of allowing the patient to become and remain independent.

Plans for discharge and procedures to be carried out in the home should be carefully and repeatedly discussed with both the patient and family prior to discharge. Instructions on wound care and general skin care should involve family members and friends whenever possible. The home program should be explicit with regard to exercises, splinting, and independent activities. Methods of carrying out procedures should be structured for convenience. Future plans for return visits or further rehabilitation should be clearly explained. After discharge, readmissions may be necessary for intense rehabilitation therapy or surgical reconstruction. If the patient and family are aware of this prior to discharge, it may decrease anxiety if readmissions are necessary.

The patient and family should be cautioned about the possibility of difficult times during the period of adjustment to home, job, school, and other daily activities. Resuming normal activities will be gradual, and the patient may become impatient and frustrated. Emotional changes, which create stressful periods, may occur in both the patient and family. They should understand that these changes are to be expected after such an injury and should be discussed openly with each other to decrease the amount of stress. If emotional stress and family crises become overwhelming, psychological intervention may be provided by the burn unit psychiatric team or a community mental health clinic.

Following recovery from a severe burn injury, adult patients often experience extreme anxiety over *resuming sexual activities.* In most instances, the patient should be able to resume sexual relations without difficulties. If the genitals or surrounding areas were involved in the injury, the healed skin may be very sensitive for a few months. Sexual activities should begin slowly and gradually increase to a level of tolerance.

Discharge planning should consider the *psychosocial environment* of the home as well as the cultural background. Instructions regarding environmental safety and precautions should be explicit. Home visits to assess the environment may be indicated, and rearrangement of the home environment may be necessary, especially when a child returns home. Costly equipment and supplies may present problems for families of lower economic status. The simpler the home care procedures, the more likely they will be carried out.

Referral agencies, such as nursing home placement, visiting nurse service, public assistance, home health care, Meals-on-Wheels, short- or long-term alcohol rehabilitation, and the like should be considered whenever there is a possibility that the patient will need such services. The intent to involve a referral agency should be thoroughly discussed with the patient and family, and approval should be received before action is taken. The patient or family may feel threatened and reluctant to agree to outside involvement. For example, it is often very difficult for the elderly patient to accept the idea of going to a nursing home. Encouragement may be required by the nursing staff as well as the family. Families may resist referrals for psychiatric therapy and may be more prone to follow through if the entire staff reinforces the need for further psychiatric care. In incidences of suspected child abuse, child protective services (CPS) or other authoritative agencies such as the juvenile court should be contacted and a referral made by the social worker, pediatrician, or another member of the staff. In most states, medical personnel are held responsible for referral if child abuse is suspected. The parents should be informed of the concern for the child's safety, the steps taken by the medical staff for intervention by the appropriate agency, and the possibility of continued follow-up.

Following a severe burn injury, there is always the possibility of *future reconstruction.* Scar revisions and release of joint contractures may require several surgical procedures to regain joint function and a more normal appearance. This is especially true of the severely burned child who may have many hospital readmissions for surgical reconstruction as the child grows and matures. Plans for future reconstruction should be a part of the discharge procedure. Although specific details cannot always be given the patient, some general information can be provided. The patient should be prepared for the fact that their scars often look worse 4 to 10 months after the injury, that the scar changes will not be complete for at least 12 to 18 months, and that reconstructive procedures are usually not planned until the scar changes are complete. This at least provides the patient with a realistic timetable on which to base future plans. Patients also need to be encouraged that their scars will eventually improve, although they also realize that scars never completely disappear. Patients should also leave the hospital with a positive but realistic attitude about cosmetic surgery. Although cosmetic surgery may be used to change a particularly obvious or worrisome scar into a less obvious or less objectionable one, it cannot be depended upon to completely remove all scars. A realistic timetable and attitude about reconstructive surgery and scar maturation provides the patient with a basis for coping with the problems of rehabilitation.

Return to the Job or School Situation

The person recovering from a burn injury may have any number of job-related concerns, including fear of acceptance by coworkers; concern over explaining the injury, treatment, and expected results; and concern over the ability to function in a previous job. Many people hesitate to return to work before they are 100 percent rehabilitated. They fear demotion or actual loss of job if they cannot perform at their preinjury level. If the accident occurred at work, the patient may be expected to experience a certain amount of apprehension upon returning to the same type of employment. Some patients experience such intense apprehension that it inhibits productivity. The patient who is worried about losing the family's only source of income may be unable or unwilling to express this fear and concern to the employer. The patient needs help in resolving these job-related concerns. It is sometimes helpful if some member of the burn team actually meets with the patient and employer. The employer may be encouraged to allow the employee to work shorter hours initially, to make a temporary reassignment, or to make specific physical changes in the work area that will allow the patient to be a productive employee. The eventual return to a job usually heralds the successful completion of rehabilitation. Even though the patient may have minor complaints or problems or may need further surgery at a later date, the return to work is a milestone in the rehabilitation process.

Some injuries may preclude the patient from returning to the same or similar employment. Since these patients may suffer further setbacks as they begin a process of vocational rehabilitation and job retraining, they should be made aware that what seems like a very negative prospect of job retraining often turns out to be a positive encounter. Through vocational rehabilitation, patients frequently find help to return to school and complete an education in a field that they rejected early in life. Although the prospect of job retraining may be formidable at first, the accomplishment of new skills leads to a more positive outlook and may aid the patient toward complete rehabilitation.

For the school-age child, the return to school represents the same milestone. Children are often fearful about returning to school because of their concern about being behind in school work, being teased by classmates because of a changed appearance, or being questioned about the accident and hospitalization, which may recall many unpleasant feelings. Again, a member of the burn team may be called upon to intervene. The nurse or social worker may correspond with the teacher or actually spend time with the child's classmates, preparing them for the child's return, presenting information to the classmates concerning the accident, and explaining the type of treatment the child had in the hospital, how the child will look upon return to school, and what problems or limitations to expect. Such information will help classmates act more positively toward the child. Also, attempts should be made throughout the hospitalization and rehabilitation period to keep the child involved in schoolwork. This gives the child meaningful tasks to accomplish while recuperating and maintains a future-oriented approach. The mere fact that the staff and family expects the child to get well and return to school has a positive effect throughout the treatment process.

THE COST OF TREATMENT AND REHABILITATION

Is the cost of treatment and rehabilitation of the severely burned individual worth it? This is, of course, a rhetorical question. Obviously, we feel it is worthwhile. Probably a more important question in light of today's rising medical costs and the increased availability of specialized burn care units in a few hospitals is, "Should a patient with moderate or major injury (i.e., greater than 20 percent TBSA, or burns involving face, hands, feet, or perineum) be cared for in expensive, specialized centers?" There is no doubt that burn care in specialized centers adds to the overall cost of medical care. The hospital bill alone may range from $30,000 to $80,000 for a patient with a 50 percent burn who is hospitalized for 4 to 6 weeks. The intensity of therapy requires many qualified staff members and usually new and expensive equipment. It also may mean that the patient has to be transported great distances to the nearest burn center at additional cost to the family. The family may also incur astronomical expenses in visiting the patient or staying in a distant city for long periods of time. This produces an added emotional as well as financial burden. So is the expertise of the center worth the additional cost? If one looks at long-term cost of a patient who is treated in a center with special expertise, it often becomes apparent that though the initial medical cost may be high, these patients generally return to work sooner, and so the total cost of care is actually less over the productive life of the individual. An exact comparison of cost versus productivity is difficult since no two injuries are alike and no two people respond to the injury in the same manner. But to answer the question, "Is the cost of burn care worth it?," one only has to see one patient return to a productive life after a terrible, disfiguring injury to answer affirmatively.

CONCLUSION: THE IMPACT OF BURN CARE ON THE BURN NURSE

We have discussed at great length the physiological and psychological needs that require diligent attention to successfully prepare the burn patient for reintegration into society. The role of the burn nurse may truly be considered unique. It demands intimate involvement on a daily basis with the family as well as the patient.

Assisting the patient and family in resolving any social and emotional conflicts that may hinder physical progress is high on the list of priorities. Often there are continued emotional interactions that may produce a great deal of stress on the nurse as well as on the patient and family. In many burn centers, it is the nurse who provides wound care including daily washing and debridement of the burn. Exercises also need to be carried out between therapy essions. An enormous feeling of guilt associated with inflicting pain has been expressed by many burn nurses. Rationalizing the necessity of performing the painful procedures to the patient and family often produces more conflicts within the nurse. The nurse who becomes detached in order to carry out these procedures may not be effective in delivering the emotional support required by the patient or the family.

Nurses working closely with severely burned children for long periods have reported developing strong emotional attachments. There is frequently a battle of wits, with the child developing manipulative behavior to avoid performing undesired activities. A behavioral modification program may need to be initiated to provide consistency of care. The success of the program requires trust, understanding, and cooperation from the family and the child. Although in most situations the families are cooperative, the nurse may find that parents are unable to cope with limit setting by the nurse. This may be especially true if the parents themselves have difficulty in setting limits for the child. The parents may be angry with their own inadequacies and project this on the nursing staff. In some cases, nurses develop a protective attitude toward their patients, which interferes with their ability to deliver appropriate care. This may lead to conflict among the nursing staff. There may be a tendency on the part of some nurses to express criticism of other members of the staff who are caring for a child. They may accuse the nurse who is able to set limits as being unfeeling or uncaring.

Caring for the elderly burned patient can also be a source of frustration. The care is extremely intense, and the patient frequently dies. Conflicts arise with the medical staff regarding the patient's right to die in a dignified manner. Often the nurse may be unable to justify the type of care being delivered to these patients, creating enormous conflicts of ideals and morals.

How do the burn nurses survive the enormous emotional pressures of burn care? In order to provide successful physiological and psychological support to the patient and family, burn nurses must be able to identify their own sources of stress and deal with them appropriately. Recognizing that a situation or patient is frustrating can minimize the emotional responses, but adequate opportunities to withdraw from the stressful setting must be available. Most burn units are aware of the extreme pressures associated with long periods in intense care. Many make a sincere attempt to change patient assignments when frustrations arise or when the nurse requests a need for change. Nurses who rotate to less intensive assignments express overwhelming feelings of relief at being removed from the burn unit environment. However, withdrawal from the situation is usually not sufficient. Most nurses feel a need to express their frustrations to "someone who understands." Many feel that their peer groups provide the best support. Group sessions in which nurses can openly express concerns or anger or frustration at the situation, patient, family, or other staff members, and can receive positive as well as negative feedback from group members, are felt to be most effective by some nurses. Although there may never be firm answers to the nurses' questions or problems, sharing these frustrations with others and gaining insight into their own feelings helps to reduce the stress for many nurses.

Even with adequate facilities and an ongoing attempt to create new methods of relieving pressure, burn nurses "burn out" fairly soon. In talking with members of burn centers across the country, the average stay of a burn nurse is 12 to 18 months. They report a 30 to 40 percent turnover rate for burn nurses each year, with the major factor being "stress." Currently, a number of burn care facilities are studying stress factors among burn nurses and methods to reduce stress or increase the nurse's ability to cope with this stress-provoking job. Will there ever be an answer to the problem? Only the future can tell.

BIBLIOGRAPHY

Alexander, J. W., R. Dionigi, and J. L. Meakins: "Periodic Variation in the Antibacterial Function of Human Neutrophils and Its Relationship to Sepsis," *Ann Surg* February: 206–213, 1971.

Baur, P. S., H. Parks, and D. L. Larson: "Healing of Burn Wounds," *Clin Plast Surg* 4(3): 389–407, 1977.

Baxter, R., J. Marvin, and P. W. Curreri: "Fluid and Electrolyte Therapy of Burn Shock," *Heart Lung* 2(5):707–713, 1973.

Bjornson, A., W. Altemeier, and S. Bjornson: "Changes in Humoral Components of Host Defense Following Burn Trauma," *Ann Surg* 186(1):88–96, 1977.

Burke, F., W. C. Quinby, and C. C. Bondoc: "Primary Excision and Prompt Grafting as Routine Therapy for the Treatment of Thermal Burns in Children," *Surg Clin North Am* 56(2):477–494, 1976.

Eriksson, G.: "Regeneration of Epidermis After Second Degree Burns," *Scand J Plast Reconstr Surg* 6:83–92, 1972.

Hamburg, David A.: "Coping Behavior in Life-threatening Circumstances," *Psychother Psychosom* 23:13–25, 1974.

Hummel, R. P., P. D. Kautz, B. G. MacMillan, and W. A. Altemeier: "Continuing Problem of Sepsis Following Enzymatic Debridement of Burns," *J Trauma* 14(7):572–579, 1974.

Jackson, D.: "Diagnosis of the Depth of Burning," *Br J Surg* 40:588–596, 1953.

Kangarloo, H., M. Beachley, and G. G. Ghahremani: "Radiographic Spectrum of Pulmonary Complications in Burn Victims," *Am J Roentgenol* 128:441–445, 1977.

Loebl, C., et al.: "Erythrocyte Survival Following Thermal Injury," *J Surg Res* 16:96–101, 1974.

Longacre, J. J.: *Scar Tissue: Its Use and Abuse,* Charles C Thomas, Springfield, Ill., 1972.

Miller, C., and D. Trunkey: "Thermal Injury: Defects in Immune Response Induction," *J Surg Res* 22:621–625, 1977.

Moylan, J. A., K. Adib, and M. Birnbaum: "Fiberoptic Bronchoscopy Following Thermal Injury," *Surg Gynecol Obstet* 140:541–543, 1974.

Muir, I. F. K.: *Burns and Their Treatment,* Year Book, Chicago, 1974.

Munster, M.: "Host Defense Mechanism in Burns," *Ann R Coll Surg* 51:69–80, 1972.

Parks, D. H., P. Bauer, and D. Larson: "Late Problems in Burns," *Clin Plast Surg* 4(4):547–560, 1977.

Steiner, Hans, and William R. Clark: "Psychiatric Complications of Burned Adults: A Classification," *J Trauma* 17(2):134–140, 1977.

Willis, B. A., D. L. Larson, and S. Abston: "Positioning and Splinting the Burn Patient," *Heart Lung* 2(5):696–700, 1973.

Wilmore, D. W.: "Nutrition and Metabolism Following Thermal Injury," *Clin Plast Surg* 1(4):603–619, 1974.

Winter, D.: "Histological Aspects of Burn Wound Healing," *Burns* 1(3):191–196, 1974.

Zawacki, B.: "Reversal of Capillary Stasis and Prevention of Necrosis in Burns," *Ann Surg* 180(1):98–102, 1974.

———, R. Jung, J. Joyce, and E. Rincon: "Smoke, Burns, and the Natural History of Inhalation Injury in Fire Victims: A Correlation of Experimental and Clinical Data, *Ann Surg* 185(1):100–110, 1977.

28
susan hillenbrand herbst

impairment as
a result of cancer

"I wanted to write a book called *Adam* which would be about the whole man, but then I decided not to write it." In these naive sounding words of a genuine sage, the whole story of human thought about man is expressed. From time immemorial, man has known that he is the subject most deserving of his own study, but he has always fought shy of treating the subject as a whole; that is, in accordance with its total character. Sometimes he takes a run at it, but the difficulty of this concern with his own being soon overpowers and exhausts him, and in silent resignation, he withdraws—either to consider all things in heaven and earth save man—or to divide man into departments which can be treated singly in a less problematic, less powerful, less binding way. (Buber, 1955)

INTRODUCTION: HOLISM

The holistic theory of health and disease provides a foundation for the nursing principles of conservation that enables them to take on new dimensions and dynamics. All nursing interventions are primarily based on the following conservation principles: (1) conservation of energy, (2) conservation of structural integrity, (3) conservation of personal integrity, and (4) conservation of social integrity (though they may not be stated in exactly these words). The uniqueness of this theory is found in the philosophical basis of holism itself (Levine, 1971).

Although indefinable in the ordinary sense of definition, holism can be stated as the interaction of a unique, dynamic person with others and with the world. Holism, by its nature, demands an approach to human beings that is at once multidimensional, open-ended, and ever-changing.

When the elements of holism are used as a foundation for the conservation principles of nursing intervention, the principles do, indeed, take on a new meaning. No longer can the conservation of energy, or of structural integrity, personal integrity, or social integrity, be seen as elements of total patient care but rather as care of the *whole* patient. A shift in emphasis takes place that, in many respects, is quite radical, that is, fundamental and, at the same time, complex.

In the theory of *total patient care*, the approach is basically simple. An objective evaluation is made of the patient, needs are determined, and then care is given within a programmed structure or schedule. Only emergency needs can upset this program. *Care* becomes the focus in this type of nursing intervention. The care that is needed is provided, and it is good care, but it often pays little attention to the person, who he or she is and what he or she likes or really needs.

Utilizing the holistic approach, the *patient* becomes the subject and care the object. All care is tailored to the individual, and everything that makes a particular patient unique is considered in planning the treatment. The patient becomes, in a real sense, part of a team that is providing treatment and a program for regaining wholeness.

At this point, one can see that the theory becomes quite complex. It does not allow for care to be strictly scheduled; it must employ a certain degree of latitude if it is to succeed. The salient point is that the conservation principles are not applied one at a time but must remain united as a whole, even if only one principle is being emphasized at a particular time. For example, the nurse must be aware not only of the fact that the individual needs a certain intervention but also that the patient is of a competitive nature, considers himself or herself to be better than others, has always been an extrovert, and is in the position of being unable even to stand up without help.

Although attention must be given to the subjective elements in the care of an individual, there remains the fact that life within a hospital or other facility must be structured or scheduled. The nurse must help the individual to realize that there are *reasons* for certain ways of doing things and then must involve the patient in these procedures. Patients must be made aware that there is a team caring for them and that they are an integral part of that team.

Levine states that nursing intervention is a

conservation of wholeness, a keeping together of the wholeness of the individual patient—his or her integrity, oneness, identity as an individual—recognizing that it is through adaptation in response to change in oneself and one's environment that wholeness is achieved (Levine, 1973).

CONSERVATION PRINCIPLES

The four major areas of care in which nursing can fulfill a conservation function are stated in the conservation principles of Levine (1973) (see Fig. 28-1):

1. Nursing intervention is based on the conservation of the individual patient's *energy*.
2. Nursing intervention is based on the conservation of the individual patient's *structural integrity*.
3. Nursing intervention is based on the conservation of the individual patient's *personal integrity*.
4. Nursing intervention is based on the conservation of the individual patient's *social integrity*.

Conservation of Energy

Life itself is a process of energy production and exchange that makes it possible for the multiple activities of the body—molecular, cellular, and organismic—to continue. Oxygen is necessary for the maintenance of life systems. It is needed to transport materials used as fuel to maintain an energy source. It must be available to the cellular components that produce the energy necessary to sustain life. Red blood cells carry oxygen to all tissues. Diet is the only means by which the patient takes in the necessary raw materials for energy production. The balance of energy input (via energy-producing nutrients) with energy output (via energy-using activities) is essential in planning nursing interventions.

Nursing assessment should include a review of the patient's oxygen supply, respiratory and hematologic status, and nutritional status. Nursing activities must be directed toward conserving patients' energy by assisting them in planning the day with periods of rest interfaced with activities of daily living (self-care, exercise, work), particularly when available energy is limited during times of stress and illness.

Conservation of Structural Integrity

The body possesses a number of exquisitely efficient defense systems that function interdependently in order to preserve and restore the anatomic and physiologic wholeness of the individual. Nursing intervention is directed toward protection of the individual whose body surface has continually been disrupted from infection. Nursing processes should be aimed at reducing the amount of skeletal-muscular restriction of movement that could result in structural damage, for example, by proper positioning of the patient on bed rest. Nursing activities are often directed toward limiting the amount of tissue involvement

Figure 28-1
Holistic nursing: The conservation principles.

HOLISTIC NURSING

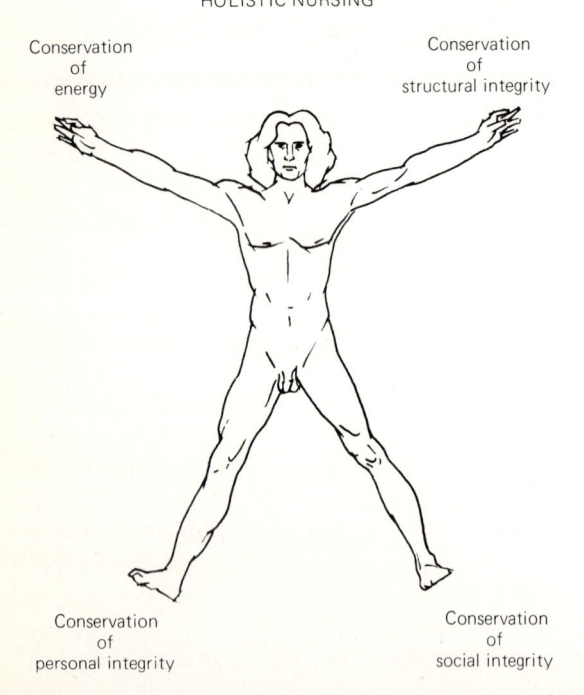

Conservation of energy

Conservation of structural integrity

Conservation of personal integrity

Conservation of social integrity

CHAPTER 28 554

in infection and disease in order to minimize scarring and promote maintenance of function of the healed body part, for the good of the whole individual.

Conservation of Personal Integrity

A person's self-esteem, sense of worth as a unique individual, and identity are among a patient's most valuable possessions. Without such self-definition, a person cannot be whole. Illness, with its concomitant dependence, is a threat to the individual's personal integrity. One's self-esteem is lowered when privacy, sense of freedom, and ability to make decisions about one's life are curtailed.

Holistic nursing interventions must begin with a recognition and acceptance of the individual's unique identity and response to illness. The physiology of a disease process may be similar in two patients, but their response to this process as human beings will always be personalized and unique. Planning must include incorporation of the individual's decision-making ability and right to continue to be involved in the direction of his or her life. Nurses are challenged to deal with the conflict of dependence–independence and to plan appropriate ways of coping with this conflict so that the patient can remain as independent in thought and action as possible.

Care must be taken to protect the individual's emotional as well as physical privacy. An attitude of respect from the nurse contributes to the patient's self-respect.

Protection of the individual's personal integrity precludes moral censure. Patients must be allowed the freedom to make decisions about their future, and these decisions must be upheld and respected, regardless of the nurse's personal response to them.

Conservation of Social Integrity

Humans, by nature, are social beings and are not meant to exist in isolation. Meaningful relationships with other human beings are necessary for the preservation of wholeness. Just as socioeconomic, religious, and cultural factors shape a person's self-definition, so too do they influence social relationships.

Recognition of and respect for these relationships must form an underlying basis for the nurse's planning with and for the individual who is ill. Too often, family and kinship ties are disregarded as a person enters the health care system. Mutual support of the patient and family depends upon the important interactions that take place between them during illness. The nurse must endeavor to include the family as well as the patient in the planning and delivery of care.

"Family," in our changing society, must be viewed from a broad base and be seen to include not only nuclear family members but also significant others in the individual's network of social ties. The nurse is also an integral part of the individual's social environment during the hospitalization period. The nurse should be committed to a warm, compassionate, human, although therapeutic, relationship with the patient and family, providing direction and support in a time of crisis.

CONCLUSION

Finally, from a holistic perspective, one must consider an episode of illness as only one part of a whole life process and hospitalization or acute care as only one segment of an entire health care system. Planning and nursing interventions should focus on continued care, either therapeutic or preventive, of the individual in the community.

There are a variety of settings in which the nurse may interact with the cancer patient. Nurses may work in teaching hospitals or in community hospitals, in a specialized oncology unit or on a general medical-surgical floor, in a community health agency or in an outpatient treatment center. The degree of involvement with the patients will depend, in large measure, upon the nurse's understanding of the special needs and problems of cancer patients and the nurse's feeling of adequacy to assess these needs and problems and follow through with the appropriate plan of intervention. A basic knowledge of the cancer disease process and the various treatment modalities is essential.

PATHOPHYSIOLOGY OF CANCER

A distinguishing characteristic of the cancer cell is its ability to multiply and invade tissues where normal cell activity is restricted. Some cancer cells may be relatively normal in appearance and organization, while others may differ greatly in size, shape, and degree of maturity from healthy, normal cells.

Mitosis of normal cells involves the division of one parent cell into two daughter cells, whereas in mitosis of cancer cells, there appears to be an abnormal regulation of this reproductive process. Any number of cells may result from one parent cell division.

Cancer cells behave as though they have an impaired sensitivity to the organizing influence of adjacent cells. They sometimes have unlimited replication ability, often at the expense of healthy surrounding tissues. The cancer cells, to a greater or lesser degree, fail to develop or maintain a fully differentiated or mature state. The less differentiated the resulting tumor is, the more rapidly it grows. Cancer cells spread either by local extension into surrounding healthy tissue or by breaking away from the primary lesion and disseminating to distant sites in the host's body via lymphatic or vascular channels. This latter process constitutes the establishment of secondary lesions or metastases. Cancers have no useful function within the host's body, and unless their growth can be arrested, they severely impair or often destroy the normal life processes of the host tissues.

Two factors can be identified in the development of cancer. One factor is a susceptible host, and the other is an agent or group of agents (carcinogens) capable of injuring cells.

There is no evidence to indicate that cancer has a single cause or is a single disease. It is, rather, a variety of diseases resulting from the interaction of many factors, some originating in the host and others originating in the host's environment. This fact makes both the etiology of cancer and the treatment of cancer more complex.

THE CELL CYCLE

In order to understand the rationale for various cancer treatment modalities, it is necessary to review the cell life cycle (see Fig. 28-2). The phases of cell reproduction are identical in normal and abnormal cells. The cell life cycle extends from the completion of one mitosis to the completion of the next. During this period, a replication of the structural elements and functional capabilities of the cell is accomplished.

In Fig. 28-2, the symbol G refers to "gap" or period of time between synthesis and mitosis in the cell cycle. G_0 represents the rest phase in a mature cell, when no activity directed toward replication is taking place. When the cell receives a stimulus, such as the death of other cells in the population, it enters the G_1 phase. During this period, RNA is manufactured as well as proteins (enzymes) needed for DNA synthesis. The S, or

**Figure 28-2
The cell cycle.**

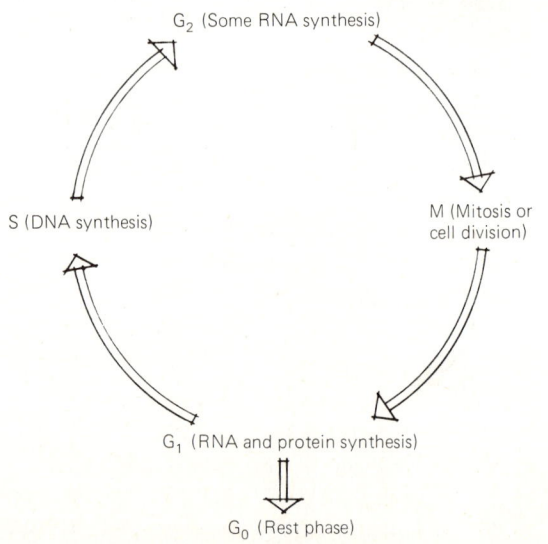

G_2 (Some RNA synthesis)

S (DNA synthesis)

M (Mitosis or cell division)

G_1 (RNA and protein synthesis)

G_0 (Rest phase)

synthesis, phase follows, and the major task accomplished is the synthesis of DNA and chromosome replication. The G_2 phase is a quiet time prior to mitosis, and it is proposed that some RNA is synthesized during this time. During the final M, or mitosis, phase, the actual division of the parent cell into daughter cells takes place. The resultant cells can then mature and repeat the cell life cycle (Marino, 1976).

TREATMENT MODALITIES

There are three major modalities utilized in the treatment of cancer patients: surgery, radiation therapy, and chemotherapy.

Surgery

Surgery has always played a primary role in the diagnosis and treatment of solid tumor malignancies. Surgical biopsies of malignant lesions can provide useful information and a positive histologic diagnosis, which is essential in order to plan the most effective treatment for a particular type of cancer.

If a cancer diagnosis can be made early in the course of the disease, surgical procedures can often be directed at cure. This objective of surgical treatment presupposes a well-defined mass of tumor that lends itself to complete resection, before the tumor has metastasized to distant sites. Improved surgical cure rates are largely the result of early diagnosis and treatment. This fact has spurred the movement, in recent years, to establish cancer detection centers and to emphasize the importance of early detection and prevention.

When cancer has disseminated beyond the limits of surgical cure, surgery can still be useful in reducing the amount of tumor bulk, thereby improving the patient's chances of responding to other therapeutic modalities, such as radiation therapy and chemotherapy. The smaller the amount of tumor in the body, the greater is the chance of destroying the remaining tumor or at least of stabilizing the disease and providing a good quality of life for the patient. Surgery can also be used to provide palliation of symptoms, such as relief of pain, bleeding, or obstruction.

Radiation Therapy

Radiation therapy has been employed in the treatment of cancer patients for many years. In the first two decades of radiation therapy, low-energy or orthovoltage machines were used. The maximum dose of radiation was delivered to the skin surface, often producing severe skin reactions, which limited the amount of radiation that could be delivered to a tumor. In the mid-1950s, supervoltage equipment was introduced. With this procedure, the dose of radiation is delivered deep into the tissues, with much less scatter to the skin, and so much higher doses of radiation can be given to deep tumors without producing such severe skin toxicity. Examples of supervoltage equipment are linear accelerators (with a neutron beam), and cobalt-60 machines (using a radioactive isotope of cobalt as the radiation source). The usefulness of radiation therapy in the treatment of any type of cancer depends, to a great degree, on that tumor's *radiosensitivity*. A radiosensitive tumor is one that is destroyed by irradiation in doses that are well tolerated by surrounding normal structures (Rubin, 1978).

Radiation therapy acts by selective destruction of tumors at the cellular (i.e., via interruption of mitosis) and subcellular (i.e., via inactivation of DNA molecules) levels. Environment also plays a role in responsiveness to radiation. Vascular, well-oxygenated tumors are most radiosensitive.

In selected types and stages of malignancies, radiation therapy is used very effectively with a curative intent. In limited Hodgkin's disease (Stages I and II), radiation therapy alone may be the treatment of choice, with a greater than 50 percent chance that the patient will respond and have no recurrence of disease. Superficial skin cancers and early carcinoma of the larynx are also treated with cure as the goal. Radium insertion followed by external radiation therapy is the treatment of choice for carcinoma in situ of the cervix.

Preoperative radiation therapy is sometimes used to destroy peripheral, well-oxygenated tumor cells around a lesion that are likely to be metastasized or to reduce the size of the tumor mass so that it can be successfully resected. Nonresectable lymph node draining in an area of tumor may be treated preoperatively.

Postoperative radiation therapy may be employed for radiosensitive tumors that cannot be completely resected (e.g., brain tumors). After mastectomy, the chest wall and axilla may be treated to prevent recurrence of breast cancer. Local control of diseases may be achieved in this situation, but radiation therapy cannot prevent or destroy distant metastases.

Radiation therapy can be used effectively in the treatment of advanced malignancies for the purpose of palliating symptoms. For example, pain resulting from bone metastases and neurologic symptoms caused by brain metastases can be alleviated rather quickly with radiation therapy.

Chemotherapy

In the last decade or so, great progress has been made in the discovery and use of chemotherapeutic agents or drugs as a major cancer treatment modality. Drugs are particularly helpful, because they are distributed via the bloodstream throughout the patient's body and are theoretically capable of destroying widely disseminated disease and even microscopic foci of tumor that might not be detected by any clinical instrumentation.

Chemotherapeutic agents work in various ways to interfere with the cell cycle. Some agents inhibit the synthesis of DNA. Others inhibit RNA and protein synthesis, thereby slowing the cell cycle. Still others damage the DNA molecule itself, destroying the cell's capability to divide. It should be obvious, then, that drugs will be most effective against tumors whose cells are less mature or differentiated, where there is a high percentage of cells undergoing mitosis.

Since all tumors are not synthesizing DNA simultaneously and dividing in synchrony, it is often advantageous to use a combination of drugs to treat a particular tumor. Each of the agents should interrupt a different phase of the cell cycle and thereby ensure a greater cell kill than if a single agent is used. The route and frequency of administration of chemotherapeutic agents varies, depending upon the goals of therapy and the type or severity of toxicity.

It is not yet possible to program drugs to seek out and destroy only tumor cells. Therefore, any of the body's highly proliferative normal cells are also targets for damage. This damage is observed clinically as any of a variety of side effects. The objective is to determine drug dosages for a particular patient in order to achieve a maximum amount of damage to tumor cells with a minimum amount of toxicity to normal cells. An effort is made in combination chemotherapy to use drugs without overlapping toxicities.

Alkylating agents (e.g., Cytoxan) interfere with mitosis by damaging the completed DNA molecule. Antimetabolites (e.g., methotrexate) block the synthesis of nucleic acids, the building blocks of DNA and RNA. Antibiotics (e.g., adriamycin) react with the DNA molecule and prevent the transcription of the genetic code onto RNA. Plant alkaloids (e.g., vincristine) destroy spindle fibers and stop cell division at metaphase. Enzymes (e.g., L-asparaginase) starve tumor cells by destroying essential amino acids. Hormones (e.g., diethylstilbestrol) create a biochemical environment unfavorable for cell growth.

Drugs are now being used in an adjuvant setting, that is, immediately after surgery for the primary cancer. In some instances, such as breast cancer, when the patient is at high risk for recurrence of disease (premenopausal, two or more positive lymph nodes), chemotherapy may be given postoperatively for a time, even in the absence of clinically detectable disease. The goal is to prevent, or at least delay, recurrence of tumor. Adjuvant chemotherapy is also being tried for other tumors (e.g., colon and gastric).

Shrinkage of tumor and palliation of symptoms are two major objectives in using chemotherapy for the treatment of cancer patients. If the tumor is responsive to drug therapy and symptoms such as pain and obstruction can be relieved, patients often have a greater sense of well-being and a better quality of life. Cancer is a chronic illness, and although cure is often not possible, if advanced disease can be controlled, the patients may have a comfortable and satisfying life whether that life is measured in weeks, months, or years. It should be noted that cure may be a realistic goal in the chemotherapeutic treatment of a small percentage of malignancies (e.g., Hodgkin's disease, some of the childhood leukemias, choriocarcinoma).

Clinical trials, often comparing two or more drug therapies for the purpose of determining their merits for treatments of specific types of tumors, are currently being conducted at most major medical centers. Many investigational drugs not yet available in general medical practive are also being studied in these clinical trials. Protocols (documents outlining the rationale, details of the study, and methodology of treatment administration and evaluation) are strictly followed. It is by means of such trials that researchers and clinicians are able to determine the best methods of treating cancer patients. The standard drug treatments used in general clinical practice have all first been through extensive clinical trials in limited settings to demonstrate their effectiveness.

CONCLUSION

Any or all of these major treatment modalities may be employed for a particular patient. In order to plan the best approach to treatment for a patient, consultation and open communication between the various disciplines are essential. This involves not only the physicians planning medical management but also, ideally, an interdisciplinary team consisting of nurses, physicians, a social worker, a dietician, a chaplain, and others dealing with the ongoing needs and concerns of the whole person, the patient. Teamwork is the best means of achieving excellence in care.

HOLISM AND THE CANCER PATIENT

The holistic viewpoint is an exceptionally fine and practical framework within which to approach the cancer patient, to assess needs, and to plan appropriate interventions. Wholeness is the name of the game in working with cancer patients. One can consider wholeness from these perspectives: wholeness of the patient, of self (the nurse), and of the disease process.

WHOLENESS OF THE PATIENT: THE CONSERVATION PRINCIPLES

How, then, do cancer patients with their altered internal environment interact with their external environment? How can one assess these individuals? The four conservation principles provide a means of doing this in an integrated manner.

Conservation of Energy

Nutrition There are many factors that interact in cancer patients to influence their level of energy. Tumor cells within the body are in competition with normal cells for nutrients that provide the raw materials for energy, for building, and for sustaining life processes. Cachexia (emaciation and weakness) is evidence of this competition.

The cachexia syndrome may be one of the most frustrating problems of the patient with advanced cancer. Cachexia is characterized by the following: (1) anorexia (loss of appetite) with a decrease in food intake, (2) a hypermetabolic state, and (3) wasting of body tissues, particularly fat and muscle.

One hypothesis to explain the cachexia syndrome is that it is caused both by direct action of the cancer on host tissues and by anorexia. Cancer changes the genetic messages in tumor cells. Polypeptides are produced that stimulate metabolic breakdown of host protein and fat. A metabolite is trapped by the tumor, which sends signals to the brain indicating a physiologic state of satiety. Further food intake is then suppressed (Cuddy, 1974).

Anorexia develops in a majority of patients with advanced malignancy. It may be correlated with abnormalities of taste sensation. Investigations by DeWys (1974) indicate two main areas of abnormal taste sensation. Patients exhibit an elevated threshold for sweet taste and an intolerance for bitter tastes; that is, a very low concentration of bitter substance produces an unpleasant reaction. It is postulated that bitter amino acids and polypeptides in meats are sensed by patients with greater intensity than normal. This is clinically correlated with the complaint of aversion to red meat voiced by many patients. Patients with an abnormality of taste have increased incidence of weight loss as compared to patients with normal taste.

Two possible explanations can be offered for an alteration of taste sensation in the cancer patient. Taste may be altered by tumor byproducts and by chemotherapeutic agents (DeWys, 1974). Regardless of the cause of abnormal taste sensation, however, the nurse is faced with a very critical clinical problem. Adequate nutritional intake enhances a positive response to chemotherapy and other treatment modalities. How does one interrupt the anorexia-cachexia syndrome and provide for adequate nutritional intake, particularly when a patient presents with altered taste sensation in addition to loss of appetite?

Awareness of the role of cachexia as a major factor influencing the patient's response to therapy, as well as the patient's prognosis and well-being, makes diet therapy and nutritional deficiencies an important focus of nursing intervention. Dietary patterns, as well as food preferences, should be incorporated into the initial nursing assessment of patients who are beginning chemotherapy or radiation therapy. Diet counseling should be an ongoing process. Nurses should be aware of specific drug regimens that have been shown to produce anorexia and/or altered taste perception.

Patients often equate reduced taste sensation with reduced appetite. To increase nutritional intake, the nurse should suggest increasing the seasoning applied to food or the selection of more highly seasoned food. It is possible to substitute poultry, fish, eggs, or milk products (including double-strength milk) for those patients who have an aversion to red meat. Some patients experience meat aversion symptoms as the day progresses, so it may be advantageous to suggest eating meat with the morning meal. Patients with an elevated sweetness threshold can be given milkshakes, eggnogs, and pastries. Frequent, small meals are often preferable to three large meals, which tend to overwhelm the patient with appetite loss. In addition, patients are more likely to eat better if they have company at mealtimes.

In the presence of normal taste thresholds, some patients experience abdominal pain and vomiting after eating, suggesting the presence of a conditioned aversion to food as the basis for loss of taste. Some form of behavior modification might be devised to interrupt this conditioned response. Premedication with an antiemetic 30 min before meals may be helpful for those patients who complain of nausea at mealtime.

Some patients state that breakfast is the best meal of the day for them and that appetite diminishes as the day progresses. In these instances, the major caloric intake might be concentrated into a nutritious breakfast, with smaller snacks or meals taken the rest of the day. Oral nutritional supplements such as Ensure, Nutri-1000, and Sustacal, taken alone or in addition to small meals, are capable of providing adequate daily caloric intake and nutritional requirements without having to be consumed in great volume.

Some patients may exhibit such severe cachexia that it is impossible to reverse the syndrome by oral diet therapy. In such situations, there are at least two available alternatives: enteral hyperalimentation and parenteral hyperalimentation.

Enteral hyperalimentation, using Vivonex-HN, has been used successfully. The solution utilizes free amino acids as a source of nitrogen, and because the ingredients are in "elemental" form, the solution requires virtually no digestion for complete absorption and thus yields negligible residue. It is administered as a continuous infusion via a #5 French feeding tube, with little discomfort to the patient, and it is useful for cachetic patients with at least minimal gut function. It normally takes 2 to 3 weeks to reverse negative nitrogen balance and achieve any appreciable amount of weight gain. Patients and/or families can be taught to prepare and administer the solutions and can carry out the procedure for an unlimited amount of time in their own homes. The level of acceptance and cooperation with home enteral hyperalimentation has been high because this approach eliminates costly, extended hospitalization.

Total parenteral nutrition (TPN), or intravenous hyperalimentation, involves the infusion of hypertonic glucose solutions with a source of nitrogen (free amino acids) via catheter directly into the superior vena cava. This form of nutrition therapy is widely used in a variety of hospital settings. Many institutions have a hyperalimentation team consisting of a physician, a nurse or nurses, and a pharmacist to ensure proper catheter insertion and care of the intravenous (IV) site, as well as proper administration of the solutions to minimize complications (sepsis, metabolic upset). Several medical centers have instituted home parenteral hyperalimentation programs for selected patients.

Studies have indicated that those patients who have received hyperalimentation prior to and during treatment often have a better tolerance for and experience a more positive response to therapy (Copeland et al., 1975). This data would support a greater utilization of either enteral or parenteral hyperalimentation for any patient experiencing significant (greater than 10 percent of ideal body weight) weight loss and loss of appetite.

Gastrointestinal Disturbances Gastrointestinal upset (diarrhea, constipation, nausea, and vomiting) is a frequent problem resulting from the disease process and/or various therapies. This can contribute significantly to nutritional and energy depletion.

Nausea and vomiting accompanying chemotherapy or radiation therapy can often be prevented or controlled by premedication with an antiemetic, and it is recommended that the patient take the antiemetic for 24 h after therapy, even in the absence of symptoms. If one antiemetic, taken either orally, intramuscularly, or as a suppository, is not effective, another should be tried. For the control of nausea and vomiting occurring *prior to* therapy, a condition that may have a psychological cause (e.g., a conditioned response triggered by the sight of a needle or the smell of alcohol), it may be helpful to investigate the use of self-hypnosis, relaxation techniques, or behavior modification. Antiemetics are not very effective in alleviating this symptom.

Appropriate interventions should be undertaken to control diarrhea, which is a side effect of certain chemotherapy drugs (e.g., fluorouracil) and of abdominal irradiation. Liberal fluid intake to prevent dehydration and a diet low in roughage are helpful. Foods high in potassium, such as bananas, help replace the potassium that is lost in large amounts when a person has diarrhea. Elemental feedings may be useful in severe cases, although the taste of these nutritional supplements may be objectionable to the patient. Lomotil or one of the opium derivatives may also control diarrhea.

Constipation is a common problem for patients who are inactive and who are taking large amounts of narcotic analgesics. It is also a possible side effect of the plant alkaloid chemotherapy drugs, which cause toxicity to the peripheral nerves innervating the bowel. Prophylactic use of stool softeners and any of the cathartics or laxatives may minimize the problem. High-fiber foods, raw fruits and vegetables, and prune juice also act as laxatives. Increased food intake and light exercise are also helpful.

Oxygen In some patients, oxygen supply can be compromised. Primary lung tumors or metastatic lung lesions can reduce available surfaces for oxygen exchange. Chemotherapy drugs may suppress the bone marrow (because the marrow contains highly proliferative normal cells), or the bone marrow may be invaded with tumor cells, reducing the number of red blood cells available for oxygen transport. In addition, the anemia caused by treatment or malignancy diminishes the amount of oxygen available to normal tissues, resulting in increased weakness and fatigue. Anemia can compromise treatment of the patient with radiation therapy. Poorly oxygenated tumor cells generally do not respond as well to radiation, and poorly oxygenated normal cells do not tolerate radiation well. Malignant pleural effusions decrease pulmonary volume and may cause moderate to severe dyspnea. Large abdominal masses, ascites, or an enlarged liver may press on the diaphragm and decrease pulmonary volume, also causing dyspnea.

A patient's respiratory and hematologic status must be assessed throughout the illness and course of treatment, and appropriate intervention such as oxygen therapy, packed red blood cell transfusions, or removal of pleural or ascitic fluid should be initiated when necessary to maximize the patient's comfort. A cool mist vaporizer in the patient's room may loosen thick secretions, making phlegm easier to raise and expectorate.

Pain The chronic pain of advanced malignancy can be a demoralizing experience, draining the patient's energy and interfering with eating, sleeping, and activities of daily living. Unlike acute pain (e.g., postoperative pain), which has a beginning and an anticipated end, chronic pain is cyclic and, at times, seems endless in its duration. Anticipation of chronic pain evokes anxiety and depression, which accentuate the physical dimension of pain. Patients have expressed a greater fear of chronic, severe pain and suffering than of death itself. Adequate control of the cancer patient's chronic pain is perhaps one of the most frustrating and challenging problems for the nurse.

Cecily Saunders speaks of the "total pain" of the cancer patient, which encompasses not only physical but also psychological, financial, interpersonal, and spiritual components. Adequate relief of this pain requires an understanding and awareness of its complex nature and an interdisciplinary approach (Saunders, 1967).

Melzack's gate control theory provides a theoretical framework for understanding cancer pain (see Fig. 28-3) (Siegele, 1974). According to this theory, there are three components to the pain experience: (1) sensory-discriminative (information about time, intensity, and duration); (2) motivation-affect (indicates the presence of an unpleasant sensation, triggering a response to alleviate the painful stimulus); and (3) evaluative or cognitive (analysis of past experience, meaning of pain, probable outcomes) (Siegele, 1974).

Malignant lesions in different parts of the body may produce pain of varying intensity and duration. Psychological elements, such as awareness of impending death, fear of the unknown, and family and financial concerns, influence all three dimensions of the pain experience.

Adequate assessment of the cancer patient's pain, its location, severity, duration, persistence, and accompanying symptoms, is an essential step in symptom control. The *McGill-Melzack Pain Questionnaire* may be a useful tool for measuring pain and its response to various interventions and could be adapted and used routinely to evaluate the pain experience. The pain questionnaire is an attempt to measure pain intensity by evaluating patient selection of qualitative words that describe the sensory (e.g., "throbbing," "sharp"), affective (e.g., "tiring," "terrifying"), and evaluative (e.g., "annoying," "unbearable") properties of pain (Melzack et al., 1976).

The physical pain of malignancy may have a variety of causes, including tumor infiltration of blood vessels or nerves, compression of nerves by tumor or fractures impinging on nerves, obstruction of a viscus, occlusion of blood vessels by an adjacent tumor, infiltration and tumor replacement of bone or tissues surrounded by pain-sensitive structures, and necrosis, infection, or inflammation of pain-sensitive structures (Murphy, 1973).

If the source of the patient's pain can be

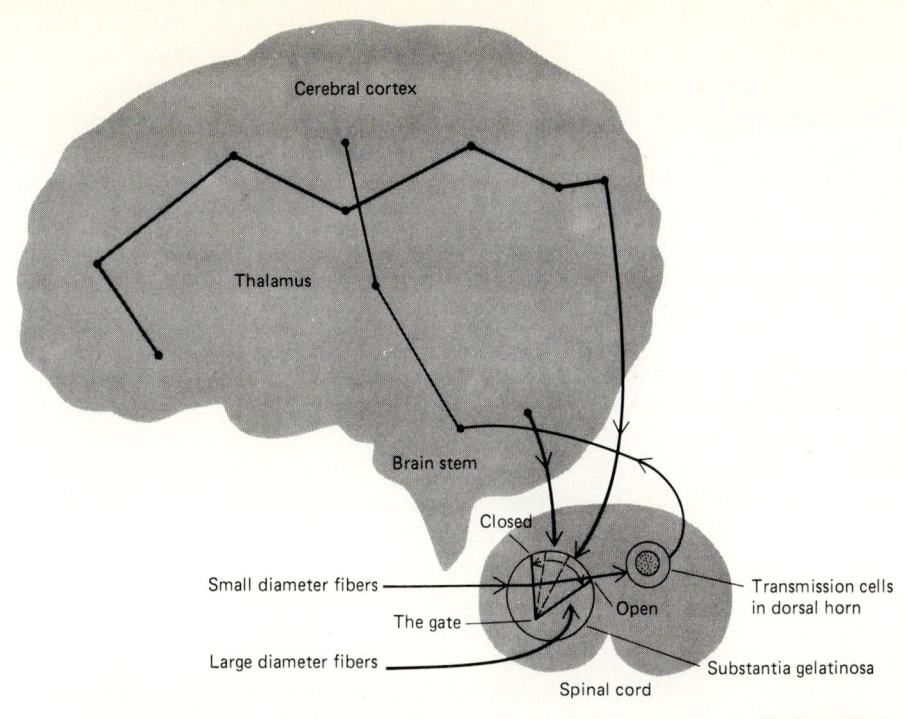

Figure 28-3

Gate control theory. Small-diameter, afferent fibers transmit painful stimuli to the *substantia gelatinosa* before transmitting them to the posterolateral horn. These impulses may be blocked at the substantia gelatinosa by stimulation of the large-diameter afferent fibers whose impulses also travel to the substantia gelatinosa and "close a gate" to the impulses from the small-diameter fibers. Also, cerebral cortical mechanisms responsible for sensory-discriminatory, motivation-affect, and cognition processes may relay impulses to the substantia gelatinosa that can close the gate. *(Adapted from Dorothy S. Siegele, "The Gate Control Theory." Am J Nurs 74:498, 1974. Used with permission of the publisher.)*

determined, there are several approaches to its relief. Any or several of the cancer treatment modalities may be used in an attempt to destroy the tumor that is causing pain (e.g., radiation therapy can be directed to osseous metastases that cause bone pain). Cancer treatment attacks pain at its source, that is, at the tumor.

The type of therapy in which the nurse plays a significant role is the use of analgesics to relieve the symptom of pain. Studies have indicated that patients with severe pain often endure needless suffering, either because inadequate analgesia is prescribed at improper intervals or because nurses tend to give less medication than is ordered. Two factors may contribute to inadequate analgesia. Health professionals may fear oversedation from the medication or addiction by frequent administration of narcotic analgesics (Marks and Sachar *973). The latter* is the factor most frequently expressed in practice, and this fear is common to the cancer patient, too. Perhaps such concerns would be valid for patients with acute postoperative pain, but certainly, for the cancer patient with intractable pain, this concern is not justified. The goals of pain relief and comfort should always take precedence over the fear of possible addiction. Cancer patients with chronic pain have a much higher tolerance for narcotic analgesics and often require much higher doses of medication at more frequent intervals to obtain relief than do patients with acute pain.

Mount and others at the Royal Victoria Hospital in Montreal have studied the chronic pain of malignancy and formulated a workable philosophy of pain control that should be given serious consideration by nurses. Prevention of pain, rather than treatment of the pain symptom, is the primary goal. Erasing the memory of pain eliminates the anxiety accompanying the *anticipation* of pain. This requires the administration of appropriate amounts of analgesics on a regular schedule rather than "as needed" (prn). Another goal is to attempt to achieve pain relief without accompanying somnolence, euphoria, or depression. Oral medication is preferable to parenteral medication, which restricts the patient's independence and mobility and which is difficult to administer over a long period to the cachectic patient who has limited muscle mass available for injection sites (Mount et al., 1976).

Brompton's solution, a mixture of morphine, cocaine, ethyl alcohol, syrup, and water, has been used successfully in the treatment of the severe pain of malignancy. The amount of morphine is in the range of 10 to 30 mg per dose and is titrated individually for each patient in increasing increments of 5 mg every 48 h until adequate pain relief is attained. Then the dose is held at this level indefinitely. Brompton's solution is a liquid and is easier to swallow than a tablet. To achieve maximum benefit, it is administered every 3 to 4h around the clock. Phenothiazines (Thorazine or Compazine syrup) are believed to potentiate the analgesic effect, contain antiemetic properties, and reduce anxiety. It is often used to give a phenothiazine with the Brompton's solution. The most common side effect of this approach to analgesia is transient sedation, lasting 48 to 72 h. As patients adjust to the medication, they normally return to an alert state. Patients have been maintained for long periods of time without progressive dose escalation or the development of tolerance. Occasionally, a mild oral analgesic (e.g., Percodan) is needed in between doses of Brompton's solution for optimal comfort (Mount et al., 1976). Recent studies indicate that cocaine does not potentiate the analgesia of morphine but only adds side effects such as somnolence in some patients. Therefore, a simple morphine syrup or morphine-water solution is currently recommended over Brompton's solution for chronic severe pain control (Lipman, 1979).

Nurses should not underestimate the effectiveness of simple comfort measures in providing relief of less severe pain. LaMaze breathing, distraction, and relaxation techniques can be taught to the patient. A supportive atmosphere with evidence of caring and concern from the staff can do a great deal to reduce anxiety and to lift the patient's spirits. This is particularly important for the patient who consciously or unconsciously may use pain for secondary gains, to get attention or alleviate fears of being alone, especially if the patient perceives that the only contact with the nurse is when medications are administered.

Patient's expressions of pain and response to pain may vary with their ethnic background and their personalities (McCaffery, 1973). For example, a patient with a quiet or a stoic personality may suffer intensely without verbalizing pain. The nurse should be aware of this fact in order to meet the individualized need for pain relief.

Activity Performance status, or activity level, influences to a great degree the individual's response to chemotherapy or radiation therapy. Activity levels are influenced by energy levels. Both the treatment and the disease process contribute to weakness and fatigue. The nurse must help the individual to conserve energy by interfacing rest periods with activity in order to get the most mileage out of the patient's energy reserves. Often, one of the most difficult challenges facing the nurse is helping the formerly very active person to accept limitations in activity and energy levels. Emphasis must be placed on finding the delicate balance between pushing oneself too hard and not pushing hard enough. Extra effort may be required on the part of the staff and family to ensure that the more debilitated patient is ambulatory and out of bed, when possible, so that the possibility of response to therapy is not compromised.

Conservation of Structural Integrity

Surgical Side Effects Therapeutic surgical interventions interrupt the body surface continuity of the cancer patient. Many of these procedures, particularly potentially curative procedures, are quite extensive and invasive, with accompanying morbidity. Adequate wound healing and the prevention of infection that could compromise healing are primary nursing care goals for the postoperative cancer patient.

Radical surgical procedures, such as pelvic exenteration, head and neck dissections, radical mastectomy, abdominal perineal resection, or amputation of a limb, result in extensive tissue invasion with possibility of infection. Attention to detail in planning care is essential in order to ensure a smooth postoperative course. For example, proper nutrition, particularly adequate intake of protein-rich foods, aids in wound healing. Strict asepsis in dressing changes, prompt removal of saturated dressings which breed infection, good oral hygiene for patients with head and neck surgery, and skin care around ostomy sites to prevent breakdown and irritation all contribute to the restoration of structural integrity.

Altered body image or self-perception after radical surgery can be very traumatic for many patients. Rehabilitation efforts directed toward the patient with physical disfigurement and change in function should ideally begin prior to surgery and continue throughout the hospital course until discharge, with a definite plan for further follow-up and instruction as needed after discharge. The interdisciplinary team approach to rehabilitation is most successful, utilizing the expertise of the ostomy specialist, the physical therapist, and speech pathologist where appropriate. In situations where such special services are not available within the institutions, referrals can be made to outside agencies. The majority of cancer patients have amazing inner strength and motivation and can be assisted in coping with their disfigurement and altered function if they participate in a well-planned rehabilitation program. There is an abundance of information in the nursing literature regarding the special needs of each type of patient who has undergone radical surgery.

Chemotherapy Side Effects Chemotherapeutic agents contribute to the disruption of the patient's structural integrity. Drugs damage highly proliferative normal cells, and the result of this damage is observed in side effects following treatment. Blood counts must be carefully monitored because bone marrow is a major target for damage by chemotherapy drugs. Some patients may experience leukopenia, which places them at increased risk for the development of either a bacterial or a fungal infection. They should be instructed to report any fever, chills, or other sign of infection. If the white blood cell count is very low (usually less than 2500), patients should be cautioned to avoid exposure to persons who have colds, flu, or other infections. In selected cases, reverse isolation, placement in a laminar flow room, or white blood cell transfusions may be indicated.

Thrombocytopenia may occur, increasing the risk of bleeding. Petechiae, spontaneous bruising, nose bleeds, and rectal bleeding are all possible manifestations of thrombocytopenia. Reporting such symptoms is essential, and patients should be told when their platelet counts are low. Most often, the platelet count recovers spontaneously without intervention, but in selected cases, administration of vitamin K or platelet transfusions may be indicated.

Mucosal toxicity resulting from the destructive action of chemotherapeutic agents on the highly proliferative gastrointestinal mucosa may take the form of mouth lesions (reddened areas inside the mouth, on gums, or tongue; canker-type lesions, or external or internal ulcerations with bleeding) or lesions along the alimentary canal to the anus. Severe toxicity may result in a slough of the entire mucosal lining. Several simple nursing interventions can relieve patient discomfort until the mucosa heals. Good oral hygiene is essential, especially when the patient has ulcerated areas, because the possibility of fungal infection is increased. **Candida albicans** is the most common fungal infection found in the gastrointestinal mucosa and has the appearance of white, cheesy patches. Cleansing of the mouth, particularly before and after meals, with a mild hydrogen peroxide solution helps to loosen debris and old blood. Soft toothbrushes or Toothettes are preferable to minimize bleeding. A Maalox-Viscous Xylocaine preparation (1:1) contains a mild topical anesthetic and is useful for the relief of mouth soreness. The patient can use either of these preparations prior to meals so that food can be swallowed comfortably. The patient should be instructed to eliminate acid-containing foods (orange juice, tomato juice) and to substitute soft foods in the diet to minimize irritation of the sore areas. If *C. albicans* is noted in the mouth or throat, mystatin (Mycostatin) solution, "swished and swallowed," can retard the fungal growth. The nurse should also be aware of the possibility of dehydration with severe mucosal toxicity.

Certain chemotherapy drugs (e.g., bleomycin, fluorouracil) can cause skin discoloration and dry skin. Use of oil-based soaps and lotions (e.g., Alpha-Keri) can relieve itching and reduce dryness and flaking skin.

Alopecia is common with many chemotherapy drugs, which block mitotic activity in the hair bulb matrix. The hair loss may be total or partial and may occur after one or several cycles of therapy. In the majority of cases, the hair loss is temporary, with regrowth occurring after several months. Generally, this side effect is accepted by the patient, especially after supportive assistance from the nurse, such as reassurance and advice about wigs or hairpieces.

Care must be taken in the administration of intravenous chemotherapy drugs because extravasation of certain drugs, especially adriamycin, into the tissues surrounding the vein can result in tissue ulceration and necrosis.

Radiation Therapy Side Effects Structural integrity can also be altered by the damaging effects of radiation therapy on normal tissues. The type of side effects observed will be related to the site irradiated, the amount and time of tissue exposure, and the dose of radiation.

Radiation to the head and neck can cause mucosal toxicity. The previously mentioned interventions, with emphasis on oral hygiene, are appropriate. When large areas of bone marrow are in the radiation field, bone marrow suppression may be a problem. Monitoring of blood counts throughout the course of therapy is important, and appropriate interventions, such as transfusions, may be initiated as indicated.

Skin reactions, similar to sunburn, may occur during radiation therapy, with or without peeling or blistering of the treated area. The skin should be washed with a mild soap, avoiding vigorous scrubbing or wiping of the affected area. Cornstarch is sometimes useful in relieving itching. Occasionally, the radiation therapist may recommend steroid creams for symptomatic relief. Permanent skin changes (discoloration) and fibrosis of tissues in the irradiated area may be observed in some patients.

Observation, creative teaching, planning, and implementation of appropriate interventions all contribute significantly to the restoration of the patient's structural integrity.

Conservation of Personal Integrity

Of all diseases, cancer constitutes one of the most violent assaults on a person's self-esteem and sense of security. Cancer patients are subjected to endless invasions of their physical and emotional privacy. Mutilative surgical procedures decrease self-esteem. An active individual is either suddenly or gradually placed in a dependent role, in which freedom and scope of activities may be limited. As an increasing number of decisions are made for these patients, they become acutely aware of diminished control over life, and this may lead to increased anxiety and frustration or to passive resignation.

Dependence–Independence The dependence–independence conflict is one of the most difficult things with which the individual has to cope. As self-worth is crushed during the disease course, the patient must be helped to recognize strengths, not limitations, and to build on these strengths. The natural tendency is to focus in on what can no longer be accomplished rather than on what *can* be accomplished. Emphasis must be placed on the life left to live and on the quality of that life.

Two general types of cancer patients illustrate the dependence–independence conflict. The first type is the one who exhibits passive resignation to illness. Over time, this patient gradually assumes less responsibility for care and becomes more dependent on others, often exhibiting regressive behavior. Beneath the surface of this dependent behavior, however, lies a measure of fear, loneliness, and the need to escape from responsibility for self.

The other type of individual is the one who exhibits increased anxiety and frustration. Often, this patient has maintained an active, responsible life-style during the course of illness until a major progression of the disease suddenly makes it impossible for self-care to be done adequately, because of either pain or generalized debilitation. The necessity of depending on others (friends, family, or health professionals) for personal care or job and household responsibilities is extremely frustrating, and the patient expends a great deal of energy verbalizing negative feelings about the situation. Patients who have been *giving* persons for a lifetime often find it most difficult to be on the *receiving* end.

There are no easy solutions to either type of patient conflict. Each patient is unique, and each situation offers a special challenge to the nurse. Consultation with other members of the staff and with the interdisciplinary team, particularly the psychologist and minister, may provide valuable insights in planning a therapeutic approach for each patient. It is most important that the nurse seek out these resources in order to facilitate patient independence, because it is often easier to take the simple way out and reinforce dependence (e.g., by doing things for the patient rather than providing opportunities for self-care) or stifle independence (e.g., by making decisions for the patient rather than by providing opportunities for freedom of choice). The greatest challenges in working with cancer patients are often in the area of interpersonal relations, and these are the challenges that the nurse may feel the least prepared to meet.

Patient Rights The issue of patient rights has been in the forum of public discussion in recent years, particularly since the publication of the Patient's Bill of Rights by the American Hospital Association. More and more nurses are becoming very vocal in defining their role as patient advocates, supporters of the rights of each patient as an individual. Some of the strongest patient advocates are the nurses who work with cancer patients.

Cancer patients, with few exceptions, have the right to know their diagnosis and to be informed throughout the course of illness about where they stand and what the chances are for response to therapy. Kübler-Ross and others have observed in their clinical practice that cancer patients **are** aware of their diagnosis, whether or not they have been told by the physician (Kübler-Ross, 1970). Sensitive, honest, and open communication with the patient about the diagnosis alleviates discomfort on the part of the patient and the staff and removes the need for both parties to "play games" with each other. Patients have verbalized the loneliness and isolation they feel when they need to "protect" their families or the staff or when they feel that information is being withheld. Use of the word *cancer* by the nurse in the normal course of conversation, rather than euphemisms such as tumor, mass, or malignancy, often assists patients in coping with their illness. Always, sensitivity to and awareness of "where the patient is" are essential in talking with the cancer patient. Patients will often give verbal and nonverbal cues about the amount and type of information they are seeking at a particular time. Overloading the patient with too much information can be as destructive as withholding information. It is also difficult to justify subjecting patients to radical surgery or toxic treatment modalities without having informed them of the diagnosis and the need for such treatment.

Informed Consent Informed consent from the patient, prior to initiating any therapy, is essential. However, whether or not it is possible to obtain *truly informed consent* from a patient is debatable. Patients, in fact, may understand and/or retain very little of the information that is presented to them prior to giving consent for a particular therapy. There are several factors that may prevent understanding or retention of information. The most important factor is probably the patient's frame of mind at the time the information is presented. So often, consent for therapy must be obtained during a period of great stress for the patient, who is already struggling to cope either with a new diagnosis or with a recurrence of cancer. The amount of information about treatment that is given to patients at this time may be more than they can absorb, either because they are already overloaded or are blocking further sensory input. A patient may seem to understand what is being explained, but questioning at a later time may reveal that, in reality, very little of the information was absorbed.

Because of the legal and moral obligations to obtain informed consent, the nurse must play an important role as patient advocate. Several nursing interventions are valuable at this time. It is important that the nurse be present, if possible, when any form of treatment is being presented to the patient by the physician. The presence of the nurse at this time serves two purposes. The nurse will know what the physician has actually said to the patient and can observe the patient's initial reaction to the information. By observing carefully, the nurse also will be able to pick up verbal and nonverbal cues regarding the patient's receptivity and understanding. These observations will be helpful later during attempts to reinforce and explain further to the patient the information that has been given by the physician. The patient needs *time* in order to give informed consent, and hopefully, the nurse will have time to spend translating and clarifying in simple language the technical and complex information. Teaching is an important role for the nurse. Patients can be given an opportunity to ask questions that they may have hesitated to ask the physician. A written informed consent that summarizes the verbal information is usually presented to the patient. The patient may also find other types of written information (e.g., drug cards that list pertinent information regarding the treatment and side effects) helpful in making a decision regarding acceptance or rejection of a particular therapy.

The nurse must always take care to ensure that the patient never feels forced to make a decision regarding treatment before feeling as comfortable as possible with that decision. In the staff's concern that the patient receive the best treatment available, subtle pressure to accept treatment may be perceived by the patient. This perception could negate freedom of choice. Decisions regarding the choice of treatment are not easy for the patient to make. Treatment risk and toxicity must be weighed against possible benefit. The health care team must present both the risks and the benefits of a particular treatment as honestly and objectively as possible so that the patient can more easily make a decision. Patients must be assured that they will not be abandoned by the health care team if they choose to refuse therapy. The fear of abandonment is a reality that is always present in the patient. Patients have no obligation to participate in research programs and should understand that they are free to withdraw from therapy without losing the care and concern of the health care team. Patients should always be active members of the decision-making team, and their decision to accept or reject treatment must be respected.

Patient Participation The more patients understand about their illness and actively participate in planning care, the more control they will retain over their lives. Many interdisciplinary teams have organized formal class sessions for cancer patients to discuss the disease, treatment, and problems of daily living with cancer. Each member of the team presents a class on a specific area of expertise, and the patients are active participants in these sessions. A lending library or learning resource center can be established, with literature and audio-visual material made available to patients and their families. These classes and learning tools provide an opportunity for patients to increase their knowledge, as well as becoming a forum for sharing with professionals and other patients.

Preservation of Personalism Whenever possible, it is advantageous to provide some consistency in follow-up for cancer patients (i.e., the same nurse and the same physician) so that they can identify with a team that knows them and respects their individuality. Patients express frustration with the impersonal and diffuse care received in many large institutional settings. The nurse's focus should be on ensuring the preservation of personalism and continuity of care. Hope and encouragement from the nurse can do much to raise the spirits of the patient and bolster efforts to continue living a fruitful life within the limitation of illness.

Sexuality Sexuality and sexual activity are integral parts of the cancer patient's life and are necessary to the preservation of personal integrity and wholeness. The issue of sexuality and sexual function is often overlooked by health professionals, either because of their own discomfort in discussing the subject or because the patient seldom raises questions pertaining to sex.

Sexual problems experienced by the cancer patient may be related to physical limitations that result from any of the various treatment modalities, to fears, and to misconceptions or misinformation (Smith, 1976). Altered body image resulting from radical surgery can affect the patient's sexual self-concept and sexual behavior and can lead to feelings of sexual inadequacy, a loss of wholeness, and depression. Feelings of emasculation or loss of femininity may be intensified by sexual dysfunction (Woods, 1979).

Four types of cancer patients present typical problems related to sexuality and sexual function: the ostomy patient, the mastectomy patient, the gynecologic patient, and the patient receiving chemotherapy or radiation therapy.

The ostomy patient often expresses concern about alteration or loss of control of the normal body function of elimination. The patient often finds the appearance of the stoma and the bag disturbing and may be concerned about the possibility of spillage of the bag's contents and the control of odor. Because the patient finds this situation distasteful, he or she may communicate this attitude to the partner or assume that the partner shares this feeling of disgust. The male patient who has undergone abdominal perineal resection or colostomy surgery involving the lower colon may be impotent after surgery as a result of surgical damage to neural pathways in the pelvis. Impotence normally creates a feeling of humiliation, rejection, and inadequacy. Male patients who experience partial or total impotence should be encouraged to explore alternate forms of sexual expression, such as oral or manual stimulation, if these forms are acceptable to both partners. Ostomy patients may experience some decrease in sexual interest and sexual function during the first year following surgery.

Support from the sexual partner in caring for the ostomy stoma and bag and making the patient feel wanted and needed can alleviate some of the stress experienced by the ostomate. If the relationship between the ostomate and spouse or partner was healthy prior to surgery, little long-term disruption of the relationship should occur after surgery. Open communication between the partners must be encouraged to clarify the misconception and feelings of rejection, which are often unfounded.

The mastectomy patient often experiences some degree of anxiety as a result of having a breast removed. The breast is laden with sexual connotations and overtones. Young women, single women, and women whose self-concept is rooted in physical appearance will be apt to experience the most anxiety. The breast connotes femininity, physical attraction, and desirability. Breast stimulation is considered by many women to be an essential part of sexual foreplay. Some women find the chest wall at the mastectomy site to be very sensitive and painful when touched.

Fear of rejection by the spouse or sexual partner is a prime concern. In reality, the incidence of rejection is low if a good relationship existed prior to surgery. The partner usually feels no less love or acceptance of the woman after breast surgery. Again, verbalization of concerns by patient and partner should be encouraged. The partner may need to reassure the patient that she is loved and still physically attractive. Sexual activity should not be decreased or less satisfying following mastectomy. Protection of the sensitive mastectomy site by a pillow or other soft object may be advisable to ensure comfort. The patient and her partner should be able to resume normal sexual activity as soon as possible after surgical recovery. Consultation with a Reach-to-Recovery volunteer may be very helpful, so that the volunteer can advise the patient regarding clothing, prosthesis selection, and other sexual concerns.

Gynecologic patients also have sexual concerns. Some women who have undergone hysterectomy express regret about future inability to have children, the cessation of menstruation, and fear of premature aging. Vaginal or cervical irradiation may cause fibrosis and strictures of the vaginal wall, making vaginal intercourse painful. Pelvic exenteration makes vaginal intercourse impossible.

Hormonal alterations after oophorectomy may result in decreased vaginal lubrication or vaginal wall thinning, causing dyspareunia (painful intercourse). Women with advanced gynecologic cancer may have fistula formations, vaginal lesions, and foul-smelling vaginal drainage, which cause discomfort, humiliation, and loss of interest in sexual activity of any kind. Vaginal dilatation and lubrication and alternative forms of sexual expression should be explored. Communication of love and support from the patient's partner is essential to the preservation of her self-esteem.

Patients who have undergone extensive radiation therapy or chemotherapy may also experience sexual dysfunction. Either form of therapy may cause sterility, cessation of menses, or impotence. This is most problematic for the young patient. The questions of pregnancy and birth control methods may be raised. Because little is known definitely about the effect of drugs or radiation therapy on the ova or spermatozoa, the advisability of having children during or after therapy is difficulty to determine. Hopefully, the physician managing the treatment of the patient will be able to give appropriate counsel regarding this important question or refer the patient for genetic counseling.

At least one member of the interdisciplinary team should assume the responsibility of exploring the sexual problems and concerns of the cancer patients. Awareness and correct information about sexual problems and interventions can enable the nurse to be effective in assisting the patient to resolve these problems.

A brief sexual assessment of the cancer patient may provide useful information for postoperative counseling. Inquiry should be made regarding biologic variables (structures and functions lost after therapy, other physical problems); psychologic variables (cognitive: patient's knowledge of surgery or other treatment, misconceptions regarding treatment; affective: value attached to lost organ or function, meaning to patient of treatment outcome, coping mechanisms prior to treatment); sociologic variables (security of relationship with partner, partner's understanding of treatment, misconceptions about partner's sexual functioning after treatment (Woods, 1979).

Time, privacy to examine and work through feelings, and a supportive atmosphere are necessary in order to provide counsel regarding sexual problems. The nurse needs to be aware of verbal and nonverbal cues indicating that a problem exists. Discussion of sexual problems should be incorporated into any pretreatment teaching program, as well as in ongoing informational and supportive programs. Partners and spouses should be asked to participate in these discussions, both individually and with the patient.

Patients need to realize that temporary loss of interest or reluctance to resume sexual activity during or after therapy is not always a sign of permanent sexual dysfunction. They should maintain the goal of having a pleasurable sexual experience, with both partners being supportive of one another, even though previous roles or methods of expression have been altered by illness (see Woods, 1979, for additional information).

Spiritual Care One must not lose sight of a very important dimension of the patient's personal integrity, namely the patient's spiritual life. There is some indication that cancer patients who have some formal or informal faith experience tend to cope more successfully with illness and death than do those who do not have such a faith experience. Religious and philosophical questions regarding the meaning of the patient's illness and destiny are raised throughout the disease course, and a supportive atmosphere in which to seek answers to these questions is essential to the preservation of the patient's wholeness. "Spiritual care includes all that we can do to bring a sense of security into the situation. Our own philosophy must never be imposed upon another person, but an unspoken conviction that there is still purpose and meaning in his life may create a climate in which he can find his own answer" (Laister, 1974).

Because religion and philosophy are viewed as "personal matters," and because staff members often feel uncomfortable in attempting to deal with spiritual and philosophical questions, this dimension of care is often neglected. Ideally, a member of the clergy should be part of the interdisciplinary team responsible for cancer patients. Ministers have expressed frustration in their efforts to respond to the spiritual needs of their patients when they have been made to feel like an outsider within health care facilities. Recognizing the importance of the relationship between minister and patient, the nurse can ensure an atmosphere of respect and privacy that is conducive to spiritual counseling.

Dying When efforts at prolonging a good quality of life have failed, the person must be allowed to make the ultimate decision: to die. The nurse has the rare privilege, if accepted, of helping the person to die peacefully and comfortably, with dignity and the final preservation of personal integrity. The desire by cancer patients to ensure a dignified death has been evidenced in the movement to make the "Living Will" a legal document (see Fig. 28-4).

Engel, Kübler-Ross, and others have written extensively about the grief process, and the subject of death and dying is discussed in volumes of literature that are available to the nurse (Engel, 1964; Kübler-Ross, 1970). It is beyond the scope of this chapter to examine in detail the theories of death and dying, but some observations that are particularly relevant to the cancer patient may be helpful.

Hospice Care The word *hospice* originated in medieval Europe. Originally, during the Crusades, a hospice was a wayside inn where travelers could pause for rest and refreshment. At the present time, the word has come to be synonymous with an approach to assisting persons with illnesses, especially cancer, who can no longer be gainfully treated to live fruitfully until they die. An interdisciplinary team provides skilled care for dying patients and their families in a loving and supportive atmosphere. Special attention is given to the physical, emotional, and spiritual needs of the patients and families, as well as to the patients' activities of daily living.

Hospice care is given in a variety of settings throughout this country, England, and Canada. Patients are cared for in the home, if this is the wish of the patient and family, by interdisciplinary

571 IMPAIRMENT AS A RESULT OF CANCER

> TO MY FAMILY, MY PHYSICIAN, MY ATTORNEY, MY CLERGYMAN
> TO ANY MEDICAL FACILITY IN WHOSE CARE I HAPPEN TO BE
> TO ANY INDIVIDUAL WHO MAY BECOME RESPONSIBLE FOR MY
>   HEALTH, WELFARE, OR AFFAIRS
>
> Death is as much a reality as birth, growth, maturity and old age. It is the one certainty of life. If the time comes when I, _____ can no longer take part in decisions for my own future, let this statement stand as an expression of my wishes, while I am still of sound mind.
>
> If the situation should arise in which there is no reasonable expectation of my recovery from physical or mental disability, I request that I be allowed to die and not be kept alive by artificial means or "heroic measures." I do not fear death itself as much as the indignities of deterioration, dependence, and hopeless pain. I, therefore, ask that medication be mercifully administered to me to alleviate suffering even though this may hasten the moment of death.
>
> This request is made after careful consideration. I hope you who care for me will feel morally bound to follow its mandate. I recognize that this appears to place a heavy responsibility upon you, but it is with the intention of relieving you of such responsibility and of placing it upon myself in accordance with my strong convictions that this statement is made.
>
> Signed_____
> Date_____
> Witness_____
> Witness_____
> Copies of this request have been given to: _____
> _____
> _____
> _____

Figure 28-4
A living will.

teams. The hospice in Marin, California, is an excellent model. Other patients are cared for at homelike hospice facilities, such as St. Christopher's Hospice in London and the Hospice of New Haven, Connecticut, which exists apart from an acute care setting. The philosophy of hospice care can also be implemented in special units within a hospital, such as the palliative care unit of Royal Victoria Hospital in Montreal, Canada.

The major goal of hospice care is to make it possible for more patients to die at home or in a homelike atmosphere, free from pain, with family and friends, living their lives to the fullest until death. The focus of hospice care is on palliation of symptoms, with family members actively involved in the care of the patient. Counseling for the patient and family and bereavement follow-up of the family after the patient has died are also provided.

Nurses will find the published report of the Palliative Care Service Pilot Project at Royal Victoria Hospital a very valuable resource to assist in implementing the hospice philosophy in their own practice. A special unit is not always necessary in order to give excellent palliative care. The major ingredient is a dedicated and motivated team that is committed to meeting the special needs of the dying patient and family.

The Grieving Family Families often need support and counseling as the patient approaches death. Although the patient frequently has accepted death and feels at peace, the family is still struggling to deny the reality of their loved one's impending death. Without intervention in this situation, such patients may feel isolated and unable to share their deepest thoughts and feelings with family because they are forced to protect the family from hurt and loss. So much sharing is lost in this way, and the family may be faced with guilt and regret after the patient dies. Individual support by the nurse may help the family members to deal with their feelings. This is not an easy task. In fact, it is physically and emotionally draining. Involvement by the family in caring for the dying patient may be helpful. Group sessions with the team psychologist may provide opportunities for the family to express feelings and gain the support that is needed to face impending death.

Bereavement follow-up after the death of the cancer patient is a very valuable service that can be provided rather simply to the family (Palliative Care Service, 1977). The nurses who have cared for the patient can send a note of sympathy immediately after death. Perhaps one or several of the nurses might attend the visitation or funeral, if this is possible. A phone call several weeks after the patient's death or on the anniversary of the death may be appreciated. Often, family members will return to the nursing unit to visit with the staff. The families find such visits useful as a means of finishing part of the grieving process. While any or all of these interventions may be helpful to the families of many patients, the nurse should be aware of the families who feel the need to separate the staff and the setting of their loved ones' illness and death. Respect for this expressed or unexpressed need may indicate *no* bereavement follow-up.

The Grieving Staff Staff members often find it difficult to cope with the deaths of their patients.

Provision of opportunities for expressing grief and for supporting one another after particularly difficult death experiences will be therapeutic for the staff and help prevent "staff burnout." Helping a patient to die well is a potentially rewarding growth experience for the nurse *and* the patient and family.

Conservation of Social Integrity

Family, friends, culture, and religion all contribute to the individual's development as a social being.

The Family and Cancer When a family member is diagnosed as having cancer and undergoes therapy, the integrity of the entire family system is threatened. Whether or not the family can successfully cope with this experience may depend, to some degree, on the support and counsel that it receives from the nurse and other members of the interdisciplinary team.

Giacquinta (1977) has proposed a model or theoretical framework within which one can view the functioning of family members of the cancer patient (see Table 28-1). Her model examines 10 phases of functioning within four stages: living with cancer, the living–dying interval, bereavement, and reestablishment. It describes the hurdles for the family to overcome and the goals of nursing intervention at each phase.

Nurses who have been actively involved in clinical practice for any length of time soon realize that the reactions of families to the illness of a family member are as unique as are the reactions of the individual patient. The previous family history and coping mechanisms will influence the response of the patient and family members to the crisis of cancer. Because the nurse is often the member of the health care team that is most intimately involved with the patient and family, he or she may be more acutely aware of the dynamics that are influencing patient–family interaction throughout the course of the illness, and the family may approach the nurse for insight and counsel. The nurse may, in fact, be not only care giver but

Table 28-1

Giacquinta Model of Families' Reactions to Cancer

POINTS OF TRANSITION FOR INDIVIDUALS WITH CANCER	FAMILY STAGE	FAMILY PHASE	FAMILY HURDLE	GOAL OF NURSING INTERVENTION
Individual receives initial diagnosis of cancer, continues to carry out role obligations with the family, and functions in varying ways as a family member.	Living with cancer	Impact	Despair	Fostering hope
		Functional disruption	Isolation	Fostering cohesion
		Search for meaning	Vulnerability	Fostering security
		Informing others	Retreat	Fostering courage
		Engaging emotions	Helplessness	Fostering problem solving
Individual with cancer ceases to perform familiar roles and is cared for either at home or in the hospital.	Restructuring in the living-dying interval	Reorganization	Competition	Fostering cooperation
		Framing memories	Anonymity	Fostering identity
Individual with cancer dies.	Bereavement	Separation	Self-absorption	Fostering intimacy
		Mourning	Guilt	Fostering relief
	Reestablishment	Expansion of the social network	Alienation	Fostering relatedness

Source: Barbara Giacquinta, "Helping Families Face the Crisis of Cancer," *Am J Nurs* 77:1585, 1977. Used with permission of the publisher.

also a friend to the patient and, in many instances, to the family or significant others. It is by being simple and human enough to share with them on a personal or social level that the nurse opens avenues of communication, builds rapport, and facilitates discussion of deeper and more problematic issues. The nurse's role involves giving support, reassurance, and listening time, as well as referring the family to other professional resources that a particular crisis may require. Care must be taken to find the delicate balance between becoming too involved and so losing objectivity and not being involved enough to provide needed support. Communication and feedback from members of the health team help to maintain this balance.

Society and Cancer Since the subject of cancer has been featured extensively by the media, society's negative attitude toward cancer is changing. The social stigma of cancer can be attributed, in part, to a lack of correct information regarding the illness, its treatment, and its prognosis. Misconceptions and fear reinforce a negative attitude.

Nurses have a role as agents of change, as teachers of the public. The public needs to be made aware of the hope that exists for the cancer patient, of the chronicity of the disease (it is not synonymous with long suffering and death), of the futility of pursuing unproven methods of cancer treatment (quackery), and of the need for regular checkups and early diagnosis to ensure a hopeful prognosis.

Cancer patients are sensitive to the negative, fearful attitudes communicated to them by family, friends, and coworkers. Those patients who are self-confident often act as agents of change in their social world, but other patients suffer needlessly in silence. In many communities, public education programs have been presented by patients and health professionals to provide opportunities for learning and dialogue, and these programs are well attended. Such forums are to be encouraged everywhere.

Economics of Care Perhaps as a result of society's negative attitude toward cancer, many patients have experienced discrimination in employment, particularly those patients who are actively undergoing treatment. Some patients find it difficult to get jobs, and others are encouraged to take an early retirement even though they are capable of working. Job insecurity creates family crises. Inadequate insurance coverage or lack of insurance places the burden of responsibility for costly treatment and supportive care on the shoulders of the family unit. The cost of long-term cancer care is skyrocketing as patients live longer and receive increasingly sophisticated treatment. Inadequate financial resources may force a patient either to refuse treatment or to barely survive as sacrifices are made to pay medical bills.

The nurse as patient advocate can assure that financial considerations are incorporated into the total patient assessment and can facilitate communication regarding finances between the patient and/or family and the hospital or clinic business office.

Community Resources With careful planning, a smooth transition can be made for the patient from health care facility to home. More patients could remain at home with their loved ones if they were aware of the resources available to them in the community. Some institutions have a home care coordinator on the staff, usually a nurse, who can assess the needs of the cancer patient and make arrangements for obtaining equipment or transportation to treatment appointments from such agencies as the American Cancer Society. Other institutions, particularly those that have palliative care units, often have a home care nurse, who follows patients in their homes after discharge from the hospital and provides necessary nursing care and psychological support. Private agencies provide registered nurses, licensed practical nurses, and homemakers to cancer patients on a fee-for-service basis. Community health nurses can be active members of the interdisciplinary team and ensure continuity of care for the patients from hospital to home. Additional community resources are available to cancer patients and their families in specific geographic areas.

Support Groups Cancer patients have much to teach and to learn from each other, and they have expressed the benefits they derive from sharing their feelings and means of coping with their illness. In recent years, support groups have been formed to facilitate such sharing. One such organization is Make Today Count, founded by Orville Kelly. The organization is intended for persons with life-threatening illnesses and other interested parties. It focuses on learning to live with illness rather than dying from it. Local chapters of Make Today Count are found throughout the United States. Other support groups have been organized in cancer outpatient treatment facilities and elsewhere. Cancer Call-Pac is another unique support service available to cancer patients in some cities. It is a telephone network of cancer patients and families who are available for support and counseling on a 24-h basis.

Reach to Recovery, Lost Cord Club, and Ostomy Club members provide preoperative and postoperative counseling, advice, and in some instances, social activities in a patient-to-patient setting. All of these efforts are valuable services that help to preserve the cancer patient's social integrity.

WHOLENESS OF SELF: THE NURSE

When considering wholeness of *self,* nurses, in order to be effective in dealing with cancer patients, must first assess themselves honestly and seriously. What qualities do nurses, as individuals, need to possess in order to work with these patients? They must be warm and kind and have a love of life, a genuine concern for persons, and be tuned in to people. They must be able to acknowledge and face personal feelings regarding some very difficult, basic, and profound issues: the value of life, the reality of death, the prospect of working with persons who have a chronic and essentially incurable illness. When these issues are confronted and when even the hostile, hopeless, and depressed feelings are recognized, the increased self-awareness will enable the nurse to face with enthusiasm the frustrating, challenging task of helping cancer patients to live fruitfully and die peacefully.

This task may be relatively easy or more difficult, depending on the nurse's own philosophical and religious beliefs, personal support systems, and the energy and motivation that can be devoted to caring for the cancer patient. The patients themselves can aid the nurse in completing this assessment. Once nurses have gotten beyond the "frightening diagnosis," they will recognize immediately that there is much to teach about the quality of life and the very basic issues that each nurse must resolve.

Once the commitment has been made to working with cancer patients, continual renewal and reinforcement are needed. The challenge is demanding, both physically and emotionally, if one dares to become truly *involved.* The support that colleagues can give one another, in formal and informal sharing sessions, cannot be underestimated. Sometimes it is easier not to share, because open expressions of feelings and reactions to situations can be painful, but the insights gained are well worth the effort. Staff support conferences with the interdisciplinary patient care team are also valuable, particularly if at least one member is skilled in facilitating communication.

An integral component of commitment is the ability to pull back from this involvement periodically, to recoup one's strength and perspective. Inner healing via rest, travel, exercise, a good talk with a friend, or an escape into a novel will ultimately renew the nurse's healing abilities with cancer patients.

Cancer patients are identical in one respect: they may share the same hopes and dreams that the nurse does, they have a very complex and profound illness, and they bring their own unique and individual selves and means of dealing with their illness. It is this uniqueness that forms the basis of approaching the cancer patient from a holistic perspective.

WHOLENESS OF THE DISEASE PROCESS

Because most cancer patients are followed over an extended period of time, the nurse must consider the "wholeness" of the disease process itself: the diagnosis, recurrence, and terminal phase. Each patient, with few exceptions, can be evaluated within this continuum, and it is a challenge for the nurse to devise an appropriate assessment of the patient, utilizing the holistic approach, at each point along the continuum.

CONCLUSION

A living organism cannot be defined by the number of cells it contains, and a human personality cannot be defined by the number of its needs, nor its life considered as an interplay of need and satisfaction. . . . For man, to be human is an existential tautology, in order to be a man, man must be more than a man. (Heschel, 1959)

This in no way disparages the success of scientists in their treatment of human beings and their problems, but their preoccupation with humans as an object of research created false views within the scientific community, which, by its very nature, should view humans as open-ended beings.

The conflicts over the quality of life and the termination of life cannot be answered within a system that is able to abstract, to dissect the human person. Human beings become, according to this viewpoint, fixed and static, that is, measurable. The moment of death can be determined; when life is human, life is measurable. However, as Robert Francouer (1970) points out, there are many questions that cannot be answered with this approach. How do we explain the effects of certain drugs on the personality? To say that they act on our body chemistry and therefore modify our personality is hardly a definitive answer.

The holsitic view of an individual is that of a "bipolar unity in process," a living person interacting with others. A human being then becomes, in holism, four-dimensional: a body, a within, a relation, and all this in process. The body, the person, and the relation to others are open-ended and dynamic, growing and evolving. To abstract one element from this view would be to destroy the individual, to fail to know him, to cause him to cease to be himself. (Francouer, 1970)

BIBLIOGRAPHY

Beland, Irene L., and Joyce V. Passos: *Clinical Nursing: Pathophysiological and Psychosocial Approaches,* Macmillan, New York, 1975.

Bouchard, Rosemary E., and Norma F. Owens: *Nursing Care of the Cancer Patient,* Mosby, St. Louis, 1976.

Buber, Martin: *Between Man and Man,* Beacon Press, Boston, 1955.

Burkhalter, Pamela K., and Diana L. Donley: *Dynamics of Oncology Nursing,* McGraw-Hill, New York, 1978.

Copeland, Edward M., et al.: "Intravenous Hyperalimentation as an Adjunct to Cancer Chemotherapy," *Am J Surg* 129:167, 1975.

Cuddy, R.: *The Role of Diet in Cancer Therapy,* National Cancer Institute, Bethesda, 1975.

DeWys, William D.: "Sytemic Effects of Cancer: Cachexia-Anorexia," *Pro XI International Cancer Congress,* 5:59, 1974.

Donovan, Marilee I., and Sandra G. Pierce: *Cancer Care Nursing,* Appleton-Century-Crofts, New York, 1976.

Engel, George: "Grief and Grieving," *Am J Nurs* 64:93, 1964.

Francouer, Robert: *Evolving World, Converging Man,* Holt, New York, 1970.

Giacquinta, Barbara: "Helping Families Face the Crisis of Cancer," *Am J Nurs* 77:1585, 1977.

Heschel, Abraham: *God in Search of Man,* Meridan, New York, 1959.

Kellogg, Carolyn J., and Barbara Peterson Sullivan: *Current Perspectives in Oncologic Nursing,* vol. 2, Mosby, St. Louis, 1978.

Kübler-Ross, Elisabeth: *On Death and Dying,* Macmillan, New York, 1970.

Laister, P.: "Symposium: Care of the Dying. The Priest's Care of the Terminally Sick," *Nursing Mirror* 139:63, 1974.

Levine, Myra E.: "Holistic Nursing," *Nurs Clin North Am* 6:253, 1971.

―――: *Introduction to Clinical Nursing,* Davis, Philadelphia, 1973.

Lipman, Arthur: "Drug Therapy in Chronic Pain: Part II," *Med Digest* September-October: 13, 1979.

Marino, Elizabeth B., and Dona H. LeBlanc: "Cancer Chemotherapy," *Nursing 76* 6(10):22, 1976.

McCaffery, Margo: "Patients in Pain," *Nursing '73* 3(6):42, 1973.

Melzack, R., et al.: "The Brompton Mixture: Effects on Pain in Cancer Patients," *Can Med Assoc J* 115:125, 1976.

Mount, B. M., et al.: "Use of the Brompton Mixture in Treating the Chronic Pain of Malignant Disease," *Can Med Assoc* 115:122, 1976.

Murphy, Terence M.: "Cancer Pain," *Postgrad Med* 53(6):187, 1973.

Palliative Care Service: Pilot Project, Royal Victoria Hospital, Montreal, 1977.

Peterson, Barbara H., and Carolyn J. Kellogg: *Current Practice in Oncologic Nursing,* Mosby, St. Louis, 1976.

Rinear, Eileen E.: "Helping the Survivors of Expected Death," *Nursing 75* (3):60, 1975.

Rubin, Philip, and Richard F. Bakemeier: *Clinical Oncology for Medical Students and Physicians: A Multidisciplinary Approach,* 5th ed., American Cancer Society, New York, 1976.

Sherman, Charles D.: *Clinical Concepts in Cancer Management (A Self-instruction Manual),* McGraw-Hill, New York, 1976.

Siegele, Dorothy S.: "The Gate Control Theory," *Am J Nurs* 74:498, 1974.

Smith, Elizabeth A.: *A Comprehensive Approach to the Rehabilitation of the Cancer Patient (A Self-instruction Manual),* McGraw-Hill, New York, 1975.

Woods, Nancy F.: *Human Sexuality in Health and Illness,* 2d ed., Mosby, St. Louis, 1979.

29
mary doherty
sue ann prato

cardiac impairment

"To Wake at Dawn with a Winged Heart and Give Thanks for Another Day of Loving."
                                           Kahlil Gibran

INTRODUCTION

What of awakening in the middle of the night with an impaired heart . . . ? The association of positive emotions with the heart in our culture is undisputable. The appreciation of the heart as the source of one's vitality is unanimous. Most would agree that the loss of significant people and relationships causes one's heart to be saddened.

Just as these associations are universal, so experience with heart disease in the United States has assumed cosmic proportions. It is the rare individual who remains unscathed, directly or indirectly, by the ravages of heart disease in our twentieth-century world. Six hundred thousand Americans die annually from coronary artery disease alone. The American Heart Association estimates the prevalence of cardiovascular diseases in the United States at close to 30 million. Rusk reports the loss of 52 million working days annually by individuals with cardiovascular disease; this, coupled with the cost of health care for these individuals, results in an estimated annual cost of $20 billion. These figures, while certainly impressive, in no way compare to the intangible losses of self-esteem, comfort, and happiness of the individuals and families affected by this epidemic.

Significant strides in dealing with the acute cardiac episode have been and continue to be made. Research in detection and, more importantly, prevention of cardiovascular diseases is of crucial importance. Rehabilitation of those who have experienced cardiac impairment must endeavor to obtain maximal cardiac function with minimal risk, enabling these individuals to perform optimally in their unique roles, relationships, and environments. And in doing so, it is essential that functional capability be congruous with perceived capability; it is clear at this time, for instance, that return to work following initial myocardial infarction has as much to do with an individual's psychological status as with physiological capabilities. How can the nurse help the cardiac-impaired person to achieve this goal?

This chapter discusses the person who has experienced cardiac impairment, the normal cardiovascular system, the most commonly occurring alterations in cardiovascular function, and the psychosocial implications and reactions. The major focus is on the nurse's role in the rehabilitation of the cardiac-impaired person.

ANATOMY

Functionally, the heart is a very simple organ, although that simplicity belies the real intricacies and fine balances that exist within the cardiovascular system. The sole function of the heart is to serve as a pump. The heart propels blood through a closed system that consists of a vast vascular network structured to deliver blood to body tissues, remove waste products, and return the blood to be reoxygenated in the lungs before it is again pumped out to body tissues dependent on aerobic metabolism. The heart is functionally divided into two halves, made up of a right atrium and right ventricle and a left atrium and left ventricle. Normally, there are no connections between the two halves, and a one-way forward flow of blood is assured via a system of valves within the heart. Blood returning from the tissues in a state of deoxygenation enters the right atrium via the superior and inferior venae cavae, crosses the tricuspid valve, and enters the right ventricle. The right ventricular output crosses the pulmonic valve to enter the pulmonary arteries and the pulmonary capillaries of the lung, where there is a release of carbon dioxide and an uptake of oxygen into the blood based on simple diffusion gradients. Oxygenated blood returns to the left atrium via the pulmonary veins, where the blood passes through the mitral (biscuspid) valve to enter the left ventricle. With contraction, the left ventricle ejects blood through the aortic valve into the aorta, through which the blood will eventually reach arteries, arterioles, capillaries, and ultimately the target tissues. The left ventricular output is referred to as the cardiac output when expressed as liters of blood per minute or as the stroke volume when referring to the amount of blood ejected with each heartbeat. It gives rise to the blood pressure as we measure it with a cuff. Obviously, the amount of blood ejected from the left ventricle per heartbeat is a function of the amount of blood present in the ventricle initially and of the amount of peripheral vascular resistance that is present against which the heart is required to work. In effect, this means that the diameter of the vessels determines the amount of pressure required to propel blood through those vessels. Should a higher pressure be required as a result of intense vasoconstriction (i.e., severely narrowed vessels resulting from an atherosclerotic process), the workload, and consequently the oxygen consumption, of the heart will be increased. All these factors become important in assessing and understanding the symptoms, treatment, and rehabilitation goals of the cardiac patient.

There are two major classifications of breakdown within the system. Since the function of the heart is to pump a certain amount of blood per unit of time to supply the body's metabolic needs, there can be either some major alteration in the volume of blood or an alteration in the pumping ability of the myocardium itself. Let us examine these two major possibilities separately with their most common causes and consequences.

DISTRIBUTION OF BLOOD VOLUME

Major derangements in blood volume occur most commonly as a result of valvular lesions such as those seen in rheumatic heart disease. Incompetent valves within the heart allow a backward flow of blood, resulting in an increase in volume work for the heart. Some portion of the same volume of blood is pumped over and over again, since ventricular emptying is incomplete. Initially, the heart speeds up its rate of contraction in an effort to expel the increasing volume. The ventricle then dilates in an effort to accommodate the increased volume. If the valve(s) become calcified and the orifice fixed, the condition is referred to as a stenotic valve and results in an increase in pressure within the heart. In this instance, the heart generates an increased contractile force in an effort to expel blood through a valve with a decreased diameter. Here the heart will actually hypertrophy; there is an increase in muscle mass in an effort to supply the increased contractile force required. Because the cardiovascular system is a closed one, a rise, or a fall, in pressure in any part of the system, if uncorrected, will be felt throughout the system.

When the major compensatory mechanisms of tachycardia, dilatation, and hypertrophy fail, as they certainly will, the patient will experience the classic symptoms of congestive heart failure, including dependent edema, dyspnea, orthopnea, jugular venous distention, and perhaps a dry cough. In severe cases, patients may exhibit hepatic enlargement and gastrointestinal disturbances secondary to a backup of blood. These patients will often do better with frequent, smaller meals, since nausea is a frequent problem.

If the cause of the congestive failure is a mechanical valvular defect such as seen in patients with rheumatic heart disease, then surgery can be performed to correct the basic defect, and an artificial valve can be implanted. Congestive heart failure is usually not a continuing problem in these patients as long as the artificial valve remains functional. These patients do need to be careful about infection of any sort, since an artificial valve can become infected. Antibiotics are taken prophylactically before any surgical procedures such as teeth extractions. The patient with a prosthetic valve will almost certainly be on anticoagulant therapy, and teaching should include the dosage, size, and color of the tablet and the purpose of anticoagulant therapy. The danger of clot formation on a prosthetic valve is a real one, and emboli are not a rare occurrence. Patients need to understand what side effects to report in terms of unusual bleeding and the importance of undergoing periodic blood tests so that a precise degree of anticoagulation can be maintained. To this end, patients are instructed to take anticoagulation medication in the evening so that if a dose needs to be altered on the basis of a clinic appointment the patient can be instructed to alter the dose that same day.

For the patient in congestive heart failure as a result of cardiomyopathy of whatever origin, treatment is generally symptomatic, and a true alteration in life-style is often required for this patient. Cardiomyopathies include a broad range of disabilities and causes and generally tend to be both irreversible and progressive, since the disease is diffuse. Cardiomyopathies have been associated with alcoholism, infectious disease processes, immune responses, and hypertrophic changes within the heart itself. Treatment is aimed at decreasing the fluid volume the heart is required to pump, primarily through the use of diuretics. Patients are taught to take the prescribed diuretic in the morning so as to not interrupt sleep when diuresis begins, and they need to be warned that an increased urine output is to be expected, for it is often initially a cause of concern. Elderly patients, in particular, may find control a problem as a result of decreased bladder tone. In such cases, they should mention it to their physician, for often a smaller dose can be prescribed to be taken twice a day in order to prevent such a vigorous diuretic response.

One of the important components of the treatment of congestive heart failure is a low-salt diet. Because the sodium ion retains water, a high intake can further complicate the volume overloading problems of the patient in congestive heart failure. The area of diet modification is a difficult one and requires a significant commitment from the patient and family. The need to prepare a separate meal for the cardiac patient can be expensive and serves to reinforce the sense of isolation, the sense of being "different," that the patient role engenders. This problem can be solved simply by having family members add salt to their food after it has been cooked. A dietician, if available, should be involved in advising the patient and family.

Another major component of therapy in congestive heart failure is aimed at increasing the contractile ability of the heart and is accomplished primarily through the use of digoxin. The usual dose is 0.25 mg and is most commonly described by patients as "my white heart pill" (Myers, Jarvetz, and Goldfien, 1976). Digoxin is taken *once* a day, most often in the morning, and patients need to be cautioned that the old maxim "if one is good, two is better" does not apply, especially with digoxin. This is a very real danger because most patients will note a definite improvement once they begin taking the digoxin. Since digoxin slows the heart rate while increasing the force of contraction, patients are generally taught to take their own pulse prior to taking the drug. However, this practice can vary with local medical custom, and the nurse should inquire regarding physician preference in any particular locale. Usually, the radial pulse is checked, but the carotid pulse may also be used provided the patient has equal carotid pulses. The most common side effects of digoxin are nausea, vomiting, yellow vision or rings around objects, and possible dizziness secondary to profound slowing of the heart.

A third treatment component commonly used with the patient in congestive heart failure is potassium replacement, which is necessary because of the potassium-wasting effect of many diuretics. The heart is also more susceptible to digitalis toxicity in the presence of low serum potassium levels. Here again, it is important to emphasize follow-up appointments to monitor the degree of heart failure present, serum electrolyte values, and periodically, the digoxin level. Because the potassium replacements commercially available are often not very palatable and the low-salt diet is difficult to follow, some use has recently been made of the fact that salt substitutes in the form of potassium chloride can be utilized to provide the potassium replacement needed. This course of action definitely requires the consultation of a dietician.

Before the patient is discharged, many nurses prepare a drug chart containing a sample of each of the patient's medications taped to a piece of cardboard beside which are listed the times of administration, the action, and the major side effects of each drug. Ideally, patients should be able to identify their medication by size, color, and shape, since many patients tend to put all of their medication into one large bottle and rely on memory to separate them again. Patients should be specifically cautioned against this practice. It is surprisingly common for patients to mistake a digoxin tablet for nitroglycerin and take perhaps three digoxin tablets in one day, with the result that they are admitted to the emergency room in digitalis toxicity.

The heart has an inherent rate of contraction that, for most adults, ranges between 60 and 100 beats per minute. Myocardial contraction results from a rhythmic depolarization of the sinus node, which is the normal pacemaker of the heart. There is no backup system for the heart should it fail to beat, and consequently, the heart has subsidiary pacemakers that are built to discharge in case the sinus node fails to fire for whatever reason. The lower subsidiary pacemakers located in the atrioventricular junction and the ventricles discharge at significantly slower rates, respectively, and are not built for long-term pacing.

Patients who can no longer rely on their sinus nodes to pace their hearts will need artificial pacemakers to supply the impetus for myocardial contraction at a rate compatible with life. Patients requiring permanent artificial pacing generally suffer either from sinus node disease, with profound slowing of the heart rate and accompanying symptoms, or from diffuse disease that causes conduction defects within the heart. Occasionally, surgical damage occurs that prevents the impulse for contraction from crossing from the atria to the ventricles; consequently, there is a loss of coordinated, sequential contractions within the heart.

Although implanting an artificial pacemaker is technically a minor surgical procedure, it can elicit strong emotional reactions in patients. Involved are issues concerning dependence on a mechanical device for life, being "part of a person," some concern about disfigurement, and questions about carrying on water-related activities, such as showering and swimming. Elderly patients, in particular, may take the stance that they have done quite well thus far and have no intention of accepting any "newfangled" devices and so refuse the procedure entirely. These patients will sometimes find it helpful to talk to other patients who have had pacemakers successfully implanted. The other end of this spectrum is the patient who has a friend or family member who has had a pacemaker implanted and who is active and doing well. These patients come to the hospital armed with information, bear a positive attitude about the procedure, and generally respond well.

It is vital that the nurse ascertain how the pacemaker is viewed by the patient and family, for it can be seen as anything from a last-ditch measure to a minor inconvenience through which the patient intends to resume life as it has always been.

Each type of pacemaker has special features, following implantation, and all patients are supplied with an information booklet from the pacemaker manufacturer. The booklet should be reviewed with the patient and family to allow them the opportunity to ask questions. Patients should be taught to take their pulse for one full minute (again either the carotid or radial artery may be used) and to immediately report a pulse rate that is below the rate the pacemaker is set for, since this is the most common indication of pacemaker failure. The predicted life of a pacemaker depends on the type of battery utilized, and this information will be contained in the booklet from the pacemaker manufacturer.

There has been some work done, especially in Europe, with nuclear pacemakers. The concept is feasible and has actually been performed, but the procedure is not cost-effective at the present time. Since nuclear pacemakers have a prolonged life expectancy, one would not be warranted in a 90-year-old patient, since the power source would long outlive the patient. A nuclear pacemaker would be more reasonable for the younger patient with a longer life expectancy. A lithium pacemaker could be used for the patient expected to live 7 to 10 years (Furman, 1978).

Patients with pacemakers will need reinforcement about keeping appointments for follow-up, usually at a pacemaker clinic, although transtelephonic monitoring of pacemakers is being done at certain institutions and will probably become more commonplace in the future. Warning devices will most likely be developed that will allow the early detection of pacemaker malfunction by both patient and physician.

ANGINA PECTORIS

The actual pumping ability of the heart muscle can be affected by ischemia, as seen in angina pectoris, by an actual destruction of some portion of functioning myocardial muscle, as seen in acute myocardial infarction, as well as by diffuse disease/infiltration of the myocardial muscle itself, which is included under the broad heading of cardiomyopathy.

It seems inconsistent that an organ that has all the blood in the body coursing through it should ever itself lack a blood supply, and yet the heart does not utilize the blood within its chambers for nourishment but depends on a separate set of vessels, called the coronary arteries, that branch off the ascending aorta. Chest pain occurs when the heart muscle requires more blood than the coronary arteries can deliver, and the condition is known as angina pectoris. Usually, it results when the atherosclerotic process occurs within the coronary arteries, thus decreasing the blood flow through those arteries.

Angina is a symptom, not a disease, that results from atherosclerotic changes, especially in the coronary vessels. Atherogenesis, with resultant narrowing of the lumen of the blood vessel, causes a disproportion between the oxygen needs of the myocardium and the ability of the vessels to deliver the required blood supply. "The underlying disorder, atherosclerosis, accounts for approximately one half of all deaths in the western world" (Kamnel, 1972).

When narrowing of the lumen of the artery becomes significant, blood flow through the vessel decreases, causing a decrease in pressure distal to the narrowing. With a drop in pressure, vascular resistance also decreases to allow maximal blood flow even when the patient is at rest. This constant dilatation of the arterioles leaves very little reserve capacity for further dilatation to meet rising O_2 demands of the heart during stress.

The large coronary arteries normally offer very little resistance to blood flow; it is the smaller arterioles that regulate the blood flow to meet the myocardial demand. Sclerosed coronary vessels cause the blood supply to become fixed regardless of myocardial O_2 demand, with resultant myocardial ischemia and the pain of angina pectoris when myocardial oxygen demand exceeds the blood vessels' capacity for delivery. Angina produces a wide range of disability depending on the amount of blood available in relation to myocardial demand.

If the constriction of the arteriosclerotic vessel develops slowly, there is a chance for collateral circulation to develop. "Collaterals are anastomotic connections between coronary arteries without an intervening capillary bed" (Braunwald, Ross, and Sonenblick, 1976). Generally, the amount of O_2 required determines the amount of vascularization. With age, the body's ability to adjust the vasculature to the needs of the body decreases. "We could, therefore, suppose that in many patients with angina, if not most, the process of collateral circulation has already de-

CHAPTER 29   584

veloped in the earlier stages of his coronary disease, and that finally he has run out of the capacity for revascularization" (Nahum, 1971).

Because the amount of coronary blood flow becomes relatively fixed as a result of the rigid arteries, the really important factor in determining the precipitation of angina is the metabolic activity of the heart. As the intensity of the cardiac workload increases, there is a corresponding increase in heart rate and blood pressure and a decrease in the time it takes to reach the critical level of angina. "The triple product (systolic blood pressure, heart rate and ejection time) at angina presumably correspond roughly to that level of myocardial O_2 demand which just exceeds the O_2 transport capacity of the narrowed coronary arteries" (Goldstein). Patients with coronary heart disease should be taught the importance of engaging in only moderate exercise with gradual increases. Physical training in and of itself is beneficial because such training results in a decrease in heart rate and blood pressure and may result in a decreased cardiac size. When physical exercise is mild enough to cause angina only after 3 or more minutes, the triple product is constant at the point of angina. In other words, anginal chest pain will develop as soon as myocardial demand exceeds the O_2 supply and serves as a warning to the patient to slow down or stop the present activity. The close relationship between the development of the critical value of the triple product (the development of myocardial demand beyond the O_2 supply) and the onset of ischemic pain does not hold for exercise that precipitates angina in less than 3 min. With short bursts of exercise, there is a time lag between the onset of ischemia and the actual anginal pain, so the critical level may be exceeded and go unnoticed for a time, possibly causing damage to the heart. Such patients need to be cautioned against short bursts of exercise (Browning et al., 1973).

Any other conditions that may adversely affect oxygen delivery and/or availability should be ruled out or treated, such as anemia, cardiorespiratory disorders that result in arterial desaturation, abnormalities of hemoglobin, aortic insufficiency, or bradycardia. In an already compromised myocardium, it is important to have maximum aeration of the blood that is delivered through sclerosed vessels.

The diagnosis of angina is based on the clinical symptoms, which is, classically, pain brought on by exertion and relieved by rest and/or nitroglycerin. The pain is usually substernal but may radiate and is described as squeezing, heaviness, choking, fullness, pressure, and occasionally as indigestion. Characteristically, there is a waxing and waning period to the pain of angina pectoris. "Pain induced by physical activity usually does not last longer than two or three minutes if the patient abandons the exertion that precipitated the pain" (Rodman, 1971).

All treatment plans for angina pectoris are aimed at increasing the blood flow to the heart, decreasing myocardial O_2 demands, or both. It is also important to relieve and/or prevent pain, deal with anxiety, and give the patient a chance to express concerns about disability and/or death. Angina is generally treated either by using medication that decreases the oxygen requirement of the heart such as propranolol (Inderal) or by using the nitrate classification of drugs (either nitroglycerin or the more long-acting Isordil) which act to dilate blood vessels and decrease workload (Meyers et al., 1976). As with all medication, the importance of taking the drug(s) as prescribed should be emphasized each time the patient receives the medication, accompanied by an explanation of what the medication is, why the patient is receiving it, the expected effects, and what untoward effects to report.

Sublingual nitroglycerin is often given routinely for the pain of angina, both as a part of the treatment plan and prophylactically. Nitroglycerin is a nonspecific smooth muscle relaxant that decreases the mean and systolic blood pressures, thus reducing cardiac preload and afterload (Braunwald et al., 1976). Nitroglycerin is useful probably because it acts to decrease oxygen consumption during exercise. If an anginal experience has warned the patient that a certain activity, such as climbing two flights of stairs, will bring on an anginal attack, the patient should be advised to take a nitroglycerin tablet before climbing the stairs. The patient should be reminded to note daily the amount, frequency, and effectiveness of nitroglycerin used. Pain that is no longer relieved by nitroglycerin should be reported to the physician. It should be emphasized that nitroglycerin is not addictive so that the patient will not try to do without it, even during chest pain, for fear of becoming dependent on or developing a tolerance to the drug. Patients are advised to keep their nitroglycerin tablets in a brown bottle without the cotton. Nitroglycerin should cause a burning/tingling sensation under the tongue and is not likely to be effective after about 6 months, at which time it should be replaced. If the patient is taking the drug for the first time, headaches and even dizziness may occur as a result of vasodilation. The patient should be told that the headaches usually diminish or disappear in time, but in the interim, they can be treated in the conventional fashion.

Nitroglycerin ointment has been in clinical use for the treatment of angina pectoris since 1955 but has only recently become a more frequently prescribed treatment modality. This form of nitroglycerin is different *only* in its duration of action. Nitroglycerin ointment has a vasodilating effect that lasts up to 5 h.

Increase in blood flow to the myocardium and subsequent relief of angina pectoris can also be accomplished by surgical revascularization of the heart. At present, this is being accomplished by surgical bypass of atheromatous areas of the coronary arteries with reversed saphenous vein grafts.

Several factors are known to precipitate anginal attacks, and these should be discussed with the patient as an integral part of any teaching plan. One of the most common factors is a cold environmental temperature that is associated with an increase in systemic arterial pressure secondary to reflex vasoconstriction. This vasoconstriction increases the total peripheral vascular resistance, which increases the myocardial afterload and myocardial O_2 consumption. Heavy meals have also been implicated in anginal attacks, possibly owing to preferential blood shunting to the digestive tract. The patient should be advised to eat frequent, lighter meals rather than eating little or nothing through the day and then a heavy meal at night, especially when alcohol is also consumed. Complete abstinence from alcohol is not necessary, but moderation is crucial. Likewise, emotional upsets have been associated with anginal pain, probably secondary to an increase in circulating catecholamines. Simply as a function of gravity, a completely supine position may occasionally precipitate angina as the venous return to the heart increases. Patients who experience this complain of being awakened from sleep by an anginal attack and often compensate by sleeping on several pillows at night. If angina patients do engage in any of the above activities (i.e., eating heavy meals, drinking too much), they should be advised not to combine any of them and to make an effort to rest after any strenuous activity. What is usually required is indeed a change in life-style, which is a difficult task regardless of one's age.

These patients need well-planned activity pacing, since the oxygen demand of the heart can be altered in other ways besides pharmacologically. If one has four different tasks to do during the day, for example, there is no reason why they must all be done before noon or done right after one another. Tasks should be done one at a time and spread over the day, with rest periods in between. Chest pain often occurs if a patient has several cocktails, eats a large dinner, and then engages in sexual activity. As an alternative, it is suggested that one can have a cocktail early in the evening, eat a moderate dinner, and perhaps engage in sexual activity the following morning.

MYOCARDIAL INFARCTION

"Acute myocardial infarction is a clinical syndrome resulting from deficient coronary arterial flow to an area of myocardium with eventual cellular death and necrosis" (Blakiston's, 1972).

Encircling the area of actual infarcted necrotic tissue is a zone of injury, the fate of which is not immediately decided following the acute episode. It is because of this zone of injury and studies done in 1929 in the length of the healing process that it became accepted practice to place patients on complete bed rest in order to avoid stress on already marginally viable heart muscle (Johnson et al., 1976). Subsequent studies have shown that cardiac workload actually increases in the recumbent position, partly as a result of increased venous return. Unconditional bed rest is no longer considered necessary, since some activities are less stressful out of bed, such as using a bedside commode instead of a bedpan (Karvonen & Barry, 1967).

Generally, the infarcted area heals in about 6 weeks, forming scar tissue. This tissue will no longer contract effectively, but adjacent cardiac muscle will compensate, and patients can do quite well, depending on infarct size and location, of course.

Since weakness is one of the most distressing aftermaths of an acute myocardial infarction for the patient, early mobilization can help to minimize this. Initially, the patient is concerned about staying alive, since as a result of public service advertisements, the Heart Association, and the epidemic proportions of heart disease, most people are acutely aware that a heart attack can be fatal. A heart attack is viewed as a major catastrophe and an assault on the self. It forces the realization that one is vulnerable and indeed mortal. "To sustain an acute myocardial infarction and not experience some depression would be unusual" (Cassem and Hackett, 1973), and consequently, the patient's rehabilitation should begin immediately and will be greatly influenced by the atmosphere the nurse creates and how apprehension and questions are handled.

This initial period is not the time for detailed answers or prolonged explanations, but short, positive answers about what has happened and what will be done are certainly warranted. A certain positivism at this stage would not be premature, since "the patient with an acute myocardial infarction who survives long enough to reach a Coronary Care Unit has a sixty to seventy percent chance of survival. With proper care and management of complications, the patient's chance of survival increases to eighty to eighty-five percent" (Grace, 1975).

The most common complication following an acute myocardial infarction is dysrhythmias; of particular concern are the ventricular dysrhythmias. Ventricular dysrhythmias are potentially lethal and are usually managed pharmacologically after treating other contributing factors such as electrolyte imbalances, hypoxia, or other drug toxicities. If the patient is to be discharged on an oral antiarrhythmic agent, the drug will most likely be procainamide (Pronestyl) (Meyers et al., 1976), disopyramide phosphate (Norpace) (Danilo, 1976), or quinidine (Meyers et al., 1976). Occasionally, diphenylhydantoin (Dilantin) or propranolol (Inderal) (Meyers et al., 1976) may be used orally in an effort to control ventricular arrhythmias, but these are used less commonly and are certainly not the first drugs of choice.

These patients need to be taught the importance of taking their medication at the designated intervals in order to maintain therapeutic blood levels of the antiarrhythmic agents. Again, instruction as to dosage, side effects, and toxic effects should be included in the teaching program. It should be stressed that the patient is not to stop taking the medication because of side effects or to skip a dose but instead to notify the physician as soon as possible so that another medication can perhaps be prescribed in place of the offending agent.

Although heart disease cannot actually be cured, neither is it without hope. The damage that occurs in an acute myocardial infarction is permanent, but there are significant compensatory mechanisms that come into play. There is also that intangible but significant element of patient determination, which helps to explain why a patient may suffer an acute myocardial infarction and afterward be in better condition than ever before. The individuals who are motivated to alter their risk factors following an infarction will often derive unexpected benefits and levels of functioning. Those who start exercising regularly, for instance, simply to regain strength and endurance following hospitalization may continue exercising until they are physically in top condition.

Many of the same suggestions for the post-hospitalization phase may be given to both the angina patient and the myocardial infarction patient. Although the life force may have been triumphant, the task of how to go about living is still in question. The family will want to protect and do things for the patient because the memory of what was almost lost remains vivid. Although the motive may be love, the effects can be devastating. The patient needs to resume activities of daily living, such as eating, dressing, walking, and a few household chores, and should engage in some purposeful activity. In the rehabilitation of these patients the focus should be on how to manage the things one must do each day rather than on what may not be done.

Eventually, the patient will again perform an activity that may have been associated with angina or perhaps the actual myocardial infarction. Since this will be a particularly trying experience and a fearful one for the patient and family, they should be prepared. At the time of the acute myocardial infarction, for example, the patient may have been carrying a grandchild, working in a garden, making love, or eating a certain food. Some patients state they simply will never again perform the activity associated with the acute event, and there is some inherent danger in this. Consider the following case.

Mr. C. was admitted to the coronary care unit with a massive anterior septal myocardial infarction that extended laterally with subsequent changes in the inferior leads as well. The patient had a stormy course, a period of cardiogenic shock, and from the night of admission to the day of his discharge from the coronary care unit a month later, Mr. C. maintained that the entire episode was caused by a corned beef sandwich he had eaten on the night of admission.

If Mr. C. is deeply convinced of this, then the logical conclusion would be never to eat corned beef again, implying that the infarction can therefore never happen again. Although this is an attempt to control the situation, it is a misdirected one, and real problems will certainly ensue should the patient fanatically avoid corned beef and yet suffer another myocardial infarction. This patient will likely despair, for although corned beef was avoided, the second myocardial infarction occurred anyway and would likely give rise to an attitude of hopelessness.

It is all but impossible to convince the patient that eating corned beef, or any specific event, probably had very little to do with the acute event, but every effort should be made to teach the patient what myocardial infarctions are, why they occur in terms of the known risk factors, and ways to control these risk factors. The importance of corned beef, for example, should be played down, but no attempt should be made to argue the point. It is terribly important to elicit the patient's perception of the illness as well as misconceptions and associations. Different teaching methods will be needed with patients who have just had their third or perhaps fourth myocardial infarction. Likewise, a patient whose father died at age 64 with a myocardial infarction will most likely be extremely anxious should the patient have an acute myocardial infarction at the same age.

There is a difference between replacing a misconception and trying to dismiss one. Patients need to alter their thinking because a more reasonable explanation or suggestion has been offered, and replacement is often a function of time and repetition.

It is the rare individual with cardiac impairment who escapes the experience of one or more episodes of acute cardiac disequilibrium. Because of the near universality of this experience, consideration of the psychological reactions to such acute cardiac episodes is essential in any discussion of cardiac rehabilitation. Largely as a result of the extensive work of Hackett and Cassem with patients hospitalized following acute myocardial infarction, the *normal* psychological responses to the acute cardiac episode have been carefully documented.

The onset of symptoms of acute myocardial

infarction is universally accompanied by the occurrence of severe anxiety. The anxiety is related to the perceived prospect of sudden death and is intensified by experiences identified by the individual as death's precursors, such as chest pain, dyspnea, and weakness. Further compounding this terror is the realization that the situation is totally beyond the patient's control, an experience that can be significantly heightened by admission to the unfamiliar world of the coronary care unit. Acute myocardial infarction is indeed a crisis, "... a sudden and unanticipated disruption of extensive and protracted significance in everyday activities, understandings and expectations ..." (Davis, 1972).

Although individual reactions to this overwhelming anxiety vary somewhat, the almost universal coping mechanism in reaction to a myocardial infarction is denial, "the conscious or unconscious repudiation of part or all of the total available meaning of an event to allay fear, anxiety, or other unpleasant effects" (Hackett, et al., 1969). The degree to which denial is used will vary with the individual. With few exceptions, denial in the acute phase of cardiac disequilibrium is an appropriately adaptive response. The effectiveness of denial is thought by Hackett to bear an inverse relationship to mortality from acute myocardial infarction. Assuming that the normal individual will set up some system of denial, it becomes the responsibility of the care givers to support, within the scope of reality, the patient's denial. The patient's description of an uncle who successfully recovered from an acute myocardial infarction should be listened to. Specific occurrences indicating stability of the patient's condition should be discussed with the patient, such as "You haven't had any extra heartbeats during the last four hours; your blood pressure has been normal every time I've checked it today." Because of the ever-present possibility of cardiac arrest in the CCU, the nurse should assure patients that each cardiac problem is different. This information is essential to patients who may witness the cardiac arrest of another patient.

No matter how effective the patient's denial mechanisms, anxiety remains a factor during the acute cardiac episode. Telling the patient that such a response is normal and expected may alleviate unnecessary expenditure of energy to mask this reaction. Judicious use of sedation during the acute cardiac episode is a most appropriate treatment modality and, if anything, is underplayed all too often.

On occasion, excessive denial becomes problematic in terms of compliance with the therapeutic regimen. Such a response is outside the realm of normal behavior and warrants attention and intervention of a more sophisticated nature. The availability of psychiatric consultation during the acute cardiac episode has become more prevalent and should be utilized in planning the management of this and other behavior problems.

The third day following an acute myocardial infarction usually heralds the onset of depression, another almost universal response to acute cardiac disequilibrium. The depression comes as a response to real and perceived losses, the focus being a fundamental threat to self-esteem. Again, this is a normal response; in the best of situations, depression represents an acceptance of the current situation and an attempt to come to terms with it. First and foremost, the patient and family need to know that this is a normal response, that grieving must be done in order to deal effectively with loss. The sadness that accompanies the restitution phase of grieving must be identified as temporary. Reflections on the successful handling of previous losses can be productive, particularly if family members can be engaged in these reflections. Helping the patient and family to maintain a future orientation can be therapeutic. Awareness that the individual with cardiac impairment is assailed with losses must be the guiding factor in planning a teaching program. Too much emphasis on *not* smoking, *not* gaining weight, and the like can be counterproductive in terms of long-range rehabilitative efforts. Individualization of teaching programs must be based on prior determination of the assigned significance of various losses to each individual and family unit; while certain assumptions can be made, it remains clear that how one *reacts* to what happens is immensely more important than what *actually* happens. Perhaps a nurse's greatest burden is to find out not what has happened to the patient, but what it means to the person and what the person intends to do about it. It is in the latter two areas that nurses often have their greatest impact. Human nature is such that most of us do not readily reveal our innermost doubts and concerns to another. As nurses interested in rehabilitation, we need to determine what meaning the patient attaches to experiencing cardiac impairment. This is asking for very private, personal information, and consequently, it is important that the person attempting to elicit the information be a consistent presence in the patient's environment and viewed by the patient as one who is truly interested. Those having only brief or sporadic involvement with the patient can only hope to begin the process of rehabilitation. Finally, in the realm of anticipatory guidance, the individual and family need to be assisted in realizing that transition through the various stages of the recovery process may revive the feelings of loss; a renewed experience with depression, for instance, is a normal reaction immediately following hospital discharge.

The patient may exhibit anxiety, bitterness, anger, clingingness, depression, hopelessness, and occasionally a seemingly genuine acceptance of whatever is to come. The latter is most often seen in the elderly person who talks freely about not really minding whether the acute cardiac episode is fatal or not. These are the patients who seem to have come to terms with their life's work, have families who are flourishing, and say that if they do survive they will enjoy their grandchildren a bit longer, and if not, they will have enjoyed life thus far and it has been enough.

Fortunately, for the majority of persons with cardiac impairment, depression is resolved by the passage of time, accompanied by real as well as perceived progress in the recouping of losses by return to familiar territory with a specifically prescribed program for reinstitution of important activities and relationships.

Most rehabilitative nursing activity should be directed to the teaching component of patient care. The teaching plan, to be at all effective in restoring the individual to optimal levels of functioning, self-esteem, and compliance, must be individualized to reach each unique individual while general enough to provide the information necessary for attaining maximal cardiac function with minimal risk.

PATIENT TEACHING

Nurses must assume the responsibility for patient teaching as an integral part of care delivery. The art and science of our profession equips us to aid the patient in returning to a state of health according to individual capabilities, but the patient's cooperation is essential to any maintenance of that state of health. "Perhaps a universally useful description of health is that of a state in which a person may live a satisfying life which makes a contribution to his society" (Kintzel, 1971). Essentially, nurses should help patients give up the patient role and teach them ways to avoid assuming that role again in the future. One must realize that the patient with an uncomplicated hospital course will have a relatively brief stay, perhaps 2 to 3 weeks. During this brief time, the patient will have suffered the acute phase, the accompanying emotional reactions, and the psychological impact and is expected to have begun the rehabilitation/planning phase that is an integral part of the teaching plan. It is important to note that it is the patient, as well as the nurse, who experiences a great deal in a short period of time. Ideally, in order to help the patient during this time, one nursing staff member should assume responsibility for the implementation of the teaching plan. For the majority of patients, learning needs will extend into the posthospitalization phase, and appropriate referrals to community resources should be considered. Before rehabilitation can begin, some degree of assessment must be made of the patient's background, the meaning of the present condition to the patient, and what lies within the realm of the reasonable and the possible for each patient. As William Osler once said, "It's more important to know what sort of patient has a disease than what sort of disease a patient has" (Slay, 1976). Table 29-1 is an example of a patient assessment guide that addresses the major points that should be considered in patient teaching.

The patient's age should be considered in any teaching program because as people get older, the rate at which they learn decreases. Ethnic groups are not easily absorbed, nor are cultures readily diluted. Some patients may have learned only enough English to ensure survival in our portion of the world but may do better if explanations and instructions are given in their primary language so examples can be utilized.

Information regarding a patient's previous hospitalization is important to screen out problem areas, as well as those topics to which the patient may have already had exposure. Mental acuity at the time of the planned teaching activity is of obvious importance. In teaching, we hope to

Table 29-1

Patient Assessment Guide

CATEGORY	EXAMPLE OF NOTATION
Age:	52-M
Language ability:	English, no hearing impairment
Previous hospitalizations:	Yes, MI 2 years previously
Mental acuity:	Alert, cooperative, inquisitive
Apparent degree of illness:	No acute distress, comfortable
Present emotional state:	Anxious to know results of angiography, wants bypass surgery
Patient's and family's perception of illness and treatment:	The patient has had a steadily decreasing exercise capacity; knows he is hospitalized for evaluation for coronary bypass; does not understand ASHD and anginal pain nor what a bypass involves
Cultural differences:	None, citizen by birth
Educational level:	Intelligent, completed high school, and worked with space program until retirement; seems mechanically inclined
Active family member:	Married, lives with wife; relationship seems good; active with children and grandchildren
Socioeconomic status:	Retired, good pension
Physical environment:	In bed 2 by window, roommate ambulates out of room frequently

affect the patient's attitudes, knowledge, and in some cases skill, all of which require, at the very least the patient's cooperation, but ideally we strive for intellectual agreement, assuming compliance will ensue. Attention is altered drastically by many factors, for example pain, which would make it necessary to assess the patient's apparent degree of illness before planning a teaching program. A patient who has a fever, is nauseated, still has chest tubes in place, or is just managing to control existing anxiety will not be amenable to lengthy, involved teaching attempts, if indeed the patient will care to talk at all.

Items 6, 7, and 8 on the patient teaching assessment guide center on the point from which one begins teaching. If the patient is a science professor, for example, then the nurse can shorten the anatomy explanations and spend more time on the possible modalities of therapy. Should the patient be a construction worker who refuses to admit that the acute myocardial infarction occurred, then the thrust of the teaching program will be altered. If a patient happens to believe that the current state of illness is God's will and is to be accepted as such, he or she will accept very little teaching. This patient sees the condition as unchangeable and indeed one that should not be changed even if it were possible.

Likewise, the nurse should ascertain whether the patient's family views the patient as terminal and in need of care or as having a reasonable chance of resuming purposeful activity with help. Whoever the active family member happens to be, that member should be included in the teaching program, for one loving, well-meaning family member can unwittingly undo a great deal of progress and teaching in a short time. It is a mistake to assume that the significant other is a spouse, for marriages can be held together by forces that defy labels. Often, one can simply ask, "Who do you see as the most important person in your life?" If that person is a child, grandchild, cousin, neighbor, or spouse, every effort should be made to include those who are most important to the patients and to the life they are to lead in the future. If the person who suffered the cardiac impairment is intellectually unable to comprehend the essential components of a teaching plan, the significant others assume an even more crucial role.

The patient's educational level needs to be considered, obviously, but this information is often difficult to elicit tactfully. Asking "What is the highest grade you completed in school?" puts whatever answer is given in a more positive light and seems to work well in obtaining the information without putting the patient on the defensive. Depending on the patient's educational level, the problem can be described as "increasing myocardial oxygen consumption" or simply as "making the heart work too hard." The art of patient teaching lies in striking a chord familiar enough in the patient to prompt future recall.

Since most people are somewhat easily distracted, the nurse should select a location for patient teaching that is out of the mainstream of traffic and that is cheerful and private, or at least open only to those with similar interests and concerns. It is also essential to create an atmosphere that allows questions to be asked.

In using the patient assessment guide, the patient's previous hospitalization and perceptions of the illness and treatment will determine the teaching needs. The patient's language ability, mental acuity, present emotional state, cultural differences, and educational level will determine the content of the teaching program. The actual presentation is determined by the patient's language ability, mental acuity, degree of illness, and physical environment.

As a general rule, patients tend to ask what they need to know, hear what they can handle, and assimilate what makes sense to them. Practically speaking, individual teaching is not done on a large scale but is handled primarily in a group setting. Patients find it comforting to share their experiences with each other, which often acts to decrease the sense of isolation. This brings us to the first pitfall in patient teaching—that of making dogmatic pronouncements. When we presume in youth and health to tell others of their fate and offer advice, we run the risk of being totally dismissed. How patients often feel toward us as teachers was eloquently stated by Job in the Bible, when he said: "I also could talk as you do, were you in my place." Our only real contribution is the knowledge we possess, and we must impart that knowledge in such a way that it becomes a part of the lives and one of the driving forces behind the future actions of those we teach. If we do not do so, we fail in teaching.

Any information given to a patient should be based on information the patient already has, for according to Jost's law, older associations are strenghtened by practice rather than newer ones. Whatever information the patient specifically asks for will have the biggest impact, so every effort should be made to answer questions reasonably and as they are asked.

A final rule of thumb in teaching centers on the fact that any information that is given will be retained longer the more senses that are involved in the learning process. Consequently, posters, pictures, models, pamphlets, and/or tape recordings are all helpful. However, the authors have found that, in practice, the large-scale, color-coded heart models are sometimes difficult to teach with for several reasons. Some patients find the model distasteful, some models are often larger than life size, and patients often get distracted by the intricate, albeit accurate detail. It is difficult to teach a class in anatomy while also explaining blue pulmonary arteries, red pulmonary veins, or the fat globules often pictured on the surface of the heart. A poster with basic heart structures, that is, one showing the four heart chambers, the valves, and the outflow tract of each ventricle, is often more helpful. Most teaching programs discuss anatomy, diet, physical activity, and the patient's emotional reactions on separate days to avoid bombarding the patient with too much information at one time.

Most of the difficulties one encounters in a teaching program center on patient unwillingness to hear what the nurse has to say, difficulty by the nurse in imparting the information, patient misunderstanding, or the patient's confusion about what to do with the information. These difficulties imply a need to review some of the initial groundwork, but they are by no means insurmountable problems.

While the patient's friends and family are relieved to know simply that the patient will live, it is the patient who is plagued by the unanswered question of *how* one is going to go on living. As President Johnson stated during an interview with Walter Cronkite, "Once you've had a heart attack it's always there." Patient teaching is aimed not at making the patient forget but at answering the "how" of going on with life. It is a common phenomenon for patients to separate time into two segments—before myocardial infarction and after the infarction, with the presumption that afterward, things can no longer be the same. A teaching plan is aimed at emphasizing those things that can remain the same while educating the patient and family about the risk factors, especially those that can be controlled.

RISK FACTORS

No program designed for rehabilitation of the person who has experienced cardiac impairment should fail to attend to the risk factors, those factors which, if present, make an individual more prone to development of atherosclerosis and therefore to heart disease. Certainly, educating the public regarding the risk factors is an essential task and clearly within the realm of all health professionals. Dietary, exercise, and smoking habits are learned in childhood. Emphasis in this area is clearly more successful than attempting to change long-established "bad habits." Prevention of atherosclerosis can certainly be seen as early rehabilitation. Information about these risk factors, as well as assistance in changing one's behavior in the appropriate areas, must be provided in the context of the overall teaching program for cardiac-impaired individuals and their families. Risk factors can be thought of as falling into two general categories, those that are unchangeable and those that are subject to change. Unalterable risk factors are heredity, increasing age, and being of the male sex.

Clearly, none of these factors are within an individual's control, but awareness of these risk factors can affect the individual in terms of possible increased motivation to deal with those risks over which control is possible. In any discussion of risk factors, those that can be controlled should be emphasized, such as cigarette smoking, hypertension, diabetes, obesity, sedentary life-style, elevation of blood cholesterol and/or triglycerides, and response to stress.

"Warning: The Surgeon General has determined that cigarette smoking is dangerous to your health." Since 1964, Americans have been acquainted with the relationship of coronary atherosclerosis and smoking. The scientific data at this time strongly *suggest* that cigarette smoking increases the incidence of atherosclerosis; the data *indict* cigarette smoking in increasing the complications of atherosclerosis. Clearly, the Surgeon General's report, again updated in 1979, has had its positive effects on the smoking behavior of Americans, although certainly not to the extent that it should have had. A significant number of persons suffering from cardiac impairment are predictably smokers. Without exception, these individuals must be advised to avoid cigarette smoking. Nicotine is known to increase the heart rate, and it also causes sympathetic stimulation. Probably more harmful than tar and nicotine is the inhalation of carbon monoxide in cigarette smoke. Carbon monoxide decreases the oxygen-carrying capacity of the blood, thus further compromising coronary blood flow. The most effective method for stopping smoking varies among individuals; approximately one in three individuals who make a systematic effort to stop smoking will succeed (McIntosh et al., 1978). The support of a group effort in changing behavior such as smoking should be noted. Whether it be family members or friends who "quit" together or participation in a more formalized group such as the American Cancer Society's "I Quit" clinics, all available supports must be rallied in an effort to effect this very necessary change in behavior.

Hypertension and diabetes are unquestionably linked to increased risk of development of atherosclerosis. The clear relationship of peripheral vascular resistance to cardiac work has been described earlier in this text. The effect of therapeutic control of these accompanying chronic diseases must be stressed to the cardiac-impaired individual. Whether this control is within the realm of dietary intake alone or in conjunction with adherence to a medication regimen, the individual and family members must be given the necessary dietary information and assistance. As with any of the risk factors that require modification of previously pleasant but maladaptive behavior patterns, change will result only if the individual identifies some significant benefits of the change. Initial motivation may well be the strictly negative factor of fear brought on by the acute episode; for long-term behavior modification to occur, this fear must be replaced by more positive reinforcers, such as "feeling better," enhanced self-esteem resulting from ability to control behavior, and the like. It is likewise essential to make compliance with the medication regimen as feasible as possible. If two drugs are available with similar pharmacological effects but different costs, the patient is more likely to continue to take the less expensive of the drugs.

Closely linked to control of diabetes and hypertension are the other diet-related risk factors, obesity and elevation of blood cholesterol and/or triglycerides. Clearly an extensive topic of and by itself, the dietary implications of cardiac disease are more appropriately treated in a text that emphasizes the intricacies of such treatment modalities. Though still controversial, at this time a diet low in cholesterol and saturated fats is being recommended for diminution of the dietary risks for atherosclerosis. Control of caloric and sodium intake is also recommended in reducing risk from hypertension and obesity. Suffice it to say that patients and their families must be provided with a dietary prescription that is clear, palatable, and realistic. Attention must be given to the patient's financial resources, cultural dietary habits, and life-style if the dietary prescription is to be followed over time.

The relationship of a sedentary life-style to

increased risk for atherosclerosis is well documented. It is likewise clear that regular, graded exercise alone has a favorable impact on reduction of other risk factors. The specifics of exercise programs are treated elsewhere in this text.

Finally, it is clear that individual style of responding to stress affects one's risk for development of atherosclerosis. To propose that an individual living in the twentieth-century American culture avoid stress is foolhardy. To counsel people to deal more effectively with the inevitable stress of our society is essential. Again, it is not the stressful stimulus as much as the reaction to it that takes its toll on our cardiovascular well-being. Acquaintance with Friedman's work on the coronary-prone individual's response to potential stress provokers is essential for nurses in their counseling efforts.

Individual and group discussions with cardiac-impaired persons and their families can be very productive both in provision of necessary information and in dealing with feelings about the need for change in behaviors and life-styles. Written information about alteration of risk factors should be included in teaching programs. References to this material following discharge can be invaluable in reinforcing learning, as well as in answering questions that arise at a time when the individual lacks direct access to health care professionals. Numerous pamphlets written for the public on risk factors are available through local chapters of the American Heart Association.

ACTIVITY-EXERCISE CONSIDERATIONS

Any teaching program for persons with cardiac impairment must include a detailed activity-exercise component. Given the multitude of variables, such as the particular cardiac impairment, the psychologic reaction of the individual and family, the possibility of other superimposed medical problems, the various cultural, socioeconomic, and religious considerations, how does one proceed with the business of setting up an activity-exercise program for the person experiencing cardiac impairment?

The initial consideration in cardiac rehabilitation must be a determination of the actual limitations imposed on the individual by his or her cardiovascular status—no small task nor by any means a static criterion. This involves placing the individual into a functional classification such as that developed by the New York Heart Association (see Table 29-2). Determination of an individual's functional class requires a great deal of clinical skill and acumen and, other than for episodes of acute cardiac disequilibrium, tends to be situationally variable. The person with mitral stenosis may be functionally Class II with deterioration to Class III during episodes of upper respiratory infection. A construction worker may be functionally Class II when working at his trade but Class I when changed to a less strenuous type of work.

An understanding of ergometry in relation to functional classification allows for meaningful translation of cardiovascular capabiliies to functional activities. The measure of energy cost of any activity can be expressed in terms of the metabolic equivalent (MET). One MET is equivalent to 3.0 to 4.0 mL of oxygen consumption per kilogram of body weight per minute (VO_2), or the energy expended when at rest in the supine, sitting, or standing position (Rusk, 1977). Walking at 3.5 miles per hour expends 5.5 METs. As indicated in Table 34-2, the functional classification can be further characterized by the maximal METs that will be tolerated by the individual in a given category.

A more scientific and individualized determination of activity tolerance of the individual with cardiac impairment is possible with the use of the multistage exercise test. The specifics of exercise testing are available in other texts; briefly, the cardiovascular capabilities of the individual can be measured by subjecting an individual to graded levels of controlled exercise, most commonly walking on a treadmill, while continuously monitoring ECG heart rate, blood pressure, and subjective awareness of such things as fatigue, chest pain, and palpitations. The results of the exercise test determine the workload at which the oxygen transport system comes

Table 29-2

New York Heart Association Classification: Sustained and Intermittent Workloads

FUNCTIONAL CLASSIFICATION	PHYSIOLOGICAL SYMPTOMS	MAXIMAL cal/min SUSTAINED	MAXIMAL cal/min INTERMITTENT	MAXIMAL MET
I	Persons with cardiac disease but without resulting limitations of physical activity; ordinary physical activity does not cause undue fatigue, palpitation, dyspnea, or anginal pain.	5.0	6.6	6.5
II	Persons with cardiac disease resulting in slight limitation of physical activity; they are comfortable at rest; ordinary physical activity results in fatigue, palpitation, dyspnea, or anginal pain.	2.5	4.0	4.5
III	Persons with cardiac disease resulting in marked limitation of physical activity; they are comfortable at rest; less than ordinary physical activity causes fatigue, palpitation, dyspnea, or anginal pain.	2.0	2.7	3.0
IV	Persons with cardiac disease resulting in inability to carry on any physical activity without discomfort; symptoms of cardiac insufficiency or of the anginal syndrome may be present even at rest; if any physical activity is undertaken, discomfort is increased.	1.5	2.0	1.5

Source: Howard A. Rusk, *Rehabilitation Medicine,* Mosby, St. Louis, 1977.

close to its capacity without the occurrence of pathologic responses. Based on these measurements, the individual can be given specific information about activities that are likely to be tolerated (see Tables 29-3 and 29-4). This information is reliable to the degree that any given activity is the sole user of energy at a given time, that is, driving a car requires expenditure of 2 METs, but fuming behind the wheel in a traffic jam increases the energy expenditure considerably.

A given workload requires a given amount of energy; it is conceivable, then, that equally efficient individuals of the same weight performing the same task will require the same amount of oxygen. In reality, the well-conditioned individual will be able to work at much higher intensities than the poorly conditioned person. This increased tolerance is related to the fact that a well-conditioned individual works with a slower heart rate, pumping more blood with each beat—hence the value of exercise programs for the person who has experienced cardiac impairment. The exercise program for each individual must be based on a specific prescription and must be subject to periodic reevaluation by the physician.

It is a definite advantage that in this era, it is really not necessary to "sell" the idea of exercise, for exercise is very much in vogue. The concept of physical fitness itself is appealing; the idea of not being "soft" is an image represented by such organizations as the President's Council on Physical Fitness. Exercise is vital to any reducing plan,

Table 29-3

Metabolic Costs of Occupational Activities

ACTIVITY	MET	V_{O_2} (mL/kg per min)
Sitting: light or moderate work		
Sitting at desk, writing, calculating, etc.	1.5	4.25
Driving a car	1.5	4.25
Using hand tools, doing light assembly work, radio repair, etc.	1.8	5.30
Driving a truck	1.8	5.30
Working heavy levers, dredge, etc.	2.0	7.0
Riding mower, etc., as individual work	2.5	8.75
Sitting, e.g., for a crane operator's job	2.5	8.75
Driving heavy truck or trailer rig (must include getting on and off frequently and doing some arm work)	3.0	10.5
Standing: moderate work		
Standing quietly, assembling light or medium machine parts where speed is not a factor, working at own pace or a moderate rate	2.5	8.75
Just standing, e.g., bartending	2.5	8.75
Using hand tools (gas station operator, other jobs where these are used other than assembly work all day)	2.7	9.45
Scrubbing, waxing, polishing (floors, walls, cars, windows)	2.7	9.45
Assembling or repairing heavy machine parts such as farm machinery, plumbing, airplane motors, etc.	3.0	10.5
Light welding	3.0	10.5
Stocking shelves, packing or unpacking small or medium objects	3.0	10.5
Sanding floors with a power sander	3.0	10.5
Janitorial work	3.0	10.5
Kneeling or squatting while doing light work	3.0	10.5
Assembling light or medium machine parts on assembly line or working with tools on line when objects appear at an approximate rate of 500 times a day or more	3.5	12.25
Working on assembly line when parts require lifting at about every 5 min or so; lifting involves only a few seconds at a time (parts weigh 45 lb or less)	3.5	12.25
Same as above (parts weigh over 45 lb)	4.0	14.0

Table 29-3 (continued)

Metabolic Costs of Occupational Activities

ACTIVITY	MET	V_{O_2} (mL/kg per min)
Cranking up dollies, hitching trailers, operating large levers, jacks, etc.	3.5	12.25
Pulling on wires, twisting cables, jerking on ropes, cables, etc., such as rewiring houses	3.5	12.25
Masonry, painting, paperhanging	4.0	14.0
Walking: moderate work		
Walking 3.0 mph	3.0	10.5
3.5 mph	4.0	14.0
Carrying trays, dishes, etc.	4.2	14.70
Walking involved in gas station mechanic work (changing tires, wrecker work, etc.)	4.5	15.75
Standing and/or walking: heavy arm work		
Lifting and carrying objects		
20–44 lb (9–20 kg)	4.5	15.75
45–64 lb (20–29 kg)	6.0	21.0
65–84 lb (30–38 kg)	7.5	26.25
85–100 lb (39–45 kg)	8.5	29.75
Heavy tools		
Pneumatic tools (jackhammers, drills, spades, tampers)	6.0	21.0
Shovel, pick, runner bar	8.0	28.0
Moving, pushing heavy objects, 75 lb or more		
Desks, file cabinets, heavy stock furniture, such as moving van work. Also, pushing against heavy spring tension, as in boiler room, etc.	8.0	28.0
Pushing a cart or dolly with objects weighing	4.2	14.70
Less than 75 lb		
75 lb or more	4.5	15.75
Other responses		
Laying railroad track	7.0	24.5
Cutting trees, chopping wood		
Automatically	3.0	10.5
Hand axe or saw	5.5	19.25
Carpentry		
Activities involved in interior repair or remodeling (laying of tile, painting, etc.)	4.0	14.0

Table 29-3 (continued)

Metabolic Costs of Occupational Activities

ACTIVITY	MET	V_{O_2} (mL/kg per min)
Building and finishing interior of house or garage	4.5	15.75
Putting in sidewalk (digging, carrying concrete, etc)	5.0	17.5
Exterior remodeling or construction of house or garage (hammering, sawing, planing, etc.)	6.0	21.0
General heavy industrial labor Handyman work, some moving, some heavy work, such as shoveling, carpentry, etc.	5.0	17.5

Source: Based on material from M. J. Karvonen and A. J. Barry (eds.): *Physical Activity and the Heart,* Charles C Thomas, Springfield, Ill., 1967 (Supplemental Readings #9). Used by permission of the Charles C Thomas Company.

and again, it is fashionable to be thin. Any cardiac patient who is overweight will be instructed to lose weight in an effort to control obesity, one of the recognized risk factors of coronary artery disease. We are becoming a health-conscious people as a whole and are seeing a surge of interest in participation in sports, health clubs, and exercising equipment.

The exercise program may involve individual activities or group exercise. The important factor is adherence to the exercise program at regular intervals, usually at a minimum of three times per week. Whether an exercise training program can prolong the life of the cardiac-impaired individual remains to be determined; it is clear, however, that regular exercise enhances the quality of life of such individuals.

Enough for the generalities. What specific counsel regarding activity-exercise do the cardiac-impaired persons and their families require? First and foremost, the cardiovascular capacity must be determined, either empirically or on the basis of an exercise test. Activities predicted to be within the realm of tolerance may then be listed for the individual either in verbal discussion or by providing a list such as those in Tables 29-3 and 29-4. To predict each and every activity that any individual may engage in is virtually impossible. Having the individual compile a list of questions, a prediction of a "typical" day's activities, a description of the physical home environment, and a listing of social support persons can be invaluable prior to developing an individualized activity plan. Involvement of the person in planning the activity program is also likely to achieve increased investment in and subsequent compliance with the plan.

The individual living in a walk-up apartment who must climb three flights of stairs faces a set of issues different from the suburban, trilevel home dweller. The young woman recovering from surgical mitral valve replacement while assuming the sole responsibility for the care of her pre-school children needs to make entirely different plans than the elderly man who is welcomed into the home of his adult children

Table 29-4

Average Metabolic Costs of Leisure Activities

ACTIVITY	MET	V_{O_2} (mL/kg per min)
Car driving, flying, model ship building	1.5	4.25
Darts, motorcycling (pleasure)	2.0	7.0
Model plane flying, mowing lawn (riding mower), power boating, shooting (rifle or pistol), shuffleboard, woodworking	2.5	8.75
Car washing, croquet, mechanical work on car	2.7	9.45
Billiards, pool, bowling, canoeing (2.5 mph), fishing (from boat, bank, or ice), horseshoe pitching, plane building, shopping, wood cutting (power equipment)	3.0	10.5
Boat racing, driving a horse (sulky), horseback riding, ice boating, sailing (handling the boat)	3.5	12.25
Archery, baling hay, caring for horses, cycling (5.5 mph), farm work (sporadic), golf, table tennis, tetherball	4.0	14.0
Military marching, mowing lawn (power mower, not riding)	4.5	15.75
Gardening (weeding, hoeing, digging, spading), lawn work (raking, digging, filling), social dancing, softball or baseball (nonteam, nongame, officiating)	5.0	17.5
Cycling (9.4 mph), fishing (wading in stream), hiking (cross-country), hunting, mowing lawn (push mower), shoveling (10/min–9 lb), softball or baseball (team game), square dancing, water skiing, water volleyball	6.0	21.0
Badminton, canoeing (4.0 mph), scuba diving, tennis	7.0	24.5
Basketball (nongame), basketball (officiating), football (touch), motorcycling (endurance runs), mountain climbing, snow skiing, soccer (nonteam)	8.0	28.0
Swimming		
Backstroke 40 yd/min	8.0	28.0
Breaststroke 40 yd/min	9.0	31.5
Crawl 45 yd/min	9.5	3.25
Cycling (13 mph), shoveling (10/min—14 lb)	9.0	31.5
Fencing, football (competition), gymnastics, snow sledding, tobogganing	10.0	35.0

Table 29-4 (continued)

Average Metabolic Costs of Leisure Activities

ACTIVITY	MET	V_{O_2} (mL/kg per min)
Basketball (game play), canoeing or rowing (competition), hockey (ice), judo, handball, paddleball, soccer, space ball, squash, trampolining, wrestling	12.0	42.0
Shoveling (10/min—23 lb)	15.0	26.25

Source: Based on material from M. J. Karvonen and A. J. Barry (eds.): *Physical Activity and the Heart,* Charles C Thomas, Springfield, Ill., 1967 (Supplemental Readings #9). Used by permission of the Charles C Thomas Company.

while recuperating from an acute myocardial infarction. Examples such as these could be provided ad infinitum; suffice it to say, the closer the teaching plan is to the real-life situations of the individuals involved, the greater will be the learning that occurs.

Almost as significant as the actual activity is the *timing* of the activity. A realistic plan of activity interspersed with rest periods should be discussed. Meals should be considered as an activity and should always be followed by a short period of rest. In addition, an individual's personal preferences should be determined; a person with limited cardiovascular capacity may, for instance, prefer a brief shopping expedition over showering.

Somehow, the person must develop the confidence of feeling in touch with his or her body. Patients often ask, "How will I know if I'm doing too much?" Measurable parameters of cardiovascular status should be taught; for example, most adults are able to learn to count their radial pulse. Weakness and fatigue, while notably very subjective parameters, can be valuable guideposts in evaluating one's own response to activity. The person being discharged from an acute hospital episode needs to be assured, however, that the initial weakness is usually more a result of the deconditioning effects of bed rest and hospitalization than an actual indicator of cardiovascular fitness and that the weakness will gradually subside. Certainly, symptoms such as chest pain, palpitations, and dyspnea occurring with an activity should alert the individual to the possibility of cardiovascular strain, and if such symptoms are unusual, they should be reported to the physician.

SEXUAL ACTIVITY

In discussing activity-exercise tolerance and recommendations for the person who has experienced cardiac impairment, one specific area seems to require special attention—sexual activity. Few individuals with cardiac impairment leave the health care setting uninformed about the dos and don'ts of walking up the stairs, driving a car, or shoveling snow. Similar counsel must be provided in the area of sexual activity. Fear, ignorance, and misinformation regarding sexual activity can do nothing but contribute to the feelings of anxiety and depression so universally experienced by the cardiac-impaired individual.

The great majority of cardiac-impaired individuals are able to engage in normal sexual activity (Scalzi and Dracup, 1978). This finding is based on numerous studies indicating that cardiac work and oxygen consumption associated with sexual intercourse with a familiar partner are of moderate intensity in the middle-aged adult (Hellerstein and Friedman, 1970). For middle-aged men, cardiovascular response to sexual intercourse is considered similar to responses to brisk stair climbing (Hellerstein and Friedman). The time for resumption of sexual activity following an acute cardiac episode should be determined by the physician and communicated to the patient, and to the patient's sexual partner when possible. Generally, sexual activity may be resumed within 2 months after an acute myocardial infarction.

Discussion of sexual activity in a private setting by a nonjudgmental, knowledgeable individual will allow questions, fears, and misconceptions to be presented. When appropriate, both partners should be included in such a discussion. Resumption of sexual activity should occur in the least stressful way possible, in familiar and comfortable surroundings, and with a familiar partner. As with other exercise, sexual activity should be reserved for a time in which no other demands are being placed on the cardiovascular system. For instance, 3 h should elapse between eating a heavy meal or consuming alcohol and engaging in sexual intercourse. Foreplay should be encouraged, as it gradually prepares the heart for the increased demands of intercourse. Positions for intercourse should be based on the preferences of the individuals, provided breathing remains unrestricted. Oral-genital sex should place no excess strain on the cardiovascular reserve of the cardiac-impaired individual. Anal intercourse does increase stress to the heart and should be specifically discussed between patient and physician. The individual should be cautioned to allow for a period of rest after engaging in sexual intercourse. Showering immediately before or after intercourse should be avoided.

Information regarding problems occurring in association with sexual intercourse must also be discussed and must be presented in a way that will not unduly alarm the individual. The patient should notify the physician of the following: (1) rapid heart and respiratory rate lasting more than 20 min after sexual intercourse; (2) chest pain during intercourse; (3) palpitations lasting more than 15 min following intercourse; (4) sleeplessness following intercourse; or (5) unusual fatigue the day after intercourse.

Participation in graded exercise programs will, as discussed, increase activity tolerance over time by increasing cardiovascular fitness. For these individuals, the increased cardiovascular capacity may lead to improved sexual functioning.

Intolerance of sexual activity, whether as a result of symptoms, arrhythmias, and/or fear on the part of either partner, presents a significant dilemma, and one that goes beyond the limits of this text. Individuals with such problems should be referred to appropriate counselors.

As significant as the cardiac-impaired individual's ability to be sexually active is the threat to sexual identity and role that frequently accompanies cardiac impairment. Christopherson (1968) discusses this threat in terms of role modification: "After acquiring a disability, he finds much of the structure of his world has changed. The new structure requires new status. Each status will yield different privileges, expectations, rewards, and deprivations and will require assuming new or modified roles." In our society, such role modification tends to be more problematic for men than for women.

Problems with the assumption of new and altered roles in the cardiac-impaired person may be aggravated by the lack of visibility of the cardiac impairment. Society sanctions role modifications of the physically disabled much more readily when the disability is visible. The person who fails to return to work following amputation of a limb is more socially acceptable than the person with seriously compromised cardiovascular capacity who fails to resume a role as "breadwinner."

Cardiac disability can be a particular threat to self-esteem when it causes a change in the traditional sex role. "The sex role image of the American male, which serves as a major referent for his self-concept is that of a fully employed, ablebodied man who assumes all or most of the support of his family" (Christopherson, 1968). The current redefinition of some aspects of traditional sex roles in our society can do nothing but diminish some of these threats. The fact that many individuals with cardiac disability have made constructive sex role modifications indicates the feasibility of such a process with the proper guidance and support.

Often closely linked to the sex role modification is the need to alter the occupational role of the person with severe cardiac impairment. Social service and vocational counselors can be of great assistance in this area and should be involved in cardiac rehabilitation as appropriate. It is hoped that employers who refuse to allow the cardiac-impaired person to continue working will respond, in time, to increased attempts at public education regarding heart disease. Willingness to continue employment of the cardiac-impaired person, even if a change in the type of work assignment is required, will hopefully become more prevalent as more effective cardiac rehabilitation programs become available.

CONCLUSION

Our discussion of the patient who has some degree of cardiac impairment has raised several medical, ethical, and moral decisions that have already begun to demand our attention. Any discussion gives rise to questions and unexplored avenues of thought that lend themselves to consideration. We live in a time when the advances of science have outstripped our ability to contain them, and science has presented us with problems that defy our efforts to label them and solve them with conventional solutions.

Current medical therapy of the cardiac patient has come under discussion in regard to how long the patient requires bed rest, observation, and indeed hospitalization. Attempts at revascularization of the myocardium through coronary artery bypass grafts have become relatively common, and yet the conditions under which surgery is done, the type of patient who will benefit the most, and some evaluation of the efficacy of these grafts in actually prolonging life are being evaluated on a long-term basis.

There is a good chance that it will become standard practice in the future for third-party payers to cover at least part of the cost of patient teaching. At that point, we will have to document the effectiveness of our efforts to control the known risk factors of heart diseases, explore methods of promoting patient compliance, and perhaps consider the value of inpatient rehabilitation of the cardiac patient in a rehabilitation facility.

There is a subset of patients within our population who may require special teaching approaches with special emphases. These are the patients who have had a cardiac arrest and have survived to suffer the so-called Lazarus complex referred to by Hackett and Cassem (1973) and described in detail by Druss and Kornfeld in 1967. In an era when we are redefining the scope of life as well as death, we have a group of patients who feel they have experienced both.

Because of the intricacies involved and the vast knowledge base from which we draw to teach patients, a multidisciplinary approach is encouraged. Ideally, a rehabilitation program would involve a chaplain, physician, nurse, physical therapist, dietician, social worker, occupational therapist, and of course, the family.

What is required of the cardiac patient during rehabilitation is perhaps a strange combination of philosophy, sociology, religion, and hopefully intellectual agreement. The change in life-style or just the possibility of change requires of the patient and family a reconciliation between what is desired and what is possible. The end product comes from the patient, from the patient's beliefs, and from the supports the patient has in life. The nurse's role in all of this is to be there and to care enough to offer knowledgeable guidance. "If he is indeed wise he does not bid you enter the house of his wisdom, but rather leads you to the threshold of your own mind" (Gibran 1970).

BIBLIOGRAPHY

Abraham, A. S., Y. Sever, M. Weinstein, et al.: "Value of Early Ambulation in Patients with and without Complications after Acute Myocardial Infarction," *N Engl J Med*, 292: 719, 1975.

Acker, J. E.: "Are We Mobilizing Early Enough?," *Bibl Cardiol*, 36:50, 1977.

Anagnostopoulos, C. E.: *Acute Aortic Dissections*, University Park Press, Baltimore, 1975.

Baker, K. G., and P. L. McCoy: "Group Sessions as a Method of Reducing Anxiety in Patients with Coronary Artery Disease," *Heart Lung* 8:525–530, 1979.

Bayer, Mary: "Anger in Illness," *Supervisor Nurse*, 8:64–65, June 1977.

Beland, Irene L., and Joyce Passos (eds.): *Clinical Nursing: A Pathophysiological and Psychosocial Approach*, 3d ed., Macmillan, New York, 1975.

Berra, Kathy A., et al.: "The Role of Physical Exercise in the Prevention and Treatment of Coronary Heart Disease," *Heart Lung*, 6: 288, 1977.

Billie, Donald A.: "The Role of Body Image in Patient Compliance and Education," *Heart Lung*, 6:143, 1977.

Blakiston's *Gould Medical Dictionary*, 4th ed., McGraw-Hill, New York, 1979.

Braunwald, Eugene, John Ross, Jr., and Edmund H. Sonenblick: *Mechanisms of Contraction of the Normal and Failing Heart*, Little, Brown, Boston, 1976.

Brest, A. N.: "Management of Refractory Heart Failure," *Prog Cardiovasc Dis*, 12: 558–567, May 1970.

Browning, R. A., et al.: "Angina Pectoris: Recent Advances in Understanding and Implications for Management," *Mo Med*, 70:235–242, April 1973.

Cassem, N. H., and Thomas Hackett: "Psychiatric Consultation in a Coronary Care Unit," *Ann Intern Med*, 75:9–14, July 1971.

———— and ————: "Psychological Rehabilitation of Myocardial Infarction Patients in the Acute Phase," *Heart Lung*, 2:382–387, 1973.

Christopherson, Victor A.: "Role Modifications of the Disabled Male," *Am J Nurs*, 66:290, 1968.

Cole, Collier, et al.: "Brief Sexual Counseling during Cardiac Rehabilitation," *Heart Lung* 8:124–129, 1979.

Cook, Rosa Lee: "Psychosocial Responses to Myocardial Infarction," *Heart Lung* 8:130–135, 1979.

Danilo, Peter, Jr., and Michael R. Rosen: "Cardiac Effects of Disopyramide," *Am Heart J*, 92(12):532–536, October 1976.

Davis, Marcella Z.: "Socioemotional Component of Coronary Care," *Am J Nurs*, 72:705, 1972.

DeBusk, Robert F.: "How to Individualize Rehabilitation after Myocardial Infarction," *Geriatrics*, 77:77, 1977.

Druss, R. G., and D. S. Kornfeld: "Survivors of Cardiac Arrest: Psychiatric Study," *JAMA* 201(5):291–296, 1967.

Exercise Equivalents, Colorado Heart Association, Denver.

Exercise Testing and Training of Apparently Healthy Individuals, American Heart Association, New York, 1972.

Furman, Seymour: "Recent Development in Cardiac Pacing," *Heart Lung* 7:813–826, 1978.

Gardner, Daniel, and Nancy Stewart: "Staff Involvement with Families of Patients in Critical Care Units," *Heart Lung*, 7:105–110, January–February 1978.

Gardner, Daniel, Zane Parzen, and Nancy Stewart: "The Nurse's Dilemma: Mediating Stress in Critical Care Units," *Heart Lung* 9(1):103–106, 1980.

Garrity, Thomas F., and Robert F. Klein: "Emotional Responses and Clinical Severity as Early Determinants of Six-Month Mortality after Myocardial Infarction," *Heart Lung*, 4: 730–737, September–October 1975.

Gentry, W. Doyle: "Emotional and Behavioral Reaction to an Acute Myocardial Infarction," *Heart Lung*, 4:738, 1975.

Gibran, Kahlil: *The Prophet*, Knopf, New York, 1970.

Gilston, Alan, and Leon Resnekov: *Cardio-Respiratory Resuscitation,* F. A. Davis, Philadelphia, 1971.

Glover, Benjamin H.: "Sex Counseling of the Elderly," *Hosp Practice,* 12:109, June 1977.

Goldstein, R. E., et al.: "Medical Management of Patients with Angina Pectoris," *Prog Cardiovasc Dis* 14:360–398, 1972.

Gotz, B. E., and V. P. Gotz: "Drugs and the Elderly," *Am J Nurs* 8:1347–1351, 1978.

Graboys, Thomas: "Clinical Pharmacology of Antiarrhythmic Agents," *Heart Lung* 8:706–710, 1979.

Grace, William J.: "Guide to the Management of the Complications of Acute Myocardial Infarction," *Hosp Med,* 6:27, October 1975.

———, James E. Crockett, and Sylvan L. Weinberg: "Intermediate Care after Myocardial Infarction," *Heart Lung,* 1:818–820, November–December 1972.

Griffith, George C.: "Sexuality and the Cardiac Patient," *Heart Lung,* 2:1, January–February 1973.

Gronim, Sara: "Helping the Client with Unstable Angina," *Am J Nurs* 10:1677–1680, 1978.

Hackett, T. P., et al.: "Detection and Treatment of Anxiety in the Coronary Care Unit," *Am Heart J,* 78:727, 1969.

Hakkila, J.: "The Pros and Cons of Organized Rehabilitation on the Basis of Repeated Short-term Supervised Programs," *Bibl Cardiol,* 36:102, 1977.

Hansen, M. S., S. L. Woods, and R. E. Wills: "Relative Effectiveness of Nitroglycerin Ointment According to Site of Application," *Heart Lung* 8:716–720, 1979.

Harper, I. E., W. T. Connor, M. Hamilton, et al.: "Controlled Trial of Early Mobilization and Discharge from the Hospital in Uncomplicated Myocardial Infarction," *Lancet,* 2:1331, 1971.

Hellerstein, H. R., and E. H. Friedman: "Sexual Activity and the Post-coronary Patient," *Arch Intern Med,* 125:992, 1970.

Hoffman, Margaret, Susan Donchers, and Martha Hauser: "The Effect of Nursing Intervention on Stress Factors Perceived by Patients in a Coronary Care Unit," *Heart Lung,* 7:804–809, 1978.

Johnson, Barbara L., et al.: "Eight Steps to Inpatient Cardiac Rehabilitation," *Heart Lung,* 5:97, 1976.

———, et al.: "Sexual Activity in Exercising Patients After Myocardial Infarction and Revascularization," *Heart Lung,* 7:1026–1031, 1978.

Kamnel, William B., and Thomas Dawber: "Contributors to Coronary Risk Implications for Prevention and Public Health: The Framingham Study," *Heart Lung,* 1:6, November–December 1972.

Karvonen, M. J., and A. J. Barry (eds.): *Physical Activity and the Heart,* Charles C Thomas, Springfield, Ill., 1967.

Kellerman, Jan J., et al.: "Cardiocirculatory Response to Different Types of Training in Patients with Angina Pectoris," *Cardiology,* 62:218, 1977.

Kintzel, Kay C. (ed.): *Advanced Concepts in Clinical Nursing,* Lippincott, Philadelphia, 1971.

Lee, Robert E., and Patricia A. Bael: "Some Thoughts on the Psychology of the Coronary Care Unit Patient," *Am J Nurs,* 75:1498, 1975.

Manwaring, Mary: "What Patients Need to Know about Pacemakers," *Am J Nurs,* 77:825, 1977.

McHenry, Paul L., et al.: "Stress Testing in Coronary Heart Disease," *Heart Lung,* 3:83, 1974.

McIntosh, Henry D., et al.: "A Symposium on Risk Factors in Coronary Artery Disease," *Heart Lung,* 7:126, 1978.

McNeer, I. F., A. G. Wallace, G. S. Wagner, et al.: "The Cause of Acute Myocardial Infarction: Feasibility of Early Discharge of the Uncomplicated Patient," *Circulation,* 51:410, 1975.

Meyers, F. H., E. Jarvetz, and A. Goldfien: *Review of Medical Pharmacology,* 5th ed., Lange, Los Altos, Calif. 1976.

Moore, Karen, et al.: "The Joy of Sex after a Heart Attack," *Nursing '77,* 77:53, 1977.

Nahum, L.: "Angina Pectoris and Coronary Collaterals," *Conn Med* 35:573–574, 1971.

Perloff, J. K., Keith M. Tindgren, and Berton M. Groves: "Uncommon or Commonly Unrecognized Causes of Heart Failure," *Prog Cardiovasc Dis,* 12:5, March 1970.

Physicians' Handbook for Evaluation of Cardiovascular and Physical Fitness, Tennessee Heart Association, Nashville, 1972.

Puksta, Nancy S.: "All About Sex . . . after a Coronary," *Am J Nurs,* 74:1623, 1974.

Preston, Thomas A.: "Future Trends in Pacing," *Heart and Lung* (5):781–782, 1978.

Redman, Barbara Klug: *The Process of Patient Teaching in Nursing,* Mosby, St. Louis, 1972.

Rodman, Morton J., and Dorothy W. Smith: *Pharmacology and Drug Therapy in Nursing,* Lippincott, Philadelphia, 1968.

Rose, G.: "Early Mobilization and Discharge after Myocardial Infarction," *Mod Concepts Cardiovasc Dis,* 41:59, 1972.

Rusk, Howard A.: *Rehabilitation Medicine,* Mosby, St. Louis, 1977.

Scalzi, Cynthia C.: "Nursing Management of Behavioral Responses Following an Acute Myocardial Infarction," *Heart Lung,* 2:1, January–February 1973.

Scalzi, Cynthia, and Kathy Dracup: "Sexual Counseling of Coronary Patients," *Heart Lung,* 7:840, 1978.

Sivarajan, Erika S., et al.: "Low-level Treadmill Testing of Forty-one Patients with Acute Myocardial Infarction Prior to Discharge from the Hospital," *Heart Lung,* 6:975, 1977.

Slay, C. L. "Myocardial Infarction and Stress," *Nurs Clin North Am* 11(2):329–338, 1976.

U.S. Department of Health, Education, and Welfare (Public Health Service): *Smoking and Health: A Report of the Surgeon General,* U.S. Government Printing Office, Washington, D.C., 1964, 1979.

Vincent, Pauline: "The Sick Role in Patient Care," *Am J Nurs,* 75:1172, 1975.

30
linda mills hennig

rheumatic disease

INTRODUCTION

Rheumatic diseases are among the leading causes of incapacity in the United States. Over 100 of these diseases have been recognized and classified by the American Rheumatism Society (Blumberg et al., 1964).

Rheumatic diseases take several forms. They can affect only the joints or muscles, be systemic and involve other organs, be systemic and produce arthralgia without pathologic changes, or be "diffuse connective tissue diseases that affect the musculoskeletal system, skin, and internal organs of the body" (Katz, 1977). Pain, stiffness, and swelling that is referable to the musculoskeletal system are commonalities among the diseases.

Connective tissues provide the supportive framework and protective covering of the body. Bone, periosteum, cartilage, tendon, tendon sheath, ligament, dermis, fascia, and the major part of the blood vessels are classified as connective tissue. Connective tissue diseases are also called collagen diseases, but the former term is currently preferred. The list of connective tissue diseases includes nine rare genetically determined diseases and about nine more common, acquired conditions (*Primer on the Rheumatic Diseases,* 1973).

Most rheumatic and connective tissue diseases are chronic in nature. Chronic diseases are of long duration, often become progressively worse, and may produce irreparable damage to body tissue. Recurrent symptoms may be periodically life-threatening or may necessitate only slight variation in daily activities.

This chapter addresses rheumatoid arthritis, juvenile rheumatoid arthritis, degenerative joint disease, and ankylosing spondylitis. All are rheumatic and chronic diseases. The adult and juvenile forms of rheumatoid arthritis are also classified as connective tissue diseases. Because of the widespread prevalence of rheumatic diseases, nurses in all delivery systems and specialty areas are likely to encounter a person in need of knowledgeable intervention.

Pathophysiology, current medical management, nursing management, and psychological impact on the person will be presented separately for each of the above conditions. The nursing care of patients with selected arthritis surgical procedures, unorthodox treatment, future outlook, and sexual problems are also included.

Although each disease is discussed separately, the reader should bear in mind the one common thread among the majority of persons with these diseases: pain. The experience of chronic pain is very private. It evokes a variety of individual physiological and psychological responses. The reader is referred to other chapters in the text that deal specifically with pain, coping mechanisms, adjustment, and sexuality of persons with disabling conditions.

RHEUMATOID ARTHRITIS

Rheumatoid arthritis (RA) is a connective tissue disease that can affect many tissues of the body. The predominant clinical feature is the presence of inflammation of the joints, producing joint stiffness and pain, that can lead to the destruction of the structural components of the joint. Other symptoms include intermittent fever, fatigue, malaise, and weight loss. The exact incidence of the disease is not known, but the Arthritis Foundation estimate is 6.5 million in the United States (*Data Sheet,* 1978). It strikes women more frequently than men.

The cause of the disease is unknown. Infections, genetic disorders, endocrine disorders, and immunopathogenesis are suspected causes, and yet the role of these factors in producing a pathological condition has not been demonstrated. Some authorities contend that the concept of a single cause for rheumatoid arthritis may be too restrictive (Person & Sharp, 1977). Recent emotional or physiological stress is often documented as a predisposing factor to the onset of symptoms; however, the mechanism of this factor is also unknown.

PATHOLOGY

The disease begins as inflammation of the synovial membrane of a joint, which produces edema, vascular congestion, fibrin exudates, and cellular infiltrate. The synovial fluid often increases in volume, decreases in viscosity, and its cushioning and lubricating effects are lessened. Repeated synovitis and swelling stretches and weakens tendons, ligaments, and supportive structures, leading to joint laxity, instability, and eventual subluxation or dislocation. Pannus, prolific granulation tissues, forms over the surface of the cartilage and often burrows into subchondral bone (*Primer on the Rheumatic Diseases,* 1973).

Any joint can be affected by the rheumatoid process, although it most frequently occurs in joints with a synovial lining. The small joints of the hands and feet are very often involved, and the pattern is usually symmetrical (Katz).

Development of subcutaneous nodules is another common feature. These generally occur over the olecranon and along the ulnar side of the forearm, but they can occur over tendons and in bursae, adhere to periosteum, or develop in the lung or other organs (Katz).

Other extra-articular manifestations include involvement of the heart, lungs, spleen, skin, blood vessels, bone, muscles, nerves, lymphatic system, and eyes. Cysts may develop in the popliteal, antecubital, or para-articular areas. Tenosynovitis is also common, particularly in the hands.

Rheumatoid arthritis is usually not life-threatening; however, certain sequelae of the disease can pose emergency situations. Cervical spine involvement can lead to atlantoaxial subluxation and possible compression on the spinal cord, especially with forceful flexion of the neck. Vasculitis, inflammation of the blood vessels, can produce neuropathies, digital gangrene, and visceral ischemia. Sepsis of a joint also requires aggressive emergency treatment (Goldenberg and Cohen, 1977).

The American Rheumatism Association has adopted diagnostic guidelines entitled "Criteria for Diagnosis and Classification of Rheumatic Diseases" (*Primer on the Rheumatic Diseases,* 1973). These criteria, when met, confirm the diagnosis of either definite, probable, or possible rheumatoid arthritis and aid in differentiation between RA and other rheumatic and connective tissue disorders. Accurate diagnosis for RA is essential in order to initiate appropriate management to reduce inflammation and to combat joint destruction and disability.

DIAGNOSTIC TESTS

Roentgenograms do not necessarily reflect the extent of the disease or the severity of the symptoms. In the early stages of the disease, there may be no abnormalities seen on x-ray. Findings, such as soft tissue swelling, subchondral osteoporosis, joint space narrowing, erosion of joint margins, and joint deformity, corroborate the diagnosis.

No single laboratory test is specific for rheumatoid arthritis, although several are useful in supporting the diagnosis. The erythrocyte sedimentation rate is one of the most important tests for assessing the degree of disease activity. It aids in confirming the presence of a systemic inflammatory process and is a rough index of the degree of involvement (Biundo and Cummings, 1977). A positive serum rheumatoid factor does not confirm rheumatoid arthritis, nor does a negative test rule out the diagnosis; other criteria must be met. Approximately 20 percent of persons who meet American Rheumatism Association (ARA) criteria for rheumatoid arthritis are seronegative for the rheumatoid factor. Approximately 20 percent will have a positive test for antinuclear antibodies. The complete blood count often reveals leukopenia and anemia. An elevated serum enzyme (SGOT) level may be a clue to acute onset of arthritis or may be seen in rheumatic conditions with liver involvement (Biundo and Cummings). Various laboratory analyses may also be done on body tissue and synovial fluid.

COURSE AND PROGRESSION

The onset and progression of RA take many forms. Symptoms may be mild or severe; progression may be insidious or rapid. The individual may experience numerous exacerbations and remissions, either of which may last weeks to years. Short-lived disease activity and spontaneous remission are not uncommon. The term *monocyclic* is used to describe one period of acute disease with a gradual tapering off or "burning out." Residual impairment may be present. *Polycyclic* refers to repeated exacerbations and remissions over time with residual damage. The progressive form of the disease is unrelenting and worsens throughout the life span. A remission does not mean the absence of pain or dysfunction.

Criteria for "Determination of Progression of Rheumatoid Arthritis and of Functional Capacity of Patients with the Disease" have also been adopted by the American Rheumatism Association (*Primer on Rheumatic Diseases,* 1973). These criteria are useful for monitoring the progression of the disease and changes in functional abilities. Other functional classification systems have been developed which more clearly specify the functional level of the patient (Convery et al., 1977; Swezey, 1978).

MEDICATIONS

Numerous medications are used in the management of rheumatic diseases. The drugs can be divided into three major categories: (1) *anti-inflammatory* agents that inhibit inflammation, (2) *analgesics* that relieve pain, and (3) *antirheumatic* drugs that control the systemic features of the disease, such as fatigue, stiffness, anemia, organ involvement, and fever.

Anti-inflammatory Agents

Aspirin (acetylsalicylic acid) is considered to be the drug of first choice in nearly all rheumatic diseases, as it has both analgesic and anti-inflammatory properties. Aspirin is a potent drug and must be used with caution. Some individuals require 4 to 6 g per day. Dosages sufficient to maintain a plasma level of 15 to 30 mg per 100 mL are needed to provide a measurable decrease in inflammation and symptoms. Levels in excess of 30 mg per 100 mL can cause toxicity (Kantor, 1977). Aspirin should be taken daily at regular intervals to maintain an adequate blood level. Timed-release aspirin is beneficial for nighttime use to decrease morning stiffness and pain and to promote rest and sleep. Numerous forms of salicylates are commercially available. Aspirin combined with other substances, such as caffeine, phenacetin, buffering agents, propoxyphene, and other analgesics, is also available. Gastric irritation is the most common adverse reaction. While food in the stomach may retard absorption, it does reduce such gastric distress. Acetaminophen is often prescribed for persons allergic or intolerant to aspirin; however, it has not been demonstrated to have an anti-inflammatory effect.

Indomethacin is a nonsteroidal anti-inflammatory drug that decreases joint inflammation and some systemic symptoms. Response is variable in patients. Some may respond promptly, while others may not see relief for 2 to 3 weeks. This drug is used for symptomatic relief of rheumatoid arthritis, gout, ankylosing spondylitis, and degenerative joint disease; however, it does not alter the disease processes. "The chief problem with indomethacin is that toxicity is closely related to the effective therapeutic range" (Kantor). The most common adverse reaction to this medication is gastrointestinal irritation; therefore, it should be taken with food or milk. Nausea, headaches, and peptic ulcers are frequent side effects. Indomethacin is rarely used in combination with salicylates, for the ulcerogenic effect is potentiated. Ocular disturbances can also occur, thus regular ophthalmologic examinations are indicated in long-term use.

Ibuprofen is a nonsteroidal, anti-inflammatory, and analgesic drug, useful for both rheumatoid arthritis and degenerative joint disease. It does not alter the course of the disease but is helpful for pain relief and reduction of swelling and inflammation. The most common side effect is gastrointestinal intolerance, usually more nausea and indigestion than ulceration. It is reported to be less irritating to gastric mucosa than aspirin. Urticaria and skin rashes are also common side effects. Persons with rheumatoid arthritis usually require higher dosages of the drug than do those with degenerative joint disease. The lowest effective dose is preferred to reduce side effects. It should be taken with food or milk and is not to be taken in combination with aspirin.

Phenylbutazone and oxyphenbutazone are potent anti-inflammatory, analgesic, and antipyretic drugs used to manage acute inflammatory conditions, including rheumatoid arthritis, degenerative joint disease, bursitis, tendinitis, psoriatic arthritis, acute gout, and ankylosing spondylitis. Cutaneous, hematologic, gastrointestinal, and cardiovascular side effects are common and warrant discontinuance of the drug if they appear. These two drugs are most useful for acute inflammatory responses when taken for a period of about 1 week. They are rarely used for long-term management of rheumatic disorders. The hypertensive patient should be monitored closely, as these drugs may cause a rise in blood pressure. Phenylbutazone and oxyphenbutazone potentiate the effect of narcotics and anticoagulant drugs. Bone marrow depression and salt retention are possible severe side effects.

Numerous other compounds are presently used for the treatment of arthritis. These nonsteroidal anti-inflammatory drugs include naproxyn, fenoprofen, tolmetin, and sulindac.

Analgesics

While aspirin is used for the anti-inflammatory effect, it also has anlgesic properties. Propoxyphene is commonly prescribed when aspirin or acetaminophen is insufficient to control pain. Propoxyphene should never be taken with central nervous system depressants, including alcohol, tranquilizers, and sedatives. It is estimated to be the sixth most abused drug in the United States, and overdoses can be fatal (*FDA Drug Bulletin,* 1978).

Codeine may be prescribed alone or in combination with acetaminophen or aspirin for severe pain. Narcotics are best avoided in the management of the arthritides because of the chronic nature of the conditions.

Antirheumatic Agents

When conservative measures and drugs fail to provide adequate control of symptoms, antirheumatic compounds are usually tried. Drugs in this category include gold salts, D-penicillamine, corticosteroids, and antimalarials.

Gold salts have been used for over 50 years in the treatment of rheumatoid arthritis, and yet the exact mechanism of action is still unknown. This drug can produce long-sustained remission when continued indefinitely. If discontinued, there is usually a recurrence of the inflammation. Gold salts are used for persons with persistent rheumatoid activity and for those who do not respond to more conservative drugs. It is available only in injectible form and must be administered into a large muscle. Injections begin with a low dose, 25 mg weekly. If tolerated, dosage is increased to 50 mg weekly for about 6 months or until remission occurs. The frequency of injections is then gradually *decreased* to every 2 weeks, then to every 3 weeks, and eventually to once a month. The lowest possible dose to sustain remission is used. Careful recording of cumulative dosage should be done at each visit. Side effects and toxicity can occur, producing mainly renal, hematologic, and cutaneous problems. A complete blood count and urinalysis are done before each injection. The drug is withheld if the test results are abnormal. The patient should be advised to report any skin rashes, mucosal ulcers, hematuria, and metallic taste in the mouth.

Gold thioglucose is supplied in oil suspension, whereas gold sodium thiomalate is in a solution. A nitritoid crisis can occur following an injection of gold sodium thiomalate. This is a transient phenomenon with symptoms of dizziness, flushing, visual blurring, arthralgia, and a sensation of warmth. The patient should be observed for at least 1 h following the first injection of this drug. Reaction rarely occurs following gold thioglucose.

D-Penicillamine is a compound that has been demonstrated to provide improvement of systemic manifestations of rheumatoid arthritis in some patients. It is especially effective for the severe vasculitis that may be present with RA. The exact mechanism of the drug is not understood. Dosage is started low, 250 mg daily in a single oral dose. Dosage is increased as tolerated every 2 to 4 weeks and given four times a day. Rarely is more than 1000 mg daily prescribed, and the maintenance dose is usually much lower. Absorption of the drug is best when taken about 1 1/2 h after a meal. It should be separated from administration of other drugs by approximately 1 h. Response may take 3 months or longer, and thus other drugs for arthritis are continued until marked improvement is noted. Hematologic, cutaneous, and renal problems are the most frequent results of toxicity. Complete blood count and urinalysis should be done every 2 to 4 weeks to monitor for proteinuria and leukopenia with thrombocytopenia. The patient should be instructed to report any occurrence of fever, skin rash, oral ulcers, loss of taste, or diarrhea.

Adrenocorticosteroids are drugs used to suppress systemic inflammation. Exogenous corticosteroids suppress the ACTH-releasing factor from the hypothalmus which suppresses the production and release of ACTH from the anterior pituitary gland. The long-term result is tissue atrophy of the adrenal cortex and a suppression of cortisol production (Kantor, 1977). Normally, the adrenal cortex produces steroidal hormones. A corticosteroid is any steroid that has the properties characteristic of the hormone of the adrenal cortex, whether natural or synthetic. A corticosteroid is rarely the drug of first choice in arthritis, being used only after an unsuccessful trial of conservative drugs or when there is severe systemic involvement. After control of inflammation, the dosage should be reduced to the lowest possible maintenance dose and discontinued, if feasible. A single daily dose, preferably in the morning, is usually prescribed. Additional amounts of the drug are required during periods of stress, such as emotional trauma and surgery, when endogenous steroid production is suppressed.

Major side effects include gastrointestinal ulceration, osteoporosis, susceptibility to systemic infection, fluid retention, skin lesions, arteritis, thrombus formation, and psychosis. Aseptic necrosis, especially of the femoral head, can follow long-term use of high doses. Prednisone and prednisolone are the two most commonly used agents in this category, as they produce fewer side effects.

There have been reports of onset of symptoms of organic brain syndrome in patients on a steroid withdrawal program. The neuropsychiatric symptoms cleared with reinstitution of corticosteroids (Gupta and Ehrlich, 1976).

Intra-articular Injections

A corticosteroid combined with a local anesthetic may be injected into the joint or para-articular structures. It provides local, not systemic, reduction of inflammation and relief of pain. It is indicated when only one or two joints are severely painful. Intra-articular injections are contraindicated when there is joint infection, fracture, or severe osteoporosis. Preparation of the skin prior to injection should be meticulous to avoid introducing bacteria into the joint. The injection site is scrubbed with antibacterial soap and rinsed, and a topical antiseptic liquid is applied and allowed to dry. Sterile technique is used for the injection. Excess synovial fluid may be aspirated prior to injecting the medication. The injection usually provides immediate relief. However, there may be an increase in inflammation for the first 24 h. If there is discomfort, the patient should be advised to apply ice to the joint for 15 min of every hour as needed. A convenient method is the use of a semifrozen towel. A wet towel that is squeezed of excess water can be folded into the desired shape and placed in the freezer. Within an hour, it will be icy but flexible. It can then be placed directly on the site and repeated as the need arises. If ice bags or cold packs are used, a layer of cloth should be placed next to the skin to prevent burning. Heat is *not* recommended after an intra-articular injection. Once pain is absent, there may be a tendency to overuse the joint, and thus the patient should be cautioned that such overuse can cause further damage.

Antimalarials

Chloroquine and hydroxychloroquine have been demonstrated to have some antirheumatic effects. Results, however, are not usually seen until approximately 1 month after initiation of the drug. Severe side effects often outweigh the clinical results of antimalarials when compared to other available drugs. Skin eruptions, visual disturbances, nausea, leukopenia, and peripheral neuropathy can occur but usually are reversible if the drug is discontinued. Retinopathy and pigmentary changes in the retina are *not* reversible toxic reactions.

Experimental Drugs

Although immunosuppressive drugs per se are no longer classified as experimental, their use in nonmalignant disease is still under study. These agents are being tested in patients with connective tissue diseases with severe extra-articular manifestations. The three major classes of compounds in most common use are alkylating agents, purine analogs, and folic acid antagonists.

Dimethyl sulfoxide (DMSO), a commercial solvent derived from the paper manufacturing industry, is a drug under research. In the solvent form, it has the ability to penetrate the skin. Interest in this substance originated in the early 1960s, and it was tested on animals as well as humans with selected conditions such as arthritis, herpes zoster, scleroderma, sprains, bursitis, and urticaria. Pharmaceutical companies halted tests in 1965 at the request of the Food and Drug Administration as a result of reported adverse reactions, particularly ocular, hematologic, and cutaneous. Tests were resumed in 1968 on individuals with persistent conditions for which there was no satisfactory treatment. Presently, several investigational programs are under way with administration of intravenous, topical, and oral preparations (Wetherell, 1978; *FDA Fact Sheet,* 1973). The efficacy and safety of this drug for arthritis is undetermined at present.

As long as a cure is not in the immediate future, new drugs will continue to be developed and tested to treat the symptoms. It is hoped that researchers will discover agents that will alter the course of the disease.

THERAPEUTIC MANAGEMENT

The basic conservative program for management of rheumatoid arthritis includes salicylates, exercise, rest, application of heat or cold, and patient education. Treatment goals are to reduce inflammation and pain, maintain function, and prevent deformities. Additional drugs and therapy are added to the basic program as indicated. The patient's attitude can be a deterrent to the conservative approach if that approach appears to the patient to be too simple (Engleman, 1972). Smith (1972) has outlined a pyramidal plan, with the above program as Level I on the foundation of a schematic pyramid. Level II is utilization of anti-inflammatory drugs, intra-articular injections, intensive occupational and physical therapy, orthopedic devices, and stronger analgesics. Level III includes oral steroids and other remitting drugs, preventive surgery, and hospitalization. Reconstructive surgery and treatment at a rehabilitation center are on Level IV. Level V is experimental drugs, treatments, and surgery. Similar plans, which move from conservative to more aggressive treatment, are used by many practitioners. Treatment approaches and sequences may change periodically in light of new drugs and research in the field of rheumatology.

Exercises to maintain range of joint motion and strengthen muscles are mandatory, since muscle atrophy is a common sequela of rheumatoid arthritis. A total exercise program that includes all joints is recommended twice daily. Several short sessions are better than one long one. If severe inflammation is present in a joint, gentle, passive range of motion may be done to tolerance. Vigorous, active exercise of inflamed joints is contraindicated. Isometric exercises allow for muscle strengthening without joint trauma.

Use of local heat or cold for relief of discomfort is also indicated. These modalities may be in the form of paraffin, a Hubbard tank, a bathtub, a basin of hot water, heat packs, or cold packs. The use of moist heat is more beneficial than dry heat. Deep heating, such as shortwave diathermy or microwave, is not used extensively, as symptoms may be aggravated by deep heating in acute inflammation (Feibel & Fast, 1976). Heat or cold is beneficial when used just prior to the exercise program.

Resting splints may be provided for the hand, wrist, and fingers (Fig. 30-1), or for the lower extremities. These splints are nonfunctional and are designed to immobilize and support an inflamed joint. Resting splints may be worn continuously or intermittently during the day or night. Stretch gloves worn while sleeping aid in reducing swelling and morning stiffness of the hands.

Functional upper extremity splints are used to stabilize and support joints that are painful during certain activities. For example, a painful wrist limits hand function. A small wrist splint that stabilizes the wrist facilitates finger pinch or grasp. For standing and ambulating, splints or braces for the lower extremities provide joint stability. Cervical collars to restrict neck motion and supportive or corrective shoes may also be prescribed.

Ambulation aids such as crutches, canes, and walkers provide external support to protect the joints of the lower extremities and provide safety. However, each of these push the fingers in an ulnar direction and cause stress on the small joints of the fingers. For many patients with hand involvement, platform crutches with a forearm trough are preferred as weight-bearing is transferred to the forearm and elbow (Fig. 30-2).

Techniques to protect the joints and to conserve physical energy are emphasized throughout the therapy program (Table 30-1). The person with arthritis must learn to do daily activities in a different way in order to maintain independence and prevent joint trauma. Dressing aids, built-up utensils, adaptive devices, safety bars, electric appliances, and raised toilet seats are just a few of the available devices. Numerous

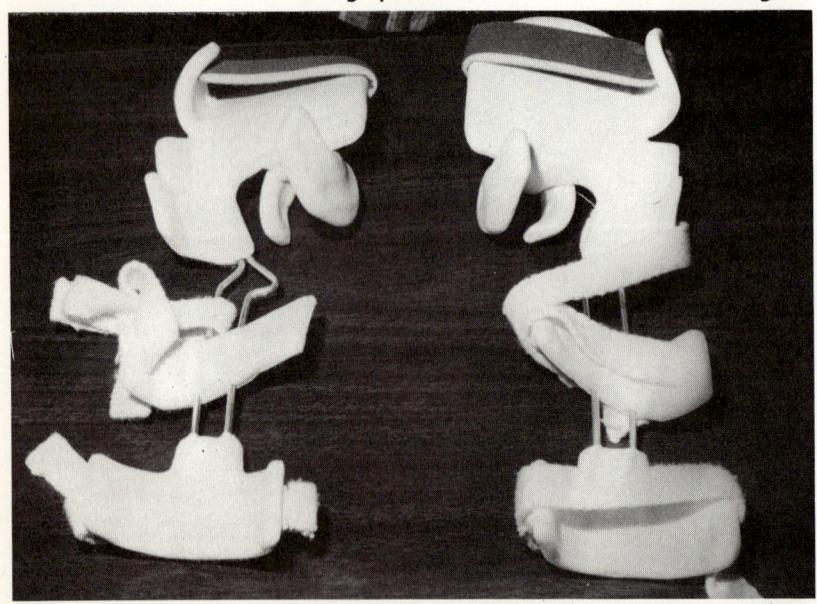

Figure 30-1
Resting splints for the hand, wrist, and fingers.

resources that describe equipment and techniques for activities of daily living are available to patients and professionals (Klinger, 1974; McKenzie et al., 1976; Watkins and Robinson, 1974).

NURSING INTERVENTION

The professional nurse can achieve positive results of intervention with the person who has rheumatoid arthritis. Such interventions require

Table 30-1

Suggestions for Joint Protection and Energy Conservation

Avoid positions of deformity	Rest chin on open palm rather than on fingers Do not put pillows under knees when lying down Avoid sitting on low, soft chairs
Avoid external pressure on small joints	Squeeze water from clothes rather than wringing Stir foods counterclockwise rather than clockwise Use commercial jar opener rather than fingers
Use strongest joints for the job	Carry purse on forearm rather than on fingers Carry objects in palms of both hands rather than with fingers
Avoid static positions of joints	Use card holder, book holder, built-up utensil or pencil Stop and stretch fingers frequently
Avoid lifting heavy objects	Fill large pots with small measuring cup or ladle Tilt coffee pot or pitcher to pour rather than lifting
Avoid stress on hips and knees	Sit in high, straight-back chair Use tub seat
Sit when at all possible	Use bar stool at kitchen sink and for job activities; use riding mower
Use mobile carts instead of carrying items	Use utility cart for setting table, gardening
Use electrically powered equipment	Electric can opener, electric blender, food chopper, mixer, typewriter
Eliminate unnecessary motions	Use lazy Susan; pegboards for utensils and tools; shop by phone; buy permanent press clothes

Source: Mary W. McKenzie, Linda M. Hennig, and Maureid McGill: *Arthritis Learning Notebook,* Mississippi Methodist Rehabilitation Center, Jackson, 1976.

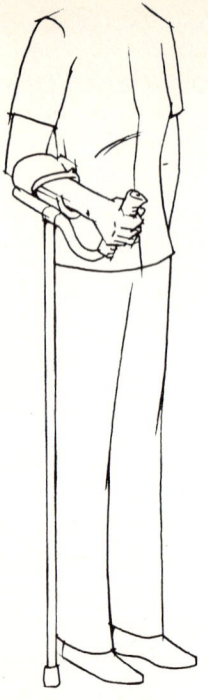

Figure 30-2
A platform crutch with a forearm trough. (Redrawn from M. McKenzie, L. Hennig, and M. McGill, Arthritis Learning Notebook, Mississippi Methodist Rehabilitation Center, Jackson, 1976.)

patience, creativity, and a willingness to accept limitations and small gains. Actions must be based on thorough assessment. The entire nursing process—assessment, planning, implementation of the plan, and evaluation of actions—is necessary for effective management. The evaluation on initial contact and data collected on subsequent contact are the bases for all nursing care, teaching, and continued support. Whether the patient is first seen in the home, in the ambulatory unit, or in the hospital, the assessment areas are the same. The setting, however, may dictate the depth of initial assessment.

The evaluation of the patient by the nurse must include physical symptoms, onset, joints affected, other organ involvement, and the presence of deformities. The patient should describe usual time, type, and duration of pain and how it is controlled. Note all medications presently taken, the patient's knowledge of their action, dosage, and side effects, and the time of the last dose. Include any medications previously taken for arthritis and the reasons they were discontinued. The assessment should also include concomitant diseases, current health practices, understanding of pathological conditions, and the patient's expectations of health care providers. Other areas of assessment to explore include how the condition has affected mobility, ability to care for self and/or others, vocation-/avocation, family relationships, sexual function, and sleep pattern. It is helpful to ascertain present stresses in life, coping mechanisms, family composition, and living arrangements. All body systems should be evaluated, with particular attention to nutritional status, skin condition, elimination, and ability to perform self-care activities. Specify any equipment or assistive devices used by the patient.

Following assessment, a plan of care can be designed and implemented. The patient's care plan should also reflect data obtained from the medical record. Specific areas for nursing intervention include pain management, nutrition, skin care, positioning, self-care, elimination, health education, rest and relaxation, sexuality, and psychological support. Systematic evaluation of the results of nursing action is needed to continue the plan or try alternative approaches.

Pain Management

Phrases such as "You'll have to learn to live with the pain" and "Grin and bear it" are frequently communicated to the person with arthritis. Although cure is not yet possible and discomfort will be present much of the time, there is no reason for the person to suffer needlessly with excruciating pain. Pain and stiffness are often most severe upon arising. It may take the person several hours just to "get moving." This is due, in part, to static positioning of the joints while sleeping and to lowered levels of medication in the blood. A brief period of exercise while still in bed will help loosen joints. Anti-inflammatory

CHAPTER 30 616

drugs should be taken immediately after awakening.

Patients are often quite concerned about becoming dependent on drugs. Medications of some type most likely will be needed throughout the lifetime. Anti-inflammatory drugs must be taken daily at regular intervals in order to maintain sustained levels of the medication in the blood. Safety caps on prescription bottles are often difficult to manipulate if hands are painful or deformed. Pharmacists will usually provide regular caps upon patient or physician request.

Medication is but one aspect of pain control. The importance of appropriately spacing activities, getting adequate rest, and supporting inflamed joints to reduce and/or prevent discomfort cannot be overemphasized. The modalities of heat and cold are helpful adjuncts to pain management.

Techniques to achieve relaxation are being used with success for persons with chronic pain. Some techniques include a light hypnotic trance, while others use pleasant memories, mantras, or fantasies to achieve total body relaxation (French and Tupin, 1974; Grzesiak, 1977). Goals are to reduce anxiety and pain and/or to induce sleep. The beauty of such techniques is that, once learned, relaxation can become self-induced. Relaxation in this manner is noninvasive and is of benefit to the total organism. Professional nurses can acquire training in these methods and can use them in a therapeutic manner with patients. The nurse can also use many other methods such as touch, back rubs, soft music, diversionary activities, and conversation to reduce anxiety, to provide tranquility, and to help the person focus on something other than pain. Behavior modification is also a useful approach.

Nutrition

There is no special diet to control arthritis. There has been some investigation into the role of food allergies in producing joint pain, but most authorities support the concept of a well-balanced diet without restrictions.

Supplemental vitamins may be indicated for the person with poor nutritional status. Vitamin C aids in reducing cutaneous bruising, which commonly occurs in persons with RA and in persons receiving long-term steroid therapy. The hemolytic anemia of rheumatoid arthritis does not respond to hematinic drugs, but if iron deficiency anemia is a result of gastric bleeding secondary to drug therapy, supplemental iron salts may help (Engleman, 1972).

The health practices of the individual with regard to diet, dietary supplements, religion, and culture should be evaluated when planning interventions. Available finances for food purchases is also a major consideration. Functional limitations may influence the ability to prepare meals and may lead to a preference for frozen, canned, or processed foods. Processed foods are often lower in nutritional value and higher in cost than fresh and home-prepared foods. Special dietary needs of the other family members may affect the patient's dietary intake. If temporomandibular joint pain is present, chewing may be difficult.

While weight loss is often a symptom of persons with rheumatic disease, obesity is not uncommon, especially after the disease becomes inactive. Weight gain frequently accompanies middle age and decreased activity. Even mild obesity can cause stress on joints, especially those of the lower extremities, spine, and hands. If weight is within normal limits, maintenance of that weight should be emphasized. The lower limits of "ideal" weight ranges are desirable. Mobility and other activities of daily living will be easier if joints do not have to carry excess weight. In addition, there probably will be a decrease in fatigue and pain, as well as an improvement in overall health. Caloric intake is evaluated in relation to the person's level of activity.

A satisfactory weight does not necessarily reflect good nutritional status. The patient's knowledge and ability to follow a well-balanced diet should be explored. Whenever possible, a dietician should be consulted to assist in diet education and meal planning. A patient may have difficulty in planning and following a therapeutic diet if other diseases requiring dietary modification are present along with the arthritis. Goals for weight reduction should be realistic and easily attainable. Losing 1 or 2 lb per week is a safe goal and provides frequent, positive reinforcement.

Skin Care

Several factors, both endogenous and iatrogenic, affect the patient's overall skin condition. The disease process of rheumatoid arthritis can involve the blood vessels, causing vasculitis, digital gangrene, or localized ulcerations. Antiarthritic drugs may produce allergic or toxic reactions such as urticaria, rashes, and ulcerations. Long-term systemic steroid therapy takes its toll on the skin, often causing the epidermis to become very friable and the capillaries very fragile. The skin will often have the appearance of "tissue paper," and ecchymosis can occur from even minor pressure.

If anemia is present, cellular metabolism will be affected, and the healing of lesions or incisions will be retarded. Dietary intake, the body's ability to utilize nutrients, and the circulatory system also affect skin condition. Subcutaneous nodules seen in rheumatoid arthritis, although usually not painful, are often located along the forearm or at the elbow and are subject to frequent bumping.

Limited range of joint motion may prevent satisfactory skin hygiene. Urine, feces, soap, and perspiration that are not removed can cause maceration and severe irritation. Ulcerations on the lower extremities can result from the pressure of poorly fitted shoes or braces, poor hygiene, and/or inadequate circulation. Hand splints, especially if applied to correct deformities, may create skin problems if not removed at regular intervals.

Nursing personnel must be attuned to all factors that can affect skin condition. Monitoring nutrition, positioning, providing hygiene, preventing injury, and inspecting the skin are nursing functions that must be performed for the patient if he or she is unable.

Positioning

When pain or stiffness is present, the person will usually assume a position of comfort. Unfortunately, this may be a position that fosters deformity. For example, if knee extension produces pain, it will be kept in the flexed position. If movement of a painful joint is avoided, the full range of joint motion quickly decreases. Regularly placing rolls or pillows under the knees when lying, as shown in Fig. 30-3a, will ultimately result in flexion deformities. When supine, the trunk and extremities should be in full extension, with only a small flat pillow under the head. Figure 30-3b illustrates the correct supine position.

The prone position should be integrated into the daily positioning program. Since many persons with arthritis may be unaccustomed to this position, a gradual program to increase tolerance is needed. A satisfactory proning program can be achieved by starting with 15 min daily, or for as long as can be tolerated, and increasing by 30 min daily. Eventually, this position can be tolerated for the duration of rest periods and for a large percentage of the nighttime sleep.

The technique of bridging (Stewart and Wharton, 1976) with pillows and foam pads (Fig. 30-4) can be modified to compensate for existing deformities and to promote comfort. Proning helps prevent hip and knee joint tightness and aids in the skin care program, the respiratory toilet, and the drainage of urine from the kidneys.

The side-lying position is permitted if the joints are kept in good alignment. Figure 30-5 illustrates the *incorrect* side-lying position.

A firm mattress is needed to support the entire body. Lightweight covers or an electric blanket create less pressure on painful joints than do heavy blankets. Covers should be loose rather than tightly tucked to prevent ankle plantar flexion and pressure on toes.

Rest and good alignment are especially important when joints are inflamed. Too much activity of involved joints can increase the inflammation.

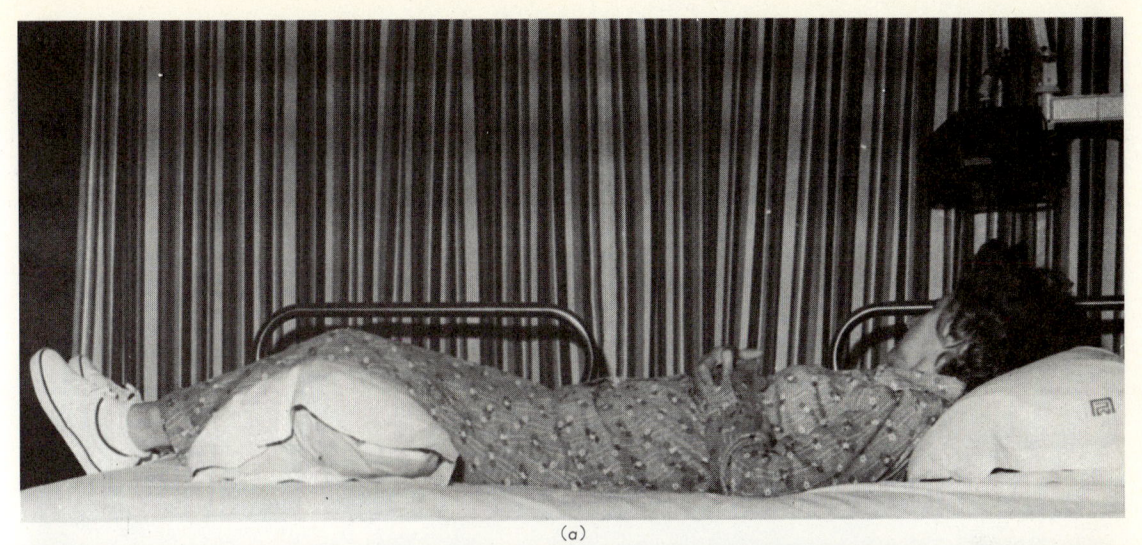

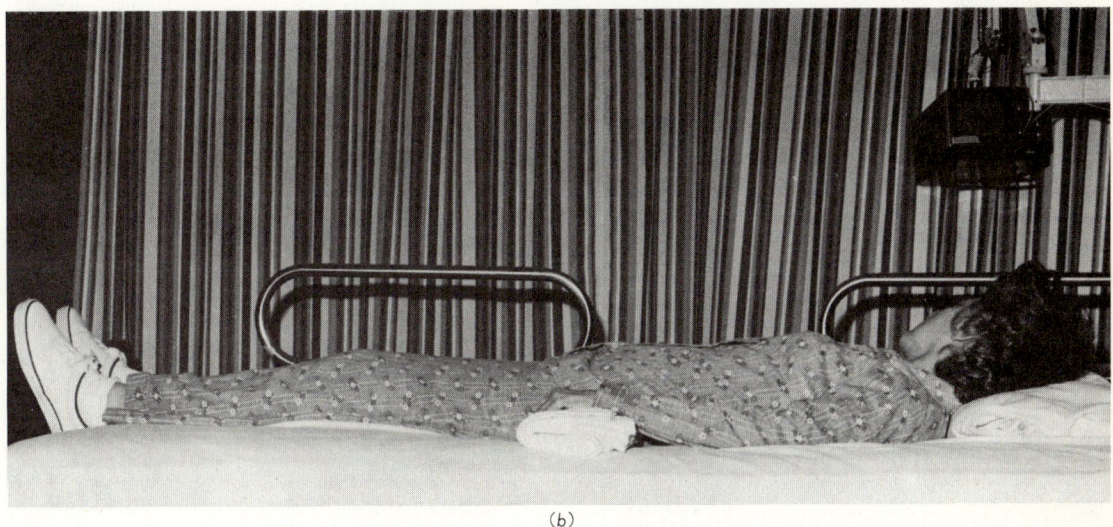

Figure 30-3
(*a*) Regularly placing pillows beneath the knees for comfort will ultimately lead to flexion deformities. (*b*) The correct supine position.

Nursing personnel must be knowledgeable in the application of functional and resting splints. Splints need to be removed every few hours and the underlying skin inspected for signs of pressure.

Attention should also be given to the sitting position and the standing posture. Chairs should have a straight back and be of a height and seat depth appropriate for the person. A foam cushion is needed if ambulation or the ability to shift weight when sitting is a problem. Sitting on soft, low couches or chairs should be avoided because they allow for a poor sitting position and require additional stress on the joints when the individual attempts to stand.

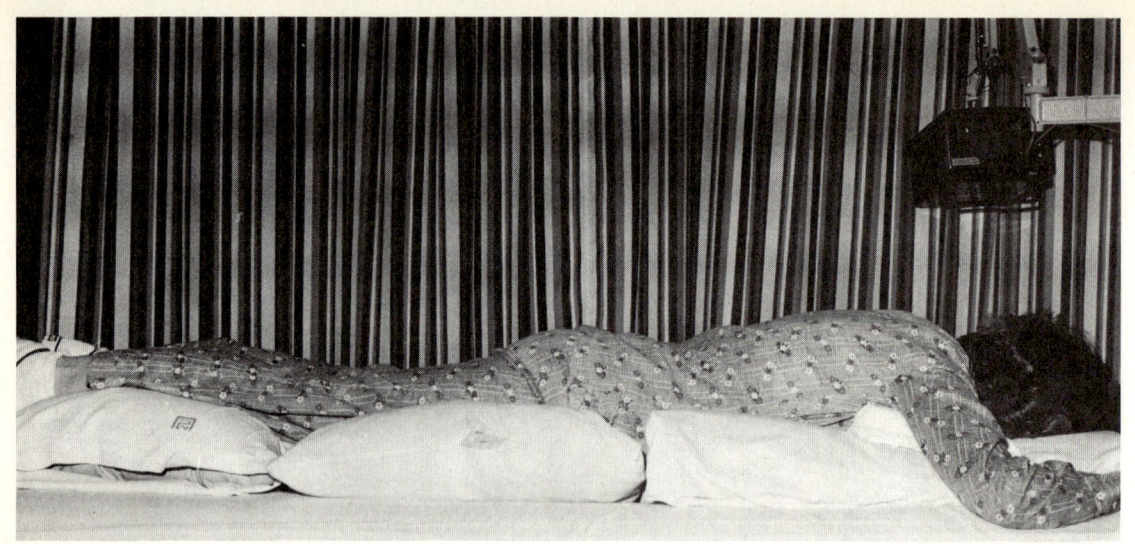

Figure 30-4
The use of pillows for support in the prone position can help compensate for existing deformities and will promote comfort.

The use of correct positions by the patient for sleep, rest, and sitting will help prevent deformity, maintain range of joint motion, and facilitate good standing posture. Any position can be detrimental if maintained for long periods. Careful positioning and repositioning will not only help prevent deformities but will also prevent unnecessary skin breakdown. The patient should be able to demonstrate techniques of achieving good alignment to all joints in all positions.

Self-care

"Self-care is the practice of activities that individuals personally initiate and perform on their own behalf in maintaining life, health, and well being" (Orem, 1971). The professional nurse needs to assess the individual's self-care requirements, the individual's ability to meet those requirements, and the need for nursing intervention. Self-care requirements may be universal, such as sleeping, eating, elimination, and bathing, or may be related to activities needed because of the disease or health deviation. Nursing action is needed when a person's self-care requirements are not equal to his or her self-care capacities (Orem). Performing necessary activities for the patient when self-care is limited is but one aspect of nursing.

The primary goals of nursing intervention should be to allow the patient to maintain and achieve as much independence as possible within the limits of the disease. Judgment is often needed in deciding to assist individuals with arthritis in one activity so that they can perform some other activity independently. For example, a patient may need some assistance with dressing and hygiene in order to conserve enough energy to participate in an exercise program. Family members may need to do the shopping so the homemaker with arthritis will have the energy to prepare meals.

Occupational and physical therapists should be consulted to provide appropriate splints and supportive and adaptive equipment. In addition, the therapists should design an exercise program and teach techniques of performing activities of daily living with an emphasis on joint protection and conservation of physical energy. Nursing personnel must be knowledgeable about these techniques and treatment methods in order to follow through with the treatment program, to assess the patient's use of the established tech-

CHAPTER 30 620

niques, and to communicate the patient's performance to the therapist. Teaching the patient how to modify activities of daily living becomes the responsibility of the nurse when other specialists are not available for collaboration.

Elimination

Problems with bladder and bowel elimination can occur for several reasons. Some medications used for arthritis may decrease gastric motility and/or have a constipating effect. Bathroom facilities may not be easily accessible for the person with reduced mobility and joint contractures. With the geriatric patient, slower gastric motility and urinary system problems may be present as a part of the normal aging process. Bedpans are an unnatural method of elimination but may have to be used for patients on bedrest. The use of a bedside commode, especially at night, would be preferable if ambulation is a problem. A urinal for males may be indicated for safety reasons.

Independence in elimination can be preserved by designing a program of regulated fluid intake and regular bathroom habits. Assisting the person to the toilet before and after every meal helps decrease urinary urgency or incontinence. A schedule of urinating every 2 to 3 h is usually satisfactory. The frequency, however, is determined by the amount of fluid intake and urinary bladder capacity.

A bowel program of daily elimination is preferred, and greater success is achieved if elimination is carried out at the same time every day. A bolus of liquid or food will stimulate the gastrocolic reflex. It is helpful to drink a cup of warm liquid about 15 min before the scheduled time or to attempt bowel elimination immediately after a meal. Firmly massaging the abdomen in a clockwise motion while on the toilet will also help evacuation. Natural laxatives and bulking agents in the diet are used to prevent constipation. A stool softener or laxative may be indicated to manage chronic problems, but natural approaches should also be used.

After elimination, the person may need assistance with perineal hygiene if contractures limit this function. A plastic perineal bottle filled with water can aid the female in washing the perineum while sitting on the toilet. A disposable sitz bath that fits in the toilet or a bidet is another alternative. An elevated toilet seat, safety rails, or grab bars help reduce stress on the joints and make toileting easier.

Figure 30-5
An *incorrect* side-lying position. *(Redrawn from M. McKenzie, L. Hennig, and M. McGill, Arthritis Learning Notebook, Mississippi Methodist Rehabilitation Center, Jackson, 1976.)*

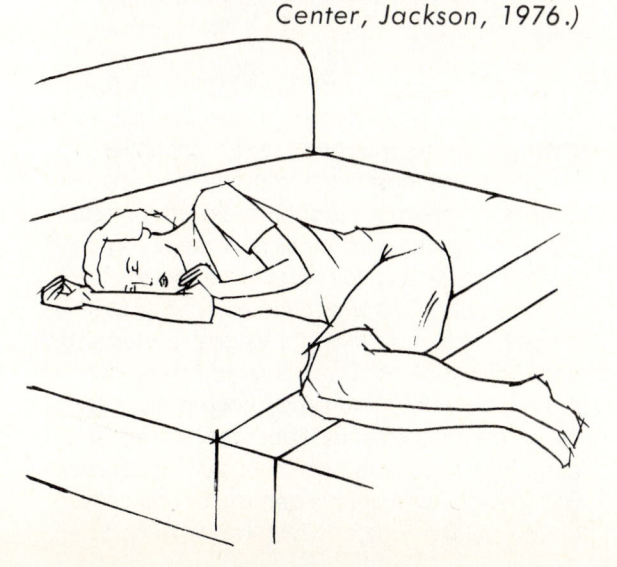

Health Education

Assessment of the individual's ability to see, hear, read, and comprehend is a prerequisite to initiating any learning activities. Methods of teaching must be geared to the individual's capacities. Health education is primarily focused on helping the person learn about the disease process and find out ways in which to meet self-care requirements. Family members and other significant persons are encouraged to participate in the educational program. Group classes are an excellent approach in that patients and families are able to share common experiences and exchange solutions to problems.

Thorough instruction regarding drugs, actions, schedules, side effects, and methods to evaluate efficacy are important. Drugs that interact with present medications should be identified. It is helpful to review and compare the previous drug regimen and to instruct the patient to discard prescriptions not included in the present plan.

Family members often tire of complaints of pain and may tend to ignore the person experiencing it. An understanding of the disease process, the effects of medication, the techniques of joint protection, and the exercise program can help family members give more support and encouragement to an individual to follow through with the prescribed program. The family may also need assistance in finding ways to restructure their life-style in such a way as to not place excessive physical demands on the person with arthritis.

The reader is encouraged to contact the Arthritis Foundation, 3400 Peachtree Road, N. E., Atlanta, Georgia, 30326 (or the local or state chapter) for a listing of patient education pamphlets. Also available is an excellent guidebook for establishing a patient education program, titled *Patient Education in Arthritis—How-To Packet.*

The Arthritis Information Clearinghouse is a service of the National Institute of Arthritis, Metabolism, and Digestive Diseases of the National Institutes of Health. It is designed to help health professionals identify print and audiovisual materials concerned with arthritis and related musculoskeletal diseases. Interested individuals need only write Arthritis Information Clearinghouse, P. O. Box 34427, Bethesda, Maryland, and request that their name be placed on the mailing list. There is no charge for this service.

Patient education manuals, such as those by McKenzie, et al. (1976) and Watkins and Robinson (1974), are available from individual treatment centers.

Rest and Relaxation

The person with arthritis requires intermittent periods of rest or inactivity to avoid fatigue and overuse of affected joints. Rest can be systemic, psychological, or apply to a single joint. Complete bed rest is rarely indicated. Remaining active does help minimize disability, but all activity must be balanced with appropriate periods of rest. The individual who feels good one day and performs many strenuous tasks may suffer an acute exacerbation for several days afterward. An often expressed fear of patients is that going to bed is synonymous with "giving in" to pain. The nurse needs to frequently reinforce the need for rest and provide alternatives to the bed. Other nursing actions include assisting with the application of resting splints and providing an atmosphere of peace and tranquility. Reading, watching television, listening to music, and playing quiet games can be incorporated into the home or hospital setting. When a patient is hospitalized, rest is often difficult or impossible because of the frequency of meals, treatment, therapies, medications, and visitors. The nurse needs to be the patient advocate in coordinating nursing care and the treatments by other professionals so as to allow the patient time for rest. The use of relaxation techniques as described for pain control are applicable for rest and relaxation.

A balanced activity schedule is one that alternates rest with activities requiring energy output and use of several joints. Table 30-2 presents an example of a balanced activity schedule.

Psychological Support

The psychological needs of the person with chronic disease may wax and wane over the life span. The onset of symptoms and exacerbations in rheumatoid arthritis are often associated with psychologic conflicts. While commonly referred to, a "typical arthritic personality" has not been identified and validated. Spergel (1977) suggests, instead, that there are patterns of personality in persons with chronic disease. While individuals with arthritis may have maladaptive behaviors and personality disorders, the traits are often seen in persons with other chronic diseases. Each person has a unique personality and pattern of coping. The way in which a person handled

Table 30-2

Balanced Activity Schedule

6:30 A.M.	Take arthritis medications
7:00	Do exercises in bed (*activity*)
7:15	Warm shower or bath (*activity*)
7:30	Dress (*activity*)
8:00	Read paper, have coffee (*rest*)
8:15	Prepare breakfast (*activity*)
8:30	Eat (*rest*)
9:00	(*Activity*)
9:45	Plan dinner, read (*rest*)
10:30	Do total exercise program (*activity*)
11:00	Rest
11:45	Prepare lunch (*activity*)
12:15 P.M.	Eat (*rest*)
1:00	Activity
1:45	Rest
2:30	Activity
3:30	Rest
4:00	Do total exercise program (*activity*)
4:30	Rest
5:15	Prepare dinner
6:00	Eat (*rest*)
7:00	Activity

stress and problems prior to the disease is a major factor in coping with the disease.

Loss of bodily function, mobility, or one's role within the family or society can lead to a grief process similar to that experienced with the loss of a loved one. One aspect of grieving in a chronic disease is that it may span a lifetime, and the stages of adjustment may be reactivated with each exacerbation.

Nursing intervention should be aimed at facilitating the patient's expression about self and the impact of the disease. Patients and family members must be allowed to grieve and move through the stages of adjustment. Chronic pain evokes many psychological reactions. Not being able to see a future role—except that of illness—often potentiates depression. Empathy, understanding, and kindness, combined with firmness, are needed on the part of the nurse to help the patient move toward adjustment and maximum independence. Pity has no therapeutic value in nursing management. Positive reinforcement by members of the health team and family, for even minor accomplishments, can help build the patient's self-esteem.

A psychological evaluation should be obtained for persons with overt problems or abnormal behavior patterns. A team approach should be used with all patients to identify psychosocial factors and to develop a plan of management for the total person and significant family members.

SURGICAL INTERVENTION

Surgery is no longer the final resort in treatment of arthritis. While some procedures may be classified as salvage, most are performed for prophylactic, reparative, or reconstructive reasons. Prophylactic procedures include synovectomy and osteotomy. Reparative procedures include tendon repair, tendon transfer, tenolysis, neurolysis, and release of nerve entrapment. Total or single joint replacement is a reconstructive procedure. Conservative surgery, such as prophylactic and reparative procedures, is performed in the early stages of diseased joints. Preservation of bony stock is important, especially in younger persons. Reconstructive procedures are usually done after advanced joint destruction.

Relief of pain, improvement of motion and function, prevention of further destruction, stabilization of a joint, and correction of deformity are indications for surgery. The majority of procedures are elective. The patient's motivation, goals, financial resources, rate of progression of the disease, and life expectancy must be taken into consideration when planning surgery. When multiple joints are involved, it may be necessary to stage procedures over a number of years.

Reconstructive Hip Surgery

Total hip arthroplasty is one of the most common and successful of the arthritis operations. It is indicated for rheumatoid arthritis, degenerative joint disease, congenital disorders, traumatic conditions, and failed previous hip surgery. The procedure is usually not performed on children but may be used in selected young adults with severe destruction of the hip.

The total hip prosthesis consists of an acetabular cup and a femoral stem and head. The acetabular cup is made of either metal or high-density polyethylene and cemented into place with methylmethacrylate. The femoral component is made of metal and is also cemented into the femoral shaft with methylmethacrylate. A metal-to-polyethylene articulation produces less friction than does metal-to-metal and thus is called a low-friction arthroplasty. The concept of low friction, as well as the procedure and design of the prosthesis, was pioneered by an English orthopedic surgeon, Sir John Charnley. The Charnley prosthesis and the modified Charnley-Müller prosthesis are commonly used in the United States. Numerous other prostheses of varying shapes, sizes, and materials are currently available.

A resurface prosthesis for the hip joint, developed in Germany, is available for persons with severe osteoarthritis. The acetabulum and femoral head are shaved of diseased bone and resurfaced with alloplastic implants that are cemented with methylmethacrylate. The femoral head and neck are preserved, and a complete joint replacement can be performed at a later age, if indicated. This option provides pain relief and improvement of function for younger persons in whom a total hip replacement is not indicated.

The type of prosthesis selected depends on the degree of pathology within the joint, the desired result, and the preferences of the surgeon. The type of incision, postoperative nursing care, and therapy protocols are determined by the prostheses, procedure, and surgeon. While each surgeon may have postoperative protocols, what is discovered and done at the time of surgery, plus the patient's overall condition, may dictate variation. The incision is usually lateral or lateroposterior. If the greater trochanter is removed for better visualization and insertion of the prosthesis, it is reattached with wires.

Total Hip Arthroplasty

Preoperative Nursing A general nursing assessment, as outlined earlier, is needed for the patient preparing to undergo surgery. In addition, it is essential to determine the patient's expectations with regard to care, length of hospitalization, therapy, and results of surgery. Discussion of preoperative anxiety and fear should be initiated by the nurse. The patient may have concerns about family relationships, finances, or employment while in the hospital. The anticipated destination after discharge, necessary family or attendant care, and the expected home modifications and/or equipment need to be ascertained and discussed prior to surgery.

The general and preoperative nursing assessment gives the nurse a data base upon which to plan a nursing program, not just to include preoperative teaching but also to manage the problems of the arthritis preoperatively and postoperatively. Instructions given the patient by the surgeon are reinforced by nursing personnel. In addition, the patient must be prepared for tests, procedures, preoperative preparation, and medication. Events that will occur in the recovery room and the expected postoperative care should be explained. The physical, occupational, and respiratory therapists collaborate with the nurse before the patient goes to surgery to teach any postoperative exercises and to explain treatments.

Postoperative Care Immediate postsurgical observation and nursing care would be the same as for almost any other major surgery. The primary goals for this patient are:

Prevent wound infection
Prevent hip dislocation
Control pain
Prevent thrombophlebitis
Prevent respiratory complications
Prevent skin breakdown
Promote adequate nutrition

Provide psychological support
Maintain adequate elimination
Maintain functional abilities for self-care
Prevent further disability

The most serious complications are wound infection, hip dislocation, and thromboembolic phenomenon. Sepsis of the joint usually necessitates eventual removal of the prosthesis and performing a Girdlestone procedure, which is the formation of a pseudoarthrosis with significant shortening of the extremity. Rarely is another arthroplasty performed.

Meticulous care is to be given by all personnel. Washing the hands before and after contact with the patient is vitally important. The patient should not share a room with another patient who has any type of infection nor be cared for by personnel with infections. Dressings are to remain intact, unless contaminated, until removed by the surgeon. The hemovac drainage tubes must be kept patent until removed.

Some surgeons routinely administer prophylactic antibiotics after surgery or may irrigate the incision and wound with an antibiotic solution during surgery. Laminar air flow or "clean air" operating suites are used in some hospitals to further reduce wound contamination.

Arthroplasty of the hip requires abduction of the hips postoperatively. This position puts less stress on the joint capsule and provides the best anatomical alignment or "seating" of the head of the prosthesis into the acetabular cup. Dislocation is least likely in this position. Hip adduction and the extremes of flexion and internal and external rotation must be avoided. An abduction pillow or splint is used to maintain abduction (Fig. 30-6). The patient may be turned on the unoperated side, prone and supine, provided hip abduction is maintained during and after the process of turning.

Sitting with 45 to 60° of hip flexion is permitted. The possibility of dislocation and pain is greater with increased hip flexion. Weight bearing on the operated extremity for short periods may begin as early as 3 days postoperatively.

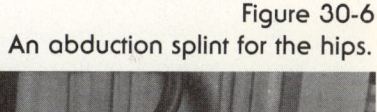

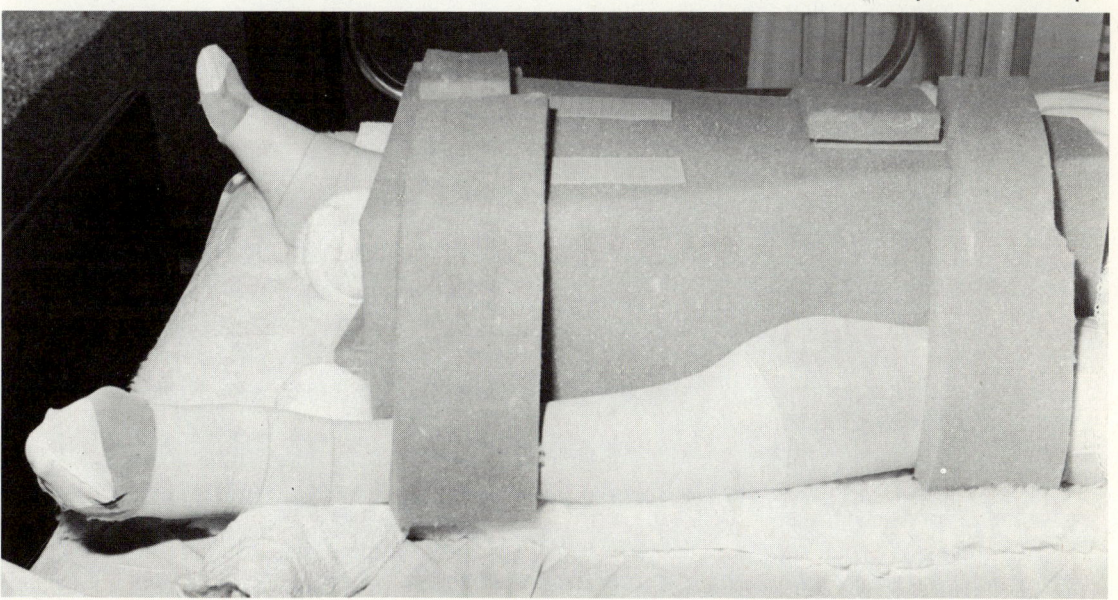

Figure 30-6
An abduction splint for the hips.

Medications following surgery will generally include narcotics, but they should be used judiciously so as to be continued no longer than necessary. Anti-inflammatory and/or antirheumatic drugs need to be restarted as soon as possible after surgery for systemic relief. For persons who have been habituated to narcotics, withdrawal from these drugs following joint replacement is usually possible. Once the source of severe pain is removed, the need for narcotics is gone. Many patients express relief after surgery, stating they feel incisional pain, but the former excruciating pain in the joint is no longer present.

A thrombus formation and embolus can be life-threatening. The use of anticoagulants following hip surgery is common, but the danger of hematoma within the wound is possible. Measures to prevent venous stasis, such as exercises, antiembolus stockings, and early ambulation, are routinely employed. One simple exercise that can be done every hour while awake is dorsiflexion and plantar flexion of the ankle. The frequency can be decreased once the patient becomes ambulatory. Postoperative edema in the leg is common and can be reduced with elastic stockings. Poorly fitted or improperly applied elastic stockings or Ace bandages can do more harm than good. Stockings are worn in bed until frequent ambulation begins, and then they are worn when the leg is in a dependent position. At least two pairs are needed for daily changing and washing.

Coughing, deep breathing, frequent repositioning, and satisfactory fluid intake are the best preventive measures to maintain respiratory function. Family members can participate in care by frequently encouraging the patient to do respiratory exercises. The frequency of repositioning is determined by skin tolerance of the patient, degree of comfort, and total physiological needs. The time spent in any one position should not exceed 2 to 3 h. An alternating pressure mattress, sheepskin, or foam mattress can be used as an adjunct to the skin care program. Equipment does not take the place of frequent turning and skin care.

Other complications that can follow hip arthroplasty are loosening of the implants, wound hematoma, and spontaneous fracture, usually along the shaft of the femur. The bones may be softer in persons with rheumatoid arthritis as a result of accompanying osteoporosis or long-term steroid therapy.

Precautions to prevent dislocation and measures to promote healing must be followed by the patient for about 8 weeks after surgery. Tables 30-3 and 30-4 present examples of postoperative and discharge instructions used by one hospital for persons who have had a Charnley-Müller total hip arthroplasty.

Table 30-3

Physical Therapy Program after Total Hip Replacement

Precautions and special instructions

Lie as flat as possible at all times except when eating, then the head of your bed should not be raised higher than 60 degrees.

You will be given a pillow that you must keep between your legs at all times. You may sleep on your back, or unoperated side, but the pillow must be kept between your legs.

When you are lying on your back in bed, your toe should always be pointing toward the ceiling. When walking, the toe should point straight ahead. At no time should you let your toe point to the outside of your foot.

Your doctor or physical therapist will advise you when you may begin sitting in a chair. The length of sitting time will be gradually increased.

You should not sit in any way that causes your hip to bend more than a right angle (90°).

You should not cross your legs.

All exercises should be done *slowly* and *carefully*.

Exercises

These first three (3) exercises should be done ten (10) times each; *every hour*.

Squeeze the muscles of both buttocks. Hold for a count of 5. Relax. Repeat.

Keep your leg straight. Push the back of your knee down into the bed and, at the same time, tighten the muscle on top of your leg. Hold for a count of 5. Relax. Repeat.

Draw a large circle with your big toe, moving the whole foot. Repeat 10 times clockwise and 10 times counterclockwise.

These exercises should be done ten (10) times each, three (3) times a day.

Move the ———— leg straight out to the side of the bed, hold for count of 5, then bring it back to the pillow. Remember to keep the toes pointing toward the ceiling.

Bend the ———— hip and knee, sliding the foot along the bed. Now keeping the hip bent, raise the foot up until leg is straight, then lower the straight leg to the bed. Keep legs spread apart and do not allow the knee to roll outward. (Keep toes pointing toward the ceiling.)

Source: M. McKenzie, L. Hennig, and M. McGill: *Arthritis Learning Notebook,* Mississippi Methodist Rehabilitation Center, Jackson, 1976.

Table 30-4

Home Instructions and Activities

Exercises
   Continue to do all the exercises you've learned two times a day, just as your therapist has shown you.

Bilateral support
   For 3 months after surgery, you must continue to use some type of support when walking. This may be either crutches, walker or a cane. Also you must not stand without support or with all your weight on the operated hip and leg.

Sitting
   You will receive instructions for sitting from your physical therapist. For at least 6 weeks after surgery, you should sit in a "slouched" position with a pillow behind your hips. You will be given further instructions at your outpatient clinic visit.

Side lying
   To lie on your side, lie on the unoperated side with 1 firm pillow between the legs. If you've had surgery on both hips, you must get your doctor's permission to lie on your side.

Pillow
   You will be seen in outpatient clinic approximately 4-6 weeks following discharge. At this time, it may be decided that you can discontinue using the pillows between your legs while lying on your back. You will still need to use them if you lie on your side.

Raised toilet seat
   You will receive a toilet seat extension (raised toilet seat) to use after you are discharged. This keeps the hip from bending past a right angle (90°) when you sit on the toilet.

Sexual activities
   When you feel your hip motions are strong and you are not having muscle pain, sexual activities may be resumed. You should discuss different positions with your nurse or therapist.

Driving
   After you are seen for your first outpatient clinic appointment, your physician will decide whether you may begin driving. If you have had a left total hip and have a car with an automatic shift, you may drive if you have your physician's permission. If you have had a right or both total hip(s), you may eventually be able to drive depending on how well the physician feels your hip(s) are working.

Sports
   After your first clinic check-up swimming may be encouraged. Any sports that may cause you to fall on your hip or cause a pounding of the joint are to be avoided; sports such as tennis, skiing, jogging or running are not recommended.

Shoes and socks
   Since you should not bend your operated hip more than a right angle (90°), you should not bend to put on your shoes and socks. A sock cone and long shoe horn should be used for dressing. (Your occupational therapist will give you this equipment and show you how to use it as well as give you tips on how to make other parts of dressing easier.) Three months after surgery the physician may allow you to increase the amount you can bend at the hip.

ADL
   Standing for long periods of time isn't a good idea. Activities which require you to stand, such as cooking, washing dishes, ironing, etc. may be done while sitting on a high kitchen chair or bar stool. This kind of chair allows you to sit while working without bending your hip more than 90°.

Source: M. McKenzie, L. Hennig, and M. McGill: *Arthritis Learning Notebook,* Mississippi Methodist Rehabilitation Center, Jackson, 1976.

Reconstructive Hand Surgery

Arthroplasty of the metacarpophalangeal (MP) joints and proximal interphalangeal (PIP) joints with flexible Silastic implants offers pain relief, restoration of function, and improved appearance for persons with arthritis or traumatic conditions affecting the hands. Prior to the advent of finger joint implants, the major procedures available were for pain relief but rendered the joints unstable (resection) or fused (arthrodesis).

Also available are thumb metacarpophalangeal implants, trapezium implants, carpal scaphoid and lunate implants, radiocarpal flexible hinged implants, ulnar head implants, radial head implants, great toe implants, and shoulder and elbow implants. The design and development of materials, surgical techniques, and postoperative therapy are largely the result of many years of study by Alfred Swanson and his coworkers.

Metacarpophalangeal Implant Arthroplasty

Gross subluxation, abnormal mechanical forces of tendons, ulnar deviation, pain, or ankylosis of joints leaves hands deformed and nonfunctional (Fig. 30-7). MP arthroplasty offers restoration of function and a more normal appearance but requires intensive postoperative therapy and a home therapy program. Patient motivation and compliance are major considerations for performing surgery.

Usually two to four of the joints are replaced at the same time. At surgery, the joint capsule and diseased bone are resected to make room for the implant. The intramedullary canal is reamed to receive the stem of the prostheses. Tendons and ligaments may need repair or release to avoid abnormal forces after surgery. The flexible hinge is interposed between the bone ends to serve as a dynamic spacer. Cementing agents are not needed, as the body eventually encapsulates the prosthesis with collagen and scar tissue. Adequate muscle and tendon support is needed to achieve the desired results, as are functional proximal joints such as the wrist.

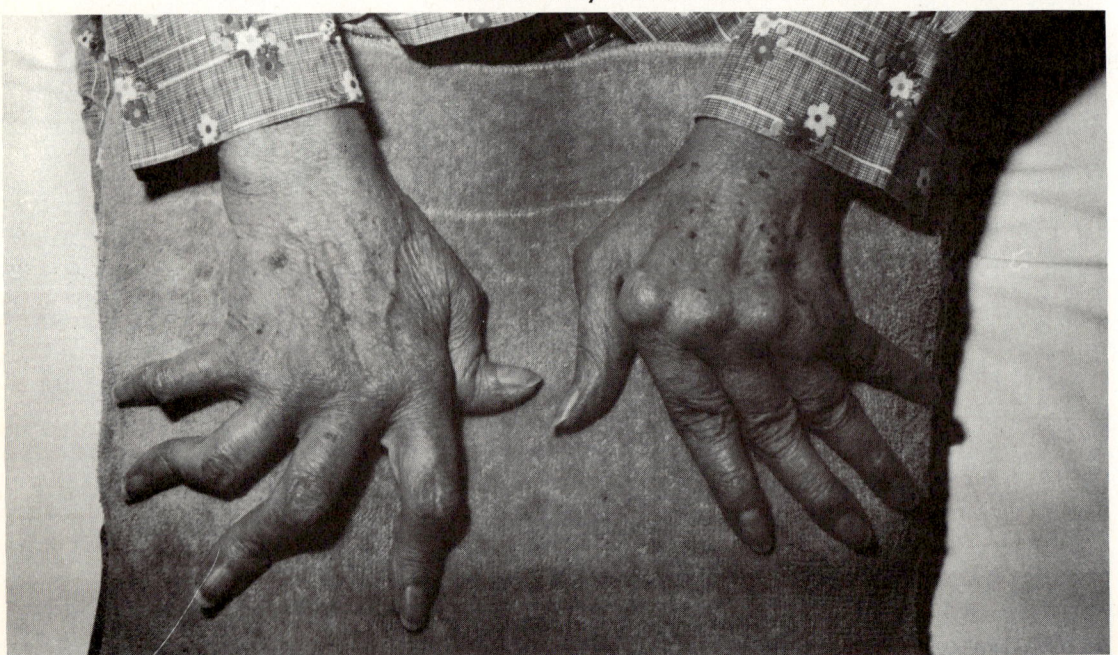

Figure 30-7
Arthritis may leave hands deformed and nonfunctional.

Postoperative Care Following MP implant arthroplasty, the patient enters a comprehensive program of exercises to help mold the capsule around the prosthesis and to achieve desired range of motion. The usual home program requires about 3 months of therapy.

In the immediate postoperative period, the nursing care is the same as for any patient returning from surgery. Special concerns for this patient are to observe and check for sensation and circulation in the fingers. The hand must be elevated above the level of the heart at all times, except for repositioning and performing the exercise program. The elbow may rest on the bed or be elevated on a pillow for comfort. Securing the hand to an intravenous stand assures a constant elevation and prevents the hand from accidentally falling off pillows.

Postoperatively, the nursing personnel must perform daily care for the patients, as there will be greater limitations after surgery than before surgery. The patient should be encouraged and allowed to do as much self-care as is feasible. Antiarthritic drugs are restarted as soon as possible to control inflammation in other joints. Generally, the patient can be out of bed the first or second day following surgery, with the arm elevated.

The postoperative hand dressing is bulky and is usually left in place for 4 to 5 days. Ice packs can be applied for the first 24 h to aid in reducing edema, but care should be taken that the dressing does not become wet. Continuous elevation of the hand is essential until the compression dressing is removed. Thereafter, the amount of elevation is based on the degree of swelling. After removal of the dressing, the forearm and hand are positioned in the dynamic splint (Fig. 30-8). The splint covers the dorsum of the wrist and has an outrigger with rubber bands and individual finger loops to keep the MPs in a neutral position of extension with the phalanges supported but loose enough to allow 70° of active MP flexion. The outriggers should be adjusted to pull the fingers in a radial direction to prevent ulnar drift. This positioning is crucial while the collagen and scar tissue are modeling around the prosthesis.

The nurse should observe for edema, pressure from the splint, and alignment of the joints. During the first week, the splint may require frequent adjustment by the therapist. The nurse should be instructed in proper application and adjustment of all parts of the splint.

On about the fifth postoperative day, the patient removes the splint for 2 or 3 h daily for active flexion and extension exercises of the MP joints. A flexion outrigger of the dynamic splint may be used later in the program if flexion is not achieved with ease. Hooks are glued onto the fingernails and/or an outrigger with rubber bands is attached to pull the fingers into flexion. A flexion cuff may also be used alternately with the extension outrigger. The crucial time for maximum results is between the second and third week, as the joint begins to tighten significantly at this time (Buchanan & Swanson, 1975). The extension portion of the dynamic splint is worn continuously for about 6 weeks postoperatively, then at night for about the next 6 weeks, and thereafter as prescribed by the physician and therapist. Splinting programs may vary considerably among patients. Daily, the patient must perform active flexion and extension of the MP joints, flexion and extension against resistance, radial deviation of all digits, especially the index finger, total flexion of fingers into the distal palmar crease, and active range of motion of the wrist, elbow, and shoulder. When exercising the MP joints, immobilization of the other joints is important in order to have true motion at the MPs.

While sutures are intact or the wound is open, the hand can be cleaned with a damp cloth. The sutures should not become wet. The hand must be thoroughly dry before applying the dynamic splint. The skin *around* the incision should be massaged several times a day with a circular motion. After sutures are removed, the hand is cleaned normally and the suture line massaged several times a day with cocoa butter or vitamin E oil. Press firmly in a circular motion or use a kneading motion. This will help prevent adhesions and minimize the scar.

After the first 3 months, the hand can be used

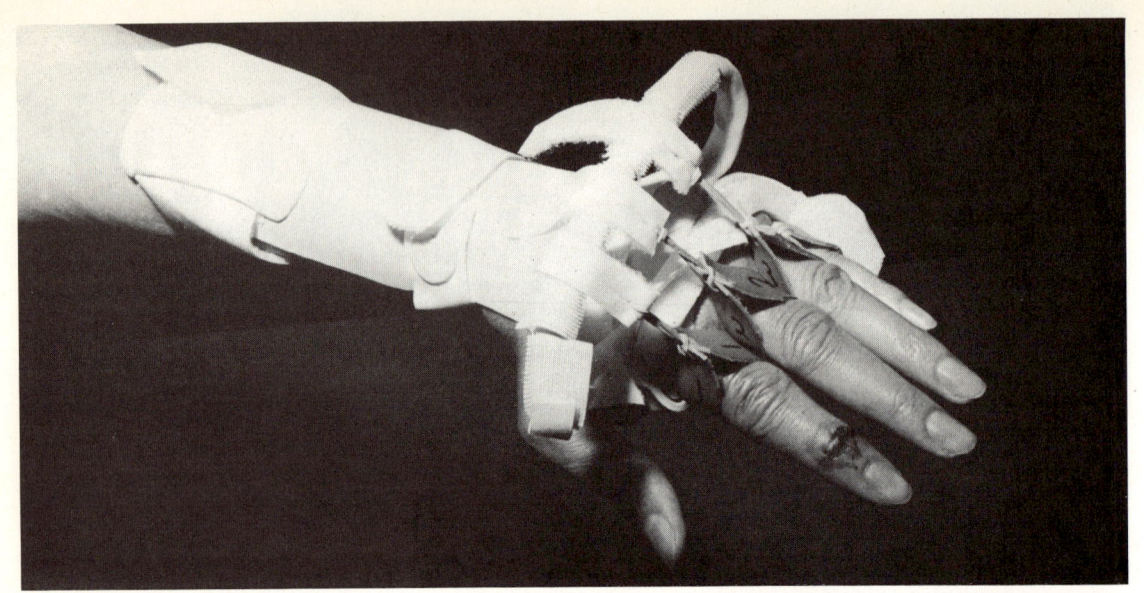

Figure 30-8
Positioning of the hand and forearm in a dynamic splint.

for light activities of daily living and job skills, except those that would traumatize the joints. Exercises and splinting of some type may be recommended for as long as 1 year postoperatively. A resting hand splint is usually provided after 3 months. The surgery provides good pain relief, good anatomical alignment, and restoration of function.

SEXUAL FUNCTION

The expression of sexuality is a natural function. A multitude of factors affect sexual expression, fulfillment, and adjustment. Cultural and religious factors influence attitudes and practices. Sexual activities and feelings are highly personal, and discussion about them is not usually within the realm of social interaction. Even within a health care setting, patients are often inhibited in initiating discussion about sexual matters. For the person with a chronic disabling disease, the ability to engage in sexual activities may be significantly altered. A sexual history is an essential part of patient evaluation, not only on initial contact but also throughout the course of management. Regardless of age, a sexual history should be obtained except for children who have not reached puberty. The patient's premorbid pattern of sexual expression is usually a good indicator of future adjustment to sexual problems. Teenagers may require special attention and assistance as they seek to achieve sexual identity.

Sexual assessment, subsequent discussion of alternatives, and guidance and counseling can be done by any health professional who understands the problems, is knowledgeable about the disease process and alternatives, and possesses the necessary counseling skills. Persons with overt psychological problems should be referred to a psychologist or psychiatrist for appropriate therapy.

Pain, limitations in range of joint motion, and fatigue are the most common physical barriers to engaging in sexual activity for persons with arthritis. Psychological factors such as depression, loss of self-esteem, poor body image, and fear of pain or pregnancy add to existing physical components and may decrease libido or cause sexual experiences to be unenjoyable or unfulfilling. Aversion to the person with disability by the sexual partner can reduce interaction. In addition, some analgesics and corticosteroids are reported to depress libido.

Other barriers to intercourse include genital problems associated with many connective tissue disorders. Behçet's disease causes ulceration on the genitalia that can be painful as well as aesthetically unpleasant. Reiter's syndrome is a triad of urethritis, arthritis, and conjunctivitis. A urethral discharge or unpleasant burning sensation of the urethra may be present. Sjøgren's syndrome is often seen in persons with rheumatoid arthritis and other connective tissue diseases. It is characterized by abnormal or absent secretions of mucous or serous glands of the body. The vaginal secretions are diminished, which can cause dyspareunia unless artificial lubricants are used (Ehrlich). With the aged female, there may also be decreased vaginal secretions that necessitate artificial lubrication.

An analgesic drug, taken 30 to 60 min prior to engaging in sexual activity, is helpful to decrease pain. A warm bath is also beneficial. Perineal hygiene may be difficult to perform if motion is limited in the hips or hands. A bath prior to intercourse would ensure cleanliness as well as relieve discomfort.

Suggestions regarding positioning for intercourse to alleviate discomfort should be provided (Onder, Lachniet, and Becker, 1973; Katz, 1977). The individual should strive to assume positions that will protect the joints as well as allow for desired movement for sexual activities. For upper extremity pain, contractures, and loss of strength, the side-lying position is preferred. Limitations in hip abduction or hip and knee flexion contractures may necessitate side-lying or kneeling in a comfortable position for rear entry intercourse. Persons who are unable to read or who have poor comprehension may benefit from viewing pictures showing various positions.

The emphasis should be on experimentation to find a satisfactory position and method of expression rather than focusing on inability to perform. Vibrators are a useful aid for total body, as well as genital, massage for patient or partner, especially if upper extremities are involved.

First and foremost in sexual guidance should be attempts at improving body image and self-esteem. Individuals with arthritis will not be able to attract or retain sexual partners if they dwell on pain and inability. Whenever possible, partners should be included in sexual counseling. It is also helpful to talk with the partner separately to seek out any underlying feelings, fears, or questions.

Repeated exacerbation and/or hospitalizations can cause financial as well as interpersonal strain within a family unit. The person may be perceived in a "sick" role, and sickness and sexuality rarely go hand in hand. In addition, separation of a couple removes the opportunity for sexual expression. Hospitalized patients often express concern that the mate will seek other sexual partners during the period of separation.

Fertility is not usually affected by the arthritis, but pregnancy often poses problems for the female patients. While many women experience a remission of the disease or, at least, less severe symptoms during pregnancy, other women may experience acute exacerbation. The initial onset of symptoms of RA often follows pregnancy (Persellin, 1977).

The additional weight during pregnancy can cause stress on the joints of lower extremities, even to the point of irreversible destruction. Hip flexion or hip adduction contractures may prevent normal delivery and necessitate a cesarean section.

When contemplating pregnancy, the couple should consider whether the addition of a child to the family would create undue financial or physical stress. If a woman has difficulty meeting her own self-care requirements independently, how will she manage child care? Would pregnancy or a child necessitate outside domestic help? In addition, some medications required for disease control may adversely affect the fetus.

If contraception is desired, selection of a method should be based not only on abilities of the patient but also attitudes of both the patient and sexual partner. Because of physical limitations, a diaphragm or contraceptive foam may be difficult to use. An intrauterine device is effective but may be difficult for the physician to insert or for the patient to check placement. Birth control pills may be prescribed if there are no contraindications. For a more permanent form of birth control, a vasectomy, tubal ligation, or other forms of sterilization may be preferred.

There is no confirmed evidence that genetic factors are involved in rheumatoid arthritis. Although there is a tendency for family members to develop various forms of degenerative joint disease and ankylosing spondylitis, this is not generally viewed as a contraindication to pregnancy (Ehrlich).

In summary, satisfactory sexual expression can be achieved by the majority of persons with arthritis. However, this area may require significant attitudinal and physical alterations on the part of the individual and partner. Sexual education and/or therapy by health care providers is essential if the total person is to be treated.

UNORTHODOX TREATMENT

At present, there is no cure for any of the arthritides. Treatment is aimed at alleviating symptoms, halting the systemic manifestations, preventing deformities and complications, and improving the individual's abilities for self-care. Patient compliance with the prescribed regimen is difficult to measure. Health care providers should not assume that prescribed treatment will be followed explicitly.

Frustration over the progressive course of the disease and the inability of medical science to offer a cure may cause some patients to seek relief or treatment from sources other than a qualified physician or to shop around from physician to physician. It is estimated that over $950 million are spent annually by Americans for unprescribed or unproven medications, devices, diets and dietary supplements, treatments, and special clinics (*Data Sheet*, 1978). Some manufacturers and individuals exploit those who suffer with claims of cure or miraculous relief.

Folk medicine, herbs, and copper jewelry are believed by many to ward off or cure arthritis. Special diets, biological therapies, and vitamin therapy are purported by some to relieve symptoms or even cure arthritis (Dong and Banks, 1973; Airola, 1968; Williams, 1971). Cultural and religious beliefs may influence compliance with standard medical treatment. Treatment programs in other countries, using drugs not approved for use in the United States, appeal to some individuals, especially those with financial resources to afford the treatment.

Programs that include high doses of a corticosteroid usually provide remarkable relief, but over time the drug can cause dangerous side effects. Dimethylsulfoxide (DMSO) is reported by patients to be readily available outside the United States.

The practice of "laying on of hands" for healing or relief of symptoms has been used for centuries. The exact mechanism as to why an individual obtains relief from this act is not well documented. Whether it is due to alterations within the body or the mind, something often occurs to relieve the symptoms of the disease.

Biofeedback as a technique to reduce tension and/or control pain is being used with some success. Acupuncture and acupressure are reported by some to relieve the symptoms of pain, but results have been unpredictable, and this is not widely accepted in this country as a common approach. Transcutaneous electrical nerve stimulators (TENS) are being used for many conditions to manage pain.

What may be viewed as quackery or unorthodox today could be a standard, acceptable treatment by medical science in the future. Health professionals must often sort out what is potentially harmful to the patient and what is not. The latent harm in a seemingly innocuous practice could be that in doing so, the patient fails to seek or follow through with the prescribed medical therapy.

It is advisable for health professionals to remain informed on nonstandard or new treatment approaches so the patient can be given an objective opinion. Learning about or observing the effects of other forms of treatment reflects an open-minded attitude and aids in building trust with the patient. It must also be kept in mind that spontaneous remissions do occur in a significant number of patients with arthritis, and only a small percentage have a progressive, unrelenting course of exacerbations throughout life.

SUMMARY

The interventions that have been outlined are primarily for persons with rheumatoid arthritis, but the majority are useful in the management of other rheumatic diseases. Since rheumatic diseases are chronic in nature, continuity of health care is of utmost importance. While one nurse may not be able to manage a patient over months or years, some continuity can be provided by thorough documentation of interventions and the results of nursing care. The results of nursing actions may not be visible for months or years. A referral to a community nursing agency is beneficial for follow-up care and for the long-term monitoring of health status. The hospital nurse has a responsibility to communicate the patient's therapeutic program to the community health nurse and to likewise receive feedback on the patient's progress.

JUVENILE RHEUMATOID ARTHRITIS

The diagnosis of juvenile rheumatoid arthritis (JRA) is used for individuals with onset of rheumatoid disease prior to age 16. Although the pathology is similar to adult rheumatoid arthritis, several features are likely to be found in children that are not usually present in the adult. Persistent high fever, rash, high incidence of monarticular onset, high incidence of cervical spine and distal interphalangeal joint involvement, low incidence of serum rheumatoid factor, and chronic iridocyclitis are common in children. Micrognathia, incomplete growth of the mandible, also occurs commonly. Subcutaneous nodules occur in less than 10 percent of all children with JRA (Vanace, 1977). Iridocyclitis and uveitis are the most severe extra-articular manifestations and may go undiagnosed, since there are often no symptoms. Ocular problems have been reported to occur in approximately 22 percent of all children with JRA (Levinson, 1972).

A characteristic transient rash is seen in a high percentage of children. It is usually erythematous or salmon pink, macular, with lesions that measure about 2 to 6 cm in diameter. The thorax, neck, abdomen, thighs, upper arms, soles, and palms are the most common sites. Light scratching and fever will usually intensify the rash (Vanace).

As in adult RA, the cause of JRA is unknown. The exact incidence and prevalence are also unknown, but estimates range from 50,000 to 200,000 in the United States (Vanace). Many cases probably are not recognized, especially if there is spontaneous remission. The disease occurs most frequently in females.

CLINICAL PATTERN

Vanace has described the following forms with regard to onset and clinical pattern.

Acute Systemic Form The predominant features include fever, rash, lymphadenopathy, hepatosplenomegaly, and cardiopulmonary involvement. Arthralgia is usually present, with eventual development of polyarthritis. Approximately 25 percent of children with juvenile rheumatoid arthritis have the acute systemic form, which is also called Stills disease.

Monarticular (Nonsystemic) Form The onset may be sudden or insidious and involves a single joint swelling, usually of a large joint. Mild arthralgia may be present, but the child is not systemically ill as in the acute systemic form. Laboratory studies are usually within the normal range. There is a significant incidence of ocular involvement with this group. The monarticular form is seen in about 40 percent of the children with JRA.

Polyarticular Form There is a close resemblance of the polyarticular form to adult rheumatoid arthritis. There may be an acute or insidious onset of low-grade fever, fatigue, morning stiffness, and polyarthralgia. Polyarthritis eventually develops. Overall, the child appears chronically ill. The classic rash is rare in this group, but erythema of the palms and soles is often noted. Laboratory findings are similar to those in adult RA. An estimated 35 percent of children with JRA have this form of the disease.

In addition to articular and extra-articular manifestations, the child with JRA experiences problems in physical growth and development, socialization, personality development, schooling, and vocational pursuits. Physical growth may be retarded as a result of early closure of epiphyseal plates resulting from the disease process and/or long-term use of corticosteroids.

MEDICAL MANAGEMENT

Early diagnosis and consistent treatment obviates many complications. Acetylsalicylic acid (ASA) is the preferred pharmacologic agent. Dosage is calculated according to the weight of the child or given in sufficient quantity to maintain satisfactory blood levels. Gold salts, crysotherapy, is effective and appropriate for those unresponsive to ASA. Corticosteroids do have a place in medical management, particularly when there are severe extra-articular problems. D-Penicillamine has been demonstrated to be effective in JRA; however, side effects can occur, and the cost of the drug may be prohibitive for some families.

Indomethacin is not used for children under 12 years of age. Antimalarial drugs are occasionally used to achieve remission. Immunosuppressive drugs and cytotoxic drugs are rarely used. Intra-articular injections of corticosteriods are useful for single joint inflammation, but frequent injections in the same joint are not recommended because of possible disturbance of bone and cartilage development.

The active child needs a balance between rest and exercise. Vigorous physical activity and fatigue can produce a flare of joint inflammation. Swimming, walking, and bicycling are preferred over running and contact sports. The overactive child will require more frequent rest periods than the one who curtails activity because of pain or preferred sedentary pursuits. The treatment approaches and goals by physical and occupational therapists are the same for children as for adults, with modifications for age. The daily exercise program does not have to be an isolated event but can often be incorporated into recreational activities. Sensorimotor experiences that aid growth and development, such as activities for eye-hand coordination, perceptual visual motor control, body awareness, and gross muscle control, can be included in the therapy program.

NURSING MANAGEMENT

The key to successful management is intervention before complications occur. Assessment of needs and problems is the first step. Specific areas of nursing assessment and intervention are outlined in the section on adult rheumatoid arthritis and are equally applicable to children.

Assessment of pain is often more difficult in children than in adults. Factors such as the child's developmental level, parental attitudes, cultural influences, unfamiliar surroundings, previous experience with hospitalization, symbolic meaning of pain, and observable physiological responses should be taken into consideration (Gildae and Quirk, 1977).

Health education becomes a challenge in that methods must be geared to the child's developmental and intellectual level. There is a dearth of materials for education of the child regarding juvenile rheumatoid arthritis. The entire family must be included in the teaching program. The child should not be excluded from discussions about the disease process, medications, toxic

CHAPTER 30   634

side effects, and reasons for the therapeutic program. The use of games to facilitate learning can be an effective tool with children.

Psychological support for both the child and parents is necessary. They need an opportunity to ask questions and discuss anxieties about deformities, life expectancy, and the future outlook.

IMPACT ON THE PERSON

Psychologically, the impact may be great. Joint deformities and external appliances are difficult to hide. Concern about appearance affects body image and personality development. Children often see adults with severe deformities from arthritis and may fear a similar outcome. During exacerbations the child is ill and is treated as such. During remission, however, the attitudes of parents and friends should change, but unfortunately they often do not. Children with JRA repeatedly express the desire to be treated normally. Children should be encouraged and allowed to set their own limits for activity.

Sibling rivalry is normal, but it may intensify if one or both parents devote excessive time and attention to the affected child. Although alterations in life-style often have to be made, the parents need support in realizing they have the right and responsibility to attend to their own needs and those of other family members. Overprotection of the child with JRA by a parent can lead to marital and family strife and to an unhealthy dependence of the child on the parent.

Schooling should continue, but teachers must be informed of the limitations imposed by the disease process. Regular physical education classes may need to be waived to permit activities within the child's abilities. Frequent exacerbations during the school year may prevent the child from completing academic requirements, and grades may have to be repeated. Every attempt should be made for tutoring or planning special assignments so the child can keep up with peers in school.

The disabled teenager may not have as many opportunities for dating as others. Classmates' attitudes, fear of rejection, and inability to engage in some activities may influence dating opportunities. Even with these obstacles to socialization and maturation, marriage and child rearing are realistic goals. Frequently the disease will "burn out" or become inactive by the time the child completes the growth process. Joint replacements for functional and cosmetic reasons are not usually performed until after maturity. Other preventive and reparative procedures may be done at an earlier age.

ANKYLOSING SPONDYLITIS

Ankylosing spondylitis is a disease characterized by inflammation and calcification of the cartilagenous and fibrocartilagenous joints of the spine, the adjacent soft tissues, paravertebral ligaments, and the sacroiliac joints. Frequently involved are the hips and shoulders and, occasionally, the peripheral joints. The early pathological joint changes are similar to those seen in rheumatoid arthritis, but the disease is a distinct entity. The term "rheumatoid spondylitis" is no longer used to describe the disease. Marie Strümpell disease and Bechterew's (or Bekhterev's) disease are common eponyms.

Symptoms include back pain, stiffness of back and hips, fatigue, malaise, anorexia, weight loss, limitations in chest expansion, and low-grade fever. Changes in posture occur, giving the person a stooped appearance as a result of bony ankylosis of the vertebral joints. The lumbar curve flattens, and kyphosis of thoracic vertebrae develops. Iritis occurs in about 25 percent of individuals with the disease (Katz, 1977), and cardiac involvement is not uncommon. Since expansion of the chest wall becomes impaired, the person usually compensates with diaphragmatic breathing. The disease often goes untreated if symptoms are mild, and the symptoms can subside spontaneously for months and years.

The cause of ankylosing spondylitis is not known. It has been observed in skeletons of human beings and some animals throughout history and described in early medical writings. The exact incidence in the United States is unknown but is estimated to be 1 or 2 per 1000 males and 1 per 10,000 females (Calin and Fries, 1975). The disease most often occurs in Caucasian males during young adulthood. There appears to be an autosomal factor related to the disease. The incidence among first-degree relatives is approximately 20 times greater than the general population. An HL-A antigen, W-27, has been reported to be present in 88 percent of persons with ankylosing spondylitis. The antigen occurs only in about 8 percent of a control population (Schlosstein et al., 1973). The presence of the HL-A W-27 antigen does not definitely confirm the diagnosis of ankylosing spondylitis, but it does help differentiate it from other back disorders. The degree of association between the disease and the antigen is so marked that a possible assumption is a "very close linkage of a gene governing immunologic responsiveness to the disease with W-27 or a strong biochemical cross-reaction of the etiologic agent with the W-27 antigen" (Schlosstein et al., 1973). The serum rheumatoid factor is usually negative, and the erythrocyte sedimentation rate is usually elevated only during inflammatory stages.

X-ray changes may show vertebral osteoporosis, ballooning of disk spaces, sclerosis of apophyseal joints, a straightening of the spinal curve, and irregularity or obliteration of the sacroiliac joint. Radiographic changes may not occur until years after onset of symptoms. Late changes may reveal disk and ligamentous calcification, joint fusion, and a "bamboo" appearance in the spine.

The diagnosis is often missed, as a large percentage of the general population experience nonspecific back pain. Calin et al. (1977) consider the clinical history as a valuable tool in diagnosis. Five factors are significant in differentiating ankylosing spondylitis from back pain of a mechanical origin. These are (1) insidious onset, (2) patient younger than 40, (3) pain persisting for at least 3 months, (4) associated morning stiffness, and (5) improvement with exercise.

MEDICAL MANAGEMENT AND THERAPY PROGRAM

Acetylsalicylic acid is the primary pharmacologic agent for suppression of inflammation. Phenylbutazone is useful in acute exacerbations but may also be prescribed for long-term management. Adrenocorticosteroids are not usually employed except for persons unresponsive to more conservative drugs or when used for short periods during acute inflammation. Gold salts are not usually effective for the axial symptoms of ankylosing spondylitis (Katz, 1977). Applications of local heat and cold aid in temporary relief of pain.

The basic therapy plan includes exercises for stretching the trunk, calf, and hamstring muscles, expanding the chest, and strengthening the abdominal muscles. The program should be carried out twice daily for maximum results. Analgesics and a warm bath prior to exercising help decrease discomfort. Swimming in a heated pool is an excellent form of general exercise. Standing posture is vitally important. The person should strive at all times when standing and walking to keep the head erect, shoulders back, chest raised, spine straight, and abdominal muscles tightened. Bed positioning is aimed at trunk straightening. A firm mattress is essential, and pillows should not be used under the head. A towel or blanket roll under the lumbar spine when supine will aid in trunk extension.

The side-lying position in bed is discouraged, for it fosters spinal and hip flexion deformities. The prone position helps prevent tightness of the hip flexors and encourages spine extension. The therapeutic positioning program should be instituted slowly and increased to tolerance. Attention should be given to possible respiratory problems when prone owing to pressure of the mattress on the diaphragm.

Eight to ten hours of sleep are recommended,

as well as two or more rest periods during the day. Sitting in a recliner-type chair for long periods is not recommended. Chairs should have a straight back and be of proper height and seat depth for the particular individual. Patients often report the most discomfort after arising and at the end of their usual day. The stiffness is usually relieved by a short period of exercises that mobilize specific joints.

As in rheumatoid arthritis, emotional or physical trauma and stress can precipitate a flare of the disease process. Excessive exercise or activity can exacerbate symptoms. Pain is often more severe during cold, damp weather.

The majority of individuals with this disease do not become totally incapacitated. Functional limitations are usually in the areas of lifting, climbing stairs, squatting, sitting, and turning the neck and trunk. The spine becomes less elastic and is subject to fracture even with minor injuries. Contact sports and hazardous occupations should be avoided. A change in occupation may be needed if involved joints are subjected to trauma. Persons with this disease are usually excellent candidates for referral to vocational rehabilitation services.

If the shoulders are involved, grooming and some dressing activities may become difficult, necessitating the use of adapted equipment. Devices such as long-handled reachers, shoe horns, sock combs, and car modifications for driving should be provided. If peripheral joints are involved, additional equipment may be needed.

Pain and deformities may affect sexual function. Counseling and guidance regarding positioning techniques for patient and partner are helpful.

SURGICAL PROCEDURES

Surgical procedures for correction of deformities are available but are not commonly used. An osteotomy of selected laminae can aid in spine realignment but requires extensive hospitalization and external braces for many months postoperatively. Hip arthroplasty may be indicated if mobility is severely impaired and the surgery can provide an improvement of overall functional status. The presence of other deformities, the patient's motivation, and long-range functional goals are thoroughly evaluated prior to any surgery.

SUMMARY

Generally, with a few modifications at work and home, equipment to increase independence in activities of daily living, and a regular home exercise and positioning program, persons with ankylosing spondylitis can remain functionally independent in most areas of daily life. Once the diagnosis is made, appropriate drugs prescribed, intensive education provided, and a home exercise program developed, the burden of management rests largely upon the patient. The prevention of some of the deformities depends upon the patient's willingness to actively participate by following the therapeutic program.

DEGENERATIVE JOINT DISEASE

Degenerative joint disease (DJD) is a common, noninflammatory disorder of movable joints, characterized by erosion of articular cartilage and formation of new bone in the subchondral areas and joint margins. It is the result of some form of biomechanical or biochemical abnormality within the joint. Osteoarthritis, osteoarthrosis, hypertrophic arthritis, and senescent arthritis are terms used to designate the disease, but *degenerative joint disease* more accurately describes the underlying pathological condition.

Degenerative joint disease can be classified as primary (idiopathic) or secondary. In the primary form, there is no known specific cause of the disease. Secondary degenerative joint disease is usually related to previous trauma, dysplasias, or some mechanism of biomechanical derangement of the joint.

Primary degenerative joint disease occurs commonly in the elderly and may, in part, be related to the aging process. It is not a systemic disease. The joints most often affected are those subjected to stress, shearing forces, or excessive use. The hips, knees, spine, and interphalangeal joints are the most commonly involved. The pattern of joint involvement is usually asymmetrical. The midcervical, midthoracic, and the lumbar vertebrae are the most frequent spinal areas involved. Although DJD is usually limited to one or two joints, there is a form called *generalized degenerative joint disease* that involves numerous joints of the body and that may be inflammatory. This form more commonly affects middle-aged women.

It is estimated that 16 million people in the United States have DJD (*Data Sheet*, 1978). This figure is probably conservative, because many persons may accept joint discomfort as a normal part of growing old and may not seek medical attention or report the condition on surveys. Terms such as "lumbago," "rheumatism," and "bursitis" are often used by lay persons to describe symptoms.

PATHOLOGY

The exact mechanisms that cause erosion of the cartilage are still not well understood. Articular cartilage is highly specialized connective tissue. It is avascular and has a slow rate of regeneration. The synovial fluid supplies nutrition and removes waste products. Stress or excessive use of a joint increases the rate of erosion of articular cartilage. The degenerative rate becomes greater than the reparative rate, and the erosion often extends to the underlying subchondral bone.

The underlying bone, in attempting to repair itself, develops osteophytes (spurs) at the margins of the joint. These sharply pointed growths of bone usually follow the contour of the joint surface (called "lipping") and can adhere to supporting ligaments. New bone also forms at the base of the articular cartilage and is an attempt by the bone to remodel the contour of the joint. The marrow can also undergo degeneration, and areas of decreasing density of the bone will develop immediately beneath the joint surface. In contrast to rheumatoid arthritis, degenerative joint disease is a disease of articular cartilage, whereas the former primarily affects the synovial membrane.

CLINICAL FEATURES

The major symptoms or findings in persons with DJD are joint pain or crepitus associated with movement, joint stiffness after prolonged inactivity, aching sensation of joint during cold and damp weather, and limitation of joint motion. Other findings include spasm or atrophy of adjacent muscles, tenderness around the joint, and malalignment of the joint. The swelling that often accompanies degenerative joint disease is usually "hard," in contrast to the swelling of rheumatoid arthritis, which is "boggy." There may be associated tendinitis and bursitis, and the joint can become inflamed if traumatized.

DIAGNOSTIC TESTS

Laboratory tests do not aid in the diagnosis. Occasionally, the erythrocyte sedimentation rate is elevated. Roentgenograms may be normal in appearance or show joint narrowing, sharpening of articular margins, bony sclerosis (eburnation), osteophytes and marginal lipping, and/or bone cysts. The x-ray does not always correlate with subjective symptoms. Many patients with definite abnormalities that appear on an x-ray are asymptomatic, while others with severe pain and loss of motion may show relatively minor x-ray changes.

Unique characteristics are often noted in the hands. Swelling, which occurs at the base of one or more distal interphalangeal joints (DIP), is the result of osteophytes that have protruded into the joint margin. These are referred to as Heberden's nodes. In the early stages of formation, these nodes may be inflamed but usually are not tender. However, they may be of concern to the patient cosmetically.

When a similar process occurs in a proximal interphalangeal joint, it is referred to as Bouchard's node. Heberden's nodes are more common, and women are affected with greater frequency than men.

MEDICAL MANAGEMENT

Some of the medications used for rheumatoid arthritis are effective for degenerative joint disease. Analgesics are preferred, often in combination with muscle relaxants. Nonsteroidal anti-inflammatory agents relieve symptoms in some patients. Local intra-articular injections with adrenocorticosteroids have an important place in the treatment of DJD when used as described previously for RA.

Systemic steroid therapy is not usually indicated in degenerative joint disease, since it is not an inflammatory systemic disease. Phenylbutazone drugs may be prescribed for short-term management if there are signs of local inflammation or associated tendinitis or bursitis.

The most common surgical interventions are for joint fusion, osteotomy or realignment, debridement, joint resurfacing, or total replacement of the diseased joint.

THERAPY MANAGEMENT

The modalities of heat and cold are useful for local relief of pain. The goals of physical and occupational therapy programs include maintaining range of joint motion, muscle strengthening, and providing assistive devices for ambulation and the activities of daily living. Techniques of joint protection and energy conservation are as essential for persons with this condition as they are for persons affected by rheumatoid arthritis. Resting the painful joint is one of the most effective ways of relieving pain.

IMPACT ON THE PERSON

A predominant concern among individuals with degenerative joint disease is that it will progress to other joints and produce crippling deformities as in rheumatoid arthritis. Knowledge that it is not systemic is usually a relief. Even though the disease may be limited to one or two joints, the resultant pain and limitation of motion can lead to loss of function, disability, and some deformity. Accurate diagnosis and prognosis are essential so that these patients can have some knowledge regarding the expectations of the physical effects that will be imposed on them by the disease in the future.

RESEARCH AND THE FUTURE

The National Arthritis Act of 1974 was signed into law on January 4, 1975 and became PL 93-640. Monies are alloted each year by Congress for support of nine institutions for direct arthritis-related research.

The Arthritis Foundation was founded in 1948 and joined with the American Rheumatism Association in 1965. The latter is the largest rheumatism society in the world. The Arthritis Foundation and the American Rheumatism Association carry out professional and public educational programs, as well as supporting research and treatment facilities through the awarding of grants.

The National Institute of Arthritis, Metabolism and Digestive Diseases (NIAMDD) is one of the National Institutes of Health of the United States Public Health Service. It was established in 1950 and presently contributes more to arthritis programs than any other institute or organization.

Future goals for health professionals in addition to supporting arthritis research should include changing public attitudes toward the disabled, eliminating architectural barriers in building, housing, and transportation, and providing public and professional education about arthritis treatment.

In the field of medicine, rheumatology is a subspecialty of internal medicine and requires board certification. Interest and research in the field are increasing rapidly. Nurses interested in specializing in arthritis can pursue several avenues. An arthritis or rheumatology clinical nurse specialist holds a master's degree in nursing and should have extensive clinical experience in the field. Arthritis nurse clinicians usually hold a bachelor of science in nursing (B.S.N.) degree, have had extensive experience with rheumatology patients, and have acquired additional knowledge through continuing education. With the establishment of arthritis centers and arthritis units within hospitals and rehabilitation centers, there is a definite need for nurses to specialize in this area.

CONCLUSION

Rheumatoid arthritis is a chronic systemic disease that can result in severe disability. Early accurate diagnosis is important for appropriate management and patient education. Pharmacologic agents, early splinting, external supports, therapeutic exercises, joint protection techniques, adaptive devices, health teaching, and surgery offer the individual a life with far less complications and disability than in years past.

Juvenile rheumatoid arthritis is a disease resembling the adult form that strikes children before age 16. It can result in severe articular disability and extra-articular problems. The child also faces problems in maturation, socialization, and schooling. JRA presents a challenge for long-term management of the entire family unit.

Degenerative joint disease is a common condition usually affecting one or two joints and is frequently seen with advancing age. Pharmacologic agents provide some relief of symptoms, therapy and adaptive devices reduce disability, and surgical intervention can restore functional abilities.

Individuals with ankylosing spondylitis experience varying degrees of disability but often remain functional with medication, regular exercises, and a few modifications in life-style and environment.

BIBLIOGRAPHY

Airola, Paavo, O.: *There Is a Cure for Arthritis,* Parker, West Nyack, N.Y., 1968.

Arthritis Manual for Allied Health Professionals, The Arthritis Foundation, New York, 1973.

Arthritis: Out of the Maze, vol. I, *The Arthritis Plan,* National Commission on Arthritis and Related Musculoskeletal Diseases, Report to the Congress of the United States, U.S. Department of Health, Education, and Welfare Publication (NIH) 76-1150, 1976.

Arthritis: Out of the Maze, vol. III, *Survey of Current Problems,* National Commission on Arthritis and Related Musculoskeletal Diseases, Report to the Congress of the United States, U.S. Department of Health, Education, and Welfare Publication (NIH) 76-1152, 1976.

Barry, Peter E., and J. Sidney Stillman: "Characteristics of Juvenile Rheumatoid Arthritis—Its Medical and Orthopedic Management," *Orthop Clin North Am* 6:641, 1975.

Bennage, Barbara A., and Marjorie E. Cummings: "Nursing the Patient Undergoing Total Hip Arthroplasty," *Nurs Clin North Am* 8:107, 1973.

Biundo, Joseph J., and Norman A. Cummings: "Biochemical, Hematologic and Immunologic Tests," in W. A. Katz (ed.): *Rheumatoid Diseases—Diagnosis and Management,* Lippincott, Philadelphia, 1977, p. 265.

Blumberg, B. S., Joseph J. Bunim, Evan Calkins, Conrad L. Pirani, and Nathan J. Zvaifler: "ARA Nomenclature and Classification of Arthritis and Rheumatism (tentative)," *Arthritis Rheum* 7:93, 1964.

Bowden, Susan Ackerman: "New Surgery for Arthritic Hands," *Nursing '76* 6:46, 1976.

Brassell, Mary P.: "Arthritis Nursing," in W. A. Katz

(ed.): *Rheumatic Diseases—Diagnosis and Management,* Lippincott, Philadelphia, 1977, p. 1000.

Buchanan, Lesley, and Alfred B. Swanson: *Home Exercise Program for Patients with Silastic Finger Joint Implants (Swanson Design),* Orthopedic Reconstructive Surgeons, Grand Rapids, 1975.

Bywaters, E. G. L.: "The Management of Juvenile Chronic Polyarthritis," *Bull Rheum Dis* 27:882, 1977.

Calin, Andrei, and James F. Fries: "Striking Prevalence of Ankylosing Spondylitis in ''Healthy'' W27 Positive Males and Females," *N Engl J Med* 293:835, 1975.

———— et al.: "Clinical History as a Screening Test for Ankylosing Spondylitis," *JAMA* 237:12810, 1977.

Carpenter, James O., and Linda J. Davis: "Medical Recommendations—Followed or Ignored? Factors Influencing Compliance in Arthritis," *Arch Phys Med Rehabil* 57:241, 1976.

Convery, F. Richard, Martha A. Minteer, Ravid Amiel, and Karen L. Connett: "Polyarticular Disability: A Functional Assessment," *Arch Phys Med Rehabil* 58:494, 1977.

Data Sheet—Arthritis Prevalence and Related Statistics, The Arthritis Foundation, Atlanta, June 9, 1978.

Dippy, J. E.: "Penicillamine in Rheumatoid Arthritis—A 2-Year Retrospective Study in 70 Patients," *Br J Clin Pract* 31:5, 1977.

Dong, Collin H., and Jane Banks: *The Arthritis Cookbook,* Crowell, New York, 1973.

Ehrlich, George E.: *Total Management of the Arthritic Patient,* Lippincott, Philadelphia, 1973.

————: "Remittive Pharmaceutical Agents," in W. A. Katz (ed.): *Rheumatic Diseases—Diagnosis and Management,* Lippincott, Philadelphia, 1977, p. 897.

Engleman, Ephriam: "Conservative Management of Rheumatoid Arthritis," in J. L. Hollander and D. J. McCarty (eds.): *Arthritis and Allied Conditions,* Lea and Febiger, Philadelphia, 1972.

Fassbender, J. G.: *Pathology of Rheumatic Diseases,* G. Loewi (trans.), Springer, New York, 1975.

FDA Fact Sheet, U.S. Department of Health, Education, and Welfare, Public Health Service, Food and Drug Administration, Rockville, Md., 1973.

Feibel, Arie, and Avital Fast: "Deep Heating of Joints: A Reconsideration (commentary)," *Arch Phys Med Rehabil* 57:513, 1976.

French, Alfred P., and Joe P. Tupin: "Therapeutic Application of a Simple Relaxation Method," *Am J Psychother* 28:282, 1974.

Gildae, Joan H., and Tina R. Quirk: "Assessing the Pain Experience in Children," *Nurs Clin North Am* 12:631, 1977.

Goldenberg, Don L., and Alan S. Cohen: "Arthritis as a Medical Emergency," in A. S. Cohen, R. B. Freiden, and M. A. Samuels (eds.): *Medical Emergencies: Diagnostic and Management Procedures from Boston City Hospital,* Little Brown, Boston, 1977, p. 245.

Grzesiak, Roy C.: "Relaxation Techniques in Treatment of Chronic Pain," *Arch Phys Med Rehabil* 58:270, 1977.

Gupta, Ved P., and George E. Ehrlich: "Organic Brain Syndrome in Rheumatoid Arthritis Following Corticosteroid Withdrawal," *Arthritis Rheum* 19:1333, 1976.

Hall, Arthur P.: "The Decision to Operate in Rheumatoid Arthritis," *Orthop Clin North Am* 6:675, 1975.

Hamilton, Ann: "The Problems of the Arthritic Patient, a Symposium on Sexual Problems of the Disabled," *Nurs Mirror* 142:54, 1976.

Hollander, Joseph L., and Daniel J. McCarty, Jr. (eds.): *Arthritis and Allied Conditions,* 8th ed., Lea Febiger, Philadelphia, 1972.

Jaffe, Israeli A.: "D-Penicillamine," *Bull Rheum Dis* 28:948, 1977–1978 series.

Kantor, Thomas G: "Anti-inflammatory and Analgesic Drugs," in W. A. Katz (ed.): *Rheumatic Diseases—Diagnosis and Management,* Lippincott, Philadelphia, 1977, p. 876.

Katz, Warren A. (ed.): *Rheumatic Diseases—Diagnosis and Management,* Lippincott, Philadelphia, 1977.

Klinger, Judith L.: *Self Help Manual for Arthritis*

Patients, Arthritis Foundation, New York, 1974.

Levinson, Joseph E.: "Juvenile Rheumatoid Arthritis," *Postgrad Med* 51:89, 1972.

MacRae, Isabel: "Arthritis: I'ts Nature and Management," *Nurs Clin North Am* 8:643, 1973.

Marbach, Joseph H.: "Arthritis of the Temporomandibular Joints and Facial Pain," *Bull Rheum Dis* 27:918, 1977.

Marmor, Leonard: *Arthritis Surgery,* Lea & Febiger, Philadelphia, 1976.

McCann, Virginia H., Cynthia A. Philips, and T. R. Quigley: "Preoperative and Postoperative Management—The Role of Allied Health Professionals," *Orthop Clin North Am* 6:881, 1975.

McDuffie, Frederic C., and Thomas W. Bunch: "Immunologic Tests in the Diagnosis of Rheumatic Diseases," *Bull Rheum Dis* 27:900, 1977.

McKenzie, Mary W., Linda M. Hennig, and Maureid McGill: *Arthritis Learning Notebook,* Mississippi Methodist Rehabilitation Center, Jackson, 1976.

Meyers, Marvin H., Dorothy B. McNelly, and Karen Nelson: "Total Hip Replacement," *Am J Nurs* 78:1485, 1978.

Millender, Lewis H., and Clement B. Sledge (eds.): "Symposium on Rheumatoid Arthritis," *Orthop Clin North Am* 6:608–906, 1975.

Moskowitz, Roland W.: "Osteoarthritis and Traumatic Conditions," in W. A. Katz (ed.): *Rheumatic Diseases—Diagnosis and Management,* Lippincott, Philadelphia, 1977, p. 581.

Onder, Jan, Donna Lachnier, and Marjorie C. Becker: "Sexual Counselling—Arthritis and Women," *Allied Health Professions Section Newsletter,* The Arthritis Foundation, 7:1, 1973.

Orem, Dorthea E.: *Nursing, Concepts of Practice,* McGraw-Hill, New York, 1971.

Persellin, Robert H.: "The Effect of Pregnancy on Rheumatoid Arthritis," *Bull Rheum Dis* 27:922, 1977.

Person, Donald A., and John T. Sharp: "Eriology of Rheumatic Arthritis," *Bull Rheum Dis* 27:888, 1977.

Primer on the Rheumatic Diseases, 7th ed., The Arthritis Foundation, New York, 1973.

"Proceedings of the Symposium on the Management of Arthritis at the 1971 Assembly of the Interstate Postgraduate Medicine Association," *Postgrad Med* 51:5, 1972.

Rosenthal, David, Michael H. Boblitz, and Vaddadi R. Roa: "Bus Use by Disabled Arthritics: Functional Requirements," *Arch Phys Med Rehabil* 58:220, 1977.

Rothermich, Norman O., et al.: "Crysotherapy: A Prospective Study," *Arthritis Rheum* 19:1321, 1976.

Schlosstein, Lee, et al.: "High Association of an HL-A Anitigen, W27, with Ankylosing Spondylitis," *N Engl J Med* 288:704, 1973.

Sculco, Cynthia, and Thomas P. Sculco: "Management of the Patient with an Infected Total Hip Arthroplasty," *Am J Nurs* 76:584, 1976.

Smyth, Charley J.: "Therapy of Rheumatoid Arthritis—A Pyramidal Plan," *Postgrad Med* 51:31, 1972.

Solomon, L.: "Patterns of Osteoarthritis of the Hip," *J Bone Joint Surg* 58-B:176, 1976.

Spergel, Philip: "Psychological Aspects of Joint Diseases," in W. A. Katz (ed.): *Rheumatic Diseases—Diagnosis and Management,* Lippincott, Philadelphia, 1977.

Stewart, Patricia, and George W. Wharton: "Bridging: An Effective and Practical Method of Preventive Skin Care for the Immobilized Person," *South Med J* 69:1469, 1976.

Swanson, Alfred B.: *Flexible Implant Resection Arthroplasty in the Hand and Extremities,* Mosby, St. Louis, 1973.

Tsang, Ian K., et al.: "D-Penicillamine in the Treatment of Rheumatoid Arthritis," *Arthritis Rheum* 20:666, 1977.

Vanace, Peter: "Juvenile Rheumatoid Arthritis and Other Rheumatic Diseases of Children," in W. A. Katz (ed.): *Rheumatic Diseases—Diagnosis and Management,* Lippincott, Philadelphia, 1977.

Watkins, Ruth A., and Dianne Robinson: *Joint Preservation Techniques for Patients with Rheumatoid Arthritis.* Medical Rehabilitation Research and Training Center, No. 20, Northwestern University-Rehabilitation Institute of Chicago, Chicago, 1974.

Wetherell, Robert C., Jr., Director, Office of Legislative Services, U.S. Department of Health, Education and Welfare, Rockville, Md., Personal communication, May 1978.

Williams, Ralph C.: *Rheumatoid Arthritis as a Systemic Disease,* Saunders, Philadelphia, 1974.

Williams, Roger J: *Nutrition Against Disease,* Pitman, New York, 1971.

Yoslow, Wilfred, Joseph Simeone, and Dawn Huestis: "Hip Replacement Rehabilitation," *Arch Phys Med Rehabil* 57:275, 1976.

Ziebell, Beth: "Psychosocial Needs of Adolescents with Arthritis," *Allied Health Professions Section Newsletter,* The Arthritis Foundation, 11,12:5, 1978.

31
irene b. alyn

pain as a result of physical impairment

INTRODUCTION

From the practitioner's perspective, pain has protective and diagnostic value and is a subjective, variously described symptom that presents an ever-present clinical challenge. Pain is initially perceived when tissue damage is occurring in the body, and it may later be evoked by a psychological event or an increase in brain activity. Pain, a subjective personal phenomenon, has been defined as an abstract concept that refers to sensation, stimulus, and response (Sternbach, 1974). McCaffery (1972) maintains that, for the clinician, pain is whatever the person experiencing it says it is and that the pain exists whenever that individual says it does.

The peripheral nerve, spinal cord, thalamus, and cerebral cortex receive, process, and cause the perception of pain. Automatically, spinal cord reflexes allow us to withdraw a hand from a hot stove and prevent further burn and pain. In this sense, pain is a protective mechanism, and without pain, we are left in a relatively vulnerable state.

For three of the leading causes of death, pain is either a very late symptom or no pain warning sign may occur at all. For example, heart attack is a leading cause of death, and pain as a warning signal comes, if at all, close to the actual event. Stroke, a second major killer, frequently results from hypertension; however, chronic hypertension usually is asymptomatic. Individuals, therefore, may not seek treatment for hypertension because they feel no discomfort or pain. A third major cause of death is cancer, and again, in the early stages of most cancers, there is little or no pain. Pain is perceived only in the advanced stages of this disease. Other chronic diseases (for example, diabetes, multiple sclerosis) do not send any early warning pain signals. In fact, people seem to pay more attention to a sunburn or splinter in the finger because these ailments hurt more than do certain illnesses of a serious nature.

THEORIES OF PAIN

SPECIFICITY THEORY

Although there are several theories about why and how we perceive pain, only two will be described in this chapter. Most practitioners are familiar with the specificity theory (Sweet, 1959) of pain, which states that nerve fibers respond to stimuli and that pain, touch, temperature, and position stimuli are transmitted through different nerve fibers. Large fibers carry touch impulses in myelinated, fast-conducting fibers to touch centers in the brain. Small fibers transmit pain impulses in unmyelinated, slow-conducting fibers to pain centers in the brain. After the specific afferent fibers carry the respective stimuli from the tissue to the dorsal column of the spinal cord, two actions occur. Impulses are relayed to the motor fibers of the reflex arc, so that specific muscles contract while other impulses cross to the opposite side of the spinal cord and are sent through the spinothalamic tract to the thalamus, where they arouse the perception of pain. These impulses are then transmitted from the thalamus to the cerebral cortex which, when activated, interprets pain impulses in terms of location, intensity, and duration. In addition, the cerebral cortex initiates efferent impulses that result in stimulation of autonomic nervous system, skeletal muscle, and psychological responses.

GATE CONTROL THEORY

In 1965, Melzack and Wall proposed the gate control theory of pain. The basic components of the gate control theory are the spinal gating mechanism, the central control system, and the peripheral response system. The spinal gating mechanism is made up of large and small fibers, substantia gelatinosa (SG), and transmission (T) cells. Peripheral afferents, the large and small fibers, pass through the SG in the dorsal horn of the spinal cord. As large fibers enter the SG, they stimulate SG activity, and entry of impulses into the T cells is inhibited, "closing the gate." Transmission from T cells is diminished, and less pain is perceived. Conversely, small-diameter fiber impulses inhibit SG activity and therefore increase T-cell transmission, "opening the gate." Thus the balance of activity of large- and small-diameter fibers is the primary determinant of T-cell activity. The central control system monitors the input from the spinal column tracts and exerts an inhibitory influence on the sensory input via descending (efferent) fibers. If pain is perceived, the net result of these interactions is a sequence of behavior responses, including reflex activities, altered physiological response, expressions of pain, and initiation of coping strategies.

Unlike the specificity theory, the gate control theory of pain has pointed to possible mechanisms of pain development in certain diseases (diabetes, alcohol neuropathy, central nervous system lesions) and has implications for pharmacological, sensory, and psychological control of pain (Melzack and Wall, 1970). The gate control theory has stimulated increased interest in the interplay of two or more impulses in the central nervous system and in counterstimulation of large-diameter fibers to block pain. The significance of the gate control theory to clinical practice is still being explored.

TYPES OF PAIN

Pain has subjectively been described as pricking, burning, or aching sensations. Pricking pain is the pain experienced by a needle prick or a cut. Burning pain is the pain of sunburn or a thermal burn from chemicals, hot water, or fire. Aching pain is pain usually arising from the viscera, for example, a stomachache or colic.

Pain has been classified by location or causal agent (six varieties of pain) as superficial or visceral pain and as acute or chronic pain. Acute pain, for example, occurs following an appendectomy or acute myocardial infarction and is relieved within hours. Chronic pain is pain sustained over long periods of time—days, months, years (i.e., low back pain, arthritis, or some types of malignancy). Superficial pain is cutaneous pain (i.e. burns) and typically initiates a sympathetic response. Visceral pain is organ pain and usually initiates a parasympathetic response.

The six varieties of pain are as follows:

1. Muscle and joint pain (arthritis or low back pain)
2. Neuralgia (variety of nerve pain)
3. Causalgia (pain due to trauma or intense physical injury)
4. Vascular pain from vasoconstriction of blood vessels (migraine)
5. Visceral pain due to tissue damage in the large body organs
6. Phantom limb pain (experienced by some persons following amputation)

Practitioners tend to categorize pain as mild, moderate, or severe. Mild pain is pain that does not interfere with the patient's ability to work and does not change behavior significantly. These are the normal pains that one suffers in daily life, and most people cure themselves with over-the-counter drugs. Moderately severe pain does interefere with a person's life, and treatment for the pain is usually a problem. Moderate pain results from headaches and bone and muscle problems and is a very difficult type of pain to treat because it continues over a long period of time, and therefore the psychological and sociocultural interplay significantly affects the individual's perception of this pain. Severe pain is pain that totally consumes the person's attention, resulting in an inability to focus on other activities of normal living. This type of pain is frequently treated by routine surgical procedure or by one of the newer experimental surgeries.

Although diagnosticians and practitioners are more interested in categorizing pain than are the patients they treat, knowledge of the type of pain is useful in directing therapy and in anticipating the types of complications (physical, psychological, cultural, economic) that might result from the pain. Even so, practitioners are continually aware of the importance of incorporating into their treatment plan the person's perception of the magnitude and significance of the pain.

TECHNIQUES FOR DIFFERENTIATING THE CAUSE OF PAIN

The history of the pain symptom is an important dimension in determining the cause of pain. At times, practitioners display a negative attitude toward patients because a patient's description of pain may not fit one of the recognized patterns. For example, if a patient complains of chest pains but the pain does not radiate to the appropriate structures, the practitioner may dismiss the pain as being insignificant. However, just because the practitioner cannot find a physical cause of an individual's pain does not mean that it is not there. The individual's history may enable the practitioner to determine whether, for example, a migraine headache is due to an organic or a psychogenic cause. If the pain results from an organic headache, the patient can describe how long ago the headache began. The patent might say, "It began 2 weeks ago when I was at the hairdresser." In a psychogenic type (no organic cause delineated, but pain is truly experienced) of migraine headache, however, the patient is usually unable to describe the exact onset (Diamond and Dalessio, 1978).

A history of the individual's sleep pattern as it relates to pain is usually helpful in determining the cause of the pain. Patients who are depressed and complain of migraine often have difficulty falling asleep and wake up two or three times during the night and/or awaken early. Sometimes, it is useful for the practitioner to ask the patient how many types of pain are experienced in order to determine whether or not the pain is a specific problem that occurs at a specific time while engaging in specific activities.

Another technique for determining the cause of pain is to know the dermatomes and referred pain patterns. In other words, in referred pain, the area that hurts is not the structure that is damaged. Most practitioners are fully aware that heart pain may be referred to the jaw, left arm, or shoulder. No one knows exactly how pain is referred, but it is believed that the phenomenon is a result of nerve fibers from certain organs that enter the main tracts to the spinal cord close to or at the same point that pain nerve fibers enter from other parts of the body. This overlapping produces or allows the referred pain to occur.

Also, in differentiating the causes of the pain, it is useful to determine from the patient what relieved the pain. Does activity relieve the pain or does rest relieve the pain? For example, while rest may relieve the pain of arteriosclerosis obliterans, activity may relieve certain muscle and joint pain.

TEMPORAL ASPECTS OF PAIN

Unlike other sensory receptors, pain receptors do not adapt over time, and in fact, pain receptors can become even less difficult to stimulate (i.e., more sensitive to painful stimuli.) Having nonadapting pain receptors affords the individual protection as long as the pain stimuli persist.

Pain is usually greater during the time when tissue damage is occurring than it is after the damage has occurred. For example, because of a lack of oxygen (hypoxemia), pain is intense during the acute phase of myocardial infarction, but later pain may be minimal. Persons who have sustained a full-thickness thermal injury frequently do not perceive as much pain as those with partial injury. The pain experienced at the time of the thermal injury may be comparable in partial and full-thickness burns, but later, owing to the destruction of free nerve endings in the skin, full-thickness injury usually does not provoke as much pain as does partial-thickness injury (Feller and Archambeault-Jones, 1973). This phenomenon may present a nursing care problem because, psychologically, practitioners tend to think that with more tissue damage there is greater pain than when minimal damage has occurred.

The timing of the initial onset of pain influences the individual's perception of pain. For example, soldiers wounded in battle in World War II felt little pain even after a very severe gunshot wound (Stiller, 1975). It was thought that being wounded signified to the soldier that he would be removed from the battle and thus survive the war. Later, in the hospital unit, these same men were reported to complain of the pricking pain caused by a simple injection of a needle into the skin.

The general body condition or what the person is doing at the time of the injury influences the pain perception. When skiing or swimming or having a pleasant time, a person may not notice an injury to the tissue and therefore not perceive pain until later, when the pleasant activity had subsided. When we are fatigued, we have less tolerance for pain and are more susceptible to increased pain caused by infection or edema.

PAIN REINFORCEMENT

Time factors affect the programming of pain reinforcers. For example, according to Pace (1976), patients with painful injuries that were satisfactorily diagnosed and treated within 6 weeks returned to gainful employment and regained their self-respect. However, persons whose pain and tissue damage persisted for up to 6 months had much more difficulty seeing themselves as useful persons, viewing themselves instead, as persons who probably would not return to successful employment. Persons whose pain persisted for over 6 months soon learned the value of the sick role and its possible compensations and began to manipulate others by use of their pain. Persons who sustained pain for over a year were extremely resistant to treatment and a relinquishment of their pain in spite of expert psychological reconditioning.

If a person has time to prepare for a painful experience, the pain perception appears to be decreased. An individual who sustains an acute myocardial infarction rarely has warning, because the injury occurs rapidly and is very painful.

These persons have no time to prepare to defend themselves against the pain stimuli and therefore experience much greater pain than persons who have had time to prepare for a painful event (Stiller, 1975). Patients who withstand repeated debridements in the treatment room of a burn unit seem, either physically or psychologically, to prepare themselves to endure these painful treatments day after day.

ANTICIPATION OF PAIN

Hilgard and associates (1974a) at Stanford University found that anticipating pain was less upsetting than anticipating no pain. They stated that uncertainty about how much pain was to be experienced increased the heart rate; conversely, the heart rate decelerated when the subject knew exactly how much pain to expect. Their conclusion was that it takes more effort to maintain analgesia than to simply accept the pain experience. These experiments by Hilgard are supportive of Jean Johnson's work.

Johnson (1973) studied patients who were to undergo endoscopy. The control group (Group 1) received only the usual or routine information about the procedure. The second group was told all about the procedure and how to behave during it. The third group was given information about what sensations to expect, and the fourth group was told how to behave and also given information about the sensation that they would feel. The patients (Group 3) who received information only about the sensations that they would feel did much better during the procedure (gagged less, needed less tranquilizers, had more stable heart rates) than the control group (Group 1) who received only standard information. Group 3 also did better than persons in Group 4, who were told how to behave as well as what sensations they should feel. It can be concluded from these experiments that by anticipating pain and discomfort, we can diminish it. Stated another way, knowledge and anticipatory thought may reduce pain perception.

TOOLS FOR THE MEASUREMENT OF PAIN

Assessment of pain is an important component of clinical management of pain. Most patients experiece pain regardless of the type of emotional or physical illness. Patients who have a physical illness seem to have difficulty describing parameters of pain and need help in selecting the specific words that help the clinician identify clearly the type of intervention needed to alleviate the pain. The artificiality of laboratory pain and respect for the dignity and suffering of clinically ill patients make the study of pain a complex undertaking. Relatively healthy persons with few emotional problems and little change in life-style as a result of the debilitating aspects of pain stop pain experiments prior to "absolute endurance," saying that pain is unbearable. However, some patients must daily experience maximal pain, extreme fatigue, and lack of sleep owing to the unrelievable nature of their pain. Many of the experiments establishing pain thresholds and pain tolerance levels have been carried out in laboratory settings rather than in a clinical setting, and the results of some of these experiments are conflicting and confusing to the clinician. In studies on the measurements of laboratory pain, persons have been exposed to a variety of noxious stimuli and asked to report when they noticed increases in the pain or experienced pain that was unbearable. The noxious stimuli have varied from heat to cold to pressure to pinpricking and to a variety of other stimuli.

Dolorimeter

Hardy, Wolff, and Goodell (1952) developed a dolorimeter to measure pain. In an effort to determine pain thresholds, they measured the amount of radiant heat that was tolerable to the patient. Other researchers have used the sphygmomanometer and asked the subjects to identify the amount of pressure that is first identified as painful to them and then the amount of pressure that is unbearable.

Attempts to measure clinical pain have included observation of behavior, number of requests for medication to relieve pain, physiological parameters (such as blood pressure and heart rates), and color or language used by patients to describe their pain. None of these methods has been completely successful.

Pain Rating Scales

The Chambers Price Pain Rating Scale (see Table 31-1) is an objective attempt to assess the amount of pain a patient is experiencing by observing behavior. The variables assessed by the Chambers Price Pain Rating Scale are attention, anxiety, verbalizations, perspiration, sounds made by the patient, nausea and vomiting, skeletal muscle movement, muscle tenseness, and facial expressions. Each behavior is rated by an observer on a scale of 1 (little or no pain) to 5 (intense pain), and a total score is obtained by adding the scores of the nine variables. Physiological parameters such as changes in blood pressure, sleep pattern, and heart rate have been observed when the patient was thought to be experiencing pain. However, there are so many other phenomena that influence these parameters that they are not reliable indices to measure the intensity of a person's pain.

Language of Pain

Melzack and Torgerson (1971) described the language used by patients to describe their pain. Patients described their pain using a variety of terms in three general classes: sensory qualities, affective qualities, and evaluative words. The McGill-Melzack Pain Questionnaire (Fig. 31-1) is a refinement of the original work. This questionnaire was sufficiently sensitive to detect differences among different methods to relieve pain and to provide quantitative information that can be used to treat patients with a variety of illnesses. If, from their work and the work of others, it seems that patients with similar diseases describe their pain using similar words, the clinician can have some point of reference to determine the actual intensity of the pain. The language of pain scale developed by Melzack and others is

Table 31-1

Objective Tool for Measurement of Pain

	5	4	3	2	1
Attention Patient directs:	almost complete attention to pain, very difficult to distract	more attention to pain, less to distraction	some attention to pain, some to distraction	little attention to pain, easily distracted	no attention to pain, no difficulty distracting
Anxiety Patient directs:	complete tension, irritability, worry	marked tension, irritability	some tension, irritability, worry	little tension, irritability, worry	no tension, irritability, worry
Verbal Patient states:	there is severe pain	there is a lot of pain	there is some pain	there is very little pain	there is no pain; asleep
Perspiration Patient has:	very marked perspiration	marked perspiration	some perspiration	little perspiration	normal perspiration
Sounds Patient:	cries out or sobs	groans, moans loudly	groans, moans softly	sighs, grunts soft	talks in normal tone, no sounds
Nausea Patient:	retches, vomits	says he or she is about to vomit	feels sick to the stomach	feels squeamish	does not mention nausea
Skeletal muscle Patient is:	very restless	markedly restless	slightly restless	very slightly restless	quiet
Muscle tenseness Patient is:	extremely tense	markedly tense	somewhat tense	slightly tense	relaxed
Facial expression Patient has:	constant frown	marked frown	some frown	little frown	no frown

Source: W. Chambers and G. Price: "Influence of Nurse upon Effects of Analgesis Administered," *Nurs Res* 16(37):228–233, 1967. Reprinted with permission.

(a)

Patient's name _____ Age _____
Hospital No. _____
Clinical category (e.g., cardiac, neurological, etc.): _____
Diagnosis: _____
_____
_____

Analgesic (if already administered):
  1. Type _____
  2. Dosage _____
  3. Time given in relation to this test _____

Patient's intelligence: Circle number that represents best estimate.
1 (low)   2   3   4   5 (high)

****

This questionnaire has been designed to tell us more about your pain. Four major questions we ask are:
  1. Where is your pain?
  2. What does it feel like?
  3. How does it change with time?
  4. How strong is it?

It is important that you tell us how your pain feels now. Please follow the instructions at the beginning of each part.

(b)

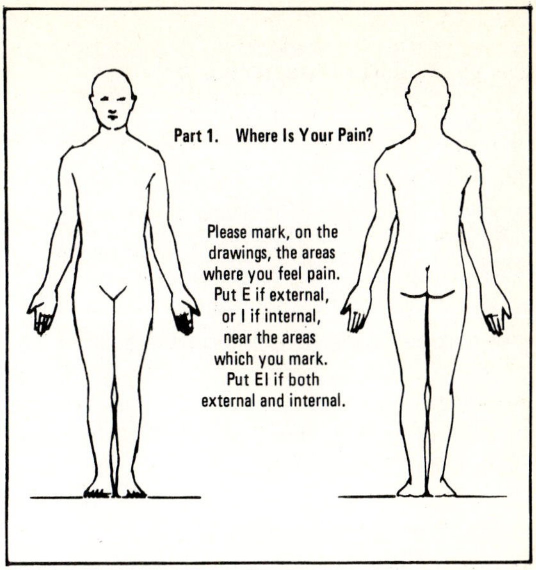

Part 1. Where Is Your Pain?

Please mark, on the drawings, the areas where you feel pain. Put E if external, or I if internal, near the areas which you mark. Put EI if both external and internal.

(c)

Part 2. What Does Your Pain Feel Like?

Some of the words below describe your <u>present</u> pain. Circle <u>ONLY</u> those words that best describe it. Leave out any category that is not suitable. Use only a single word in each appropriate category--the one that applies best.

1	2	3	4	5
Flickering	Jumping	Pricking	Sharp	Pinching
Quivering	Flashing	Boring	Cutting	Pressing
Pulsing	Shooting	Drilling	Lacerating	Gnawing
Throbbing		Stabbing		Cramping
Beating		Lancinating		Crushing

6	7	8	9	10
Tugging	Hot	Tingling	Dull	Tender
Pulling	Burning	Itchy	Sore	Taut
Wrenching	Scalding	Smarting	Hurting	Rasping
	Searing	Stinging	Aching	Splitting
			Heavy	

11	12	13	14	15
Tiring	Sickening	Fearful	Punishing	Wretched
Exhausting	Suffocating	Frightful	Gruelling	Blinding
		Terrifying	Cruel	
			Vicious	
			Killing	

16	17	18	19	20
Annoying	Spreading	Tight	Cool	Nagging
Troublesome	Radiating	Numb	Cold	Nauseating
Miserable	Penetrating	Drawing	Freezing	Agonizing
Intense	Piercing	Squeezing		Dreadful
Unbearable		Tearing		Torturing

(d)

Part 3. How Does Your Pain Change With Time?

1. Which word or words would you use to describe the <u>pattern</u> of your pain?

1	2	3
Continuous	Rhythmic	Brief
Steady	Periodic	Momentary
Constant	Intermittent	Transient

2. What kind of things <u>relieve</u> your pain?
_____
_____
_____

3. What kind of things increase your pain?
_____
_____
_____

Part 4. How Strong Is Your Pain?

People agree that the following 5 words represent pain of increasing intensity. They are:

1	2	3	4	5
Mild	Discomforting	Distressing	Horrible	Excruciating

To answer each question below, write the number of the most appropriate word in the space below beside the question.

1. Which word describes your pain right now? _____
2. Which word describes it at its worst? _____
3. Which word describes it when it is the least? _____
4. Which word describes the worst toothache you ever had? _____
5. Which word describes the worst headache you ever had? _____
6. Which word describes the worst stomach-ache you ever had? _____

Figure 31-1

The McGill-Melzack pain assessment questionnaire. (a) Cover sheet. (b) Part 1. (c) Part 2. (d) Parts 3 and 4. (Courtesy of R. Melzack.)

used to describe an emotional or qualitative aspect of the pain experience and not as a tool for measurement of pain intensity.

Pain Intensity

To determine intensity of pain, patients in a number of studies were given a sheet of paper with a straight line drawn on it (Pilowsky & Bond, 1969; Melzack & Torgerson, 1971; Berry & Huskesson, 1972). A 0 was at one end and the number 100 was printed at the other end of the line; 0 indicated no pain, and 100 represented the highest level of pain. Patients were asked to indicate where on this line their pain would fall. Johnson (1973) made a similar attempt to measure the intensity of the pain but also assessed the reaction or emotional component of the subject's pain. Two scales were presented to the patient, a sensation scale and a distress scale. Subjects cited pain ranging from no sensation (0) to maximal sensations (100). In the pain distress scale, subjects rated their reaction to the pain sensations as no distress, slight distress, moderate distress, very distressed, and extremely distressed. Johnson found that subjects could independently judge these two aspects of the pain experience.

Color of Pain

Stewart (1977) developed the Stewart Pain Color Scale and Pain Circles. The color intensity ranges on the pain color scale from yellow, representing no pain, to black, representing the worst possible pain. Patients were asked to slide the indicator on a line to the color that was most like what they sensed their pain to be. Orange or orange-reds were colors chosen for milder pain. The stronger red hues were selected to indicate increasing pain intensity. In her work, Stewart found that both black and red can represent pain and that as the pain quality or pain intensity increases, patients are more likely to select a brilliant red to describe their pain.

In the Stewart Pain Circles (Stewart, 1977), patients were asked to point to the circle that indicated or best described their current pain and then to point to the circle that best described their worst recent pain. The six circles appear on a white background, and the sizes of the red and black circles vary in each of the six circles. Patients were asked to select that circle that best represented their pain and to point to that part of the circle that best represented themselves. The choice of color seemed especially significant in patients with rheumatoid arthritis and cancer, because these patients selected a circle that had a large or thick black circle on the outside and then a smaller red circle on the inside as most representative of themselves and their pain.

Audiometer

Peck (1967) used an auditory signal to create a pain stimulus. By the use of the audiometer, Peck was able to determine the intensity of pain that subjects were able to tolerate before stopping the experiment.

Clinical versus Laboratory Pain

Many researchers and practitioners think that clinical and laboratory pain cannot be equated. They state that the difference in the meaning of the pain in the laboratory versus the clinical setting is so significant that the reaction to pain will be dissimilar. Most clinicians would agree that the individual's personality and past experiences of pain will influence either the amount (intensity) of pain experience or the perception of the pain, or both.

TREATMENT OF PAIN

The treatment of pain has varied significantly throughout recorded history. However, the most significant intervention has been pharmacological, that is, the administration of some type of drug. Other methods used in the treatment of pain are acupuncture, behavior modification, psychotherapy, hypnosis, biofeedback, electrical stimulation, neurosurgery, diet, sex, exercise, rest, x-ray, giving information about what to expect, and helping to develop skills for communication of pain.

ANALGESICS

The major categories of drugs used in the treatment of pain are the narcotics analgesics and mild analgesics (Table 31-2). The narcotic analgesics are natural alkaloids (codeine and morphine), semisynthetic compounds (hydromorphone), and synthetic compounds (meperidine). The mild analgesics are salicylic acid, acetaminophen (Tylenol), and derivatives of strong analgesics (codeine). At times, clinicians fail to evaluate the precise source of pain and administer a narcotic analgesic when a simple antacid or muscle relaxant or body position change would alleviate the pain.

Pain Cocktail

A commonly used method of administering drugs to patients for control of pain is the pain cocktail (Mount, Ajemian, and Scott, 1976). The pain cocktail is a liquid containing pain medications that are camouflaged in a flavored (frequently cherry) and colored "cocktail." Since patients cannot determine the amount of pain medication that is administered, they do not know whether or not the medication has been increased or decreased. The pain cocktail is administered at a fixed time interval, not just when the patient has pain. While "fading" the active ingredients in the pain cocktail, the practitioner hopes to encourage a relearning of patient behaviors previously associated with controlling pain. After baseline data have been recorded on the patient's pain medication behavior pattern, the active pain-relieving ingredient may be decreased (or increased) by one-tenth every 3 days over a period of 5 weeks. If the analgesic is completely removed from the pain cocktail, the patient still receives the constant volume of about 10 mL of liquid at fixed times throughout the day. The whole process of administration of the pain cocktail is discussed with the patient.

Table 31-2

Drugs to Relieve Pain

GENERIC NAME	BRAND NAME	ROUTES OF ADMINISTRATION	RELATIVE POTENCY OF ANALGESIC	RELATIVE ADDICTION LIABILITY
Narcotic analgesics				
Codeine	—	Oral, SC	+ to ++	+
Morphine	—	Oral, SC, IV	++++	+++
Heroin	—	SC, IV	++++	++++
Hydromorphone	Dilaudid	SC, Oral	++++	+++
Meperidine	Demerol	IM, Oral	+++	++
Alphaprodine	Nisentil	SC, IV	+++	+
Milder, nonnarcotic analgesics				
Acetylsalicylic acid	Aspirin	Oral	+	—
Acetaminophen	Tylenol	Oral	+	—
Phenylbutazone	Butazolidin	Oral	+	+
Propoxyphene	Darvon	Oral	+	+
Pentazocine	Talwin	Oral, IM, IV	+++	—
Ethoheptazine	Zactane	Oral	+	—
Methotrimeprazine	Levoprome	IM	+++	—

A + indicates that the drug has an analgesic or addictive effect. An increasing number of + signs indicates increasing strengths of the effect. The − sign indicates that the drug has little or no known addiction liability.

Placebo

The ethics of use of a placebo are currently under discussion. Practitioners disagree on whether or not it is ethical to administer a "pill" that looks like the analgesic that the patient has been taking but which, in reality, is a sham and contains no active pain-killing ingredient. Clinicians have held the view that if the placebo was effective, the patient was "faking the pain." This view of suffering only reveals our lack of compassion and comprehension of the psychological component of the pain experience.

ACUPUNCTURE

Acupuncture is another method used to produce analgesia for pain. As described earlier, organic pain may be referred to a distant part of the body. For example, the pain of a myocardial infarction is referred to the left shoulder or the jaw although the original site of the pain is the myocardium. This and many other examples of referred pain support the theory that there are neurological links between body sites, and it is logical that stimulation, via acupuncture, at one site could have an effect on the alleviation of pain at another. Also, the gate control theory is congruent with an explanation of acupuncture analgesia because it is thought that local intense stimulation of large-diameter fibers by needles inserted at specific body sites "closes the gate" so the pain stimuli are not transmitted to the brain.

BIOFEEDBACK

Biofeedback is a technique that has recently become very popular in the alleviation of tension, pain, and other clinical problems. Biofeedback training has several goals including increasing subjects' awareness of physiological functioning within their bodies, establishing control over these functions, and then transferring the control from the training setting into other areas of life. Patients are aided in becoming aware of their physiological function and in gaining control over these functions by use of the electroencephalogram (EEG), electromyogram (EMG), and sometimes cassette tape recordings of relaxation exercises. In stress-related disorders (i.e., migraine and tension headaches, insomnia, gastric ulcer, selected cardiovascular problems) many patients can learn to maintain physiological functioning within normal range and eliminate many symptoms of these disorders. At the present time, effectiveness of the biofeedback training in treatment of pain is enhanced when used in conjunction with other treatment modalities (Melzack and Perry, 1975).

HYPNOSIS

Hypnosis has been used in the treatment of pain with varying results. Hilgard et al. (1974b) at Stanford University has been a major proponent of the use of hypnosis in the treatment of pain. The patient is hypnotized and told to anticipate lower amounts of pain or sensations. It is thought that the hypnotic conditioning can decrease tension by allaying anxiety and increasing one's sense of well-being. Although the mechanism of action for hypnoanalgesia is not clearly understood, it is thought that in the hypnotic state the higher cortical centers can be inhibited or blocked so that pain is not consciously perceived. However, hypnosis not only alters the perception of pain but also affects its physical signs; therefore, hypnosis is best used in conjunction with medication and biofeedback, not as a substitute for them.

Melzack and Perry (1975) found that biofeedback combined with hypnosis is an effective modality for the treatment of pain. Their experiments and those of others increasingly provide strong evidence that multiple approaches are indicated in the treatment of pain, since problem pain has multiple interacting determinants.

ELECTRICAL STIMULATION

Electrical stimulation of a peripheral nerve or dorsal column of the spinal cord to relieve pain is based on the Melzack and Wall gate control theory on the mechanism of pain. Electrical stimulation is accomplished by delivering sensory input through electrodes applied to the skin (transcutaneous method), through needles or wires inserted into or near a peripheral nerve (percutaneous stimulation), or through an electrode applied during laminectomy over the dorsal column of the spinal cord (dorsal column stimulator) or implanted into a major peripheral nerve (peripheral nerve implant) (Erickson, 1975; McDonnell, 1977).

Not every person with chronic pain responds well to electrode implantation, so the effectiveness of surface electrode stimulation in allaying pain must be determined prior to surgery. If it is ascertained that implantation of an electrode will help the person with chronic pain, the electrode is implanted into the selected nerve, and the attached receiver is anchored in subcutaneous tissue. The tansmitter sends stimuli to the receiver, and these stimuli, hopefully, counteract pain impulses. The transmitter is worn externally by the patient, who can initiate stimuli as needed to relieve pain.

The amount of pain relief derived from electrical stimulation is variable. The success rate is enhanced by teaching the patient what to expect prior to and after implantation and by helping the patient to use the equipment properly.

SURGICAL INTERVENTION

Neurosurgery of many types has been used to combat intactable pain, but since nerve transection does not control the psychological contribution to pain sensation, pain may persist despite neurosurgery. Examples of neurosurgical procedures to afford pain relief are chemical nerve blocks (usually with alcohol or phenol), neurectomy, cordotomy, sympathectomy, rhizotomy, thalamotomy, lobotomy, and gyrectomy (used to treat phantom limb pain).

Even though chemical nerve block is temporary and is useful for checking potential effects of further neurosurgery, irreversible complications occur with this procedure, as they may in many of the other neurosurgeries used to combat pain. Complications such as personality changes occur with thalamotomy and lobotomy. Urinary retention and/or sexual impotence may occur with cordotomy. Changes in normal functioning of the autonomic nervous system occur following sympathectomy (McDonnell, 1977).

BEHAVIOR MODIFICATION

Behavioral methods for treatment of people with chronic pain require alteration of behavior patterns. Patients are asked to change some behaviors that they enjoyed or that had some value for them and to initiate new sets of behaviors that were not previously viewed as necessary. In attempting to disrupt or reduce the pain–medication cycle, a process of unlearning or deconditioning occurs. Stimuli or cues present when a behavior is being positively or negatively reinforced will tend to become positive or negative reinforcers of that behavior. Since we tend to associate objects, people, situations or feelings with other similar objects, people, situations, or feelings, this means that additional sources of reinforcement are potentially available.

Fordyce (1976) has successfully helped people with chronic pain to reduce or eliminate requesting and taking pain medications by using techniques of behavior modification. Upon admission to the hospital, each patient is asked to give all pain medications to the nursing personnel, who willingly give the pain medication to the patient whenever requested. The purpose of this procedure is to obtain accurate baseline data on the pain–medication patterns. The average daily intake of the medication that a patient takes is calculated, and a reproduction of the baseline intake (including all analgesics, narcotics, or tranquilizers) is prepared in a pain cocktail with a cherry syrup base. The cocktail is taken in equal doses around the clock regardless of whether or not pain behaviors are exhibited. This procedure usually controls pain because it is comparable or even stronger than the baseline dose. The dosage of analgesics is decreased (called fading), as described earlier in the chapter.

The goal in using behavior modification techniques in pain cocktail administration procedures is not merely to decrease pain medication intake but to reinforce activity and other "well" behaviors so that medication ceases to be a reward for expressing pain. Exercise routines are outlined so that patients exercise to a point below that which previously caused pain; in this intervention, rest and attention become reinforcers for activity rather than for pain.

Some clinicians are concerned that shaping (altering) behavior without informed participation of the individuals is a violation of human rights. Fordyce and associates discuss fully with patients the concept of behavior modification, including (1) why staff members may seem to be inattentive or to ignore certain of their activities (usually pain behaviors), and (2) the concept of fading active ingredients in pain cocktails.

COUNTERIRRITANTS

Counterirritants are included in the host of other remedies that have been tried to relieve both acute and chronic pain. Counterirritants (mustard plasters, flaxseed poultices, liniments) ease joint pain of rhematoid arthritis and osteoarthritis by increasing blood flow to the area, thereby causing a sensation of warmth. The increased blood supply removes noxious metabolites in the tissue, decreases muscle spasm, increases oxygenation, and increases joint mobility (White, 1973).

OTHER TREATMENTS

Application of heat and cold has been found to decrease pain sensations. Heat causes decreased gamma motor activity, which induces muscle spasm. Other "home remedies" have included exercise, rest, distraction, and sexual activity. Specific exercises for people who endured low back pain for years have been dramatically effective in reducing or alleviating pain. Persons who stopped smoking report less pain as a result of the arterial insufficiency caused by heavy smoking. More recently, nutritional aspects of pain have been investigated. It is thought that a diet low in tyramine results in decreased pain perception.

IMPLEMENTING NURSING ROLES

The reader will note that the role of the professional nurse seems to be minimal in a number of current, commonly used treatments for pain. Nurses have had a major role in the success of behavior modification implemented to ease the pain–medication cycle, and nurses have been shown to effectively decrease patients' pain by giving information to patients about sensations to anticipate while undergoing endoscopy (Johnson, 1973). Perhaps, nursing interventions, though extremely effective in alleviating pain, have not been as visible or as highly valued by the medical community as have interventions made by other health professionals.

Nurses encounter pain daily, and one cannot help but wonder what nurses feel when they are unable, as perhaps are other health team members, to relieve or ease patients' pain. At best, it may be described as frustrating, and when frustrated, most of us become irritable and angry (Larsen, 1976). Since nurses are, like all professionals, trained not to express anger at medically ill patients, this anger is either repressed or displaced. A more gratifying way of interacting and viewing this problem clearly is indicated. Research data to show the effectiveness of various nursing interventions compared with traditional drug administration or surgical intervention are needed.

If total pain relief is not possible for some patients, the nursing goal can perhaps be directed toward (1) helping patients develop skill for communicating feelings about themselves, their pain, their worth as individuals, and their roles within their families and society; (2) developing new interventions to decrease pain sensations; (3) improving the assessments of the sensations the patients call pain; (4) exploring combinations of previously tried methods to relieve pain; and (5) taking a philosophical view of the pain experience and teaching patients to live as though the pain did not exist or to not perceive the pain as pain.

TOTALING THE GAINS AND LOSSES OF THE PAIN EXPERIENCE—THE NURSING APPROACH

Previously, nurses' patterns of responding to the pain experience in the clinical setting were similar to being conditioned in a stimulus–response learning experiment. Patients stated that they had pain (stimulus), and the nurse determined when they had had their last pain medication (response). This behavior on the part of the nurse certainly reinforced the patient's view of how to obtain relief from pain. As discussed earlier in this chapter, breaking this pain–medication cycle by changing responses (reinforcers) is one goal of behavior modification. Perhaps to be more effective in interactions with the person in pain, a shift in nursing focus is needed in several areas of the nursing process: assessment, intervention, evaluation.

ASSESSMENT

Practitioners agree that assessment of clinical pain is a major responsibility of nurses. Traditionally, the primary focus in assessing pain was on the history of the pain experience and the location, intensity, and quality of the pain. In obtaining this history, the nurse established whether the pain was acute or chronic, where it began, its exact location, structures to which the pain radiated, what provoked the pain, and the character and quality of the pain. More recently, nurses have included in their assessments the nature of the patients' response to pain, the meaning of the pain, and the reactions of significant others to whom the patients "complain."

Complaint of Pain

The use of the phrase "complaint of pain" summarizes a dominant attitude toward persons with pain. Nurses "know" that specific interventions (i.e., debridement, injections, coughing, and deep breathing after cholecystectomy) cause pain in a circumscribed time period. Outlined in the nurses' thought processes (based on memory, previous experience, assessment of patients, personality, cultural orientation) is an idea of what and when pain is supposed to occur. Nurses have strong opinions about behavior that constitutes acceptable expressions of pain. Any patient who exhibits behavior or verbally expresses pain that does not fit the nurses' preconceived expectations is labeled as a "complainer" or the pain is described as "psychogenic" (even though the pain is nonetheless real). It is possible that this preset cognitive framework interferes with making the most accurate assessment of the individual and his or her pain. If the nurses' assessments are erroneous, so are the interventions and evaluations of nursing performance.

Persons who have endured a spinal cord injury and have little sensory or motor ability below their level of injury are thought to be unable to "feel pain" in that area. Thus, any expression of pain may be immediately labeled as psychogenic or as "not real pain." The overlap between psychogenic and organic pain is probably so great in most cases that nursing assessments are improved when pain is assessed as a continuum in which psychological influence on the cause, exacerbation, and/or tolerance is either minimal or great. When nurses "accuse" patients of having psychogenic pain (which nurses at times view as fake pain), the real affront to the patient may not be that so little effort has been exerted to achieve comfort but rather that the nurses do not believe the description of pain.

Temporal Aspects of Pain Assessment

After giving due consideration to biases and preconditioned reaction, the assessment of the person in pain is refined by the nurse. Temporal aspects of the pain experienced are included.

When did this pain begin? What preceded it? What initiated it? Factors that initiate pain are varied and numerous: interpersonal interactions, position changes, immobility, room temperature or humidity, arterial oxygen content, environmental noise, fatigue, and a host of other known and unknown factors. The focus at this point in the assessment phase of the nursing process is on why the patient has this particular pain at this particular time. If the type and cause of the pain have been established or are not relevant at this point in the interaction with the patient, the nurse may wish to measure the intensity of the pain using one of the tools described earlier in the chapter.

Assessing the Meaning of Pain

As the nurse talks with patients to determine how or what measures are used to relieve specific types of pain and what the patients think is the meaning of their pain at this time, an assessment is made of the response that is desired from others; in other words, what is the goal of the pain expression? Does the patient merely want to be touched, have company, have a change of position, or be given a drink of water, the bedpan, or a medication? Some of these needs (motivators, goals) will be subconscious and too frightening for direct verbalization. Both the meaning of pain and the goal of pain expression are variable and warrant periodic reassessment. In intervening with patients in pain, nurses should remember behavior modification techniques. It is easy to fall into the pattern of spending time with patients only when they request your presence because they need to tell you about their pain (suffering) and need for relief. In implementing successful pain management, it is critical that nurses spend time with patients prior to the onset of maximal pain and/or the point of a patient's inability to tolerate the pain in order to increase the individual's comfort and to decrease administration of analgesics.

Decreasing the frequency of medications is not synonymous with withholding drugs from persons in extreme pain. At times, patients require large doses of narcotic analgesics, and nurses may be reluctant to administer them (McCaffery, 1976). Each individual case is assessed and the benefit of pain relief is weighed (assessed) against the risk of narcotic administration. For example, if a patient is in the terminal stages of a disease process and is in excruciating pain, the risk of drug addiction or even decreasing blood pressure is of minimal concern. Individual comfort and dignity are of prime importance!

Communicating Pain

Just as patients communicate the response they desire from others verbally and nonverbally, they use both verbal and nonverbal behavior to communicate information about their pain experience to others. Mehrabian (1968) stated that if one total communication equals 100 percent, 55 percent of the total is communicated by the facial expression, 38 percent by the tone of voice, and 7 percent by the words used.

If the theories of communication patterns are valid for persons in pain, the large majority of what the patient tells the nurse about pain is communicated nonverbally. What should nurses assess by studying facial expressions and listening to the tone of voice, as well as the words, of a person in pain?

Facial Expression In assessing facial expressions, the nurses should note and record all of the following and watch for any change:

> hairline—Does the hair cover the forehead or not?
> forehead—Are there wrinkles? Do the wrinkles extend continuously across the forehead or are they broken? How many lines (wrinkles) are there? Are the hands holding the forehead?
> eyebrow—Are the eyebrows raised or lowered in a squint?
> eyes—Are the eyes opened or closed? Is the gaze direct or avoiding? Are the hands covering the eyes?
> cheeks—Are the cheeks flushed or pale?

lips—What color are they? Are the lips being bitten? Are the lips drawn back to show the teeth and gums?

teeth—Is a finger or some part of the hand being bitten?

mouth—Is the contour of the mouth upward, downward, or straight (horizontal)? Are the hands placed over or in the mouth?

Additional information can be obtained by studying the movement and orientation of the face. Is the neck flexed, lowering the chin to the chest, or is it extended, moving the occiput toward the scapula? Is the facial movement congruent with the rest of the body movements? That is, is the head shaking while the rest of the body is motionless or vice versa?

Tone of Voice In assessing the tone of voice, the nurse should determine and record all of the following and closely observe any change:

pitch—Is it high or low? Is it consistent? Is the same pitch used for discussion of pain as for other subjects? Does the pitch sound like whining?

volume—Does the volume decrease or increase when talking about pain? Is the volume constant or wavering?

quality—Does the voice sound more like controlled commanding or dependent, pleading whining?

Vocalizations In assessing the vocalizations, the nurse should listen to and record the following and determine whether or not a change occurs:

words—Are the sounds distinct words or utterances? If the patient is bilingual, which language is used when in pain?

patterns of words—Are the words spoken in specific repeating phrases? Are the sounds spoken aloud or distinctly formed but not projected?

As noted in each discussion of the aspects (facial expression, tone of voice, vocalization) of the communication of pain, it is important for nurses to ascertain any change in the pattern of pain expression. With practice, it is probable that most nurses will be able to contrast these communications and their changes with changing pain intensity. Development of this ability will allow the nurse to make an intervention early in the buildup of pain intensity.

Assessing the Impact of the Pain Experience

The assessment of the person is not complete until the impact of the pain experience is placed in the context of the family and/or significant others. Using the balance sheet model developed by Janis and Mann (1977), the nurse can help patients total the gains and losses of the chronic pain experience. The balance sheet has four main categories:

1. Gains/losses for self
2. Gains/losses for family or significant other
3. Approval/disapproval of self
4. Approval/disapproval of family or significant others

In each category are listed a number of items that individuals rate as positive (gain, approval) or as negative (loss, disapproval) for them or for family members and significant others.

The balance sheet developed by the author to assess the impact of pain and to facilitate decision making is presented in Table 31-3. Nurses can use this balance sheet or a modification of it to assess the individual impact of the pain experience and to stimulate patients' assessment of their pain experience and facilitate their decision making. The use of the balance sheet requires little, if any, direct nursing intervention because the process of helping the patient, family, and significant others to assess the pain experience is the best intervention. This process usually heightens mutual awareness of gains and losses, of approval and disapproval, resulting from the chronic pain experience.

Table 31-3

Balance Sheet to Assess Impact of Pain Experience and Facilitate Decision Making

Instructions: Place a positive sign (+) to the left of those items that have been gains or approvals and a negative sign (−) to the left of those things that have been losses or disapproval for you during your pain experience.

1. Gains/losses for self
    a. Pain
    b. Medication
    c. Money
    d. Love and affection
    e. Attention
    f. Self-image, self-esteem change
    g. Responsibility
    h. Anxiety, anger
    i. Social control
    j. Time for family hobbies
    k. Sexual activity
    l. Attainment of own goals

2. Gains/losses for family and significant others
    a. Money
    b. Love and affection
    c. Social control
    d. Responsibility
    e. Time with spouse/friend/family member
    f. Social image or position
    g. Sexual activity
    h. Attainment of family goals
    i. Anxiety/anger

3. Approval/disapproval of self
    a. Adjustment to pain experience
    b. Ability to readjust to premorbid role
    c. Style of pain expression
    d. Rate of change in pain intensity
    e. Amount of time spent talking about pain
    f. Amount of time directed toward self-help
    g. Role in family/society

4. Approval/disapproval of family and significant others
    a. Adjustment to pain experience
    b. Style of pain expression
    c. Rate of change in pain intensity
    d. Amount of time spent talking about pain
    e. Amount of effort directed toward self-help
    f. Current role in family and society
    g. Ability to establish premorbid role in family and society

INTERVENTIONS

Nursing interventions designed to give comfort to persons in pain can be summarized by the following list of nursing activities:

1. Communicates with the patient and family to enhance expression of reactions to or meaning of pain
2. Gives pain medication as an adjunct to but not as an exclusive intervention
3. Teaches the patient to communicate about pain more effectively
   a. Teaches the names of body parts in which pain is experienced
   b. Sharpens description of the pain by enabling the use of appropriate terms: sharp, dull, deep, superficial, aching, burning, etc.
   c. Learns from patient and others the cultural aspects of patient's pain phenomena, applies this information, and teaches it to others who interact with the patient
   d. Facilitates open expression of what is thought to be the meaning of pain and the feelings these thoughts engender
   e. Helps patients focus communications about pain experiences
      (1) Elicits from the patient the most critical or important aspect of the pain
      (2) Suggests to the patient that dwelling on or whining about pain has a negative effect
      (3) Helps the patient identify significant others who are apt to have high or low tolerance for communications about pain
   f. Persuades patient to discriminate between those sensations of pain caused by physiological changes in body tissues and those caused by anxiety, anger, or fatigue (the patient should avoid using the term "pain" to characterize everything that is upsetting)
   g. Increases patients' knowledge about body sensations that they are apt to experience during treatments, diagnostic procedures, and physiological changes in tissues
4. Assists the patient to have power over pain
   a. Increases tolerance of pain (sometimes this is accomplished by pointing out the "permanency of pain")
   b. Helps find ways to effect distraction from pain by increasing sensory input through touch, massage, or vibration
   c. Encourages self-analysis of the meaning of pain rather than immediately seeking a remedy

The selection of nursing activities is based on assessments of the individual, the individual's pain experiences, and the goals that the nurse and the individual have established. In many cases of chronic pain, total alleviation is an unrealistic goal, so the goals of distraction or increased tolerance may be set. The rationale for the selection of nursing activities is sometimes governed by the desire to do that which is humane.

For example, if for a terminally ill person it is established that specific facial expressions, voice tones, and word phrases indicate intense pain and, by use of the balance sheet, that both patient and family have a healthy grasp of the crisis, the patient, the family and significant others, and the nurse can select the goals of care. Based on these goals, the nurse determines which nursing activities are most therapeutic; that is, which are most likely to achieve the desired goals. In reference to pain, the goals vary and can range from absolute pain relief to maintenance of the status quo to no change in pain status, which may require no intervention from any health team member. When death is imminent, the goal of comfort is usually established.

Health professionals, especially nurses, often take a shortsighted view of the administration of pain medications to the terminally ill. In this chapter, giving analgesics as the only nursing activity has been criticized, but the point is not that nurses should withhold pain medications but rather that they should administer them within the framework of nursing assessments and goals of care. Again, if the terminally ill patient is expected to die within hours or days, it is ridiculous to make the person in obvious pain wait 3 or 4 h for a pain medication because of the possibility of addiction to the drug.

Finally, if the list of nursing activities should be determined to be incomplete, it may be because nurses have not done thorough, systematic assessments of persons in pain. If clear goals of nursing care are not established, assessments and nursing activities cannot be evaluated and the list of therapeutic nursing interventions in the pain experience cannot be expanded.

EVALUATION

How do nurses know that they have made the best nursing intervention in the patient's total pain experience? One criterion that is frequently used to show the effectiveness of nursing activity is that the patient stops complaining of pain and the frequency of requests for pain medication decreases. Another criterion is that the patient becomes interested in the environment (people, objects, activities) and less focused on self and on pain. Use of these criteria for evaluating nursing effectiveness in helping a person in pain is productive if the criteria are congruent with the goals of care established by nurses and patient.

Continuous assessment is necessary in any successful program of pain management. Nurses are confounded in giving care to persons in pain if a nursing activity that has been successful in meeting goals of care suddenly becomes useless. Reassessment continues to determine what factors influenced the outcome of the intervention. For example, if the patient has developed an inflammation, an infection, fatigue, or necrosis, the pain threshold may be lowered. The patient may be tense and anxious, conditions that increase pain as a result of muscle tensing. Patients in pain sometimes develop an increased sensitivity to noxious stimuli (noise, heat, cold, odors), so that presence of these in the environment should be determined before abandoning the nursing intervention. Interventions that worked during the day may be ineffective at night because of darkness and the absence of pain-distracting stimuli (music playing, people touching or talking with the patients, movement of staff members, patients' visitors engaging in various activities). Reassessment should be made of all drugs.

As reassessment continues, it is essential to consider, in addition to environmental and physiological factors, psychological factors that may be hindering the effectiveness of nursing interventions. Patients sometimes use pain to relieve guilt feelings and so may be reluctant to relinquish their pain. Others believe that it is God's will that they suffer, because illness is a result of sin. Also, an interaction may have stimulated the patient's memory of some previously painful experience that is now associated with the current situation.

CONCLUSION

People have pain, endure it (even find value in it), and develop remedies to combat it. The nurse's role is, with awareness of the health team's plan of care, to learn about the meaning of the pain and the patient's strategies for coping with pain and to teach patients refinements in communicating and alleviating pain and the suffering that it engenders.

BIBLIOGRAPHY

Berry, H., and E. C. Huskesson: "A Report on Pain Measurement," *Clin Trials J* 9:13–20, 1972.

Bonica, J. J.: "Cancer Pain: A Major Health Problem," *Cancer Nurs* 1:313–316, 1978.

Copp, L.: "The Spectrum of Suffering," *Am J Nurs* 74:491–495, 1974.

Davis, A. J.: "Brompton's Cocktail: Making Goodbyes Possible," *Am J Nurs* 78:610–612, 1978.

Diamond, S. M., and D. J. Dalessio: *The Practicing Physicians Approach to Headache,* 2d ed., Williams & Wilkins, Baltimore, 1978.

Erickson, D. L.: "Percutaneous Trial of Stimulation for Patient Selection of Implantable Devices," *J Neurosurg* 43:440–444, 1975.

Feller, I., and C. Archambeault-Jones: *Nursing the Burned Patient,* Institute for Burn Medicine, Ann Arbor, 1973.

Fordyce, W. E.: *Behavioral Methods for Chronic Pain and Illness,* Mosby, St. Louis, 1976.

Gaarder, K. R., and P. S. Montgomery: *Clinical Biofeedback: A Procedural Manual,* Williams & Wilkins, Baltimore, 1977.

Goth, A.: *Medical Pharmacology,* 8th ed., Mosby, St. Louis, 1976.

Guyton, A.: *Medical Physiology,* Saunders, Philadelphia, 1976.

Hardy, J. D., H. G. Wolff, and H. S. Goodell: *Pain Sensations and Reactions,* Williams & Wilkins, Baltimore, 1952.

Hilgard, E. R., H. McDonald, G. Marshall, and A. Morgan: "Anticipation of Pain and of Pain Control Under Hypnosis: Heart Rate and Blood Pressure Responses in the Cold Pressor Test," *J Abnorm Psychol* 83:561–568, 1974(a).

———, A. H. Morgan, A. F. Lange, J. R. Lenox, H. MacDonald, G. D. Marshall, and L. B. Sach: "Heart Rate Changes in Pain and Hypnosis," *Psychophysiology* 11:692–702, 1974(b).

Janis, I., and I. Mann: "Coping with Decisional Conflict," *Am Sci* 64:657–667, 1977.

Johnson, J.: "Effects of Structuring Patient's Expectations on Their Reactions to Threatening Events," *Nurs Res* 21:499–504, 1972.

———: "The Effect of Accurate Expectations about Sensations on the Sensory and Distress Components of Pain," *J Pers* 27:261–275, 1973.

Larsen, K. S.: *Aggression: Myths and Models,* Nelson-Hall, Chicago, 1976.

McCaffery, M.: *Nursing Management of the Patient with Pain,* Lippincott, Philadelphia, 1972.

———: "Undertreatment of Acute Pain with Narcotics," *Am J Nurs* 76: 1586–1591, 1976.

McDonnell, D.: "Surgical and Electrical Stimulation Methods for Relief of Pain," in A. Jacox (ed.): *Pain: A Sourcebook for Nurses and Other Health Professionals,* Little Brown, Boston, 1977, pp. 169–207.

Mehrabian, A.: "Communication without Words," *Psychol Today* 2:53–55, September 1968.

Melzack, R.: "The McGill Pain Questionnaire: Major Properties and Scoring Methods," *Pain* 1:277–299, 1975.

———: "Using the Language of Pain," *Curr Concepts Pain Analgesia* 2:1–3, 12–13, 1976.

———, J. G. Ofiesh, and B. M. Mount: "The Brompton Mixture: Effects on Pain in Cancer Patients," *Can Med J* 115:125–129, July 17, 1976.

———, and C. Perry: "Self-regulation of Pain: The Use of Alpha-Feedback and Hypnotic Training for the Control of Chronic Pain," *Exp Neurol* 45:452–469, 1975.

———, and W. S. Torgerson: "On the Language of Pain," *Anesthesiology* 34:50–59, 1971.

———, and P. D. Wall: "Pain Mechanisms: A New Theory," *Science* 150:971–979, 1965.

———, and ———: Psychophysiology of Pain," *Int Anesthesiol Clin: Anesthesiol Neurophysiol* 8(1):3–34, 1970.

Mount, B. M., J. Ajemian, and J. F. Scott: "Use of the Brompton Mixture in Treating the Chronic Pain of Malignant Disease," *Can Med J,* 115:122–124, July 17, 1976.

Nathan, P. W., and P. Rudge: "A Flaw in the Gate Control Theory?," *J Neurol Neurosurg Psychiatry* 37:1366–1377, 1974.

Pace, J. B.: *Pain: A Person Experience,* Nelson-Hall, Chicago, 1976.

Peck, R. E.: "A Precise Technique for the Measurement of Pain," *Headache,* 6:189–194, 1967.

Pilowsky, J., and M. R. Bond: "Pain and IB

Management in Malignant Disease," *Psychosom Med* 31:400–404, 1969.

Sternbach, R. A.: *Pain Patients: Traits and Treatment,* Academic Press, New York, 1974.

Stewart, M. L.: "Measurement of Clinical Pain," in A. Jacox (ed.), *Pain: A Source Book for Nurses and Other Health Professionals,* Little Brown, Boston, 1977, pp. 107–137.

Stiller, R.: *Why It Hurts, Where It Hurts, When It Hurts,* Nelson, New York, 1975.

Strauss, A., S. Y. Fagerhaugh, and B. Glaser: "Pain: An Organization-Work. Interactional Perspective," *Nurs Outlook* 22:560–566, 1974.

Sweet, W.: "Pain," In J. Field, M. W. Magoun, and V. E. Hall (eds.): *Handbook of Physiology,* section 1, vol. 1, American Psychological Society, Washington, D.C., 1959, pp. 459–506.

Villarerde, M., and C. W. MacMillan: *Pain: From Symptom to Treatment,* Van Nostrand, New York, 1977.

Weisenberg, M.: *Pain: Clinical and Experimental Perspectives,* Mosby, St. Louis, 1975.

White, J. R.: "Effects of a Counterirritant on Perceived Pain and Hand Movement in Patients with Arthritis," *Phys Ther* 53: 956–960, 1973.

Wiener, C. L.: "Pain Assessment on an Orthopedic Ward," *Nurs Outlook* 23:508–516, 1975.

Woodforde, J. M., and H. Merslay: "Some Relationships Between Subjective Measurements of Pain," *J Psychosom Res* 16:173–178, 1972.

Wylie, N. A.: "Victoria General Hospital: A Nursing Model," in G. W. Davidson (ed.): *The Hospice: Development and Administration,* Hemisphere Publishing, Washington, D.C., 1978, pp. 21–39.

Zborowski, M.: *People in Pain,* Jossey-Bass, San Francisco, 1969.

PART FOUR

THE WORLD OUT THERE

32

susan m. povse
mary e. keenan

discharge planning
for the transition
from a health care facility
to the community

INTRODUCTION

The primary goal of our national health care system today is disease prevention and health promotion and maintenance. Numerous programs have evolved in health care institutions and schools to facilitate this "healthful" emphasis. Legislation and planning committees have been established at the local and national levels to examine and set standards for costs, accessibility, utilization, availability, and quality.

It has been suggested that a partial remedy to the deficiencies in the American health care system could be accomplished by establishing systems for better continuity of patient care, with the major focus on discharge planning (Stroman, 1976; Zeigler, 1974). In the context of this chapter, we refer to *discharge planning* as the planned events that occur in one setting that prepare for the orderly transition of the patient to another setting, whether it be institutional or community. The immediate goal of this preparatory process is to ensure continuous and uninterrupted health care services to meet both actual and anticipated patient needs. In addition, and equally as important, it is believed that this process should assist the patient to develop and nurture positive health attitudes and behaviors. Patients are encouraged to be active participants in their own health care as well as in the health care delivery system.

Who needs discharge planning? We believe all people, of all ages, in all settings, regardless of diagnosis, have a right to discharge planning. And what does discharge planning involve? It involves coordination, communication, and collaboration between the patient/family unit and the health care team. The responsibility lies within this network of people to improve not only their own situation but also the local, state, and national situation as it relates to the achievement of continuity of care.

What are the anticipated benefits of discharge planning? Clearly, the benefits are as follows:

- The promotion of optimal health and, hopefully, disease prevention
- A decrease or elimination of complications
- A decrease in the number of admissions and readmissions
- The assurance that services are available and appropriate to meet needs
- Provision for a connection between services
- Identification of resources still needed in the system
- Protection against duplication of services
- A reduction in the cost of care if the above benefits are accomplished

In 1972, Friedson addressed the referral system within hospital settings. Today, we are still attempting to assist the individual to maneuver successfully through the matrix of the health care system. Figure 32-1 serves to illustrate this phenomenon over time.

Consumers, that is, patients, are never absent from the health care system. In many instances, they enter it before birth. Degrees and frequencies of one's involvement vary through the life continuum. The influencing variables are numerous, and selected ones are discussed in this chapter.

The chapter depicts only one segment of the life continuum of the patient: planning for the transition from a health care facility, where rehabilitation has been the primary emphasis, to the community. We will discuss the individuals involved in this process, focusing primarily on the rehabilitation nurse and the patient/family unit, and their interactions.

The purpose of this discussion is to identify nursing responsibilities in the process and to provide helpful information in achieving those critical responsibilities. Even though this chapter addresses the patient leaving a rehabilitation hospital or unit, the principles of discharge planning are applicable to all health care facilities, and the process always begins at the patient's point of entry.

Figure 32-2 depicts the segment of the patient's life that we will be addressing in this chapter. A crisis event, resulting in a physical disability, has precipitated a higher degree of involvement with the health care system (see

Health Care Resources

People:
  Health professionals
  Informed public
  Legislators
  Providers and officials of health related programs

Places:
  Clinic–physician's office
  Ambulatory care setting
  Home
  Hospital
  Emergency room
  Long-term care facility
  School
  Community health center

Events:
  Lecture
  Group courses
  Legislation
  Screening programs
  Innoculation programs

Things:
  Medications
  Supplies
  Equipment
  Literature

LIFE CONTINUUM

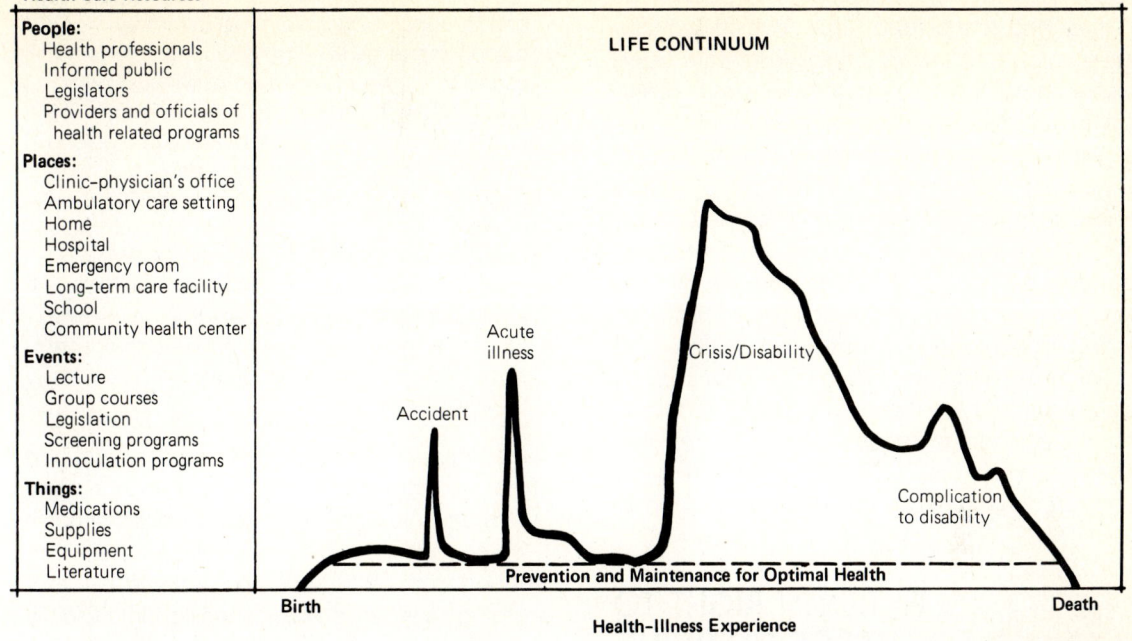

Accident
Acute illness
Crisis/Disability
Complication to disability

Prevention and Maintenance for Optimal Health

Birth — Death

Health-Illness Experience

Figure 32-1

Figure 32-2

669 DISCHARGE PLANNING

Fig. 32-1). Within the institution, the people, activities, and interactions result in a logical progression of events toward the goal of satisfactory transition back into the community with continuation of the patient's health care plan. The objective is that the patient/family unit will learn how to interrelate with the health care system—knowing what the system is and how it can work for them, and knowing when to exert independence and at the same time being comfortable with some necessary dependency on others. Health care in a community setting takes on dimensions different from those that occur in an institution; nevertheless, Fig. 32-2 still applies, for there continue to be people, actions, and interactions. Figure 32-2 will be further operationalized throughout the context of this chapter.

PATIENTS' RIGHT TO DISCHARGE PLANNING

Discharge planning is a priority and a right for all patients, of all ages, regardless of diagnosis. In November 1972, the American Hospital Association included the following in the Patients' Bill of Rights:

> The patient has the right to expect reasonable continuity of care. He has the right to know in advance what appointment times and physicians are available and where. The patient has the right to expect that the hospital will provide a mechanism whereby he is informed by his physician or a delegate of the physician of the patients' continuing health care requirements following discharge. (American Hospital Association, 1972)

Although not speaking specifically to the concept of discharge planning, Dr. Scott K. Simonds, in a more individualizing tone, summarized the idea of patients and their rights by suggesting that the patient should

> be respected and cared for as a human being . . . be recognized as having a unique sociopsychological, cultural and familial background relevant to his condition and to communicating with him concerning his condition . . . have access and opportunity to obtain the information and guidance that he sees as needed to care for his condition . . . be provided an active and participating role in his own care to the extent that he chooses and is able . . . be stimulated and guided through effective educational means to acquire new knowledge, attitudes, and actions that will promote his ability to care for himself more adequately and to maintain his health at an optimum level, and . . . be cared for through services designed and organized to promote and support learning ad behavior that are appropriate to his care and to the maintenance of his health. (Shapiro, 1972)

Discharge planning is a basic and integral part of patient care and therefore should not stand out as a single entity, for then it appears that it is being provided over and above the other planned care. It is common knowledge that anything considered extra or nonstandard usually is not a priority and therefore does not get done, or if it is accomplished, it appears last on a checklist of items to consider the day before the patient leaves the institution. The elements of the discharge planning process should begin on the day of admission in conjunction with the immediate therapeutic goals of the health team. In some cases, this process is initiated by an agency prior to admission to the immediate setting.

RESOURCE BANK

An effective discharge plan depends on the availability of resources. In the context of this chapter, the resource bank is the composite of people, places, things, and events that can be instrumental to planning.

THE PATIENT AND THE FAMILY UNIT

The patient and the family unit bring an array of personal resources to a situation. These resources should not be underestimated or overlooked, for in so doing, one may well miss some resources and qualities that can greatly strengthen the discharge plan.

According to Reinhardt (Reinhardt and Quinn, 1973), the following should be looked for when assessing the family unit:

- Types of relationships between parents and children
- Distribution of work activities
- Pattern of decision making
- Authority pattern in the home
- General attitude about health and medical care
- Level of comprehension of health practices
- Degrees of closeness among family members
- Which family members work together and which do not
- Certain family values that are important to understand
- General pattern of family activities—who does what, when, and where

The resources may include friends, neighbors, church members, work associates, schoolmates, and fellow members of social or fraternal organizations.

INSTITUTIONAL SETTING

Only a small portion of health care actually occurs in a hospital setting. Structurally and organizationally, however, these settings may be better equipped to effect and promote a patient's transition within the health care system. According to Imirie (1974), the following are characteristics a health care agency assumes if it is a leader in this area:

- A leadership and participative role
- Responsibility to develop resources
- Continuation of the provision of services
- Maintaining contact with dischargees
- Auditing the discharge plan
- Provision to meet new needs
- Avoidance of depersonalization and fragmentation of the care plan
- A comprehensive discharge service
- A comprehensive plan for solutions, both medical and nonmedical

The concentration and availability of health care workers in these hospital settings, representing multiple disciplines, are also adjuncts to comprehensive planning. The focus must extend out from the institutional boundaries into the community setting, looking beyond immediate care needs.

The team is a given in all settings. If the team is formalized, accountability related to the process is defined and shared. Rehabilitation hospitals or units traditionally utilize the formalized team with a wide representation of health care professionals, such as the physician, nurse, occupational therapist, physical therapist, speech therapist, social worker, psychologist, vocational counselor, recreational therapist, chaplain, and the patient/family unit. If the team is informal in structure, for example, consisting of a nurse and the resource people that the nurse calls in as needed, the teamwork is staggered and depends to a great extent on a central communication source if effective discharge planning is to occur. Teamwork is an imperative, regardless of structure.

In examining what a particular institution has to offer in discharge planning, the following questions are pertinent:

- What is the philosophy of patient care services?
- Is there a formal written protocol for discharge planning?
- Is discharge planning included in orientation programs?
- What is the status of the nurse as a member of the team?
- Who is accountable for keeping the internal system updated by being aware of what is occurring in the community and in legislation?
- What freedom does the nurse have to plan and act creatively?
- What is the communication and feedback

system between the institution and the resources in the community so that experiences are utilized for future patients and benefit the system as a whole?

Who are the resource people available, and is there a formal or informal team system of interaction and support?

COMMUNITY

Health care resources tend to be plentiful in urban areas; rural areas may leave much more to the resourcefulness of the patients and their personal resources. With the aid of this knowledge, the nurse can more effectively plan with the patient modes of intervention that get to the specific problems. Since the availability of resources is ever-changing, this section will list by service rendered those that are most commonly found in urban communities and are, for the most part, tax supported or funded by voluntary contributions and services.

Home Care Nursing

Home care nursing agencies provide professional nursing visits into the home to teach, assess, support, and give direct service. These nurses provide supervision for nonprofessionals or for family members who are providing direct patient care in the home. The agencies most often involved are visiting nurse associations, public health nurses (county and municipal) and hospital-based home care programs. Many of these agencies provide an array of health care services, including physical, speech, and occupational therapy, social work, nutritional counseling, and home health aides. Therapy may be given in the home on a regular basis by a registered therapist, but it is often supervised or carried out by the nurse, with the therapist as a consultant. These agencies are also instrumental in the coordination of other community-based resources, such as medical care and counseling agencies. In fact, the nurse from the involved agency is often the primary coordinator of the community-based plan that has been initiated.

Private Medicare home health agencies can provide most of the above services. These fall under Medicare regulations covering home health care and primarily serve the Medicare patient. Therefore, eligibility for services and length of time the service can be provided can be issues if this resource is selected.

Social and Counseling Agencies

The trend today is toward agencies that provide comprehensive services, preferably at the neighborhood or community level. Typical of some services offered are housekeeping and homemaking services, individual and family counseling, vocational guidance, financial and legal assistance, and other social and recreational programs in keeping with the needs of the population of the area. Mental health, drug abuse, and alcohol treatment centers may also be found in most communities, with services consisting of emergency treatment and detoxification programs, counseling, and in some cases, inpatient treatment programs. Many of these social and counseling agencies are supported in full or in part by public funds, while others are supported by some of the voluntary organizations, such as Jewish Family Services, Catholic Charities, and the Salvation Army. The Easter Seal Society maintains centers in many communities and offer various services such as physical therapy, occupational therapy, speech therapy, and counseling on an outpatient basis, equipment loan pools, and homebound programs.

Other Services

Transportation and meal service in the home can be found in communities and is usually sponsored by special programs for the elderly, ill, and handicapped.

Health screening clinics, educational materials, information resources for specific questions, and some personal services are offered by a variety of voluntary organizations, for example, the Heart Association, Multiple Sclerosis Society, Arthritis Foundation, Diabetic Association, and the Cancer Society.

Special services are also offered to the handicapped population by various fraternal organizations such as the Shriners, Lions, and Rotary clubs. In addition, volunteer services can be found within some neighborhoods and community groups. These services tend to be spotty and of a very short-term nature, as such services are dependent on the availability of volunteers, but they can be approached for occasional transportation needs and for short-term relief of a caretaker, such as for shopping.

Resources for emergency care that the nurse may wish to consider when making plans with the patient and family would be the local police and fire departments. They will certainly be a resource for emergency transportation and may also need to be alert to the fact that there is a physically disabled person in the home.

Support and Special Interest Groups

Support and special interest groups may consist of formal or informal gatherings for the disabled and/or their families and may serve as support, social, educational, or action groups. Some examples of such groups are Make Today Count, coronary clubs, and the National Paraplegic Foundation.

Resources for Medical Care

If the patient does not have a private physician in the community, then a neighborhood clinic may be the resource used to meet the patient's general medical needs. These may be located through the Public Health Department, voluntary agencies, or hospital ambulatory care clinics.

Medical supplies and nonspecialized equipment can usually be obtained from most retail pharmacies and retail medical supply and equipment vendors. Community hospitals and, on occasion, community-sponsored equipment pools may be additional resources.

Finding the Resource

It is to be hoped that there is a mechanism within the system that can provide quick identification of resource availability. Such help may be provided by a discharge planning coordinator, a directory compiled for use in the institution, or listings of multiple community agencies put together for use in social work departments. Other possibilities would be the visiting nurse associations and public health nurses in the area, a nurse or social worker who is involved in discharge planning within the community hospital, and of course, the patient and family.

What One Needs to Know about the Agency

In selecting the resource, it will be important to have the following data, and these could well be the questions which the nurse or the patient or family would pose to the agency:

- What is the population served by the agency?
- What are the boundaries served by the agency?
- What are the eligibility requirements?
- What are the fee scales?
- What are the services available from the agency?
- What body governs standards?
- Does the agency coordinate multiple services in the community?
- Is the service accessible to the patient if it is not a home-based service?
- What is the system of feedback and communication with the referring agency?

RESPONSIBILITIES OF THE NURSE IN DISCHARGE PLANNING

The nurse plays a vital role in formulating a viable discharge plan. The responsibilities of the nurse in discharge planning are identified in the following sections. These points can be adapted to any individual situation despite the variables in the community or institutional setting, type and size of the setting, and the system of discharge planning available to the nurse. The responsibilities discussed are those that are already within the standards of care of nursing practice; most of the tools and processes suggested are those that are universally used, although there is some variation in format.

COORDINATION

The number of people and decision-making actions that take place in the transition planning of a patient can be overwhelming. In order to facilitate the development of a smooth, concerted discharge plan, coordination of efforts is essential.

Nurses are in a position to witness the overall performance of the patient and implementation of the plan because they are constantly in contact with the patient, have access to the central data base of the patient, and are in continual contact with other members of the health care team involved with the patient either as a result of their consultations with patients or through conferences set up to discuss individual patients. For these reasons, coordination of the transition planning logically becomes the responsibility of the nurse.

COMMUNICATION

Coordination demands communication. This can be a major task because, according to Bergman (1977), there are three major systems of interpersonal relations in health care: the client-practitioner relationship, which incorporates the individual/family/group and caregivers; interdisciplinary relationships, which are the various disciplines of health professionals; and intradisciplinary relationships, which would be the levels of nursing hierarchy and peer relationships. All of these people, if they are involved in the patient's care, must be informed. Of course, this does not mean that the nurse bears the full responsibility, but nursing personnel are responsible for initiating and/or taking an active part in those situations that enhance communication and thus the planning process. Team conferences, patient/family meetings, and nursing rounds are some examples of communication methods.

Effective documentation methods can promote information exchange, save much time, and provide for accuracy of the information transmitted. For efficient and effective recording, one should consider the following:

- What are the minimum data that can be recorded and still be meaningful?
- What is the significant information required for other team members, for third-party payment?
- What data can be coded? Be sure all disciplines can gain information from your records.
- What tools need to be developed? For example, nursing history form, patient care plan, interagency form, teaching checklist, nursing interim summary format.
- Are these important records accessible to interdisciplinary team members?

TEACHING

All disciplines have an area of responsibility and accountability for patient and family teaching. However, nurses must be aware of what is being taught to ensure that the information is carried through on the care unit and to coordinate their own teaching with that which is occurring with other disciplines. It is the nurse's responsibility to develop, coordinate, and implement a teaching plan with the patient and family. The teaching process is a vital part of a patient's hospitalization, for success or failure in learning affects the quality of the outcome of the discharge plan.

Individualized teaching objectives should be developed with the patient. This is an extremely important step. Objectives help to clarify what is to be accomplished, and if well formulated, they give direction and serve as a very important key to the evaluation process. The content material can be devised into a checklist format, which helps to standardize content somewhat and also facilitates documentation. There should be a place on the checklist to state the goals to be achieved, since this operationalizes and individualizes the plan.

PRACTICE

The accountability of the nurse to the patient is described in the standards of nursing practice. This accountability defines the nurse's relationship to and responsibility as a significant member of the therapeutic team. The nurse's expertise as a practitioner and the ability to articulate planning efforts with the patient can greatly effect the quality of the outcome of the discharge plan.

The area of nursing represented (acute or chronic or a speciality or general area), the level of nursing represented (staff nurse, head nurse, clinical specialist), and the method of nursing practice (primary or functional) govern the constants that are available to the nurse for planning. Variables that affect the planning process include:

- The length of time one has to work with the patient
- The authority over and level of responsibility for the patient
- The style of record keeping and freedom to create new methods
- Amount of autonomy as to place and time
- The availability of personal and professional resources for planning and support

The method of approach to the development of the discharge plan is accomplished by means of the stages of the nursing process. To begin, the initial data base (referral material, history and physical, nursing history) gathered on admission gives clues to the discharge plan. From this initial assessment, plans are developed and goals are jointly established. These plans are implemented by means of care delivery, teaching, and intrainstitutional referral and are then evaluated by formal and informal methods. Thus the process continues in an open-ended cyclical fashion until actual components to the final discharge plan begin to evolve. The final assessment that occurs toward the end of the patient's stay is for the purpose of taking one last critical look to ensure that all bases have been covered by the final plan. The final assessment, finalization of the plan, and implementation of referral will be discussed at length.

The following case studies illustrate how nursing responsibilities that are critical to effective discharge planning can be put into operation.

Mr. and Mrs. B. are a couple in their early seventies. Mrs. B. was admitted to a rehabilitation hospital following a cerebrovascular accident (CVA) resulting in right hemiplegia and expressive aphasia.

Mrs. B. had a long history of illness. She was diabetic for years, and subsequent complications necessitated bilateral amputation of the lower extremities. Following these crises, Mrs. B. was fairly independent from a wheelchair, and she and Mr. B. managed at home quite well with the support and help of Mrs. B.'s daughter (from a previous marriage), who lived in the neighborhood, and Ms. D., a nurse from the Visiting Nurses Association (hereafter referred to as VNA).

At this time, however, the CVA had left Mrs. B. almost totally physically dependent, and some perceptual and intellectual losses eliminated any possibility of her safely managing any aspect of her care needs. To further complicate the situation, Mr. B. and Mrs. B.'s daughter were involved in a conflict, and the daughter was withdrawing any support and assistance as a result.

Mr. B., being very lonely, spent long hours at the hospital, and the nurses involved him in teaching and assisting with the care of Mrs. B. Despite his willingness and need to care for his wife, it became obvious that he was not physically able to render some of the care, such as transfers, nor was he able to safely carry through more complex skills, which was especially obvious in regard to insulin dosage and injections. These facts were presented to Mr. B., along with the need to look at the alternatives. He became very distressed and verbalized that staff members and his stepdaughter were trying to keep him from taking his wife home.

It was then decided by the nurse to look at the positive skills that Mr. B. demonstrated and to allow him to participate fully in these care areas, while resources to meet other care needs were being examined by the team.

The visiting nurse, Ms. D. was then consulted and was invited to participate in a planning conference. Ms. D. was able to bring forth information related to the strengths in the family that had not been apparent, such as the strong likelihood that the daughter would stay involved despite the message she was now giving. A plan was set up by the team and Ms. D. for Mr. B. to take his wife home on an overnight pass. From this home experience, it was hoped that Mr. B. would be able to get a more realistic picture of what it would be like to be totally in charge of his wife's care when alone and in the home environment and that upon return to the hospital, he would participate in setting up an alternative to his desired, but unsafe, plan. The daughter was notified of the planned overnight pass and of her stepfather's strong desire to manage his wife alone in the home.

Mr. and Mrs. B. left in the early evening. Transportation was provided by an ambulance service, thus eliminating any need for Mr. B. to do transfers. Ms. D., the visiting nurse, scheduled her visit for early morning for the purpose of giving the insulin and observing Mr. B.'s ability to manage the other aspects of care. Upon the nurse's arrival, she found Mrs. B.'s daughter assisting Mr. B. with the care. The results gained from the home visit were not as anticipated, that is, the realization of a need for a more workable plan by Mr. B., but instead it brought the daughter back on the scene in a supportive and helpful role, thereby allowing Mr. and Mrs. B. to remain in their home.

The patient was a 70-year-old Jewish man with right hemiplegia and severe expressive aphasia. Prior to the disability, he had been the dominant family figure. His wife was, and continued to be, passive and frail in character. The married daughter took on the responsibility for her mother and father since his illness, and she exhibited a very aggressive and highly anxious personality, verbally expressing the attitude, "I must fight for my father, for he can no longer fight for himself." After several weeks and many attempts at teaching, it was determined that neither the wife nor the daughter exhibited the capacity to assimilate information related to the patient's capacity to function after his stroke, nor could they recognize his progress. They blamed him for not trying, and they blamed the health team for not accomplishing anything with him. Thus, all attempts at planning for discharge with the family and at helping them to follow through with steps to achieve a goal were met with resistance and challenge.

Recognizing heightened frustrations and dissonance between the family and members of the health team, the nurse arranged for a meeting with the family and key team members. At the meeting, the disability was reexplained, the progress the patient made was reemphasized, and options for the final discharge plan were openly discussed. The family did finally communicate that they were going to take their father home after discharge.

In the days following the meeting, the family's behavior remained unchanged. However, the team was able to rekindle their direction and use a consistent approach with the family, for all team members had the same degree of understanding of what information the patient and family had been given and how the patient and family were coping with the situation, and all were aware of abilities and capacities of the patient and family.

Prior to discharge, the nurse initiated a referral to the Jewish Family Services and the Visiting Nurses Association, including the interagency referral form the significant information pertaining to the specific approach required for dealing with the family in the home setting.

After discharge, and in the home environment, the family seemed to relax. They provided care that they had previously refused to do and were thus able to participate in further upgrading the patient's independence.

THE DISCHARGE PLAN: REFINEMENTS AND IMPEDIMENTS

The discharge plan evolves with increasing clarity as short-term goals are achieved and new goals are set, as long-term goals become more evident, as teaching is accomplished and the results evaluated, as joint discussions and planning occur in patient care conferences, nursing rounds, and family meetings, and as the patient and family have had opportunities for situational experiences that simulate the setting to which the patient will be discharged.

Plans do not always move forward. The patient and/or the family may refuse or avoid participation in active planning. Extremes of behaviors related to the adjustment process are frequently the source of the obstacle. Anger can be the most stifling block to any attempt at long-range planning. A patient often projects anger toward staff members, hospital facilities, and/or family members. This anger is often expressed in such comments as "I'm not leaving here until I am well, you haven't done anything for me." A second behavior that often emerges is denial. Denial of any possible permanency of the disability is a common reaction. A remark such as "Why do you want me to have a visiting nurse when I'm going to be well within a few weeks?" reflects the denial the patient is manifesting. Passivity is a third behavior capable of severely hindering progress toward a reasonable discharge plan. This behavior may be demonstrated by the patient agreeing with a given plan but taking no initiative toward actively implementing the plan. A fourth behavior that is equally difficult to work with is depression. When patients are emotionally "down," lack energy, and/or are highly anxious, certain steps must be taken by the team to actively and constantly guide these patients to a more productive use of their intact energy. During this period, only short-term goals and very specific information should be presented. It is not uncommon for a patient to demonstrate one type of behavior while a family member demonstrates another. The interaction of such divergent behaviors results in conflict and in consistent goals, reflected in the failure to move ahead with plans for a reasonable discharge.

A strategy helpful in dealing with some of these behaviors is a joint planning conference with the patient, family, and key team members. This type of meeting allows everyone to hear the same information related to needs, prognosis, and long-term plans. It will likely force communication between the patient and family, who may have been avoiding open discussion. It will clarify any gaps in the team's communication and approaches and promote mutual decisions. Finally, it will demonstrate the team's support of and concern for the patient and family.

Another useful strategy would be to set one desirable and attainable goal and work toward that goal until it is accomplished. For example, if the goal is setting a definite date for the first daytime pass[1] to the patient's home; the patient and family should be informed of the specific steps necessary to reach that goal, such as attending teaching and therapy sessions and practicing needed skills, and of the need for a mutual commitment in order to perform the steps.

Another impediment to the progression of the discharge plan is often found within the professional team. A team member who has lost objectivity and is not seeking counsel or direction, a controlling team member who is unwilling to share planning, poor communication among team members, poorly defined accountability, and a failure to carry out responsibilities are some examples of how a professional can cause barriers that will affect the entire plan despite the best efforts of the patient, family, and the remainder of the team.

Value systems that are not understood or considered by professionals can have a detrimental effect on any aspect of discharge planning. In addition to interaction patterns within a family unit, the nurse and the professional team need an understanding and appreciation of the attitudes, beliefs, and customs of the patient, of the immediate and extended family, and of the community that will influence long-term health care and reentry of the patient into the family and community. Whether the values are based on past experience, culture, religion, or environmental influences, the following questions deserve exploration when considering the immediate and long-term effects on the patient and family:

How are illness and disability viewed?
How do these views affect the adjustment process and therefore realistic planning?
What is the effect of placing the expectation

---

[1] A pass constitutes an authorized leave of absence from the hospital. Rehabilitation settings commonly use this type of leave to enhance evaluation, practicing of skills, and community reentry for the patient.

for care giving on a particular family member?

What will be the effect of the attitude of many of the urban poor toward planning ahead and determining priorities?

If there is no alternative to long-term care-facility placement, what will be the effect?

How will this circumstance affect the patient's ability to accept help or strive for physical independence?

Several years ago, a university professor became paraplegic as the result of an automobile accident. Complete physical independence, though attainable, was not his major goal; instead, it was to return as quickly as possible to his position at the university and to fulfill his role of teacher, lecturer, and author. He has very successfully maintained these positions and continues to receive help in some care programs and, to use his words, in "the housekeeping chores." This physical assistance enables him to direct his energy and time toward continued achievement in his professional role.

FINAL ASSESSMENT: PATIENT AND FAMILY STATUS AND NEEDS

The purpose of the final assessment is to evaluate what problems and needs still exist and to what degree. From this assessment, it is important to determine if these problems can be managed by the personal resources of the patient and family or if a formal or informal referral is necessary to provide interventions in the following areas:

Direct services for upgrading, prevention, and maintenance
Support and counseling
Teaching and/or review of past learning

When assessing for referral, the needs and problems of both the patient and the family must be considered. Their level of knowledge, abilities, and attitudes should be in harmony if conflicts and/or unrealistic expectations are to be avoided. For example, a referral may be made to coordinate the level of a significant family member's understanding of the disability with that of the patient if continued progress is to occur.

The parents of Mike, an adolescent boy with paraplegia, continually sought "cures and miracles" for him, often bringing into the hospital related newspaper clippings and magazine articles to discuss with professionals. Mike was adjusting well to the loss, making excellent progress, and had realistic hopes and goals for his future. However, these demonstrations by his parents were a constant source of embarrassment to him. His reaction was to retreat from any communication with them about the entire issue. However, this added to the problem, because it resulted in a loss of much-needed parental support and enouragement.

FUNCTIONAL CAPACITY AND ABILITY

In assessing functional capacity and ability, one must determine the extent of the physical impairment as it affects the patient's ability to functionally perform in a manner that is sufficient to meet needs and prevent problems. When assessing functional performance, one must consider the degree, frequency, and quality of assistance needed in such areas as self-care routines, mobility, home management, shopping, general safety, and nutritional and medication needs.

Are environmental factors a problem in the home, school, or work situation?

Who is advising and counseling the patient and family in planning for modifications that will allow for optimal physical functioning?

Is relocation indicated, and what plans have been made in that direction?

Is the care giver physically capable of managing the care? Consider health status, age, and size of the patient and care giver when making this assessment.

What is the backup system for the care giver? The ideal situation has more than a single family member prepared to give any aspect of care, with the details of responsibilities clearly outlined.

What are the other alternatives that can provide this relief? Will a home health aide come in several times a week for a few hours, or does the care giver prefer relief in the area of homemaking or child care?

Another important area for evaluation and planning is the availability of the care giver in relation to the needs of the patient. Although the plan to meet the routine needs may be sound, one must also account for unplanned events. For example, a quadriplegic patient may well be able to manage for a number of hours once basic care is given and he or she is in a wheelchair, but what if an emergency occurs, such as a plugged catheter or a bowel accident? Is there a neighbor available, willing, and knowledgeable who can come to the rescue or will it be necessary to call a parent or mate away from work or social event? If the latter is the plan, it might be very wise to encourage other alternatives.

TEACHING AND LEARNING COMPONENTS

In all cases, it must be assumed that teaching has occurred with the patient and family, that the content was presented in an understandable manner, and that experiences were provided to utilize the learning. Based on the patient's and family's abilities for learning, their knowledge base, their response to learning, and their demonstrated ability to utilize information, one can determine if resources will be needed in the community setting.

Because of various factors, there may be little indication that learning has occurred. This may be related to denial, depression, poor intellectual functioning, or a value system that does not include prevention as a priority. Or this may be related to a poor teaching plan, an inaccurate assessment of readiness for learning, or a poor selection of teaching method. Failure to learn, when the patient and family do have the ability, is a phenomenon that is very difficult to accept, and the discharge plan will certainly be less than ideal. It then becomes extremely important to assess the deficits, identify the best resources to bridge the gap, and accurately convey the problem to the referral resource.

Evaluation of the following situations will help to assess more reliably the patient's and the family's initiative and ability to utilize learning:

- Situations set up within the patient care unit whereby the caretakers participate and/or have responsibility for care routines for an extended period of time, such as overnight or for a weekend
- Day, weekend, or a more extended leave of absence to the home, which can also be incorporated with a home visit by team members and/or a community health nurse
- Situations set up on the patient care unit whereby the patient assumes responsibility for care routines or, if not physically independent, directs all aspects of care
- Formal or informal testing situations that provide opportunities for the patient to display knowledge and/or problem-solving abilities

If the patient and family has had a variety of situational experiences in which to practice learned skills, these not only enhance the assessment of their abilities but also provide them with an added degree of confidence and a realistic awareness of the future.

Another important area when considering the status of learning and need for continued teaching is the nature of the disability. Is it a permanent condition, or is it likely to improve or deteriorate? The very nature of a progressive disease, in most people, will require ongoing support, teaching, and assistance in adapting care routines as change occurs. For example, the patient with multiple sclerosis is probably faced with remissions and exacerbations that may alter basic bodily functions, requiring changes in management programs. Initial teaching about the disease process will have prepared the patient somewhat to recognize change, but it is not likely that even basic information related to management of changes will have been assimilated or retained.

Other questions that will assist the nurse when making the final assessment of learning include the following:

- What has been the participation of family members with other disciplines? Have they attended therapy sessions?
- Has the patient and family availed themselves of other information sources such as special interest groups?
- If the patient is being discharged to a long-term care facility, are staff skills sufficient to carry out highly technical care routines such as the use of specialized equipment? What is the plan for teaching the agency staff if there is no alternative to that particular placement? Has the patient or family been adequately counseled regarding the role they must assume in directing the agency staff and the right to expect high-level care?
- If care is to be given by a private attendant, have arrangements been made with the patient and/or family to have this person participate in care routines and therapies prior to discharge? Will the attendant require supervision in the home by a community health nurse?
- Do family members have the knowledge and skills sufficient to assist the physically independent patient in the event of an emergency or illness, including instructing staff regarding care routines if hospitalization should be necessary?

Upon discharge, the patient and family will need written information to serve as a guide and/or a reminder in the many areas that have been the focus of teaching. The following are some examples of the information they will need:

- General information related to the disease process or disability, such as home care manuals and information available from various voluntary organizations such as the Diabetic Association and the American Heart Association.
- Specific programs individualized to the patient, including medication schedules, supplies and equipment used, and care techniques. If the patient is being discharged to a long-term care facility and a procedure is highly individualized, it is advisable that this information be sent in writing along with the nursing interagency form.
- Written instructions for maintaining equipment, including safe methods for cleaning, which may allow for reuse.
- Written home programs from other therapists involved in the patient's rehabilitation program, such as speech, physical, and/or occupational therapists

SOCIAL AND EMOTIONAL COMPONENTS

Evidence of social or emotional problems demonstrated by the patient or significant family member may be the basis for a referral upon discharge. Any degree of difficulty in these areas can impede an effective transition back into the community.

In assessing social and emotional states, the nurse should consider behaviors the person has displayed since injury or by history. This would include problems in adjustment to the disability, such as severe or prolonged depression, denial, or anger; drug or alcohol abuse; psychotic behavior; poorly developed social behaviors; or an unresolved crisis affecting the functioning of the family unit as a whole. Depending upon the degree of the problem, it may require only the support and surveillance of the community health nurse. If the problem has overtly interfered with care and progress, then referral to a psychiatrist or a mental health clinic may be necessary. The person within the system who is responsible for recommendations and referrals for continued management should be notified.

Often, patterns of interaction within the family unit interfere with the reentry of the patient back into that unit. These same patterns of interaction can also interfere with basic needs of the involved family members. Examples of these are as follows:

Overprotecting or overhelping the patient
Lack of willingness to ask for or accept relief for caretaking responsibilities
Inability to become creative or flexible in adapting care routines around other family or social needs
Impossible demands made by the patient upon the time and energies of the caretaker and/or family
Unrealistic expectations for recovery placed upon the patient by a significant family member
Family members who exhibit resentment at being placed in the role of caretaker
The disabled family member demonstrating or verbalizing discomfort with family members involved in personal care

These interactions may not be amenable to change but certainly warrant the consideration for a referral for continued counseling and possible alternatives.

Other factors to consider with the patient, family, and team for a satisfactory transition are as follows:

Who will provide for the relief of the caretaker in event of illness and to allow for social and emotional needs? Many care needs do not require expert skill or extensive teaching and thus can easily be shared with or delegated to friends and relatives.
Who is taking charge of financial counseling, and are there deficits that may likely produce stress and affect care and health needs?
What will be the long-term impact on the family unit of a patient who cannot safely function alone for even minimal periods of time?
Have the recreational needs of the patient been considered, including participation with peers and socialization away from the home?
If the patient will not be actively involved in vocational or educational pursuits, what are the avocational interests that will provide stimulation and satisfaction? Are there programs within the community that can serve as a resource?
Who will provide financial support if the disability requires that the patient make a significant change in vocation?
Have spiritual or religious needs been considered? What is planned for meeting these needs?
What is the interest of the patient in neighborhood or community organizations? Is an interest being supported and encouraged if feasible?
What is the understanding within the family unit of personal and privacy needs being respected?

SAFETY

The idea of safety means protection from aspects of self or the environment that could result in harm to the individual. In most settings, several disciplines play a part in this assessment. The following questions should be asked:

Does the patient have an impairment in intellectual functioning, judgment, memory, or behavior? If so, what type and amount of help would be needed for the patient's safety?
Does the patient have a communication disorder? Can he or she call for help?

Has the telephone been adapted for use by a patient with poor hand function?

Are there any aspects in the home environment that could be hazardous to the individual with poor mental functioning, such as steps and unlocked doors?

Are there any aspects in the home environment that could be hazardous to the individual with altered physical functioning, such as throw rugs, stairs without railings, a bathtub without grab bars?

In the event of fire, will the lack of mobility on the part of the patient and/or the lack of easy accesss out of the home be a problem? If so, the police and fire departments should be notified in advance that a disabled individual is in the home.

Factors to consider when planning for emergency care include the following:

What resources will be used in an emergency, for example, the facility, type of transportation, and medical resource?

Is the potential for an emergency situation great enough to warrant some preplanning with the emergency room staff and school or work associates?

Should the patient wear or carry identification that identifies a condition or a significant medication, such as diabetes, hyperreflexia, epileptic seizure, pacemaker, coumadin therapy.

MEDICAL CARE

This section is concerned with examining the types of medical management needed in the areas of maintenance and prevention as they relate to general health and to those special needs that arise as a result of the disability. Some questions that the patient and/or the family may need guidance in resolving are as follows:

What "kind" of a primary physician does the patient need, that is, a generalist or specialist?

If the discharging physician is not the primary physician, does the patient and/or family know what this implies?

What is the role of the discharging agency in providing follow-up?

If the discharging physician is not primary, how does this follow-up interface with that of the primary medical resource?

Will pertinent medical information be communicated to the physician?

Where are clinics located when there is no primary physician?

How soon should an appointment be made with the primary medical resource?

Are there specific recommendations for future diagnostic tests that need to be communicated to the primary physician?

MEDICATIONS, MEDICAL SUPPLIES, AND EQUIPMENT

At the time of discharge, the patient may need to be supplied with medications, prescriptions, and an understanding of which of the medical resources will assume responsibility for future prescription renewals if there is more than one physician involved. In making a final assessment of medication and equipment needs and management, the following should be considered:

What is the status of knowledge related to the regime? Is there a likelihood of mismanagement or noncompliance?

Can the patient safely and functionally manage the administration? Is there a need for adaptations such as special containers?

Are there financial concerns? Does the patient and family understand the system of public funding or eligibility for reimbursement through special insurance programs? Has the necessary paperwork been processed?

Does the program include medications that require close monitoring by laboratory tests, and if so, what is the need and the plan?

- What is the status of specialized equipment such as hospital bed, wheelchair, commode chair, special mattresses? Who on the team is assuming responsibility for identifying and coordinating these needs?
- What does the patient and family understand about care, maintenance needs, and replacement sources?
- Have the patient and family been able to use the identical equipment while in the hospital?
- If the equipment is quite complicated, should the use be reviewed in the home setting by a visiting nurse or a manufacturer's representative?

When identifying the ongoing medical supply needs with the patient and family, consider not only the items and quantities but also what is economical and practical in the home situation. Patients become so accustomed to the disposable items in hospitals that it is often very difficult for them to adapt to other methods. It is essential that the nurse plan with them and provide information for conservation, safe cleansing, and sterilization methods and perhaps even alter a program so that it still meets the need but stays within the realm of economic feasibility. By the time of discharge, the patient and/or family should already have selected a resource for maintenance of medical supplies and verified with the resource that all the needs can be met. It will probably be necessary upon discharge to send along sufficient supplies to allow for time in making this connection.

The nurse must convey to a patient and/or family the importance of maintaining adequate supplies and medications if the patient is to function optimally and maintain good health. This can be especially difficult with some families if planning ahead has not been their style. Over time, this problem may improve through the intervention of the community nurse.

NEGOTIATING RESOURCE SYSTEMS

Another area of assessment is the ability of the patient and family to successfully negotiate and work with systems to their own benefit. This applies not only to those public funding resources but also to any resource available to them. Working with multiple systems can often become confusing, frustrating, and sometimes demeaning, but it is important that the patient or family have some preparation, for the inability to persist appropriately or to be assertive in their own behalf will often result in needs not being met. It is important to identify who in the system is providing the patient and family with this information and counseling.

Premorbid behaviors, such as the ability to set priorities and be assertive, can indicate the strengths that the patient and family may have in order to negotiate systems after discharge. A clue to their abilities in this area may be elicited by looking at how effectively they utilized resources of and negotiated the hospital system!

Another area of assessment is the knowledge required by the patient and family if the resources are to be fully utilized. What do they understand about:

- What a resource does in general and what it can do specifically for them
- How to contact a resource and who at the agency to contact
- The method in which the agency will help them, understanding the concept of "doing for" versus "helping you to do for yourself"
- When to involve a resource
- How one resource interfaces with other resources
- How the resource will be financed
- Rationale and goals for the referral
- Anticipated duration of time of the service

REFERRAL TO THE COMMUNITY AGENCY: COMMUNICATION AND COORDINATION

By this time, the patient's needs will have been identified and the selection made for appropriate resources with the patient and family. To ensure

683 DISCHARGE PLANNING

continuity of care, the referring institution must communicate to the referral resource *specific* needs, problems, and goals of the patient. In some cases, there may already have been communication with the agency in planning around a specific problem. The nurse may have asked their assistance in the home assessment or invited their participation in a predischarge planning conference.

The formal referral is made before the patient is discharged. Agencies vary in their requirements for written referral information and often have specific forms that include demographic data, brief medical history, and specific treatment orders to be carried out. In most cases, these orders will require the signature of the referring physician. All significant written information should be available to the agency at the time of the first visit.

Required information is generally minimal; therefore, it is the responsibility of the nurse who has worked closely with the patient and family to provide the added written communication that will be referred to as the nursing interagency form. Uninterrupted services during the transition can only occur if the interagency form is current and truly reflects the abilities, strengths, and limitations of the patient and family. Table 32-1 presents suggestions for what to include on a nursing interagency form.

Table 32-1

Suggested Content for Nursing Interagency Form

AREA	SPECIFICS
Demographic data	
Medical information	Diagnosis—primary and secondary
	Date of onset
	Brief and pertinent medical history
	Brief summary of clinical course and progress
	Significant diagnostic data
	Patient and family understanding of diagnosis and related teaching completed
Psychosocial information	Patient adaptation to the disability
	Family response to the disability
	Support structures and primary care giver(s)
	Coping and interaction patterns
	Significant premorbid and postmorbid behaviors
	Sexuality issues
Learning aptitude	Patient and family abilities for learning
	Response to teaching
	Significant problems
	Recommended approaches
Communication	Ability to send and receive messages
	Reliability of communication
	Problem areas
	Recommended approaches
Safety	Losses and deficits affecting safety, including intellectual, perceptual, physical, sensory, medical, and behavioral abilities
	Patient and/or family understanding of the problem(s)
	Recommended management and approaches

Table 32-1 (continued)

Suggested Content for Nursing Interagency Form

AREA	SPECIFICS
Perceptual-sensory	Losses and deficits
	Effect on performance and safety
	Patient and/or family understanding of the deficit(s)
	Suggested approaches
Care programs	Consider under each program:
Skin	Current status
Musculoskeletal	Specific programs of management
Bladder	Level of independence
Bowel	Special or adaptive equipment used
Respiratory	Complications—current, past, or potential
Rest and sleep	Teaching completed with patient and family
Nutrition and fluids	Response to teaching
ADL, including hygiene, bathing, mobility, transfers, dressing, and light homemaking abilities	Compliance with program
	Current and future goals
Discharge plan	Patient destination and environmental assessibility
	Primary care giver(s)
	Agencies and resources to be involved after discharge
	Plan for follow-up from the discharging institution, including clinic dates
	Community medication and supply source and funding
	Primary medical resource

Some of the areas listed as essential content in the interagency form have been the responsibility of other disciplines, such as mobility, communication, and certain activities of daily living (ADL). Ideally, there is a mechanism within the system that places accountability on other team members to provide timely written information to the agency, such as problems, progress, recommendations, and goals. If, however, the mechanism is ill defined and left to chance, then it becomes the nurse's responsibility to include the information. This information can be gained from observations, progress reports, and conferences, and its inclusion will ensure that the interagency form is as comprehensive as possible under the circumstances.

If the patient is to be transferred to an acute care hospital, either for an elective or an emergency situation, the information contained on the interagency form must be shared with the nurses involved in the care of the patient. This not only allows for the continuity of care but also conveys the status of the discharge plan.

For the patient returning to school or work situations, it may be necessary and beneficial to the patient to convey pertinent information related to health problems and self-care abilities, but this should only be done with the patient's knowledge and consent, and rights to privacy and confidentiality must be respected.

FOLLOW-UP FROM THE REFERRING AGENCY FOR EVALUATION AND COORDINATION

Follow-up from the referring institution is necessary for evaluating the effect of services provided before discharge, the soundness of the discharge plan, and the adequacy of services provided by the resources selected in the discharge plan, for identifying deficits in the community resource system, and for revising the plan if new or unmet needs are identified. Highly specialized agencies often assume a more significant role in providing direct services, including health maintenance and educational opportunities, and may even coordinate services.

Follow-up can be accomplished in several ways, the best being direct contact with the patient, which enhances verification of actual patient status. Other methods of follow-up and evaluation include surveys, questionnaires, phone contact with the patient and/or family, and feedback and communication from involved agencies in the community.

Communication with the involved community agencies not only provides an adjunct to evaluation but also clarifies patient needs, problems, and services provided, thereby avoiding duplication of services, decreasing confusion and gaps, and providing an opportunity for mutual setting of goals and approaches with the patient and family.

DISENGAGEMENT

In several areas, this chapter has touched upon the necessity for the patient and family to "take over." Because this concept is so significant to successful transition planning and thus to an individual's success in living within the community, it will now be discussed in more detail.

The process of "taking over" entails transfer back to an independency state, given the patient's capacity to do so. Capacity is determined by premorbid characteristics that are affected by and combined with postmorbid characteristics. It includes functional capacity, motivation, personal resources, and resourcefulness. This process will be referred to as disengagement, although it is realized that in sociological data, this term is usually used in conjunction with discussion of the gerontological patient.

The process of disengagement does occur in stages, but the stages do not usually follow a chronological order. Instead, the disengagement process follows a progression based on the patient's need, readiness, and willingness for autonomy.

When does the disengagement process begin? Signs of "taking over" may be evidenced very early, even before knowledge related to the effects of the disability is assimilated. More realistically, it is likely to begin when the patient begins to achieve short-term goals and demonstrates the ability to manage certain areas, such as a basic care activity. It is a gradual process, with each experience building one onto the other. As the patient masters certain areas, more complex ones are introduced.

Staff members must be able to recognize environmental conditions and set up conditions that assist and allow the patient to move forward in the process. Some examples would be:

Staff attitudes that allow, promote, and reward independence in the patient
Rewards within the system for independence
A physical environment conducive to learning and utilizing skills
Awareness and skill of staff in utilizing techniques of interaction that foster progress toward autonomy, such as involving the patient in problem solving, choices, bargaining, and use of resources and, on occasion, allowing a failure
Setting up an independent living situation within the care unit

Disengagement is an important issue to rehabilitation nursing and often becomes a complex one. These patients have usually experienced life-threatening and/or life-altering events. The severity of the loss promotes a vulnerable and dependent role, as does the long-term hospitalization. The primary nursing method of care delivery in conjunction with the lengthy hospital stay contributes to the development of deep relationships. It is also not

CHAPTER 32   686

uncommon for the nurse to develop a strong identity with the patient because of age and lifestyle similarities or an arousal of unresolved experiences or crisis, such as death of a parent.

The intensity of the demands placed upon the nurse may evoke many types of feelings that are quite normal and need to be recognized as such. According to Gunther (1977), "Some staff distress is an inevitable, normally occurring feature of the intense, complex relationships that any dedicated professional staff develops with severely damaged, long term patients."

The dedication mentioned by Gunther is well exemplified in the following: "Nurses are human; it is difficult to believe but at last I have found it to be true. I even found that orderlies are human; and the aides. The only people in a hospital who are no longer human are the patients; and I will not mention the doctors. Sometimes I think that the doctors, nurses, orderlies, and aides care more than the patients do." This message was written by a patient in a rehabilitation hospital while practicing typing skills and was later found by a nurse.

There is often a feeling of sadness and loss on the part of the nurse when the patient is about to be discharged. There may be anger toward self, patient, and/or family when, for some reason, plans that seem ideal become disrupted. Nurses often feel they have failed when the patient or family, by choice and despite attempts at interventions, continue on a less than ideal course toward discharge.

Continuous support and objectivity from peers and other team members can assist the nurse in dealing with these feelings. Invaluable assistance can be gained from experienced peers and team members who have dealt with the struggles of the process and have had an opportunity to gain more insight into the process.

If the disengagement process does not seem to be progressing satisfactorily, an objective reexamination of the situation is in order. Consider the following:

- Does the patient always seek the nurse out to solve problems, or does staff always send the patient back to the nurse? Has delegation of responsibilities to peers been attempted when dependency on the nurse seems prolonged?
- Where are the patient and family in the adjustment process? Do they have the capacity to begin taking on aspects that require emotional or physical independence?
- Is it possible that levels of independence for the patient are being expected prematurely?
- Have the patient's personal resources been involved, and have creativity and resourcefulness been encouraged?
- Is there a conflict in goals between the nurse and patient or other team members?
- Have resources outside the institutional setting been introduced?
- Are there premorbid characteristics that indicate that the patient has not usually valued or strived for an independent role?

CONCLUSION

All patients have the right to discharge planning. The ultimate goal of such planning is to attain and maintain optimum health and functioning and to prevent health problems. Nurses, often in collaboration with other peer professionals, assist in coordinating and communicating the planning, utilizing the steps of the nursing process to achieve the final plan. Upon the initiation of referral, a different set of events unfold in the community, but the familiar steps of the process continue.

BIBLIOGRAPHY

American Hospital Association: *A Patient's Bill of Rights,* 1972.

Bergman, Rebella: "Interpersonal Relations in Health Care Delivery," *Int Nurs Rev* 24: 104–107, 1977.

Bristow, O., C. Stickney, and S. Thompson: *Discharge Planning for Continuity of Care,* National League for Nursing, New York, 1976.

Dubos, Rene: *Man Adapting.* Yale University Press, New Haven, 1965.

Freidson, Eliot: "Client Control and Medical Practice," in E. Gartly Jaco (ed.): *Patients, Physicians, and Illness,* 2d ed., Free Press, New York, 1972, pp. 214–221.

Gunther, Meyer S.: "The Threatened Staff: A Psychoanalytic Contribution to Medical Psychology," *Compr Psychiatry* 18(4):386, 1977.

How to Select a Nursing Home, Division of Long-term Care, Public Health Service, U.S. Department of Health, Education, and Welfare, Washington, D.C., 1976.

Imirie, John F., Jr.: "The Role of the Hospital Administrator as It Relates to Discharge-Referral Planning," in *Patient Discharge and Referral Planning: Whose Responsibility?,* National League for Nursing, New York, 1974, p. 10.

Jennings, Carole: "Discharge Planning and the Government," *Supervisor Nurse* March: 48–52, 1977.

Kratzer, John: "What Does Your Patient Need to Know?," *Nursing 77* December: 82–84, 1977.

LaMontagne, M., and K. McKeehan: "Profile of a Continuing Care Program Emphasing Discharge Planning," *J Nurs Admin* October: 22–23, 1975.

Leininger, Madeleine: "An Open Health Care System Model," *Nurs Outlook* 21:171–175, 1973.

——— (ed.): *Health Care Dimensions, Spring 1975: Barriers and Facilitators to Quality Health Care,* Davis, Philadelphia, 1975.

———: *Transcultural Health Care: Issues and Conditions,* Davis, Philadelphia, 1976.

———: *Transcultural Nursing Concepts: Theories and Practices,* Wiley, New York, 1978.

Lewis, Charles, Rashi Fein, and David Mechanic: *A Right to Health: The Problem of Access to Primary Medical Care,* Wiley, New York, 1976.

McAtee, Patricia: "Poverty, Relevance, and Program Failure," *Nurs Outlook* September: 56–58, 1969.

Monaco, Judy Tincher, and Barbara Lang Conway: "Motivation: By Whom and Toward What?," *Am J Nurs* 69:1719, 1969.

National League for Nursing: *Continuity of Nursing Care from Hospital to Home: A Study in a Voluntary General Hospital,* National League for Nursing, New York, 1966.

National League for Nursing: *Patient Discharge and Referral Planning: Whose Responsibility?,* National League for Nursing, New York, 1974.

Peitchinis, Jacquelyn A.: *Staff-Patient Communication in the Health Services.* Springer, New York, 1976.

Pender, Nola: "A Conceptual Model for Preventative Health Behavior," *Nurs Outlook* 23: 385–390, 1975.

Rancho Los Amigos Hospital: *Guidelines for Discharge Planning.* Rancho Los Amigos Hospital, Downey, Calif., 1968.

Redman, Barbara Klug: *The Process of Patient Teaching in Nursing,* Mosby, St. Louis, 1976.

Reinhardt, Adina M., and Mildred D. Quinn (eds.): *Family-centered Community Nursing: A Sociocultural Framework,* Mosby, St. Louis, 1973.

Role and Responsibility of Hospitals in Home Care, American Hospital Association, 1976.

Shapiro, I. S.: "Health Education Horizons and Patient Satisfactions," *Am J Public Health,* 62:229–232, 1972.

Standards of Rehabilitation Nursing Practice, American Nurses Association, Division on Medical-Surgical Nursing Practice, and the Association of Rehabilitation Nurses, 1977.

Stroman, Duane F.: *The Medical Establishment and Social Responsibility,* National University Publications Kennikat Press, Port Washington, N.Y., 1976.

Weller, Miriam D., D. Henry Ruth, and Robert H. Seller: "Effective Use of Patient Resources: A

Training Guide for Family Physicians," *Family Prac,* 4:515–519, 1977.

Will, Marilyn B.: "Referral: A Process, Not a Form," *Nursing 77* December: 44–45, 1977.

Wright, Beatrice A.: *Physical Disability: A Psychological Approach.* Harper, New York, 1960.

Yura, Helen, and Mary B. Walsh: *The Nursing Process: Assessing, Planning, Implementing Evaluating,* 3d ed., Appleton-Century-Crofts, New York, 1978.

Zeigler, Deloris N.: "Overview of the Discharge Referral Planning Problem: What Is Being Done Locally and Nationally?," in *Patient Discharge and Referral: Whose Responsibility?,* National League for Nursing, New York, 1974, pp. 6–8.

33
patricia booth
jack mason

vocational rehabilitation

Many health care professionals are unaware of the vocational rehabilitation services that are available to the disabled and are thus unable to advise their patients as to what kind of help to seek in returning to a job or entering the employment market. This chapter presents an overview of vocational rehabilitation in order to give the nurse a general introduction to the field as it exists today.

Vocational counseling, vocational evaluation, work evaluation, vocational work evaluation, and job placement are all terms nurses will encounter in various combinations in the rehabiliation setting. All refer to the services offered to help disabled persons prepare for employment.

The field, as a profession, is relatively new and thus is growing and changing. There is as yet no commonly accepted approach, department structure, or personnel delineation. However, generally there will be a vocational counseling/evaluating component with provisions for job placement. One person may provide all these services, or, depending on the facilities' size, funding, caseload, and philosophy of rehabilitation, a division of staff with specialities in counseling, evaluation, and job placement will exist.

Whatever the personnel involved, the goal of the vocational rehabilitation unit is to assist the client in becoming employed. The processes in reaching this goal include counseling; assessing or evaluating interests, skills, and abilities; predicting vocational potential and options; and locating employment opportunities.

As already suggested, opinions vary as to what functions should be included in each process. In general, however, the counseling component is concerned with locating persons who might benefit from vocational rehabilitation and determining their eligibility for the programs available. In doing this, the counselor utilizes and thus must have a good knowledge of community resources and occupational information. The counselor is reponsible for finding and arranging for the funding source used to purchase the vocational service for the client. Overall, the counselor is the manager of the case, coordinating the services and funds and ensuring that the process runs smoothly. Initially, the counselor and the client work together to arrive at a rehabilitation plan or goal. The counselor then determines what diagnostic services are necessary to facilitate this plan, such as vocational or work evaluation, interest testing, psychological testing, and occupational or physical therapy evaluation. The counselor further performs what is perhaps thought of as the "classic" counselor role by supporting and encouraging the client during the process of following the plan. The counselor is responsible for interpreting the findings of the various diagnostic procedures for the client. The two continuously reassess the plan based on these interpretations.

> The counselor establishes a professional relationship with the client, continuing from the onset or recognition of disability to the attainment of greatest competitive capacity. The counseling relationship is a dynamic, ongoing process in which the personalities of the counselor and the client interact in such a way as to maximize present vocational assets and foster realistic self-acceptance in the client. The counselor's counseling responsibilities may include work with various members of the client's family. (Sink and Porter, 1978)

It always includes knowledge of and coordination with the medical, psychological, and social aspects of the client's situation. Vocational counselors generally use one of the five following counseling models: trait-factor, client-centered career, psychodynamic, behavioral, or developmental.

The trait-factor model takes an authoritative approach in addressing the matter of vocational choice. The counselor is very directive, specifically leading the client through the testing, occupational investigation, interviewing, and placement process. Vocational choice is made in a logical, straightforward manner from the test results. Placement is specific and selective.

The client-centered career model uses the seven-stage Rogerian process, which allows clients to actualize their own potential. The model emphasizes development of the self-concept and implementation of that concept in work.

The psychodynamic model focuses on preferred ways of need gratification to affect a positive work personality change. This involves exploring the client's personal decision-making factors and how they affect vocational problems, plus analyzing job duties or tasks as to what needs they gratify.

The behavioral model aims to reduce client anxiety and to foster client acquisition of decision-making skills. This model specifically addresses such problems as decision/indecision, anxiety in making job choices, unrealistic job expectations and vocational goals, and choice conflicts arising for the multipotentialed client.

The developmental model faces the issue of vocational maturity. Through a series of interviews using a combination of directive and nondirective counseling techniques, the counselor determines the client's level of vocational development and guides the client to the next stage.

Assessing the client's vocational skills and abilities is the function of the evaluation component of vocational rehabilitation. The evaluator is responsible for determining the evaluation procedures that will be used to diagnose the appropriateness of the plan as developed by the client and the counselor. The evaluator decides which techniques, be they established systems, self-developed means, or a combination, will best answer the questions raised by the plan. These questions vary widely, depending on the case, but are all concerned with the client's physical ability, mental ability, social and behavioral appropriateness, and general "readiness" for meeting the vocational goal. The evaluator administers the procedures and measures the results against competitive employment standards. The resultant information is used in the process of predicting vocational potential and options. The counselor, evaluator, and client reassess the vocational plan and determine what other services, such as school, training, continued therapy, occupational information, job-seeking skills, if any, will be required to facilitate meeting the goal.

The four methods presently being used in work or vocational evaluation for assessing and predicting a client's vocational potential are (1) mental and or psychological-psychometric testing, (2) job analysis, (3) work sampling, and (4) situational assessment, which can include a job trial or work station approach (Neff, 1969).

Mental and/or psychological testing is possibly the most well known method of testing vocational abilities. Walter S. Neff, a leading psychologist in the rehabilitation field, dated the inception of this method at the turn of the twentieth century in the work of Binet and Spearman. He indicates that the primary qualities of the psychological test as a vocational tool are that it is quick, easy, and inexpensive to administer, it is objective, and it is reliable (Neff, 1968). However, much controversy has resulted from the use of psychological testing as an indicator of vocational skills and abilities, primarily because it often requires cognitive abilities rather than psychomotor abilities which are related more closely to most industrial sites, and it is ineffective in evaluating a large minority of the disabled population who have low literacy levels and an unsatisfactory experience with such tests in school (Sax, 1973). Also, the differences between the test site situation and the actual job site can affect job performance and invalidate predictions of job success based solely on such tests. The use of psychological testing may improve in the future through more investigative studies into its technical aspects.

Job analysis is the process of breaking down a specific existing job into its component parts, analyzing those parts to determine what skills and abilities are required to do the job, and then testing the client to determine if he or she has the needed skills and abilities. This method usually involves the use of job analysis techniques that were devloped within industry about the same time as were mental testing methods (Neff, 1968). Presently, there is a developing interest in job analysis as a basis for job restructuring. In this process, job analysts go into industry and select a job to bring back into the laboratory and then redesign, adapt, or modify it so that a person with a handicap, for example, a person who is quadriplegic, could be afforded the opportunity to compete for the job. This is an extremely expensive and time-consuming method that requires a degree of specialization not common in most vocational rehabilitation personnel. It is becoming more prevalent for engineers, job designers, and vocational/work evaluators to combine forces to develop new jobs to meet the needs of the handicapped person, usually with the aid of funding from special grants.

The third approach, *work sampling,* has become one of the most significant methods of vocational work evaluation in predicting and assessing the vocational potentials of rehabilitation clients. Work sampling is largely a post-World War II phenomenon (Neff, 1968). Task Force #3 of the Vocational Evaluation and Work Adjustment Association (1975) defines the work sample method as a specific work activity involving tasks, materials, and tools that are identical or similar to an actual job or cluster of jobs. It is used to assess an individual's vocational aptitude, worker characteristics, and vocational interests. It gives the following five classifications of work samples:

- indigenous work samples—Represent the essential factors of an occupation as it presently exists in one community.
- job sample—Work samples that in their entirety are replicated directly from industry and include the equipment, tools, raw materials, exact procedures, and work standards of the job.
- simulated work sample—Work samples that attempt to replicate a segment of the essential work-related factors and tools of the job as it is performed in industry.
- single trait work sample—Work samples that assess a single worker trait or characteristic such as finger dexterity, color discrimination, or clerical perception. They may have relevance to a specific job or many jobs, but they are intended to assess a single, isolated factor.
- cluster trait work sample—A single work sample developed to assess a group of worker traits. It contains a number of traits inherent in a job or a variety of jobs. Such a sample is based on an analysis of an occupational grouping and the traits necessary for successful performance therein. It is intended to assess the client's potential to do a variety of jobs.

In general, the work sample is as close an approximation of the reality of work as can be achieved in a rehabilitation facility. It provides exposure to and experience in a wide variety of jobs and requires performance identical to work. Besides assessing skills, the sample can also reveal aspects of the client's personality, interest, and attitudes toward the type of work. Certain clients often respond more naturally to hands-on work-related tasks than to abstract intellectual tasks and can thus be tested more accurately with the work sample. Also, cultural, educational, and language barriers can be eliminated. Many prospective employers of the handicapped are more receptive to reports of positive work sample performance than to predictions of employee success based on other performances. However, the work sample method has disadvantages. Developing samples for all jobs is not feasible, and keeping them up to date is usually economically impossible for the market sample systems. The trait samples are less vulnerable to becoming obsolete, but the other types of samples face this possibility.

The fourth method of assessing and predicting a client's vocational potential is situational assessment. *Situational assessment* is defined as a "clinical assessment method utilizing systematic observational techniques in established or created environments. Situational assessment includes evaluation in vocational training setting, job tryout, on the job evaluation, production work evaluation, simulated job station and work samples" (Vocational Evaluation and Work Adjustment Association, 1975). The idea behind this method is that to really evaluate a person's vocational potential, one must duplicate as closely as possible the job as it really exists or even allow the client to do the job for a period of time. Situational assessment is the newest method of work evaluation, beginning in the early 1950s (Neff, 1968). The essence of situational assessment answers the following questions: Can the client do what the system has predicted? How well does the client do it according to the competitive standard? If the client cannot perform as predicted, what are the problems? This method tends (as does job analysis) to be expensive and time-consuming, often requiring more preparation, personnel, and follow-up than can be economically justified by the funding source.

Of the four methods of work evaluation—mental and psychological-psychometric testing, job analysis, work sampling, and situational assessment—surveys indicate that work sampling is the method used most often by evaluators across the nation.

There are currently available 11 work-sampling systems. They are designed to serve a varied population, including those with low learning capabilities, the mentally ill, the culturally deprived, the disadvantaged, the physically disabled, the industrially injured, the professional and nonprofessional, the skilled and unskilled, those with or without work histories, and the minimally educated.

Two of the oldest work-sampling systems were developed with primary financing by the federal government. TOWER, the oldest system, developed by the Institute of the Crippled and Disabled (ICD), was funded by the Vocational Rehabilitation Administration in 1954. JEVS was developed by the Philadelphia Jewish Vocational Service and was funded by the United States Labor Department. Numerous systems have developed since TOWER and JEVS, but their means of funding has been, for the most part, independent of federal financial assistance.

In the development of a work sample system, the most commonly used basis is the *Dictionary of Occupational Titles* (DOT), which was first published in 1939. This book was developed by the United States Employment Service as an occupational information source, and it has been used by rehabilitation workers for many years. Worker Trait Groups: Data, People, Things and Aptitude Clusters, which are delineated by the DOT, are the major categories that provide the basis for 5 of the 11 commercial work-sampling systems. Using the DOT as a basis has the advantage of eliminating the need for job analysis and thus saving time. Usually, the work sample based on DOT will resemble actual jobs rather closely. However, the DOT has the disadvantage or limitation of being revised only every 10 years, and thus any information regarding occupational changes or new occupations is not provided until the next revision. This, along with the fact that most occupational work samples focus on entry-level jobs, limit the assessment of workers with skills that would allow them to work at higher positions; in addition, many of the jobs listed in the DOT are ones that people acquire after years of learning and experience.

The JEVS system makes vocational recommendations that are directly related to the DOT. It was developed for a target group of disadvantaged persons. It consists of 28 samples that take 6 to 7 days to administer. The client's work behavior is observed closely, and performance is scored on time and quality of work against a norm base of other clients.

The TOWER system was developed to assess the physically and emotionally disabled. It is made up of 93 samples that take 3 weeks to administer. The client is scored on the time it takes to complete each sample and the quality of work. The scores are compared to other client scores. Work behavior is observed and noted, but this observation is not emphasized. The vocational recommendations, which the system offers based on results, are limited to the jobs directly related to the samples.

MICRO TOWER, which is a newer system sponsored by the ICD Rehabilitation and Research Center and is targeted for the rehabilitation clients of the facility, has 13 samples that take 15 to 20 h to complete. Quality of performance is emphasized, and norms are based on the performance of a variety of groups. The client's behavior is frequently observed and noted. Resultant recommendations are related to the DOT.

McCarron-Dial, devised by L. T. McCarron and J. G. Dial, and VIEWS, from the Philadelphia JEVS, are both systems developed to evaluate the mentally retarded. The former has 17 samples that take 2 weeks to administer. The latter has 16 samples that can be completed in 20 to 35 h. Both are normed against clients, and both require behavioral observations. McCarron-Dial emphasizes quality in scoring and makes vocational recommendations for one of five particular programs. VIEWS emphasizes time and quality equally and makes vocational recommendations based on the DOT.

TAP, developed by Talent Assessment Programs, and WREST, developed by the Guidance Associates of Delaware, Inc., takes $2^1/_2$ and $1^1/_4$ h to administer, respectively. Both systems emphasize time in scoring and do not require behavioral observations. TAP norms against seven different groups and relates results to specific jobs. WREST norms against different age groups and employed workers but does not make specific vocational recommendations. Neither system was developed for a specific target group.

The COATS system was developed by Prep Inc. for Manpower, secondary education, and rehabilitation clients. It has four components: job matching, employability, work samples, and living skills. It is estimated to take 28 to 60 h to complete. Scoring is based on quality and is normed against the scores of students who have taken the sample. Behavioral observations are not emphasized. Specific jobs are recommended based on results.

The Singer system, sponsored by Singer Education Development, has 20 samples. They were not developed for a specific target group, and the results usually indicate a direction for training rather than employment. The samples take 3 weeks to complete and emphasize quality of client work in completing the sample, with extensive behavioral observations by the evaluator. The results are normed against "more than 100 individuals" who have taken the samples.

Valpar, by the Valpar Corporation, was developed for the industrially injured. It has 16 samples, with more in the developmental stages. The 16 samples take 12 to 15 h to complete. Time and quality are equally important factors in scoring, and behavioral observation is important. Results are normed against a variety of groups, including employed workers and mentally retarded clients. The vocational recommendations are general and are based primarily on DOT.

The Hester system, from Goodwill Industries of Chicago, was developed specifically for rehabilitation clients, that is, the physically disabled, the socially maladjusted, and the educable mentally handicapped. Its vocational recommendations are completely related to the DOT. The system has 28 components and also uses psychological and psychophysical tests. The developers state that these tests negate any need for behavioral observations. The samples take approximately 5 h to complete. Scoring is based on time. There is little information supplied by the developers on the norm base.

At the present time, no single system is comprehensive enough to meet the total needs of vocational work evaluation. Because the clientele of most facilities is so varied and the services offered so individual, most major vocational work evaluation facilities find it necessary to use two or more different work-sampling systems in order to derive maximum benefit from the work sample method. Also, because of the unique nature of each case, the evaluator may use only certain samples from different systems and frequently may choose not to give the entire battery of samples in the system. Further development of work samples and research in their utilization are becoming major goals of many work evaluation specialists.

The final process in vocational rehabilitation, that of locating the employment opportunities, is becoming the responsibility of all personnel involved in the other processes discussed above, including the client. In some facilities, however, a job placement specialist may exist. This person is responsible for gathering current occupational information, keeping abreast of the needs of the job market, and feeding this information into the counseling and evaluation process. The specialist maintains and develops the contact with business and industry in a constant effort to be aware of and foster job opportunities for the rehabilitation clients. The specialist serves to educate employers to the special skills, abilities, and needs of the handicapped worker and is frequently involved in facilitating the return of injured employees to their former employers.

The vocational rehabilitation unit, whether made up of specialists in the three basic processes or of generalists who perform counseling, evaluation, and placement, tends to flex and change depending on the client needs and the developing professional and educational theories of the field. New systems and ideas are arising rapidly. The situation is complex, and although it is not the purpose of this chapter to examine this complexity, it is important to realize that there is extensive variety in the field. The nurse, as a resource person to the patient, should be aware of the different types of vocational rehabilitation facilities in the area. With a basic knowledge of what these can offer, the nurse will be better able to advise the patient in the vocational rehabilitation process.

BIBLIOGRAPHY

Botterbusch, K.: *A Comparison of Four Vocational Evaluation Systems,* University of Wisconsin-Stout, Stout Vocational Rehabilitation Institute, Materials Development Center, Menomonie, Wis., 1977.

Neff, W.: *Work and Human Behavior,* Atherton, New York, 1968.

——: "Problems of Work Evaluation," in R. Sankovsky, G. Arthur, and J. Mann (eds.): *Vocational Evaluation and Work Adjustment: A Book of Readings,* Auburn University, Alabama Rehabilitation Media Service, Auburn, 1969, p. 20.

Pruit, W.: *Vocational (Work) Evaluation,* Author, Menomonie, Wis., 1977.

Pruit, W., and R. Pacinelli, (eds.): *Work Evaluation in Rehabilitation,* Association of Rehabilitation Centers, Washington, D.C., 1969.

Sankovsky, R., G. Arthur, and J. Mann (eds.): *Vocational Evaluation and Work Adjustment: A Book of Readings,* Auburn University, Alabama Rehabilitation Media Service, Auburn, 1969.

Sax, Arnold B.: *Vocational Evaluation and Work Adjustment Project,* Materials Development Center, Univ. of Wisconsin, Stout, Wis., 1973, p. 2.

Sink, J., and T. Porter: "Convergence and Divergence in Rehabilitation Counseling and Vocational Evaluation," *J Appl Rehabil Counseling* 9(1):5–20, 1978.

Vocational Evaluation and Work Adjustment Association: "Task Force #7: Vocational Evaluation Project Final Report," *Vocational Evaluation and Work Adjustment Bulletin* 8:91–93, 1975, special edition.

34
betty goldiamond

resocialization

RESOCIALIZATION: AN ESSENTIAL ELEMENT IN COMPREHENSIVE REHABILITATION

Literally, *resocialization* refers to the "refriending" or "reassociating" of the patient, which begins, consciously or not, immediately after a major disease or catastrophic injury interrupts the patient's everyday life and activities. In some contexts, resocialization is seen as an important goal of the total rehabilitation process, one that can serve as an indicator of the quality of life attained by the individual. That is, it is possible to find objective answers to questions such as the following: Is the patient working or attending school? Is the family intact? Does the patient have friends, belong to social groups, participate in recreational activities with others? In addition, patients can be asked to report on the degree of satisfaction they experience in the various areas of life.

In other contexts, resocialization is used to indicate the process through which the patient is integrated into relevant social systems, some of which are totally new, some are carry-overs from pretrauma social life, while others are modifications of preexisting social networks. Here the concern is to answer questions such as these: Has the community environment, both physical and social, been made accessible to the patient? Has the patient been taught how to take advantage of the range of options made available? Does the patient make efforts to reenter normal community life and are these efforts supported? In this chapter, we will consider resocialization both as goal and as process.

The nurse and other health professionals who work with severely ill or injured patients in any medical setting are deeply involved in the process of patient resocialization, whether or not they recognize the significance of their daily interactions with these patients. The student nurse who tries to make conversation with a 50-year-old accident victim by casually inquiring, "What *were* you, Mr. Jones?" is affecting the resocialization process just as surely as is the more sensitive nurse who offers to arrange for a better light so that Mr. Jones can get back to doing some of his work while he is confined to bed. Unfortunately, what Mr. Jones makes of his new life as a paraplegic may be determined as much by the words of the first nurse, who takes it for granted that his career identity has been destroyed, as by the actions of the second, who knows that lives and careers can be rebuilt.

All too often, members of patients' families may have little insight into the possibilities for successful rehabilitation, and thus their initial reaction to a traumatic event may be overwhelming grief or desperate behavior. An extreme example of this occurred in New Jersey, on the night of June 20, 1973. At that time, Lester M. Zygmanik, a 23-year-old construction worker, visited the intensive care unit of the hospital to which his brother George had been admitted 3 days earlier following a motorcycle accident during the celebration of Father's Day on the Zygmanik family farm. As a result of the accident, George was paralyzed from the neck down. Lester carried with him a loaded, 20-gauge, sawed-off shotgun. Withdrawing the gun from beneath his raincoat, he pointed it at George's head from a distance of about 4 ft and fired it. George died 2 days later. According to Lester's own testimony, he had said to his brother, "I am here to end your pain, George. Is it all right with you?" George is said to have nodded his assent.

After the shooting, Lester testified, "I said goodby and pulled the tube out of his neck. I did that because my brother didn't like that tube." Lester was later tried on charges of first- and second-degree murder, and a sympathetic jury found him not guilty on the basis of temporary insanity (Johnson, 1973; Mitchell, 1976).

Whereas most people react to catastrophic events in a far less dramatic manner than did the Zygmanik brothers, the fear of pain and helplessness, the sense of loss of all that one is and does, and the abandonment of hope for a normal life in the future are always there to some degree and must be dealt with during the period of rehabilitation. The basic medical care elements of the rehabilitation system are rapidly being put into place. Technology to preserve life is improving at an exponential rate, but the structures and techniques through which patient resocialization can be successfully accomplished remain relatively weak components in the rehabilitation process. In the past, health professionals have been taught to save lives, not to ask "What kind of life can this person have now?" or "How can the patient achieve a good life?" But these questions must be asked by a caring society, and answers must be found.

THEORETICAL PERSPECTIVES ON PATIENT RESOCIALIZATION

Before proceeding with our consideration of some of the specifics of patient resocialization, it may be useful to examine the concepts underlying this approach. According to DiRenzo, the socialization of its members is commonly thought of as a functional requirement of society in general or of any specified social subsystem (DiRenzo, 1977). From the viewpoint of the system, individuals must be assigned statuses and taught roles that are essential to system function and maintenance. In this approach, socialization is understood as the transmission of necessary knowledge about the culture to the individuals who belong to the society and who assume the roles established within the social system. It is the process through which people learn the rules of the game. Full resocialization of members of the group who become handicapped may be viewed as one of the courses of action that a society can employ when its stability is threatened by the presence of large numbers of persons who are unable to carry out their usual social roles in the prescribed manner. Clearly, alternative courses of action can be followed, and have been, in many instances.

From the viewpoint of the individual, the socialization task is one of learning to assume the social roles and behave in the ways that society either requires or permits. Gewirtz (1969) has attempted to cast the phenomena dealt with by social learning approaches into a consistent, operational, and parsimonious framework. Rather than emphasizing global concepts like social environments or individual traits, which summarize stimuli or responses through lengthy time spans, his approach calls for an in-depth analysis of stimuli, responses, their interchange at a particular moment, and the sequences of such interactions across successive moments. Gewirtz believes that it is reasonable to conceive of social behavior as following the general laws of behavior, but with the relevant stimuli mediated by the behavior of persons rather than by other environmental sources. Thus, his approach to the study of social learning proceeds in the same way as does the study of other behavioral categories, that is, by detailed analysis of the variables provided by the social environment, both in the present and in the past, that control behavior change. Such an approach provides a flexible model for ordering the complex developmental patterns characterizing early socialization, socialization in later years of life, or resocialization under conditions such as those experienced by victims of accident or disease.

Although students of social learning originally tended to emphasize socialization during the first few years of life, there has been a trend in recent years to extend the study of socialization practices and their consequences for personal development to encompass the entire life cycle (Neugarten, 1968). It is no longer taken for granted that the personality is formed immutably during early childhood. Instead, it is suggested that persons are continually resocialized, with consequent personality change, as they leave earlier social statuses and are inducted into new roles, for example, as they move from bachelorhood to marriage and parenthood, or from marriage to widowhood, or from career involvement to retirement.

Similar changes can be assumed to occur when persons who have previously been healthy experience the unaccustomed physical limitations created by severe, long-lasting disease or injury. The transition from being healthy to being a patient involves numerous changes, including the loss of some previous valued social roles, the entrance into an unfamiliar and, to some, frightening new medical environment that makes unaccustomed demands on the patient, sometimes the loss of capacity to respond voluntarily to either the old or the new environmental agents, and frequently, deprivation of the reinforcers that had functioned to maintain behaviors in the past.

Although the process of patient resocialization may be especially difficult in some cases for reasons that will be discussed in greater detail later, it nevertheless bears analogies to resocialization processes in other situations. For example, the problems of adjustment faced by a newly handicapped person are similar in some ways to those that confront the freshman on a university campus, the immigrant from a country with very different customs, or the young woman entering the army. A new way of life must be learned, and learned as rapidly and gracefully as possible if the novice is to survive and participate in the new society. The individual's old behavioral repertoire is likely to be inappropriate or insufficient, and the new social group may reserve its low status roles for its most recent recruits. However, in spite of the commonalities in resocialization process and problems, there are some significant differences, especially in that the assumption of student, immigrant, or military roles usually has voluntary elements and occurs subsequent to some planning and preparation on the part of the novice. By contrast, it is only the rare rehabilitation patient who has ever imagined being the victim of a catastrophic disease or accident and living for perhaps 30 years thereafter with a handicap. Induction into the role of patient is likely to be unexpected, involuntary, and sudden, and the relevant social environment may be similarly unprepared to undertake the adjustments necessary to the everyday functioning of the chronic patient.

In spite of the recognition that patient resocialization differs in certain important ways from other instances, the kind of analysis that is otherwise employed in the study of resocialization may be helpful to the rehabilitation nurse who is trying to develop plans for individual patients. That is, at a minimum, the following questions should be considered:

1. What kinds of social roles is the society prepared to offer this patient as options?
2. What social knowledge or material elements of the culture can be employed to assist the patient in the effort to achieve a satisfactory way of life?
3. What outcomes does the patient want, and what is the patient capable of learning and doing?
4. What methods of teaching can be used to facilitate progress toward those outcomes?
5. Which other persons who have a relationship to the patient can be taught how to help?
6. What are the consequences that can be employed to maintain the patient support system? That is, what will the social system get out of resocializing the patient?
7. What consequences will reinforce patient behavior and maintain it as time passes? What will the patient get out of making the required efforts?

Although it is not to be expected that the nurse can find detailed answers to all these questions for each patient, the list may provide rough guidelines for orienting interventions. The basic assumption is that the patient is not merely a patient but a person who can be a contributing and, we hope, a happy member of society, given the right help at the right time.

MEASURING THE NEED FOR RESOCIALIZATION

Number of Disabled Persons

When the Congress of the United States authorized President Carter to call the White House Conference on Handicapped Individuals of 1977, it found that there was a need for such a public policy forum because "there are seven million children and at least twenty-eight million adults with mental or physical handicaps." Other estimates of the size of the handicapped population vary somewhat, since surveys have used different definitions of disability and diverse methods of data collection. At the present time, there are no generally accepted exact data on incidence and prevalence of the various impairments.

In 1975, the Urban Institute conducted a comprehensive needs study of the *most* severely handicapped for the Secretary of the Department of Health, Education, and Welfare, who was directed to make such a survey under the provisions of the Rehabilitation Act of 1973 (PL 93-112) (Urban Institute, 1975a). The institute estimated that in 1975 there were more than 10 million persons who should be classified as most severely handicapped. Approximately four-fifths of these were not living in institutions. They found that the severely disabled noninstitutional population contains disproportionate numbers of older persons, women, nonwhites, the less well educated, and Southerners and that the severely disabled are more likely to have multiple impairments than are the less severely disabled. The most frequent disabilities are musculoskeletal and cardiovascular impairments, followed by mental and nervous system disorders.

Further, the Urban Institute estimated that by 1984, the total number of severely disabled and moderately disabled individuals will increase to 38,648,000, of whom almost 13 million will be severely disabled (Urban Institute, 1975b).

In their effort to organize the sometimes contradictory information about the prevalence of certain chronic conditions in the United States, the Urban Institute concluded that the most common conditions are respiratory (46.9 million persons), circulatory (36.5), skin (25.2), and musculoskeletal (25.4). About 17 million persons have digestive disorders, 14.5 million have hearing disorders, and 9.6 million have visual defects. At least 4 million have convulsive disorders, including epilepsy, 1 million have cancer; and one-half million have multiple sclerosis. There are more than 6 million retarded persons. The Urban Institute survey found that about 1.9 million persons are receiving institutional care, and of these, more than 93 percent are severely handicapped. There has been a decrease in the number of persons in mental hospitals, institutions for the retarded, and chronic disease hospitals, since many community-based and outpatient facilities have been developed during the past decade. However, the number of persons in nursing homes has increased. The nursing home population is drawn primarily from the aged group and consists largely of the severely disabled.

Are All Health Problems Handicaps?

Althogh the extent of health problems as sketched out in the foregoing paragraph is alarming, it is wise to bear in mind that individuals with impairments are not necessarily severely handicapped in their daily lives, nor are they candidates for resocialization efforts. The National Rehabilitation Association sponsored a seminar in 1975 with the avowed purpose of discussing and possibly achieving a consensus with regard to the definitions of "pathology," "impairment," "functional limitation," and "disability." The participants emphasized that it is important for rehabilitation research and practice to distinguish between an "impairment," that is, a physiological, anatomical, or mental loss, other abnormality, or both, and a "disability," which they define as a form of inability or limitation in performing roles and tasks expected of an individual within a social environment (Whitten, 1975). The distinction is clarified by reference, for example, to the individual with a severe visual *impairment* whose eyesight can be corrected by properly fitted eyeglasses or contact lenses in such a manner that no *disability* in carrying on a normal life is suffered. Similarly, compensation for many other impairments is a relatively simple matter.

The Urban Institute engaged in a similar effort to clarify the terminology identifying categories of persons with health problems. They arrived at a three-term rubric as follows: (1) an *impairment* is the residual limitation resulting from a congenital defect, disease, or injury; (2) a person with an impairment may or may not have a *disability,* that is, an inability to perform some important life activities; and (3) a *handicap* exists when the disability interacts with the environment to impede the individual's accomplishment of goals for work, education, or other major life activities. Significantly, they note that "there are severely handicapping environments as well as impairments" (Urban Institute, 1975a).

With the recognition of this conceptual distinction, it is obvious that we have no single, reliable estimate of need for patient resocialization. Although it is possible to count the number of persons with impairments and/or chronic diseases, it is not a simple matter to determine whether the interaction between impairment and environment has resulted in a handicap requiring societal intervention. When handicap does exist, a two-pronged resocialization process may be the answer. That is, environmental accommodation may be as critical to resocialization as is new learning and adaptation on the patient's part. The Seeing Eye dog and braille maps and markers for the blind student on a large urban campus will not be sufficient solutions to the student's problems, but they may well be necessary.

A LOOK AT HARD PROBLEMS

When it becomes obvious that a patient's personal life is in crisis and that something must be done to reduce the social discontinuities that are producing suffering, attention must be paid to patient, to environment, and to the interactions between these. Every effort must be made to identify the strengths and weaknesses on both sides and to review and evaluate the options that can be made available. This section describes some of the problems that may complicate or limit possible actions. It is important that they be recognized, because interventions can only proceed on the basis of what actually exists in the patient's own social world; there is no magic—and very few miracles.

PATIENT PROBLEMS IN RESOCIALIZATION

Necessity for Unlearning

On arrival for rehabilitation, the patient does not appear as a *tabula rasa,* a clean slate. Patients arrive with ideas about themselves and their particular environments and with ways of doing things that they have learned in their premorbid lives. Unfortunately, some of these ideas and behaviors may be inappropriate under the changed circumstances of the patients' lives and may interfere with the learning of new behaviors. Such interference, sometimes called proactive inhibition, has been a major topic of research on learning (Hilgard and Bower, 1975). Patients may have to unlearn much that has previously been "second nature" to them, and that task may be far more difficult than the original learning. For instance, hemiplegics, amputees, or paraplegics capable of ambulating with braces and crutches each have a personal way of walking. In trying to master a new procedure for getting from one place to the other, they must, in the beginning at least, deal with the interference created by deeply ingrained habits.

In roughly the same manner, the patients' former ways of fulfilling various social roles may be inappropriate and may interfere with adaptation to the impairment. Much of the past experience gained in being an executive, a spouse, a parent, a student, or whatever may have to be unlearned before the patient can successfully redefine the social roles to be undertaken and learn behaviors appropriate to the new conditions. Heart patients who have been accustomed to giving orders may have to learn first to hold their tongues and then to delegate responsibilities; burn victims who have relied mainly on physical appearance in relating to others may have to learn the hard way that their good looks will no longer work but that other things will.

Disturbances of Sensation and Response

When psychologists speak of learning, they are referring to the "change in a subject's behavior to a given situation brought about by his repeated experiences in that situation, provided that the behavior change cannot be explained on the basis of native response tendencies, maturation, or temporary states of the subject (e.g., fatigue, drugs, etc.)" (Hilgard & Bower, 1975). Although there are various theories of learning, the two major paradigms currently in use that will concern us here are respondent, or classical, conditioning and operant conditioning.

Classical conditioning follows the familiar S → R model (stimulus elicits response). To establish conditioning, a conditioned stimulus is presented to an experimental subject just slightly before the presentation of an unconditioned stimulus during a series of discrete learning trials. In time, the subject "learns" to make the same response to the conditioned stimulus that had been previously elicited only by the unconditioned stimulus. Early Pavlovian experiments involved conditioning dogs to salivate to an arbitrary stimulus such as a light or a bell. To accomplish this, the ringing of a bell is paired with, say, the placing of meat powder in the mouth of a hungry animal. The drops of saliva elicited are measured carefully. Originally, the dog salivates only when it tastes the food (the unconditioned stimulus), but after a series of conditioning trials, the saliva begins to flow as soon as the bell (the conditioned stimulus) sounds. The dog has been conditioned, or has learned, to respond to a stimulus to which it had not responded earlier. Using this procedure, behavior change is observable and reliable.

Operant conditioning, most frequently associated with the contributions of B. F. Skinner (1953), follows an R → S model (response leads to reinforcing stimulus). The experimental subject (Skinner frequently used the pigeon) emits a preselected response, perhaps a peck at a disk, and thereafter the reinforcing stimulus or reinforcer (grain) is made available to the subject. The subject's response is called an operant, because it operates on the environment. Presentation of the reinforcer is contingent upon occurrence of the response; if the response does not occur, the reinforcer is not made available. With continued repetiion of the R → S sequence, the rate of occurrence of the operant increases, and the behavior can be easily maintained or altered at will by manipulating the schedule of reinforcement. Sometimes a three-term contingency is established, that is, the model S^D → R → S^R is employed. In this procedure, the S^D (discriminative stimulus) sets the occasion on which the response will be reinforced; in the absence of the discriminative stimulus, the response is not reinforced. For example, a monkey can "learn" very quickly that when a red light is on, a bar press will produce a food pellet but that when a green light is on, the same bar press will not be followed by reinforcement. The contrast in response pattern on the animal's cumulative record reveals clearly that the animal discriminates between the colors red and green. With the red light, the monkey works at a steady rate, but with the green, it rests from its bar-pressing activity.

Both respondent and operant conditioning are demonstrated daily in laboratory experiments with both animal and human subjects, and they are easily observed in everyday life. In a rehabilitation setting, many examples of these types of conditioning can be seen. When a physical therapy room is decorated in a bright and pleasant manner, it is hoped that the cheerful responses the room elicits will be conditioned to the exercise equipment itself through the process of respondent conditioning. On the other hand, operant conditioning may be used in teaching upper extremity amputees to manipulate their prosthetic devices to move food from plate to mouth, for example. Praise may be given as each part of the complex sequence of behaviors is mastered, and the proper placement of food in the mouth at last acts as the primary reinforcer. Sometimes, the training is explicitly planned as part of the patient's rehabilitation program, and sometimes new ways of responding are simply learned by the patient during repeated attempts to solve recurring problems of daily living.

Reflection upon the foregoing discussion of

the two major types of learning makes it apparent that any disturbance either of perception of environmental stimuli, such as occurs with deafness, blindness, or paralysis, or of responding to such stimulus input, as is the case with amputations and diseases that restrict muscular movements, will function as a limitation on the retraining that can occur. With sensory impairments, the effort is frequently made to compensate for the input deficit by using another sensory modality. For example, the blind person is taught how to respond to what is heard or can be felt with parts of the body. Pareplegics, who cannot feel their legs being sunburned, are taught to examine the skin for changes in color. Similar compensations may have to be made when the sensory deficit affects the reinforcement characteristics of stimuli. If food tastes "bad" to a patient, other reinforcers that will maintain desired patient behavior, such as socializing with others, must be used. If patients refuse to go to the cafeteria to eat, for instance, perhaps they can be persuaded to go there in order to listen to music.

When patients are able to perceive stimuli but cannot respond to them in the accustomed manner, efforts must be made to facilitate responses that use whatever systems remain intact. If the patients cannot speak, perhaps they can write or use gestures. If they cannot walk, they may nevertheless be able to crawl or scoot across the floor. With encouragement, patients will either discover substitute ways of getting things done or will adopt suggestions made by those who have greater experience with the particular response handicap. Regardless of whether the patients' deficits are sensory, responsive, or both, the trained professional should be familiar with the many assistive devices that can also be used to supplement intact human resources and facilitate relearning.

Emotional Problems

The resocialization of seriously ill or injured persons can be hindered by problems that are not caused by the physical changes but are instead produced by emotional reactions to the disease or injury. In discussing a research project on patients' reactions to the news that they have cancer, Abrams (1974) noted that the initial response of 56 out of 60 patients was anger and rage, directed either at themselves or at others. Gunther (1969), in attempting to organize his impressions of emotional reactions to spinal cord injury, has suggested that the patient may go through several stages as time passes after an accident. First, the reaction may be one of shock, with the patient appearing numb, confused, and remote. After that, there may be a stage of partial recognition and recovery, followed by a superficial reconciliation to the situation. As time passes and as society makes greater demands on the recovering patient, a regression may occur; that is, the patient may display anxiety and distress through expressions of self-pity and egocentric demands. After this kind of regression, the patient may take any one of several pathways. There may be a continuing denial of personal responsibility, leading to paranoia; there may be depression, with thoughts of suicide or somatization of complaints; or, in the usual case, there is a gradual social recovery, with a shifting of psychic energy to the establishment of normal relations and interactions with the outside world (Gunther, 1969).

On the other hand, it is not unheard of for a person who has survived a serious accident, myocardial infarction, or extensive surgery to experience elation, that is, a sense of joy at the "miracle" of survival. Individual differences in response to trauma are very great, and the same patient may display a wide range of emotional reactions on different days, or to different people, or in different situations. While the nurse must be aware of the possibility that depression and other types of emotional distress can produce a lack of patient cooperation in rehabilitation programs, the continued existence of such problems should not be taken for granted. In many instances, the emotional state is reversible. Careful attention to the individual's comfort, a joke shared at the right moment, or a friendly gesture signaling recognition of some small achievement may do as much to set the patient back on the road to recovery as any medicine.

ENVIRONMENTAL AGENT PROBLEMS IN PATIENT RESOCIALIZATION

Lack of Awareness and Information

Persons who constitute the social environment of a patient may act in inappropriate ways simply because they are unaware of, ignorant about, or insensitive to the patient's changed capabilities. Some problems, such as a bad heart, diabetes, high blood pressure, and epilepsy, are invisible or have minimal overt effects. In these, as in other cases where the impairment is more readily apparent, environmental agents may lack information about what the patient is capable of doing, what the limitations are, or what assistance is needed. Without guidance, they may hesitate to undertake a relationship with the disabled person. If patients can be encouraged to initiate social interactions and to take responsibility for explaining their condition and what they need to significant persons in their environments, the chances are excellent that they will be met at least halfway.

Albrecht (1976a) has recently reported on a study of helping behavior offered to the physically disabled in public places and of situational variables that affected the helping relationship. Although several previous studies had found that members of the able-bodied public were likely to react to a person with visible disability in an uncomfortable and inhibited manner, if at all, Albrecht's findings lend support to a more optimistic view. Over a period of several months, he conducted a series of 102 trials of the following experiment. The "stimulus subject," a wheelchair-bound 25-year-old white male, wheeled down a city sidewalk until he reached a curb bordering an alley, where by prearragement in accordance with the experimental design matrix, he stopped his chair where the curb was either high, medium, or low. Then he either looked down at the curb (the not-agitated condition) or moved his wheelchair back and forth as one would in an effort to negotiate the curb (the agitated condition). The subject stayed in that position until he was helped across the alley.

Videotape operators concealed across the street recorded each trial. At the conclusion of each trial, interviewers who had been out of sight earlier approached passersby, whether they helped the subject or not, and interviewed them, if they were willing, with regard to their attitudes toward the handicapped.

This carefully controlled research produced several results that were at variance with earlier findings about helping behavior. A question of primary interest was the length of time it would take for the disabled person to receive help; the astounding fact was that the mean time for receiving help was only 33.3 s and that the longest time that the subject waited for help was just over 4 min. Situational variables were the best predictors of total length of time until help was forthcoming. That is, when crowd density was great, help occurred more quickly than when there were few passersby. The subject received help more rapidly when he was in the agitated condition (ie., when his actions showed he needed help) than when he was motionless on the sidewalk. And when the subject had taken his position at the high curb, where he had the greatest disadvantage, he was helped more quickly than when he was at medium or low positions. Attitudinal variables were not predictive of the behavior of passersby, since there were no statistically significant differences in attitude between helpers and nonhelpers. For both groups, attitudinal scale scores were quite positive, but they revealed a lack of specific knowledge about the disabled and their needs. In the discussion of his findings, Albrecht recommended, among other things, that the disabled should be encouraged to go out in public places and that they should be taught to control how other people react to them. He concluded that the positive public attitudes toward the physically disabled are there already but that what is lacking is information about when and how to give assistance. This can often be supplied by the handicapped person, who can be taught how to function in public by rehabilitation professionals.

The disabled persons who know their own needs can, and should, resolve the ambiguities inherent in many encounters. Although Albrecht's research dealt only with interactions involving strangers, there is no obvious reason that his recommendations should be limited in that manner. Family members and friends also find many situations involving the disabled individual to be ambiguous, and they, too, need guidance about how to help.

Overgeneralization, Spread, and Labeling

The development of satisfactory relationships between handicapped and able-bodied individuals may be impeded by certain psychological and societal processes that have been most thoroughly studied with regard to interactions between members of different races or other groups of unequal status or between social deviants of any type and the "normal" members of society.

Overgeneralization occurs when inferences are made about a total population based on observation of a nonrandom sample. The tendency to classify persons about whom one has limited information according to certain distinguishing criteria, such as sex, race, age, or handicap, and then to ignore or fail to discriminate individual differences in other characteristics is very strong indeed. It can interfere with the resocialization of the disabled. The middle-aged couple who is having trouble with an infirm, aged parent may begin to assume that all old people are "like that," or the nurse who has a run of bad luck with several difficult stroke patients may infer that stroke victims inevitably have quarrelsome dispositions. The fact is that the main thing all old people have in common is their chronological age and that the only certain shared characteristic of stroke patients is the stroke. When similar behaviors are observed in members of such classes, it may be that commonalities in the current environment are interacting with the old persons' or the stroke patients' changed physical condition to produce those behaviors. Once environmental agents recognize that the individual characteristics that made one person different from another before adversity occurred still exist, they can program environmental options that will encourage the disabled to exhibit a much wider range of behaviors.

Overgeneralization is essentially an error in logic, one in which we "go beyond the data." Social psychologists have called attention to some related psychological processes. In her emphasis on *spread,* Wright (1977) has been concerned with the emotional valence that may color our perceptions of a person once we have had a positive or negative reaction to some characteristic of that person (such as lameness or physical beauty) which, for us, is dominant. The term "halo phenomenon" refers to the positive aspects of this process. If one is favorably impressed by another's beauty, it is easy to believe that the person has other positive attributes, such as good character and intelligence. By the same token, if one is disturbed or repelled by the appearance of a person with cerebral palsy, one may ascribe to the person other negative attributes, such as emotional instability or intellectual limitations. The health professional must learn to be on guard against the spread of negative affect, which can interfere with accurate observation and evaluation of patient potentialities. Sometimes, the most annoying, most demanding, and angriest patient can be the one who otherwise has exactly what it takes to achieve an excellent recovery.

Societal reaction theorists have been concerned with the personal and societal consequences of the formal *labeling* of patients by the health institutions responsible for treatment and rehabilitation (Becker, 1963; Goffman, 1961). They argue, for example, that the primary determinant of the resocialization process for a former mental patient is not the occurrence of the mental deviancy itself but is, instead, the labeling process. This includes the routing of the individual through treatment deemed appropriate for one who has been thus labeled, which produces changes in the patient's self-image and later behavior. Former patients are likely to be "stigmatized"; that is, in dealing with patients, environmental agents both inside and outside the institution may overgeneralize and express the spread of negative affect that they experience. Patients' social role options may be restricted to those considered appropriate to their disability, without regard to the strengths they also possess. Thus, they may be resocialized, perhaps irreversibly, to assume a devalued status in the larger society.

On the other hand, health professionals view the labeling of the patient somewhat differently. They are likely to see such labeling simply as the patient's ticket to treatment. In a society with finite resources that perforce establishes treatment and rehabilitation priorities and then develops a network of specialized facilities, the labeling of the patient as "orthopedically handicapped," "schizophrenic," or whatever expedites access to the health care system at the proper point. Nevertheless, the criticisms of societal reaction theorists deserve attention. It seems clear that health personnel must be continually vigilant in order to guarantee that efficiency not become the excuse for institutional depersonalization of patients, that treatment be individualized and continuity of care assured, and that the patients be, to the fullest extent possible, active participants in making decisions about their own treatment programs. Whatever can be done to reduce stigma and to open opportunities for patients must be done.

Competing Behavior

In addition to being hampered by a lack of knowledge or emotionality, environmental agents may find it difficult to assist in patient resocialization because the agent and the patient are, as a matter of course, engaged in competing behaviors. Helping a wheelchair-bound person across a street takes very little time or effort, but care-giving during a lengthy recovery period requires that the primary helpers find ways to eliminate many behaviors that interfere with patient care, often including some role of critical importance, like work. To free themselves to function in a supportive manner, they may have to reorder personal priorities and rethink the customary ways of carrying out their own necessary activities. The rehabilitation nurse and other health personnel may be able to offer many practical suggestions that will make adjustments easier for the primary care-giver as well as for the patient. However, since the pressures of other social roles and responsibilities can be devastating in spite of the best efforts to organize the use of time and energy, the care-giver may need to build a backup resource network that can be drawn upon as needed.

DESIRED OUTCOMES OF REHABILITATION

Most individuals who survive the occurrence of severe disease or trauma but are left with lifelong limitations and health management problems accomplish some type of resocialization. There are exceptions, however. For example, gerontologists have long been aware that there is an uncomfortably large and probably growing number of social isolates among our aged population. These people, frequently the victims of debilitating progressive disease, have often survived their spouses, have been forced to retire from work, and have lost track of children and other relatives who may live far away. As they become more disabled, they give up friendships and drop out of social activities, and they may be housebound except for trips to the mailbox, clinic, and grocery store. If they are not identified and helped by social agencies, they may demonstrate almost complete *disengagement* rather than any level of resocialization (Cumming and Henry, 1961).

Perhaps no other category of the disabled falls so completely beyond the boundaries of our rehabilitation systems as do the socially isolated, frail, elderly. However, many other persons with disabilities assume a "sick" or "dependent" role while, at the same time, they disengage from most social systems. The Rehabilitation Institute of Chicago conducted a follow-up study of the 512 accident-disabled persons who had been patients during the years 1958–1969. Of these, 463 were located, 47 of whom (10 percent) had died. Of the remaining 416, 400 participated in the follow-up study. Seventy-five percent of the sample were male, and the majority were less than 55 years old. Just under half were either paraplegic or quadriplegic, while others were burn victims, amputees, or other patients. The survey showed that nearly all had returned to their predisability living arrangements, with only 6 percent living in nursing homes; that 77 percent performed self-care activities independently, while an additional 18 percent did so with assistance; and that 35 percent were employed, 22 percent were students, and the rest were unemployed. However, the former patients were found to be making minimal use of social and recreational services in their communities, with only 4 percent reporting participation in church groups, 5 percent ever using the public library, and 3 percent using city park facilities (DiAngelo et al., 1974).

How should such outcomes be evaluated? Lacking any measures of the patients' subjective evaluation of their own progress in resocialization, we may ask the question, "How do these outcomes compare with what would have happened to the same persons in the absence of rehabilitation training?" It seems a safe guess that without rehabilitation, many more would have died or ended up in nursing homes, many more would be completely or partially dependent in activities of daily living, and many more would be numbered among the unemployed. Any way one looks at it, however, the former patients made a disappointing showing on the indicators of resocialization into the larger community.

If, instead of the above question, we ask, "How do these outcomes compare with the outcomes of rehabilitation and resocialization training we would desire for ourselves?," we are bound to conclude that, even given the severity of the disabilities, there is much room for improvement.

GOALS ESTABLISHED IN PUBLIC POLICY

For all but the very wealthy or the exceptionally well insured, our framework of public health and social welfare policies is the primary determinant of the limits within which decisions about rehabilitation goals for individual patients must be made. Clearly, the outcomes that are possible differ with different diseases and traumas, at different stages of the life cycle, and under different socioeconomic conditions. Having recognized that all things are not possible for everyone, let us examine the ideal as expressed in a recent United Nations document (United Nations, 1977).

At its thirtieth session in 1975, the General Assembly adopted a Declaration on the Rights of Disabled Persons [General Assembly Resolution 2445 (XXX)]. The declaration proclaims that "these rights shall be granted to all disabled persons without any exception whatsoever and without distinction and discrimination." It further states, among other things, that "disabled persons have the inherent right to respect for their human dignity"; that they "have the same civil and political rights as other human beings"; that they "have the right to economic and social security and to a decent level of living . . . , to secure and retain employment or to engage in a useful, productive and remunerative occupation and to join trade unions." It adds that "no disabled person shall be subjected, as far as his or her residence is concerned, to differential treatment other than that required by his or her condition or by the improvement which he or she may derive therefrom" and that "disabled persons shall be protected against all exploitation, all regulations and all treatment of a discriminatory, abusive or degrading nature."

Similar principles have been enunciated in laws passed during this decade by the Congress of the United States. The first White House Conference on Handicapped Individuals was authorized by PL 93-516. Title III of that act declared, "It is of critical importance to this Nation that equality of opportunity, equal access to all aspects of society and equal rights guaranteed by the Constitution of the United States be provided to all individuals with handicaps." The White House Conference, which took place in May 1977, brought together both handicapped individuals and providers of rehabilitation services in a mission that had three goals: to provide a national assessment of problems and potentials of individuals with mental or physical handicaps, to generate a national awareness of these problems and potentials, and to make recommendations to the President and to Congress that, if implemented, will enable individuals with handicaps to live their lives independently, with dignity, and with full participation in community life to the greatest degree possible (White House Conference, 1976).

While there is not as yet an equal rights amendment for the handicapped, and although the handicapped have not been included as a category in the Federal Civil Rights Act of 1964, progress is being made in that direction. The Rehabilitation Act of 1973 (PL 93-112) is the federal law that comes closest to the nature of a civil rights statute for the handicapped. Sections 501–504 of Title V of that act forbid discrimination against handicapped persons in any federally funded institution or program. Section 501 requires affirmative action in federal agencies; Section 502 authorizes the Architectural and Transportation Barriers Compliance Board to ensure that buildings are made accessible to the handicapped; Section 503 requires all contractors and subcontractors with federal contracts of $2500 or more to take affirmative action to employ and promote qualified handicapped individuals (approximately half of all businesses in the United States are covered under this section); and Section 504 forbids discrimination against the handicapped in all public and private agencies that receive funds from the federal government.

The Department of Health, Education, and Welfare was given responsibility for coordinating the Section 504 enforcement effort, and regulations were issued in June 1977. The Rehabilitation Act of 1973 was the first to mandate that both the Department of Health, Education, and Welfare and the state vocation rehabilitation agencies provide services on a top-priority basis to those with severe handicaps. It also requires vocational rehabilitation agencies in the states to develop individualized written rehabilitation programs for each client, working in conjunction with the client, and to make periodic reviews of each program.

Important federal laws that move our society in the direction of significant environmental modification for the benefit of disabled persons are the Education of All Handicapped Children Act of 1975 (PL 94-142), which provides financial assistance to the states in return for assurances that the state maintain a policy mandating the right to free, appropriate public education for all handicapped children and requiring the development of individualized educational programs; the Architectural Barriers Act of 1968 (PL 90-480), which states that all federal buildings, as well as any buildings constructed or leased in whole or in part with federal funds, must be made accessible to and usable by the physically handicapped; the Federal Aid Highway Act of 1973 (PL 93-87), which forbids the Secretary of Transportation to approve any state highway program that does not provide for adequate and reasonable access for the safe and easy movement of the physically handicapped across curbs; and the Urban Mass Transportation Act (PL 91-453), which states that elderly and handicapped persons have the same right as other persons to utilize available mass transportation facilities and services.

Many states and local communities have followed suit, requiring nondiscriminatory treatment of the handicapped in specified institutions within their jurisdictions. State and federal courts have been moving in the direction of clarifying the right of the mentally ill, the mentally retarded, and physically handicapped persons who are institutionalized to be treated in a minimally restrictive environment.

DISCRIMINATORY LAWS

The hard struggle for equal rights that has been carried on by articulate handicapped individuals and their advocates for many decades has finally begun to have its effects. A social revolution is under way. However, we are still a long way from establishing equal rights for the handicapped as a universal principle. For example, about half the states have involuntary sterilization statutes, and several of those laws include persons with epilepsy, as well as the mentally ill and the mentally retarded. Many states have prohibitions on marriages between handicapped persons, and most states forbid marriage where one of the persons is mentally ill or retarded. Some also limit the right of physically handicapped people to marry, and at least 17 states have prohibited marriage by epileptics. Several states restrict or deny the right of mentally handicapped persons to make contracts. The right to vote is denied citizens with mental handicaps in some states, and in most, orthopedically handicapped and blind persons find it difficult to use the booths or machines and almost equally difficult to secure absentee ballots. Very little state legislation has been enacted specifically for the purpose of aiding the handicapped who need and want either automobile or health insurance; this is an area in which disabled individuals are very much disadvantaged.

Rigdon (1976) has called attention to a group of bizarre provisions discriminating against the physically handicapped, which he calls "ugly laws." Until recently, the Chicago Municipal Code provided that

> no person who is diseased, maimed, mutilated or in any way deformed so as to be an unsightly or disgusting object or improper person to be allowed in or on the public ways or other public places in this city, shall therein or thereon expose himself to public view, under a penalty of not less than one dollar nor more than fifty dollars for each offense.

Rigdon notes that Columbus, Ohio; Omaha, Nebraska; and other cities still have similar ordinances in effect.

UNSETTLED QUESTIONS RELATING TO DESIRED OUTCOMES

Legitimacy of Self-care as Opposed to Solely Vocational Goals

Throughout our history, beginning with the 1798 act of Congress that established a marine hospital fund to care for disabled seamen, there has been conflict between humanitarian and utilitarian positions with regard to the desired outcomes and purposes of publicly supported rehabilitation efforts. Up to and including the present, utilitarian arguments have prevailed; we rarely rehabilitate because need exists and it is "right" to help. Some laws benefiting the handicapped have been passed primarily because cost benefit analysis demonstrates that it costs society more to support the dependent disabled entirely than to rehabilitate them, particularly if they can be returned to gainful employment or trained in the activities of daily living so that primary care givers can be released to join the labor force. One important consequence of the emphasis on rehabilitation-for-work is that access to the comprehensive services provided through vocational rehabilitation agencies has been limited to those judged to have employment potential, and the sifting and sorting decisions may be influenced by variables that have nothing to do with the applicant's impairment or the extent of need. For example, Safilios-Rothschild (1970) has claimed that the disabled poor, blacks, and women have often been barred from vocational rehabilitation programs as "bad rehabilitation risks." Recently, in describing the findings of a just-completed study conducted by the U.S. Commission on Civil Rights on discrimination against the elderly in federal programs, the chairman of that Commission, Dr. Arthur S. Flemming, charged that older Americans are almost completely neglected by vocational rehabilitation agencies (U.S. Bias, 1978). They, too, are assumed not to warrant the investment, even though it is estimated that about 20 percent of the disabled who are over 55 would prefer to continue working.

Many rehabilitation professionals continue to maintain, as they have argued in past years, that they can provide services that will be of great value to disabled persons who may never make the grade in competitive employment, as well as to those others, like housewives and retired persons, who do not wish to be trained for gainful work.

In an awareness paper prepared for the White House Conference, Fay (1976) estimates that there are millions of severely disabled persons among the 2 million who are housebound, the 4 million in nursing homes, and the 2 million in institutions who could benefit from rehabilitation services that would enable them to meet, without assistance, the normal demands of daily living. Their needs may eventually be met to some extent through the implementation of 1978 amendments to the Rehabilitation Act of 1973 which authorized federal support for "independent living" rehabilitation.

Normalization or Segregated Special Care?

In past years, we took pride in building special facilities for the care and training of the blind, deaf, and orthopedically handicapped, as well as institutions where the mentally retarded and mentally ill could live, separate from the rest of society. More recently, the principle of *normalization* has been put forth by behavioral scientists and rehabilitation professionals. According to this principle, disabled persons should be treated the same as the nondisabled, except with regard to specific needs arising from their deficit or disability (Strubbins, 1977). Thus the desired outcome of rehabilitation efforts would be the integration of the handicapped into normal society to the fullest extent possible. The principle has become familiar to us, especially as it is exemplified in the mainstreaming of physically disabled and retarded youngsters in the regular school system and in the deinstitutionalization of mentally disabled persons. The sheltered workshop is another example of efforts to normalize life activity, as is the new emphasis on placing the handicapped in the least restrictive environment.

Although the principle seems straightforward enough, applications have produced many difficulties and honest differences of opinion. For example, there is controversy over subsidized special housing for group living for the severely disabled. Some maintain that it is in compliance with normalization because it provides the means for near-normal living otherwise denied to the severely disabled. Others say that it violates the principle of normalization because of the segregation involved and the subsidization not available to other disadvantaged persons.

In instances where the disabled have had special prerogatives as a result of their disability, such as a pension, an educational grant, preference in employment, or a tax break, the principle of normalization may require foregoing those privileges based on diagnostic labeling. Thus, some advocates of the disabled have come to regard the movement toward normalization as a mixed blessing. Differences of opinion are especially keen with regard to the mainstreaming of handicapped children in the public schools. The advantages to which the handicapped had become accustomed in special education classes, including small class size, specially trained teachers, counseling services, specially constructed buildings, and free transportation to school, are not likely to be so efficiently provided when the students are integrated in the regular school system. However, the social cost of special education was segregation throughout the grade school and high school years. By the time handicapped young people were ready for college, they were usually tremendously disadvantaged socially, and in fact, many found it impossible to make a successful transition to a competitive environment. Although it is hoped that normalization in early education will facilitate the integration of the youthful handicapped into adult society, nevertheless, it must be admitted that there is a price to be paid for the experiments in mainstreaming, and the results are not yet in.

Another experiment in normalization, the deinstitutionalization of the mentally disabled, has been subjected to sharp criticism, mainly as a result of haphazard program implementation. Before the 1960s, mentally disabled persons who could not afford private care had to rely primarily on large, public institutions. Such institutions became overcrowded, treatment programs were limited, few educational or recreational activities were available, and individual privacy was lacking. In short, the mentally disabled were, for the most part, simply warehoused and provided with custodial care.

Beginning in 1963, the federal government embarked on an approach to improve the care and treatment of the mentally retarded and the mentally ill that has been termed *deinstitutionalization.* The program is based on the principle that mentally disabled persons are entitled to live in the least restrictive environment necessary and lead as normal and independent a life as possible. There are three major objectives: to prevent unnecessary admission to and retention in institutions; to find and develop appropriate alternatives in the community for housing, treatment, training, education, and rehabilitation of the mentally disabled who do not need to be institutionalized; and to improve conditions, care, and treatment for those who need institutional care.

There have been numerous successes, and many former patients have become less dependent on public support or family members for their needs and have learned to live normal or nearly normal lives. However, it is the failures that usually come to public attention, and they have been widespread and appalling. Many former state hospital patients have ended up in nursing homes that were less adequate than their original institutional placement; some have been placed in group homes, foster care homes, and other residential facilities that are substandard and provide few needed services; others have been returned to state institutions because of the total lack of community-based outpatient health services in their areas.

In reviewing the deinstitutionalization programs, the United States Comptroller General has pointed out the lack of a comprehensive and clearly defined national plan to achieve the goals, as well as the meager funding that has been provided for the development of the projected community services and facilities. He has proposed an overall national management system to implement the program by rationalizing the roles of the various agencies that could, and should, be contributing to the effort (U.S. General Accounting Office Report, 1977). Whether his recommendations and those of other critics will be followed remains problematic, but the current deinstitutionalization program is certain to undergo modifications in the near future.

INEQUITIES IN ACCESS TO THE REHABILITATION SYSTEM

The inequities in access to publicly supported health care systems in the United States are very great. By necessity, they influence the planning that the rehabilitation nurse can do with individual disabled patients and the services that the nurse can provide or refer the patient to. The public role in health care systems has grown by slow accretions, which, in the main, reflect compromises between organized special interest groups, including those taxpayer lobbies opposing social programs, the medical society lobbies, hospital and insurance industry associations, organizations representing private service providers, and of course, the specialized consumer organizations like the Paralyzed Veterans of America, the National Federation of the Blind, the National Association for Retarded Citizens, the National Council of Senior Citizens, and many others. In the past, research, training, and facility construction for acute care have been emphasized, to the detriment of long-term care and rehabilitation systems, which are only now beginning to be placed among the high-priority public concerns.

At the present time, access to our rehabilitation systems and services, and hence to the full range of desirable outcomes, continues to be greatly restricted. Although private health insurance varies in the adequacy of its coverage, it is usually designed to cover costs in hospitals and, perhaps, in skilled nursing facilities but not the costs of the lifelong outpatient care needed by some disabled persons, of attendants, of equipment, or of environmental modifications. Many of the handicapped are forced to rely upon public health and service systems, where one person is pitted against another according to criteria for which there are various justifications, none of which make sense to the persons who fall between the cracks.

In the section above entitled "Legitimacy of Self-care as Opposed to Solely Vocational Goals," differential access to vocational rehabilitation programs was discussed. Those fortunate enough to be judged as having rehabilitation potential may have available to them a full range of services, including counseling and guidance; physical and mental restorative services, including medical and surgical treatment; hospitalization; prosthetic, orthotic, and other assistive devices; physical and occupational therapy; psychological services; training, including personal and work adjustment; maintenance; transportation; reader, orientation, and mobility services for the blind; interpreter services for the deaf; and postemployment services.

Persons under 65 who have been working under Social Security long enough and recently enough prior to the occurrence of the disability may receive Social Security Disability Insurance monthly cash payments when they suffer an impairment that has lasted or is expected to last 12 months or more and that prevents substantial employment. Other members of the family of insured workers may also be eligible for direct benefit in case of disability. After being entitled to disability payments for 24 consecutive months, the disabled person is eligible for Medicare.

Medicare, enacted in 1965, was originally designed to provide hospital insurance for Social Security and railroad retirement beneficiaries (or dependent spouses or survivors) who are age 65 or over, but coverage was extended in 1974 to include long-time Social Security Disability Insurance beneficiaries and persons with permanent kidney failure who need maintenance dialysis treatments or a transplant. This is a non-income-tested program, providing hospital and posthospital services in a skilled nursing home or other extended care facility and home health services for the housebound. The Medicare beneficiaries who elect to enroll in Part B of the program, Supplementary Medical Insurance, receive partial reimbursement for physicians' and surgeons' services, regardless of where they are provided; home health services, without a prior hospitalization; outpatient hospital services and physical therapy; certain medical supplies, equipment, and prosthetic devices; and limited ambulance services.

The Social Security system also provides Supplemental Security Income (SSI) direct payments to persons who are over the age of 65, or blind, or totally disabled and who, on the basis of their monthly income and assets, are below a certain level of support. Those eligible for SSI payments qualify also for Medicaid, but the Medicaid benefits differ greatly from state to state, as do the SSI state supplementation programs themselves (Rigby and Morrison, 1975).

Workers who suffer from occupational disease or injuries incurred on the job may be eligible for rehabilitation services through the workmen's compensation agency in their state. This system aims to compensate for disability, to restore physical function, and to "return the worker to gainful employment and to his place in the community" (Ross, 1976). Thus the various state workmen's compensation agencies pay weekly compensation benefits and provide medical treatment for the disabling condition, and they are beginning to develop rehabilitation programs, frequently in conjunction with vocational rehabilitation agencies. Presently, 19 state workmen's compensation agencies provide direct rehabilitation services, of which the most common is counseling and guidance, followed by vocational training or retraining.

Disabled veterans, especially those who have a severe handicap and those whose disabilities are service-connected, are eligible for substantial benefits and services through the Veterans' Administration and other federal and state agencies. These benefits may include comprehensive health and medical care, including hospitalization, outpatient medical and dental treatment, and prosthetic appliances; disability compensation and pensions; nursing home and domiciliary care; aids and guide dogs for the blind; vocational rehabilitation and educational training; specially adapted housing assistance; funds for the purchase of an automobile and adaptive equipment; mortgage insurance, property tax abatement, and commissary privileges; allowances for aid and attendance if needed; and special consideration and services in job placement.

The major programs providing either cash benefits or in-kind services for specified groups of handicapped individuals were listed in the preceding paragraphs. However, there are at least 70 other federal programs that have the primary mission of serving the handicapped; 6 programs that emphasize service to handicapped persons although they also serve others; and 45 additional programs serving disabled persons on the same bases as others. As these programs have proliferated, the difficulties of coordinating the delivery of services, identifying gaps and overlaps, and ensuring access to services by persons in need have become major problems. In an effort to reduce the confusion, Congress in 1979 enacted legislation which established a new cabinet level, Department of Education, in which there is an assistant secretary for Special Education and Rehabilitation. This office centralizes responsibility for the activities of the Rehabilitation Services Administration, the new National Institute of Handicapped Research, and the Bureau of Education for the Handicapped. This administrative consolidation is expected to strengthen federal programming and improve service delivery.

Reorganization of existing federal programs, with their various eligibility criteria, is not likely to bring us substantially closer to the goal of equity of access, however. It is for this reason, among others, that several national health insurance plans are now under consideration in the Congress. The same concern underlies the interest and support for health maintenance organizations, community health centers, and other new and innovative service delivery models. Although we have a long way to go before we establish the principle of universal entitlement to health services and are prepared to fully honor the entitlement by expanding the provider agencies, we are on the way. The trend is clear (Anderson, Kravits, and Anderson, 1975).

RESOCIALIZATION AGENTS

HEALTH PROFESSIONALS AND FELLOW PATIENTS

Newly disabled patients rarely have much information about rehabilitation options and the whole new environment that is being shaped by both public and private agencies for the benefit of the handicapped. At a later stage of recovery, they will discover the benefits of curb cuts, braille signs, captioned news, and other aids. Initially, however, their horizons may extend no further than the walls of the hospital room. The agents of early resocialization are those who enter therein, that is, hospital staff members and aides, family, and close friends.

Later, as patients move out into rehabilitation facilities, they discover that there is a whole community of fellow patients, some of whom have impairments from which they will secretly rejoice that they have been spared. There they will also discover that among the disabled are many persons who display grace, great courage, and ingenuity as they learn to cope with the problems of living with an impairment. Although the patients may hang back a bit when they are newcomers, some of the earlier initiates into this strange and exclusive society are likely to draw them into their social group. Such a group provides affectional supports, much good-natured reinforcement for efforts to improve, and perhaps most important, a thorough introduction to the lore of the handicapped centering around the personal issues they face. While group members may not have pieced together a comprehensive picture of what disabled persons can do with their lives or what options the larger society provides, they will have put together many questions and many answers that will help novices begin to develop their own perspectives and plans if they have not done so already.

The good rehabilitation facility makes sure that its personnel are trained to recognize the importance of the patients' early efforts to reassociate themselves with the world of the living and to reinforce their steps along the way. Such an institution is also formally structured to encourage resocialization, both in its physical features and in time-and-activity scheduling. Private areas are provided where patients and family members or friends can have time alone together, and public areas are made as cheerful and attractive as possible. Visiting hours are generous. Time off from therapy schedules is deliberately arranged so that patients will have time for informal socializing and either work or personal avocations that interest them. Both individual and group trips to restaurants, movies, concerts, and other normal recreational events of the outside world are encouraged. In addition, vocational counseling and rehabilitation are important offerings in the comprehensive program.

The rehabilitation personnel play a major role not only in the early resocialization of the patients but also in that of the entire family if the patients have families to which they are returning. Both patients and primary caregivers must understand how to carry out health maintenance and everyday living procedures, and they should also know why the procedures are done as they are and how they may need to be adjusted according to changes in the patient's condition. They need to know what constitutes an emergency and how to get the appropriate help when it is needed. Such information eases anxieties within the family group and facilitates planning for the handicapped person's reintegration into family and community living.

Of equal importance is the need for help in modifying the home environment. Rehabilitation institutes usually arrange for a gradual transition to the home, permitting the patient to leave the facility for only a few hours on the first trip, then perhaps for a full day and night, and, finally, for several weekends in succession prior to actual discharge from the institute. On each of these occasions, patient and family gradually discover which features of the physical and social environment are going to make life difficult. Sometimes they themselves can figure out how the necessary changes can be made, and sometimes they return to the institute with many worries about how they can possibly work things out. It is at this point that rehabilitation personnel make one of their greatest contributions to the transition home. They have heard the problems before, and they can apply their information about possible solutions to the specific situation. The aim, of course, is to assist in the creation of an individualized prosthetic environment within the patient's home.

THE PATIENT TAKES CHARGE

At some time during the rehabilitation period, and this may vary greatly from patient to patient, disabled persons reach the point where they wish to become the primary agents in their own resocialization. On the basis of an extensive study of paraplegics from the time of injury to the time they resumed roles in the community, Cogswell (1977) has described what she calls self-socialization, the readjustment of paraplegics in the community. Pointing out that in the first phase of rehabilitation, medical personnel are available for teaching the physical skills necessary for independent living, and that in the final phase, rehabilitation counselors are there to assist with occupational choice, training, and placement,

Cogswell draws attention to a middle phase of rehabilitation—the period after patients have left the hospital and before they resume full-time work or student roles. During this period, no professional assumes explicit responsibility for assisting paraplegics to learn the social skills necessary to relate successfully with nondisabled in the community. They are on their own, and they become their own socializing agents.

Cogswell found that for the paraplegics she studied, the middle period of rehabilitation began with a self-imposed moratorium during which the former patient remained at home. During the first few weeks, friends and neighbors would come to visit, but this activity often was not sustained. If family members and friends encouraged outings without getting a positive response from the paraplegic, their overtures ceased. The paraplegics themselves described this period as a time of social isolation and inactivity. When asked, "Who do you see?," they answered, "Nobody." When asked, "What do you do?," they repied, "Nothing."

Gradually, the former patients began to reenter the community, but on their own terms. The return was structured simultaneously in two ways: by sequential choice of social settings and by sequential choice of associates. They tended to enter first those social settings that were most easily accessible and that provided the greatest possibilities for making a hasty retreat, like public streets, and only much later to move into settings requiring greater physical effort and more intimate personal contacts, for example, parties. The workplace was the community setting entered last by most of the subjects. The sequence of associates followed a discernible pattern in which the paraplegics first phased out and seldom resumed relationships with pretrauma friends; next, they began to associate with individuals of lower social status; and, finally, they began to associate with new individuals of equal status.

While it would be a mistake to assume that every newly handicapped person goes through identical stages of self-socialization, something similar to the social withdrawal and then the tentative rebuilding of social relationships that Cogswell describes probably does occur in many cases of severe disability. Certainly for some, the family may play a more prominent part in reducing social discontinuities and smoothing the patient's way back into work and community life.

THE FAMILY

During the early years of our history, the family had primary and virtually sole responsibility for the care of its disabled members. Patients usually remained in the home, although some ended up in prisons or on poor farms. Subsequently, we passed through a period in which public and private specialized institutions, with names like the Home for Incurables or the Hospital for Destitute Crippled Children, were built to provide restorative and custodial care for persons with severe impairments. When institutionalizations were lengthy, ties with home and family were often broken, never to be resumed.

At the present time, a new trend is taking shape, one in which the patient's family is again seen as a major health care resource, especially when the prognosis is for permanent or severe disability. Although specialized community agencies are being developed to assist patient and family in many areas of need, the home is considered to be the most appropriate living setting for many categories of long-term disabled individuals. The family itself forms a first line of social support, and it can also serve as a vital link between patients and the larger community. Family members can be major agents of resocialization, along with the patients themselves.

It is difficult to make generalizations about the impact of major illness or long-term disability upon the patients' families, because most of the existing research is limited to study of single types of disability; or is cross-sectional, describing family reactions at one phase of illness or rehabilitation; or is concerned with effects on behavior patterns within the family when the patient has a particular role within the group, such as child, breadwinner, wife, or grandparent. In an effort to develop a conceptual approach of general applicability to the many and heterogeneous situations in which the family experiences the disability of one of its members, Cogswell (1976) has proposed that the family be viewed as a group, a small system in process of change. She developed a working analytic framework that permits longitudinal comparisons of a single family system as it changes or cross-sectional comparisons of different families, and she applied it in the study of 12 households, each of which had a severely disabled member, over a 2- to 3-year period.

Cogswell found that in the process of adaptation, each family passed at its own pace through broad stages, which she defined as the crisis, transition, temporary stabilization, and readaptation stages. At each of these stages, changes were occurring in family system properties, including general system characteristics, structures, goals, roles, and boundaries. Commonly, family members initially responded to the occurrence of the acute illness or injury with the assumption that the patient would either die or make a complete recovery. Only in the later stages did family members seriously consider the possibility of permanent disability. Acceptance of the family member as disabled developed gradually during the last stages of adaptation.

When the patient returned home, almost all family members over the age of 6 contributed to personal care. Definitions of how to manage this care were usually diffuse until the stage of temporary stabilization, when the performance of the necessary tasks became better defined and routinized. A single family member, always a woman if that was possible, took over as caretaker. At that point, family concern began to focus on the handling of financial problems, the social and psychological consequences of permanent disability, and the more usual concerns of other family members. However, the disabled member and the caretaker remained the hub around which other members of the family organized their own activities.

The readaptation stage was reached when the family made a partial return to the precrisis situation, with more individual priorities being taken into account and precrisis roles resumed. There was then less help and attention from outsiders, a tighter family interaction system, and greater apparent competence in achieving group goals, such as the care of the disabled member.

Regardless of the many variations among the study families prior to the disability, Cogswell found similar changes occurring within all family systems, although the timing of changes differed from one family to another; this, in spite of the curious fact that when the families were asked directly about changes resulting from the disability, the consistent answer was "Nothing has changed." Most of the families showed evidence of residual change in role flexibility; group cohesiveness, direction, and goals; and more problem-solving and self-regulatory behavior. All but one of the 12 families exhibited considerable role flexibility at all stages of adaptation, with young children taking on household tasks and sex role boundaries being crossed when necessary. Those families in which precrisis entry boundaries were very open to visitors seemed to experience social adjustment to disability more quickly and easily than those that had closed entry boundaries. Casual visiting in the home tended to enhance the social rehabilitation of the disabled member by reducing social isolation and providing opportunities to acquire techniques of stigma management in a protected situation.

Although the study described above intentionally remained at a macroanalytic level, the conceptual framework developed may have utility for the rehabilitation nurse who is trying to assist real patients and real families as they go through the process of mutual resocialization. Too much attention has been focused on the assumed devastating psychological and social effects of trauma and too little on the growth that many patients and their families exhibit under stress. In those instances in which the family home is to be the living setting of the disabled patient, rehabilitation workers may help by arranging meetings where members of different families can exchange practical information about the ways they are accomplishing various tasks. Meetings of this type are especially useful if the professionals make sure that family members are acquainted with the local vocational rehabilitation and educational facilities, employment opportunities, and the network of other helping agencies. These, then, can be drawn upon as social resources in addition to the informal network of kin, neighbors, or friends that the family may already have established.

AGENCIES IN THE LARGER COMMUNITY

Relatively few handicapped persons go directly from a hospital or rehabilitation center to a nursing home. An increasingly large number of those who, through choice or necessity, do not return to their nuclear families live either independently in the community or in some type of congregate housing arrangement. For persons who are on their own, a variety of housing options and supportive services of all types are in process of development. A recent directory listed more than 200 national organizations, both public and private, that are interested in the handicapped (*Directory,* 1976). Some of these are devoted to the needs of a single category of disabled persons, while others carry out activities of general utility. Many either are run entirely by handicapped persons or incorporate them in advisory, policy-making, or service delivery roles. However, since there is a great deal of organizational variation from community to community at the present time, rehabilitation professionals and the handicapped must map out and evaluate in each situation the facilities that are actually available to help with special needs.

Those who choose independent living are most often young adults or elderly widowed persons who were living alone prior to trauma. They usually prefer to return to their own house or apartment. Sometimes, assistance in making modifications in the home is all that is required, but in other cases, it becomes apparent that new housing must be sought. Federal and federally assisted housing may provide suitably accessible units, or, if the housing must be found in the private market, local organizations for elderly or handicapped citizens may be able to provide lists of appropriate units.

The disabled persons living alone in the community differ in their level of functional independence. A lucky few make an immediate return to their pretrauma occupations. Although some may be able to manage entirely on their own once their home is prepared, others may need to take advantage of homemaker or chore services (provided without charge to the needy handicapped in California and a few other states), Meals-on-Wheels or congregate dining programs, and publicly supported special transportation facilities. They may seek special vocational retraining or job placement assistance and may find this through a variety of public and private agencies. The United States Employment Service and the Veterans' Administration provide special counselors for the handicapped, and, of course, local departments of vocational rehabilitation can be helpful. Most public school systems have a staff of teachers who specialize in education for the housebound, and many community colleges have developed special curricula and educational aids for disabled students. All institutions of higher education that receive federal funding are now in the process of making their programs accessible to the handicapped. In addition, federally supported libraries and recreational and leisure-time facilities are making the necessary changes to offer their services to the disabled. Local religious groups frequently provide excellent activities for the handicapped or offer special assistance through volunteer programs.

When attendant help is needed, this is available through public agencies in some states. In other cases, such help may be privately supplied or must be purchased. Communities differ also in the amount and kind of medical and rehabilitation help they provide for handicapped persons who have returned to their homes. Sometimes, continuing medical care, physical and other therapies, and day care centers are made available in community clinics; many local government units provide visiting nurses and physical therapists who go to the patient's home. In addition, there are demonstration follow-along projects in a few communities, in which rehabilitation nurses or social workers assume responsibility for assuring continuing care and surveillance of handicapped individuals living independently (*Research Directory,* 1975).

While many of the programs that have been mentioned in the preceding brief review may be available to aid in the resocialization of disabled persons living with their families, certain of them are of critical importance to the quality of life that can be attained by those living alone. Without them, independent living would be an impossibility for many.

For persons who are not quite able to be on their own, congregate living facilities of various types are available. Again, these are not to be found in every community. Although some of the residential alternatives are for-profit enterprises created in the private sector, many depend for their funding on federal or local housing authority or other aid. They provide nonmedical care in a structured, supportive environment, but they do not always provide additional rehabilitative programs on their own premises. They generally aim to help clients participate in community life to the fullest degree that they are able, and some do, indeed, serve a transitional function, preparing patients for independent living. Foster homes, sheltered apartments, and boarding homes usually serve a small clientele, but halfway houses, long-term care facilities, and nursing homes may have larger numbers of residents. The congregate facilities vary along a continuum in terms of their suitability for residents at different functional levels, from the nursing homes that have been developed for patients who are at a low level and need regular supervision to the cooperative apartment arrangements for those who are nearly independent and need minimal supervision and assistance.

Some of the most successful models for independent or congregate living have been developed in conjunction with university programs for disabled students. The University of Illinois at Champaign-Urbana and Southern Illinois University at Carbondale pioneered in the development of facilities and programs of all types for the handicapped and gained much experience that is now being put to use throughout the country as other institutions of higher education prepare to integrate disabled persons.

The Berkeley Center for Independent Living (CIL), which grew out of the Physically Disabled Students' Program at the University of California, has developed rapidly into a community-based consumer organization that presently serves over 3000 disabled, blind, deaf, and elderly persons. Already, several spin-off centers have been established in California and elsewhere in the United States, some by former CIL members. The Center for Independent Living is completely controlled and partially staffed by the handicapped members themselves. Although CIL does not provide housing, it offers a wide variety of services in the area of housing by operating a resource directory for apartments, attendants, and cooks, as well as offering expert consultation services with regard to environmental modifications and assistive devices. The CIL has also developed peer counseling; offers several courses of study that prepare severely handicapped persons for responsible jobs; carries on research and legal advocacy, especially in the areas of financial support, health and social services, employment, environmental barriers, and transportation; and publishes a quarterly journal. In addition, CIL provides self-help education in such problem areas as health, sex, finances, and wheelchair and appliance repair. It encourages the disabled to participate in many available leisure-time activities, such as horseback riding, white-water canoeing, skiing, and camping. Many of its members now hold full-time, responsible jobs in Berkeley or surrounding areas and participate in the life of the total community, as well as in the activities of the Center for Independent Living. They thus exemplify the kind of community integration that remains a somewhat distant goal for many of the handicapped individuals elsewhere. The Berkeley Center for Independent Living is demonstrating in a most impressive manner the many ways in which handicapped persons, as a group, can achieve improvements in the quality of life for the individual.

METHODS TO FACILITATE RESOCIALIZATION

BEHAVIORAL ORIENTATIONS

The rehabilitation nurse, reading the foregoing, may feel like commenting, "Oh, that's all well and good.... There've always been a few Helen Kellers and Franklin Delano Roosevelts here and there. But what does all that have to do with *my* patients? They don't want to get up in the morning, refuse to learn catheter care, and will do anything in the world to get out of going down to physical therapy." It may be some comfort to be reminded that in every acute-care hospital and rehabilitation center in the country, the majority of severely disabled, early post-trauma patients act like anything but candidates for total resocialization. More than likely, most of the handicapped individuals now identified with the Center for Independent Living were not much different from the rest. Indeed, one of the early CIL leaders has written about his near-successful suicide attempt, which occurred about a year after a diving accident made him a quadriplegic and before he finished college with a Phi Beta Kappa key in his possession, went off to graduate school at the University of California, and then continued on to a career in the computer sciences (Luebking, 1977). What distinguishes the CIL activists from many others of the disabled is that they are rapidly learning how to join together to manipulate the environment so that it works for them.

The problem of patient inactivity is usually considered to be the result of depression or lack of motivation. However, a group of behavioral psychologists whose work is heavily influenced by B. F. Skinner's contributions in the field of learning (see the earlier section on disturbances of sensation and response) have begun to develop a different way of viewing the problem, which leads to new approaches to intervention at every level of rehabilitation. One major concern is to develop teaching methods that will help turn reluctant rehabilitees into self-starters. The scientific foundation of the approach is usually called the experimental analysis of behavior, and relevant applications, which by now have been made in many different situations, are perhaps most commonly referred to as behavior modification, programming, or programmed instruction.

Fordyce, who was one of the first psychologists to recognize the contributions that the experimental analysis of behavior might make to the field of physical rehabilitation, has carried out major research programs designed to determine ways of influencing the level of patient participation in the rehabilitation process. He points out that in the past, it has been assumed that the primary source of influence on participation is patient motivation, something assumed to be located *within* the person as part of a fixed personality. Under this assumption, if the motivation to participate is lacking, the nurses and other professionals have little recourse other than reason, persuasion, and threat. Fordyce suggests a different model. Instead of focusing on the allegedly lasting behavioral predispositions a patient is assumed to *have,* he shifts the focus to what the patient *does* and to the interaction between the patient's behavior and the immediate environment. He says, "... the immediate and systematic consequences in the environment to a person's behavior have a great deal of effect on what the person subsequently does. ... Simply stated, the behavioral conceptualization of what influences people's actions attributes to the immediate environment considerably more impact and potentiating effect than does the more traditional motivational model" (Fordyce, 1975).

The institutional intervention problem then becomes one, not of how to change the psychological characteristics of the patient, but of how to change the environment. What is required is an examination and reprogramming of the interactions between patient behavior and environmental response or consequence. Under this assumption, the nurse no longer exhorts patients to behave differently. Instead, the nurse arranges the environment in such a way that patients are likely to exhibit behavior that is appropriate to recovery goals and then makes sure that when the behavior occurs, it is strongly and immediately reinforced.

Once patients begin to progress, the intervention strategy shifts to enlist their active participation in the setting of goals and to teach them to observe and analyze their own interactions with the environment in terms of behavior/consequence contingencies. Eventually, patients are led to the discovery that they can exert control over the environment that is controlling them. According to I. Goldiamond (1974), a major outcome of behaviorally oriented interventions should be that **both** health professional and patient gain insight into the contingencies that govern the patient's repertoires, as well as how to assess them and change them. When patients understand the conditions under which their coping and adaptive behaviors will be reinforced and maintained, they can then construct their own prosthetic environments that will support the behaviors they desire to undertake in order to reach their goals.

TEACHING PROCEDURES

While behavior modification can become quite complex, requiring much ingenuity in certain difficult cases, the basic principles of operant learning on which it rests can be stated rather simply. When the purpose is to *strengthen* a behavior, reinforcement is presented contingent on the occurrence of that response and not otherwise. The reinforcement does not have to be continuously delivered but may be scheduled for delivery after a specified number of responses or when the correct response occurs after the passage of an interval of time. Once a behavior has been established, it can be maintained on a schedule in which reinforcers are infrequently delivered, but, for maintenance, reinforcement must occur.

When the purpose is to weaken, or *extinguish*, an undesirable behavior, reinforcement is not presented after that behavior occurs. Gradually, the behavior will extinguish, although, paradoxically, the rate of occurrence may increase during the period immediately following the introduction of extinction procedures. To hasten the extinction process, the procedure of strengthening an incompatible behavior is sometimes followed. For example, a person who is singing will not be smoking simultaneously.

The procedure of *behavior shaping* can be of great assistance in rehabilitation nursing. There are two elements involved in shaping behavior: differential reinforcement is employed, and the behavioral requirement for reinforcement is increased through a process called successive approximation. For example, a therapist may be concerned with increasing the verbal repertoire of an aphasic stroke patient. A decision is made to work on a limited vocabulary including words that can be used to satisfy basic needs, beginning with "water." At first, the therapist may bring in a glass of water and model the word "water"; then the therapist reinforces the patient's lip movements and, finally, efforts at vocalization of any type. On later teaching trials, the therapist will reserve praise for a "wa" sound and, still later, will reinforce "wa-wa" and, eventually, will withhold the reinforcer until the word the patient says closely resembles the sound of "water." The same procedure may be patiently followed as other words are introduced to build up the verbal repertoire.

Another kind of rehabilitation activity in which behavior shaping is frequently employed at present is physical therapy. When a patient who must remain in bed needs exercise and is given 2-lb wrist-encircling sandbags and asked to practice raising the arms from the bed, the patient may be able to move them only a few inches at the first try. Reinforcement is given immediately. On subsequent trials, the behavioral requirement for reinforcement is increased very gradually until, finally, through the procedure of successive approximation the patient is making exactly the desired arm movements.

A slightly more elaborate procedure that involves establishing a *behavior chain* can be employed in teaching many self-care activities. Let us suppose that the patient is an elderly woman who must learn how to put on elasticized, antiembolism stockings if she is to return alone to her apartment, and yet lectures on the hazards associated with poor venous return have had no effects on her performance. Should one try more lectures? Hardly. Should one put the stockings on for her? That will not produce the desired behavior. How, then, should teaching proceed?

What might be done is to establish a behavior chain, using a backwards program in which props are provided initially and are then faded out. On the first trial, the nurse pulls the stockings up to the point where the patient can easily complete pulling them up toward the knee successfully, and abundant praise of that behavior is given. The next time, a bit more of the pulling-up job is left for the patient to complete, and praise follows. Eventually, the patient pulls the stockings all the way up from the ankle and, then, the next day gets them up from the instep. Finally, the patient is able to position the stockings at the toes correctly, wiggle them over the foot, slide them into place properly at the heel, and slowly get them unrolled and pulled up exactly right. By that time, the nurse's praise will not be necessary; the achievement of the task will be reward enough.

The essential elements of the procedure of *programming* are as follows: (1) a goal is established; (2) the patient's relevant behavioral repertoire is assessed; (3) a program is devised, beginning with a behavior already present in the repertoire and proceeding through small, discrete steps until the goal is reached; and (4) reinforcers are provided as each step in the program is completed successfully. Programming can be used to shape complex social, intellectual, or other behaviors, as well as the simpler type of self-care chain described in the foregoing example.

The importance of individualizing the program cannot be overemphasized. The most successful programs are those in which the patients participate in the choice of the goals, help assess their own relevant repertoires, and help analyze what steps must be taken to get from where they are to where they want to be. In addition, reinforcers must be individualized. Some people dislike verbal praise, especially if they detect artificiality, but they may put out substantial effort for a smile or a gesture from the right person. Sometimes, persons will work at something they do not enjoy in order to get the opportunity to do something else that they really like to do, for example, rest quietly, watch TV, or play a game. The use of opportunity to engage in a high-frequency behavior as a reinforcer for low-frequency behavior is common; the employment of this type of reinforcement is called the Premack principle (Premack, 1965). Some individuals need extrinsic reinforcement, like tokens or perhaps gold stars placed on a wall chart, or favorite foods, whereas the behavior of others can be maintained at a high rate by the intrinsic reinforcement that performance of some tasks provides. In each case, the determination of adequacy of reinforcers is a matter for empirical discovery.

Some psychologists believe that one of the most important functions of reinforcement is that it provides feedback to the person trying to learn or do something. Delivery of the reinforcer carries the information that the behavior exhibited is up to specification, or, if the reinforcer is not presented, the learner knows that the response must be made differently. Because it is difficult to evaluate the adequacy of one's own responses, and machine definition is not a possibility for many of the behaviors that a patient will want or need to learn, the role of the teacher (or reinforcing agent) may have to be transferred to others when the patient is leaving the rehabilitation center. Family members and friends can be invited to observe the procedures used in teaching while the disabled person is still an inpatient and encouraged to try behavioral methods under guidance. They may then be able to continue the approach in the home setting, using reinforcement appropriately to maintain the behavior that has been acquired earlier and developing new programs to establish the different skills needed at home and in the community.

A COMMUNITY APPROACH

In 1972, the Training in Community Living Program was developed at Mendota Mental Health Institute in Madison, Wisconsin (Test and Stein, 1977). Although this program was concerned with a psychiatric population only, certain of the procedures used there would seem to be applicable, with minor changes, in planning resocialization programs for other categories of disabled persons who need supportive services. The project had two major purposes: to reduce or eliminate institutionalization in the mental hospital and to improve the quality of life for psychiatric patients. For experimental purposes, 130 persons seeking psychiatric hospital admission were randomly assigned to either the experimental or the control group. Those who were in the experimental group received the Training in Community Living Program, while the control subjects were usually admitted to the Mendota Mental Health Institute, a state hospital, given progressive short-term in-hospital treatment, and then linked to community aftercare services. All were evaluated on an array of assessment instruments at the time of admission to the experimental or control program and again after 4, 8, and 12 months by an independent research team. The course of treatment for all was followed throughout the first year.

The experimental treatment included work with patients, with their families, and with the community. Immediately after a patient was assigned to this treatment, a member of the experimental staff interviewed the patient and made a decision as to whether hospitalization was necessary. Only those who were imminently suicidal or homicidal or required high dosages of medication were hospitalized; the instances when this was necessary were rare and of short duration. Most patients were taken directly from the hospital admissions office to the Training in Community Living staff office to begin in-community treatment. They were informed that they would be given intensive assistance but were told that the "best place to treat these problems is in the community rather than in the hospital," and they were then familiarized with the operations of the new treatment program. Initial assessment was carried out through formal evaluation procedures and through informal interactions. By the end of the first day, the patient was started on medications, if appropriate, and a decision was made about where the patient should live. Fairly independent settings, such as a room or apartment or the residential section of the YMCA or YWCA, were selected over sheltered ones in order to provide the patient with healthier models and to maximize community requirements for responsible behavior.

During the initial days in the program, patients were given as much support as was needed to reduce symptoms and to gain comfort in the community. In some cases, this meant 6 h or more of staff time daily in the patient's home or neighborhood; later, staff time could be reduced. However, throughout the patient's involvement in the program, 24-h telephone contact with staff members was available. A staff member worked with the patient on such things as grooming, shopping, learning about the neighborhood, and setting up a schedule with persons like occupational therapists and vocational rehabilitation counselors. Within the first few days, a plan was developed with the patient for the in-community program, and a daily schedule for work, leisure activities, and personal needs was prepared.

From then on, the focus was directly on teaching of copying skills in real-life situations. Staff members went with the patients to carry on daily activities of living, gave sustained assistance in finding a job or sheltered workshop placement, and then continued daily contacts to make sure the patient was performing as planned and had assistance available when needed. Staff members found it important not only to give continuing support but also to be assertive in making behavioral requirements. They utilized a variety of individualized behavioral contingency programs.

Work with the families was primarily directed toward breaking pathological dependency ties and realigning relationships. Gradual resumption of patient contacts with intimates proceeded in accordance with carefully planned programs designed to help the patients behave and be treated as responsible adults. Work with the community involved thorough preparation to ensure understanding of the aims of the program and to establish close working relationships. The major effort was to influence landlords, employers, the police, and others in contact with the patients to respond to them in a manner that would promote responsible behavior rather than reinforce maladaptive modes of coping.

Data from the first 12 months of the research showed that an unselected group of patients seeking in-hospital admission can be treated almost entirely in the community. In terms of every measure employed, the experimental subjects had the advantage over the control subjects. As a group, they experienced many fewer days of hospitalization or readmission; they spent less time unemployed and earned significantly more income; they belonged to and attended activities of social groups significantly more often than did the controls; they ranked higher on a life satisfaction self-report scale; and they showed significantly less severe symptoms on the Short Clinical Rating Scale. Cost-benefit analysis of the program showed that, in monetary terms, the experimental program cost more than the conventional program but yielded greater benefits. Added benefits more than offset added costs.

The Mendota research group has succeeded in formalizing an in vivo resocialization program that works for many psychiatric patients. It offers an alternative to chronic institutionalization that may serve as a model for health planners who are primarily concerned with physically impaired patients. If the kind of environmental modification and the programming of social learning that goes on within rehabilitation centers can be extended into the patient's natural environment during the reentry transition period, there will be many advantages for the patient and for the larger society.

CONCLUSION

Literally, resocialization refers to the "reassociating" of patients that begins immediately after a serious accident or the onset of chronic disease disrupts their everyday activities and their normal social relationships. In assigning statuses and roles in the community to the physically and mentally impaired, the larger society has a range of possible options that it can employ to maintain its equilibrium. In past years, we have often segregated handicapped individuals, sometimes providing completely separate institutional facilities for their housing, education, and employment, or sometimes relegating them to low-status, dependent roles within the community. During the 1970s, however, a new public policy was adopted, perhaps, in part, because the number of the severely impaired who live for many years is steadily increasing as a result of improvements in medical technology and the strain that such a large dependent population places on the total society is growing greater, and perhaps, in part, because of genuine humanitarian concern for the quality of life of chronic patients. Whatever the reasons may be, present national policy recognizes that handicapped citizens have the same rights as the able-bodied and forbids discrimination in federal and federally assisted employment, education, transportation, public facilities, and other areas of community life.

Implementation of the goal of resocialization for full and equal participation in society is proceeding slowly and with many inconsistencies. In addition, there are persistent inequities in access to helping systems. However, through the efforts of both handicapped persons themselves and of rehabilitation professionals, the impetus is building. Every community still retains many barriers, both attitudinal and physical, that impede integration. Nevertheless, many are becoming more hospitable to the handicapped and are making new opportunities of all kinds available to them. Health care professionals are deeply involved in efforts to prepare their patients to take full advantage of the options that exist in their own communities, and supportive systems to facilitate resocialization are now evolving as important elements in comprehensive rehabilitation.

BIBLIOGRAPHY

Abrams, Ruth D.: *Not Alone with Cancer,* Charles C Thomas, Springfield, Ill., 1974, p. 15.

Albrecht, Gary L.: "Helping the Physically Disabled in Public Places: An Experimental Design Study," in *Annual Progress Report Number Nine,* U.S. Department of Health, Education, and Welfare, Office of Human Development, Rehabilitation Services Administration Medical Rehabilitation Research and Training Center No. 20, Northwestern University–Rehabilitation Institute of Chicago, Chicago, 1976(a), pp. 79–109.

——— (ed.): *The Sociology of Physical Disability and Rehabilitation,* University of Pittsburgh Press, Pittsburgh, 1976(b).

Andersen, Ronald, Joanna Kravits, and Odin W. Anderson: *Equity in Health Services: Empirical Analyses in Social Policy.* Ballinger, Cambridge, Mass., 1975, p. 266.

Becker, Howard: *Outsiders: Studies in the Sociology of Deviance,* Free Press, New York, 1963.

Berni, Rosemarian, and Wilbert E. Fordyce: *Behavior Modification and the Nursing Process,* Mosby, St. Louis, 1973.

Cobb, A. Beatrix (ed.): *Medical and Psychological Aspects of Disability,* Charles C Thomas, Springfield, Ill., 1973.

Cogswell, Betty E.: "Conceptual Model of Family as a Group: Family Response to Disability," in Gary L. Albrecht (ed.): *The Sociology of Physical Disability and Rehabilitation,* University of Pittsburgh Press, Pittsburgh, 1976, pp. 139–168.

———: "Self-socialization: Readjustment of Paraplegics in the Community," in Joseph Stubbins (ed.): *Social and Physiological Aspects of Disability,* University Park Press, Baltimore, 1977, pp. 123–130.

Cumming, Elaine, and William H. Henry: *Growing Old: The Process of Disengagement,* Basic Books, New York, 1961.

DiAngelo, Eleanor, Byron B. Hamilton, Paul S. Swarts, and Henry B. Betts: *Rehabilitation Follow-up of the Accident-Disabled,* Rehabilitation Institute of Chicago, Chicago, May 1974.

Directory of Organizations Interested in the Handicapped, Committee for the Handicapped/People to People Program, Washington, D.C., 1976.

DiRenzo, Gordon J.: "Socialization, Personality, and Social Systems," in Alex Inkeles, James Coleman, and Neil Smelser (eds.): *Annual Review of Sociology,* Vol. 3, Annual Reviews, Palo Alto, Calif., 1977, p. 268.

Fay, Frederick: *Problems of the Severely and Multiply Handicapped,* awareness paper prepared for the White House Conference on Handicapped Individuals, Washington, D.C., 1976, p. 20.

Fordyce, Wilbert E.: "Research on Influencing Level of Patient Participation in the Rehabilitation Process," in Marcus J. Fuhrer (ed.): *Selected Research Topics in Spinal Cord Injury Rehabilitation,* Rehabilitation Services Administration, Office of the Assistant Secretary for Human Development, U.S. Department of Health, Education, and Welfare, Washington, D.C., July 1975, p. 59.

———: *Behavioral Methods for Chronic Pain and Illness,* Mosby, St. Louis, 1976.

Gewirtz, Jacob L.: "Mechanisms of Social Learning: Some Roles of Stimulation and Behavior in Early Human Development," in David A.

Goslin (ed.): *Handbook of Socialization Theory and Research,* Rand McNally, Chicago, 1969, pp. 57–212.

Goffman, Erving: *Asylums: Essays on the Social Situation of Patients and Other Inmates,* Anchor Books, Garden City, N.Y., 1961.

Goldiamond, Israel: "Towards a Constructional Approach to Social Problems," *Behaviorism* 2(1):30, Spring 1974, University of Nevada, Reno.

Gunther, Meyer S.: "Emotional Aspects," in Daniel Ruge (ed.): *Spinal Cord Injuries,* Charles C Thomas, Springfield, Ill., 1969, pp. 93–108.

Hilgard, Ernest R., and Gordon H. Bower, *Theories of Learning,* 4th ed., Prentice-Hall, Englewood Cliffs, N.J., 1975.

Ince, Laurence P.: *Behavior Modification in Rehabilitation Medicine,* Charles C Thomas, Springfield, Ill., 1976.

Johnson, Richard J. H.: " 'Mercy Killing' Defendant Tells of Shooting Brother, *New York Times,* November 1, 1973; and " 'Mercy Killer' Acquitted on Insanity Plea," *New York Times,* November 6, 1973.

Luebking, Scott: "Getting There Is Half the Fun: The Sexually Active Quad," *The Independent* 3(4):20–21, Spring 1977, Center for Independent Living, Berkeley.

Michael, Jack L.: Rehabilitation, in Charles Neuringer and Jack L. Michael (eds.): *Behavior Modification in Clinical Psychology,* Appleton-Century-Crofts, New York, 1970.

Mitchell, Paige: *Act of Love: The Killing of George Zygmanik,* Knopf, New York, 1976.

Neff, Walter S. (ed.): *Rehabilitation Psychology,* American Psychological Association, Washington, D.C., 1971.

Neugarten, Bernice L. (ed.): *Middle Age and Aging: A Reader in Social Psychology,* University of Chicago Press, Chicago, 1968.
———, and Robert J. Havighurst (eds.): *Social Policy, Social Ethics, and the Aging Society,* Committee on Human Development, University of Chicago, Chicago, 1976.

Premack, David: "Reinforcement Theory," in D. Levine (ed.): *Nebraska Symposium on Motivation, 1965,* University of Nebraska Press, Lincoln, 1965, pp. 123–180.

Research Directory of the Rehabilitation Research and Training Centers, Fiscal Year 1975, Rehabilitation Services Administration, Office of Human Development, U.S. Department of Health, Education, and Welfare, Washington, D.C., 1975, pp. 142–143.

Rigby, Donald E., and Malcolm H. Morrison: *The Supplemental Security Income Program for the Aged, Blind, and Disabled: Selected Characteristics of State Supplemental Programs,* U.S. Department of Health, Education, and Welfare, Social Security Administration Office of Research and Statistics, HEW Publication No. (SSA) 76-11975, Washington, D.C., 1975.

Rigdon, Louis T.: *Civil Rights,* awareness paper prepared for the White House Conference on Handicapped Individuals, Washington, D.C., 1976, p. 2.

Ross, Eleanor Mayo: *Workmen's Compensation Rehabilitation of Injured Workers in the United States and Member Jurisdictions of the International Association of Industrial Accident Boards and Commissions,* IAIABC, Des Moines, 1976, p. 1.

Safilios-Rothschild, Constantina: *The Sociology and Social Psychology of Disability and Rehabilitation,* Random House, New York, 1970.

Skinner, B. F.: *Science and Human Behavior,* Macmillan, New York, 1953.

Stubbins, Joseph: "Introduction to Part IV, Normalization of Disabled Persons," in J. Stubbins (ed.): *Social and Psychological Aspects of Disability: A Handbook for Practitioners,* University Park Press, Baltimore, 1977.

Test, Mary Ann, and Leonard I. Stein: "A Community Approach to the Chronically Disabled Patient," *Social Policy* 8(1):8–16, May/June 1977.

United Nations Department of Economic and Social Affairs: *Social Barriers to the Integration of Disabled Persons into Community Life,* Report of an Expert Group

Meeting, Geneva, June 28 to July 5, 1976, United Nations, New York, 1977, p. 3.

Urban Institute: *Report of the Comprehensive Service Needs Study,* prepared under contract to the U.S. Department of Health, Education, and Welfare, Washington, D.C., June 23, 1975(a).

──: *Modeling and Forecasting Disability Information,* Working Paper 0981-02, submitted to the U.S. Department of Health, Education, and Welfare, June 9, 1975(b).

"U.S. Bias Against Elderly Told," *Chicago Tribune,* January 14, 1978.

U.S. General Accounting Office Report to the Congress by the Comptroller General of the United States: *Summary of a Report—Returning the Mentally Disabled to the Community: Government Needs to Do More,* Washington, D.C., January 1977.

The White House Conference on Handicapped Individuals, No. 0-218-920, U.S. Government Printing Office, Washington, D.C., 1976.

Whitten, E. B. (ed.): *Pathology, Impairment, Functional Limitation, and Disability—Implications for Practice, Research, Program and Policy Development, and Service Delivery,* Report of the First Mary E. Switzer Memorial Seminar, National Rehabilitation Association, Washington, D.C., 1975, pp. 1–2.

Wright, Beatrice A.: "Spread in Adjustment to Disability," in Joseph Stubbins (ed.): *Social and Psychological Aspects of Disability: A Handbook for Practitioners,* University Park Press, Baltimore, 1977, pp. 357–365.

35
barbara l. allan
robert e. small

the environmental situation

INTRODUCTION

What do individuals need in order to allow maximum use of the physical environment? Obviously, the needs are many and varied. A mountain climber or a scuba diver might need more strength and endurance, coupled with certain skills, knowledge of the territory, and perhaps some special equipment. These elements combine to maximize the individual's performance in those specific situations. Human beings adapt and adjust to the natural elements they wish to surmount. But what about the man-made environment? Do such human adaptations need to be made to cope with it? Or can criteria be applied to make the environment more adaptable to human performance? Does the man-made environment currently reflect the accelerated adaptability of the human beings for whom it was presumably made? Have planners and designers kept pace with advances in rehabilitation and related medical technology? Let us explore the issue.

Designers and builders have generally considered "averages" in planning and construction, and this is reflected in our existing buildings, site developments, and equipment. But these "averages" are clearly shifting. Our concepts have expanded to include people formerly thought to be outside this average in terms of ability to function in or through the community. It is gradually being recognized that a liberation movement has been taking place among people once thought of as needing full-time care. Advancements in technology, rehabilitation, and medicine, as well as attitudinal changes, have contributed to this shift. People with physical disabilities are moving up and out of this cared-for category. More and more, they are recognizing their abilities and skills and particularly their right to be included as users of the man-made environment. Such recognition has already been translated into various laws and mandates. But planners and designers, as well as the public in general, are still largely unaware that they continuously place unnecessary obstacles, both physically and psychologically, in the path of countless people. There is still much education needed about what constitutes these barriers and the need for their removal.

To enable more users to function independently in society, certain needs must be considered in planning and design. The physical elements restricting free passage for people with physical disabilities are identified typically as curbs, stairs, narrow doorways and aisles, steep ramps, inaccessible restrooms, unreachable telephones, heavy doors, hard-to-grasp hardware and handrails, inadequate information, warning or cuing systems, and lack of rest areas or supports. These unnecessary obstacles combine to curtail or discourage the mobility of people with various physical limitations. It is the modification or removal of such environmental barriers that is increasingly being promoted and mandated. It must be emphasized that such modification and barrier-free designing benefits *all* users, not just people with disabilities.

Inseparably related to the physical barriers are the still prevalent attitudinal restrictions and myths. In fact, if it were not for the mental restraints, it is doubtful that the physical ones would dominate. It is clear, from prevailing designs, that there is little awareness of the wide range of needs. The stereotyped term "handicapped" conjures up only a few generalized images. This term is now generally being replaced by the more preferred (by some) term "disabled." It should be pointed out, however, that a person *with* a disability is by no means a **disabled person.** Yet stereotypical thinking still categorizes and stigmatizes such individuals as fitting only designated and preconceived roles, such as "wheelchair people" or "the blind." The broad array of physically limiting conditions, seen or unseen, is largely unrecognized. This lack of recognition prevails in spite of continued efforts to educate and sensitize. However, there is an encouraging growth of interest and awareness of the general problem. Access to the environment and its relationship to the quality of life— for all people—remain something of an enigma to most. The need to educate and sensitize must be given much more attention and allocation of resources.

PEOPLE AFFECTED

MORE THAN STATISTICS

Understanding the need for a barrier-free environment means understanding the related needs of people with mobility and functional problems. While such understanding is more important than the knowledge of statistical data, planners and politicians require data to justify the allocation of resources. Although there are many sources of statistical information regarding the disabled population, most are geared to a particular segment; a more comprehensive total assessment and study is still needed. Moreover, there are problems in accurately gathering such data, resulting in part from the reluctance of many people to identify themselves as "disabled" or "handicapped." It is hoped that the 1980 census will provide a more accurate statistical base. In the meantime, estimates generally utilized are those given by the President's Committee on Employment of the Handicapped, the Architectural and Transportation Barriers Compliance Board, and the National Center for a Barrier Free Environment. These all conclude that approximately 10 percent of the entire population of the United States have physical limitations that significantly affect mobility. While this is considered by many to be a conservative estimate, it is nonetheless conclusive evidence of a need.

Beyond the figures is the need for an understanding of what they are composed of. This is essential to the accomplishment of effective solutions. Individual worth remains more important than statistics. The value in maximizing opportunities for independence and self-sufficiency of the individual should be evident. This concept is being promoted through current mainstreaming and normalization efforts. Such efforts seek to assist in releasing the potential of people formerly restricted by misconception of both their abilities and their needs. As a result of such efforts and the gradual shift in thinking, these misconceptions are being replaced by a more positive view of the capabilities of these individuals.

FUNCTIONAL ASPECTS

The functional or performance capacities of people with disabilities vary greatly. For this reason, it is almost impossible, if not unjust, to generalize on types of disabilities. Each individual is unique and therefore has unique abilities—and needs. However, the main consideration here is how such functions relate to the man-made aspects of the environment. For the purpose of relating basic functional needs to the design of various elements or components of the physical environment, key categories are useful.

The scope and complexity of disability types are much greater than is generally recognized and extend considerably beyond the usually identified categories of the "handicapped," that is, those in wheelchairs, the blind, the elderly, or the mentally retarded. For the purposes of planning environments, persons with disabilities that affect their related function and mobility can be grouped within the categories given in Table 35-1. Within these generalized categories exist wide variations of visible and nonvisible restrictions.

In planning for the needs of persons with these various levels of physical functioning, certain design standards based on studies of these levels are useful. Data collected from such studies have attempted to standardize specific design requirements to meet as broad a range of these needs as seems reasonable and cost-effective.

There are obvious differences in levels of physical functioning. These are based not only on the type of disability and the particular category mentioned but also on the skills, training, ability, and even attitude of the individual. In spite of these divergencies, there are basic considerations that generally benefit all users. For the most part, people with ambulatory restrictions will benefit from the same considerations used for people in wheelchairs. Floor sur-

Table 35-1

Disability Categories for Environmental Planning

The ambulant disabled	Persons with problems of coordination, strength, stability or stamina, or those whose movements may be slow or restricted but who do not require the use of assistive devices
The semiambulant	Persons who use assistive devices such as canes, crutches, walkers, or braces
The nonambulant	Persons who are unable to walk and whose mobility is accomplished by means of a wheelchair or similar device
The manipulatory impaired	Persons with limited manual dexterity or restricted use of their arms or hands
The sensory impaired	Persons with sight or hearing impairments

faces should be smooth and slip-resistant. They should be free from obstructions that might cause tripping, slipping, catching of cane or crutch tips, imbalance, or difficulty in navigation. Space requirements for necessary maneuvering must be provided for both groups, and are welcomed by able-bodied users as well. Doorway clearances with minimum width of 32 in allow arm maneuvering room and passage for both crutch and wheelchair users. Doors and openings must also allow for extremely tall persons and should be free of obstructions or protrusions hazardous to visually impaired persons. A minimum width of 36 in along aisles and walkways provides sufficient allowance for movement on the open path of travel.

Other functional design considerations include those of travel distance between areas of rest, which should be minimized for persons who are easily fatigued. For people who find bending or stooping a problem, equipment and controls should be located within an optimal range of reach of both standing or seated persons. Also, many ambulant disabled and those with restricted balance or stamina need to have support and balance assists such as grab bars and handrails. People with manipulatory impairments that affect the arms and/or hand dexterity are greatly assisted by hardware or controls that enable their use without precise movements such as pinching, grasping, twisting, or pressure.

Persons with sensory impairments are aided by unobstructed pathways and cuing devices. Paths of travel should be free of protrusions such as benches, light standards, receptacles, or other street furnishings, including low hanging signs or overhanging stairways. Tactile cuing along pathways to indicate direction or hazards is also helpful. Many partially sighted persons can read signs if they are of adequate size and have a high contrast between background and foreground. Signs should be free of glare, and lettering and images should be simple and bold. Persons with hearing impairments need adequate visual warnings and directions. Signs should be clear and easily located. Some telephones, at least, should be provided with amplification devices for those with partial hearing.

BEYOND MOBILITY

In addition to design aspects that allow for increased mobility, there is a need to optimize independent functioning for people. We recognize and support the inherent value of individuals by enabling them not merely to function but also to grow and be enriched by a variety of experiences. Optimizing independent function in the physical environment is a primary need in order to foster this growth and development. People who have been forced to function within the limits of an institutional setting or who have little or no access to public transportation or to their surrounding, larger environment are thus deprived of the opportunities it offers.

Independent function is also increased through better communication networks. Information must be presented in multimodal systems to allow for variations in interpretation and different levels of comprehension. The blind need cuing by way of tactile or audible signals. Those with slow or limited comprehension are aided by visual directness and clarity. The deaf also benefit from clear visual information, as well as from such assistive devices as TTYs (teletypewriters that transmit audio information to a visual display readout). Incorporating these systems into planning and design enables more users to benefit with greater freedom and safety. It opens the environment to wider usage and opens the doors to growth and advancement through increased participation and interaction.

REHABILITATED AND NONREHABILITATED CONSUMERS

In planning and designing for greater functional use, it should again be pointed out that there are great differences among individuals in their ability to function and negotiate the environment. This is the result not only of the particular physical or emotional limitation of the individual but also of the adaptive skills that may or may not have been acquired and the devices used for assistance. Those who have been through an established physical rehabilitation program are benefited by being taught how to adapt to their environment, as well as being equipped, where needed, with appropriate assistive devices. Many undergo rigorous training before coping on their own. Even then, however, few, depending on the severity of their limitation, are adequately prepared for the real test that independent functioning presents. Most must further explore and experience on their own, before becoming more innovative in coping with the challenges thrust upon them. Obviously, some individuals are more responsive than others. Those with readily available assistance by way of friends or family may, in fact, become lazy or at least less adventuresome in coping with the environment. The fragile elderly may naturally seek a more protected and less stressful life-style. But often the younger and more vigorous wish to participate and have their "piece of the action." They are apt to be more daring and energetic in their pursuits to utilize the many resources of the community, with or without the benefits of a rehabilitation program.

Many people, however, do not undergo any special rehabilitation or training and must learn through experience, or the lack of it, their own way of functioning or adapting. For this reason, it is difficult to plan or design within any standard mode. While variations of need are numerous, they must at least be considered. Design standards have to be sufficiently flexible to allow for continued changes in the abilities and functioning of people, as well as for related technological developments. They must allow for greater adaptability so that building and construction design may be more readily modified as society's needs change. Certainly people with disabilities have already grown and progressed as a result of advances in rehabilitation and technology. Design of the physical environment to incorporate these changes must keep pace.

TRANSITIONAL ADJUSTMENT

An individual's adjustment to a disability may be a complex one, depending upon both the severity and the initiation of it. Those with restrictions dating from birth or early childhood adjust somewhat gradually, often depending on the protection of the home environment and parental attitude. If they are overly sheltered, attend "special schools" for the handicapped, and have limited experiences, they are further handicapped by these added limitations when obligated or desiring to function independently. Those who become limited later in life as a result of injury or disease may find the adjustment process more difficult and sometimes traumatic. Accidents frequently thrust people into a new role with cataclysmic immediacy—and the psyche often rebels at accepting it. Degrees of adjustment thus vary, depending on these and many other factors.

SUPPORTIVE TO "HOSTILE" ENVIRONMENT

If the transition is one from a hospital or rehabilitation setting, it may sometimes be likened to moving from a supportive to a comparatively "hostile" environment. Severely disabled persons, and often even the less disabled, may find they are faced with more adjustments than anticipated. The transition from a setting in which support and assistance are available to one fraught with hitherto unnoticed "barriers" can be a frightening and discouraging experience. It is generally a step-by-step discovery, both of the barriers in the environment and the individual's ability to cope with them. Some perceive such barriers as challenges to be overcome and learn to be more innovative in dealing with them. Others become so discouraged that they give up and stop trying or at least greatly curtail their activities and pursuits. Thus the transitional adjustment to the man-made environment is widely varied and individualized. Individuals' own attitude toward their disability and their resultant estimate of self-worth are key factors in their adjustment. These influence their acceptance by others and their relative adjustment process. They must learn to bridge the gap and to communicate their needs in an effective manner.

Rehabilitation programs can help bridge this gap through various means of preparation, even beyond the valuable physical skills they teach. Many do indeed provide preparatory information and assistance in the necessary adjustments of housing, transportation, employment, recreation, and even sexuality. It is evident from those who have benefited from such recent and enlightened programs that the individual success rate is proportional to the opportunities available in such programs.

TYPES OF ACCESSIBILITY CONSIDERATIONS

We have discussed what may or may not be accomplished on the part of the individual adapting to the environment. Now let us view some of the adjustments needed to adapt the environment to more aptly fit its users. The gaps that must be bridged here, too, are many. In the physical environment, they include many facets that must be linked to provide a total network for balanced living. These elements include transportation, housing, education, employment, recreation, services, and social needs. All are interrelated with total functioning in the environment and must be provided with accessible linkages.

Transportation

Perhaps the key element of this linkage is that of transportation. Public transportation systems have been notably lacking in any provisions of adequate access for people with physical mobility limitations. Buses, trains, planes, and ships all present access problems. High steps, difficult entries, narrow doors and aisles, and inadequate signs and information systems continue to hamper or restrict the disabled traveler. Without access to public transportation, these individuals are frequently unable to utilize other environmental provisions or have other experiences. Their world shrinks to their immediate surroundings or to the limits of their financial resources to pay for private transportation.

In the community there is a universal need for access to services, but for the physically disabled person the need is much greater. Access to shopping, medical, and other support services is crucial. Yet few advancements in accessible transportation that links such services have been made. The considerable demand for change has been met with equal resistance and lethargy toward specific developments. An amendment to the Urban Mass Transportation Act of 1964 made it a "national policy" for elderly and handicapped persons to have the same rights to use mass transportation as others. Other legislation has been equally general.

The Urban Mass Transportation Act (UMTA) has funded some research on access, notably the Transbus project to develop a bus of the future. Specific access provisions for the Transbus were addressed by three subcontractors. Handicapped groups across the country tested the three prototypes developed. The basic criteria for greater accessibility were lower floors, smaller steps, wider doors and aisles, ramp or lift systems, and space to accommodate wheelchairs. Consumers offered suggestions, and in 1976, the UMTA issued a policy statement that barely satisfied expectant consumers. As a result, a federal suit was filed by a coalition of handicapped citizens against the UMTA, charging failure to require all federally assisted purchasers to purchase only the accessible Transbus. In May 1977, then Secretary of Transportation Brock Adams announced his decision to require all new public buses purchased with Department of Transportation grants to be designed for easy access by elderly and handicapped persons. All buses offered for bid after September 1979 were required to use the new accessible bus specifications. As stated by Adams, "I believe it is my responsibility to insure to the extent feasible that no segment of our population is needlessly denied access to public transportation. It is now within our technological capability to insure that elderly and handicapped persons are accorded access to urban mass transit buses. This access is fundamental to the ability of such persons to lead independent and productive lives. We cannot deny them rights that so many others enjoy, when it is within our ability to accord them such rights."

Interstate bus companies are beginning to make at least some effort by way of offering assistance to travelers, such as Greyhound's Helping Hand Service, which allows handicapped travelers to be accompanied, free of charge, by someone to assist them. The Interstate Commerce Commission has recently issued rules stipulating that all new or renovated bus stations must offer facilities like ramps, wheelchairs, lowered telephones, and restrooms that are accessible to the physically disabled. Carriers may not deny transportation to anyone with a physical disability and must allow Seeing Eye dogs free passage with blind passengers.

Airline regulations have progressively been eased and modified as handicapped travelers have demonstrated their desire and ability to travel independently. Many airport terminals have made considerable efforts to improve their accessibility, even though the air carriers they service have not. Many airports offer guidebooks of their facilities for handicapped travelers. In spite of some improvements, however, persons with limited mobility still experience difficulties in air travel. In 1974, the Federal Aviation Administration proposed regulations for amending criteria for transporting handicapped persons on civil air carriers. Because of the negative response, largely from the disabled community, these regulations were not issued, and recommendations were instead to be issued by individual carriers.

Amtrak, the national railroad system, has long had a "policy" of accommodating disabled persons, and there is beginning evidence of this. Plans for the provision of special, accessible cars as equipment is replaced makes improvement a slow process. Some railroad stations have been remodeled to include access features, but these are relatively limited.

There is also the need for small vehicle transportation to serve people who are physically, mentally, or financially unable to operate their own automobile. Door-to-door transportation service seems economically unfeasible and would require considerable subsidization. However, this method is preferred by many planners to that of incorporating needed accessibility changes into existing public transportation systems. Many disabled consumers believe such separate-but-equal options would be detrimental to the concept of integration and mainstreaming they are seeking. Experiments in Dial-a-Ride or demand responsive systems continue. There seems no easy or immediate solution.

Thus, in spite of some isolated improvements, transportation remains a critical issue for people with limited mobility. Their access to the network of available goods and services demands vital advances in this linkage system.

Housing

Accessible housing is another missing element in the network of balanced living. Historically, people with disabilities have been segregated, institutionalized, or just plain forgotten. Until recently, few able-bodied persons even considered that people with severe physical limitations might want or be able to "fend for themselves." Hence, options for independent living by the provision of accessible design and support services have been almost nonexistent. Because of the lack of such options, many capable people have been forced to live in restrictive housing situations and have thus been hampered in their growth and development.

Such needless segregation is finally being addressed in recent legislation and in the promotion of the concepts of normalization and mainstreaming. It is becoming increasingly clear that dependency fostered by needless institutionalization or other types of isolation is detrimental not only to the individual but also to society as a whole. Medical and technological advances have enabled people to overcome, in ever-increasing degrees and numbers, dependence on being cared for by others. Instead, life is being prolonged and self-care advanced. The need for a variety of independent living options has been steadily growing. Ranges in housing type, price, and degree of support services available should be provided. Congregate facilities, with and without care, are the most common. Less common are the alternatives for independent self-care facilities with easy access to supportive services or attendant care. Inadequate provisions for attendant care itself can be a major obstacle to independent living for many disabled individuals who need some degree of occasional assistance. Some experiments in shared living arrangements with shared attendant care have proved successful. Unfortunately, all forms of subsidized housing and assistive care programs are severely limited by shortages of money and skilled personnel.

Housing accessibility needs are obviously unique to the user and ideally should be specifically tailored to meet individual needs. However, there are basic access considerations that can be easily and inexpensively incorporated into most new living facilities. These include accessible linkage from the public way or allotted accessible parking area through the site to a level entry, doorways that are wide enough to accommodate crutch and wheelchair users, and units that include sufficient maneuvering space and reach considerations, particularly in the kitchen and bathroom (see Figs. 35-1, 35-2, and 35-3).

At the White House Conference for Handicapped Individuals held in May 1977, Patricia Harris, then Secretary of the Department of Housing and Urban Development, announced the establishment of a new Office of Independent Living for the Disabled. This was felt to be a major step forward in comparison to the former passive approach to considerations for disabled persons. Progress and assistance from this new office are eagerly anticipated by waiting disabled consumers.

While various federal laws mandate certain housing provisions for disabled and elderly persons in federally assisted projects, most building codes, both state and national, fail to require housing accessibility features of any kind. North Carolina and recently Washington State have both incorporated at least minimal access provisions in their building code requirements for apartment buildings over 10 units in size. These minimal provisions are those of basic access mentioned above. It is hoped that more state codes will follow and that increased access requirements will increase the options available.

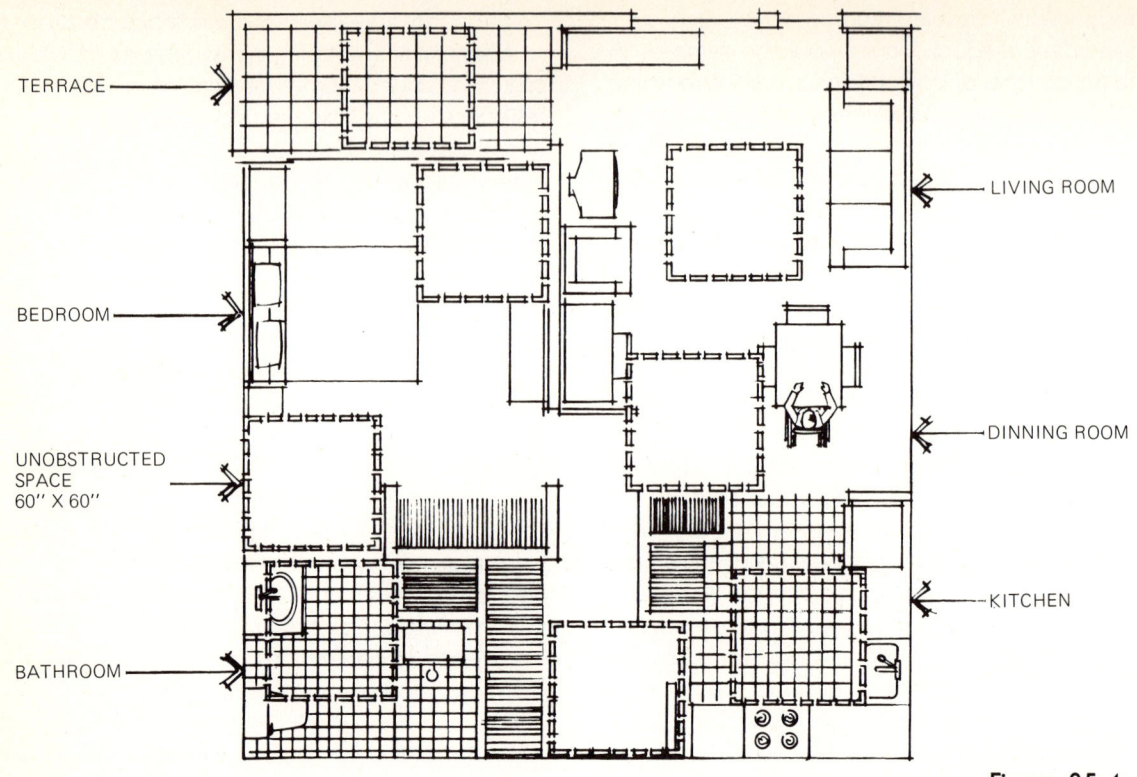

**Figure 35-1
A dwelling unit.**

Labels: TERRACE, BEDROOM, UNOBSTRUCTED SPACE 60" X 60", BATHROOM, LIVING ROOM, DINNING ROOM, KITCHEN

Education

Access to education has been given a major thrust by way of the recently enacted Section 504 regulations of the Vocational Rehabilitation Act of 1973. These regulations affect most major educational facilities, since most receive at least some amount of federal assistance. These regulations prohibit discrimination on the basis of physical or mental handicap in programs receiving federal assistance. Although the regulations deal primarily with programming aspects, physical accessibility is closely allied. The regulations state that "no otherwise qualified handicapped individual shall, solely by reason of his handicap be excluded from participation in, be denied the benefits of, or be subjected to discrimination under any program or activity receiving federal financial assistance." Accessibility provisions of this section, as well as those of the affirmative action Section 503, have already effected changes in educational facilities and are requiring many more institutions to comply with standards in both existing and new facilities.

In addition, PL 94-142, the Education for All Handicapped Children Act, which was signed into law in 1975, has also been a landmark piece of legislation affecting education for the disabled. Among its many requirements for more equalized educational opportunities for handicapped children is the stipulation that assures them of such education in the "least restrictive" environment.

This mandate and recognition for inclusion of disabled children and adults into our educational networks is long overdue. The potential impact of these two pieces of legislation is just beginning to be understood. They will provide for many needed changes in our educational system for years to come.

Employment

Both of the mandates mentioned above will, of course, greatly affect employment possibilities for individuals who are disabled. Sections 503 and 504 already do, and PL 94-142 certainly will. Employers must think beyond the immediate effects and consider the potential long-range impact. Presently, largely as a result of the above-mentioned provisions of the Vocational Rehabilitation Act, as well as other employment-related legislation, employers are recognizing their responsibility to make "reasonable accommodations" for disabled employees. Such accommodations include access to personal offices as well as individualized accommodations on the job, if needed. Federal contractors with contracts of $2500 or more must have affirmative action clauses in their contracts for hiring disabled people. Those with contracts or subcontracts of $50,000 or more and having at least 50 employees are required to develop and maintain affirmative action programs.

Another piece of legislation affecting accessibility in employment is the Tax Reform Act of 1976. This law allows for tax deductions of up to $25,000 per year for expenses incurred in the removal of qualified architectural and transportation barriers. This deduction is allowed for the purpose of making any facility or public transportation vehicle that is owned or leased by the taxpayer for use in his or her trade or business more accessible to or usable by handicapped persons. Effective January 1977 to continue for 3 years, it was extended through 1982.

Although the above measures are significant in effecting needed change, much remains to be accomplished in implementing these laws as

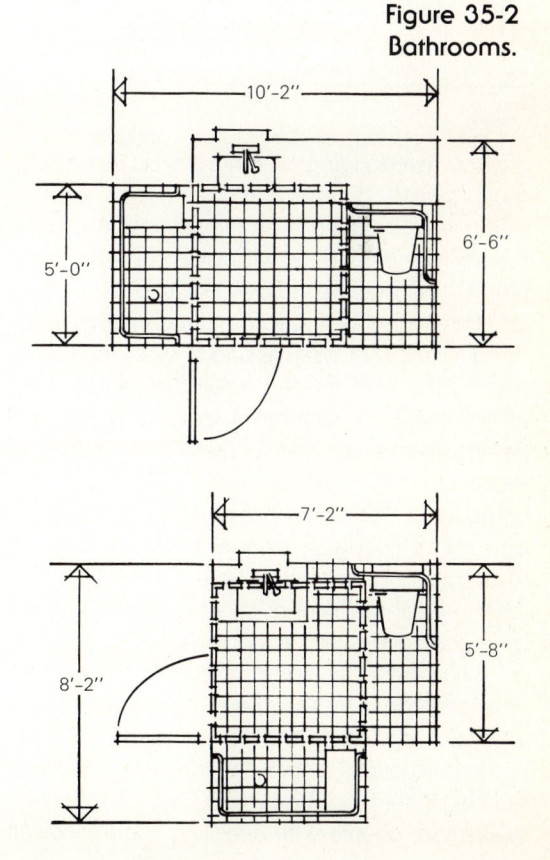

Figure 35-2
Bathrooms.

Figure 35-3
Kitchens.

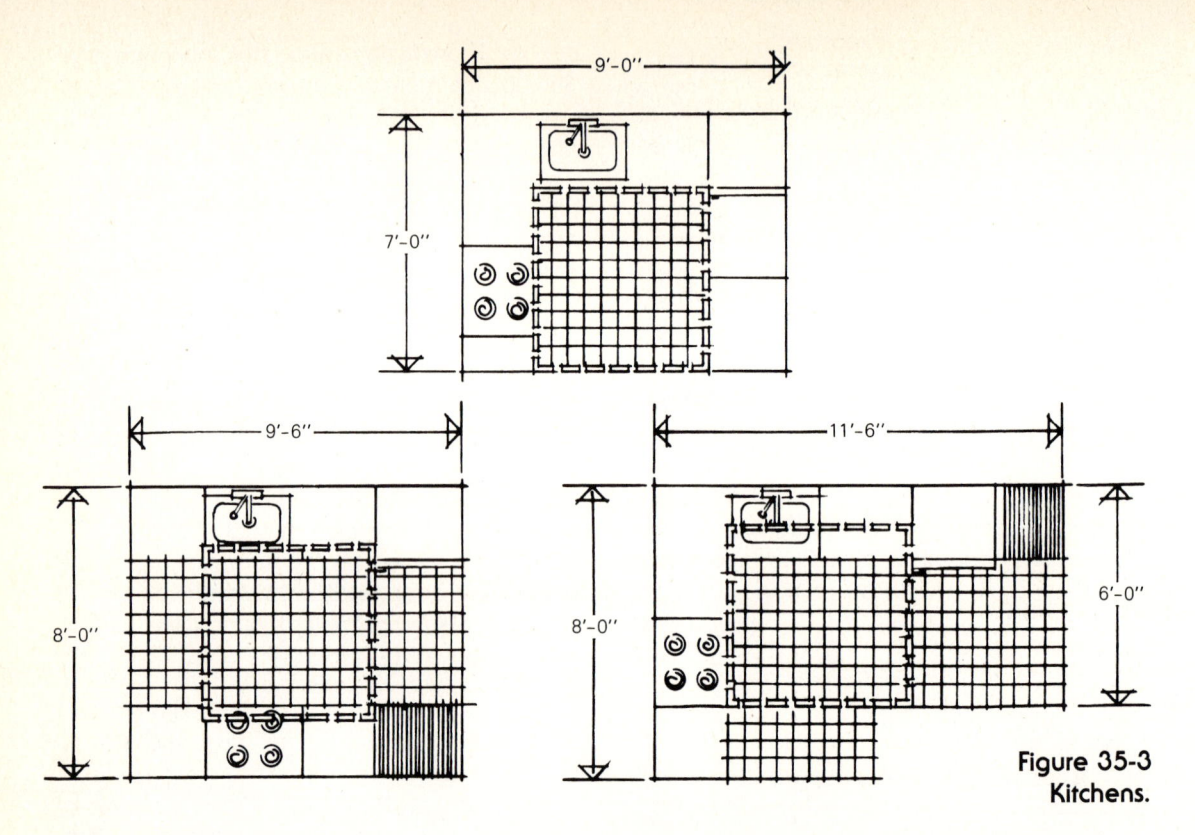

well as in changing of attitudes of those who must comply. There is a continued need to sensitize and educate employers regarding the capabilities of people with physical limitations. Employers must be made aware of the many advances in rehabilitation and technology. They need to know of systems and devices that allow many otherwise limited individuals to function effectively and to perform jobs once thought to be impossible for them. They must begin to recognize that major structural changes for accessibility are seldom necessary, and frequently, only minor changes or none at all are required to accommodate even a severe disability problem. Special equipment can often be provided by organizations other than the employer. Employers are merely being required to give equal consideration to prospective qualified employees who are disabled and to make reasonable accommodations where and if needed. Without such consideration, understanding, and affirmative action, people with disabling conditions will continue to be discriminated against in employment practices.

Recreation and Socialization

Recreation and socialization are additional elements of the network where opportunities are limited by problems of access and attitudinal restraints. Like anyone else, people with mobility problems desire and need recreation and socialization.

Park and recreational services are beginning to incorporate access features in their planning and design. The publication *Barrier-Free Site Design,* which was developed by the American Society of Landscape Architects Foundation (1971) and funded by the U.S. Department of Housing and Urban Development, has offered much useful information and assistance regarding access features.

Opportunities for socialization and cultural experience are still minimal. Theaters and museums have long been inaccessible to many disabled people. Yet the exposure to such avenues of expression is vital to enhancing the quality of life. Fortunately, accessibility to the arts has recently been furthered through a project jointly sponsored by the National Endowment for the Arts and the Educational Facilities Laboratories. Their National Arts and the Handicapped Information Service provides useful information for making arts programs and facilities more accessible to persons with disabilities. It provides information on facilities for educational, social, and cultural services. Such provisions allow for enlarged participation in and appreciation of the arts by disabled persons.

To summarize, the combined network of *all* these individual elements calls for a system of linkages for its proper utilization. Not only must each element be accessible within its own framework, but since they interrelate, they must also be connected by an accessible linkage system. Transportation as well as pedestrian access to sites and buildings form the basis of this system. To provide an improved and enhanced quality of life to people with physical restrictions, these elements must be incorporated into planning and designing of the entire community.

BARRIER-FREE PLANNING AND DESIGN

EVOLUTION AND DEVELOPMENT

The barrier-free movement began in the late 1950s. Following World War II and the Korean war and the resultant growth of rehabilitaion programs for the many disabled veterans, it became evident that those emerging from such programs were being hindered in their continued rehabilitation by man-made obstacles in the environment. They could learn new skills for adapting to their disability and could cope with certain aspects of their surroundings, but few could be prepared for the alarming number of obstacles newly discovered through their forced change of perspective. Parts of the landscape formerly taken for granted assumed new and formidable proportions from the vantage point of a wheelchair or other restricted mobility position. A formerly insignificant curb was as effective a barrier as a stone wall; steps, in effect, meant "keep out"; items formerly reachable were now out of reach. The continuous barrage of frustrations was annoying and discouraging.

In view of the need for modifying and eliminating such barriers, a liaison between the National Easter Seal Society and the President's Committee on Employment of the Handicapped was formed to study the problem and propose some action. As a result, in 1961 the National Easter Seal Society funded a research grant to the University of Illinois to develop building accessibility standards for the physically handicapped. From this research emerged a set of standards known as "Specifications for Making Buildings and Facilities Accessible to, and Usable by, the Physically Handicapped." These standards included basic minimum specifications for accessibility and considered such elements as exterior grading, walkways, and parking; access to and through buildings by way of ramps, entries, doorways, stairs; and interior facilities such as floor surfaces, restroom requirements, drinking fountains, telephones, elevators, and some reference to hardware and identification systems. A national program to educate the building and design professions on these standards was then undertaken.

LEGISLATIVE EFFORTS

Legislation to provide for accessibility in buildings constructed with federal financial assistance was passed as PL 90–480 in 1968 and incorporated the use of these standards (ANSI A117.1) for accessibility. Gradually, states began to adopt, in some form, the ANSI standards, generally relating to state-funded buildings. In many cases, this appeared to be a token effort and few or no attempts were made toward compliance at either the national or state levels.

Figure 35-4
Community access.

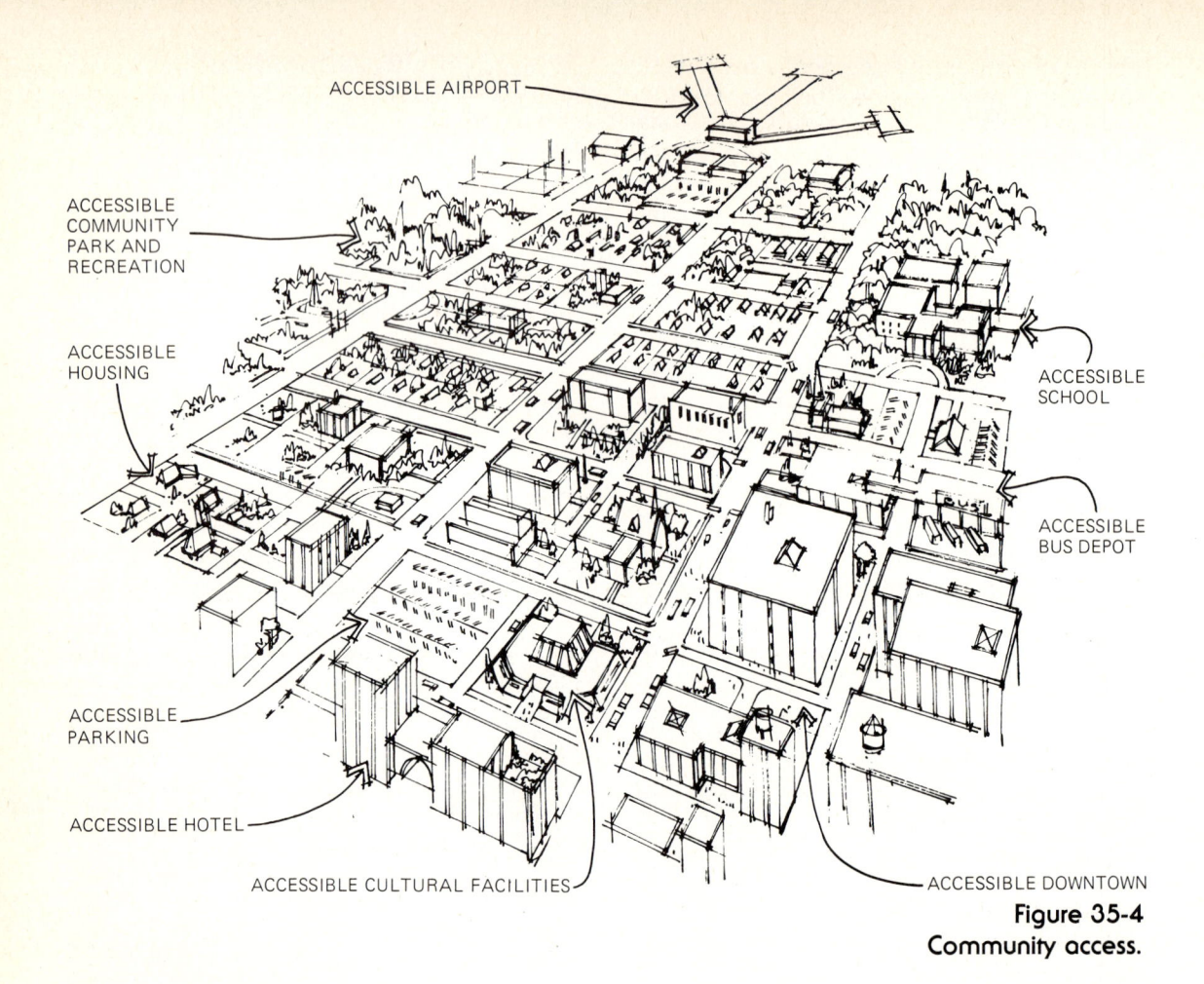

It became apparent that besides the need for greater awareness and education further legislation was required to assure compliance and enforcement. The most important response to this recognized need was embodied in provisions of the Rehabilitation Act of 1973. Several sections of this act had direct and major impact on access, but Section 502 dealt specifically with the enforcement and compliance problems. This section established the Architectural and Transportation Barriers Compliance Board specifically to enforce standards of accessibility required under PL 90–480.

Since the development of the original ANSI standards for accessibility, there has been a growing awareness and with it a more acceptable climate for needed changes. The early requirements, based on strict minimums and suited to the times, have become inadequate in view of the many changes that have occurred since their initiation. New legislation and methods of rehabilitation, the technological changes previously mentioned, as well as the moves to integrate and mainstream people have all combined to prove the need for revising and updating the former standards. Consequently, in 1974, the Department of Housing and Urban Development sponsored a 2-year research and development grant to Syracuse University to revise and update the ANSI A117.1 standards and to include residential provisions as well. This study, now completed, has been approved by the American

CHAPTER 35   740

National Standards Institute and is expected to serve as a much needed unifying force for change in the existing proliferation of nonuniform regulations and standards that are so confusing to builders and designers.

ACCESSIBILITY—THE BROADER VIEW

Beyond the particularized standards and regulations dealing primarily with buildings and their components lies the needed broader view—that of basic access to the community as a whole. This view relates all the major components and their individual elements and ties them together with necessary linkage systems. The major components are the community and its transportation network; individual sites and their related exterior networks, composed of approach, parking, walkways, and entry systems; the buildings themselves and their interior networks of corridors, rooms, and facilities; and finally, equipment and fixtures, including built-in furnishings, surface treatments, and signs.

To accomplish this accessibility linkage means providing selected accessible routes of travel through the environment that connect accessible transportation, public rights of way, sites, buildings, and facilities. The major components to be interconnected are the community, sites, buildings, facilities, and equipment.

Community Access

Access to the community as a whole is, for people with mobility limitations, primarily dependent on public or private transportation and to some degree on the pedestrian right of way. This network includes considerations of loading and unloading areas and overlaps the site considerations of rest, waiting areas, and parking. Access to this network affects access to the elements within the community it serves (see Fig. 35-4).

Site Access

The elements of site access are the next major component in the sequence of network linkages. This component includes public and private property, such as streets, parks, and recreation sites. Its network is composed of the site entrance and walkways, including ramps, curb cuts, stairs, and handrails; parking areas, unloading zones, and waiting and rest areas; site facilities such as swimming pools or site furnishings; and site illumination and signs. These combined elements must also be planned for accessibility in order to provide selected routes of travel linking the major facilities. For example, arrival at a site should provide adequate information as to parking and direction to the accessible entrance. Where parking is provided there should be designated accessible parking spaces displaying the International Symbol of Access and marked "reserved for disabled" (Fig. 35-5). These spaces should be at least $12^1/_2$ ft wide to allow space for wheelchair loading and unloading and should have ramped or open access to an adjacent walkway that connects to the accessible route of travel. Such spaces should be located as near as possible to the building entrance (Fig. 35-6).

A designated or clearly recognizable route of travel should be provided from the site entry or entries to the accessible primary building or facility entry, allowing the person with limited

Figure 35-5
International symbol of access for the handicapped. Designed for display in any suitable size or material on public buildings, hotels, motels, theaters, restaurants, stores, parking lots, conveniences, and transportation facilities of all kinds that are fully accessible for use by wheelchair users and other persons with limited mobility.

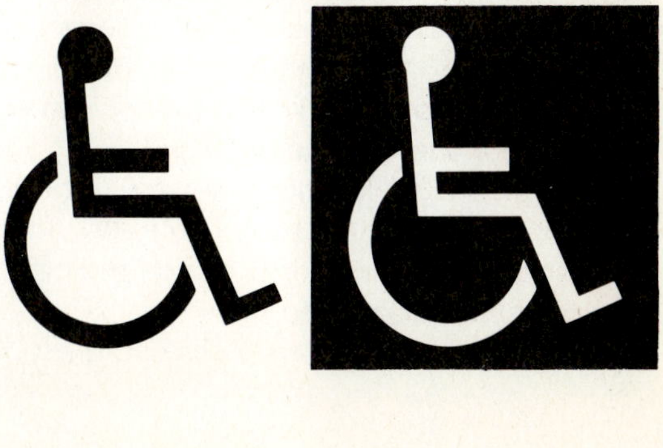

Figure 35-6
Site access.

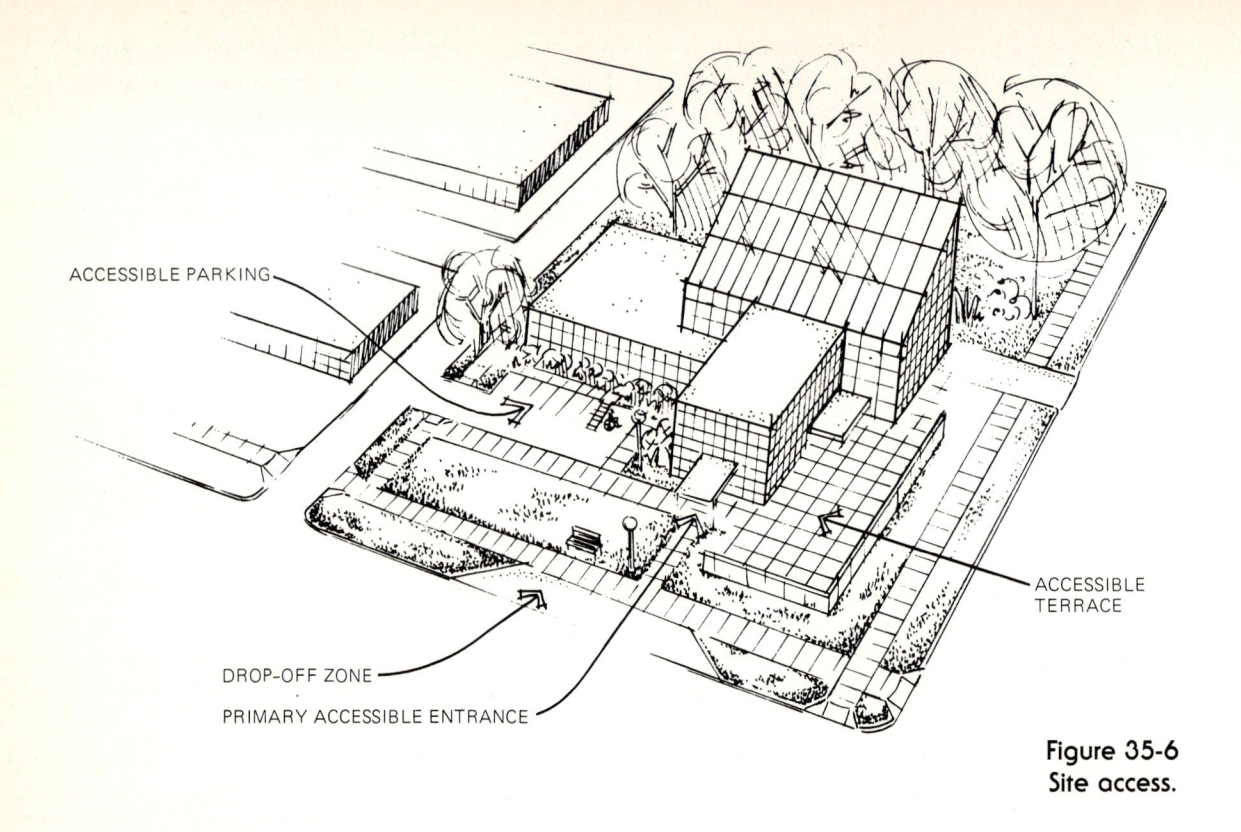

mobility a safe and unobstructed passage. Walkways need to be firm, slip-resistant, and basically level. They should be free of obstructions or protrusions such as site furnishings, signs, or tree limbs. Walks should be at least 48 in wide and avoid abrupt edges or changes in height greater than 1/2 in. Where ramps or curb cuts are provided, the slope should not exceed a ratio of 1:12, or 8 percent, and should preferably be less. Ramps should be clearly designated by contrast from the surrounding surface. Curb cuts should be marked with textured strips to warn the blind or visually impaired or be placed adjacent to (where possible) rather than within the direct line of travel. Ramp length should not exceed 30 ft without a level rest area (Fig. 35-7).

Site signs should identify accessible facilities and routing information where necessary. They should be well illuminated, with large characters on contrasting background.

Building Access

At least one primary public entrance to a building should be accessible, which means that it must have a level landing of at least 5 square ft and be connected by a level or ramped approach or walkway. Entry doors should have at least 36 in clear opening and be easily operable, preferably with a pressure of less than 8 lb. Automatic doorways are of great benefit to many people, as are lever handles. Thresholds should be beveled and no greater than 1/2 in in height, and kickplates at least 12 in high should be provided. A space at least 18 in wide on the strike jamb side of the door allows space for positioning outside the door swing when opening the door from a wheelchair or when on crutches (see Figs. 35-8, 35-9, and 35-10).

Once inside the building, clear directional information should be easily located. The accessible route of travel through the building itself would include connecting the major spaces or components and accessible facilities. In large buildings, these elements may need to be designated by floor location on its directory.

Vertical access by stairs, ramps, or elevators

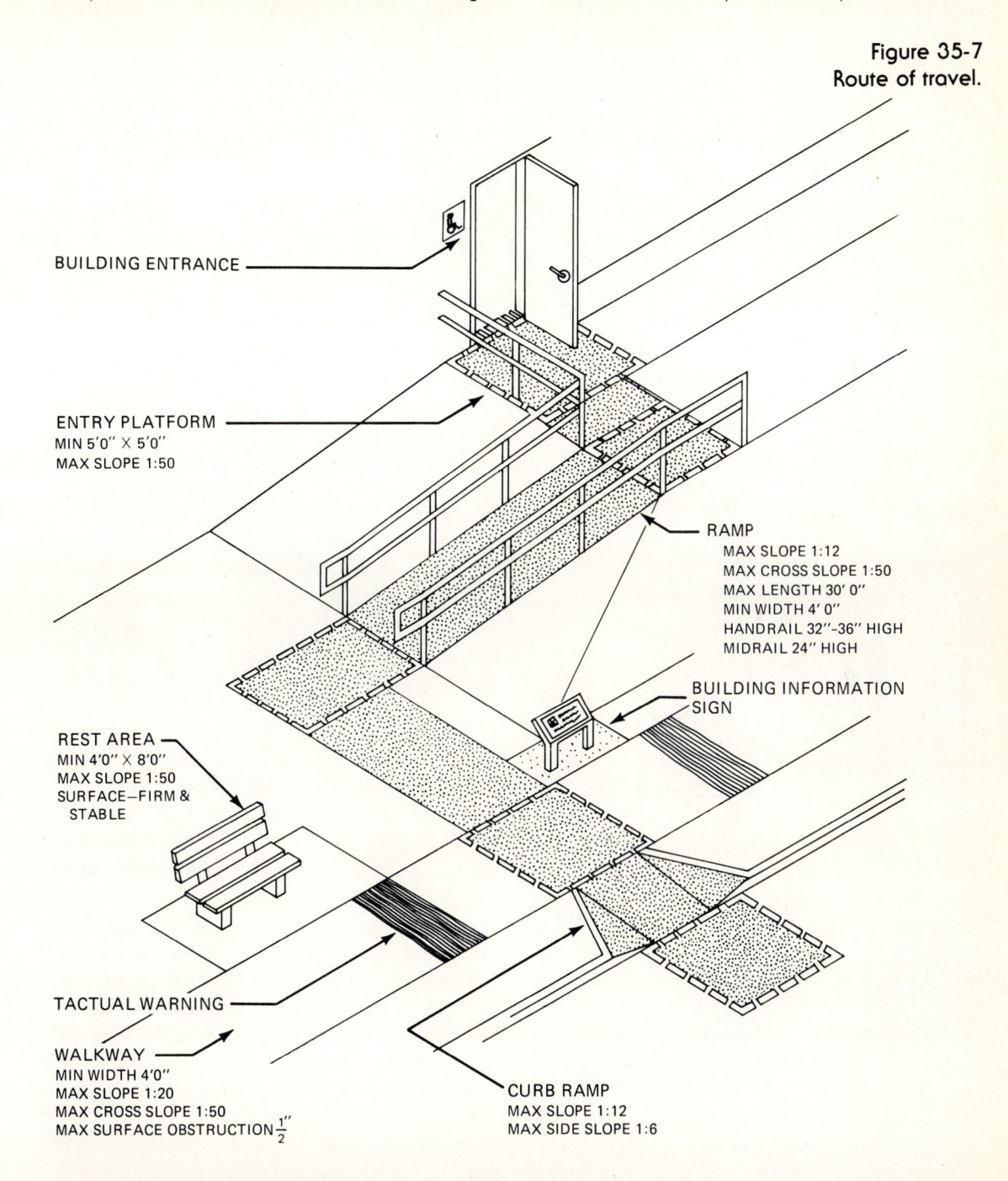

Figure 35-7
Route of travel.

BUILDING ENTRANCE

ENTRY PLATFORM
MIN 5'0" X 5'0"
MAX SLOPE 1:50

RAMP
MAX SLOPE 1:12
MAX CROSS SLOPE 1:50
MAX LENGTH 30' 0"
MIN WIDTH 4' 0"
HANDRAIL 32"-36" HIGH
MIDRAIL 24" HIGH

BUILDING INFORMATION SIGN

REST AREA
MIN 4'0" X 8'0"
MAX SLOPE 1:50
SURFACE—FIRM & STABLE

TACTUAL WARNING

WALKWAY
MIN WIDTH 4'0"
MAX SLOPE 1:20
MAX CROSS SLOPE 1:50
MAX SURFACE OBSTRUCTION $\frac{1"}{2}$

CURB RAMP
MAX SLOPE 1:12
MAX SIDE SLOPE 1:6

743 THE ENVIRONMENTAL SITUATION

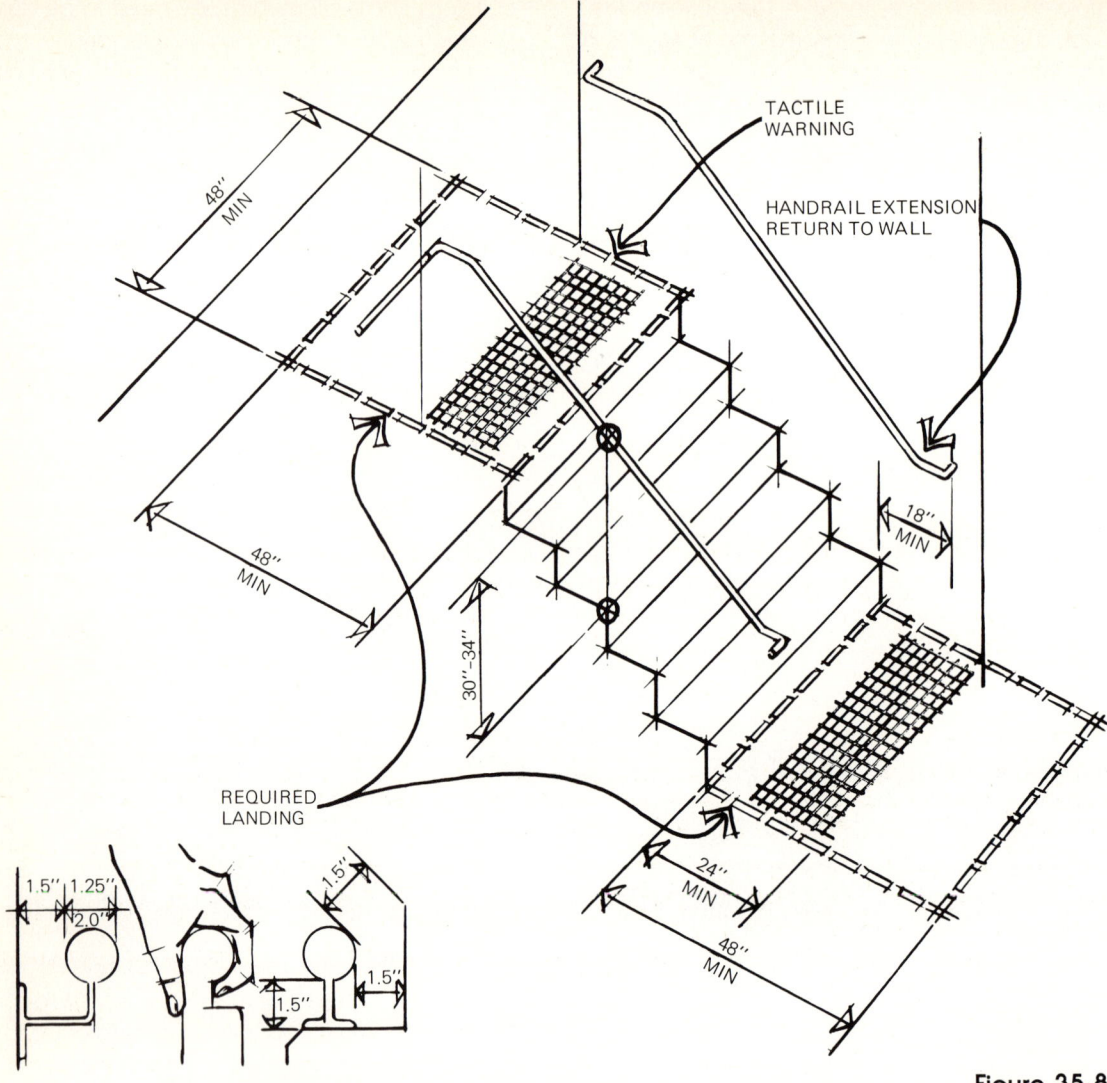

Figure 35-8
Stair and handrail.

must also be properly designed and located. Stairs adjacent to the accessible route of travel (which may be preferred to ramps by some ambulatory disabled) should avoid overhanging or open risers that cause tripping. They should also have securely mounted handrails that can be easily grasped. Ramps, as mentioned above, should not exceed 8 percent in slope and must also provide properly designed handrails. Elevators should be located as near as possible to the accessible primary entry. The elevator cab should be large enough to allow a person in a wheelchair to turn around, and all control buttons should be within reach of a seated person. Control panels should provide tactile identification for the sight disabled by way of raised or recessed lettering or braille markings. Buttons should not be flush with the panel but should instead protrude. Elevator directional signals should be audibly and visually discernible.

CHAPTER 35

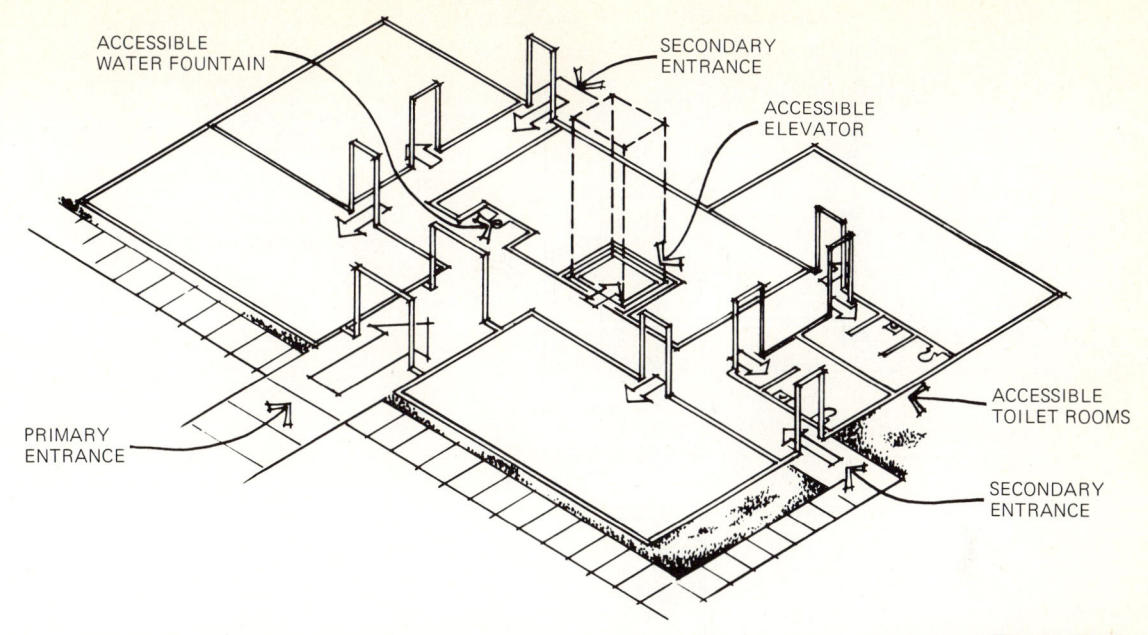

Figure 35-9
Route through building.

Corridors and aisles must be wide enough for wheelchair and pedestrian passage and should also provide wheelchair turning space at reasonable intervals. Doorways should have at least a 32-inch-wide clear opening. Vestibules need to be deep enough and wide enough to allow a person in a wheelchair sufficient space to maneuver without becoming trapped between doors.

Facilities Access

Facilities within the building that should also consider access features include public assembly areas, restrooms, public telephones and drinking fountains, and kitchen and bath facilities in apartments and hotels.

Public restrooms should have adequate maneuvering space for a wheelchair, and facilities such as towel dispensers, mirrors, and shelves should be placed within easy reach. Sinks need to have wheelchair maneuvering space beneath them, and hot water pipes should be protected or insulated. Toilet compartments for the disabled need to provide sufficient space for transfer from the wheelchair. Although the most common method is for a lateral transfer, space provided, as shown in Fig. 35-11, will allow for different positioning of the wheelchair. Compartment doors should swing out, be self-closing, and have lever-type hardware.

Equipment Access

Equipment access includes considerations of hardware, such as door and window operators, plumbing fixtures, switches, thermostats, alarms, and dispensers. Some percentage of fixed furnishings, including drinking fountains, telephones, seating, tables, and counters must be accessible to disabled individuals. Especially important is the ability to manipulate controls and hardware by persons with manipulatory impairments. Lever hardware or controls that are easily operable without precise movements are recommended.

We have already touched upon sign requirements and surface treatments. In addition, floor coverings such as carpeting can be a hindrance to many disabled people. If carpeting is used, it

Figure 35-10 Door.

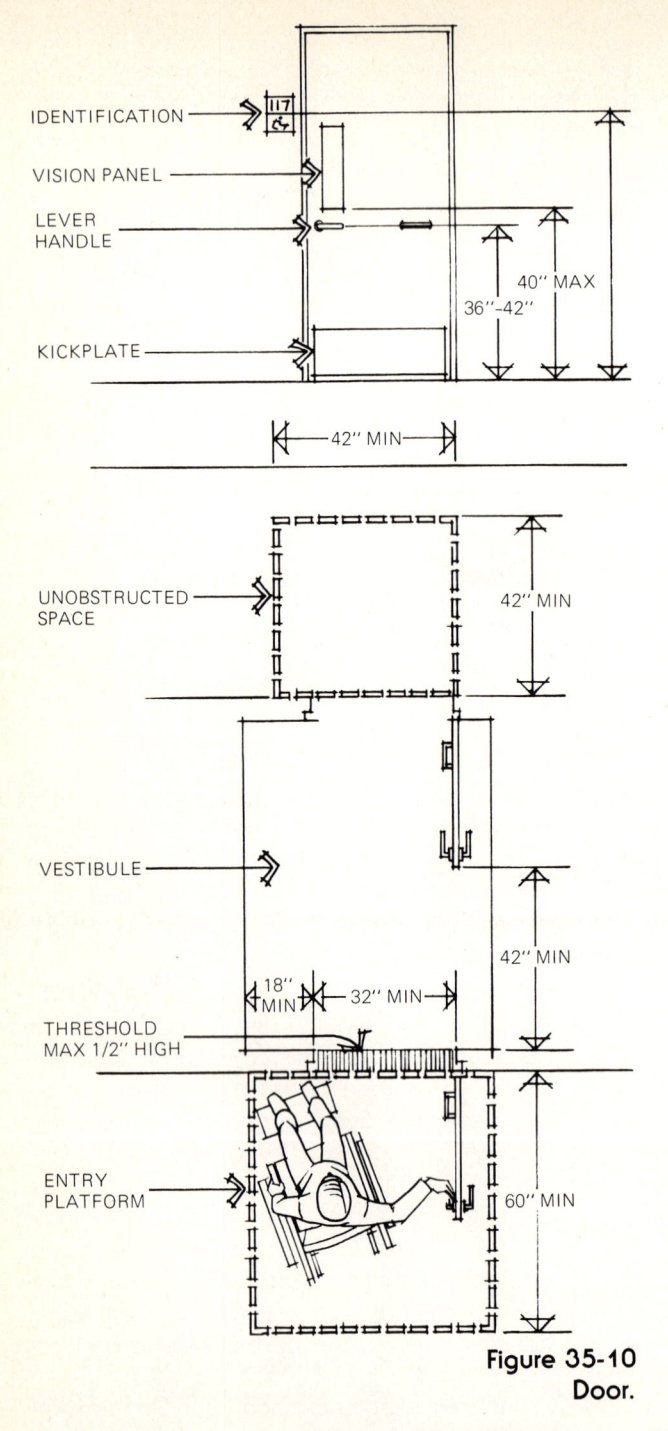

should have a tight weave, a low pile, and preferably be unpadded and glued down or firmly anchored.

This combination of accessible elements and the importance of relating them is what makes the whole composite picture work. The com-

CHAPTER 35   746

ponents of community, site, buildings, facilities, and equipment, together with their linkage systems, compose the overall network of relationships that must be considered by planners when designing to include the disabled population. Planners and designers must begin to

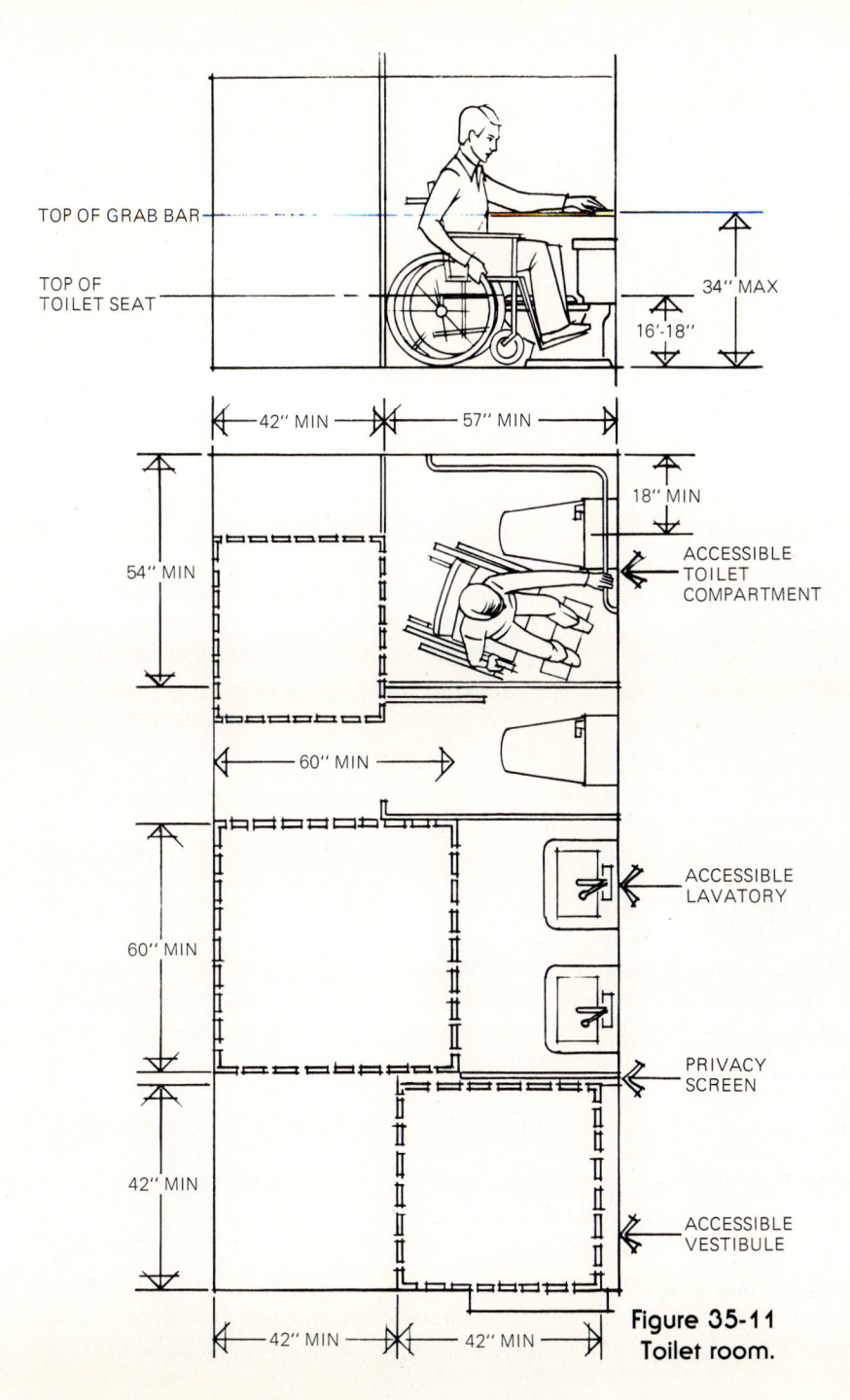

Figure 35-11
Toilet room.

747 THE ENVIRONMENTAL SITUATION

recognize the need for such a network of relationships and thus grow beyond segmental and segregating design. Until this happens, people will continue to encounter needless roadblocks to their progress and to their individual growth development.

ACCOMPLISHMENTS AND PROGRESS

As a result of the continued efforts of the many organizations that assist disabled people, but particularly by the direct and increasing involvement of consumers themselves, progress is being made. Organizations of and formed by disabled people are taking a lead in determining needed direction and change. Notable in this respect was the history-making involvement of over 2000 leaders and representatives of disabled people in the White House Conference for Handicapped Individuals held in Washington, D.C. in May 1977. This conference, authorized by PL 93-516, stated in part: "It is of critical importance to this Nation that equality of opportunity, equal access to all aspects of society and equal rights guaranteed by the Constitution of the United States be provided to all individuals with handicaps." The conference was further authorized to "... develop recommendations and stimulate a national assessment of problems, and solutions to such problems, facing individuals with handicaps." These recommendations have been published and should offer valuable suggestions toward solutions of the identified goals. It is hoped that the momentum generated by this conference, and the national awareness it created of the problems and potentials of handicapped individuals, will continue to effect needed changes.

This gathering, more than any other, crystallized the variety of areas that affect the quality of life for disabled people. The resulting recommendations are far reaching, and the impact of this and other movements is accelerating the changing perspectives of planners and designers. It is slowly being realized that accessibility benefits everyone and that the provision for greater opportunities for advancement and increased quality of life for persons with physical limitations improves the quality of life for us all.

EXISTING NEEDS

At the White House Conference, the specific plea, in terms of barrier-free design, was for better implementation and enforcement of existing statutes. Much progress has been made in legislative mandates, as well as in increased awareness of the need for such design, and perspectives are changing. But there are still many unmet needs. The continuing education of architects and planners is of particular importance. Courses on barrier-free design are still greatly needed in the curricula of schools of architecture and landscape architecture. More continuing education workshops and seminars for architects, builders, planners, and building officials to explain the laws, code requirements, and methods for more innovative design are also needed. Strengthening of existing legislation and enforcement has already been mentioned. And, as previously discussed, we are just beginning to scratch the surface regarding the major needs of housing and transportation.

FUTURE EXPECTATIONS

Largely as a result of legislative measures, as well as related education and awareness, the future outlook seems favorable and promising. The direct and growing involvement of affected users has been a significant influence toward the furthering of accessibility goals and objectives. But much continued effort is needed to reach the ultimate goal of total accessibility for all.

CONCLUSION

The environmental situation as related to persons with limited mobility is a multifaceted one. Positive solutions depend on an understanding of user needs within the overall context of a relationship of networks and components. Newly emergent users, in their mainstreaming and normalization efforts, should be willing to accept the allied responsibility for extending their own capabilities and skills in coping with existing barriers. They should be willing to help bridge the gaps in planning and design by their own efforts and involvement. But planners and designers must also be willing to at least meet this effort part way, in innovative and responsible design and construction. By such mutual extensions, the access gaps in transportation, housing, education, employment, recreation, and socialization can be bridged. Through the combined efforts of consumers, planners, designers, legislators, and others, we are witnessing moves in this direction. Such moves must be assisted by continued awareness and sensitization efforts. Enforcement, education, and innovative design all play an important role in this ongoing movement. By encouraging and participating in such developments, we can assist in making *life* more accessible.

BIBLIOGRAPHY

American National Standards Institute: *Specifications for Making Buildings and Facilities Accessible to and Useable by the Physically Handicapped,* New York, ANSI A117.1, 1980.

American Society of Landscape Architects Foundation: *Barrier-Free Site Design,* U.S. Department of Housing and Urban Development, Washington, D.C., 1975.

Bedner, Michael J. (ed.): *Barrier-Free Environments,* Dowden, Hutchinson and Ross, Stroudsburg, Pa., 1977.

Cotler, Stephen R., and Alfred H. DeGraff: *Architectural Accessibility for the Disabled of College Campuses,* State University Construction Fund, Albany, 1976.

General Services Administration, Public Buildings Service: *Design Criteria: New Public Building Accessibility,* 1977.

Goldsmith, Selwyn: *Designing for the Disabled,* 3d ed., Royal Institute of British Architects, London, 1976.

Harkness, Sarah P., and James N. Groom, Jr.: *Building without Barriers for the Disabled,* Whitney Library of Design, New York, 1976.

Mace, R. L., and B. Laslett (eds.): *An Illustrated Handbook of the Handicapped Section of the North Carolina State Building Code,* North Carolina Department of Insurance, Raleigh, 1974.

McGaughey, Rita: "From Problem to Solution: The New Focus in Fighting Environmental Barriers for the Handicapped," *Rehabilitation Literature* 37:1, 1976.

Small, Robert E., and Barbara L. Allan: *An Illustrated Handbook for Barrier-free Design of the Washington State Rules and Regulations,* Washington State Office of Community Development, Olympia, WA, 1978.

36
sandra mock
jeanette taylor

the future:
commitment to
the disabled?

THE FUTURE

FROM "HANDICAPISM" TOWARD EQUALITY

"Handicapism" is a dirty word. It is a subtle state of discrimination, oppression, and paternalism. Only when it pertains to oneself, a friend, or a family member or when one works in the field does one begin to recognize the complex and interrelated maze of barriers that someone in a wheelchair has to deal with on a daily basis.

Handicapism is stereotyped thinking. In a restaurant, a waiter may ask anyone accompanying a person in a wheelchair what that person would like, as if the person were unable to speak or were a child. This is typical of the handicapped person's daily encounters with the uninformed public.

Handicapism means barriers and disincentives. Architecturally, economically, and therefore socially, society is ill equipped to deal with the physically impaired person who has goals of work and independence.

THE CONSUMER MOVEMENT AND MAINSTREAMING

Current discussion regarding the disabled population covers the issues of normalizing and mainstreaming or integration. Rehabilitation facilities are the front line of resocialization and normalizing. Patients use the rehabilitation facility as a mirror in terms of assessing themselves and redefining their identity. The process of community reintegration begins here; the hospital is a microsystem of society itself.

The consumer movement also helps with the process. The movement provides an opportunity for the newly disabled to share common experience; it interprets the environment and its demands. If the newly injured individual can identify with the disabled community, a great deal of learning can take place, and thus mainstreaming can be accelerated.

Part of the present consumer rights movement is a growing effort to protect the rights of patients in hospitals, nursing homes, and mental institutions. A national organization has been formed by patient representatives. Both the U.S. Department of Health, Education, and Welfare (DHEW) and the American Hospital Association (AHA) have developed standards for the protection of patients. In 1975, the American Civil Liberties Union (ACLU) published a pioneering study, *The Rights of Hospital Patients* (Foster and Pearman, 1978).

"Leaflets listing patients' rights, now given to patients in most hospitals and nursing homes, are an outgrowth of a statement prepared by the AHA (*A Patient Bill of Rights*), the report of the DHEW Secretary's Commission on Medical Malpractice, and the DHEW regulations on patients' rights in skilled nursing facilities" (Foster and Pearman). The AHA statement expresses rights that a patient can now invoke in litigation but is really a prescription for voluntary compliance. Several states have already enacted statutes that contain a patient's bill of rights.

The concern for patients' rights has stimulated the development of patient representatives in many hospitals in various areas of the country. The role of the patient representative, or hospital ombudsman, is that of advocate and patient-grievance mechanism. The patient can speak to this individual about the barriers and problems within the system, and the representative can recommend changes in hospital policies and procedures so that services become more responsive to patient needs and the like. In some hospitals, social workers incorporate this as part of their role, acting as a professional liaison between the patient and the system, but sometimes the social worker's role as a member of the health care delivery team or system is in itself a conflict or barrier to the best interests of the patient. Many malpractice suits could be avoided if patients felt they were respected and that the facility cared. Because institutions can be dehumanizing and demoralizing, the patient representative provides warmth and understanding and improves the hospital's image.

There are now more than 700 patient representatives in the health care system, primarily around the larger metropolitan areas such as New York and Chicago. These are not true patient advocacy programs, however, because the representatives are employed by the hospital and cannot truly represent the patient. They also are not involved in policy making that would affect quality of care or protect patient rights. Experts working in the area of civil liberties and consumer rights recommend patient rights advocates who know both law and medicine and who would be hired by and accountable to the patients they serve. Careful attention must be given to statutory wording to ensure legal rights for patients. Adequate enforcement mechanisms are needed.

What are patients' rights?

1. Informed consent. This is the cornerstone that supports other specific rights. Any medical procedure performed on the patient's body without his or her permission is, in common law, a case of battery constituting both a crime and a tort subject to civil damages.
2. The right to refuse treatment.
3. The right to considerate and respectful care.
4. The right to refuse to participate in experimental research projects.
5. The right to privacy, both personal and informational.
6. The right to confidentiality of records.
7. The right to explanation and planning before transferral.
8. The right to staff indentification.
9. The right to continuity of care.
10. The right to full explanation of hospital bill.
11. The right to knowledge of institution's rules and regulations.
12. The right to private and unrestricted communication.
13. The right to freedom from mental and physical abuse and from physical or chemical restraints.
14. The right to have a written list of rights. (Foster and Pearman, 1978)

LEGISLATIVE CONCERNS AND ISSUES

The White House Conference on Handicapped Individuals, held in May 1977, highlighted concerns and issues to be resolved. Consumers spoke about health, social, economic, and educational concerns. The need to expand research facilities and dissemination of information were discussed. Expansion of health resources was recommended. In the area of health, attention was focused on several factors. One important factor was prevention, with educational programs and media campaigns directed toward schoolchildren. The additional training needs of service providers (physicians, physical therapists, occupational therapists) was another issue. These providers need to have some interaction with consumers who can help to identify needs. The conference recommended training in the areas of research and technology and recruitment of persons who have some commitment as researchers, trainers, and providers. Greater access to health care at an affordable cost was also recommended. Robert R. Humphreys, Commissioner of HEW's Rehabilitation Services Administration, recommends a nationwide service network that will provide a continuum of care for disabled citizens.

Insurance companies make it difficult for the handicapped to obtain personal and automobile coverage. These companies are being urged to get involved in prevention education. Educational mainstreaming is a priority issue for the consumer. Education for the general public, children, and teachers is beginning. Raising the public's awareness level and modifying attitudes are two future goals. Education of clients in terms of their rights and training them to become more critical and assertive consumers are also important.

The law now states that educational facilities, not only buildings but also programs, must be accessible. Universities must explore the best ways to provide programs for special groups. The teaching of sign language to the non-hearing impaired is at least beginning in experimental programs in some institutions. The systematic education for "independent living" is a great need that is being met in a few facilities around the country.

Changing the social scene means preparing teachers to become "change agents." The disabled need to be depicted more often as "normal" in the media and in textbooks. Self-advocacy is being promoted; in 1977, an office was set up as part of the Department of Health, Education, and Welfare to help deal with the issue nationwide. A consumer holds the position of Special Assistant to the Commissioner of Rehabilitation Services. The disabled want to establish lobbies in Washington and speak for themselves. A barrier-free environment as a reality must continue to be pushed for in terms of access in areas such as building codes, transportation, reserved parking, and interpreters for the deaf in hospitals, courts, and police stations. The disabled are concerned about economic disadvantages and want enforcement of equal employment opportunity laws, strengthened affirmative action programs, subsidized attendant and rent programs, aid for structural modifications, travel considerations, more liberal tax deductions, guaranteed minimum income for all persons who cannot work, establishment of independent living centers, and deinstitutionalization of the handicapped.

The whole area of an individual's rights is made up of multiple, interdependent issues. For example, all the rights of a free individual, such as the right to vote, work, learn, and engage in socialization, are based on the assumption that an individual is mobile. If that assumption is incorrect, as it often is in the world of the handicapped person, then it diminishes that individual's capacity to pursue those rights. It is not so much a matter of individual withdrawal because of socialization problems as it is the lack of freedom that service deficits, such as inadequate transportation, make a reality. The lack of low and moderate accessible housing, independent living centers, and home care programming are also part of this double message regarding free choices and independence. There is a growing recognition of the problems and solutions, but legislative action and programs have been slow to develop.

The disabled are increasingly taking up their own cause locally and nationally in such organizations as American Coalition for Handicapped Citizens and Mainstream Inc., a national nonprofit agency to promote affirmative action for the handicapped. The Center for Independent Living in Berkeley, California, is an outstanding example of what is going on in the area of independent community living. This program performs several essential functions: (1) it is active and influences legislation; (2) it knows community resources and mobilizes them on behalf of consumers in the areas of employment, housing, finance, and health; (3) it provides an information service and a quarterly publication of excellent quality; and (4) it offers concrete services, such as counseling, equipment repairs, and an attendant pool. This organization is organized by and for the consumers themselves.

Another program deserving mention is New Options, a project sponsored by the Texas Institute for Rehabilitation and Research in Houston. It is a 6-week live-in program designed to enable severely handicapped persons to acquire skills necessary for integration into the community. It is geared to teach skills for management in all areas, including social, educational, vocational, and independent living training. An impressive aspect of the program is the structured contacts with active and independent severely disabled persons in the community.

The state of Alabama, because of Governor George Wallace, has an excellent Homebound Rehabilitation Program that is financed by the state. All severely disabled persons confined to home are eligible; they receive such services as attendant care, home modifications, equipment and supplies, and services of a home health team.

Special programs focusing on skills, such as attendant management (locating and training an attendant), financial management (programs of assistance and money management), mobility, educational and vocational opportunities, self-care, social skills and/or assertiveness training, and human sexuality hold promise for the increased independence of the physically impaired.

WHAT THE HEALTH PROFESSIONAL CAN DO

Today's consumers of health care services often complain that professionals do not help them in the most effective ways. Rehabilitation is a multifaceted, individual endeavor that touches all aspects of a person's being; it is a point on a continuum, a life experience. In order to be most helpful, professionals must remember this and also that they are part of people's lives for a very brief period and need to focus heavily on activities and techniques that relate to living fully and achieving maximum independence. Independence for all persons actually means a smooth working interdependence, just as everyone needs someone else in some way.

KNOWLEDGE AND UNDERSTANDING

The first step in applying the science and art of rehabilitation to an individual is knowledge and understanding of that person. The person is part of many systems that influence what one is and how one does in rehabilitation. Often, patients cannot articulate their values or the values of their systems and how they came by them, but that does not lessen the importance of those values.

One technique that can be employed for increased understanding is doing a sociological profile of a patient. The social worker asks the patient to list all the groups of which he or she has ever been a member. Nearly everyone lists at least 10 groups; active persons may list three times that many.

Membership in groups may be determined by sex, age, education, religious upbringing, marital status, political affiliation, number of children in family of origin, occupation, place of birth, or present residence. These basic demographics may already be listed on the medical chart. However, hundreds of other groups contribute to and affirm the value system of any individual. Being a Cub Scout, a sorority or fraternity member, an Ivy League graduate, an athlete in a particular sport, a health food enthusiast, a gay man or woman, an environmentalist, or a liberated feminist tells certain things about a person. A group has enormous power of support, pressure of conformity, and influence.

Performing this exercise with a patient provides a way of beginning discussion. The main purpose is to achieve rapport, to give permission for someone to talk in a meaningful way about themselves. Listening to a patient or to family members is a major way of communicating caring. No other factor seems as vital to persons in institutions as to be really heard. Professional staff members must believe that their listening to and caring about what patients say makes a big difference in the patients' perception of their experience, their general satisfaction, and the way they respond to their treatment.

Empathy is an essential skill for a health care professional to develop. Empathy, as defined here, is the ability to imagine "walking in someone else's shoes," to consider how an experience would seem for that person and not in terms of one's own values. To be empathetic, one must learn to listen in a concentrated, feeling way, trying to understand something from another person's point of view. The easiest beginning exercise in learning empathy can be tried with a colleague. One person makes a statement. The other rephrases that statement in a way that is accepted by the first as catching its meaning. The second person then responds to the statement. The most difficult part of empathy is that all persons are so programmed to have their own ideas of what is right and to state their opinions directly or indirectly that it is hard to understand someone else's thinking and to *really* hear and communicate.

COMMUNICATION SKILLS

People communicate best when they speak the same language. The use of medical or psychological terminology or acronyms that are unfamiliar to patients is a barrier to communication. Unless health professionals explain or interpret their meaning to the patient, they may lose the patient's interest as well as rapport. This often results in alienation and is a frequent consumer complaint. Most persons enjoy acquiring new knowledge, and there is no medical information that cannot be communicated adequately to the nonprofessional.

It is the health professional's responsibility to help facilitate learning and to remove barriers. For this reason, the health care team member must learn to view the family in a dual context of resource and client. If family members sense how important their input is and that they have power in decision making, they will be better able to express their concerns, identify their problems, and work toward solutions.

If health care professionals do not establish rapport and meet the needs of the family members, they cannot be expected to perform as caretakers. For example, if a woman is overwhelmed and anxious because of her husband's stroke, her ability to learn will be affected. She will resist taking her husband home on weekend passes because she wants to put off the reality she hates facing.

Both the patient and the family must be taken "where they are" and led down a road of structured education and training that has built-in allowances for less than expert coping and totally stabilized emotions. Fears must be taken seriously and nonjudgmentally, and conditions that enhance basic trust must be established. For example, patients who have lapses of incontinence, or who masturbate in public, or who swear profusely must be dealt with calmly and nonpunitively. It is sometimes necessary to explain to families why a particular behavior is occurring and what to expect. Family members who resist learning how to care for the patient or maintain that they were not meant to "become nurses" have to be accepted, helped to look at all alternatives, and taught when they are ready.

Any information that the patient and family have no control over is usually more sensitive and subject to conflict and resentment. If a decision about a discharge date or the need for a surgical procedure or consultation is brought up casually and from an unexpected source, patients and families feel confused and even angry that "things are being sprung on them" and that they have little control. This is why utilization review discharges are almost always traumatic disasters.

If a patient's or family's responses are extreme or maladaptive, the social worker should try to outline concrete behavioral alternatives that might be helpful and give a rationale for them. The point is not to attack defenses but to give universal guidelines, with support and understanding.

THE HEALTH PROFESSIONAL AS TEACHER

A definition of the health professional's role is in order before she or he begins to teach. Also, it is important to have some understanding of what people expect and to clarify this as necessary. Resistance to change and denial is part of the coping process. In rehabilitation, there needs to be less distance between the expert and the learner (patient and/or family) in order to decrease controls and help facilitate independence. Because a large part of rehabilitation takes place outside the institution, it is reasonable to state that the best role for the professional is that of consultant and teacher. If patients are aware of their condition, their sense of being in control of their lives increases, thereby making them feel as if they can succeed.

Theoretically, there is high correlation between positive rehabilitation outcomes and subjective emotional states such as high self-esteem, feelings of sexual attractiveness, and self-regard. Theory also stresses the influence of the interpersonal environment as detrimental to coping. What it is helpful to teach an impaired patient is that persons who know little about physical impairment may react irrationally and unrealistically to impairment. It is their psychological problem, not the problem of the person with the impairment. Patients should learn to recognize this irrational behavior, attempt to educate and change the views of others, and not devalue themselves because of someone else's discomfort. The reason this is so important is that people's attitudes about themselves really do influence their ability to deal constructively with changes in their lives and the challenges that living offers.

Persons who are happy with themselves are consciously able to avoid habits that are destructive physically and emotionally. Persons who feel good about themselves do not turn, for any period of time, to excessive eating, drinking, and the use of mind-stultifying drugs.

Awareness of oneself and a curiosity about one's condition and treatment should be encouraged. To teach people how to exercise their freedom and their rights is to help them control their lives. One of the most popular ways of controlling illness is with the use of drugs; certainly more difficult and less quantifiable is habit and life-style change. Drugs have side effects and often do not change the problem but only modify or temporarily control it. No one should throw away medication, but everyone should be aware of and try to understand one's body, its needs, and the treatment possibilities. This should be as important as knowing one's job.

The point here is to promote physical and emotional independence in as many ways as possible. An attitudinal change for staff members may be needed. At all times, to the extent possible, all persons should be part of any decision making that concerns their bodies and care. Obtaining informed consent and giving full information to patients and families are part of this issue. Patients may learn their own care only to have this knowledge minimized at a later point. Professionals gradually have to give up control and see themselves as partners with their patients.

Patients and families who seek to be educated in new skills may be ambivalent because of stress and coping. This affects their ability to learn. Everyone requires reinforcement (it is not possible to say "well done" often enough), as well as permission to express feelings about what has happened. Patients and families may feel helpless and inadequate at some point. They may need to borrow temporarily from a professional's "strength," and that professional should be available to teach specific skills when necessary.

Sometimes, a patient or a family member may be so angry, depressed, or generally upset that staff members have a hard time understanding the meaning of the behavior and react in a way that creates more problems rather than solving the initial one. In dealing with this, the first thing to do is to accept that the behavior has meaning for those concerned, even though the meaning is not clear to staff members.

To understand this attempt to adapt, it is necessary to ask three questions:

1   What is the person or family trying to accomplish?
2   What meaning does the attempt at solution have for the individual(s)?
3   Why does this solution seem to offer the best answer at the time?

Sometimes, a patient's presentation of herself or himself is disturbing to the extent that professionals do not value or respect the person. A problem can occur when the values of the health care team members are different from those of the patient. Self-examination is essential. It is difficult, if not impossible, for people to communicate respect if they do not feel it. In such instances, health professionals should either transfer the case or work on their feelings. Sol Gordon, a psychologist, suggests that staff members "burn out" in rehabilitation work principally because of working with clients they do not really value. It is a team member's personal right to make this kind of decision, but professionally, it has to be recognized that it is not possible to work effectively with a person about whom one has strong negative feelings. Such feelings can apply to a whole system with a particular patient and family.

TWO TREATMENT CONCEPTS

Social workers have historically been involved with the "person-in-situation." The goal of such practice is the enhancement of the quality of life. This practice model is very appropriate for working as part of a team to facilitate successful rehabilitation. The social worker performs roles as advocate, mobilizer/broker, educator, and counselor.

- advocate—Is committed to serving individuals who are victims of social injustice.
- mobilizer/broker—Assembles and energizes groups, resources, organizations, and structures to create new ways of dealing with problems that exist or to prevent problems from occurring.
- educator—Interprets details and implications of roles that are desired or expected to be assumed when there is inadequate role preparation or lack of role perception; provides structured learning experiences; gives information; designs growth experiences; acts as a model; and provides feedback.
- counselor—Enables client to cope effectively with the physical and human environment. (Brashear, 1976)

A final suggestion is a treatment concept borrowed from Meyer Gunther, the psychiatric consultant for the Rehabilitation Institute of Chicago. Illness is like adolescence in that it is a time of disequilibrium when things are changing or have changed and emotional reactions are trying to catch up to physical changes and realities such as role changes. So, like adolescents, patients have mixed feelings and needs about dependency-independency issues and are extremely sensitive about what they want to do for themselves and what to expect from others.

The treatment approach is simple:

1. Recognize and acknowledge feelings. Do not confront, as it is not important to be "right."
2. Support achievements toward independence and productiveness and allow for lapses.
3. Give enough structure and thought to interaction so that "acting out" possibilities are minimized and are not destructive.

In all of this, health care professionals are working toward positive functioning, as defined by the patient, and are saying that they are there to help. In order to do this, the team members must feel a sense of wholeness about themselves and impart this feeling to patients and families. Team members must also be equipped with broad theoretical knowledge and be able to consider each theory a resource that has use in particular circumstances.

CONCLUSION

The growing technological ability to sustain life has great implications for impaired individuals. Society has an increased obligation to provide the handicapped with a quality of life and some social programming equivalent to the technological improvements. It is also hoped that more and more persons will take responsibility for their health, not just demanding their rights as health care consumers but also seeing their responsibility for themselves.

The handicapped have a right to their basic civil rights, "the right to vote, the right to gainful employment, the right to equal educational opportunities and freedom of movement" (Douglas, 1976). Many environmental barriers have been legally eliminated to increase the mobility of the handicapped. Attitudinal barriers are more difficult to remove in a society where "rugged individualism" is valued rather than social interdependence (Park, 1977). Societal attitudes can be improved, however, through the use of educational experiences that include both personal contact and dissemination of information. Opportunities for this kind of learning experience should be extended to potential employers and to the community at large by health care professionals and rehabilitation agencies.

How can barriers be removed to bring millions of disabled citizens into the mainstream of American society? Priority status is recommended in three areas:

1. Self-help groups directed toward social action and advocacy. There is renewed interest in this approach and recognition of its effectiveness.
2. Inclusion of social skills or assertiveness training programs in rehabilitation facilities and services.
3. Continued development of coalitions around specific issues where there is mutual interest between consumers, professionals, and the community.

Our futures are tied together, the disabled and the nondisabled. We all have a responsibility to grow if we are to remove the barriers to normality.

BIBLIOGRAPHY

Anthony, W. A.: "Societal Rehabilitation: Changing Society's Attitudes Toward the Physically and Mentally Disabled," in R. P. Marinelli, and A. E. Dell Orto (eds.): *The Psychological and Social Impact of Physical Disability,* Springer, New York, 1977, pp. 194–205.

Brashear, Diane B.: *The Social Worker as Sex Educator,* Sex Information and Education Council of U.S., 1976.

Buscaglia, Leo: *The Disabled and Their Parents: A Counseling Challenge,* Slack, Thorofare, N.J., 1975.

Cobb, A. Beatrix: *Medical and Psychological Aspects of Disability,* Charles C Thomas, Springfield, Ill., 1973.

Collins, Alice H., and Diane L. Pancoast: *Natural Helping Networks: A Strategy for Prevention,* Pub. No. CBC-070-C, National Association of Social Workers, Washington, D.C.

Douglas, William O.: *Gazette* 19:46, 1976.

Foster, Marion G., and William A. Pearman: "Social Work, Patients' Rights and Patient Representatives," *Social Casework,* February 1978.

Gellman, W.: "Projections in the Field of Physical Disability," in R. P. Marinelli and A. E. Dell Orto (eds.): *The Psychological and Social Impact of Physical Disability,* Springer, New York, 1977, pp. 34–48.

Jacques, Marceline E., and Kathleen M. Patterson: "The Self-Help Group Model: A Review," in R. P. Marinelli and A. E. Dell Orto (eds.): *The Psychological and Social Impact of Physical Disability,* Springer, New York, 1977, pp. 270–281.

Lane, Helen, J.: "Working with Problems of Assault of Self-Image and Life Style," *Social Work in Health Care* 1:191–218, 1975.

Park, Leslie, D.: "Barriers to Normality for the Handicapped Adult in the United States," in R. P. Marinelli and A. E. Dell Orto (eds.): *The Psychological and Social Impact of Physical Disability,* Springer, New York, 1977, pp. 25–33.

Perkins, Robert A., Jack B. Parker, and Barry M. Daste: "Multiple-Influence Paradigms in Illness," *Social Casework* 56(9):531–537,

Romano, M.: "Social Skills Training with the Newly Handicapped," *Arch Phys Med Rehabil* 56:559, 1976.

Safilios-Rothschild, Constantina: "Disabled Person's Self-Definition and Their Implications for Rehabilitation," in Garl L. Albrecht (ed.): *The Sociology of Disability and Rehabilitation,* University of Pittsburgh Press, Pittsburgh, 1976, pp. 39–56.

Sussman, Marvin B.: "The Disabled and the Rehabilitation System," in Garl L. Albrecht (ed.): *The Sociology of Disability and Rehabilitation,* University of Pittsburgh Press, Pittsburgh, 1976, pp. 223–246.

The White House Conference on Handicapped Individuals: *Final Report,* Vol. II, Part A, U.S. Government Printing Office, Washington, D.C., 1977.

37

helen m. degner

the insurance industry as a support structure

INTRODUCTION

Philosophically and historically, the insurance industry has been vitally interested in achieving the optimum recovery and rehabilitation of disabled persons. Although rehabilitation efforts are seen in all areas of insurance, this chapter will focus upon workers' compensation insurance as one example of the effective application of rehabilitation concepts within the insurance industry.

HISTORY OF WORKERS' COMPENSATION AND REHABILITATION

In 1911, the first workers' compensation laws, as we now call them, were enacted in the United States. These laws directed industrial employers to assume the cost resulting from occupational disability regardless of any fault involved. Insurance programs were thus able to provide a method whereby employers could relieve themselves of the logistic responsibilities that liability under the law imposed upon them. Under present law, employers may be permitted, under certain circumstances, to insure their own risks, or they may be compelled to insure through a compensation system administered by the state, or they may continue to have the opportunity to obtain coverage through a private insurer.

Rehabilitation of employees who are physically disabled as a result of work-related injuries has always been recognized as one of the primary goals of the workers' compensation system. The experience of insurance companies in the area of physical and vocational rehabilitation has been of major significance to industry and other agencies now active in the rehabilitation field. Employers Insurance of Wausau, Liberty Mutual Insurance Company, Michigan Mutual, Texas Employers' Insurance Association, and Aetna Life and Casualty are prominent among insurers that pioneered in rehabilitation efforts and in some cases provided direct assistance before the inception of the public Vocational Rehabilitation Program in 1918.

In 1928, when only a few public or private agencies were active in rehabilitation throughout the country, Employers Insurance of Wausau established a pilot rehabilitation center in Wausau, Wisconsin, to demonstrate what could be accomplished in restoring disabled workers to a productive role in society. As time passed and similar services gradually became more broadly available throughout the nation, the Wausau pilot rehabilitation center was closed, having fulfilled its original purpose.

Until the early 1940s, rehabilitation was primarily concerned with acute medical and surgical aspects of an individual's physical restoration. Since World War II, rehabilitation has come to mean "the process of decreasing dependence of the handicapped or disabled person by developing to the greatest extent possible, the abilities needed for adequate functioning in the individual situation" (Krusen, Kottke, & Ellwood, 1971).

Minor injuries or illnesses that are to varying degrees self-limiting and therefore of some concern to the insurer represent only a small portion of the problem to be addressed. The major social concern is the assumption of responsibility by employers for those who are disabled as a result of injury on the job. Effective intervention almost always results in shorter periods of disability, less residual disability, and less expense.

George P. Sawyer, Vice President, Liberty Mutual, summarizes the concern of the insurer in this way:

> As a matter of practical economy, we want to limit the effects of injury . . . the measure of good medical care is not the amount of the fee, but the quality of results for the patient. Medical science has progressively reduced lost time due to injury or illness. Techniques now available save the lives of many that normally would not have survived the initial impact of trauma. Patients with injuries that were once totally disabling can now return to many kinds of gainful employment. This gives an incentive to push the rehabilitation effort beyond the primary curative stages of medicine. No longer can we be concerned only with restoring the body, but now we must teach

people to lead useful lives within the limits of their ability. The patient who returns to work earlier or with a smaller residual impairment is better off, and so are we (Sawyer, 1975).

The insurance industry takes all the aspects of rehabilitation seriously. The insurer's responsibilities for effective medical coordination, cost control, and sound rehabilitative efforts are necessitated not only by internal interests but also by society's funding mechanisms and social conscience. The dimensions of the problem are more clearly seen when one realizes that

> Three out of four people will suffer an industrial injury before they retire.
> One disabling injury occurs every 3 min.
> Approximately $20 billion is spent for compensation each year.

THE TEAM CONCEPT APPLIED TO THE INSURANCE INDUSTRY

The team concept has long been stressed in care of the disabled, and the insurer's approach to rehabilitation is based on this concept: a group of individuals working closely and cooperatively together to achieve a common goal. Each member adds knowledge and skills to the effort, enabling the team to tackle and solve problems in the most effective way.

A simplistic representation of the team approach to rehabilitation that can be applied to any line of insurance can be obtained by dividing the approach into three segments—the claimant's team, the therapeutic team, and the insurance team.

CLAIMANT'S TEAM

The disabled individual is the rehabilitation team's most important member, as only the claimant can be rehabilitated. Other important members of the claimant's team obviously include family members, friends, coworkers, and perhaps the claimant's attorney.

THERAPEUTIC TEAM

The therapeutic team consists of all those health professionals who can provide curative or functional restoration services required by the claimant. Members may include physicians, nurses, physical and occupational therapists, and others with specific skills who join the team as needs are defined, such as social workers, prosrthetists, psychologists, vocational evaluators, and rehabilitation counselors.

The therapeutic team must realize that the insurer will be working with many claimants for the remainder of their lives, and there must be continued planning to maximize abilities and prevent further disability. Only by establishing a good and continuous relationship can the insurer fulfill its proper role and meet fully its obligations. This calls for close and continuous teamwork, as well as clear and prompt communication concerning information, problems, observation, goals, solutions, decisions, and accomplishments. The sense of a common goal to be accomplished must be sustained through a systematic flow of effective communications.

INSURANCE TEAM

The insurance team is defined by the insurer; it may well include medical coordinator, claim supervisor, representative or adjuster, certified rehabilitation counselor, safety consultant, and of course the insurance nurse. The claimant's employer is also an important member of this team through such representatives as personnel department staff, occupational health nurses, and union representatives.

THE NURSE WITHIN THE INSURANCE INDUSTRY

The insurance industry's nursing services have broadened and changed substantially through the years since Metropolitan Life launched a home nursing program for policy holders in

1909. Metropolitan continued this service for 44 years and then shifted the voluntary responsibility to the appropriate professional and community organizations that had by then been developed and expanded to meet various health needs. In 1928, Employers Insurance of Wausau became the first workers' compensation insurer to provide industrial nursing service to policyholders. Over the years, this service expanded into areas of employee health, occupational health, and insurance nursing.

Although recognizing the need for long-term professional services, the recent increase of nurses within the insurance industry has been nothing short of phenomenal. Liberty Mutual Insurance Company, Employers Insurance of Wausau, Hartford Insurance Group, CNA/Insurance, Fireman's Fund Insurance Companies, Industrial Indemnity, and Texas Employers' Insurance Association are a few of many insurers that employ their own rehabilitation nurses. In the private sector, such agencies as International Rehabilitation Associates and Homemakers-Upjohn have developed programs on a contractual basis. The Industrial Commissions in some states, such as Florida and North Carolina, have established their own units of rehabilitation nurses to work in liaison with workers' compensation insurers.

INSURANCE NURSE ACTIVITIES

As the purpose of the rehabilitation center may be considered to be the bridge between the acute-care hospital and the home, the role of the nurse within the insurance industry may be viewed as a bridge between the onset of the disability and the long-term integration of the disabled client into his or her former roles. The insurance nurse is at once afforded the luxury and responsibility of being the health professional who follows the client from the onset of the disability through resolution and assimilation of the disorder. The insurance nurse is relied upon to assume responsibility for maintaining nursing standards by actions with and through others to provide coordinated service to the patient for the achievement of rehabilitation goals. The nurse also brings about the integration of medical and ancillary service by providing meaningful exchanges of information among patient, physician, family, employer, and attorney. The nurse's role is that of a health professional who is not directly involved in claim handling; as such, the nurse can provide an active and positive force for the client.

PERCEPTION OF THE INSURANCE NURSE BY NURSING COLLEAGUES

It is not unusual for the insurance nurse to be viewed suspiciously and be received negatively by nurses in acute hospitals or rehabilitation agencies when these nurses have had no prior working relationship with insurance nurses. In an attempt to "protect the patient" from the insurance nurse who only "wants to save the insurance company money," efforts will be made to hide information, and in other ways, to hinder communication regarding the patient's situation. By so doing, services to the patient are at best slowed and at worst seriously damaged.

While all nurses must vigilantly protect the privacy and confidentiality of their clients, nurses also have the equally important responsibility to foster appropriate communication when it is in the client's best interest. The insurance nurse must, of course, be appropriately identified. It is also helpful if the nurse can be introduced by a hospital or rehabilitation agency nurse with whom the insurance nurse has had a prior effective working relationship.

EARLY INTERVENTION

The earlier the insurance nurse becomes involved, the better will be the potential outcome for the client. Promptness is the most essential item in medical treatment and rehabilitation services. The nurse must be able to recognize and evaluate chronic illness or disability at the onset. Too often, the acute medical aspects of an injury or illness are treated without consideration for long-term rehabilitation goals.

Reliance upon the insurance nurse for assuming responsibility for guiding a client's rehabilitation program is based upon the nurse's abilities. For insurance nurses to function effectively as members of the insurance team, they need actual experience in following and practicing rehabilitation procedures for medically diagnosed categories such as spinal cord injury, brain damage, amputation, and burns. Professional skills obviously must be updated regularly.

There is constant need to look ahead and formalize the course of action involving the claimant, the insurance team, and the therapeutic team. Delay and duplication of effort can be eliminated by planning, which also assures the efficient use of personnel and skills, and this, in turn, helps to minimize medical and vocational costs.

BROAD SCOPE OF RESPONSIBILITIES OF THE INSURANCE NURSE

The insurance nurse's responsibility to assess the total situation, arrive at a nursing diagnosis, counsel, develop goals, and provide close follow-up of cases presents the best of all worlds. There are few positions in nursing that offer the opportunity for practice in acute-care facilities, in the home, in industry, and in the community. Following are just a few of the diverse tasks of the insurance nurse:

- Reviewing claim files to evaluate medical and related data
- Hospital visits to assist in early discharge and referral to home care services where indicated
- Physician contacts to confirm and discuss the treatment regime, as well as short- and long-range plans
- Evaluation visits and referrals to rehabilitation facilities
- Employer visits to assess employment opportunities
- Family visits to help achieve optimum development of personal resources
- Surveys of home or plant to evaluate accessibility and recommend alterations to remove or reduce obstacles and increase mobility of the disabled.

A collection of data on the return of rehabilitation patients to work revealed that of all individuals returning to the job, 77 percent had been assisted by an insurance company's nurse at some stage of the rehabilitation process and that 93 percent of those in retraining programs had been assisted by insurance nurses (McKay, 1976).

VOCATIONAL CONSIDERATIONS

All of our medical management, cost control, and rehabilitation efforts ultimately have the goal of returning the patient to work or to some vocationally oriented alternative. Aggregate experience has taught the insurance industry that individuals with minor injuries and minimal handicaps should, wherever possible, be returned to work immediately. The two most important factors in such a decision are the severity of the injury and the individual's job requirements. An office worker with a fractured leg in a long leg cast is capable of full-time sedentary work, but such an injury to a construction worker precludes employment until the person is substantially returned to the physical status enjoyed before the injury.

Industrial rehabilitation cases are highly specialized and should be considered differently from those involving similar but non-work-related injuries. For example, in a recent review of 200 low back injuries seen at the Industrial Injury Clinic in Neenah, Wisconsin, by Dr. William F. Kennedy, only 17 percent of the cases involved disability for purely physical reasons.

Most employers realize that good personnel practices are the key to rehabilitation, and they are genuinely interested in taking the individual back in their employ. In order to achieve this,

38

john a. mcwethy

going back to work:
a personal recollection

Never will I forget the day I returned to work. Eight months before, an auto accident had severed my spinal cord, paralyzing me from the shoulders down. In the hospital, I often dreamed of returning to my job as an editor of the *Wall Street Journal* and just as often doubted I'd ever make it back.

Had I suffered the injury a few years earlier, prior to the advent of modern rehabilitation medicine, the nursing and other medical care I received would not have existed, and the chances of resuming my old position would have been nearly nonexistent.

In this chapter, I will tell the story of how I managed to resume a useful life. I will relate what happened at the Rehabilitation Institute of Chicago (R.I.C.), where doctors, nurses, and therapists gave me the know-how and helped me generate the determination that enabled me to wheel back to my desk and job at the paper. I will discuss my initial experiences when I resumed my position as an editor and continue with details of the many and significant adjustments I made over the ensuing 7 years until I reached the age of 65 and retired.

My experience has much in common with other spinal cord cases, amputees, the blind, and others who have overcome severe physical disabilities and yet returned to work or obtained a job. The difficulties I encountered, my approach to them, and the way I handled them will, I hope, enable nurses and others who may read this account to better understand those going through rehabilitation and thus help them cope with the problems of employment.

It all began on a cold afternoon in late February 1971. The car I had rented inexplicably careened off Interstate 70 west of St. Louis, flipped over, and ended upside down. Hours later, I regained consciousness in the intensive care unit of St. John's Mercy Hospital. My fifth and sixth vertebrae had scissored across each other 2 inches, severing my spinal cord.

A decision that proved crucial for my return to work was made before I left the hospital in St. Louis. Looking back from the perspective of time, it seems to me the decision was one of the wisest my wife and I made. Should I stay in St. Louis for the rehabilitation, or would further hospitalization at the prestigious Craig Rehabilitation Hospital in Denver work better? We also considered rehabilitation at highly recommended institutions in California and Boston. Our choice of R.I.C. was dictated by a number of considerations, but the one that proved of greatest value in relationship to my position with the *Wall Street Journal* was that it was close to my job. This did much to enable me to keep closely in touch with those who worked for me and with business friends in Chicago.

My rehabilitation began in earnest on April 4, 1971, the day I was flown from St. Louis to Chicago in a jet ambulance plane. After the customary questioning and tests, R.I.C. subjected me to a coaching program fully as painstaking as that of a professional football player. My coaches, however, were the nurses, therapists, doctors, and supporting staff at R.I.C.

The approach R.I.C. took was one it customarily follows. As soon as the staff had appraised my condition and needs, I was placed on a regular "PT" and "OT" schedule. At first I did not even know the meaning of the letters, but they quickly became my major concern, the path over which I might return to something at least approaching a normal life. PT, of course, is physical therapy, and OT is occupational therapy.

Over the next 6 months, I wheeled down to PT morning and afternoon, 5 days a week. Little by little, I was able to sit up without becoming intolerably dizzy. The therapists taught me how to propel my wheelchair and directed me in exercises to strengthen those muscles that had not been deadened by my accident. Mostly, these were the muscles in my shoulders and arms. Initially, I could not sit for more than a few minutes without the skin on my buttocks turning red, threatening to deteriorate into a pressure sore. But my sitting tolerance lengthened as the skin toughened, so that by the time I left R.I.C., I was able to remain in the chair for 6 h with several brief lifts by my attendant during that period. For much of my hospitalization, I used a heavy wheelchair with a back that could be lowered by an aide to relieve dizziness. But as the day of my discharge neared, the doctor and therapists switched me to a lighter chair with a rigid back and prescribed this model for my permanent use.

Experiences that were not part of these formal rehabilitation procedures played a key role in my getting back to work. One of them took place while I was in a regular PT session. It made a deep impression on me. For the sessions at PT, I was dressed in old, rumpled clothes like most of the patients. They were easy to put on and readily washed if there was a catheter failure. Keeping urine off the skin is fundamental to avoiding skin problems that could rapidly end one's employment. I looked like someone's gardener rather than an editor of a major newspaper. Clothes may not make the man, but I found they had a lot to do with the image I had of myself.

I looked up from the mat where my young, athletic-looking therapist was bending my legs up and down in a range of motion routine. Rolling our way was a well-dressed, middle-aged man. He looked like he had come right out of my old world of business and finance. The startling discovery I made was that he, too, was a quad. More surprising to me was that he had "graduated" from R.I.C. and obtained a job as an architect working for the city of Chicago. If he could do it, I reasoned, I could too! The impression he made on me was deepened because it was unrehearsed and happened at precisely the point in my stay at R.I.C. when I sorely needed inspiration and goals.

Incidents like this, some entirely by chance and others contrived by people on the R.I.C. staff, did much to prepare me for the long jump back to my job. Rehabilitation medicine, it seems to me, should be very flexible and adapted to the diverse needs of those who benefit from it. I found that flexibility present in abundance at R.I.C.

The occupational therapists assigned to me had more to work with than their colleagues in PT. My brain and head were not paralyzed. Fred Taylor, who was managing editor of the *Wall Street Journal* at the time of my injury, put it graphically in a letter he wrote to me in the summer of 1971, when my mood was still dark:

> As you must know, but I think it bears stating, your value to the *Journal* lies not in your ability to hop, skip or jump, but in your judgment of people and news, which has proved over the years to be high. We can always hire someone to hop, skip and jump if we need those activities.

Those words were very encouraging, but it took the occupational therapists to help me find ways to bridge the gaps opened by my handicap. As an editor, I needed to use the telephone, type, write, and dictate. So we began experimenting. It took alterations in equipment and seemingly endless practice, patience, ingenuity, and stubborn determination.

The therapists pointed the way, but I was able to find a number of practical adaptations for the techniques they taught me that made them much more workable for a newspaper editor. The telephone is indispensable to an editor of a wide-ranging newspaper like the *Wall Street Journal*. It's doubly so for one who cannot walk or readily go to see people.

With no use of my fingers, I could not pick up the phone to talk or listen. The therapists fitted me with hand braces utilizing my wrist extensors, muscles that were not destroyed, so I was able to grip the instrument. But my arm was so weak, I could not hold it up to my ear for even a minute. By putting a stick or pencil in the brace, I could come close to pushing the Touch-Tone buttons but did not have quite the strength to handle the operation.

I related my frustrating experience with the telephone to my assistant at the *Wall Street Journal*, Harlan Byrne. "I'll talk to Joe O'Brien at Illinois Bell Telephone Company," he said. "Maybe he'll have some ideas for helping you." Joseph P. O'Brien is an assistant vice-president of the Illinois Bell Telephone Company, and an old friend.

The next day, Joe came to see me at R.I.C. The day after that, two engineers from his

CHAPTER 38   768

company appeared. They fitted my phone with a metal gooseneck that held the instrument up to my ear, loosened the push-button springs so I could activate them, and found a toggle switch to turn the phone on and off. The toggle switch, which I could operate by striking it with the side of my hand, led to other applications for the device. I obtained similar switches that I now use for such purposes as turning on my electric typewriter, lights, and radio.

The telephone illustrates not only how I was able to go beyond routine procedures to fit them to my work needs but also how I turned back to my associates at the *Wall Street Journal* and to business friends for help. I could not have done this had I been in a hospital remote from my place of employment.

Proximity to the *Wall Street Journal* again was important in enabling me to cope with dictating. My therapist suggested that a dictating machine would facilitate my going back to work. Instead of typing or writing longhand, why not talk into a machine and have a secretary transcribe it? So we tried a number of different kinds of tape recorders and dictating machines. My therapist helped me adapt this kind of equipment so I could use it, but I found I was so in the habit of thinking with a typewriter that my efforts at dictating were discouragingly poor.

So again I turned to my employer. My secretary came over to R.I.C. with a huge stack of letters that needed replies, and I dictated answers. Gradually my dictating improved. It was good enough when I returned to work so I could do passably well.

There was yet another way that our choosing Chicago for the long hospital period of rehabilitation paid off. I was placed in a room at R.I.C. with Dr. Israel Goldiamond, a professor of psychology at the University of Chicago. His wife, Betty, wrote another chapter in this book, the one on resocialization. Dr. Goldiamond suffered a spinal cord injury several months before mine. Evenings and weekends, when not engaged in therapy, I noticed many of his students called on him, and soon he was conducting seminars from his hospital bed. So I copied him. Before long,

reporters from my paper began calling. Seldom did a day pass that I did not see or talk with one of my *Wall Street Journal* associates. This keeping in touch with my job, which would not have been possible at a distant hospital, was very effective in enabling me to resume my preinjury position at the paper.

Extension of routine occupational therapy in another direction also facilitated my return to work. The public relations department and one of the directors of R.I.C. put me to a test that helped my typing and editing and, most of all, gave me a shot of much-needed self-confidence. The director, Maurice B. Rotman, a skilled Chicago public relations practitioner, visited me one afternoon as I rested in my hospital bed. I had known him for years, so he was acquainted both with my rehabilitation case and my basic journalistic skills.

He suggested that I prepare the dedication message for the $26 million building R.I.C. was about to begin constructing. At first, I thought he didn't mean it but was trying to make me feel good. I did not think I could possibly handle the task. It was to prove one of the most difficult jobs I ever undertook. I could barely write with a ballpoint pen. My typing was exasperatingly slow and crammed with errors. I could not think well when typing with my arms, sticks, and hand braces. But Maurie, the public relations director for R.I.C., and my occupational therapist persuaded me to tackle the task of writing the dedication.

Those 250 words took me nearly a month to compose in readable, literate form. I thought about it at night when I couldn't sleep. I typed at it in OT. I took it home two weekends and labored with ballpoint pen to edit my rough versions. Back at R.I.C., I finally typed it in fairly good form on a typewriter in OT. What I had written was read at the dedication ceremonies and printed for wider distribution. It demonstrated to me that I could type and write reasonably well. Perhaps I could manage to go back to work.

Developing self-confidence, however, went much beyond composing the dedication message. Everything certainly did not work in that direction. As the end of my stay at R.I.C. approached, I had an experience that made me doubt I could ever surmount the obstacles involved in going back to work.

Nursing assistants, that is, aides and orderlies, were an integral part of my rehabilitation experience. They dressed me, changed my catheter, told me about other quads, handled my bowel care, bathed me, and before I could again use a spoon and fork, fed me. My relationship with them was as intimate as that between a baby and its mother.

By far the most experienced and efficient of the nursing assistants was a middle-aged orderly whose regular job had for years been in the paraplegic ward of one of Chicago's large veterans' hospitals. At R.I.C., he moonlighted during the evening shift. He could straighten a pair of trousers better and in less time than anyone else. At bathing me and handling my bowel care, he had no equal. He had a ready answer to explain my wide variety of aches and pains. Naturally, I had develped great faith in his wisdom. So his comment one evening on my ambition to go back to work struck me hard and has remained vividly in my mind. "I have known dozens of quads like you," he told me, "and none of them was able to work. You will never make it back to the *Wall Street Journal*."

Other experiences I was having, some meticulously planned by R.I.C. and others fortuitous, worked in the opposite direction. Our youngest son, Jack, decided to get married in July, after I had been at R.I.C. about 3 months. Should I attempt to attend? Could I make it? My wife, my brother-in-law, who is a surgeon, my son, and the staff at R.I.C. made up my mind for me. They dressed me in sport jacket, colorful tie, and my best wool slacks. An orderly wheeled me to the ambulance entrance, and I was loaded in the car for the hour-long drive to Crown Point, Indiana. At a motel on the edge of town, I was unloaded and stretched out on the bed so I could remain up for the ceremony without developing skin problems. Then on to the wedding. I could not restrain a flood of tears. And tears did and still do make my nose run. My wife wielded the handkerchief. Then came a huge backyard reception with dozens of our close friends, a flood of champagne, heaps of food, and a torrent of talk. The trip back reversed the outward journey and was uneventful.

The wedding gave me some insight into how difficult it is for one in a wheelchair in large crowds. This was to help me when I was back at work. I am 6 ft 4 in tall and was accustomed to looking down on most people. In a wheelchair, I come up to most people's hips. I'm often ignored in crowds. Weeping and a running nose, I discovered, are serious problems. I'd have to solve them before I could handle my job well. But I managed the test of participating in the wedding, and my confidence rose.

The recreational therapy department at R.I.C. bolstered my confidence, too. I attended a number of motion pictures with its help, went to a ballet, and one evening got to a performance by Beverly Sills, the opera coloratura.

The nurses at R.I.C. were the glue that held the foundation for my return to work together. Skin care, bowels, catheters, leg bags, sleeping, diet, and a host of other aspects of helping a quad return to a somewhat normal life came under the aegis of the nursing staff. But the best nurse has turned out to be my wife. The staff at R.I.C. taught her the fundamentals of caring for a quad. The divorce rate among quads is about 90 percent. The nursing and other help I have had from my wife put her in that small minority who have stuck with their mates. Weekends, as my discharge approached, she drove me home to suburban Western Springs, and we practiced going it alone without R.I.C. staff help.

Life began again for me on November 1, 1971. That was the day I returned to work, 36 weeks after my injury. It took all I had learned at R.I.C., the continuing loving and courageous backing of my wife, and a great many concessions and much encouragement from the people at the *Wall Street Journal* to get me through that first terrifying, trying day and the many that followed.

A 9 months' vacation might be restful or make

CHAPTER 38 770

one better fitted to carry on with work. But being hospitalized for that length of time did not have that effect on me. As the months dragged slowly by, I increasingly felt that returning to my old job was beyond the possible. How could I physically get to work? Before my injury, I walked briskly the half mile to the train, read three newspapers en route to the city, walked to our office, and by 9:30 was at my desk, sleeves rolled up, telephone ringing, and people clamoring for decisions. What would reporters who worked for me think if the catheter I now depended on twisted and burst? I could not bend down to empty the leg bag that catches my urine. So how was I to empty it during my working day? Before my injury, I would pound out a page on my typewriter in 3 or 4 min. With hand braces and two pencils, it took me an hour to turn out that much.

Relive that initial working day with me. It began at 7 A.M., the same time I rolled out of bed before my injury. That was one of the few aspects of my day that was unchanged. My 19-year-old attendant, Bruce Addleman, whom we had hired a week prior to my discharge from R.I.C., teamed up with my wife to dress and transfer me to my wheelchair. He wheeled me to our kitchen, where I shaved, brushed my teeth, and had breakfast.

My preinjury overcoat was too long for a wheelchair. So we dug out a corduroy jacket my son had used in college and discarded. An old golf hat kept my head warm. Then Bruce wheeled me to the car and transferred me into the seat for the 45-min drive through thick expressway traffic to my office. I quickly found it took great willpower to let him drive and not be a "backseat driver." It was a severe test of nerves to sit in my own $5000 car, keeping quiet while a teen-ager, who thought he had mastered all there was to know about driving, snaked in and out of traffic.

We arrived at the office about 10 o'clock and Bruce put me back in the wheelchair. As I wheeled through the familiar press room, with its giant machines and printing ink odor, I choked back tears. Then we rode the elevator to the block-long newsroom on the second floor. I mumbled a few words to reporters and others who had worked for me and went on up to my old desk, only to find that my knees would not fit under it.

Our production manager, Gene Arehart, rallied to my aid. He found tables that would accommodate my wheelchair and fastened my gooseneck attachment for the telephone to it. Prior to my injury, I had a spacious, walnut-paneled office with fireplace, davenport, and a rich, Oriental rug. The rug, I discovered, was so heavy I could barely move the wheelchair on it. So they rolled the rug up and placed it in storage. They put blocks under the davenport so I could be transferred to it for 15 min to ease pressure on my skin. The threshold into the office was so high I could not get over it. They removed it.

By noon I was exhausted. So we traced our course back home. It was an abbreviated day, but I had made it. Gradually, as the months went by, I built up my tolerance so I could work 6 hours or longer, but I was not able to equal my old schedule of 8 or more hours. Little by little, many other aspects of my job and life also changed as I was able to adjust to my handicap. Rehabilitation, I found, did not end when I was discharged from R.I.C. I continued to visit and consult with R.I.C. But much of this on-the-job rehabilitation is highly individualistic. My transportation to and from the job altered drastically. We found many better ways of locating and training attendants. Such work essentials as handling the problem of incontinence, business lunches, and such a seemingly small thing as reading a newspaper came under better control. The changes also affected the way I dealt with people, my mental attitude, and my view of religion.

Getting to a job is, of course, fundamental for anyone who is working, but it poses staggering problems when you are a quad. So we tackled this problem while I was still at R.I.C. My wife went car shopping, but instead of checking colors and horsepower, she measured leg room, door width, and roof height of different makes of cars. Being very tall, it was hard to fit into most models.

771   GOING BACK TO WORK: A PERSONAL RECOLLECTION

We also figured that a six-way electric seat would facilitate transfers and possibly make it feasible for me to drive. So we finally selected a Ford LTD, which came closest to meeting our goals, and traded in our old compact car. Then we bought a Hoyer hydraulic lift for the top of the car.

The Hoyer, it turned out, was an obstacle rather than an aid in transfers. My attendant tried the Hoyer but found he could make the transfers better and faster with a transfer board. My wife, too, soon stopped using the Hoyer, so we moved it from the car. The next thing to go, after about 2 years, was the transfer board. Then I decided it was time to learn how to drive. So I took three lessons in a two-door model equipped with hand controls. Had I persisted, I perhaps could have learned how to drive with these controls, but instead I decided to stick with an attendant and concentrate my energy on my job.

The most drastic change in my mode of transportation came 4 years after my injury. Over this span of time, huge improvement was made in vans modified to carry wheelchairs. We investigated and tried all the different types we could find. Ultimately, we purchased a Volkswagen van with the center section lowered about 9 in. Because of the closeness to the ground, the slant of the ramp that lets down at the side is small. Very little strength is required to push a wheelchair up into the van. I no longer had to be bodily transferred in and out of the car, greatly reducing the chance of catheter failure. It made it possible for someone of far less strength and experience to drive me, vastly broadening my ability to go places.

In a scale of importance of the essentials for returning to work and successfully continuing on the job, my attendant would rate up at the top, with transportation. I had to have an attendant and a good one. It was a need I did not have or could not even imagine before my injury. We have hired and used 14 different attendants since 1971. Our first attendant quit in 3 months; the last one prior to my retirement worked for us over 2 years. That's one measure of the progress we made. One of our early attendants failed to show up for work; we located him in jail 150 miles from home.

When we began searching for our first attendant, we tried friends, our minister, high schools, colleges, the state employment service, and nursing agencies. We received many suggestions but no suitable candidates for the job. So we tried classified ads in the local newspapers.

I had earned my living as a reporter and editor for years but discovered that my ability at composing classified ads was not very great. Our first classified yielded an attendant, but our results were much better as we gained experience. Again, I was able to obtain invaluable assistance from the *Wall Street Journal.* The manager of our classified department reworked my ad to appear to a broad cross section of possible candidates. Our ad pictured the advantages of the job and succinctly described our needs. It was amazingly effective. Over 90 phone calls resulted, and we interviewed a score of candidates. I have hired many professional journalists, but that task is simple compared to finding a good attendant.

One hurdle I faced when returning to work was handling the problem of being incontinent. When I left R.I.C., I was equipped with an external catheter and leg bag, or urine collector. But I could not bend over to empty it and regain sitting position. I had the largest size I could buy, about a quart, but had no control over when it would fill. In my mind, I could imagine how embarrassed I would be if the leg bag overflowed or the catheter twisted and burst. Few things I can imagine would be more out of character for a managing editor.

The possibility of a catheter failure will always be a hazard for me, but after a few months, I was able to work out a solution to the problem. I meticulously regulated my intake of fluids, cutting way down early in the day. When I returned home late in the afternoon, I drank liquids heavily. At night, my wife connected my catheter to a gallon jar. That was adequate to handle my output of urine.

Eating may not seem an essential part of one's

job, but I found it took a mixture of ingenuity and perseverance to fit lunching into my working day. For a time at R.I.C., I was what the nurses labeled "a feeder"—I could not feed myself. By the time I returned to work, I could handle a spoon, fork, and tumbler half full of liquid. But eating and my job went far beyond that. I took care of my own lunch and my shortened day by bringing a sandwich and thermos of coffee. I ate at my desk and tried to finish in 5 or 10 min, stretching out my working time. Others in the office spent an hour or more at lunch.

Prior to my accident, however, lunch had not only been an enjoyable but also an integral and productive part of my day. Sometimes I lunched with a reporter or one of my superiors from New York. At other times, it was with the president of a large corporation, a stockbroker, or a banker. Lunches helped iron out employee problems, turned up ideas for stories, and helped keep my paper and its readers on top of what was happening in the world of business and finance.

The idea that solved this problem was not mine. It came from Mary, my wife. "The executives you used to lunch with at their fancy clubs would come to your office and eat a sandwich with you, if you asked them," she said. "Try it. I'll fix the sandwiches."

She pressed me to experiment. I had visions of an overturned glass of coffee, a blown catheter, or a sudden dizzy spell. There was the frightening thought of the reaction of a $200,000-a-year executive to munching a peanut butter sandwich. Add to that the fact that we did not have a dining room or cooking facilities at the paper.

To my surprise, the executives liked the idea. We eventually developed more elaborate meals, but they were simple fare compared to that served in expensive restaurants and clubs. Those who came to lunch included such key executives as the president of International Harvester Co., the chairman of Chicago's biggest bank, and other top corporate officials from as far as Minnesota and Michigan. The president of one Midwestern company that does over $1 billion worth of business a year lunched with me three times in one year at these affairs in the office. In many respects, they were more productive than the usual business lunches.

Reading, particularly newspapers, was another key part of my position. Prior to my injury, I read eight newspapers every day, a number of magazines, and page after page of typed copy by reporters. This kind and volume of reading is crucial for a newspaper editor. You must know what other publications are saying. Reading is essential for developing ideas for features your staff can expand. How could I keep up with the printed page when I could not hold a newspaper and could turn pages only painfully slowly.

I did not manage to accomplish the quantity of reading I had formerly done, but I learned how to be more selective. I edited my reading. First, I figured how to cope with my own paper. I had the advantage of knowing exactly where to find different subjects. In a well-edited paper, the headlines enable you to sift out the stories you don't need and guide you to those you find necessary to read. I coupled this with improving my reading and scanning speed. I also became more attentive to suggestions from others about material I should read. So I slashed the quantity of my reading and upgraded the quality.

My relationship with the people I worked and dealt with during the business day gradually changed. As a newspaper editor and, before that, a reporter, I am interested in people. When I was in R.I.C., I discovered that if I listened to others and expressed interest in them, they liked to talk with me. Perhaps I was exercising my reporter's instincts. One of the secrets of a good reporter is simply being a good listener. So I attempted to learn the names and interests of as many patients, nurses, aides, and orderlies as I could.

When I returned to the *Wall Street Journal,* I did much the same thing. This refined curiosity about others helped me in discussing story ideas with reporters. When one of our employees had a health or family problem, he was more likely to talk it over with me. I found my handicap repelled some but made it easier to get along with others. This knowledge was useful in getting a helping hand when I needed one and increased my effectiveness in administering the Chicago bureau. I did not have a formal rating system but generally found that women were more compassionate than men, blue collar workers more so than white collar, and blacks more than whites. People with a handicapped dependent or friend were similarly more understanding than those without such experience.

As I was reestablishing myself in my job, my wife and I struggled to resume our social life. This helped me act naturally toward others, bolstered my self-confidence, and kept me from stagnating when not at work. We had people in for dinner, played bridge in the evening, went to the theater, attended church, and in many ways attempted to live as we did prior to my injury.

Mental attitude is one of the keys to a handicapped person getting back to work and staying there. I developed an obsession about getting to work. Over my 6 years as an editor after returning to work, I did not miss a day—a better attendance record than most of the nonhandicapped people who worked for me. If it was 10° below zero, I went to work. Mornings when I was so dizzy I couldn't clearly distinguish the trees at the side of the road, I persisted in going to my job. On more than one occasion, my catheter failed downtown when I was transferred from my car to the wheelchair. I had my attendant drive me the 20 miles back home, my wife met us at the door, the two of them changed the catheter and my clothes, and back I went to the *Wall Street Journal*. I would be nearly 2 hours late and mentally shaken by the experience. It never failed to be humiliating. But after it was over and I was behind my desk with phones ringing and the comforting office bustle, I was glad I had returned and not buckled after the mishap. My attitude became one of always trying to outperform the nonhandicapped.

Self-pity is something I learned to fight. People, I found, don't like to hear about how your legs hurt—mine do most of the time—or about your trouble in getting to work, your indigestion, or your tough luck at being in a wheelchair. So when I feel sorry for myself, I don't talk about it. That isn't easy when someone you envy for his physical condition fusses to you about some ailment that appears minor compared to your own.

I adopted a "one day at a time" attitude when things seemed roughest. Some days, when I felt particularly bad, that state of mind helped get me through. The same was true when my attendant failed to show up in the morning, and I worried that I would not be able to get out of bed or that my wife would attempt to get me in my wheelchair and strain herself.

As time progressed, I probably became less self-centered and developed a stronger interest in attempting to help others. My ambition to rise in the company was dulled, and instead I was thankful to have a job. Working was much more fun and more interesting than vacations.

Plain, unadulterated luck was part of the recipe I used to get and hold my job. It was luck that helped us finance the overwhelming cost of rehabilitation and the costs we incurred after I went back to work. Because I was injured while working, I have been covered by workers' compensation insurance. Under this coverage, the insurance pays the medical costs related to my spinal cord injury. This includes hospital expenses during rehabilitation, drugs, and the wages of our attendants. This coverage will continue as long as I live. Currently, these costs run about $1000 a month. During the period from the time of my injury in 1971 to my retirement at the close of 1977, payments under this coverage by Liberty Mutual Insurance Company totaled $137,000.

My religion has time and time again helped my wife and me over rough spots. Prior to my injury, we were average churchgoers, but I was not above playing golf Sunday morning, and I did not teach Sunday school. Our religion has provided answers to many of our questions that seem unanswerable. One of them, "Why did God pick on me?," came up frequently. The answer is He didn't. The injury probably deepened and broadened our religion, which most assuredly was a significant factor in my return to work and in my being able to continue in my job.

Officially, I retired on December 31, 1977, 2 months less than 7 years after my car edged onto that median strip outside St. Louis. Actually, I continued working through October 2, my sixty-fifth birthday. The *Wall Street Journal* kept me on the payroll for 3 extra months. On October 4, we departed for Sun City, Arizona, and a new round of "rehabilitation" as I learn to live in retirement in a totally new environment.

Index

Page numbers in *italics* indicate tables or illustrations.

Acceptance of disability, 300, 380, 477
Activities of daily living, 299–339
   after amputation, 502
      bathing, 330
      dressing and undressing, 326–327
      eating, 310–312
      hygiene, 317, *318*
      toileting, 334, *335*
   assessment of skills for, *296*
   after head injury, 393
   in hemiplegia, 306–307, 312–313, 319, 323, 328–331
   in multiple sclerosis, 410–415
   in rheumatic disease, 614–615
      bathing, 330
      dressing and undressing, 326
      eating, 310
      hygiene, 317
      toileting, 333–334, 621
   after spinal cord injury, 460–462, 482–484
      bathing, 329–330
      dressing and undressing, 323–326
      eating, 307–310, 437
      hygiene, 313–316
      toileting, 331–333
   after stroke, 374–378
   training for, 299–339
      factors affecting success of, 300
   (*See also* Functional skills)
Acupuncture, 632, 654
Addiction, 563–564, 626, 658, 661–662
Adjustment to disability, 22, 117–119, 122
Adolescent, 32, 213, 398
   patient compared to, 757
   pressure sores and, 248, 255, 265
   responses of, to rheumatoid arthritis, 630, 635
   scoliosis in, after spinal cord injury, 488
   sexuality of, 90–91, 630
Affect, liability of:
      in multiple sclerosis, 405, 413
      in stroke, 366, 380
Aged persons, 707
   burn injuries of, 524, 534, 549
   response of, to myocardial infarction, 590
Agnosia, 142, 158
Alcohol (beverage), 12–13
   and heart disease, 586
   and sexual functioning, 89, 92
   use of, in rehabilitation hospital, 480–481
   withdrawal from, after hospital admission, 442
Alternating pressure mattress, **256,** 257

Ambulation:
  after amputation, 510, 511, 514–515
  after stroke, 373, 374
American Academy of Orthopaedic Surgeons, range-of-motion assessment system of, 278–279
American Cancer Society, 575, 594, 672
American Coalition for Handicapped Citizens, 753
American Diabetes Association, 680
American Heart Association, 169, 580, 595, 672, 680
American Hospital Association, 567, 670, 751
American Rheumatism Society, 608–610, 639
American Speech-Language-Hearing Association, 169, 349
Amputation, 493–505, 507–519
  exercises following, 500, 508–509, *510–513*
  and family involvement in rehabilitation, 499, 504, 516, 517
  of lower extremity, 507–519
    dietary and fluid requirements after, 509–510
    mobility after, 510–511, 514–515
  motivation for rehabilitation following, 515–517
  positioning after, 305–306, 508, 511
  response of patient and family to, 498–499, 504, 509
  sexuality after, 518
  teaching of patient or family about, 507–515
  of upper extremity, 493–505
    compared to lower extremity, 493
    types of, 494–495
  (*See also* Activities of daily living, after amputation; Pain, phantom; Prosthesis; Stump care)
Amputee clinic, 494, 500, 502–504
Anal reflex, 189, 227, 231, 426
  urinary function and, 189
  (*See also* Saddle sensation)
Anal sphincter:
  neurologic assessment and, 426
  (*See also* Saddle sensation)
Anger:
  in aphasia, 154, 157
  toward self, 476, 544
  toward staff, 299–300
    after burn injury, 544
    discharge planning and, 676–677
    management of, 756
    in multiple sclerosis, 414
    after spinal cord injury, 476–477
Angina pectoris, 584–586
Ankylosing spondylitis, 635–637
Anomia, 153–154

Anosognosia, 362–364
Aphasia, 151–161
  anomic, 156–157
  assessment of, 157–159
  Broca's, 152–156, 161, 359–360
  in childhood, 342–346, 348
  classification of, 152–157
  cognition and, 138–140, 142
  conduction, 156
  definition of, 152
  global, 157, 159
  after head injury, 397
  nursing care in, 167–170
  prognosis in, 159
  transcortical, 157
  treatment of, 159–161
  Wernicke's, 154–156, 360
Apraxia, 142, 177
  of speech, 153, 154, 158, 161, 342
Architectural Barriers Act of 1968, 709
Architectural design for handicapped, 730–732, 739–748
Architectural and Transportation Barriers Compliance Board, 709, 730, 740
Arthritis, 608–643
  (*See also* Ankylosing spondylitis; Degenerative joint disease; Rheumatoid arthritis)
Arthritis Foundation, 608, 622, 639, 672
Arthritis Information Clearinghouse, 622
Arthroplasty, 623–630
Assertiveness, patient, 70, 483
Assessment of Children's Language Comprehension, 344
Attendant, care by, 753, 772
Attitudes toward impaired persons (*see* Impaired persons, interactions of able-bodied persons with)
Autonomic hyperreflexia (*see* Dysreflexia)

Balance, assessment of, 291
Bargaining as patient reaction, 117, 299
Barriers:
  physical, 729–749
    in employment settings, 737–738
    in homes, 482, 715
    in public places, 18, 415, 737–748, 709
    in schools, 736
  psychosocial, 17, 18, 705–708, 729–730
Bathing, 329–330
Baxter formula, 522

INDEX 778

Bechterew's disease, 635
Behavior:
   equity theory of, 43–45, 47
   toward impaired persons (see Impaired persons, interactions of able-bodied persons with)
   reactance theory of, 42
Behavior modification:
   application to rehabilitation, 65–66, 160, 162, 720–723
   with burned children, 549
   with cancer patients, 560, 561
   ethics of, 37, 656
   and normalization, 16
   for pain control, 617, 655–658
   principles of, 16, 36–37, 702–704
Bender Visual-Motor Gestalt Test, 141
Biofeedback, 166, 632, 654
Bladder:
   normal function of, 188–190, 192–193
   surgery of, 216–219
   (See also Incontinence, urinary; Neurogenic bladder; Urinary function)
Bladder outlet dysfunction, 198–199
Bladder training, 202–206
   after head injury, 396
   after spinal cord injury, 436–437, 453–456, 467–470
   after stroke, 378–380
   teaching of patient or family about, 219–220
Body image, 23, 72, 103
   after burn injury, 540
   after cancer surgery, 565, 569
   in juvenile rheumatoid arthritis, 635
   in multiple sclerosis, 414
   proprioceptive disturbances and, 284, 285
     (See also Visual neglect)
   sexuality and, 95, 414, 569, 631
   after stroke, 380
Boston Diagnostic Aphasia Examination, 158
Bowel, function of, 223, 241
   alterations in, 226–241
   assessment of, 228–232
   normal, 225–226
   nursing research needed about, 226, 240
   (See also Constipation; Diarrhea; Incontinence, bowel; Neurogenic bowel)
Bowel program, 223–241
   after head injury, 396
   in multiple sclerosis, 412
   after spinal cord injury, 438, 452–453, **455**, 465–467

   after stroke, 378
Brace (see Orthesis)
Brain, functions of hemispheres of, 177, 182, 359, 360
   (See also Brain damage, right hemisphere; Hemiplegia, left; Hemiplegia, right)
Brain damage, 353–385, 387–399
   and cognition, 137–147, 343
   nursing care in, 137–147, 167–170
   nursing research needed about, 145–146
   recovery from, 138–140, 162, 389–391
   right hemisphere, 161–162, 168–169, 342–343, 346–348
   from stroke, 353–385
   from trauma, 387–399
   (See also Head injury; Stroke)
Brompton's solution, 564
Brunnstrom hemiplegia evaluation system, 288–291
Bureau of Education for the Handicapped, 714
Burn injury, 521–551
   assessment of, 542–544
   cardiovascular function after, 521–523
   contractures after, 527, 530–532, 535–538
   discharge planning after, 544–548
   fluid therapy for, 522
   infection after, 524–525, 532–534
   nursing goals for patients with, 524
   nutritional requirements after, 526–527, 532
   physiologic responses to, 521–530
   positioning after, 524, 530–531, 535–538
   pressure garments for, 537–538, **540, 541**
   prevention of deformity and disability from, 530–548
   psychosocial responses to, 539–546
   pulmonary function in, 523–524
   range-of-motion exercises after, 524, 530–532, 537
   renal function in, 521–523
   scarring after, 529–530, 535–538, 547–548
   sexual function after, 545, 547
   shock after, 521, 522, 525
   skin grafting for, 529, 534–535
   surgical treatment of, 523, 527–529
   teaching of patient and family after, 537, 538, 543, 546–548
   wound healing after, 525, 527

Cancer, 553–578
   anorexia and cachexia in, 559–561
   body image in, 565, 569

Cancer (*continued*)
   death and dying and, 571–573
   diagnosis of, informing patient about, 567–568
   family responses to, 573–574
   gastrointestinal disturbances in, 561
   nutrition in, 559–561
   oxygen exchange in, 561–562
   pain in, 562–564
   pathophysiology of, 556–559
   patient rights in, 567–568, 571
   sexuality in, 569–571
   societal attitudes about, 574–575
   support groups for patients with, 575–576
   treatment for, 557–559
      side effects of, 565–566
Cane, selection of, 374
Cardiac status:
   assessment of, 291–293
   and exercise tolerance, 291–293, 595–601
Catheter, external, 206–208, 332–333, 379
Catheterization:
   indwelling, 214–216, 468
   and infection, 199, 213–216
   intermittent, 201, 204, 208–214, 468–469
   (*See also* Self-catheterization)
Center for Independent Living, 719, 720, 753
Central nervous system:
   anatomy of, 421, **423**
   assessment of, 285–291
   functions of, 291
Cerebrovascular accident (CVA) (*see* Stroke)
Cervical collar, 432, 614
Cervical fraction, 427, **430**, 431–432
Chambers Price Pain Rating Scale, 649, **650**
Chemotherapy, 558–559, 565–566
Chewing and swallowing, 164, 165, 171–185, 343, 407
   (*See also* Dysphagia; Eating; Swallowing)
Child:
   with amputation, 504
   with arthritis, 633–635
   with bowel function alteration, 230
   with burn injury, 524, 528, 531, 534, 549
      metabolism in, 526
      scarring in, 530, 547
      and separation from parents, 542
   care of, by handicapped parent, 378
   with central nervous system impairment, 285
   curiosity of, about amputation, 517
   handicapped: normalization of, 16, 711–712, 732–733
      social status of, 16–17
   with hemiplegia, 358
   language development of, 341–342
   motor development of, 291
   pressure sores and, 255
   right brain damage in, 342–343
   scoliosis in, after spinal cord injury, 488
   speech and language disorders in, 341–350
   with urologic problems, 187, 192, 206
      intermittent catheterization for, 209, 211
      leg bag for, 216
Child abuse, 544, 547
Chronaxie studies, 285
Cine-esophagram, 176, 182
Circ-o-lectric bed, **256,** 257, 434
Clubs for patients, 66, 758
   with cancer, 575–576
   with multiple sclerosis, 414, 415
   with stroke, 169, 381
   (*See also names of specific organizations*)
Cognition, 137–147, 285
   assessment of, 137, 140–144, 146
   after brain damage, 137–147, 162
   in childhood, 343
Collagen disease, 608
Collar, cervical, 432, 614
Communication:
   impairment of, 335–338, 443
      after head injury, 397
      in multiple sclerosis, 415
      nursing care in, 167–170, 335
      research about, 170
      (*See also* Alphasia; Speech and language)
   problems in, of nursing staff, 542–543, 591
   (*See also* Team, rehabilitation, communication within)
Community, return to, 668–689, 698–727, 751
   preparation for, 187, 252, 382, 672–673
   variables predicting success in, 69–84, 299, 338, 477
   (*See also* Resocialization)
Compliance, 13, 52–67
   assessment of capacity for, 64–65
   definition of, 54
   excessive, 300
   factors affecting, 55, 57–63
   measurement of, 56–57
   promotion of, 63–67
   research about, 55–63
Concussion, 387–388
Conditioning:
   classical, 703–704

Conditioning (*continued*)
  operant, 703–704, 721–723
Conformer, *531*, 535
Congestive heart failure, 581–584
Connective tissue disease, 608
Conservation principles, 553–555
Constipation, 230, 234, 236–239
  in cancer, 561
  in multiple sclerosis, 412
  in rheumatoid arthritis, 621
  in spinal cord injury, 466
Contraception, 478–479, 570, 631–632
Contract between patient and professional, 65–66
Contractures, 366, 397, 487–488
  after amputation, 508, 511
  after burn injury, 527, 530–532, 535–538, 547–548
  in rheumatoid arthritis, 618
Contrecoup head injury, 388
Contusion, brain, 388
Coordination, assessment of, 291
Coping, 21–38
  assessment of, 29–31, 34–35
  belief systems and, 25, 28, 29
  classification of, 24–26
  definition of, 22, 23
  facilitation of, 34–38
  failure and, 507
  grief and, 32–33, 319
  illness or disability and, 29–30, 32–34, 76, 119
  patterns of, 25–26
  steps of, 26–29, 34
  successful, 31–32
Coping strategy, 23, 32–34, 413
Corpus callosum, 359
Cost of rehabilitation (*see* Rehabilitation, cost of)
Cough, assisted, 435, 458
Counseling (*see* Sex education and counseling; Vocational counseling)
Coup head injury, 388
Credé method of manual bladder emptying, 190, 196, 197, 205, 212
Crisis:
  identity, 95, 96
  rehabilitation as, 79, 450–451
Cultural differences, 542–543
Cystometry, 192

Death, 571–573
  preferred to disability, 116
  right to choose, 550, 571
  (*See also* Grief)
Declaration on the Rights of Disabled Persons, U.N., 708
Degenerative joint disease, 637–639
Denial, 104, 116–119, 299–300
  and burn injury, 540
  and disability from stroke, 374, 380
  and discharge planning, 677
  and multiple sclerosis, 413
  and myocardial infarction, 589
  and spinal cord injury, 442–443, 476–477
Dependence, 41, 48–49, 78
  in cancer, 566–567
  and holism, 555
  after spinal cord injury, 441, 482–484
  (*See also* Independence; Interdependence)
Depression, 105, 117, 118, 299–300
  and aphasia, 154, 157, 159
  and body image, 569
  and discharge planning, 677
  after head injury, 398
  after myocardial infarction, 587, 589–590
  and pain, 562
  and pressure sores, 255, 260, 261
  after spinal cord injury, 443, 464, 476–477
Detroit Test of Learning, 142
Development Sentence Analysis, 344
Developmental Test of Visual-Motor Integration, 344
Diagnosis, right of cancer patient to know, 567
Diarrhea, 230, 234, 239
  in cancer, 561
  after head injury, 396
  after spinal cord injury, 467
Dictionary of Occupational Titles, 694
Diet:
  after amputation, 509–510
  and bowel function, 226, 231, 234
  after burn injury, 526–527, 532
  in calculus uropathy, 201–202, 437
  in cancer, 559–561
  in dysphagia, 184
  after head injury, 396–397
  in heart disease, 581, 582, 586, 594
  in multiple sclerosis, 404, 406–407
  pressure sores and, 254, 262–263
  in rheumatoid arthritis, 617–618
  after spinal cord injury, 437, 440–441, 466, 470
  after stroke, 375
Digital stimulation of bowel, 235, 238–239, 438, 453

Digital stimulator, 332–333, 465
Disability:
  acceptance of, 300, 380, 477
  adjustment to, 22, 117–119, 122
  definition of, 12, 701–702
  functional categories of, 730–731
  incidence of, 4–5, 700–701, 761
  (See also Handicap; Impairment)
Discharge:
  from acute care to rehabilitation center, 445, 450–451
  anxieties about, 544–545
  of high risk patient, 264–265
  planning for, 668–689
    after burn injury, 544–548
    after head injury, 398–399
    impediments to, 676–678, 680–681
    nursing responsibilities in, 673, 676
    referral in, 683–685
    resources pertinent to, 670–673, 683–685, 718
    right of patient to, 670
    after spinal cord injury, 462–464, 471–475, 488–489
    after stroke, 382–383
Discrimination against impaired persons, 11, 12, 575, 710
Disfigurement:
  from burn injury, 539–541, 543–545, 547–549
  from cancer surgery, 565
  from cranial surgery, 392–393
Divorce rate among quadriplegics, 770
Dressing and undressing, 319, 323–327, 376
Driver education, 383, 772
Drug use, illicit:
  and coping, 12–13, 31, 480–481
  in the rehabilitation center, 480–481
  and sexual functioning, 89, 93
  withdrawal from, in the rehabilitation center, 442
Dysarthria, 163–166, 361–362
  assessment of, 164–165
  in childhood, 343, 347, 348
  differential diagnosis of, 163, 164
  treatment of, 165–166, 169, 347, 348
Dysphagia, 174–185, 407
  assessment of, 175–178, *179*
  causes of, 174
  differential diagnosis of, 175–177
  mechanical, 178–180, 185
  paralytic, 181, 185
  pseudobulbar, 177, 182–183, 185

  rehabilitation in, 176, 178–185
Dysreflexia, 194–196, 456, 470, 479
  causes of, 194–195, 466
  definition of, 194
  prevention of, 195–196, 235
  signs and symptoms of, 195, 235, 239–240, 466
  treatment of, 195, 240, 466–467

Eating, 306–312, 437
  independence in, 177, 306–312
  (See also Chewing and swallowing; Diet; Dysphagia)
Eating Aid, 308
Ectopic bone, 487
Education of All Handicapped Children Act of 1975, 709, 736
Electromyography, 193, 271, 285
Emotional lability, 366, 380, 413
Emotional problems, 393, 413–414
Employment:
  as requirement for rehabilitation, 710–711
  resumption of, 16, 691–696, 736–738, 760–761
    by cardiac patient, 580, 603
    concerns of patient about, 548
    personal report about, 767–775
    views of insurance companies about, 760–761, 763–764
  (See also Vocational counseling)
Environment, modification of, 724, 729–749
  (See also Vocational counseling)
Equity theory of behavior, 43–45, 47
Erection, penile, 444, 478, 479
Eschar, 523, 527–528
Ethics of rehabilitation:
  financial considerations, 5–6, 446, 710–711
  value of disabled person, 4–9
  (See also Patient rights)
Evers-Root diet, 407
Exercise testing, 291–295, 595–601

Family:
  assessment of, 81
    for discharge, 670–671, 678–683
  definition of, 80, 555
  functions of, 46–47, 80–82
  grief of, 573
  as participant in care, 66, 82, 224, 398, 555
  as patient, 122–123

Family (*continued*)
  problems of, following impairment, 96, 119, 681, 698–699, 707
  relationships with rehabilitation staff, 76, 80–82, 543
  roles in, 80, 96, 118, 475
    revision of, following disability, 96, 118, 475, 545, 717
  stages of response to disability, 716–717
  (*See also* Teaching of patient or family)
Family systems theory, 81–82
Federal Aid Highway Act of 1973, 709
Fertility, 478–479, 569–570
Financial considerations in rehabilitation, 5–6, 446, 710–711
Fisher-Logemann Test of Articulation Competence, 344
Flaccidity, 286, 288, 289
Flex-a-lace, 322
Flotation devices for prevention of pressure sores, **256,** 258, 261
Functional Communication Profile, 158–159
Functional limitation, 12
Functional skills, 269–297, 678–679
  (*See also* Activities of daily living)

Gait analysis, 281, **282,** 286
Gastrostomy, 183, 396, 437
Gates-MacGinitie Reading Tests, 345
Gel pads, **256,** 258
Girdlestone procedure, 625
Glossectomy spoon, 178, *180*
Glossopharyngeal breathing, 471
God:
  as resource for patient, 31, 48, 51
  thoughts of patient about, 132, 374, 571, 592, 662
  (*See also* Religion, role of, in rehabilitation)
Grief:
  after amputation, 504
  after burn injury, 539–540
  in cancer, 571, 573
  and coping, 32–33
  after myocardial infarction, 588–590
  of nurses, 573
  in progressive disease, 338
  in rheumatoid arthritis, 623
  after spinal cord injury, 441–442, 460, 475–477
  stages of, 74, 103–105, 116–119, 299–300
  after stroke, 380

  (*See also* Loss)
Guilt feelings, 544, 549
Gunshot wounds, 389

Halo phenomenon, 706–707
Halo traction, 427, 431
Hand, arthroplasty of, 628–630
Handicap, 15, 702
  (*See also* Disability; Impairment)
Handicapism, 11, 751
Harrington rod, 427, 436
Head injury, 387–399
  assessment following, 390–391
  classification of, 387–389
  incidence of, 387
  nursing process in, 390
  philosophy of rehabilitation in, 390, 391
  prognosis for recovery from, 138–140, 162, 389–391
  sequelae of, 391–393, 395–397
  sexuality after, 394–395
Health, definition of, 590
Health belief model of behavior, 62–64
Hearing, 344
Heart, anatomy of, 580–581
Heart disease, 578–606
  activity and exercise in, 595–601
  coronary (*see* Angina pectoris)
  functional classification of, 595, **596**
  goals of rehabilitation in, 580
  incidence of, 580
  risk factors for, 593–595, 599
  sexuality in, 586, 601–603
  teaching of patient or family about, 581–586, 590–603
  (*See also* Myocardial infarction)
Heart valve, prosthetic, 581–582
Help, 39–52
  ability to accept, 49
  decision to provide, 44–46, 48, 50, 705–706
  eliciting, 46–49, 51
  need for, 44–51
  unwanted, 48, 49
Helping, 39–52, 705–706
  motivations for, 43–46, 48
  process, 46–51
Helplessness, 39–52, 79
  development of, 41
  gratification and, 41, 42, 51
  hopelessness and, 41

Helplessness (*continued*)
    learned, 42, 46, 51
    manifestations of, 41–42
Hematoma, 389
Hemianopsia:
    definition of, 363
    self-care neglect in, 312
    self-feeding in, 307, 375
    in stroke, 363, 364
Hemiparesis, 142, 155, 157
Hemiplegia:
    assessment of, 288–291
    Brunnstrom evaluation system for, 288–291
    communication problems in, 335–336
    left, 362–363
    positioning in, 301–303
    right, 359–362
    stages of recovery from, 289–291
    (*See also* Activities of daily living, in hemiplegia)
Heterotopic bone, 487
Heterotopic ossificans, 487
Hip, arthroplasty of, 623–627
Holism, 553–556
    cancer patient and, 559–577
    nurse and, 576
Homebound Rehabilitation Program, 753
Homemaking after stroke, 378
Homosexuality, 89, 94
Hook (terminal device), 497–498, **542**
Hospice care, 571–573
Hospitalization, responses to, 7–8, 450–451
Housing for impaired persons, 718–719, 735–736
Hoyer hydraulic lift, 772
Hubbard tank, 614
Hydronephrosis, 199, 471
Hygiene, 312–317, *318*
Hyperalimentation, 560–561
Hyperkinesia, speech patterns in, 164
Hyperreflexia (*see* Dysreflexia)
Hyperthermia:
    in head injury, 391
    in multiple sclerosis, 405, 406, 408
    in spinal cord injury, 431, 485
Hypnosis, 561, 654
Hypotension:
    postural, 370, 435, 485–486
    in spinal cord shock, 425
Hypothermia, 485

Identity crisis, 95, 96
Illinois Test of Psycholinguistic Abilities, 345

Impaction, fecal, 239, 438
Impaired persons:
    community integration of, 17, 698–727
        (*See also* Normalization; Resocialization)
    discrimination against, 11, 12, 575, 710
    housing for, 718–719, 735–736
    interactions of able-bodied persons with, 11–18, 96, 705–706, 756, 773–774
    isolation of, 11, 13–14, 18, 707–708
    self-presentation of, 12–14
    stereotype of (*see* Stereotype, of impaired persons)
    transportation for, 733–735, 737, 771–772
    understanding of, by professional, 754–755
        (*See also* Nurses, feelings of, toward patients)
Impairment:
    definition of, 11, 701–702
    (*See also* Disability; Handicap)
Incontinence:
    bowel: causes of, 224
        control of, 224, 232–238
        social consequences of, 224, 452
    and pressure sores, 255
    urinary: diagnostic evaluation of, 192
        social consequences of, 187
        surgical interventions for, 216–219
        types of, 190
Increased intracranial pressure, 391
Independence, 79, 187
    criteria of, 483
    development of, 41
    in holism, 555
    (*See also* Activities of daily living; Interdependence; Self-esteem, and independence)
Independent living unit of hospital, 483
Infant:
    care of, by handicapped parent, 378
    motor development in, 291
Informed consent (*see* Patient rights)
Institute of the Crippled and Disabled, 694
Insurance:
    coverage for handicapped persons, 713, 752
    nursing services provided by, 761–764
Insurance industry, role of, in rehabilitation, 760–765
Insurance nurse, 761–764
Intelligence testing, 141–142
Interdependence, 41, 48, 77, 754
International Rotary, 673
Interpersonal relations:
    between impaired and nonimpaired persons, 11–18, 705–706, 756, 773–774
    need for, 103

Intracranial pressure, increased, 391
Isolation, social:
    of bedridden persons, 409
    of brain-injured persons, 139–140
    of incontinent persons, 187
    self-imposed, 716
Isometric exercise, 293, 508, 516, 613–614

Jejunostomy, 183
Jewish Family Services, 676
Jobst elastic garments, 537–538, **540**
Joint, assessment of, 273–281
Juvenile rheumatoid arthritis, 633–635

Keane Roto-Rest bed, **256,** 257, 434
Keloids, 529
Kineplasty, 500, 502
Kno-bows, 322

Labeling of individuals, 11, 12, 50, 706–707
Language (see Speech and language)
Laws, 710, 739–741
Lazarus complex, 603
Learning, 702–704
    (See also Teaching of patient or family)
Learning theory, 36–37, 160, 162, 702–704
Left brain:
    functions of, 177, 182, 359, 360
    symptoms of damage to, 177, 182, 359
Leg bag (see Urine-collecting devices, external)
Lhermitte's sign, 409
Limb synergies, 289
Lions Club, 673
Living Will, 571, **572**
Locus of control, 29, 73, 255–256, 265
Loss, 103–105, 115–123
    disability and, 116, 117, 299, 358, 380
    (See also Grief)
Lost Cord Club, 575–576
Lumex bath bench, 329

McCormick loop, 304
McGill-Melzack Pain Questionnaire, 562, 649, **651,** 652
Mainstream, Inc., 753
Mainstreaming (see Normalization)
Make Today Count, 673

Marie Strümpell's disease, 635
Marijuana, spasticity and, 404
Masturbation, 89, 94, 394
Meals-on-Wheels, 547, 718
Medicaid, 713
Medic-Alert bracelet, 467
Medicare, 713
Medications, teaching of patient or family about, 381, 382
Melodic Intonation Therapy, 161
Memory loss, 141–142, 342–343, 364–366
Menstruation, 444, 478, 570
Minnesota Test for Differential Diagnosis of Aphasia, 158
"Miracle" cure, 132, 374, 405, 632–633
Mobility:
  assessment of, 288–291
  maintenance of, in multiple sclerosis, 408–410
  restoration of, 370–374, 510–511, 514–515
Motivation:
  for activities of daily living, 299, 300, 312
  for rehabilitation, 145, 146, 515–517, 543–544, 587–588
  role of, in rehabilitation, 721
  for self-catheterization, 210–213
Motor development, assessment of, 291
Motor-Free Visual Perception Test, 344
Motor vehicle, retraining for operation of, 383, 772
Motor vehicle accidents, 5, 6, 387, 419
Mourning (see Grief; Loss)
MUD bed, **256,** 259, 261
Multiple sclerosis, 400–417
  cause of, 401–403
  communication in, 415
  diagnosis of, 402–404
  diet in, 404, 406–407
  exacerbations of, 402, 405–408
  family relations in, 413–414
  incidence of, 401–402
  medical management of, 404–405
  mobility in, 408–410
  nursing management of, 405–415
  nursing research needed about, 416
  psychosocial functioning in, 405, 408–409, 413–415
  sexuality in, 414–415
  signs and symptoms of, 401–403, 406, 412
  skin care in, 407
  stress and, 402, 406–408, 412–414
  vision in, 409–410

Muscle function, assessment of, 271–272, **274–279**, 286–288
Muscle tone, assessment of, 286–288
Muscle weakness, causes of, 271
Musculoskeletal system, assessment of, 270–281
Myelography, 427
Myocardial infarction, 586–590
    activity and exercise following, 291–293, 587, 595–603
    dysrrhythmias following, 587
    family responses to, 588
    patient responses to, 588–590
    patient teaching in, 587–589, 590–603
    prognosis following, 587
    rehabilitation following, 292–293, 586–590
Myositis ossificans, 487

National Arthritis Act of 1974, 639
National Arts and the Handicapped Information Service, 739
National Association for Retarded Citizens, 712
National Center for a Barrier Free Environment, 730
National Council of Senior Citizens, 712
National Easter Seal Society for Crippled Children and Adults, 169–170, 739
National Federation of the Blind, 712
National Institute of Arthritis, Metabolism, and Digestive Diseases, 622, 639
National Institute of Handicapped Research, 714
National Institute of Neurological Disease and Stroke, 420
National Multiple Sclerosis Society, 402, 404, 415, 672
National Paraplegic Foundation, 673
National Rehabilitation Association, 701
Needs assessment, 50, 51
Nerve conduction studies, 285
Nervous system:
    assessment of, 281–291
    (*See also* Central nervous system; Peripheral nervous system)
Neurogenic bladder, 193–198, 202–221
    autonomous, 196, 204
    mixed, 197
    motor paralytic, 196–197
    patient teaching about, 202–216, 219–221
    reflex, 194, 203, 206
    sensory paralytic, 197
    treatment of, 193, 198, 202–219
    uninhibited, 197, 206, 379
    voiding facilitation techniques for, 203–206

Neurogenic bowel, 226–241
    autonomous, **227**, 228, 233, 235–236
    classification of, 227
    management of, 232–241
    motor paralytic, **228**
    reflex, **227**, 228, **233**, 234–235
    sensory paralytic, **228**
    uninhibited, 227, **233**, 236–237
Neurologic status, assessment of, 281–291
    (*See also* Spinal cord injury, assessment of)
New Options, 753
Normalization, 16–17, 730, 735, 751
    versus segregation, 711–712, 732–733
    (*See also* Resocialization)
Nurses:
    anxieties of, 111–113, 549–550
    communication of, with patients, 542–543, 591, 744–756
    empathy of, 109, 111, 113, 686–687
    employee turnover of, 109, 550
    feelings of, toward patients, 107–108, 110–111, 420–431
        anger, 477, 687
        attachment, 480, 549, 686–687
        devaluation, 756–757
        expectation for rehabilitation, 698–699
        failure, 687
        guilt, 421, 549
        identification, 686–687
    grief of, 573
    group work with, 112, 550, 687
    in insurance industry, 761–764
    role of, on rehabilitation team, 6–7, 128–130, 133, 355, 420
    stresses on, 101–114, 549–550, 656, 687
Nursing history:
    on admission to rehabilitation center, 451–452
    of burn patient, 542–544
    of cardiac patient, 590–593
    of rheumatoid arthritis patient, 616
Nursing research, recommendations for:
    about bowel function, 226, 240
    about cognition, 145–146
    about multiple sclerosis, 416
    about pain, 656
    about positioning, 446
    about pressure sores, 254, 256, 259, 260, 264
    about rheumatic disease, 639
    about sensory alterations, 446
    about stroke, 383
    about teaching, 446

Nutrition (see Diet)
Nutrition history, **229**, 231

Obesity:
    and bowel function, 230
    and cardiac risk, 599
    and rheumatoid arthritis, 617
    and spinal cord injury, 434
    and stroke, 370
Occupational therapy, 131, 299–339
Office of Independent Living for the Disabled, 735
Organizations for patients, 66, 758
    cancer, 575–576
    multiple sclerosis, 414, 415
    stroke, 169, 381
    (*See also names of specific organizations*)
Orgasm after spinal cord injury, 478
Orthesis (orthosis):
    lower extremity, 322–323
    spinal, 323, **430–433**, 464
    upper extremity, 301–310, 313–316, 332–333, 337
Osteoarthritis, 637
Ostomy, 219, 565
Ostomy Club, 575–576

Pacemaker, cardiac, 583–584
Pain, 645–664
    assessment of, 649–652, 657–660
    in cancer, 562–564
    causes of, 562, 647
    classification of, 646–647
    communication of, 658–659
    definition of, 645
    measurement of, 649–652
    nursing care of patient with, 656–662
    phantom, 485, 509, 646, 655
    referred, 509, 647, 654
    research about, 649–652, 656
    in rheumatic disease, 608, 616–617, 622, 623
    after spinal cord injury, 485
    theories of, 645–646
        gate control, 562, 645–646, 654, 655
        specificity, 645
    treatment of, 564, 652–656, 662
Pain cocktail, 653, 655–656
Paralyzed Veterans of America, 712
Passes from hospital:
    costs of, 481
    debriefing after, 381, 482

    preparation for, 381–382, 462–464, 481–482, 677
    as preparation for discharge, 398, 482, 677, 715
    responses of patient and family to, 482
Patient:
    contract between professional and, 65–66
    as member of rehabilitation team, 128, 160, 293, 553
        most important, 132, 483, 761
    as participant in care: in decision making, 443, 707
        in discharge planning, 668
        in goal setting and intervening, 66, 67, 78, 132, 250
        in planning, 35, 54, 132, 569
        in responsibility for care, 132, 240, 265
    as participant in team conferences, 134, 483
    (*See also* Organizations for patients; Teaching of patient or family)
Patient rights, 550, 567–568, 670, 708–712, 751–752
    (*See also* Ethics of rehabilitation)
Patient's Bill of Rights, 567, 670, 751
Peabody Individual Achievement Test, 345
Perception:
    assessment of, 177, **178**, 285, 344–345
    deficits in: in childhood, 342
        communication and, 335
        eating and, 177, 307
        hygiene and, 312, 313
        left brain damage and, 362
        right brain damage and, 162
Peripheral nervous system, 284–285, 421
Phantom pain, 485, 509, 646, 655
Phantom sensation, 429, 509
Pharyngostomy, 183
Phrenic-nerve stimulator, 458–459
Physical therapy, 131, 269, 297
    after amputation, 502
    in bowel program, 224
    after burn injury, 505
    in cancer, 565
    in rheumatoid arthritis, 620
Physician, role of, in rehabilitation, 128–130, 133–134
Picture Story Language Test, 345
Placebo, ethics of using, 654
Porch Index of Communicative Ability, 158
Positioning:
    after amputation, 305–306, 508, 511
    in ankylosing spondylitis, 636–637

Positioning (*continued*)
   after burn injury, 524, 530–531, 535–538
   in hemianopia, 375
   in hemiplegia, 301–303
   in multiple sclerosis, 408
   in rheumatoid arthritis, 304–305, 618–620, **621**
   in spinal cord injury, 303–304, 431–436, 456–457, 472–475
      immediately after accident, 424–428
   after stroke, 366–370
   in wheelchair, 373
Posture:
   assessment of, 281, **283**, 295
   central nervous system damage and, 287
Pregnancy:
   after cancer treatment, 570
   and exacerbation of multiple sclerosis, 402, 408
   in rheumatoid arthritis, 631
   after spinal cord injury, 444, 478–479
Prejudice, 11, 14, 130
   (*See also* Stereotype)
Premack principle, 722
President's Committee on Employment of the Handicapped, 730, 739
President's Council on Physical Fitness, 596
Pressure sores, 242–268
   causes of, 244–245, 253–256, 369, 438–439
   classification of, 245, 247
   high-risk factors associated with, 243–244, 248, 264–265
   nursing research needed about, 254, 256, 259, 260, 264
   prevention of, 243, 247–248, 250–260, 264–265
      assessment of patient for, 248–250
      devices for, 256–259
      in multiple sclerosis, 408
      in rheumatoid arthritis, 618, 619
      after spinal cord injury, 431, 438–440, 456–457, 472–475
      after stroke, 369
   treatment of, 243, 260–264
Prism glasses, 433, 443
Progressive disease, 338, 679–680
Prostate, 198, 218
Prosthesis, 305, 317, 517, 539
   care of, 330, 513, 514
   fitting for, 500, **501**, 512
   hip, 624
   selection of, 317
   self-feeding with, 310–312
   skill, 393
   stump care preceding application of, 499–500
   types of, 495–498, 508, 512–515, **542**
   upper extremity, 493–504
Prosthetist, 493, 513
Pulmonary status, assessment of, 293–295, 426
Pylon, 512

Radiation therapy, 557–558, 566
Rancho flotation bed, **256,** 259, 261
Range of motion:
   assessment of, 272–281, 286
   exercises to maintain: after amputation, 500, 508–509, *510–513*
      after burn injury, 524, 530, 531–532, 537
      after head injury, 397
      in multiple sclerosis, 408
      in rheumatoid arthritis, 613–614
      after spinal cord injury, 436
      after stroke, 366, 368–369
Reach to Recovery, 570, 575–576
Reactance theory of behavior, 42
Reading and writing:
   in aphasia, 154–156, 161, 342–345
   in hemiplegia and spinal cord injury, 336–338
Recreational therapy, 131, 355
Reflex:
   anal, 189, 227, 231, 426
   bulbocavernosus, 192–193, 227, 230
   cough, 176, 178
   deep tendon stretch, 285–287
   duodenocolic, 225
   gag, 176, 182, 396
   gastrocolic, 225, 412, 465, 621
   labyrinthine, 286
   spinal, 225
   swallow, 174, 175, 181, 396
   tonic neck, 287
Reflex sweating, 484–485
Regression, 104, 108–110
   after burn injury, 540
   in cancer, 567
   after head injury, 393, 398
   after spinal cord injury, 464
Rehabilitation:
   access to, inequities of, 712, 714
   admission to center for, 445, 450–451
   cost of, 5–6, 71, 419, 548–549
      versus cost of not rehabilitating, 5–6, 710–711
   as crisis, 79, 450–451
   definition of, 760

Rehabilitation (*continued*)
  goal of, 70, 146, 187, 524
  motivation for, 145, 146, 515–517, 543–544, 587–588
  philosophy of, 390, 391, 420–421
  responses of patient and family to, 445, 450–451
  role of nurse in, 128–130, 133
  role of physician in, 128–130, 133–134
  success of: criteria for, 70–71, 541
    defined, 70
    factors associated with, 71, 73–78, 128–135, 379, 460
  (*See also* Team, rehabilitation)
Rehabilitation Act of 1973, 701, 709, 711, 740
Rehabilitation Services Administration, 420, 714
Relaxation techniques, 561, 617, 622
Religion, role of, in rehabilitation, 132, 134, 374, 774–775, 571
  (*See also* God)
Research (*see* Nursing research, recommendations for)
Resocialization, 70, 362, 380–381, 698–727
  community approach to, 723–724
  definition of, 698
  facilitation of, 720–724
  peer influences on, 714–715
  problems in, 702–707
  teaching of patient or family about, 721–723
  (*See also* Community, return to; Normalization)
Respirator, discontinuation of, 435
Respiratory function, assessment of, 293–295, 426
Rheumatic disease, 608–643
  (*See also* Activities of daily living, in rheumatic disease; Ankylosing spondylitis; Degenerative joint disease; Rheumatoid arthritis)
Rheumatic heart disease, 581
Rheumatoid arthritis, 608–635
  activity and rest in, 622
  assessment in, 616
  diagnosis of, 609
  incidence of, 608
  juvenile, 633–635
  medications for, 610–613
  nursing intervention for, 615–635
    after surgery, 624–630
  nutrition in, 617–618
  pain in, 608, 616–617, 622, 623
  pathophysiology of, 609
  positioning in, 304–305, 618–620, **621**
  range-of-motion exercises in, 613–614
  responses of patient and family to, 622–623, 635

  sexuality in, 630, 632
  signs and symptoms of, 608–610
  skin care in, 618, 619
  teaching of patient and family about, 621, 622
  treatment of, 610–634
    levels of, 613
    surgical, 623–630
    unorthodox, 632–633
Right brain:
  function of, 177, 182, 359
  signs and symptoms of damage to, 359
    in childhood, 342–343
  treatment for damage to, 346–348
Rigidity, 286
Role play, 36, 161
Roles:
  resumption of, 380
  revision of, 118, 380, 602–603
    in family, 96, 118, 475, 545, 717
  sex, 96
  traditional, 80, 96
Rorschach Projected Drawing Test, 142
Roto-Rest bed, **256,** 257, 434

SACH (stable ankle, cushioned heel) foot prosthesis, 513 *514*
Saddle sensation:
  and bowel dysfunction, 227, 230–231
  and urinary incontinence, 189
Safety, patient, 363–364, 382, 409, 681–682
School, return to, 397, 548, 685, 718, 736
  (*See also* Vocational counseling)
Scoliosis, 488
Segregation, normalization versus, 711–712, 732–733
Seizures, 382, 395–396
Self-care, 299–399
  (*See also* Activities of daily living; *specific health problems*)
Self-catheterization:
  indications for, 196, 197, 202–204, 206
  procedure for, 210–214, 333
Self-esteem:
  in cancer, 566–567
  and compliance, 62
  and coping, 23, 24
  and grieving, 118
  and independence, 41, 48, 338, 483, 555
    in dressing, 319
    in hygiene, 312, 313

Self-esteem (*continued*)
   and sexuality, 95, 444, 570
   and social skills, 70, 380
Self as therapeutic tool, 112
Sensation, assessment of, 284–286
Sex education and counseling, 90–91, 98, 381
   after amputation, 518
   in cancer, 570–571
   after head injury, 394–395
   in rheumatoid arthritis, 630–632
   after spinal cord injury, 444, 477–480
Sexual response cycle, 87–89
Sexuality, 16, 85–99
   after amputation, 518
   after burn injury, 545, 547
   in cancer, 569–571
   developmental stages and, 90–93
   differentiated from sexual function, 93–94, 444
   after head injury, 394–395
   and heart disease, 586, 601–603
   and marital harmony, 16
   in multiple sclerosis, 414–415
   in rheumatoid arthritis, 630–632
   societal expectations about, 86–87
   after spinal cord injury, 444, 477–480
   after stroke, 381
   uncertainties of impaired persons about, 96–97, 381, 444, 477–480
Shock, 391, 521, 522, 525
   (*See also* Spinal cord shock)
Shriners, 673
Sick role, 13, 590, 631, 648, 707–708
Skeletal system, assessment of, 272–281
Skin care (*see* Pressure sores)
Skin grafting, 529, 534–535
Smoking, 594, 656
Social activity, resumption of (*see* Resocialization)
Social interaction theory, 11
Social isolation (*see* Isolation, social)
Social relationships (*see* Impaired persons, interactions of able-bodied persons with)
Social Security Disability Insurance, 713
Social support, 61–62, 66, 76, 78
Social work, 71, 132, 757
Spasticity, 288, 289
   definition of, 286
   after head injury, 397
   marijuana and, 404
   in multiple sclerosis, 404, 408, 409
   after spinal cord injury, 484, 487–488
Speech and language, 149–171, 341–350
   assessment of, 157–159, 162–165, 177, 343–345
   after brain trauma, 143–144, 149–172, 359–362, 397
   and cognition, 138–140
   normal, 150–151
   development of, in childhood, 341–342
   (*See also* Aphasia; Communication)
Sphincterotomy, 218, 469
Spinal cord injury, 419–448, 450–491
   acute abdomen in, 488
   assessment of, 424–426, 428–431
      on admission to rehabilitation center, 451–452
      at time of injury, 424–426, 444
   bladder program and, 436–437, 453–456, 467–470
      (*See also* Neurogenic bladder)
   body temperature regulation after, 431, 485
   bowel program and, 438, 452–453, **455**, 465–467
      (*See also* Neurogenic bowel)
   cause of death in, 199, 453, 471
   communication problems in, 336–338
   divorce rate after, 770
   gastrointestinal system and, 431, 437–438
   incidence of, 5, 419–420
   neurological deficit, prevention of, 432–435
   nutrition and, 437, 440–441, 466, 470
   philosophy of care after, 419–421
   positioning after, 303–304, 424–428, 431–436, 456–457, 472–475
   prognosis of, 4, 5, 419, 422–423, 441
      informing patient and family about, 442, 459
   respiratory assessment after, 426
   respiratory care after, 435–436, 457–459, 471–472
   responses of patient and family to, 442–444, 459–461, 475–477
   sexuality after, 444, 477–480
   skin care after, 255, 431, 438–440, 456–457, 472–475
   teaching of patient and family about, 462–464, 470
   thromboembolic disease after, 430, 478, 486
   treatment of, at time of injury, 424–426, 444
   types of, 421, 433
   (*See also* Activities of daily living, after spinal cord injury; Spinal cord shock)
Spinal cord shock, 255, 422–425, 464
Spinal Injury Learning Series, 219–220
Spiritual care, 571

Splints:
  after burn injury, 531, *532–533*, 535
  (*See also* Orthesis)
Stereognosis, 285
Stereotype:
  of impaired persons, 706–707, 729, 751
    counteracting, 17, 76–77
  sexual, 86, 91, 96–97
Stewart Pain Circles, 652
Stewart Pain Color Scale, 652
Still's disease, 633–635
Stimulation, requirements of brain-injured persons for, 138–140, 144, 168, 393–394
Stimulator:
  digital, 332–333, 465
  phrenic-nerve, 458–459
Stoke-Manville-Egerton Turning Bed, 434
Stones, urinary, 191, 200–202
  diet for prevention of, 437, 440, 470
Strength-duration curve, 285
Stress, 101–114
  coping and, 23–26, 35, 36
  definition of, 23
  and multiple sclerosis, 402, 406–408, 412–414
  for nursing staff, 100–114, 549–550
  as predisposition to rheumatoid arthritis, 608
  and rehabilitation outcome, 76
Stress ulcer, 431, 437
Stroke, 353–385
  affective lability after, 366, 380
  assessment after, 355, 358
  causes of, 354
  cognition after, 137–148
  factors contributing to, 354
  incidence of, 354
  nursing research needed about, 383
  positioning after, 366–370
  prevention of, 453
  psychological responses to, 380
  seizures after, 382
  sexuality after, 381
  (*See also* Brain damage)
Stryker frame, *256,* 257, 424, 427, 432–434
Stump care, 503, 507–509
  exercises: of lower extremity, 508–509, *510–513*
    of upper extremity, 500
  before prosthesis is applied, 499–500, 507–509
Stump socks, 503, 514
Suicide, 104–105, 118, 442, 704
Supplemental Social Security, 713
Suppository, rectal, 235–239, 453, 466

Suppository inserter, 332–333
Suprapubic cystostomy, 217
Surgi-Fix, 262
Swallowing:
  anatomy and physiology of, 174–175
  bypass surgery and, 183–184
  perceptual and language deficits and, 177
  (*See also* Chewing and swallowing; Dysphagia)
Sweating, reflex, 484–485
Synergy of limbs, 289

Taste, 174–175, 181, 182, 560
Tax Reform Act of 1976, 737
Teaching of patient or family, 755–757
  after amputation, 507–515
  about bladder training, 219–220
  about bowel program, 232
  after burn injury, 537, 538, 543, 546–548
  after communication impairment, 169–170
  about dressing and undressing, 376
  about dysreflexia, 467
  about heart disease, 581–586, 590–603
  about medications, 381, 382
  after memory loss, 365–366
  about pass or discharge, 462–464, 481–482, 674–675, 679–683
  about pressure sores, 248–250, 439
  about resocialization, 721–723
  about rheumatoid arthritis, 621, 622
  about seizures, 382, 395–396
  about sexuality (*see* Sex education and counseling)
  after spinal cord injury, 462–464, 470
  about transfers, 372
Team, rehabilitation:
  collaboration within, 292, 355, 428, 507, 671
  communication within, 133–134
    about activities of daily living, 304, 307, 310
    about cancer patient, 559
    about multiple sclerosis patient, 406
    about spinal cord–injured patient, 445
    about stroke patient, 355
  conferences of, 133–134, 445, 483, 677
  leadership in, 129, 131
  membership of, 128–135
    in amputee clinic, 494
    in bowel program, 224
    in discharge planning, 671
    in heart disease, 603
    in stroke, 355

791 INDEX

Team, rehabilitation (continued)
    (See also Patient, as member of rehabilitation team)
    role of nurses on, 6–7, 128–130, 133, 355, 420
Telephone, use of, 337, 415, 443, 769
Temperature, body:
    and exacerbation of multiple sclerosis, 405, 406, 408
    after head injury, 391
    regulation of, after spinal cord injury, 431, 485
Terminal device, types of, 497–498, *542*
Test for Auditory Comprehension of Language, 344
Thematic Apperception Test, 142
Thromboembolic disease, 430, 478, 486
Toileting, 330–334, *335*, 372, 621
Toothettes, 566
Tracheostomy:
    care of patient with, 471
    discharge from hospital with, 471, 472
    discontinuation of, 392
    in dysphagia, 183–184
    in spinal cord shock, 435
Traction, cervical, 427, *430,* 431–432
Transfers:
    after amputation, 511
    for bathing, 328, 329, 377
    from bed to chair, 371
    from chair to bed, 372
    role of physical therapist in, 372
    for toileting, 330, 331, 334, 372
Transportation for impaired persons, 733–735, 737, 771–772
Transurethral resection:
    of bladder neck, 218
    of prostate, 218
Trauma:
    psychic, 103
    (See also Head injury)
Typewriter, use of, 337–338, 769

Ulcer, stress, 431, 437
Unconscious mental processes, 102
United Nations Declaration on the Rights of Disabled Persons, 708
Urban Mass Transportation Act, 709, 734
Urethral pressure profile, 193
Urethral strictures, 198

Urinary diversion, 219
Urinary function, 186–222
    abnormal: assessment of, 187–193
        causes of, 187
        infection and, 199–200
        nursing care in, 187–219
        surgical treatment of, 216–219
    assessment of, 187–193, 453–456
Urine-collecting devices, external, 206–208, 216

Valsalva maneuver:
    and bowel evacuation, 226, 236–238
    and cardiovascular disease, 370
    and initiation of voiding, 190, 205
Valsalva phenomenon, 293
Value clarification, 98
Vesicoureteral reflux, 199
Veterans Administration, 420, 493, 714, 718
Vineland Maturity Scale, 141
Vision, 363–364, 409–410
    (See also Hemianopia; Visual neglect)
Visiting Nurses Association, 220, 676
Visual neglect, 162, 168, 307, 312, 362
Vocational counseling, 132, 691–696, 718
    after burn injury, 548
    after head injury, 397
    in heart disease, 580, 603
    in multiple sclerosis, 415
    after stroke, 383
    (See also Employment, resumption of; School, return to)
Vocational Evaluation and Work Adjustment Association, 693
Vocational Rehabilitation Act of 1973, 736
Vocational Rehabilitation Administration, 694
Voiding, 190, 469
Voiding facilitation techniques, 203–206

Water Pik, 377
Wechsler Adult Intelligence Scale, 141, 142, 163
Wheelchair, selection of, 373, 408–409
White House Conference on Handicapped Individuals, 700, 708, 735, 748, 752
Work simplification, 338
Workers' compensation, 713–714, 760, 761
Writing (see Reading and writing)

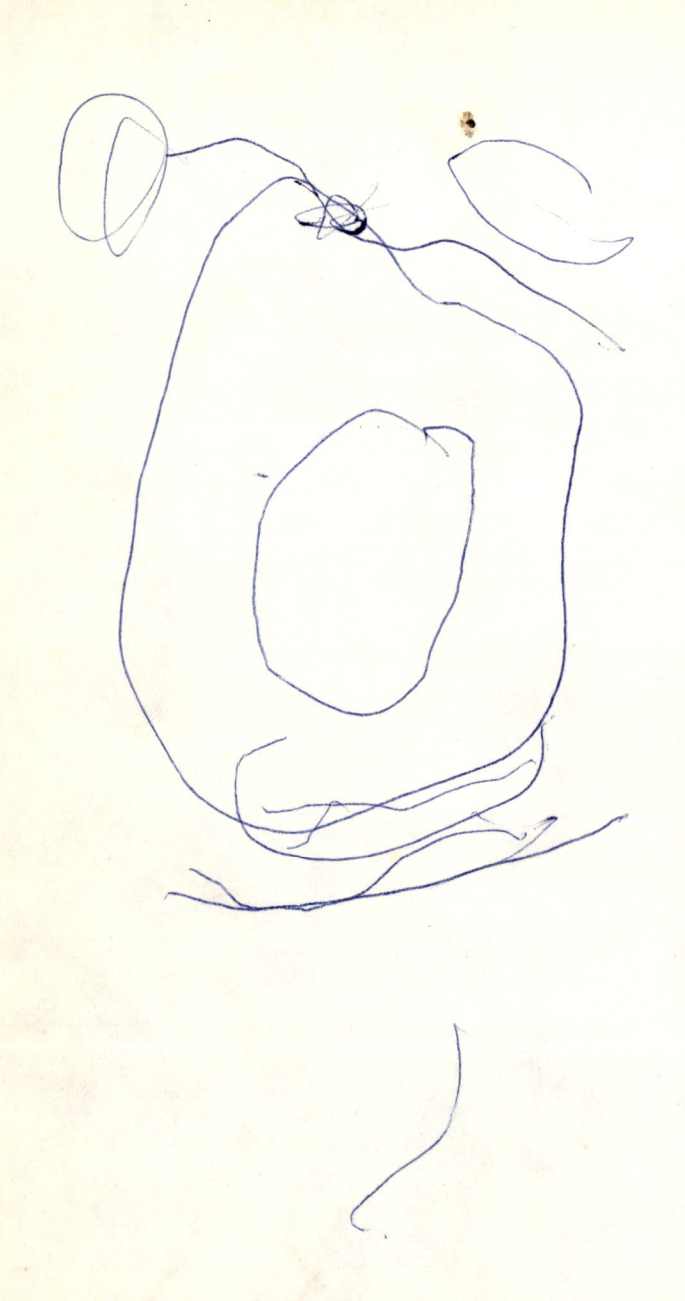